TEXTBOOK OF CORONARY THROMBOSIS AND THROMBOLYSIS

Developments in Cardiovascular Medicine

M.LeWinter. H. Suga and M.W. Watkins (eds.): *Cardiac Energetics: From Emax to Pressure-volume Area.* 1995   ISBN 0-7923-3721-2

R.J. Siegel (ed.): *Ultrasound Angioplasty.* 1995   ISBN 0-7923-3722-0

D.M. Yellon and G.J. Gross (eds.): *Myocardial Protection and the Katp Channel.* 1995   ISBN 0-7923-3791-3

A.V.G. Bruschke. J.H.C. Reiber. K.I. Lie and H.J.J. Wellens (eds.): *Lipid Lowering Therapy and Progression of Coronary Atherosclerosis.* 1996   ISBN 0-7923-3807-3

A.S.A. Abd-Elfattah and A.S. Wechsler (eds.): *Purines and Myocardial Protection.* 1995   ISBN 0-7923-3831-6

M. Morad, S. Ebashi, W. Trautwein and Y. Kurachi (eds.): *Molecular Physiology and Pharmacology of Cardiac Ion Channels and Transporters.* 1996   ISBN 0-7923-3913-4

A.M. Oto (ed.): *Practice and Progress in Cardiac Pacing and Electrophysiology.* 1996   ISBN 0-7923-3950-9

W.H. Birkenhager (ed.): *Practical Management of Hypertension. Second Edition.* 1996   ISBN 0-7923-3952-5

J.C. Chatham, J.R. Forder and J.H. McNeill (eds.): *The Heart In Diabetes.* 1996   ISBN 0-7923-4052-3

M. Kroll, M. Lehmann (eds.): *Implantable Cardioverter Defibrillator Therapy: The Engineering-Clinical Interface.* 1996   ISBN 0-7923-4300-X

Lloyd Klein (ed.): *Coronary Stenosis Morphology: Analysis and Implication.* 1996   ISBN 0-7923-9867-X

Johan H.C. Reiber, Ernst E. Van der Wall (eds.): *Cardiovascular Imaging.* 1996   ISBN 0-7923-4109-0

A.-M. Salmasi, A. Strano (eds.): *Angiology in Practice.*   ISBN 0-7923-4143-0

Julio E. Perez, Roberto M. Lang, (eds.): *Echocardiography and Cardiovascular Function: Tools for the Next Decade.* 1996   ISBN 0-7923-9884-X

Keith L. March (ed.): *Gene Transfer in the Cardiovascular System: Experimental Approaches and Therapeutic Implications.* 1997   ISBN 0-7923-9859-9

Anne A. Knowlton (ed.): *Heat Shock Proteins and the Cardiovascular System.* 1997   ISBN 0-7923-9910-2

Richard C. Becker (ed.): *Textbook of Coronary Thrombosis and Thrombolysis.* 1997   ISBN 0-7923-9923-4

TEXTBOOK OF CORONARY THROMBOSIS AND THROMBOLYSIS

Edited by

Richard C. Becker, M.D.
Director, Cardiovascular Thrombosis Research Center
Director, Coronary Care Unit

University of Massachusetts Medical School
Worcester, Massachusetts

Springer Science+Business Media, LLC

Library of Congress Cataloging-in-Publication Data

Textbook of coronary thrombosis and thrombolysis / edited by Richard
C. Becker.
     p. cm. -- (Developments in cardiovascular medicine)
     Includes index.
     ISBN 978-1-4757-7078-0   ISBN 978-0-585-33754-8 (eBook)
     DOI 10.1007/978-0-585-33754-8

     1. Coronary heart disease. 2. Thrombosis. 3. Thrombolytic
therapy. I. Becker, Richard C. II. Series.
     [DNLM: 1. Coronary Thrombosis--drug therapy. 2. Myocardial
Infarction--drug therapy. 3. Thrombolytic Therapy. 4. Fibrinolytic
Agents--therapeutic use. WG 300 T355 1997]
     RC685.C61375 1997
     616.1'23--dc21
     DNLM/DLC
     for Library of Congress   97-16368
                                                  CIP

Copyright 1997 by Springer Science+Business Media New York
Originally published by Kluwer Academic Publishers in 1997
Softcover reprint of the hardcover 1st edition 1997

Printed on acid-free paper.

Dedicated to Clinton Frederick, Gillian Martha, and Kristian Charles Deiter — "Seek the truth and devote yourselves to those that have not."

Dedicated to my colleagues at the Cardiovascular Thrombosis Research Center — "Keep asking questions."

Dedicated to my soulmate — "Inspiration knows no boundaries and manifests itself in many wonderful and loving ways."

ABBREVIATED CONTENTS

CONTENTS

PREFACE

Teleologically, the hemostatic mechanism is among the most fundamental yet complex physiologic processes in humans. Early scientists and physicians were fascinated by the blood's ability to remain in a liquid state only to clot in response to vascular injury. The cellular and noncellular components of normal hemostasis took centuries to discover, and the intricacies of their delicate interactions are still being unraveled today. As is so often the case, an in-depth appreciation of physiologic hemostasis, representing a basic life-sustaining sequence of events, paved the way for understanding abnormal hemostasis or pathologic thrombosis. Aristotle, Malpighi, and Osler, representing but a few of the founding fathers in the field, would undoubtedly be honored to see their observations form the template for lifesaving treatments.

The evolution of thrombocardiology, a hybrid of cardiology, hematology, and pathology has proceeded at an extraordinary pace. Fueled by a seemingly insatiable sense of enthusiasm and a "need to know" attitude, modern-day pioneers and visionaries have taken on the challenge of defeating coronary arterial thrombosis, a leading cause of death, disability, and healthcare expenditures in the United States and other industrialized nations worldwide. Now, more than ever before, the timeless links between cellular biology, vascular biology, and the practice of medicine are being recognized and justly exploited through basic investigation and clinical research endeavors, providing answers to fundamental questions and sparking new hypotheses, with the ultimate goal of developing universally applicable and affordable therapies as well as practical guidelines for their use.

The *Textbook of Coronary Thrombosis and Thrombolysis*, in essence, represents a heartfelt gift of knowledge from a dedicated group of scientists and clinicians, who collectively have set out on a mission to minimize the societal impact of "hemostasis in the wrong place." The book is divided into four distinct sections: Part 1, Scientific Principles, lays down the supporting foundation; Part 2, Clinical Application of Scientific Principles, places the knowledge base in a working perspective, directly applying science to patient care; Part 3, New Dimensions, provides a glimpse of tomorrow. Steering the field clear of self-proclaimed victory and the dangers of complacency as we move into the 21st century, Part 4, Evolution of Thrombocardiology, focuses on laboratory standards, clinical trials, and drugs in development.

These major sections are systematically divided into smaller sections, each with a composer who has been asked to assemble the works of the finest scientific minds in the world. When brought together and conducted well, this orchestra plays a symphony for all the world to hear. It is this spirit of coordinated research and clinical practice that has captured the pain of human disease and suffering, and is rising swiftly to meet the needs of humanity in the global village. The *Textbook of Coronary Thrombosis and Thrombolysis* represents the culmination of a long journey designed solely for the purpose of serving basic scientists, clinician-scientists, and practicing clinicians intimately involved with seeking truth through pointed investigation and unconditional clinical application of current concepts in thrombocardiology.

Richard C. Becker, M.D.

FOREWORD

Eric J. Topol

In looking back over the past decade, the progress made in the treatment of patients with acute coronary syndromes has been enormous. The use of intravenous thrombolysis for acute myocardial infarction was first approved by the United States Food and Drug Administration in late 1987, and was implemented in clinical practice over the next 2–3 years. Intravenous heparin was shown to change the natural history in patients with unstable angina, and aspirin was demonstrated in 20 randomized trials to provide important protection from death and myocardial infarction in patients with acute myocardial infarction, unstable angina, and those undergoing percutaneous coronary intervention. In aggregate, in this discipline of cardiovascular medicine — the treatment of patients with acute manifestations of ischemic heart disease — we have been on a steep, ascending climb, acquiring new and vital information, and, coincidentally, it has led to a major transformation in clinical practice. Most of us who cared for these patients before this time fully recognize that this represents a true revolution in medicine.

While our therapies have indeed improved, there are major residual shortcomings. With the most potent thrombolytics available today, nearly half of patients are left without prompt restoration of infarct vessel patency 90 minutes into therapy. Reocclusion, a manifestation of rethrombosis, occurs in up to 25% of patients within a year from the index event. Furthermore, in patients receiving aspirin, there is an incomplete effect on inhibiting platelet aggregation, and with heparin there is an inconsistent effect owing to lack of inactivation of clot-bound thrombin and the natural inhibitors of heparin, such as platelet factor 4. Accordingly, there is a major gap between the actual therapies of today and, their ideal improved and optimized forms in the future.

The number one killer, the most important manifestation of heart disease today, is still coronary thrombosis. Fundamental to more effectively addressing its treatment in the years ahead is an improved understanding of its principles and the thrombotic process. In the *Textbook of Coronary Thrombosis and Thrombolysis*, Richard Becker has organized a superb and comprehensive examination of all the relevant basic and clinical information in the field.

In the first section on scientific principles, the leading international authorities have reviewed each major building block in coronary thrombosis and clot lysis, including detailed reviews of the coagulation cascade, platelets, plasminogen activators, atherosclerosis, thrombosis, plaque rupture, and vascular biology. This is followed in Section II by a review of the central concepts pertaining to clinical applications, which include thrombolytic agents, the pathophysiology of the acute coronary syndromes, prehospital and early in-hospital therapy, coagulation and myocardial necrosis serum markers, the use of coronary angiography and percutaneous interventions, along with a systematic review of the complications of therapy and the futuristic approach of gene therapy. These sections are followed by a section dedicated to the future directions of basic and clinical investigation, along with another that provides an exhaustive glossary of relevant clinical trials, terms, and drugs that are in development but not yet commercialized.

Dr. Becker has done a masterful job of soliciting outstanding input from so many of the leading authorities on this subject. The superb content of the book is a direct reflection of the top-notch authors who have contributed to it. All of the pivotal aspects of coronary thrombosis are at least touched on, if not fully reviewed, in this textbook.

The future of improved therapies directed against coronary thrombosis in the years to come is predicated on enhanced understanding of the current state of the art with a visionary eye toward where the field is headed. In this textbook, both of these notable objectives are fully met. There is no other book available that ties together this important wealth of information, and undoubtedly this monograph will prove useful for not only cardiologists but also trainees and internists caring for patients with ischemic heart disease.

CONTRIBUTING AUTHORS

Dr. George S. Abela
Division of Cardiology
Michigan State University
Department of Medicine
B-208 Clinical Center
East Lansing, MI 48824

Dr. Dana Abendschein
Cardiovascular Division
Washington University School of Medicine
St. Louis, MO 63110

Dr. John A. Ambrose
Cardiac Catheterization Laboratory
The Mount Sinai Medical Center
One Gustave L. Levy Place
New York, NY 10029-6574

Dr. Felicita Andreotti
Istituto di Cardiologia
Policlinico A. Gemelli
Largo F. Vito, 1
00168 Roma
Italy

Dr. Alfred Arnold
Department of Cardiology
Medical Center Alkmaar
P.O. Box 501
1800 AM Alkmaar
The Netherlands

Dr. James M. Atkins
University of Texas Southwestern Medical School
5323 Harry Hines Boulevard
Dallas, TX 75235-8890

Dr. Richard C. Becker
Cardiovascular Thrombosis Research Center
University of Massachusetts Medical School
55 Lake Avenue North
Worcester, MA 01655

Dr. Narinder P. Bhalla
Cardiac Catheterization Laboratory
Brooklyn Hospital Center
New York University Medical Center

550 First Avenue
New York, NY 10016

Dr. Christoph Bode
Medizinische Klinik III (Kardiologie)
Bergheimerstrasse 58
69115 Heidelberg
Germany

Dr. Eric Boersma
Department of Cardiology
Medical Center Alkmaar
P.O. Box 501
1800 AM Alkmaar
The Netherlands

Dr. Peter Carmeliet
Center for Transgene Technology and Gene
    Therapy
Vlaams Interuniversitair Instituut voor
    Biotechnologie
Campus Gasthuisberg
O&N, Herestraat 43
B-3000 Leuven Belgium

Dr. Steffen P. Christow
Virchow Hospitals of the Humboldt University
at Berlin
Franz-Volhard-Hospital
Wiltbergstrasse 50
D-13125 Berlin
Germany

Dr. Richard Cohen
Evans Memorial Department of Clinical Research
Department of Medicine
Boston University Medical Center
Boston, MA 02118

Dr. D. Collen
Center for Molecular and Vascular Biology
Campus Gasthuisberg, O&N Herestraat 49
University of Leuven
B-3000 Leuven
Belgium

Dr. David P. de Bono
Department of Medicine

University of Leicester, LE3 9QP
UK

Dr. Marco Diaz
Sections of Cardiology and Vascular Medicine
Evans Memorial Department of Clinical Research
Department of Medicine
Boston University Medical Center
Boston, MA 02118

Dr. Sanjay Dixit
Cardiovascular Division
Department of Medicine
State University of New York Health Science Center
   at Syracuse
Syracuse, NY 13210

Dr. Paul R. Eisenberg
Cardiac Care Unit
Washington University
School of Medicine
660 South Euclid Avenue
St. Louis, MO 63110

Dr. Daniel Eitzman
University of Michigan Medical School
1301 Catherine Road
Medical Science Building I
Ann Arbor, MI 48109-0624

Dr. Christopher J. Ellis
Cardiologist and Senior Lecturer in Cardiovascular
   Medicine
Auckland Hospital
Private Bag 92 024
Auckland 1030
New Zealand

Dr. Mark L. Entman
Section of Cardiovascular Sciences
Department of Medicine
Baylor College of Medicine
The Methodist Hospital and the DeBakey Heart
   Center
Houston, TX 77030-3498

Dr. William P. Fay
University of Michigan Medical School
1301 Catherine Road
Medical Science Building I
Ann Arbor, MI 48109-0624

Dr. James Ferguson
Cardiology Research MC 1-191
Texas Heart Institute

P.O. Box 20345
Houston, TX 77225-0345

Dr. Nikolaos G. Frangogiannis
Section of Cardiovascular Sciences
Department of Medicine
Baylor College of Medicine
The Methodist Hospital and the DeBakey Heart
   Center
Houston, TX 77030-3498

Dr. David Ginsburg
University of Michigan Medical School
1301 Catherine Road
Medical Science Building I
Ann Arbor, MI 48109-0624

Dr. Robert J. Goldberg
Department of Medicine
University of Massachusetts Medical School
55 Lake Avenue North
Worcester, MA 01655

Dr. Paolo Golino
Division of Cardiology
University of Naples "Federico II"
via S. Pansini 5
80131 Naples
Italy

Dr. Dietrich Gulba
Virchow Hospitals of the Humboldt
University at Berlin
Franz-Volhard-Hospital
Wiltbergstrasse 50
D-13125 Berlin
Germany

Dr. Robert Harrington
Duke Clinical Research Institute
2024 West Main Street
Durham, NC 27705

Patricia K. Hodgson
Department of Medicine
Duke University Medical Center
Durham, NC 27710

Dr. Kurt Huber
Department of Cardiology
University of Vienna
Wahringer Gurtel 18-20
A-1090 Vienna
Austria

Dr. Jeffrey M. Isner
Tufts University School of Medicine
136 Harrison Avenue
Boston, MA 02111

Dr. Allan S. Jaffe
SUNY HSC at Syracuse
750 E. Adams Street
Syracuse, NY 13210

Dr. John F. Keaney, Jr.
Evans Memorial Department of
    Medicine
Cardiology Section Room W507
80 E. Conccord Street
Boston, MA 02118

Dr. Bruce A. Keyt
Genentech, Inc.
Department of Cardiovascular
    Research
460 Point San Bruno Blvd.
South San Francisco, CA 94080

Dr. Reza Khoshnevis
Cardiology Research
MC 1-191
Texas Heart Institute
P.O. Box 20354
Houston, TX 77225

Dr. Benedikt Kohler
Medizinische Klinik III (Kardiologie)
Bergheimerstrasse 58
69115 Heidelberg
Germany

Dr. Willemein J. Kollöffel
Pharmacy of St. Anna Hospital
P.O. Box 90
5660 AB Geldrop
The Netherlands

Dr. H. Joost Kruik
Department of Cardiology
University Hospital St. Radboud
Nijmegen, P.O. Box 9101
6500 HB Nijmegen
The Netherlands

Dr. Costas Lambrew
Maine Medical Center
Division of Cardiovascular Medicine
22 Bramhall Street
Portland, ME 04102-3175

Dr. L. Veronica Lee
Washington University School of Medicine
    Cardiovascular Division
660 South Euclid Avenue
St. Louis, MO 63110

Dr. H. Roger Lijnen
Center for Molecular and Vascular
    Biology
University of Leuven, Campus Gasthuisberg
O&N Herestraat 49
B-3000 Leuven
Belgium

Dr. Joseph Loscalzo
Boston University School of Medicine
Evans Memorial Department of Medicine
Center for Advanced Biomedical Research
700 Albany Street
Boston, MA 02118

Dr. Douglas W. Losordo
St. Elizabeth's Hospital of Boston
736 Cambridge Street
Boston, MA 02135

Dr. Ted W. Love
Genentech, Inc.
Department of Product Development
460 Point San Bruno Blvd.
South San Francisco, CA 94080

Dr. Elizabeth G. Nabel
Division of Cardiology
University of Michigan Medical School
MSRB III 7220
1150 W. Medical Center Dr.
Ann Arbor, MI 48109-0644

Dr. Thomas K. Nordt
Medizinische Klinik III (Kardiologie)
Bergheimerstrasse 58
69115 Heidelberg
Germany

Dr. Patrick O'Gara
Brigham and Women's Hospital
75 Francis Street
Boston, MA 02115

Dr. Joseph P. Ornato
Internal Medicine Section of Emergency Medical
    Services
Virginia Commonwealth of Virginia
Richmond, VA 23298

Dr. Voula Osganian
New England Research Institute
9 Galen Street
Watertown, MA 02172

Dr. Mary Ann Peberdy
Medical College of Virginia
P.O. Box 525, MCV Station
401 North 12th Street
Richmond, VA 23298-0525

Dr. Linda R. Peterson
Division of Cardiology
Washington University School of Medicine
660 S. Euclid Avenue, Box 8086
St. Louis, MO 63110

Dr. Hans J. Rapold
Basel University Medical School
Urichstrasse 27
D-79618 Rheinfeiden
Germany

Dr. Robert Roberts
Department of Medicine
Section of Cardiology
6550 Fannin, MS SM 677
Baylor College of Medicine
Houston, TX 77030

Dr. Arie Roth
Intensive Cardiac Care Unit
Tel Aviv Medical Center
Ichilov Hospital
6 Weizman Street
Tel Aviv 64239
Israel

Dr. Una S. Ryan
Vice President of Research
T Cell Sciences, Inc.
115 Fourth Avenue
Needham, MA 02194-2725

Dr. Pamela A. Sakkinen
University of Vermont
Aquetec Bldg. T205
55A South Park Drive
Colchester, VT 05446

Dr. Harsch Sanchorawala
Evans Memorial Department of Medicine
Cardiology Section, Room W507
80 E. Concord Street
Boston, MA 02118

Dr. William P. Santamore
Division of Thoracic and Cardiovascular Surgery
Department of Surgery
University of Louisville
Louisville, KY 40292

Dr. Harry P. Selker
New England Medical Center
Health Services Research
750 Washington Street
Boston, MA 02111

Dr. Maarten L. Simoons
Department of Cardiology
Medical Center Alkmaar
P.O. Box 501
1800 AM Alkmaar
The Netherlands

Dr. Richard Smalling
Division of Cardiology
University of Texas Medical School at
    Houston
6431 Fannin, Room 1.246 MSB
Houston, TX 77030

Dr. Frederick A. Spencer
Thrombosis Research Center
University of Massachusetts Medical School
55 Lake Avenue North
Worcester, MA 01655

Dr. David Stump
Genentech, Inc.
I DNA Way
South San Francisco, CA 94080

Dr. Melvin E. Tan
Duke Clinical Research Institute
Division of Cardiology
Duke University Medical Center
Durham, NC 27710

Dr. Cynthia M. Thaik

Dr. Mark C. Thel
Division of Cardiology
Department of Medicine
Duke University Medical Center
Durham, NC 27710

Dr. Russell P. Tracy
University of Vermont
Aquatec Building, T205

55A South Park Drive
Colchester, VT 05446

Dr. Maureen van der Vlugt
Department of Cardiology
Medical Center Alkmaar
P.O. Box 501
1800 AM Alkmaar
The Netherlands

Dr. Steven Vanderschueren
Center for Molecular and Vascular Biology
University of Leuven
Campus Gasthuisberg
O & N, Herestraat 49
B-3000 Leuven
Belgium

Dr. Freek W.A. Verheugt
Department of Cardiology
University Hospital St. Radboud, Nijmegen
P.O. Box 9101
6500 HB Nijmegen
The Netherlands

Dr. W. Douglas Weaver
Division of Cardiology
Henry Ford Hospital
Detroit, MI

Prof. Harvey D. White
Coronary Care and
Cardiovascular Research
Green Lane Hospital
Private Bag 92 189
Auckland 1030
New Zealand

Dr. James M. Wilson
Cardiology Research MC 1-191
Texas Heart Institute
P.O. Box 20345
Houston, TX 77225-0345

Dr. Robert J. Zalenski
Emergency Medicine and Medicine (Cardiology)
School of Medicine
Wayne State University/The Detroit Medical Center
Detroit, MI 48201

PART A: SCIENTIFIC PRINCIPLES

SECTION I: THE BIOCHEMISTRY OF THROMBOSIS

Richard C. Becker

Hemostasis, the prompt cessation of hemorrhage at a site or vessel wall injury, is among the most fundamental and vital physiologic defensive mechanisms in humans. From a teleologic point of view, vascular hemostasis represents a series of biochemical events that has allowed natural evolution through even the most primitive (and traumatic) periods. The rapid transition of fluid blood to a gel-like substance (clot) has been a topic of great interest to philosophers, scientists, and physicians dating back to the days of Plato and Aristotle. However, it was not until the beginning of the 18th century that blood clotting was appreciated as the means to stem blood loss from wounds. As with other major developments in science and medicine, the microscope played a pivotal role in our understanding of coagulation. It was soon learned that individual components within the blood (cells, serum, fibers) and vessel wall were involved in the process and that intricate regulatory mechanisms were at play. Developments in the mid-19th and early 20th centuries paved the way toward a more complete understanding of coagulation at the biochemical level.

1. BIOCHEMISTRY OF INTRAVASCULAR CLOTTING: FOCUS ON THE PROTHROMBINASE COMPLEX

Frederick A. Spencer and Richard C. Becker

Prothrombinase Complex — Assembly and Function

The prothrombinase complex plays a pivotal role in the coagulation cascade. It is responsible for the proteolytic conversion of prothrombin to thrombin, which in turn is involved directly in the formation of fibrin, activation of platelets, and feedback activation of other components of the cascade. It is among the most thoroughly studied coagulation processes, and some have suggested that the mechanisms of prothrombinase assembly can serve as a model for understanding other components of the coagulation system. Prothrombinase assembly requires a platelet surface in vivo; thus, this stage of clotting involves a unique interaction between the protein-based coagulation cascade and platelet activity. Accordingly, the investigation and development of antithrombotic compounds has recently been directed toward prothrombinase. In this chapter we summarize the current understanding of prothrombinase assembly and function.

Prothrombinase

Prothrombinase is similar to other coagulation enzyme complexes and is composed of a vitamin K–dependent serine protease (factor Xa), a protein cofactor (factor Va), a membrane surface, and divalent ions (Ca^{2+}). The assembly of prothrombinase on a membrane surface adjacent to membrane-associated prothrombin results in conversion of the prothrombin substrate to thrombin (factor IIa; Figure 1-1). Furthermore, a marked enhancement (~300,000-fold) in this conversion has been noted in reactions involving prothrombinase compared with those involving the serine protease factor Xa alone [1].

Factor X/Xa

Factor X is a vitamin K–dependent zymogen that has structural similarity to factors II, VII, and IX and to protein C. It is a 59,000-d glycoprotein that is synthesized as a single polypeptide chain but circulates as a two-chain protein following postsecretion proteolysis. Its serine protease resides at the COOH terminus, and the *GLA domain* is found at the NH_2 terminus (on the light chain). The GLA domain consists of 9–12 glutamic acid residues that are carboxylated in a vitamin-K–dependent post-translational modification. This modification is necessary for factor X/Xa activity in vivo. Between the serine protease and GLA domain is the *EGF domain*, containing two *epidermal growth factor–like* regions [2,3] (Figure 1-2).

Membrane Binding

The GLA domain (also present in factors II and VII, and in protein C) is important for Ca^{2+} binding [4], which in turn induces conformational changes in the proteins that are required for membrane binding [5]. In factor X this domain contains approximately 20 Ca^{2+} binding sites. Multiple studies have shown that Ca^{2+} binding results in conformational changes in *both* the heavy and light chains of factor X/Xa that are necessary for the binding of Xa to acidic phospholipids. Alteration or deletion of GLA domains results in an inability of factor Xa to bind phospholipid surfaces. The factor X–membrane interaction has been shown to have a dissociation constant of 0.19 μmol/L [1]. Interestingly, this correlates with the reported plasma concentrations of factor Xa (~0.17 μmol/L).

Activation

The production of Xa from factor X can occur via one of two pathways (Figure 1-3). The first is mediated by

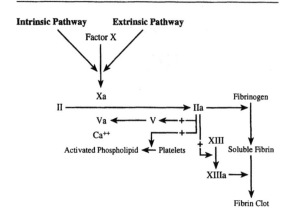

FIGURE 1-1. Prothrombinase complex consists of serine protease factor Xa, protein cofactor Va, a phospholipid membrane surface, and calcium ions. This complex promotes the conversion of prothrombin to thrombin, which acts as a final mediator in both physiologic hemostasis and pathologic thrombosis.

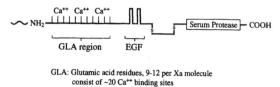

GLA: Glutamic acid residues, 9-12 per Xa molecule
consist of ~20 Ca^{++} binding sites

EGF: Epidermal growth factor domain
similar to that seen in factors VII, IX, protein C

FIGURE 1-2. Illustration of the structural features of factor X. The carboxyglutamic acid domain (GLA region) consists of 9–12 such residues per Xa molecule and provides approximately 20 Ca^{2+} binding sites. The epidermal growth factor–like region (EGF Domain) is structurally similar to that seen in factor VII, factor IX, and protein C. The serine protease domain found at the carboxyl terminus is a highly conserved region found in all of the vitamin K–dependent zymogens.

the action of an *intrinsic Xase* complex, consisting of factor IXa, factor VIII, Ca^{2+}, and a phospholipid membrane. This complex effects a proteolytic cleavage of factor X at a specific site (Arg^{51}–Ile^{52}) to produce Xa [6]. It should be noted that there are many structural and functional similarities between intrinsic Xase and the prothrombinase complex.

The second pathway is determined by the action of an *extrinsic Xase* complex composed of tissue factor (TF) associated with factor VII/VIIa and Ca^{2+} ions. The factor VIIa-catalyzed activation of factor X is dramatically enhanced by tissue factor. At plasma concentrations of factor X, the rate enhancement due to TF has been calculated to be ~16,000-fold [7]. Extrinsic Xase also acts by cleavage of factor X at Arg^{51}–Ile^{52} to produce factor Xa.

As noted in the review by Krishnaswamy et al. [8], the rate constant for activation of factor X by factor VIIa–TF is approximately 50 times lower than that for activation by the intrinsic Xase complex. Accordingly, although factor VIIa–TF acts as the initiating catalyst for hemostasis by activation of factor X (as well as activation of factor IX), it is likely that intrinsic Xase acts to propagate coagulation by continued production of factor Xa.

Factor V

Factor Va serves as a protein cofactor in the prothrombinase complex. It is derived from factor V,

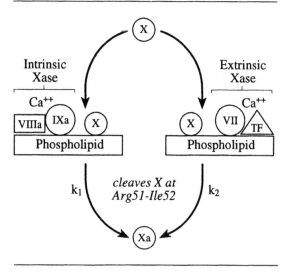

FIGURE 1-3. Schematic representation of factor X activation. Factor X may be converted to factor Xa by peptide bond cleavage at Arg^{51}–Ile 52 from either the intrinsic Xase complex (factor VIIIa–IXa) or the extrinsic Xase complex (factor VIIa–tissue factor).

a single-chain glycoprotein of MW 330,000 d [9] and is composed of three A domains at the NH$_2$ terminus, two C domains at its COOH terminus, and a connecting B region. Factor V is similar in structure to another plasma cofactor, factor VIII (Figure 1-4).

It should be noted that 20–25% of blood factor V is stored within the α granules of platelets as multiple

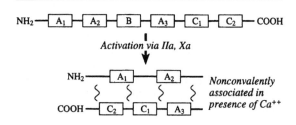

FIGURE 1-4. Factor V is similar in structure to another plasma coagulation cofactor–factor VIII. During the formation of factor Va from factor V in the presence of factor IIa or factor Xa, a large portion of the central connecting region is released as activation fragments. The resulting two subunits are held together by noncovalent associations in the presence of calcium ions.

peptides [10]. As a result, a large portion of factor V in vivo is highly concentrated in <0.2% of blood volume [11]. It is not completely clear to what extent the roles of plasma and platelet factor V overlap. There is indirect evidence that platelet factor V plays a significant role in hemostasis. A study by Rand et al. showed that platelet factor Va is the major phosphoprotein secreted and phosphorylated after α-thrombin stimulation of platelets [12]. It has been demonstrated that α-thrombin activation of platelet factor V results in a heavy/light chain complex similar to that derived from plasma factor V. Finally, multiple studies have linked a deficiency of platelet factor V to a hemorrhagic diathesis [11,13].

Binding Characteristics

Unlike factor X/Xa, the binding of factor Va to membrane phospholipid is a Ca^{2+}-independent process. Interestingly, factor Va's binding affinity for phospholipid surfaces is ~10 times greater than that of factor Xa or thrombin [14]. Several authors have determined that binding of factor Va to the platelet membrane involves the cofactor's light chain [14–16]. A study by Kalafahs et al. delineated this interaction further [17]. Their findings suggest that two regions of factor Va's light chain interact with the platelet membrane's lipid bilayer. The first binding site is a 30,000-d fragment of factor Va on the A_3 domain. This region interacts with phospholipid vesicles containing neutral phospholipid (i.e., phosphatidylcholine). The second site is a 46,000/48,000-d fragment at the COOH terminal portion. This

region interacts with membranes consisting of both/either anionic or neutral phospholipids. Thus the A_3 domain of factor Va is responsible for the interaction of the molecule's light chain with the lipid bilayer, involves hydrophobic interactions, and requires neutral phospholipids. The COOH-terminal site may be responsible for absorption of the light chain to the bilayer, involves Ca^{2+}-independent electrostatic interactions, and is independent of phospholipid composition.

Stop-flow kinetic studies examining the binding of factor Va to phospholipid vesicles found that this reaction occurred at a rate close to the diffusional controlled rate and had a very high collisional efficiency [18]. Similar observations have been reported with the binding factor Xa to phospholipid membranes [19]. Accordingly, it has been proposed that the rate-limiting step for prothrombinase complex formation is protein–membrane interactions (rather than the protein–protein interactions) [20]. This is discussed in a subsequent section on complex assembly.

Activation

Factor Va is derived by proteolysis of factor V. It has been well established that thrombin is a potent activator of factor V and results in a 20- to 80-fold increase in cofactor activity [21–23]. Once generated, factor Va, in turn, enhances the rate of prothrombin conversion by a factor of ~13,000. Factor Va is a two-chain molecule that is noncovalently associated in the presence of Ca^{2+} ions [18,22,24,25] with a dissociation constant of 5.9×10^{-9} mmol/L [26]. The heavy chain (105,000 d) contains the NH_2 terminus and includes the $A_3 C_1 C_2$ domains.

Given that factor Va (as part of prothrombinase) is required for thrombin generation in vivo, the question that arises is, How is factor Va generated initially if thrombin is not present? Prior work by Nesheim et al. demonstrated that factor V has 1/400 the activity of activated factor Va. Thus, it is possible that factor V acts as cofactor initially and generates enough thrombin to start feedback activation of factor V to Va [23]. Another possibility is that other activators of factor V exist in vivo. This concept has been addressed by Foster et al. [27]. Cofactor V activation was assessed by monitoring the conversion of prothrombin 1 to thrombin in the presence of 5-dimethylaminonaphthalene-1-sulfonylarginine-n-(3-ethyl-1,5-pentanediylamide) (DAPA). DAPA can act as a fluorescent marker for the production of thrombin in various reactions. In this instance, it also acted to attenuate feedback activation of factor V by even small amounts of thrombin formed within the system.

The authors proposed that factor Xa may, in fact, be responsible for initial activation of factor V to Va. In an elaborate series of experiments, factor V was incubated with Xa in the presence of phospholipids, Ca^{2+}, and DAPA. Immunoabsorption was used to clear the system of factor Va and thrombin. It was determined that the addition of factor Xa affected conversion of factor V to Va with a rate constant of 0.14 mol factor Va/min/mol of factor Xa. A value of 11.9 mol of factor Va/min/mol, using thrombin for conversion, was found under similar conditions. Thus factor V activation by thrombin is ~100-fold faster than factor Xa.

However, it was also shown that in the absence of thrombin, factor Xa is solely responsible for factor Va production. As thrombin is generated it gradually assumes the role of a factor V *activator*. It should be noted that while most of the products of factor Xa–catalyzed activation of factor V differ from those of thrombin-mediated activation, there is one component (94,000 d) produced by both. Immunoprecipitation experiments suggest that this component is one of the two subunits of factor Va. Lastly, it is important to acknowledge that whichever protein produces factor V to factor Va activation (factor Xa or factor IIa), the resulting product is equally effective as a cofactor in the prothrombin 1 to thrombin conversion.

Phospholipid Membrane

The structure, binding, and activation of factors V/Va and X/Xa have already been discussed. It is important to appreciate that the phospholipid membrane surface is an integral part of the prothrombinase complex; without it the catalytic efficiency/function of this enzyme would be lost. Early studies by Barton and Hanahan illustrated the importance of the clinical and physical properties of membranes in coagulation reactions [28]. Subsequent experiments by Higgins et al. examined the influence of membrane fluidity on prothrombinase complex assembly using phospholipid vesicles with high- and low-phase transition temperatures [29]. It was found that prothrombin activation lagged when measured in a system using nonfluid phospholipids. This lag was eliminated by preassembling the enzyme complex prior to initiation with prothrombin, suggesting that complex assembly can be rate limiting.

It has also been shown that the assembly and activity of prothrombinase is dependent on the presence of acidic phospholipids at the membrane site. In vivo

the cellular membrane surfaces do not naturally offer an acidic phospholipid surface; this must occur by translocation of acidic phospholipid head groups after cell activation [6]. Once a coagulation reaction has generated small amounts of thrombin, platelets are activated and produce the required acidic phospholipid environment. Mechanically injured endothelial cells also express an acidic phospholipid surface.

A number of possible cellular sites for prothrombinase assembly have been identified [30,31]. Monocytes, lymphocytes, neutrophils, and platelets are as kinetically efficient as phospholipid vesicles in supporting prothrombinase assembly. Endothelial cells can also support assembly, but quantitatively endothelial cell prothrombinase activity is modest relative to its membrane area [32]. Therefore, initiation of thrombin activation can occur on endothelial membranes, but it is unlikely that this surface supports propagation of the process.

Prothrombinase Complex Assembly

The interaction of each individual component of the prothrombinase complex has been a subject of intense research over the past two decades. Understanding the events is important because prothrombinase, once fully assembled, is approximately 300,000 times more active than factor Xa alone for the conversion of prothrombin to thrombin. Therefore, relevant activation of thrombin in vivo occurs only in the presence of a fully assembled prothrombinase complex (Table 1-1).

Studies of prothrombinase complex reconstituted from purified components indicated that it consists of 1 mol factor Xa to 1 mole of factor Va on a phospholipid vesicle surface in the presence of Ca^{2+} ions [23,33–35]. As previously discussed, factor Xa binds to the membrane expressing acidic phospholipid in a Ca^{2+}-dependent fashion. Factor Va binds to the membrane in a Ca^{2+}-independent manner.

To fully understand prothrombinase assembly and activity, the mechanics of factor Xa and factor Va interactions, the role that each plays in membrane binding, and how the complex interacts with its substrate, thrombin must first be understood. It has been clearly demonstrated that factor V is required for the binding of factor Xa to platelets because platelets treated with factor Va antibody or platelets from factor V–deficient individuals show decreased factor Xa binding. A study by Kane et al. used DAPA to prevent thrombin-induced platelet activation during factor Xa–platelet binding [36] studies. They determined that nonactivated platelets would not bind

TABLE 1-1. Relative rates of prothrombinase activation in the presence of various combinations of the components of prothrombinase complex

Components present[a]	Relative rate (%)[b]
factor Xa, Ca²⁺, phospholipid, factor Va	100
factor Xa, Ca²⁺, factor Va	0.13
factor Xa, Ca²⁺, phospholipid	0.008
factor Xa, Ca²⁺	0.0007
factor Xa	0.0003

[a] Proteins were present at potential physiological concentrations: prothrombin, $\sim 10^{-6}$ mol/L; factor V, $\sim 10^{-8}$ mol/L; factor Xa, $\sim 10^{-9}$ mol/L. Phospholipid is present at a concentration adequate to saturate the reaction.
[b] Expressed in comparison with prothrombinase.
Reprinted with permission from Mann et al. [6].

factor Xa, even in the presence of exogenous factor V. However, unstimulated platelets incubated with bovine factor Va will bind Xa with the same affinity and number of binding sites as thrombin-stimulated platelets. The investigators concluded that factor V activation is necessary for platelet factor Xa binding and that the sites required for binding are present on unstimulated platelets.

Thrombin stimulation of platelets promotes factor Xa binding by activation of factor V to Va, *not* by new expression of a unique platelet Xa binding site. A number of studies have suggested that factor Va may act as the receptor for factor Xa on the platelet surface [37–40]. Investigators at the University of Vermont set out to determine if factor Va could truly act as the "receptor" for factor Xa binding. Their prior work had already delineated the binding of factors V and Va to platelets [41]. They found ~800–900 high-affinity factor Va binding sites (dissociation constant, $\sim 4 \times 10^{-10}$ M) and also a class of lower affinity binding sites (dissociation constant, $\sim 3 \times 10^{-9}$ M) shared by both factors V and Va. Platelet activation was not found to have any effect on the binding of factors V or Va to platelets.

To delineate if factor Va was the receptor for factor Xa binding, a series of simultaneous binding measurements of bovine factor Va and factor Xa to unstimulated platelets, immunochemical assays of the reaction, and kinetic studies were performed [31]. They found that factor Xa receptor sites were present on unstimulated bovine platelets, that factor Va and factor Xa interact with platelets in a 1:1 stoichiometry (and with high affinity), and that high-affinity factor Va platelet sites likely represent factor Xa binding sites (if not an actual receptor per se). They also determined that unactivated factor V will pro-

mote the binding of factor Xa to platelets, albeit at a reduced level. The authors point out this would be physiologically important because factor V is likely to be associated with unstimulated platelets at plasma concentrations of factor V [41,42]. Thus, factor V platelet sites may bind small amounts of factor Xa, and, as suggested earlier, factor Xa could, in turn, activate factor V to Va. Following this, increased amounts of factor Xa would be bound, more factor Va could be generated, and thrombin would be produced. Eventually enough thrombin would be produced to take over the role of activation of factor Va and the reaction would be able to proceed at full force.

In summary, while the binding of factors Va and Xa to the membrane surface can occur as independent events, interaction between the two (protein–protein) within the prothrombinase complex increases the affinity of each factor's interaction with the membrane ~100-fold [43]. Similarly, the interaction between factor Va and factor Xa may be strengthened by the presence of membranes. Binding studies of prothrombinase assembly give a dissociation constant for factor Va and factor Xa interaction on membranes of ~1 nmol/L [23,31,44], which is 1000 times greater than that of factor Va and factor Xa in solution [43].

There is compelling evidence from kinetic and equilibrium studies for the existence of the prothrombinase complex. However, experiments detecting direct physical interactions between factors Xa and Va and a phospholipid surface have only recently been performed. Studies conducted at the University of Vermont made use of a potent irreversible inhibitor of factor Xa, dansyl-glutamylglycl arginylchloromethyl-ketone (DEGR) [45]. This agent also acts as a fluorophore, and thus allows the use of fluorescence polarization to investigate the actual assembly of prothrombinase.

In brief, factor Xa–DEGR produces a characteristic fluorescence excitation spectra, whose intensity at certain wavelengths is altered with the addition of factor Va to mixtures of DEGR, factor Xa, Ca²⁺, and phospholipid. Previous work had demonstrated no such changes in intensity with "intermediate" mixtures of components (i.e., DEGR.Xa, DEGR.Xa plus Va, DEGR.Xa plus phospholipid, etc.), which do not result in prothrombinase formation. Changes in fluorescent intensity result on assembly of the prothrombinase complex due to perturbation in the fluorophore (DEGR.Xa). Because DEGR is known to be covalently incorporated into factor Xa's active site, this suggests that this site is detectably *altered* on incorporation of factor Xa into prothrombinase.

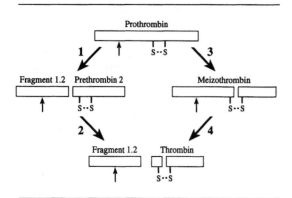

FIGURE 1-5. Schematic representation of the pathways for prothrombin activation. The activation of prothrombin to α-thrombin involves the cleavage of two peptide bonds in the zymogen. A reaction proceeding via steps 1 and 2 (cleavage at Arg^{274}–Thr^{275} followed by cleavage at Arg^{323}–Ile^{324}) yields prethrombin 2 and fragment 1.2 as intermediates. A reaction proceeding via steps 3 and 4 (cleavage at Arg^{323}–Ile^{324} followed by cleavage at Arg^{274}–Thr^{275}) yields meizothrombin as an intermediate. Prothrombin activation catalyzed by solution-phase factor Xa proceeds exclusively via steps 1 and 2, while the reaction catalyzed by prothrombinase proceeds via steps 3 and 4. (Reprinted with permission from Mann et al. [3].)

Thus using DEGR.Xa as a fluorescent "reporter" for the actual assembly of prothrombinase, the kinetics of assembly were systematically studied. Specifically, stopped-flow kinetic studies of assembly using saturating concentrations of Ca^{2+} ions, phospholipid vesicles, factor Va, and DEGR.Xa were performed. The rate of actual complex formation was found to depend on the premixing protocol used to initiate assembly. The most rapid assembly was obtained mixing factor Va with preformed DEGR.Xa–phospholipid. The rate of assembly was limited by the initial reaction between factor Va and the available combining sites on the vesicle (dissociation constant, $5.7 \times 10\,m^{-1}s^{-1}$) followed by very rapid reactions between phospholipid-bound DEGR.Xa and phospholipid-bound factor Va (dissociation constant, $>1 \times 10^{-9}\,m^{-1}s^{-1}$). Reaction rates by reacting DEGR.Xa with preformed Va–phospholipid complex or by reacting phospholipid vesicles were lower and were inhibited by increasing concentrations of factor Va. The authors thus conclude that the formation of a separate factor Va–phospholipid complex and a separate DEGR.Xa–phospholipid complex were prerequisites for prothrombinase assembly. A model of prothrombinase assembly complex assembly was then proposed as follows.

Assembly proceeds via formation of separate factor Xa–phospholipid and factor Va–phospholipid complexes, with the association of factor Xa or factor Va with phospholipid acting as the limiting step. Rates of these association/dissociation reactions indicate that formation of these initial complexes proceeds at near diffusion-limited rates (Figure 1-5) [45] and at high collisional efficiency (almost every factor Xa or factor Va collision with a phospholipid vesicle leads to a productive protein–membrane complex). Following these reactions, it is proposed that the separate complexes react by as yet unspecified rearrangements of factor Va and factor Xa on the vesicle surface.

This model is attractive for several reasons: (1) It suggests that prothrombinase assembly occurs in a highly localized manner on a membrane site, thus enhancing catalytic efficiency; (2) constituents do not need to detach and reattach from the membrane's surface for successive reactions; and (3) constituents of the reaction are relatively protected from high plasma concentrations of coagulation inhibitors.

In an attempt to expand knowledge of how prothrombinase assembles in vivo, Swords and Mann studied its assembly on adherent platelets [46]. They hypothesized that in vivo platelets function by first adhering to a damaged vascular site and that study of platelets adherent to immobilized van Willebrand factor was a reasonable simulation of this process. Using fluorescent probes, total internal reflection spectroscopy, and electron microscopy, a number of important observations were made regarding the mechanics of prothrombinase assembly. It was determined that factor Va binds to adherent platelets and activated adherent platelets with a similar dissociation constant of ~58 nmol/L. However, factor Xa displayed only minimal platelet binding prior to platelet activation. Once platelets were stimulated with thrombin, factor Xa binding markedly increased and, in fact, was not saturable. As might be expected, the binding of factor Xa to unstimulated adherent platelets was dependent on the presence of added factor Va (thus, adherence alone did not cause release of platelet factor Va). After thrombin stimulation, factor Xa bound readily without the addition of exogenous factor Va.

Direct observation of complex assembly on membranes was achieved through detection of energy transfer between fluorescein-labeled factor Va and rhodamine-labeled factor Xa. An estimated dissociation constant of 4 nmol/L for the factor Va–factor Xa interaction on platelet membrane surfaces was determined. Thrombin stimulation of platelets prior to assembly resulted in a slight decrease in energy

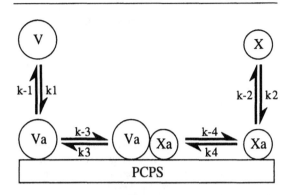

FIGURE 1-6. Schematic representation of the reaction steps required for prothrombinase assembly. Prothrombinase assembly on the phosphatidyl choline-phosphatidyl serine (PCPS) vesicle surface proceeds after initial reactions that yield separate factor Xa–PCPS and factor Va–PCPS binary complexes on the same membrane surface. The PCPS-bound proteins then react rapidly on the vesicle surface to form prothrombinase. (Reprinted with permission from Krishnaswamy et al. [8].)

transfer, possibly secondary to competition of the exogenous fluorescent-labeled factor Va and endogenous platelet Va for factor Xa. Overall, it appears that adherent platelets and thrombin-stimulated adherent platelets support equivalent binding of the prothrombinase complex. It is still not known if the activity of prothrombinase is *dependent* on platelet activation in vivo; this has been reported for human platelets in suspension [31]. Use of these techniques may help answer this important question.

Prothrombin Activation

As previously discussed, the interaction of fully assembled membrane-based prothrombinase and membrane-based prothrombin results in increased catalytic efficiency for the conversion of prothrombin to α-thrombin. It should be noted that prothrombin activation may proceed by several pathways (Figure 1-6). It has been determined that activation of membrane-bound prothrombin by membrane-bound prothrombinase appears to follow the second pathway depicted, specifically cleavage at Arg 323 followed by cleavage of Arg 274, with meizothrombin as the intermediate product. This is opposed to findings of earlier studies in which factor Xa (in solution) was reacted with prothrombin and subsequent activation followed the first pathway. Interestingly, the pathway

by which prothrombin is activated depends not only on prothrombinase as the effector but also on the membrane-based characteristics of prothrombin. Prothrombin with altered membrane binding properties (achieved via deletion of greater than two carboxygluthamic acid residues) will be activated by prothrombinase via the first pathway only.

The actual interaction of prothrombin and prothrombinase on the membrane surface remains to be delineated. Many of the techniques used to unravel the interaction of factor Va, factor Xa, Ca^{2+}, and membrane to form prothrombinase can be applied to answer this question as well. As reviewed by Mann et al. [43], a point of contention is whether prothrombin binds to the membrane prior to interaction with prothrombinase or is delivered directly to the enzyme complex from plasma.

In summary, assembly of the prothrombinase complex requires a series of interactions between the activated state of its major components — serine protease Xa, protein cofactor Va, and an acidic phospholipid surface. Extensive studies of the mechanics of this process favor a model in which factor Va and factor Xa each bind the phospholipid surface immediately prior to their interaction, to form prothrombinase. However, these binding events are by no means independent of each other. Kinetic analyses of the reactions involved reveal a marked codependency, that is, the rate of factor Xa–phospholipid binding is enhanced by the presence of factor Va and vice versa. Similarly, the reaction rate between factor Va and factor Xa is negligible without a phospholipid surface.

Following formation of prothrombinase, prothrombin can be converted to thrombin at a 300,000-fold increased rate compared with conversion with factor Xa alone. Analogous to prothrombinase assembly, this reaction requires a prothrombinase–phospholipid and prothrombin–phospholipid complex prior to any significant interaction between the two. Indeed, several investigators have suggested that understanding the mechanics of prothrombinase assembly may provide the key to understanding several other key coagulation complexes.

With increased knowledge of the assembly and function of prothrombinase has come an interest in new agents that can act specifically at this step to inhibit coagulation. Such agents would exert their effect at a point prior to the generation of substantial amounts of thrombin. In theory, this would markedly reduce the effect of thrombin's positive feedback/amplification on the coagulation cascade. Unlike thrombin-specific agents, incorporation, and thus protection, of the intended substrate into a clot would not be a concern.

References

1. Mann KG, Lawson JH. The role of the membrane in the expression of the vitamin K-dependent enzymes. Arch Pathol Lab Med 116:1330, 1992.
2. Doolittle RF, Feng DF, Johnson MS. Computer-based characterization of epidermal growth factor precursor. Nature 307:558, 1984.
3. Mann KG, Nesheim ME, Church WR, Haley P, Krishnaswamy S. Surface-dependent reactions of the vitamin K-dependent enzyme complexes. Blood 76:1, 1990.
4. Church WR, Boulanger LL, Messier TL, Mann KG. Evidence for a common metal ion-dependent transition in the 4-carboxyglutamic acid domains of several vitamin K dependent proteins. J Biol Chem 264:17882, 1989.
5. Malhotra DP, Nesheim ME, Mann KG. The kinetics of activation of normal and gammacarboxyglutamaic acid-deficient prothrombins. J Biol Chem 260:279, 1985.
6. Mann KG, Krishnaswamy S, Lawson JH. Surface dependent hemostasis. Semin Hematol 29:213, 1992.
7. Silverberg SA, Nemerson Y, Zur M. Kinetics of the activation of bovine coagulation factor X by components of the extrinsic pathway. J Biol Chem 252:8481, 1977.
8. Krishnaswamy S, Jones KC, Mann KG. Kinetic mechanism of enzyme assembly on phospholipid vesicles. J Biol Chem 263:3823, 1988.
9. Nesheim ME, Myrmel KH, Hibbard L, Mann KG. Isolation and characterization of single chain bovine factor V. J Biol Chem 254:508, 1979.
10. Viskup RW, Tracy PB, Mann KG. The isolation of human platelet factor V. Blood 69:1188, 1987.
11. Nesheim ME, Nichols WL, Cole TL, Houston JG, Schenk RB, Mann KG, Bovie EJW. Isolation and study of an acquired inhibitor of human coagulation factor V. J Clin Invest 77:405, 1986.
12. Rand MD, Kalafatis M, Mann KG. Platelet coagulation factor Va: The major secretory platelet phosphoprotein. Blood 83:2180, 1994.
13. Tracy PB, Giles AR, Mann KG, Elde LL, Hoogendourn H, Riourd GE. J Clin Invest 74:1221, 1984.
14. Bloom JW, Neisheim ME, Mann KG. Phospholipid binding properties of bovine factor V and factor Va. Biochemistry 18:4419, 1979.
15. Higgins DL, Mann RG. The interaction of bovine factor V and factor V-derived peptides with phospholipid vesicles. J Biol Chem 258:6503, 1983.
16. Tracy PB, Mann KG. Prothrombinase complex assembly on the platelet surface is mediated through the 74,000 dalton component of factor Va. Proc Natl Acad Sci USA 80:2380, 1983.
17. Kalafahs M, Rand MD, Mann KG. Factor Va membrane interaction is mediated by two regions located on the light chain of the cofactor. Biochemistry 33:486, 1994.

18. Krishnaswamy S, Jones KC, Mann KG. Prothrombinase complex assembly on kinetic mechanism of enzyme assembly on phospholipid vesicles. J Biol Chem 263:3823, 1988.
19. Krishnaswamy S, Field KA, Edgington TS, Morrissey JH, Mann KG. Role of the membrane surface in the activation of human coagulation factor X. J Biol Chem 267:26110, 1992.
20. Pryzdial EL, Mann KG. The association of coagulation factor Xa and factor Va. J Biol Chem 266:8969, 1991.
21. Esmon CT. The subunit structure of thrombin-activated factor V. Isolation of activated factor V, separation of subunits, and reconstitution of biological activity. J Biol Chem 254:964, 1979.
22. Nesheim ME, Mann KG. Thrombin-catalyzed activation of single chain bovine factor V. J Biol Chem 254:1326, 1979.
23. Nesheim ME, Taswell JB, Mann KG. The contribution of bovine factor V and factor Va to the activity of prothrombinase. J Biol Chem 254:10952, 1979.
24. Foster BW, Neisheim ME, Mann KG. The factor Xa catalyzed activation of factor V. J Biol Chem 258:13970, 1983.
25. Monkovic DD, Tracy PB. Activation of human factor V by Xa and thrombin. Biochemistry 29:1118, 1990.
26. Krishnaswamy S, Russell GD, Mann KG. The reassociation of factor Va from its isolated subunits. J Biol Chem 264:3160, 1989.
27. Foster WB, Nesheim ME, Mann KG. The factor Xa catalyzed activation of factor V. J Biol Chem 258:13970, 1983.
28. Barton PG, Hanahan DJ. Some lipid protein interactions involved in prothrombin activation. Biochem Biophys Acta 187:319, 1969.
29. Higgins DC, Callahan PJ, Prendergast FG, Newsheim ME, Mann KG. Lipid mobility in the assembly and expression of the activity of the prothrombinase complex. J Biol Chem 260:3604, 1985.
30. Tracy PB, Mann KG. In Wolmsen H (ed). Platelet Responses and Metabolism. Boca Raton, FL: CRC Press, 1986:297.
31. Tracy PB, Nesheim ME, Mann KG. Coordinate binding of factor Va and factor Xa to the unstimulated platelet. J Biol Chem 256:743, 1981.
32. Newroth PP, Hundley DA, Esmon CT, et al. Interleukin induces endothelial cell procoagulant activity while suppressing cell-surface anticoagulant activity. Proc Natl Acad Sci USA 83:3460, 1986.
33. Nesheim ME, Kettner C, Shaw E, Mann KG. Cofactor dependence of factor Xa incorporation into the prothrombinase complex. J Biol Chem 256:6537, 1979.
34. Nesheim ME, Eid S, Mann KG. Assembly of the prothrombinase complex in the absence of prothrombin. J Biol Chem 256:9874, 1981.
35. Krishnaswamy S, Church WR, Nesheim ME, Mann KG. Activation of human prothrombin by human prothrombinase. Influence of factor Va on the reaction mechanism. J Biol Chem 262:3291, 1987.

36. Kane WH, Lindhout MJ, Jackson CM, Majerus PW. Factor Va dependent binding of factor Xa to human platelets. J Biol Chem 255:1170, 1980.

37. Miletich JP, Jackson CM, Majerus PW. Properties of the factor Xa binding site on human platelets. J Biol Chem 253:6908, 1978.

38. Miletich JP, Majerus DW, Majerus PW. Patients with congenital factor V deficiency have decreased factor Xa binding sites on their platelets. J Clin Invest 62:824, 1978.

39. Miletich JP, Kane WH, Hoffman SL, Stanford N, Majerus PW. Deficiency of factor Xa-factor Va binding sites on the platelets of a patient with a bleeding disorder. Blood 54:1015, 1979.

40. Kane WH, Lindhout MJ, Jackson CM, Majerus PW. Factor Va-dependent binding of factor-Xa to human platelets. J Biol Chem 255:1170, 1981.

41. Tracy PB, Peterson JM, Nesheim ME, McDuffie FC, Mann KG. Interaction of coagulation factor V and factor Va with platelets. J Biol Chem 254:10354, 1979.

42. Tracy PB, Peterson JM, Nesheim ME, McDuffie FC, Mann KG. In Taylor FB Jr, Mann KG (eds). The Regulation of Coagulation. New York: Elsevier, 1980:237.

43. Mann KG, Nesheim ME, Church WR, Huley P, Krishnaswamy S. Surface-dependent reactions of the vitamin K dependent enzyme complexes. Blood 76:1, 1990.

44. Krishnaswamy S. Prothrombinase complex assembly: Contributions of protein-protein and protein-membrane interactions towards complex formation. J Biol Chem 265:3708, 1990.

45. Krishnaswamy S, Jones KC, Mann KG. Kinetic mechanism of enzyme assembly on phospholipid vesicles. J Biol Chem 263:3823, 1988.

46. Swords NA, Mann KG. The assembly of the prothrombinase complex on adherent platelets. Arterioscleros Thrombos 13:1602, 1993.

2. PLASMA COAGULATION FACTORS

Pamela Sakkinen and Russell P. Tracy

Overview

The role of thrombosis in precipitating acute cardio-vascular disease (CVD) events has been well known since the early 1970s [1]. It is now becoming increasingly apparent that thrombosis may also be involved with the chronic development of CVD [2–4]. Clot formation or thrombosis can be conceptualized as a balance between procoagulant and anticoagulant and fibrinolytic forces [5] (Figure 2-1). Although some factors, such as thrombin, may have more than one role, this "pseudoequilibrium" provides a schema for assessing the relative coagulant balance.

Traditionally the hemostatic system has been divided into intrinsic and extrinsic pathways, which come together at the prothrombinase complex in a common pathway. The components of the intrinsic system are contained entirely within the vasculature, whereas the extrinsic system involves components from both the blood and the vasculature itself. There are interactions between components of the *intrinsic* and *extrinsic* pathways, however, and this division does not exist strictly in vivo. Tissue factor (TF)–factor VIIa complex, the major trigger to coagulation, activates small amounts of both factor IX of the intrinsic pathway and factor X of the common pathway [6] (Figure 2-2A). Activation of factor X to factor Xa and of prothrombin to thrombin results in autoamplification through activation of the obligate cofactors, factors V and VIII, of factor VII by thrombin, and of factor Xa. Thrombin further activates platelets to provide cellular binding sites for the assembly of vitamin K–dependent protein (VKDP) complexes and catalyzes activation of factor XIII. Measurements of prothrombin fragment 1–2 (F1–2), thrombin–antithrombin complexes (TAT), and fibrinopeptide A (FPA) provide indices of thrombin generation, neutralization, and action, respectively. Activation peptides, released when a zymogen is activated to an enzyme, can also be quantitated as measures of enzymatic activity [7].

While the classic model of the clotting cascade has provided a logical understanding of hemostasis, it is evident that it does not account for various clinical coagulation pathologies, for example, the bleeding diatheses experienced by hemophiliacs. A study attempting to simulate in vivo conditions has proposed that factor Xa produced on the phospholipid surface has a different role than factor Xa produced by the TF–factor VIIa complex [8]. The inactivation of factor Xa by tissue factor pathway inhibitor (TFPI) has also been postulated to interfere with the extrinsic pathway in vivo [9]. Alternatively, Mann and colleagues have proposed a model of factor X activation based on kinetic experiments in systems containing elements of both pathways, which provides a plausible explanation for the bleeding that occurs in the factor VIII and IX deficiencies (Figure 2-2B) [10]. The key to this model is the activation of factor IX through an inactive intermediate, factor IXα. Factor IXα is initially produced by the small amount of factor Xa formed by the TF–factor VIIa complex. Once factor IXα is formed, it becomes the preferred substrate of TF–factor VIIa. Action of TF–factor VIIa on the intermediate factor IX produces factor IXa (factor IXaβ). From this point on, the factor IXa–factor VIIIa complex exceeds the TF–factor VIIa complex in the generation of factor Xa. Therefore, deficiencies of factors IX or VIII under normal physiological conditions would result in inadequate hemostasis.

A common theme in major reactions of the coagulation cascade is the role of the phospholipid surface [11]. The Xase complex (factor IXa–factor VIIIa), as well as the prothrombinase and protein case reactions, are localized to a phospholipid surface. The components of the reaction include a vitamin K–dependent (VKD) enzyme, a cofactor protein that binds the enzyme, lipid surface, and ionized calcium (Figure 2-3). Although the components of each reaction are substrate specific, they assemble in similar patterns and provide the same advantage — amplified kinetic rates of reaction through a localized reaction complex protected from plasma dilution and plasma inhibition factors [12,13] (Figure 2-4). It is thought that physiologically the Xase and prothrombinase reactions occur on the same phospholipid surface, with the

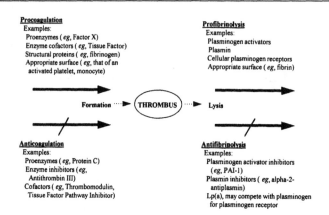

FIGURE 2-1. Thrombosis as a pseudoequilibrium between pro- and anti-coagulant and fibrinolytic factors. Increases in procoagulant or antifibrinolytic factors favor thrombosis, whereas anticoagulant and profibrinolytic factors prevent clot formation and enhance clot dissolution, respectively.

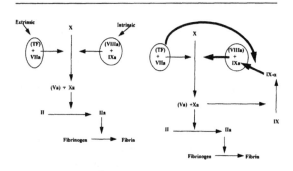

FIGURE 2-2. A: The traditional view has the intrinsic and extrinsic pathways coming together at the activation of factor X. Newer information suggests that TF–factor VIIa activates factor IX to factor IXa as well. The model of Mann and colleagues (B) proposes that an intermediate form of factor IX (factor IX α) is preferred by TF–factor VIIa over factor X. The action of factor IXα results in the formation of factor IXa. Factor IXa is then responsible for the majority of factor Xa formed. Obligate cofactors are shown in parentheses.

product of the first reaction becoming the enzyme of the second, but this has not been demonstrated in vivo [13].

The major role of thrombin as a procoagulant is to enhance the hydrolysis of fibrinogen to form fibrin. Thrombin acts sequentially at the amino terminus of fibrinogen, initially cleaving the two A-α chains of fibrinogen, followed by excision of terminal peptides of the two B-β chains, releasing FPA and FPB peptides, respectively. Although other enzymes, such as tissue plasminogen activator (t-PA), can catalyze the site-specific hydrolysis of fibrinogen, resulting in formation of fibrin monomer I, they do so relatively

slowly, and the measurement of FPA is felt to be specific for thrombin activity. Fibrin monomer II can be crosslinked by factor XIIIa to form stable fibrin strands [14].

Fibrin polymerization occurs in sequential steps. First, exposure of the new N termini results from cleavage of the A-α and B-β chains of fibrinogen in the central region of the molecule. These new N termini bind weakly to the terminal D domains of the fibrin II monomers. Factor XIIIa catalyzes bond formation between terminal D domains. The final step of fibrin polymerization is covalent crosslinking of the α chains.

There are four major proteins involved in the regulation of coagulation: TFPI, protein C, its cofactor protein S, and antithrombin III (AT III; Figure 2-5). In vitro studies have demonstrated that TFPI inhibits factor Xa, and TF–factor VIIa in a factor Xa-dependent reaction [15], and animal studies have shown that decreased levels of TFPI predispose to coagulation [16,17]. Measurement of levels in human populations in various states of health and disease, however, have been less straightforward in defining an in vivo anticoagulant role for TFPI. Whereas some studies have shown an elevation of TFPI in procoagulant states [18–20], suggesting TFPI increases to compensate for increases in procoagulant activity, others have shown decreased or normal levels of TFPI in thrombotic disease [20–22]. Recent data from cross-sectional analysis are consistent with TFPI

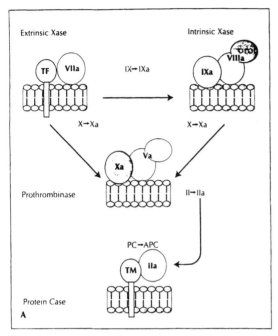

FIGURE 2-3. Major reactions of the coagulation cascade and the role of the phospholipid surface. The Xase complex, prothrombinase, and protein case reactions are localized to the phospholipid surface. (From Bovill E, Mann K, Lawson J, et al. Biochemistry of vitamin K: Implications for warfarin therapy. In Ezekowitz M (ed). Systemic Cardiac Embolism. New York: Marcel Dekker, 1994: 31–54, with permission.)

B. RATES OF PROTHROMBIN ACTIVATION IN PRESENCE OF VARIOUS COMBINATIONS OF THE PROTHROMBINASE COMPLEX

COMPONENTS PRESENT*	RATE OF ACTIVATION[†]
Xa	0.004
Xa, Ca^{++}	0.01
Xa, Ca^{++}, phospholipid	0.09
Xa, Ca^{++}, Va	1.55
Xa, Ca^{++}, phospholipid, Va	1210.00

*Proteins are present at potential physiologic concentration: prothrombin ~ 10^{-6} M; factor Va ~ 10^{-8} M; factor Xa ~ 10^{-9} M. Phospholipid is present at a concentration adequate to saturate the reaction.

[†]Rates are expressed as moles of thrombin/min/M of factor Xa.

FIGURE 2-4. Influence of selected elements of the prothrombinase complex on the rate of activation of factor Xa. (From Mann K. The assembly of blood clotting complexes as membranes. Trends Biochem Sci 12:229–233; 1987, with permission.)

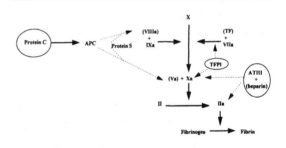

FIGURE 2-5. The anticoagulant proteins: Protein C (actually the activated form, activated protein C or APC), tissue factor pathway inhibitor (TFPI), and antithrombin III (ATIII) inhibit thrombin and factor Xa generation. APC with protein S acts through inhibition of cofactors Va and VIIIa, while TFPI inhibits factor Xa directly and factor VIIa–TF in a factor Xa–dependent manner. ATIII, in the presence of cellular heparans or exogenous heparins, inhibits both factors Xa and IIa directly. The obligate cofactors are shown in parentheses. Inhibition is indicated by dotted lines.

functioning as an inflammation-sensitive protein, as well as an anticoagulant protein (P Sakkinen, manuscript in progress).

Thrombin binds thrombomodulin, and this complex (the protein case complex) activates protein C to activated protein C (APC) [23]. APC then inactivates Factors Va and VIIIa. Protein S circulates in an active free form and an inactive form bound to C4B-binding protein of the complement system. The active free form functions as a cofactor for APC [23]. Plasminogen activator inhibitor-3 (PAI-3) of the fibrinolytic system, α_2–macroglobulin, and α_1–antitrypsin are all capable of inactivating APC. AT III, as previously noted, inactivates predominantly factors Xa and thrombin, in a heparin- or cellular-heparan–dependent manner.

We have observed elevated protein C and AT III levels with active heart disease in cross-sectional analysis (P Callas, manuscript in progress), as have others [24]. It seems likely that they are upregulated through a homeostatic mechanism in procoagulant states. Although this reasoning is intriguing, a mechanism has not yet been defined.

Deficiencies of protein C, Protein S, and AT III, in contrast to TFPI, are clearly associated with an increased risk of venous thromboembolism in population studies [25,26]. In normal nondiseased arteries, the rapid blood flow dilutes coagulant factors, as well as the anticoagulant proteins, so that deficiencies of anticoagulant proteins have been associated with venous thromboembolism, and not arterial thrombosis. Factors that lead to disturbed arterial flow or result in endothelial damage have been associated with an increased risk of arterial thrombosis.

The most common cause of hereditary thrombophilia, resistance to APC, was described in 1993 [27,28]. APC resistance is a laboratory finding in which there is less prolongation of the clot time with added APC than might be expected. Most cases of APC resistance are due to factor V Leiden, a mutation of the second domain of the factor V gene (base substitution of G to A at nucleotide position 1691) [29], resulting in markedly decreased degradation of plasma factor V [29,30], and platelet factor V [31] by APC. This mutation theoretically results in a biological picture similar to protein S or protein C deficiency, with the caveat that factor VIII degradation is not impaired with factor V Leiden. Similar to deficiencies of the anticoagulant proteins, prospective and cross-sectional studies have demonstrated no associations between factor V Leiden and ischemic myocardial or stroke events [32–35]. Interestingly, a recent abstract reported an association between arterial thrombosis and APC resistance in patients negative for the factor V Leiden mutation [36]. This suggests that sources of APC resistance, other than factor V Leiden, may play important roles in arterial disease.

However, many patients heterozygous for protein C deficiency or factor V Leiden exhibit no thrombophilic manifestations. Heterozygous protein C deficiency has a prevalence of 1 out of 200 healthy asymptomatic donors [37], heterozygous factor V Leiden a prevalence of approximately 5 out of 100 [28,38]. Bovill et al. examined a kindred of 184 members, which included a number of members heterozygous for protein C deficiency [25]. They found positive thrombotic histories in only 13 of 46 family members with biochemical deficiencies of protein C, and in 5 of their unaffected relatives. There was no significant difference in the prevalence of protein S or AT III deficiency between members with thrombosis and those who were asymptomatic. These results led them to suggest that although heterozygous protein C deficiency is a risk factor for venous thrombosis, additional factors (e.g., an endothelial cell defect leading to decreased production of thrombomodulin; or diminished activity of the fibrinolytic system) may be required for expression of the thrombophilic phenotype.

Regarding factor V Leiden, phenotypic heterogeneity has been reported among homozygous subjects, as well as heterozygous carriers. One family with four homozygous siblings reported that half had experienced no thrombotic disease by approximately 30 years of age, while the other two had experienced severe thrombotic disease [39]. Among heterozygous patients who had experienced prior thrombosis, a recent retrospective study examining the recurrence of thrombosis in patients with and without factor V Leiden found no significant difference in recurrence of events between patients heterozygous for factor V Leiden and control patients [40]. Further work is needed to establish the influence of factors that predispose patients to express thrombophilia in order to adequately counsel patients and their families on the full implications of their genotype.

Structural Considerations

The vitamin K–dependent factors (VKDF: Factors II, VII, IX, and X; protein C and protein S) are structurally similar [41] (Figure 2-6). The amino terminus of each factor contains 9–12 glutamic acid residues, which undergo posttranslational gamma carboxylation (GLA modification). The GLA domains mediate calcium-dependent binding to the phospholipid membrane by allowing conformational changes in the amino terminus (amino acids 1–35) [12,42]. Warfarin, an oral anticoagulant, interferes with carboxylation of the glutamic acid residues by inhibiting vitamin K reductase and limiting the supply of reduced vitamin K [43] (Figure 2-7). Uncarboxylated VKDFs have limited clotting activity, dependent on the number of carboxylated GLAs. A reduction in only three GLA residues results in a marked reduction in the biological activity of the VKDFs [44–47].

Paradoxically, initiating warfarin therapy causes a temporary thrombotic state, due to the differential half-lives of the VKDFs. Protein C and factor VII have the shortest half-lives (6 hours), followed by factor IX, factor X, and finally prothrombin (half-life, 60–72 hours) [48]. The initial effect of warfarin may be thrombotic in some people due to the reduction in protein C levels occurring faster than the reductions of the procoagulant factors. There is evidence that suggests reduction in prothrombin is responsible for the majority of the antithrombotic effects of warfarin [49,50]. Because prothrombin levels are not reduced to less than one half of normal until day 4 of therapy, this provides a rationale for cotreating with heparin during the first days of anticoagulation.

An uncommon complication of warfarin, warfarin-induced skin necrosis, is related to the initial hyper-

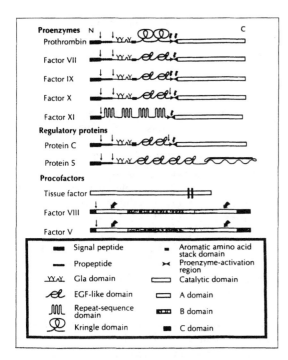

FIGURE 2-6. Schematic of the various domains comprising the proenzymes, regulatory proteins, and procofactors. (From Furie B, Furie B. Molecular and cellular biology of blood coagulation. N Engl J Med 326:800–806, 1992, with permission.)

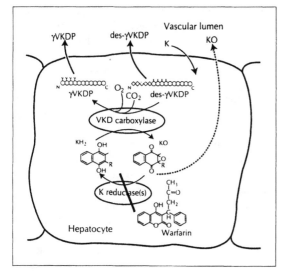

FIGURE 2-7. Vitamin K metabolism and the role of warfarin. (From Mann K. The assembly of blood clotting complexes as membranes. Trends Biochem Sci 12:229–233, 1987, with permission.)

coagulability that occurs when instituting warfarin therapy [48]. It occurs in 1/1000 to 1/10,000 of treated patients. Histological examination reveals thromboses of subcutaneous and cutaneous venules. Warfarin-induced skin necrosis typically presents as painful red plaques in fatty areas of the body within 3–5 days after initiating therapy, classically in an obese woman in the sixth to seventh decade of life, and in patients given high loading doses of drug (i.e., >10 mg). One quarter of patients who develop skin necrosis have active infection [51], and one third have a deficiency of protein C [52]. It has been suggested that infection contributes to hypercoagulability through cytokine-mediated increases in acute-phase reactants, such as C4B-binding protein and PAI-1, which reduce levels of protein S and plasmin, respectively [48]. Because the majority of patients with protein C deficiency tolerate warfarin therapy successfully, it is likely that other factors that contribute to the disease pathogenesis remain to be resolved.

Prothrombin contains Kringle domains with binding properties for factors Va and Xa of the prothrombinase complex [53]. The remaining VKDP proenzymes and protein C contain an EGF-like domain, which similarly facilitates the binding of substrate-specific factors [54]. Factor XI contains a repeat sequence domain [41]. The VKDP zymogens and factor XI share a similar signal peptide region and propeptide region, as well as a catalytic serine protease domain at the C terminus. The signal peptides and propeptides are cleaved intracellularly. In the circulation, cleavage at the activation region results in release of an activation peptide and formation of the active enzyme.

Thrombin and factor Xa are inactivated by a heparan-enhanced AT III reaction. Exogenous heparin or endogenous heparans facilitate anticoagulation by AT III, by providing a negatively charged template to enhance complex formation of factor Xa and thrombin, as well as factors XIIa, XIa, and IXa, with AT III. Heparin is a heterogeneous mixture of disaccharides that range in size and variably contain a specific pentasaccharide site that binds AT III [55]. Carbohydrate chains greater than 18 units in length allow sufficient surface for the binding of thrombin and AT III. Because heparin needs only to bind AT III to facilitate anticoagulation of factor Xa, heparin chains less than 18 units (i.e., low molecular weight heparin [LMWH]) that contain an AT III binding domain are effective at inhibiting factor Xa [56].

There is evidence in vitro and in experimental animal models that suggests LMWHs may cause less bleeding than standard heparin, while providing an equal or more effective antithrombotic effect [57–

62]. Multiple clinical trials have supported an effectiveness of LMWHs similar to standard heparin in the prevention of venous thrombosis in both surgical and medicine patients [63–67]. In addition, many studies report that LMWHs do not demonstrate an increase in major bleeding compared with placebo [68–71]. LMWHs may also be more effective than standard heparin in decreasing the size of an established thrombus with less bleeding [72,73]. The advantages of LMWHs over standard heparin are related to the thrombin–factor Xa difference described earlier, as well as differences in interactions with platelet function [74] and vascular permeability [75], and major differences in bioavailability and pharmokinetics [76].

Standard heparin, to a greater degree than LMWHs, is bound to plasma proteins (histidine-rich glycoprotein [HRGP]), PF4, vitronectin, fibronectin, and von Willebrand factor [vWF] [77,78], and endothelial cells and macrophages [79]. This results in dose-dependent recovery and clearance of standard heparin [80–82]. Conversely, the recovery and clearance of LMWHs is dose independent, and LMWHs have a longer half-life [83]. In addition, the binding of vWF, in particular, interferes with platelet function, and there is evidence that standard heparin may also contribute to an increased risk of bleeding by inhibiting collagen-induced platelet aggregation and increasing vascular permeability [74,75]. Therefore, the anticoagulant response of LMWHs compared with standard heparin may be more predictable, with the possibility of less frequent administration and laboratory monitoring. The effectiveness of LMWHs preoperatively remains to be evaluated, as do questions regarding the use of LMWHs in pregnancy, in patients with a history of heparin-induced thrombocytopenia, and the risk of osteoporosis in long-term users [56].

Cofactors V and VIII are homologous in structure, activation sequences, and function, although they circulate in different forms and have different activation sites. Factor VIII is bound to vWF in plasma, while factor V circulates in a free form. Both share a triplicated A domain, duplicated C domain, and variable B domain [12]. The B domain is excised during activation of the cofactor and is, therefore, homologous to the activation peptides of the zymogens. Factors Va and VIIIa provide mechanisms to link factors Xa and IXa to the phospholipid surface. Binding of the phospholipid membrane is mediated through the A3 domain [12]. Tissue factor and thrombomodulin, as cofactors, are different in this respect because they are integral membrane proteins. Tissue factor, for example, consists of a cysteine cytoplasmic domain, a transmembranous domain, and an extracellular macromolecular ligand binding domain, which is expressed on extravascular cells and monocytes [84–86].

New Perspectives

There is evidence to support the hypothesis that thrombogenic risk factors become more important in the progression of atherosclerotic cardiovascular disease with age [87] (Figure 2-8). Thrombotic risk factors are defined as hemostatic factors (procoagulant or fibrinolytic), which when elevated (or decreased) tip the hemostatic pseudoequilibrium toward thrombosis. Also, this category includes markers of coagulant or fibrinolytic activity. Although this definition includes thrombolytic factors such as PAI-1 and t-PA, the majority of work has focused on the coagulant factors, fibrinogen and factor VII.

Prospective studies have demonstrated that increased levels of fibrinogen are associated with an increased incidence of ischemic heart disease. Meade initially demonstrated this relationship [88]. Since that time, fibrinogen has been shown to be an independent risk factor in the prediction of ischemic cardiac events at a level similar to that of low density lipoprotein (LDL) cholesterol [89–93]. Four nonexclusive pathophysiological mechanisms relating fibrinogen to heart disease have been described. The first involves the kinetics of the fibrinogen-to-fibrin reaction. Increased fibrinogen (i.e., substrate) should lead to increased fibrin production, because the Km for this reaction is near the average plasma concentration of fibrinogen [94]. The second hypothesis suggests that because fibrinogen effectively aggregates activated platelets through the GPIIb-IIIa receptor, higher levels of fibrinogen may predispose an individual to increased platelet aggregation [95]. The evidence for this mechanism is not definitive because the dissociation constant for this reaction is much lower than the average plasma concentration of fibrinogen [96].

Third, an increased fibrinogen concentration results in increased plasma viscosity, and increased viscosity has been related to an elevated risk of cardiovascular disease [97]. Results of a multivariate analysis, however, suggest fibrinogen and plasma viscosity may make independent contributions to the prediction of ischemic heart disease [92]. Finally, because atherosclerotic disease has an inflammatory aspect [98–104], elevations in fibrinogen may reflect, rather than regulate, thrombosis. There is a large body of evidence to support the position that this last "mechanism" is true. Currently, the issue is whether or not any of the previous three "causal" mechanisms

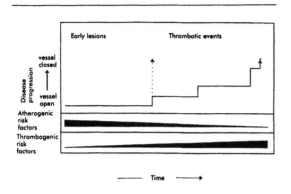

FIGURE 2-8. Schematic diagram illustrating the change in the relative importance of coronary vascular disease risk factors with increasing age. (Modified with permission from Fuster V, Badimon L, Badimon J, et al. N Engl J Med 326:242–250, 310–318, 1992; Fuster V, Stein B, Ambrose J, et al. Circulation 82:II47–II59, 1990. Tracy RP, Bovill EG. Hemostasis and risk of ischemic disease. Epidemiologic evidence with emphasis on the elderly. In Califf RM, Mark DB, Wagner GS (eds). Acute Coronary Care. 2nd ed. St. Louis, MO; Mosby-Year Book, 1995: 27–43.)

(or some unknown mechanism) actually come into play. Future research with experimental models should help in this regard.

Factor VII is the only other procoagulant factor that has been studied extensively in relationship to CVD. The association of factor VII with incident CVD is less defined than that of fibrinogen. In the Northwick Park study, factor VII was prospectively correlated with CVD events in middle-aged men, independent of fibrinogen and cholesterol [89,105]. This finding has not been confirmed in further prospective studies. The PROCAM study (Prospective Cardiovascular Munster Study) of middle-aged male industrial workers of West Germany reported no significant difference in mean factor VII levels in those who developed incident coronary heart disease or stroke [106]. Nor was there a significant relationship between factor VII levels and incident ischemic events in a preliminary report from a community-based biracial study of middle-aged men and women in the United States (the Atherosclerosis Risk in Communities Study) [107].

Despite the lack of confirmation of the findings of the Northwick Park study in other prospective trials, numerous cross-sectional studies have shown significant correlations between factor VII and men with CVD [108]; men with CVD risk factors such as smoking and hyperlipidemia [109–111]; and pa-

tients with peripheral vascular disease [112]. However, again, not all have done so [113,114]. Part of the ambiguity of the relationship between factor VII and CVD may be explained by the multiple circulating forms of factor VII, as well as the correlations of factor VII with plasma lipids, also independent risk factors for CVD [108,110,111,115–118]. The majority of CVD studies have used factor VIIc (a one-stage clotting assay of factor VII using factor VII–deficient plasma) as an indicator of in vivo factor VII levels, which is dependent on the relative amounts of activated factor VII (factor VIIa) and total factor VII protein (factor VIIag) [117]. Some forms of this assay, for example, those that using bovine thromboplastin instead of human, may be more sensitive to factor VIIa than others [119]. The recent development of a direct assay for factor VIIa may be helpful in defining the role of factor VII in CVD [120].

Less is known about the relationships between measurements of ongoing processes, such as activation peptides, and CVD. Correlates of thrombin generation or activity (prothrombin fragment F1–2 and fibrinopeptide A, respectively) have been demonstrated to be increased in many hypercoaguable states; for example, active angina [121], acute myocardial infarction [122,123], deep venous thrombosis (DVT) [124], and peripheral vascular disease (PVD) [125]. A report on correlates of thrombin generation and activity (prothrombin fragment F1–2 and fibrinopeptide A, respectively) in a healthy elderly population (Cardiovascular Health Study) was recently published [126]. They demonstrated significant associations between these markers of hemostasis and traditional cardiovascular risk factors, such as age and smoking. Another study of correlates of selected hemostatic factors with traditional CVD risk factors in male and female plasma donors reported relationships between CVD risk factors and F1–2, even closer than those observed for fibrinogen and factor VII [127]. These studies suggest that activation peptides, especially of thrombin generation, may help determine which patients will develop ischemic disease. A recently published abstract on treated hypertensive men aged 56–77 years has, in fact, shown F1–2 to be an independent predictor of congenital heart disease and mortality after adjusting for pre-existing CVD at baseline, age, diabetes mellitus, and smoking [128]. Further prospective studies are currently ongoing.

Factor VIII is a known acute-phase reactant, as well as a cofactor in the intrinsic Xase complex. In contrast to factor VII, factor VIII has been less strongly correlated with modifiable risk factors in cross-sectional studies [114]. However, factor VII has been confirmed as a risk factor for ischemic disease. The

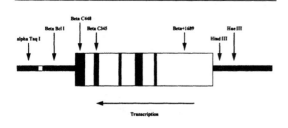

FIGURE 2-9. Beta-fibrinogen gene. Exons are indicated by black bars; introns by white bars. Arrows indicate locations of selected common polymorphisms. The figure is not drawn to scale. (Modified from Behague I, Poirier O, Nicaud V, et al. Circulation 93:440–449, 1996.)

Northwick Park study reported factor VIII levels were higher at baseline in patients who died from CVD compared with those who survived [88,89], and factor VIII levels have been shown to be predictive of ischemic events in patients with vascular disease [129] and in middle-aged subjects in the ARIC study [130]. Recently it has been reported that factor VIII remained a significant predictor of ischemic events in the elderly, even after adjusting for the presence of other CVD risk factors [131]. This suggests that factor VIII may have a predictive role in thrombotic disease, independent of its inflammatory component.

There is evidence to suggest that genetic heritability may play a role in explaining the variance of both fibrinogen and factor VII. The heritability estimate for fibrinogen has ranged from very weak to over 50% [132,133], possibility due to different populations. Fibrinogen itself is composed of three pairs of polypeptide chains (Aα, Bβ, and γ), each encoded by discrete genes on the long arm of chromosome 4 [134,135]. Most investigations into the genetic variability of fibrinogen have focused on the β gene, because formation of the β polypeptide is the rate-limiting step in fibrinogen synthesis [136–138]. Figure 2-9 illustrates several known fibrinogen genetic polymorphisms. In 1987 it was reported that restriction fragment length polymorphisms (RFLP) of the β gene (G $\Rightarrow$ A^{-455} [Hae III], C $\Rightarrow$ T^{-148} [Hind III] identified by Humphries et al. explained approximately 3% of the variance of fibrinogen levels [139]. This RELP was second only to smoking in predicting fibrinogen levels in a multivariate analysis. Since that time numerous polymorphisms have been identified; most, but not all, relate to fibrinogen concentration [133,140–146]. In addition, some studies have re-

ported interactions between the β fibrinogen gene and smokers, particularly the Hind III and Hae III polymorphisms [145,147,148]. It is hypothesized that these alleles may mediate a smoking interaction through an interleukin (IL)-6 response sequence adjacent to the Hind III allele [147].

Fibrinogen polymorphisms have also been correlated with atherosclerosis. The β-gene Bcl I polymorphism, for example, has been related to the presence of PVD [140] and the severity of CAD [145]. Notably, neither of these studies demonstrated a concurrent association with fibrinogen levels, even though the β bcl I polymorphism has been previously correlated with fibrinogen concentration. An alternative mechanism proposed that the β Bcl I polymorphism, located downstream of the β gene, may affect function, rather than quantity of gene transcribed, or may serve as a marker of a gene that affects function. Interestingly, a high degree of linkage disequilibrium has been reported between the polymorphisms, implying the potential for functional interrelationships within the haplotype [145]. Establishing a link between the presence of a polymorphism, fibrinogen levels, and atherosclerotic disease will be useful in untangling the role of fibrinogen in CVD. Furthermore, study into the interactions of the genes with modifiable risk factors will undoubtedly prove useful in determining patients who would most benefit from behavioral modifications.

Concerning factor VII, a single base substitution of G to A in the factor VII gene has been identified. This is a common polymorphism, which results in a change in amino acid 353 from arginine to glutamine [149], and in decreased factor VII levels (heterozygote expression of factor VII decreased by 20–30% of normal, and homozygote expression decreased by 40–60% of normal) [150]. Interestingly, differences in relationships between CVD risk factors and factor VII levels stratified by genotype have been reported. One study has reported no significant associations between cholesterol and triglycerides with factor VII of people with the glutamine allele [150], and another report suggested that levels of factor VII in women with the glutamine allele did not exhibit an elevation with menopause and the use of hormone therapy [151]. This mutation may therefore have implications for defining the relationship between factor VII and lipids, as well as factor VII and CVD.

This is a time of growth in our understanding of coagulation factors, and their physiologic and pathophysiologic roles. Further advances are being made in understanding the mechanisms of coagulation as they truly exist in vivo, as well as the relationships of hemostatic factors to the progression of atherosclerotic disease. Both will have great impact on the promotion of health and the treatment of disease.

References

1. DeWood M, Spores J, Notske R, Mouser L, Burroughs R, Goldens M, Lang H. Prevalence of total coronary occlusion during the early hours of transmural myocardial infarction. N Engl J Med 303:897, 1980.

2. Harker LA, Hanson SR, Runge MS. Thrombin hypothesis of thrombus generation and vascular lesion formation. Am J Cardiol 75:12B, 1995.

3. Fuster V, Badimon L, Badimon J, Chesebro J. The pathogenesis of coronary artery disease and the acute coronary syndromes: Part 1. N Engl J Med 326:242, 1992.

4. Fuster V, Badimon L, Badimon J, Chesebro J. The pathogenesis of coronary artery disease and the acute coronary syndromes: Part 2. N Engl J Med 326:310, 1992.

5. Tracy R, Mann K, Bovill E. Mechanisms of thrombolysis. In Ezekowitz M (ed). Cardiac Sources of Systemic Embolization. New York: Marcel Dekker, 1994:55.

6. Rapaport SI, Rao LVM. Initiation and regulation of tissue factor-dependent blood coagulation. Arterioscleros Thrombos 12:1111, 1992.

7. Bauer K, Rosenberg R. The pathophysiology of the prethrombotic state in humans: Insignts gained from studies using markers of hemostatic system activation. Blood 70:343, 1987.

8. Hoffman M, Monroe DM, Oliver JA, Roberts HR. Factors IXa and Xa play distinct roles in tissue factor-dependent initiation of coagulation. Blood 86:1794, 1995.

9. Rao LVM, Rapaport SI. Studies of a mechanism inhibiting the initiation of the extrinsic pathway of coagulation. Blood 69:645, 1987.

10. Lawson JH, Mann KG. The cooperative activation of human factor IX by the human extrinsic pathway of blood coagulation. J Biol Chem 266:11317, 1991.

11. Mann K, Lawson J. The role of the membrane in the expression of the vitamin K-dependent enzymes. Arch Pathol Lab Med 116:1330, 1992.

12. Mann K, Nesheim M, Church W, Haley P, Krishnaswamy S. Surface dependent reactions of the vitamin K dependent enzyme complexes. Blood 76:1, 1990.

13. Mann K. The assembly of blood clotting complexes as membranes. Trends Biochem Sci 12:229, 1987.

14. Mosesson MW. Fibrin polymerization and its regulatory role in hemostasis. J Lab Clin Med 116:8, 1990.

15. Broze G, Tollefsen D. Regulation of blood coagulation by protease inhibitors. In Stamatoyannopoulos G, Nienhuis A, Majerus P, Varmus H (eds). The Molecular Basis of Blood Diseases. Philadelphia: W.B. Saunders, 1994:629.

16. Sandset PM, Warn-Cramer BJ, Rao LVM, Maki SL, Rapaport SI. Depletion of the extrinsic pathway inhibitor (EPI) sensitizes rabbits to disseminated intravascular coagulation induced with tissue factor: Evidence supporting a physiologic role for EPI as a natural anticoagulant. Proc Natl Acad Sci USA 88:708, 1991.

17. Sandset PM, Warn-Caramer BJ, Maki SL, Rapaport SI. Immunodepletion of extrinsic pathway inhibitor sensitizes rabbits to endotoxin-induced intravascular coagulation and the generalized Schwartzman reaction. Blood 78:1496, 1991.

18. Sandset PM, Hellgren M, Uvebrandt M, Bergstrom H. Extrinsic coagulation pathway inhibitor and heparin cofactor II during normal and hypertensive pregnancy. Thromb Res 55:665, 1989.

19. Sandset PM, Sirnes PA, Abilgaard U. Factor VII and extrinsic pathway inhibitor in acute coronary disease. Br J Haematol 72:391, 1989.

20. Lindahl AK, Sandset PM, Abilgaard U. The present status of tissue factor pathway inhibitor. Blood Coagul Fibrinolysis 3:439, 1992.

21. Novotny WF, Brown SG, Miletich JP, Rader DJ, Broze GJJ. Plasma antigen levels of the lipoprotein-associated coagulation inhibitor in patient samples. Blood 1991:2, 1991.

22. Bajaj MS, Rana SV, Wysolmerski RB, Bajaj SP. Inhibitor of the VIIa-tissue factor complex is reduced in patients with disseminated intravascular coagulation but not in patients with hepatocellular disease. J Clin Invest 79:1874, 1987.

23. Esmon C. The roles of protein C and thrombomodulin in the regulation of blood coagulation. J Biol Chem 264:4743, 1987.

24. Gensini GF, Rostagno C, Abbate R, Favilla S, Mannucci PM, Serneri GGN. Increased protein C and fibrinopeptide A concentration in patients with angina. Thromb Res 50:517, 1988.

25. Bovill E, Bauer K, Dickerman J, Callas P, West B. The clinical spectrum of heterozygous protein C deficiency in a large New England kindred. Blood 73:712, 1989.

26. Pabinger I, Brucker S, Kyrle PA, Schneider B, Korninger HC, Niessner H, Lechner K. Hereditary deficiency of antithrombin III, Protein C and Protein S: Prevalence in patients with a history of venous thrombosis and criteria for rational patient screening. Blood Coagul Fibrinolysis 3:547, 1992.

27. Dahlback B, Carlsson M, Svensson P. Familial thrombophilia due to a previously unrecognized mechanism characterized by poor anticoagulant response to activated protein C: Prediction of a cofactor to activated protein C. Proc Natl Acad Sci USA 90:1004, 1993.

28. Griffin J, Evatt B, Wideman C, Fernandez J. Anticoagulant protein C pathway defective in majority of thrombophilic patients. Blood 82:1989, 1993.

29. Griffin JH, Heeb MJ, Kojima Y, Fernandez JA, Kojima K, Hackeng TM, Greengard JS. Activated protein C resistance: Molecular mechanism. Thromb Haemost 74:444, 1995.

30. Kalafatis M, Bertina R, Rand M, Mann K. Characterization of the molecular defect in factor VR506Q. J Biol Chem 270:4053, 1995.

31. Camire R, Kalafatis M, Cushman M, Tracy R, Mann K, Tracy P. The mechanism of inactivation of human platelet factor Va from normal and activated Protein C-resistant individuals. J Biol Chem 270:20794, 1995.

32. Cushman M, Bhushan F, Bovill E, Tracy R. Plasma resistance to activated protein C in venous and arterial thrombosis. Thromb Haemost 72:643, 1994.

33. Ridker P, Hennekens C, Lindpaintner K, Stampfer M, Eisenberg P, Miletich J. Mutation in the gene coding for coagulation factor V and the risk of myocardial infarction, stroke, and venous thrombosis in apparently healthy men. N Engl J Med 332:912, 1995.

34. Kontula K, Ylikorkala A, Miettinen H, Vuorio A, Kauppinen-Makelin R, Hamalainen H, Palomaki H, Kaste M. Arg506Gln factor V mutation (factor V leiden) in patients with ischemic cerebrovascular disease and survivors of myocardial infarction. Thromb Haemost 73:558, 1995.

35. Ardissino D, Peyvandi F, Merlini PA, Colombi E, Mannucci PM. Factor V (Arg506-Gln) mutation in young surviors of myocardial infarction. Thromb Haemost:701, 1996.

36. van der Bom JG, Bots ML, Grobbee DE, Slagboom PE, Haverkate F, Meijer P, Kluft C. Activated Protein C and risk of stroke and transient ischemic attack (abstr). Circulation 95:622, 1996.

37. Miletich J, Sherman L, Broze G. Absence of thrombosis in subjects with heterozygous protein C deficiency. N Engl J Med 317:991, 1987.

38. Bertina R, Koeleman B, Koster T, Rosendaal F, Dirven R, deRonde H, van der Velden P, Reitsma P. Mutation in blood coagulation factor V associated with resistance to activated protein C. Nature 369:64,1994.

39. Greengard J, Eichinger S, Griffin J, Bauer K. Brief report: Variability of thrombosis among homozygous siblings with resistance to activated protein C due to an Arg > Gln mutation in the gene for factor V. N Engl J Med 331:1559, 1994.

40. Rintelen C, Pabinger I, Knobl P, Lechner K, Mannhalter C. Probability of recurrence of thrombosis in patients with and without Factor V Leiden. Thromb Haemost 75:229, 1996.

41. Furie B, Furie B. Molecular and cellular biology of blood coagulation. N Engl J Med 326:800, 1992.

42. Soriano-Garcia M, Park CH, Tulinsky A, Ravichandran KG, Skrzypczak-Jankun E. Structure of Ca^{2+} prothrombin fragment 1 including the conformation of the Gla domain. Biochemistry 28:6805, 1989.

43. Whitlon DS, Sadowski JA, Suttie JW. Mechanisms of coumarin action: Significance of vitamin K epoxide reductase inhibition. Biochemistry 17:1371, 1978.

44. Malhotra OP. Dicoumarol-induced prothrombins. Ann NY Acad Sci 370:426, 1981.

45. Malhotra OP, Nesheim ME, Mann KG. The kinetics of activation of normal and gamma-carboxylated glutamine acid-deficient prothrombins. J Biol Chem 260:279, 1985.

46. Malhotra OP. Dicoumarol-induced prothrombins containing 6, 7 and 8 gamma-carboxyglutamic acid residues: Isolation and characterization. Biochem Cell Biol 67:411, 1989.

47. Malhotra OP. Dicoumarol-induced gamma carboxyglutamic acid prothrombin: Isolation and comparison with 6-, 7-, 8- and 10-gamma-carboxyglutamic acid isomers. Biochem Cell Biol 68:705, 1990.

48. Bauer KA. Coumarin-induced skin necrosis. Arch Dermatol 129:766, 1993.

49. Wessler S, Gitel SN. Warfarin: From bedside to bench. N Engl J Med 311:645, 1984.

50. Zivelin A, Rao VM, Rapaport SI. Mechanism of the anticoagulant effect of warfarin as evaluated by selective depression of individual procoagulant vitamin-K dependent clotting factors. J Clin Invest 92:2131, 1993.

51. Wankmuller H, Ellbruck D, Seifried E. Pathophysiologie, klinik und therapie der cumarinnekrose. Dtsch Med Wochenschr 116:1322, 1991.

52. Broekmans AW, Teepe RGC, van der Meer FJM, Briet E, Bertina RM. Protein C (PC) and coumarin-induced skin necrosis (abstr). Thromb Res 6:137, 1986.

53. Magnusson S, Sottrup JL, Petersen TE, Dudek WG, Glaeys H. Homologous "kringle" structures common to plasminogen and prothrombin. Substrate specificity of enzymes activating prothrombin and plasminogen. In Ribbons DW, Brew K (eds). Proteolysis and Physiological Regulation. New York: Academic Press, 1976.

54. Doolittle RF, Feng DF, Johnson MS. Computer-based characterization of epidermal growth factor domains. Nature 307:558, 1984.

55. Lindahl U, Backstrom G, Thunberg L. The antithrombin-binding sequence in heparin. J Biol Chem 258:9826, 1983.

56. Hirsh J, Levine M. Low molecular weight heparin. Blood 79:1, 1992.

57. Carter CJ, Kelton JG, Hirsh J, Cerskus AL, Santos AV, Gent M. The relationship between the hemorrhagic and antithrombotic properties of low molecular weight heparins and heparin. Blood 59:1239, 1982.

58. Esquivel CO, Bergqvist D, Bjork C-G, Nilsson B. Comparison between commercial heparin, low-molecular weight heparin and pentosan polysulphate

on haemostasis and platelets in vivo. Thromb Res 35:613, 1982.

59. Cade JF, Buchanan MR, Boneau B, Ockelford P, Carter CJ, Cerskus AL, Hirsh J. A comparison of the antithrombotic and haemorrhagic effects of low-molecular weight heparin fractions: The influence of the method of preparation. Thromb Res 35:613, 1984.

60. Holmer E, Matsson C, Nilsson S. Anticoagulant and antithrombotic effects of low molecular weight heparin fragments in rabbits. Thromb Res 25:475, 1982.

61. Andriuoli G, Mastacchi R, Barnti M, Sarret M. Comparison of the antithrombotic and hemorrhagic effects and a new low molecular weight heparin in the rat. Haemostasis 15:234, 1985.

62. Bergqvist D, Nilsson B, Hedner U, Pedersen PC, Ostergaard PB. The effects of heparin fragments of different molecular weight in experimental thrombosis and haemostasis. Thromb Res 38:589, 1985.

63. Kakkar VV, Murray WJG. Efficacy and safety of low molecular weight heparin (CY216) in preventing postoperative venous thromboembolism. Br J Surg 72:786, 1985.

64. Group EFS. Comparison of a low molecular weight heparin and unfractionated heparin for the prevention of deep vein thrombosis in patients undergoing abdominal surgery. Br J Surg 75:1058, 1988.

65. Bergqvist D, Burmark US, Frisell J, Hallbrook T, Lindblad B, Risberg B, Torngren S, Wallin G. Low molecular weight heparin once daily compared with conventional low dose heparin twice daily: A prospective double-blind multicentre trial on prevention of postoperative thrombosis. Br J Surg 73:204, 1986.

66. Bergqvist D, Matzsch T, Burmark US, Frisell J, Guilbaud O, Hallbook T, Horn A, Lindhagen A, Ljungner H, Ljungstrom K-G, Onarheim H, Risberg B, Torngren S, Ortenwall P. Low molecular weight heparin given the evening before surgery compared with conventional low dose heparin in prevention of thrombosis. Br J Surg 75:888, 1988.

67. Turpie AGG, Levine MN, Power PJ, Ginsberg JS, Jay RM, Klimek M, Leclerc J, Cote R, Neemeh J, Geerts W, Hirsh J, Gent M. A double-blind randomized trial of ORG 10172 low molecular weight heparinoid versus unfractionated heparin in the prevention of deep vein thrombosis in patients with thrombotic stroke. Thromb Haemost 65(Suppl):753, 1991.

68. Pezzuoli G, Neri Sernerri GG, Settembrini P, Coggi G, Olivara N, Buzzetti G, Chierichetti S, Scotti A, Scatigna M, Carnovali M. STEP-Study group: Prophylaxis of fatal pulmonary embolism in general surgery using low molecular weight heparin CY216: A multicentre double-blind randomized controlled clinical trial versus placebo. Int Surg 74:205, 1989.

69. Ockelford PA, Patterson J, Johns AS. A double-blind randomized placebo controlled trial of thromboprophylaxis in major elective general surgery using once daily injections of a low molecular weight heparin fragment. Thromb Haemost 62:1046, 1989.

70. Turpie AGG, Levine MN, Hirsh J, Carter CJ, Jay RM, Powers PJ, Andrew M, Magnani HN, Hull RD, Gent M. A double-blind randomized trial of ORG 10172 low molecular weight heparinoid in the prevention of deep vein thrombosis in thrombotic stroke. Lancet 1:523, 1987.

71. Prins MH, den Ottolander GJH, Gelsema R, van Woerkom TCM, Sing AK, Heller I. Deep vein thrombosis prophylaxis with a low molecular weight heparin (Kabi 2165) in stroke patients. Thromb Haemost 58:(Suppl):117, 1987.

72. Bratt G, Aberg W, Johansson M, Tornebohm E, Granqvist S, Lockner D. Two daily subcutaneous injections of fragmin as compared with intravenous standard heparin in the treatment of deep venous thrombosis. Thromb Haemost 64:506, 1990.

73. Duroux P, Beclere A. A randomized trial of subcutaneous low molecular weight heparin (CY216) compared with intravenous unfractionated heparin in the treatment of deep venous thrombosis. Thromb Haemost 65:251, 1991.

74. Sobel M, McNeill PM, Carlson PL, Kermode JC, Adelman B, Conroy R, Marques D. Heparin inhibition of von Willebrand factor-dependent platelet function in vitro and in vivo. J Clin Invest 87:1787, 1991.

75. Blajchman MA, Young E, Ofosu FA. Effects of unfractionated heparin, dermatan sulfate and low molecular weight on vessel wall permeability in rabbits. Ann NY Acad Sci 556:245, 1989.

76. Bara L, Billaud E, Gramond G, Kher A, Samama M. Comparative pharmacokinetics of low molecular weight heparin (PK 10169) and unfractionated heparin after intravenous and subcutaneous administration. Thromb Res 39:631, 1985.

77. Lane DA. Heparin binding and neutralizing protein. In Lane DA, Lindahl U (eds). Heparin, Chemical and Biological Properties, Clinical Applications. London: Edward Arnold, 1989.

78. Lane DA, Pejler G, Flynn AM, Thompson EA, Lindahl U. Neutralization of heparin-related saccharides by histidine-rich glycoprotein and platelet factor 4. J Biol Chem 258:3803, 1986.

79. Barzu T, Molho P, Tobelem G, Petitou M, Caen J. Binding and endocytosis of heparin by human endothelial cells in culture. Biochem Biophys Acta 845:196, 1985.

80. de Swart CAM, Nijmeyer B, Roelofs JMM, Sixma JJ. Kinetics of intravenously administered heparin in normal humans. Blood 60:1251, 1982.

81. Olsson P, Lagergren H, Ek S. The elimination from plasma of intravenous heparin. An experimental study on dogs and humans. Acta Med Scand 173:619, 1963.

82. Bjornsson TO, Wolfram BS, Kitchell BB. Heparin kinetics determined by three assay methods. Clin Pharmacol Ther 31:104, 1982.

83. Bara L, Samama MM. Pharmacokinetics of low molecular weight heparins. Acta Chir Scand 543:65, 1988.

84. Spicer EK, Horton R, Bloem L. Isolation of cDNA clones coding for human tissue factor: Primary structure of the protein and cDNA. Proc Natl Acad Sci USA 84:5148, 1987.

85. Morrissey JH, Fakhrai H, Edgington TS. Molecular cloning of the cDNA for tissue factor. Cell 50:129, 1987.

86. Wilcox JN, Smith KM, Schwartz SM, Gordon D. Localization of tissue factor in the normal vessel wall and in the atherosclerotic plaque. Proc Natl Acad Sci USA 86:2839, 1989.

87. Tracy R, Bovill E. Thrombosis and cardiovascular risk in the elderly. Arch Pathol Lab Med 116:1307, 1992.

88. Meade T, Chakrabarti R, Haines A, North W, Stirling Y, Thompson S. Haemostatic function and cardiovascular death: Early results of a prospective study. Lancet 1:1050, 1980.

89. Meade T, Brozovic M, Chakrabarti R, Haines A, Imeson J, Mellows S, Miller G, North W, Stirling Y, Thompson S. Haemostatic function and ischaemic heart disease: Principal results of the Northwick Park Heart Study. Lancet 2:533, 1986.

90. Wilhelmsen L, Svardsudd K, Korsan-Bengtsen K, Larsson B, Welin L, Tibblin G. Fibrinogen as a risk factor for stroke and myocardial infarction. N Engl J Med 311:501, 1984.

91. Stone M, Thorp J. Plasma fibrinogen — a major coronary risk factor. J R Coll Gen Pract 35:565, 1985.

92. Yarnell J, Baker I, Sweetnam P, Bainton D, O'Brien J, Whitehead P, Elwood P. Fibrinogen, viscosity, and white blood cell count are major risk factors for ischemic heart disease. Circulation 83:836, 1991.

93. Kannel W, Wolf P, Castelli W, D'Agostino R. Fibrinogen and risk of cardiovascular disease: The Framingham study. JAMA 258:1183, 1987.

94. Naski M, Shafer J. A kinetic model for the alpha-thrombin-catalyzed conversion of plasma levels of fibrinogen to fibrin in the presence of antithrombin III. J Biol Chem 266:13003, 1991.

95. Marguerie G, Plow E, Edgington T. Human platelets possess an inducible and saturable receptor specific for fibrinogen. J Biol Chem 254:5357, 1979.

96. Plow E, Ginsberg M. Cellular adhesion: GPIIb-IIIa as a prototypic adhesion receptor. In Coller B (ed). Progress in Hemostasis and Thrombosis, Vol. 9. Philadelphia: WB Saunders, 1989:117.

97. Letcher R, Chien S, Pickering T, Sealey J, Laragh J. Direct relationship between blood pressure and blood viscosity in normal and hypertensive subjects: Role of fibrinogen and concentration. Am J Med 70:1195, 1981.

98. Esmon C, Taylor F, Snow T. Inflammation and coagulation: Linked processes potentially regulatedthrough a common pathway mediated by protein C. Thromb Haemost 66:160, 1991.

99. Libby P, Clinton S. Possible roles for cytokines in atherogenesis. J Cell Biochem 16(Suppl A):2, 1992.

100. Kuller L, Eichner J, Orchard T, Grandits G, McCallum L, Tracy R, for the MRFIT Research Group. The relation between serum albumin levels and risk of coronary heart disease in the Multiple Risk Factor Intervention Trial. Am J Epidemiol 134:1266, 1991.

101. Marcus A. Thrombosis and inflammation as multicellular processes: Pathophysiologic significance of transcellular metabolism. Blood 76:1903, 1990.

102. Munro J, Cotran R. Biology of disease: The pathogenesis of atherosclerosis: Atherogenesis and inflammation. Lab Invest 58:249, 1988.

103. Schwartz C, Sprague E, Valente A, Kelley J, Edwards E, Suenram C. Inflammatory components of the human atherosclerotic plaque. In Glagov S, Newman W, Schaffer S (eds). Pathobiology of the Human Atherosclerotic Plaque. New York: Springer-Verlag, 1990:107.

104. Schwartz C, Valente A, Sprague E, Kelley J, Suenram C, Rozek M. Atherosclerosis as an inflammatory process: The roles of the monocyte-macrophage. Ann N Y Acad Sci 454:115, 1985.

105. Meade T. The epidemiology of haemostatic and other variables in coronary artery disease. In Verstraete M, Vermylen J, Lijnen H, Arnout J (eds). Thrombosis and Haemostasis 1987, Leuven: International Society on Thrombosis and Haemostasis and Leuven University Press, 1987:37.

106. Heinrich J, Balleisen L, Schulte H, Assmann G, van de Loo J. Fibrinogen and factor VII in the prediction of coronary risk: Results from the PROCAM study in healthy men. Arterioscler Thromb 14:54, 1994.

107. Folsom A, Wu K, Rosamond W, Sharrett A, Chambless L. Hemostatic factors and incidence of coronary heart disease in the Atherosclerosis Risk in Communities (ARIC) study (abstr). Circulation 93:622, 1996.

108. Dalaker K, Smith P, Arnesen H, Prydz H. Factor VII-phospholipid complex in male survivors of acute myocardial infarction. Acta Med Scand 222:111, 1987.

109. Dalaker K, Hjermann I, Prydz H. A novel form of factor VII in plasma from men at risk for cardiovascular disease. Br J Haematol 61:315, 1985.

110. Hoffman C, Miller R, Lawson W, Hultin M. Elevation of factor VII activity and mass in young adults at risk of ischaemic heart disease. J Am Coll Cardiol 14:941, 1989.

111. Hoffman C, Shah A, Sodums M, Hultin M. Factor VII activity state in coronary artery disease. J Lab Clin Med 111:475, 1988.

112. Bruckert E, Carvalho de Sousa J, Giral P, Soria C, Chapman M, Caen J, de Gennes J-L. Interrelationship of plasma triglyceride and coagulant factor VII levels in normotriglyceridemic hypercholesterolemia. Atherosclerosis 75:129, 1989.

113. Tracy R, Bovill E, Yanez D, Psaty B, Fried L, Heiss G, Lee M, Polak J, Savage P, for the CHS Investigators. Fibrinogen and factor VIII, but not factor VII, are associated with measures of subclinical cardiovascular disease in the elderly: Results from the Cardiovascular Health Study. Arterioscler Thromb Vasc Biol 15:1269, 1995.

114. Cushman M, Yanez D, Psaty B, Fried L, Heiss G, Lee M, Polak J, Savage P, Tracy R, for the CHS Investigators. Association of fibrinogen and coagulation factors VII and VIII with cardiovascular risk factors in the elderly: The Cardiovascular Health Study. Am J Epidemiol 143:665, 1996.

115. Folsom A, Wu K, Davis C, Conlan M, Sorlie P, Szklo M. Population correlates of plasma fibrinogen and factor VII, putative cardiovascular risk factors. Atherosclerosis 91:191, 1991.

116. Carvalho de Sousa J, Bruckert E, Giral P, Soria C, Truffert J, Mirshahi M, de Gennes J, Caen J, Plasma factor VII, triglyceride concentration and fibrin degradation products in primary hyperlipidemia: A clinical and laboratory study. Haemostasis 19:83, 1989.

117. Miller G, Walter S, Stirling Y, Thompson S, Esnouf M, Meade T. Assay of factor VII activity by two techniques: Evidence for increased conversion of VII to VIIa in hyperlipidemia, with possible implications for ischaemic heart disease. Br J Haematol 59:249, 1985.

118. Skartlien A, Lyberg-Beckmann S, Holme I, Hjermenn I, Prydz H. Effect of alteration in triglyceride levels on factor VII-phosphlipid complexes in plasma. Arteriosclerosis 9:798, 1989.

119. Kario K, Matsuo T, Asada R, Sakata T, Kato H, Miyata T. The strong positive correlation between factor VII clotting activity using bovine thromboplastin and the activated factor VII level. Thromb Haemost 73:429, 1995.

120. Morrissey J, Macik B, Neuenschwander P, Comp P. Quantitation of activated factor VII levels in plasma using a tissue factor mutant selectively deficient in promoting factor VII activation. Blood 81:734, 1993.

121. Theroux P, Latour J, Leger-Gauthier C, De Lara J. Fibrinopeptide A and platelet factor levels in unstable angina pectoris. Circulation 75:156, 1987.

122. Eisenberg P, Sherman L, Schectman K, Perez J, Sobel B, Jaffe A. Fibrinopeptide A: A marker of acute coronary thrombosis. Circulation 71:912, 1985.

123. Pacchiarini L, Storti C, Zuchella M, Salerno JA, Grignani G, Fratino P. Fibrinopeptide A levels in patients with acute ischemic heart disease. Haemostasis 19:147, 1989.

124. Yudelman IM, Nossel HL, Kaplan KL, Hirsh J. Plasma fibrinopeptide A levels in symptomatic venous thromboembolism. Blood 51:1189, 1978.

125. De Buyzere M, Philippe J, Duprez G, Baele G, Clement DL. Coagulation system activation and increase of D-dimer levels in peripheral arterial occlusive disease. Am J Haematol 43:91, 1993.

126. Cushman M, Psaty B, Macy E, Bovill E, Cornell E, Kuller L, Tracy R. Correlates of thrombin markers in an elderly cohort free of clinical cardiovascular disease. Arterioscler Thromb Vasc Biol 16:1163, 1996.

127. Rugman FP, Jenkins JA, Duguid JK, Maggs PB, Hay CR. Prothrombin fragment F1 + 2: Correlations with cardiovascular risk factors. Blood Coag Fibrinolysis 5:335, 1994.

128. Agewall S, Fagerberg B, Wikstrand J. Circulation 94:457, 1996.

129. Cortellaro M, Boschetti C, Cofrancesco E, Zanussi C, Catalano M, de Gaetano G, Gabrielli L, Lombardi B, Specchia G, Tavazzi L, Tremoli E, della Volpe A, Polli E, for the PLAT Study Group. The PLAT study: Hemostatic function in relation to atherothrombotic ischemic events in vascular disease patients. Principal results. Arterioscler Thromb 12:1063, 1992.

130. Folsom AR, Wu KK, Rosamond WD, Sharret AR, Chambless LE. Hemostatic factors and incidence of coronary heart disease in the Atherosclerosis Risk in Communities (ARIC) study (abstr). Circulation 93:622, 1996.

131. Tracy RP, Arnold A, Ettinger WH, Fried LP, Meilahn E, Savage PJ. Circulation 93:457, 1996.

132. Reed T, Tracy R, Fabsitz R. Minimal genetic influences on plasma fibrinogen level in adult males in the NHLBI twin study. Clin Genet 45:71, 1994.

133. Hamsten A, Iselius L, DeFaire U, Blomback M. Genetic and cultural inheritance of plasma fibrinogen concentration. Lancet 2:988, 1987.

134. Kant JA, Crabtree GR. The rat fibrinogen genes. J Biol Chem 258:4666, 1983.

135. Kant JA, Furnace AJJ, Saxe D. Evolution and organization of the fibrinogen locus on chromosome 4: Gene duplication accompanied by transcription and inversion. Proc Natl Acad Sci USA 82:2344, 1985.

136. Yu S, Sher B, Kudryk B, Redman CM. Intracellular assembly of human fibrinogen. J Biol Chem 258:13407, 1983.

137. Yu S, Sher B, Redman C. A scheme for the intracellular assembly of human fibrinogen, In Lane DA, Henshen A, Jasani MK (eds). Fibrinogen, Fibrin Formation and Fibrinolysis, Vol. 4. Berlin: de Gruytler, 1986:3.

138. Ray SM, Mukhopadtyay G, Redman CM. Transcription of HepG2 cells with B beta cDNA specifically enhances synthesis of the three component chains of fibrinogen. J Biol Chem 265:6389, 1990.

139. Courtois G, Morgan J, Campbell L, Fourel G, Crabtree G. Interaction of a liver-specfic nuclear factor with the fibrinogen and α_1-antitrypsin promoters. Science 238:688, 1987.

140. Fowkes FGR, Connor JM, Smith FB, Wood J, Donnan PT, Lowe GDO. Fibrinogen genotype and risk of peripheral atherosclerosis. Lancet 339:693, 1992.

141. Connor JM, Fowkes FGR, Wood J, Smith FB, Donnan PT, Lowe GDO. Genetic variation at

fibrinogen loci and plasma fibrinogen levels. J Med Genet 29:480, 1992.

142. Iso H, Folsom A, Winkelman J, Koike K, Harada S, Greenberg B, Sato S, Shimamoto T, Iida M, Komachi Y. Polymorphisms of the beta fibrinogen gene and plasma fibrinogen concentration in caucasian and Japanese population samples. Thromb Haemos 73:106, 1995.

143. Humphries S, Cook M, Dubowitz M, Stirling Y, Meade T. Role of genetic variation at the fibrinogen locus in determination of plasma fibrinogen concentrations. Lancet 1:1452, 1987.

144. Berg K, Kierulf P. DNA polymorphisms at the fibrinogen loci and plasma fibrinogen concentration. Clin Genet 36:229, 1989.

145. Behague I, Poirier O, Nicaud V, Evans A, Arveiler D, Luc G, Cambou J-P, Scarabin P-Y, Bara L, Green F, Cambien F. Beta-fibrinogen gene polymorphisms are associated with plasma fibrinogen and coronary artery disease in patients with myocardial infarction. Circulation 93:440, 1996.

146. de Maat MPM, de Knijff P, Green FR, Thomas AE, Jespersen J, Kluft C. Gender-related association between beta-fibrinogen genotype and plasma fibrinogen levels and linkage disequilibrium at the fibrinogen locus in Greenland Inuit. Arterioscler Thromb Vasc Biol 15:856, 1995.

147. Green F, Hamsten A, Blomback M, Humphries S. The role of beta-fibrinogen genotypes in determining plasma fibrinogen levels in young survivors of myocardial infarction and healthy controls from Sweden. Thromb Haemost 70:915, 1993.

148. Thomas A, Kelleher C, Green F. Variation in the promoter region of the beta-fibrinogen gene is associated with plasma fibrinogen levels in smokers and non-smokers. Thromb Haemost 65:487, 1991.

149. Green F, Kelleher C, Wilkes H, Temple A, Meade T, Humphries S. A common genetic polymorphism associated with low coagulation factor VII levels in healthy individuals. Arterioscler Thromb 11:540, 1991.

150. Lane A, Cruickshank J, Stewart J, Henderson A, Humphries S, Green F. Genetic and environmental determinants of factor VII coagulant activity in different ethnic groups at differing risk of coronary heart disease. Atherosclerosis 94:43, 1992.

151. Meilahn E, Ferrell R, Kiss J, Temple A, Green F, Humphries S, Kuller L. Genetic determination of coagulation factor VIIc levels among healthy middle-aged women. Thromb Haemost 73:623, 1995.

SECTION II: PLATELETS

Frederick A. Spencer and Richard C. Becker

Without normal hemostasis, one could exsanguinate following even minor trauma associated with everyday life. In contrast, untimely or excessive clotting could compromise perfusion to vital organs. Fortunately, humans have developed an integrated system of checks and balances that, under usual circumstances, allows both maintenance of blood fluidity and prompt arrest of bleeding. Platelets, found in great numbers in circulating blood, play a pivotal role in the hemostatic mechanism (primary hemostasis) and, together with coagulation proteins (secondary hemostasis) and the blood vessel itself (mediated by vasoconstriction), provide a unique, efficient, and readily available means to minimize blood loss after vascular injury. The section provides a contemporary view of platelet anatomy and biology.

3. PLATELETS: STRUCTURE, FUNCTION, AND THEIR FUNDAMENTAL CONTRIBUTION TO HEMOSTASIS AND PATHOLOGIC THROMBOSIS

Frederick A. Spencer and Richard C. Becker

Introduction

Platelets play a critical role in normal hemostasis by stopping blood loss after vascular injury. By adhering to sites of injury, recruiting other platelets and blood cells to the developing clot, and activating the plasma coagulation cascade, primary hemostasis is effected. In synchrony with the end products of the coagulation cascade, predominantly crosslinked fibrin, a more stable clot quickly forms. However, by these same mechanisms, platelets also contribute directly to pathologic vascular thrombosis. In the ongoing search for means to prevent or temper vascular thrombosis while preserving physiologic hemostasis, a better understanding of platelet structure and function is of paramount importance. In this chapter we provide a composite overview of platelets, focusing on their structure, function, and fundamental contribution to normal hemostasis and pathologic thrombosis.

Platelet Structure

Although deceptively simple in appearance, the platelet is in fact functionally complex. The structure–function relationship is simplified somewhat by dividing the resting platelet into four anatomically distinct zones [1].

PERIPHERAL ZONE

The platelet's peripheral zone consists of a membrane and its invaginations, which form the open canalicular system. It can be further divided into three distinct domains: the exterior coat, the unit membrane, and the submembrane region (Figure 3-1).

EXTERIOR COAT

The exterior coat is a 15–20 nm thick glycocalyx, rich in glycoproteins. To date nine different glycoproteins

(GPs) have been identified [2–5]. A majority serve as receptors for cell–cell and cell–vessel wall interactions. They are discussed in greater detail in sections to follow on platelet adhesion and aggregation.

PLATELET UNIT MEMBRANE

The platelet unit membrane is similar to other blood cell membranes in the following ways: (1) It is a lipid bilayer rich in phospholipid, (2) it provides a physiochemical separation between intracellular and extracellular processes, and (3) it contains anion and cation pumps (i.e., Na/K-ATPase) critical to the maintenance of transmembrane ionic gradients. The platelet membrane is an important catalyst for fluid-phase coagulation. With activation, acidic phospholipid groups are translocated to the membrane's exterior, where they serve as a surface for prothrombinase assembly [6,7]. The rate of assembly is increased substantially in the presence of a platelet membrane that fosters localization of factors V and X. See Chapter 1 for an in-depth discussion of the prothrombinase complex.

SUBMEMBRANE REGION

The area beneath the unit membrane is appropriately called the *submembrane region*. It contains a distinct network of microfilaments that are anatomically (and functionally) associated with both membrane glycoproteins and an extensive cytoplasmic filament system [8,9]. In resting platelets the submembrane region helps to maintain the platelet's discoid shape. It may also play an important role in transmembrane signaling events [10].

SOL-GEL ZONE

The matrix of the cytoplasm is called the *sol-gel zone* and consists of two fiber systems in varying states of polymerization. Just beneath the submembrane re-

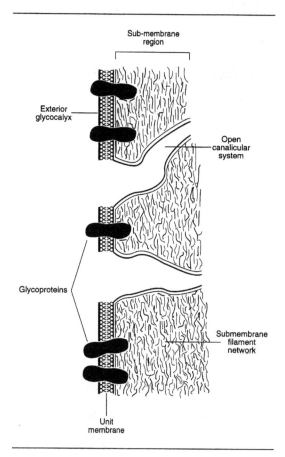

FIGURE 3-1. Peripheral zone — a schematic representation. The exterior glycocalyx is a 15–20 nm thick, glycoprotein-rich layer. The unit membrane is a lipid bilayer with invaginations that increase the membrane surface area, forming the open canalicular system. The submembrane region has a microfilament network connecting membrane glycoproteins to cytoplasmic filaments.

gion are tightly coiled microtubules that help maintain resting platelet shape [11]. Their exact role during activation is less clear. With activation the microtubules constrict into tight rings around centrally clustered organelles. Contrary to initial observations, the driving force for this contractile event is actually provided by the cytoplasmic filaments, not the microtubules [11].

The second set of fibers within the sol-gel zone is the actin microfilaments. In the resting platelet only 30–40% of actin is polymerized into filaments [12]. With activation there is an increase in polymerization, with new filaments appearing at the cell periphery and within developing filopedia [13] (Figure 3-2). This is associated with reorganization of filaments into close parallel bundles. Myoglobin binds the filaments and provides the contractile force required for platelet shape change (discoid → spherical), filopedia extension, and centralization of organelles (Figure 3-3).

ORGANELLE ZONE
The organelle zone is not, in the purest sense, a distinct zone but contains storage granules, dense bodies, peroxisomes, lysosomes, and mitochondria dispersed throughout the cytoplasm. As such this zone is centrally involved with metabolic processes and also acts as a storage site for enzymes, adenine nucleotides, serotonin, calcium, and a wide variety of proteins.

MEMBRANE SYSTEM
The membrane system constitutes the fourth and final zone. The plasma membrane and the microfilament cytoskeleton have been described previously. The plasma membrane also contains numerous invaginations that course deep within the platelet. Commonly referred to as the *open canalicular system*, these channels provide a large surface area for cellular transport and remain patent (and functionally active) throughout platelet activation, with shape change, and during the release reaction [14,15].

The dense tubular system represents a second membrane system located within the cell's interior. Derived from parent cell endoplasmic reticulum, the dense tubular system acts as a storage site for calcium as well as for the enzymes involved in prostaglandin synthesis [16,17]. The two membrane systems are in direct communication with one another, allowing for an exchange of contents.

PLATELET FUNCTION
Under normal conditions platelets circulate freely in blood vessels without interacting with other platelets or the vascular endothelium. In the presence of endothelial damage, whether from vascular injury or rupture of an atherosclerotic plaque, a chain of events is triggered, leading to platelet-rich clot formation. Depending on the initiating event, this may represent normal hemostasis or pathologic vascular thrombosis. The responsible events represent a complex series of biochemical and cellular processes that can be loosely divided into four general categories: adhesion, activation, secretion, and aggregation [18].

PLATELET ADHESION
Platelets adhere avidly to damaged, disrupted, or dysfunctional vascular endothelium. This is especially

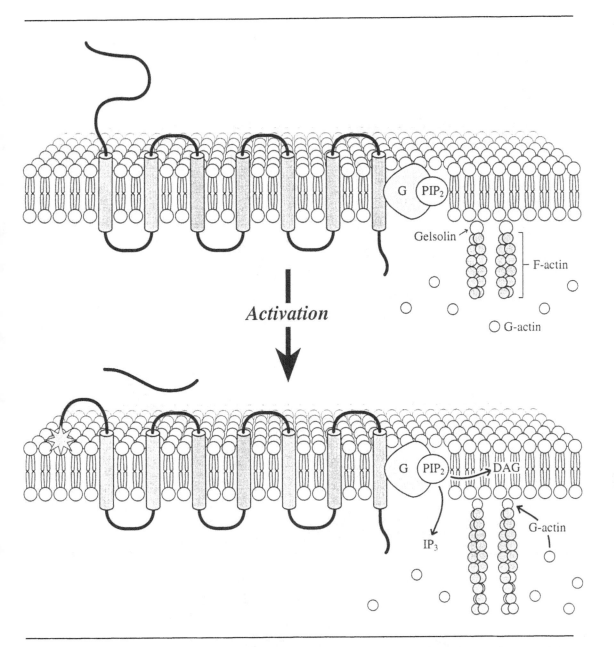

FIGURE 3-2. Increased polymerization of actin filaments occurs after platelet activation. In the unstimulated platelet (**top panel**), actin filaments are capped near the periphery by gelsolin or other capping proteins. Their release allows extension of existing filaments by actin monomers (**bottom panel**). Released gelsolin molecules may also sever existing actin filaments, which can then polymerize in the same way. These activities probably involve intracellular second messengers, particularly inositol triphosphate.

true in areas of exposed subendothelial collagen and lipid deposits, as found in ruptured or ulcerated atherosclerotic plaques. Coverage of the exposed site by platelets is mediated by adhesive proteins that are recognized by specific platelet membrane glycoproteins. These glycoproteins are also critical for cell–cell interactions (Figure 3-4).

To date nine of the predominant platelet membrane glycoproteins have been characterized [2–5]. The most common nomenclature for identification is

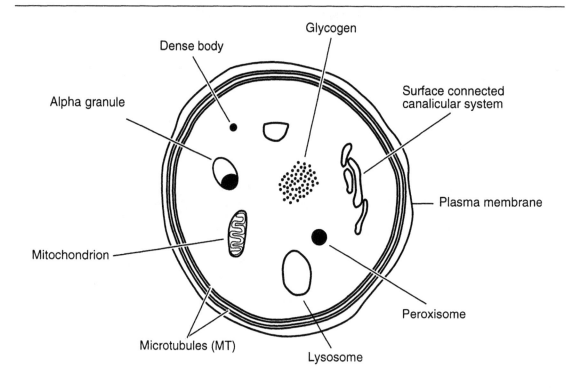

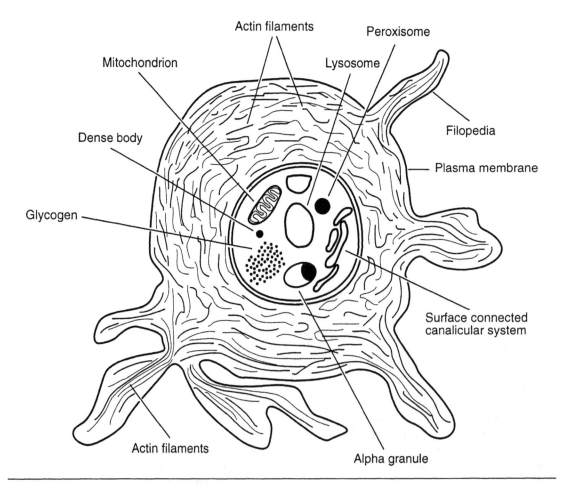

TABLE 3-1. Surface membrane glycoprotein receptors

Receptor	Ligand	Integrin components	Biologic action
GPIa/IIa	Collagen	$\alpha_2\beta_1$	Adhesion
GPIb/IX	von Willebrand factor	—	Adhesion
GPIc/IIa	Fibronectin	$\alpha_5\beta_1$	Adhesion
GPIIb/IIIa	Collagen	$\alpha_{IIb}\beta_3$	Aggregation
	Fibrinogen		(secondary role
	Fibronectin		in adhesion)
	Vitronectin		
	von Willebrand factor		
GPIV	Thrombospondin	—	Adhesion
(GPIIIb)	Collagen		
Vitronectin receptor	Vitronectin	$\alpha_v\beta_3$	Adhesion
	Thrombospondin		
VLA-6	Laminin	$\alpha_6\beta_1$	Adhesion

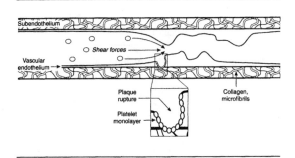

FIGURE 3-4. Platelet adhesion is the initiating step in normal hemostasis and in pathologic thrombosis. Prior to plaque rupture there is little platelet adhesion, despite the presence of shear forces generated by blood flow past the atherosclerotic plaque. With plaque rupture subendothelial collagen, microfibils, and Von Willebrand Factor (VWF) are exposed. Platelets adhere in a monolayer to the damaged site (see the text).

based on polyacrylamide gel separation, giving rise to GPI, GPII, GPIII, etc. With increasing sophistication of the gel systems, increasing separation within groups became possible, that is, GPIa, GPIb, and GPIc.

Most platelet membrane receptors consist of noncovalent complexes of individual glycoproteins. The various surface membrane glycoproteins and their

FIGURE 3-3. A: Schematic representation of a resting platelet (see the text). B: Schematic representation of the changes effected in activated platelets (see the text).

ligands are summarized in Table 3-1. It should be noted that there is considerable functional overlap because several receptors may bind the same ligand and one particular receptor may respond to more than one ligand. The receptors can also be divided into integrins and nonintegrins. Integrins are heterodimeric cell-surface molecules composed of α and β subunits. Platelets express at least two β subunits (β_1 and β_2) and five α subunits, which in varying combinations identify distinct surface receptors [19].

The initial events in adhesion is contact, a process by which an inactivated circulating platelet "stops" and "sticks" to a site of vascular damage [20]. This important event is accomplished by an interaction between the platelet glycoprotein Ib–IX complex and von Willebrand factor (vWF), a large protein synthesized by vascular endothelial cells and secreted on both the luminal *and* subendothelial surfaces. vWF also has functional domains that contribute to the binding of platelets to vessel wall constituents (collagen, microfibrils) [21,22].

A unique feature of platelet adhesion is its dependence on shearing forces. In fact, without forces of at least $600–3000\,S^{-1}$ between surfaces, platelet "contact" will not occur [23–25]. Adhesion of platelets to vascular subendothelial components represents the primary hemostatic response to vessel wall injury. It also effects a strong stimulus for platelet activation via pathways mediated by the membrane glycoprotein receptors (discussed in Alater Section).

PLATELET ACTIVATION

Platelet activation can be triggered by a wide variety of biochemical and mechanical stimuli (in addition to platelet adhesion; Table 3-2). Many of the biochemi-

TABLE 3-2. Responses of platelets to activation[a]

1. Shape change and pseudopod formation
2. Change in the conformation of GPIIb/IIIa to the form that binds fibrinogen and von Willebrand factor
3. Increase in cytosolic Ca^{2+} due to influx from the exterior
4. Cytoskeletal assembly
5. Aggregation
6. Activation of phospholipase C, producing the second messengers inositol 1, 4, 5-triphosphate (IP_3) and diacylglycerol
7. Mobilization of Ca^{2+} from internal stores by IP_3
8. Activation of phospholipase A2, leading to formation of thromboxane A2
9. Activation of protein kinase C by diacylglycerol, leading to phosphorylation of a 47-kd protein
10. Secretion of contents of α and dense granules (lysosomal granule contents secreted only upon strong stimulation)
11. Surface expression of some α-granule proteins (e.g., thrombospondin and fibrinogen)
12. Surface expression of granule membrane proteins (e.g., P-selectin, also known as GMP-140, PADGEM, or CD62)
13. Development of coagulant activity by transbilayer movement of procoagulant phospholipids
14. Inhibition of adenylyl cyclase
15. Clot retraction

[a]Thrombin can cause all of these responses, not necessarily sequentially, but other aggregating agents may induce only some of them [28, 161, 162].

TABLE 3-3. Physiologic agonists for platelet activation

Agonist	Source	Receptor(s)
Thrombin	End product of coagulation cascade	Seven-transmembrane domain receptor GPIbα
Adenosine diphosphate (ADP)	Platelet dense body	Aggregin
Collagen	Subendothelium component	GPIa/IIa GPIIb/IIIa GPIV
Serotonin	Platelet dense body	5HT$_2$ receptor
Thromboxane A$_2$	Produced by platelets after initial stimulation	PGH$_2$/TXA$_2$ receptor
Platelet activating factor	Lipid mediator produced by other cells	PAF receptor

cal agonists are produced or released by platelets themselves after vessel wall adhesion, initiating a positive feedback loop that amplifies the response to a given stimulus.

Platelet agonists bind surface glycoprotein receptors and stimulate signal transmission across the membrane via a messenger protein that, in turn, triggers one of two intracellular pathways. The phosphoinositide pathway is initiated with activation of phospholipase C. Phosphatidylinositol 4-5-biphosphate (PIP_2) is cleaved to form two secondary messengers, inositol 1,4,5 triphosphate (IP_3) and diacylglycerol [26]. IP_3 stimulates calcium mobilization from the dense tubular system. Increased cellular Ca^{2+} concentrations are required for activation of other intracellular enzymes responsible for physiologic platelet responses [27]. Diacylglycerol activates protein C, causing protein phosphorylation, granule secretion, and fibrinogen receptor expression.

The second pathway that can be initiated following platelet activation involves phospholipase A_2, which liberates arachidonate from cell membranes. Arachidonate is subsequently converted to thromboxane A_2 (TxA$_2$) by the platelet's cyclooxygenase enzyme system. TxA$_2$ is a potent platelet agonist in its own right, thus providing yet another positive feedback mechanism that promotes the thrombotic mechanism.

Platelet agonists can be classified as strong or weak (Table 3-3). Strong agonists, thrombin, for example, affect both phosphoinositide hydrolysis *and* arachidonate metabolism (via phospholipase C and phospholipase A_2). Accordingly, their ability to promote platelet activation and aggregation persists despite inhibition of one of the two pathways. Indeed, it has been shown that even low concentrations of thrombin (≤ 0.1 IU/mL) can produce platelet aggregation in the face of inhibition of platelet TxA$_2$ produc-

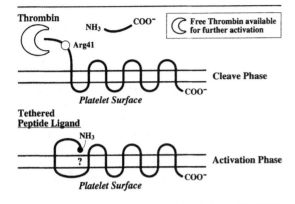

FIGURE 3-5. Thrombin binds to its platelet receptor along a lengthy extracellular amino-terminal extension. Thrombin cleaves the receptor at a specific site and exposes a new amino terminus, which then functions as a tethered peptide ligand to activate a receptor (which has not yet been identified).

tion [28]. Weak agonists (collagen and adenosine diphosphate, for example) lack the ability to trigger phosphoinositide hydrolysis and are more dependent on TxA_2 formation for their effects. Studies as early as 1977 revealed that inhibition of TxA_2 formation could reduce collagen-induced platelet aggregation [29].

THROMBIN ACTIVATION

As one of the most potent platelet agonists, thrombin deserves special attention. Following activation, platelets provide the procoagulant membrane surface and factor V necessary for prothrombinase assembly. Thus the protein-based clotting system and the platelet hemostatic response are closely linked through this unique serum protease.

To date, two separate thrombin receptors have been identified on the platelet surface — a high-affinity receptor and a moderate-affinity receptor [30,31]. The high-affinity receptor is felt to be GPIbα. Observations that Bernard Soulier platelets (congenitally deficient in GPIbα) are poorly activated by low levels of thrombin support this hypothesis [32]. Experiments in which GPIbα is cleaved also reveal an impaired response of platelets to lower (but not higher) concentrations of α thrombin [33,34].

The "moderate-affinity" receptor, now known as the *thrombin receptor*, was first cloned by Coughlin and colleagues in 1991 [35]. This receptor is a member of a G-protein–linked, seven-transmembrane do-

main receptor family and is found on platelets, endothelial cells, smooth muscle cells, and fibroblasts (Figure 3-5). Thrombin interacts with at least two sites on this receptor's lengthy extracellular amino-terminal end. The first site is a leucine-aspartic acid-proline-arginine (LDPR) sequence, and the second, nearby, is a sequence closely resembling hirudin. Thrombin cleaves the amino-terminal extension after the LDPR sequence (at Arg^{41}–Ser^{42}) to expose a new amino terminus. This new amino-terminal domain acts as a "tethered ligand," which activates platelets by binding to an as yet unidentified region of the same receptor (35–37).

It is not yet clear whether interactions of α thrombin with GPIbα or the G-protein–linked thrombin receptor or both are required for in vivo platelet activation. Liu and colleagues used a variety of proteases to cleave platelet GPIbα or anti-GPIb antibodies and then assessed the ability of α thrombin to bind to and activate platelets [38]. They found that α thrombin will bind to and cleave the G-protein–linked α-thrombin receptor (resulting in platelet activation) *and* that these processes can occur independently of GPIb. These observations do not rule out a role for GPIb in additional signal transduction resulting from α thrombin binding to platelets.

Until recently little attention had been paid to the 41 amino acid peptide (TR 1-41) cleaved from the G-protein–linked thrombin receptor with thrombin binding. Work by Furman and colleagues has shown that this peptide is, in fact, a potent platelet agonist [39]. Using whole-blood flow cytometry, TR 1-41 was more potent than thrombin receptor activating peptide (TRAP) and almost as potent as thrombin, as demonstrated by surface expression of P-selectin, increased exposure of fibrinogen binding sites on the GPIIb/IIIa complex, and increased fibrinogen binding to the activated GPIIb/IIIa complex. Further work is needed to better define the roles of GPIbα, the G-protein–linked thrombin receptor, and the TR1-41 peptide in physiologic and pathologic platelet processes.

PLATELET SECRETION

Platelet activation prompts the secretion of contents from within three different types of platelet storage granules: lysosomes, α granules, and dense bodies. The exact mechanism of granule secretion is largely undetermined, but it is felt to involve an energy-dependent contractile process, resulting in extrusion of granule contents. Fusion of α granules with each other and with deep invaginations of the plasma membrane (the open canalicular system) followed by an "emptying" of contents to the exterior has since been demonstrated [40,41]. It is unclear if other platelet granules use a similar mechanism to release their contents.

The lysosomes contain a wide variety of acid hydrolases that digest materials that have been endocytosed. Lysosome secretion occurs more slowly than does dense granule or α granule secretion [42–44]. The weaker agonists (ADP, epinephrine, TxA$_2$) are generally unable to stimulate lysosome secretion, and acid hydrolases are also more easily inhibited by metabolic blockade (e.g., decreased ATP availability) [44].

The platelet also contains a small number of osmophilic electron-dense granules, referred to as *dense bodies*. They contain a large amount of nonmetabolic adenines (ADP, GDP) as well as divalent cations (Ca^{2+}, Mg^{2+}), serotonin, and pyrophosphates. Physiologically ADP is the most important constituent of the dense bodies. As previously discussed, ADP secretion following platelet activation promotes recruitment and activation of additional platelets to the site of vascular injury. ADP has a short half-life in plasma (approximately 4 minutes); thus, one would anticipate a brief period of platelet stimulation [45]. Serotonin is also a relatively weak platelet agonist.

The platelet α granules are spherical (300–500 nm in diameter) bodies, each with an eccentric staining pattern. They contain platelet-specific proteins, coagulation factors, and a variety of glycoproteins. Among the platelet-specific proteins are a number of peptides that can modulate cell growth. Of these, platelet-derived growth factor (PDGF) is among the most extensively studied. Two distinct receptors for PDGF have been isolated on smooth muscle cells and fibroblasts [46]. It has been suggested that PDGF modulates smooth muscle cell proliferation that occurs after platelet–vessel wall interaction. Two other structurally related α-granule proteins are connecting tissue activating peptide III (CTAP III) and platelet factor-4. CTAP III is involved with fibroblast proliferation and is also a probable precursor to β thromboglobulin [47]. The physiologic effects of β thromboglobulin are less clear, but radioimmunoassays of β thromboglobulin have been developed to determine platelet activation. Platelet factor-4 binds to heparin and effectively neutralizes its anticoagulant activity. It may also participate in inflammatory reactions because it has been shown to be chemotactic for neutrophils and monocytes [48].

The α granules contain a variety of coagulation proteins. Of physiologic importance, 20–25% of blood factor V is stored within platelet α granules, and it has been demonstrated that platelet factor V is the major protein secreted and phosphorylated following α-thrombin stimulation [49,50]. Accordingly, platelet factor V is critical to the assembly of prothrombinase, which can then generate additional thrombin. Platelets also contain protein S (the cofactor for protein C–mediated factor V and VIII inhibition). Accordingly, it has been postulated that protein C may exert its anticoagulant effect largely at platelet sites [51]. Release of plasminogen activator inhibitor 1 (PAI-1) may play a role in local fibrinolytic potential [52]. Platelets also contain and release fibrinogen. Although meager in comparison with plasma levels, platelet fibrinogen is more highly concentrated, further suggesting platelets provide a site for localizing hemostatic responses [53].

Platelet α granules contain at least seven different glycoproteins; some are secreted and some are bound to the granule membrane. The major soluble glycoprotein secreted is thrombospondin. Also secreted by endothelial cells, thrombospondin is thought to play a role in the regulation of smooth muscle cell proliferation [54]. There is also an internal pool of GP IIb/IIIa within the α granules. With activation they are expressed on the platelet surface and can increase the total number of surface GPIIb/IIIa receptors by up to twofold [55–57].

PLATELET AGGREGATION

The final event requiring discussion is platelet aggregation. Indeed, this is considered the physiologic goal of platelet activation because it is through platelet aggregation that primary hemostasis can occur. As already reviewed, a variety of agonists can stimulate platelets via interaction with specific membrane receptors, followed by production of secondary messengers, which in turn promote a series of intracellular reactions. One of the most important platelet responses triggered is a conformational change in the membrane receptor GPIIb/IIIa. This allows fibrinogen and the GPIIb/IIIa receptor to interact, forming multiple crosslinks between adjacent platelets. This reaction represents the "final common pathway" for platelet activation and is a vital process in the formation of platelet-rich thrombi. Accordingly, scientific investigators have focused their attention on this basic event in attempting to develop new platelet antagonists for clinical use. Both fibrinogen and GPIIb/IIIa are discussed in greater detail.

Fibrinogen is a dimeric glycoprotein with three pairs of nonidentical subunits (Aα, Bβ, δ). It is abundant in plasma and is also highly concentrated in the α granules of platelets. Fibrinogen does not avidly bind to resting platelets, but stimulated platelets may bind >40,000 fibrinogen molecules per

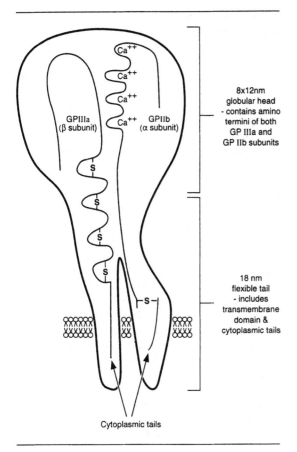

FIGURE 3-6. Schematic representation of the platelet surface membrane glycoprotein IIb/IIIa receptor. It consists of two subunits; the amino termini of both appear as a single globular head extending from the cell surface. Each subunit's carboxyl tail forms a hydrophobic transmembrane domain. (Adapted with permission from Plow and Ginsberg [19]).

cell [58,59]. Sequences of the fibrinogen molecule that bind GPIIb/IIIa have been identified on the Aα chain (RGDF) and the δ chain (RGDS) [60–62]. With a total of six potential binding sites per fibrinogen molecule, adjacent platelets may be crosslinked via their GPIIb/IIIa receptors in a variety of ways. At least initially fibrinogen binding is reversible with a dissociation constant (Kd) of approximately 0.3 μM [58,63]. Plasma fibrinogen concentration exceeds this Kd by ~30-fold, and therefore the fibrinogen binding sites are easily saturated. Following reversible fibrinogen binding, the interaction undergoes "a time-dependent" stabilization, which closely correlates with irreversible platelet aggregation [54,58,59]. At this point removal of the

stimulating agonist or the divalent ion cofactors will no longer dissociate fibrinogen from the cells (or disaggregate platelets). The mechanisms underlying stabilization have not yet been determined.

Glycoprotein IIb/IIIa acts as the platelet membrane receptor for fibrinogen. GPIIb/IIIa is a member of the integrin family of receptors, composed of α and b subunits (α_{11b}, β_3) (Figure 3-6). The α subunit consists of a heavy chain and a light chain. The heavy chain is entirely extracellular, while the light chain spans the platelet membrane, ending in a short extracellular domain [64]. The β subunit is a single polypeptide, also spanning the membrane, but with a long extracellular sequence [65,66]. Electron microscopy has shown that the GPIIb/IIIa receptor consists of an 8 × 12 nM globular head with two 18-nm flexible tails extending from one side [67]. The globular head consists of the amino termini of each subunit, while each tail represents a subunit's carboxyl terminus. The subunits are synthesized separately but rapidly complex in the presence of micromolar calcium concentrations.

With platelet activation, GPIIb/IIIa undergoes a conformational change, rendering it competent to bind protein ligands in general and fibrinogen in particular. The underlying biochemical mechanism for this transformation is not entirely clear. Electron microscopy studies of the GPIIb/IIIa–fibrinogen complex have provided several important insights [67]. The globular head of GPIIb/IIIa interacts with the distal end of the fibrinogen molecule; the tails are extended laterally at an angle of 98° to the long axis of the fibrinogen molecule. Thus with GPIIb/IIIa binding to opposite ends of a fibrinogen molecule, the tails are oriented to opposite sides, enabling a bridge to be formed between two adjacent platelets. The RGDF and RGDS sequences occur on a variety of other proteins other than fibrinogen, including fibronectin [68], von Willebrand factor (vWF) [68,69,71], and vitronectin [70]. Although each protein is capable of binding platelets via the GPIIb/IIIa receptor, fibrinogen, by virtue of its high plasma concentration, predominates in normal physiologic circumstances. However, these other ligands may play a role in stabilizing platelet adhesion because they are present in the vascular subendothelium whereas fibrinogen is not [21]. There is also evidence that vWF may play a role in platelet aggregation under conditions of high shear stress [71].

Platelet aggregation can be prevented by inhibiting fibrinogen binding. Peptides with the RGD sequence are naturally occurring (snake venoms) or can be synthesized. Monoclonal antibodies to platelet GPIIb/IIIa are currently available for clinical use.

TOOLS FOR MEASURING PLATELET ACTIVATION
With the recognition of platelet participation in physiologic and pathologic thrombosis has come an increased interest in developing ways to determine, and whenever possible to quantify, platelet activation. There has been a great deal of effort spent on developing a means of measuring plasma levels of platelet-specific proteins, particularly β-thromboglobulin (BTG) and platelet factor-4 (PF4). As discussed previously, these proteins are secreted from α granules following platelet activation. As early as 1975 a radioimmunoassay was developed for BTG in plasma [72]; a similar assay for PF4 soon followed [73]. Initially touted as markers of platelet activation and potentially as new markers for the detection of thrombotic states, many laboratories developed similar assays. Indeed, studies have reported increased plasma levels of BTG and PF4 in a number of thrombotic conditions, including venous thrombosis [72], coronary artery disease [74–76], cerebrovascular disease [77], and disseminated intravascular coagulation [78].

Unfortunately, an increase in plasma BTG and PF4 is not necessarily representative of in vivo platelet activation. The assays themselves are prone to error due to platelet activation and/or rapid leakage of proteins during preparation of platelet-free plasma [79]. Even with meticulous attention to blood collection and processing, there are a significant number of false-positive tests. There is also considerable laboratory-to-laboratory variability. In one comparative analysis, levels differed by up to 300% between laboratories for identical samples [80]. There are also increased levels of BTG antigen in renal diseases due to impaired renal catabolism. Several investigators have suggested the use of a BTG/PF4 ratio [81,82,84]. The normal ratio in properly prepared plasma is approximately 5:1. With platelet activation there is usually a small increase in PF4 with a larger increase in BTG (due to slower clearance of BTG in vivo). This results in elevated ratios of BTG/PF4 of up to 10:1. Increased BTG/PF4 ratios have been detected in a variety of thrombotic conditions, including coronary disease [83]. It is also possible to measure BTG levels in the urine, which offers the potential advantage of not being as influenced by collection technique [84].

As previously discussed, platelet activation leads to the synthesis and secretion of thromboxane A_2 (TxA_2). In plasma, TxA_2 is subsequently converted to a series of metabolites including 2,3-dinor-TxB_2 and 11-dehydroxy TxB_2; both are renally excreted. It has been demonstrated that measured concentrations of urinary 2,3-dinor-TxB_2 by gas chromatography/mass spectrometry accurately reflect TxA_2 production attributable to platelet activation [85,86]. Not surprisingly, urinary levels of 2,3-dinor-TxB_2 have also been found to be increased in a variety of thrombotic disorders [86]. Because gas chromatography/mass spectrometry is not widely available, a radioimmunoassay for urinary 11-dehydro-TxB_2 has been developed.

The development of the *platelet aggregometer* in the 1960s allowed the measurement of platelet responses to exogenous physiologic agonists in vitro [85]. Investigators have demonstrated that some patients with thrombotic conditions (acute myocardial infarction [MI], thrombotic stroke, peripheral vascular disease) have platelets that spontaneously aggregate [86]. This suggests an increased susceptibility to activation or "hyperreactivity." One prospective study was able to show that "spontaneous platelet aggregation" was a predictor of mortality in acute myocardial infarction [87]. Wu and Houk extended these observations by developing a method that measured platelet aggregates already circulating at the time of phlebotomy [88]. In the Wu and Houk method, platelet aggregates in patient samples are fixed with paraformaldehyde and then counted. A reduced ratio of aggregates in the fixed sample, compared with an unfixed sample, reflects an increase in circulating platelet aggregates. As with the other markers, the presence of increased circulating platelet aggregates has been noted in a variety of thrombotic and prethrombotic conditions [89–92,94].

One of the most promising techniques for assessing in vivo platelet activation is flow cytometry [93]. Cells in suspension are labeled with a fluorescently conjugated monoclonal antibody and passed through a focused laser beam. The fluorophore is activated at its excitation wavelength, and a detector analyzes both the emitted fluorescence and the light-scattering properties of each cell. Monoclonal antibodies can be raised against a wide variety of platelet surface antigens. The development of antibodies that recognize surface antigens expressed only after platelet activation permits the detection and quantification of platelet activation, as well as analysis of platelets under more physiologic conditions, that is, in the presence of red blood cells and white blood cells. Flow cytometry minimizes the extent of sample processing, thus reducing the potential for artifact.

In the absence of added exogenous agonists, measurement of "activation-dependent" monoclonal antibodies to platelet antigens during flow cytometry reflects the activation state of circulating platelets in vivo. Inclusion of various exogenous agonists to the assay allows analysis of the reactivity of circulating platelets in vitro. The two most widely studied activation-dependent antibodies are those (1) directed

TABLE 3-4. Activation-dependent monoclonal antibodies:
Antibodies that bind to activated but not resting platelets

Activation-dependent surface change	Prototypic antibodies
Changes in GPIIb-IIIa	
Activation-induced conformational change in GPIIb/IIa, resulting in exposure of the fibrinogen binding site	PAC1
Ligand-induced conformational change in GPIIb/IIIa	PM 1.1, LIBS1, LIBS6
Receptor-induced conformational change in bound ligand (fibrinogen)	2G5, 9F9, F26
Exposure of granule membrane proteins	
P-selectin (α granules)	S12, AC1.2
CD63 (lysomes)	CLB-gran/12
LAMP-1 (lysomes)	H5G11
Binding of secreted platelet proteins	
Thrombospondin	P8, TSP-1
Multimerin	JS-1
Development of a procoagulant surface	
Factor Va binding	V237
Factor VIII binding	1B3

Reprinted from Michelson [93], with permission.

against changes in the GPIIb/IIIa complex and (2) those directed against granule membrane proteins (Table 3-4). As previously discussed, the GPIIb/IIIa receptor complex binds fibrinogen, vWF, fibronectin, and vitronectin. The crosslinking of platelets via GPIIb–GPIIIa–fibrinogen bridges is the critical step in platelet aggregation. The monoclonal antibody PAC1 is directed against the fibrinogen binding site of GPIIb/IIIa that is exposed only after conformational changes induced by platelet activation [94]. As a result, it recognizes only activated platelets. Antibodies have also been developed that recognize the GPIIb/IIIa receptor only after its ligand has bound (ligand-induced binding sites) [95]. Conversely, antibodies to receptor-induced binding sites recognize the ligand (i.e., fibrinogen) only after it binds to the receptor [96,97].

Monoclonal antibodies have been raised against platelet granule membrane proteins that translocate to the surface after platelet activation. The most common granule membrane antigen targeted is P-selectin, which mediates adhesion of activated platelets to neutrophils and monocytes. Antibodies against P-selectin bind only activated, degranulated platelets [98].

In contrast to the GPIIb/IIIa and granule membrane, protein activation–dependent antibodies is the GPIb–IX–V (CD42)–specific antibody that actually

binds to a reduced degree with platelet activation because of its translocation to the open canalicular system [99,100]. In one study, a decrease in binding of monoclonal antibody to the GPIb–IX–V complex proved to be a more sensitive marker of platelet activation than antibodies directed against GPIIb/IIIa or P-selectin [101].

As we learn more about the changes platelets undergo with activation, additional activation-dependent monoclonal antibodies will be developed. This, in turn, will allow further delineation of the contribution of platelets in acute coronary syndromes [102,103].

PLATELET–LEUKOCYTE INTERACTIONS
It could be stated that platelets are to thrombosis as leukocytes are to inflammation. However, over the past decade there has been increasing recognition that inflammation and thrombosis are linked at several levels. Study of the modulating effects of neutrophils and platelets on one another became possible with improved methods for the preparation of platelet-free neutrophils and platelet-rich plasma (PRP) [104]. Early studies focused on the ability of platelets or neutrophils to enhance each other's response to an aggregating agonist. Reintroduction of platelets to a neutrophil preparation increased the neutrophil aggregation response to various chemotactic agents

TABLE 3-5. Platelet-derived mediators altering neutrophil function

Platelet-derived mediator	Effect on Neutrophil [134]
1. TxA_2	Enhances PMN adhesiveness [114]
	Mediates PMN diapedesis [115]
	Regulates neutrophil effect on atherosclerotic vessel
	Vasocontricts [116,117]
2. PDGF	Induces PMN chemotaxis [124]
	Stimulates PMN phagocytosis [125]
	Inhibits activated PMN O_2 release
3. PF4	Induces PMN chemostaxis [127]
	Stimulates PMN elastase release [128]
4. 12 HETE/12HPETE	Induces PMN chemotaxis [129]
	Stimulates PMN oxidative burst [130]
	Promotes PMN adhesion to endothelium [130]
	Modulates PMN stimulation with increased shear? [131]
5. Serotonin	Enchances PMN adherence to endothelium [132]
6. Adenosine	May inhibit PMN activation [133]

TxA_2 = thromboxane A_2; PDGF = platelet-derived growth factor; PF4 = platelet factor-4; PMN = polymorphonuclear leukocyte.
From Siminiak et al. [134], with permission.

[104,105]. Similarly, reintroduction of activated neutrophils to a platelet preparation caused either direct platelet aggregation or increased the response to various agonists [106–109].

Neutrophil-mediated cytotoxicity, oxidant production, lysosome release, and arachodonic acid metabolism are all increased in the presence of platelets [7–10,104,110–113]. Platelets activated by platelet activating factor (PAF) have increased calcium mobilization and thromboxane β_2 release in the presence of activated neutrophils [109]. The capacity of platelets and leukocytes to modulate one another's activity is potentially explained by one or more mechanisms: (1) release of soluble mediators, (2) metabolism of released mediators, (3) presentation of surface-bound mediators, and (4) direct cell adhesion.

PLATELET-DERIVED MEDIATORS
The release of TxA_2 from activated platelets has been found to enhance polymorphonuclear leukocytes (PMN) adhesiveness [114], to mediate PMN diapedesis (via regulation of PMN adhesion receptor C18) [115], and to regulate the effect of activated neutrophils on atherosclerotic arterial vasoconstriction [116,117]. In turn, TxA_2 inhibition has been demonstrated to decrease neutrophil accumulation in ischemic myocardium, with a subsequent reduction in experimental infarct size [118–123].

Platelet-derived growth factor (PDGF) induces PMN chemotaxis and stimulates phagocytosis [124,125]; however, it also appears to inhibit oxygen-derived free radical release from stimulated neutrophils. Plasma PDGF concentrations are depressed in patients with acute MI or unstable angina [126]. Other platelet-derived mediators shown to have effects on neutrophil function include platelet factor-4, 12-HETE/12-HPETE, serotonin, and adenosine (Table 3-5) [124–134].

NEUTROPHIL-DERIVED MEDIATORS
Oxygen-derived free radicals released by activated PMNs can have either excitatory or inhibitory effects on platelets. Superoxide anion has been shown to act synergistically with thrombin to activate platelets as well as to stimulate platelet serotonin release [135]. In contrast, there is at least one report that suggests that PMN-derived H_2O_2 can inhibit platelet aggregation [136].

Elastases secreted from neutrophils have been found to inhibit thrombin-mediated platelet activation and serotonin release, perhaps by cleaving specific platelet receptors [137]. Interestingly, platelet-derived PF4 may stimulate the release of PMN elastase [128], representing a potentially important physiologic link between platelets and PMNs.

Arachadonic acid metabolites derived from neutrophils may be utilized by platelets. Leukocyte-derived 5 HETE is the precursor for the platelet product 5,12 diHETE [137]. PMN-derived leukotrienes have been shown to enhance platelet aggregation in response to several agonists [138]. Finally, activated neutrophils can activate platelets by presenting surface-bound PAF [139]. This event requires cell–cell interaction and, in addition, may depend on direct adherence.

PLATELET LEUKOCYTE ADHESION

Platelet leukocyte adhesion is of physiologic importance for a variety of reasons. Close contact of cells ensures increased local concentrations of released mediators and provides a means of protection against circulating plasma inhibitors. Indeed, it has been shown that platelet activation by neutrophil-derived mediators is increased if neutrophils are included in the in vitro preparation [140,141]. The adhesion event itself may provide a stimulus for subsequent intracellular signaling events.

Cell–cell adhesion may be the necessary link between inflammation and thrombosis. It is well documented that neutrophils and platelets bind to regions of vessel wall damage. While they clearly interact, independent function is often required of each. It has been noted that thrombocytopenia is not, in and of itself, associated with an impaired immune response, nor is neutropenia linked with hemostatic abnormalities. Although the interaction between neutrophils and platelets may not be essential for normal physiologic function, it may play a role in the pathologic thrombosis, reperfusion injury, and chronic inflammation [142]. For these reasons, investigation of platelet–leukocyte interactions has steadily increased.

The in vitro adherence of platelets to neutrophils in ethylenediaminetetraacetic acid (EDTA) anticoagulated blood was noted as early as the 1960s and was commonly termed *platelet satellitism* [143–145]. This phenomenon was confirmed in several experiments using whole blood: Platelet agonist-induced aggregates contain both platelets and neutrophils [146], exposure of whole blood to glass causes deposition of both cell types [147], and adhesion of neutrophils to nylon fibers increases with increasing platelet concentrations [148]. Nash and colleagues observed heterotypic aggregates after mixing heparinized PRP and granulocytes [149]. Aggregation was increased if the platelets were activated, and the process was found to be calcium dependent. Neutrophil activation increases the aggregatory response but is not an absolute prerequisite.

In the late 1980s a number of investigative groups reported that platelet–leukocyte adhesion was mediated largely through expression of platelet activation-dependent granule external membrane protein (PADGEM), also known as granule membrane protein 140 (GMP-140) or CD62 [150–152]. PADGEM is an α granule membrane protein expressed on the surface of activated platelets after granule secretion. Initially felt to be platelet specific, PADGEM has also been found in megakaryocytes [153] and endothelial cells [154]. Additional studies determined that platelet binding to both PMNs and monocytes was dependent on a specific epitope of GMP-140. Unactivated platelets bind leukocytes through a divalent cation-independent receptor, but with a much decreased affinity. Interestingly, the receptor(s) mediating adhesion on unactivated platelets become nonfunctional after thrombin activation.

The dynamics of leukocyte-platelet adhesion in whole blood have been examined [156]. Using RGDS peptides to block platelet aggregation, whole blood was stimulated by thrombin. As expected, this caused increased expression of GMP-140 (platelet activation). In addition, there was a marked increase in monocyte– and neutrophil–platelet aggregates, as well as an increase in the number of platelets bound per cell. The observed increase in adhesion was blocked using a monoclonal antibody against GMP-140. With thrombin stimulation, monocytes bind more platelets, and at a faster rate, than do neutrophils. With weaker agonists (ADP, epinephrine) less GMP-140 is expressed, and whereas monocyte–platelet conjugates are present, neutrophil–platelet conjugates are not.

When whole blood is stimulated with either ADP or epinephrine in the absence of RGDS (thus allowing platelet aggregation), there is a marked decrease in leukocyte–platelet binding but an increase in pure platelet aggregates. With time (~5 minutes) the platelet aggregates spontaneously dissociate and the percentage of monocytes and PMNs with adherent platelets again increase. This subsequent "reaggregation" is also blocked by the monoclonal antibody G1, supporting GMP-140 as the putative receptor.

The leukocyte receptor required for platelet adhesion has not been identified conclusively. Evidence points to CD15, a nonsialated pentasaccharide not found on resting cells, as the leukocyte ligand for GMP-140 [157]. However, there are contrasting views [158,159]. The fact that monocytes have a competitive advantage over PMNs for platelet adherence also suggests that CD15 is *not* the major ligand, given the existence of a 30-fold lower expression of CD15 per monocyte compared with PMN [52].

There is some experimental evidence that the GPIIb/IIIa complex may play a role in the adhesion of activated platelets to leukocytes [160]. Using washed platelets that were activated with various agonists and then incubated with leukocytes, Jorgi and colleagues identified heterotypic aggregates that were then fixed in glutardialdehyde. Using a unique scoring system based on microscopic analysis, the degree of adhesion of activated platelets to leukocytes was quantified. When monoclonal antibodies to GPIIb/IIIa receptor or RGDS peptides were included in the experimental preparation, a partial inhibition of adhesion events was noted. Similarly, dissociation of the GPIIb/IIIa complex using EDTA also resulted in decreased leukocyte–platelet binding. Finally, platelets in GPIIb/IIIa-deficient patients tend not to interact strongly with leukocytes.

Our knowledge of the mechanisms behind platelet–leukocyte interactions is just now beginning to expand. Gains in this field will enhance our understanding of the relationship between inflammation and thrombosis. In turn, this may offer insights into how we may inhibit thrombosis while sparing hemostasis.

References

1. White JG. Platelet ultrastructure. In Bloom AL, Thomas DP (eds). Haemostasis and Thrombosis, 2nd ed. Edinburgh: Churchill Livingstone 1987:20.
2. George JN. Studies on platelet plasma membranes. IV. Quantitative analysis of platelet membrane glycoproteins by (^{125}I)-diazotized diiodosulfanilic acid labeling and SDS-polyacrylamide gel electrophoresis. J Lab Clin Med 92:430, 1978.
3. Nurden AT, Caen JP. Membrane glycoproteins and human platelet function. Br J Haematol 38:155, 1978.
4. Phillips DR, Agin PP. Platelet membrane defects in Glanzmann's thrombasthenia. Evidence for decreased amounts of two major glycoproteins. J Clin Invest 60:535, 1977.
5. Phillips DR, Agin PP. Platelet plasma membrane glycoproteins. Evidence for the presence of nonequivalent disulfide bonds using nonreduced-reduced two-dimensional gel electrophoresis. J Biol Chem 252:2121, 1977.
6. Mann KG, Nesheim ME, Church WR, Haley R, Krishnaswamy S. Surface-dependent relations of the vitamin K-dependent enzyme complexes. Blood 76:1, 1990.
7. Tracy PB. Regulation of thrombin generation at cell surfaces. Semin Thromb Hemost 14:227, 1988.
8. Zucker-Franklin D. The submembranous fibrils of human blood platelets. J Cell Biol 47:293, 1970.
9. White JG. The submembrane filaments of blood platelets. Am J Pathol 56:267, 1969.
10. Fox JE, Lipfert L, Clark EA, Reynolds CC, Austin CD, Brugge JS. On the role of the platelet membrane skeleton in mediating signal transduction. Association of GP IIb-IIIa, pp60c-src, pp62c-yes, and the p21ras GTPase-activating protein with the membrane skeleton. J Biol Chem 268:25973, 1993.
11. White JG. Effects of colchicine and vinca alkaloids on human platelets. I. Influence on platelet microtubules and contractile function. Am J Pathol 53:281, 1968.
12. Fox JE, Boyles JK, Reynolds CC, Phillips DR. Actin filament content and organization in unstimulated platelets. J Cell Biol 98:1985, 1984.
13. Fox JE. The platelet cytoskeleton. Thromb Haemost 70:884, 1993.
14. White JG. Electron microscopic studies of platelet secretion. Progr Hemost Thromb 2:49, 1974.
15. White JG. Identification of platelet secretion in the electron microscope. Ser Haematolog 6:429, 1973.
16. Cutler L, Rodan G, Feinstein MB. Cytochemical localization of adenylate cyclase and of calcium ion, magnesium ion-activated ATP ases in the dense tubular system of human blood platelets. Biochim Biophys Acta 542:357, 1978.
17. Kaser-Glanzmann R, Jakabova M, George JN, Luscher EF. Further characterization of calcium-accumulating vesicles from human blood platelets. Biochim Biophys Acta 512:1, 1978.
18. Weiss HJ. Platelet physiology and abnormalities of platelet function (first of two parts). N Engl J Med 293:531, 1975.
19. Plow EF, Ginsberg MH. The molecular basis of platelet function. In Hoffman R, Benz EJ, Shaltil SJ, Furie B, Cohen HJ (eds). Hematology. Basic Principles and Practice. New York: Churchill Livingstone, 1991:1165.
20. Roth GJ. Platelets and blood vessels: The adhesion event. Immunol Today 13:100, 1992.
21. Fauvel F, Grant ME, Legrand YJ, Souchon H, Tobelem G, Jackson DS, Caen JP. Interaction of blood platelets with a microfibrillar extract from adult bovine aorta: Requirement for von Willebrand factor. Proc Natl Acad Sci USA 80:551, 1983.
22. Birembaut P, Legrand YJ, Bariety J, Bretton R, Fauvel F, Belair MF, Pignaud G, Caen JP. Histochemical and ultrastructural characterization of subendothelial glycoprotein microfibrils interacting with platelets. J Histochem Cytochem 30:75, 1982.
23. Roth GJ. Developing relationships: Arterial platelet adhesion, glycoprotein Ib, and leucine-rich glycoproteins. Blood 77:5, 1991.
24. Turrito VT, Muggli R, Baumgartner HR. Physical factors influencing platelet deposition on subendothelium: Importance of blood shear rate. Ann NY Acad Sci 283:284, 1977.
25. Turrito VT, Baumgartner HR. Platelet-surface interactions. In Colman RW, Hirsh J, Marder VJ, Salzman EW (eds). Hemostasis and Thrombosis. Basic Principles and Clinical Practice. Philadelphia: JB Lippincott, 1987:555.

26. Berridge MJ. Inositol trisphosphate and diacyl-glycerol: Two interacting second messengers. Ann Rev Biochem 56:159, 1987.

27. Rink TJ, Sage SO. Calcium signaling in human platelets. Ann Rev Physiol 52:431, 1990.

28. Packham MA. Platelet reactions in thrombosis. In Gottlieb AI, Langille BL, Federoff S (eds). Atherosclerosis. Cellular and Molecular Interactions in the Artery Wall. New York: Plenum Press, 1991:209.

29. Kinlough-Rathbone RL, Packham MA, Reimers HJ, Cazenave JP, Mustard JF. Mechanisms of platelet shape change, aggregation, and release induced by collagen, thrombin, or A23, 187. J Lab Clin Med 90:707, 1977.

30. Seiler SM, Goldenberg HJ, Michel IM, Hunt JT, Zavoico GB. Multiple pathways of thrombin-induced platelet activation differentiated by desensitization and a thrombin exosite inhibitor. Biochem Biophys Res Commun 181:636, 1991.

31. Greco NJ, Jamieson GA. High and moderate affinity pathways for alpha-thrombin-induced platelet activation. Proc Soc Exp Biol Med 198:792, 1991.

32. Jamieson GA, Okumura T. Reduced thrombin binding and aggregation in Bernard-Soulier platelets. J Clin Invest 61:861, 1978.

33. Wicki AN, Clemetson KJ. Structure and function of platelet membrane glycoproteins Ib and V. Effects of leukocyte elastase and other proteases on platelets response to von Willebrand factor and thrombin. Eur J Biochem 153:1, 1985.

34. Cooper HA, Bennett WP, White GC, Wagner H. Hydrolysis of human platelet membrane glycoproteins with a *Serratia marcescens* metalloprotease: Effect on response to thrombin and von Willebrand factor. Proc Natl Acad Sci USA 79:1433, 1982.

35. Vu TK, Hung DT, Wheaton VI, Coughlin SR. Molecular cloning of a functional thrombin receptor reveals a novel proteolytic mechanism of receptor activation. Cell 64:1057, 1991.

36. Vu TKH, Wheaton VI, Hung DT, Charo I, Coughlin SR. Domains specifying thrombin-receptor interactions. Nature 353:674, 1991.

37. Coughlin SR, Vu TKH, Hung DT, Wheaton VI. Characterization of a functional thrombin receptor. Issues and opportunities. J Clin Invest 89:351, 1991.

38. Liu L, Freedman J, Hornstein A, Fenton II JW, Ofusu FA. Binding of thrombin the G protein linked receptor and not to glycoprotein 1b, precedes thrombin-mediated platelet activation. Unpublished data.

39. Furman MI, Benoit SE, Liu L, Barnard MR, Becker RC, Michelson AD. The cleaved peptide of the thrombin receptor is a strong platelet agonist. Unpublished data.

40. Stenberg PE, Shuman MA, Levine SP, Bainton DF. Redistribution of alpha-granules and their contents in thrombin-stimulated platelets. J Cell Biol 98:748, 1984.

41. Ginsberg MH, Taylor L, Painter RG. The mechanism of thrombin-induced platelet factor 4 secretion. Blood 55:661, 1980.

42. Holmsen H, Day HJ. The selectivity of the thrombin-induced platelet release reaction: Subcellular localization of released and retained constituents. J Lab Clin Med 75:840, 1970.

43. Kenney DM, Chao FC. Microtubule inhibitors alter the secretion of beta-glucuronidase by human blood platelets: Involvement of microtubules in release reaction II. J Cell Physiol 96:43, 1978.

44. Holmsen H, Robkin L, Day HJ. Effects of antimycin A and 2-deoxyglucose on secretion in human platelets. Differential inhibition of the secretion of acid hydrolases and adenine nucleotides. Biochem J 182:413, 1979.

45. Holmsen H. Platelet secretion. In Colman RW, Hirsh J, Marden Vj, Solzman EW (eds). Hemostasis and Thrombosis. Basic Principles and Clinical Practice. Philadelphia: JB Lippincott, 1987:606.

46. Heldin CH, Westermark B. Platelet-derived growth factor: Three isoforms and two receptor types. Trends Genet 5:108, 1989.

47. Wenger RH, Wicki AN, Walz A, Kieffer N, Clemetson KJ. Cloning of cDNA coding for connective tissue activating peptide III from a human platelet derived lambda qt II expression library. Blood 73:1498, 1989.

48. Deuel TF, Keim PS, Farmer M, Heinrikson RL. Amino acid sequence of human platelet factor 4. Proc Natl Acad Sci USA 74:2256, 1977.

49. Viskup RW, Tracy PB, Mann KG. The isolation of human platelet factor V. Blood 69:1188, 1987.

50. Rand MD, Kalafatis M, Mann KG. Platelet coagulation factor Va: The major secretory platelet phosphoprotein. Blood 83:2180, 1994.

51. Schwarz HP, Heeb MJ, Wencel-Drake JD, Griffin JH. Identification and quantitation of protein S in human platelets. Blood 66:1452, 1985.

52. Erickson LA, Ginsberg MH, Loskutoff DJ. Detection and partial characterization of an inhibitor of plasminogen activator in human platelets. J Clin Invest 74:1465, 1984.

53. Keenan JP, Solum NO. Quantitative studies on the release of platelet fibrinogen by thrombin. Br J Haematol 23:461, 1972.

54. Majack RA, Goodman LV, Dixit VM. Cell surface thrombospondin is functionally essential for vascular smooth muscle cell proliferation. J Cell Biol 106:415, 1988.

55. Woods VL Jr, Wolff LE, Keller DM. Resting platelets contain a substantial centrally located pool of glycoprotein IIb-IIIa complex which may be accessible to some but not other extracellular proteins. J Biol Chem 261:15242, 1986.

56. Niija K, Hodson E, Bader R, Byers-Ward V, Koziol JA, Plow EF, Ruggri Z. Increased surface expression of the membrane glycoprotein IIb/IIIa complex induced by platelet activation. Relationship to the

binding of fibrinogen and platelet aggregation. Blood 70:475, 1987.

57. Savage B, Hunter CS, Harker LA, Woods Vl Jr, Hanson SR. Thrombin induced increase in surface expression of epitopes on platelet membrane glycoprotein IIb/IIIa complex and GMP–140 is a function of platelet age. Blood 74:1007, 1989.

58. Bennett JS, Vilaire G. Exposure of platelet fibrinogen receptors by ADP and epinephrine. J Clin Invest 64:1393, 1979.

59. Marguerie GA, Edington TS, Plow EF. Interaction of fibrinogen with its platelet receptor as part of a multistep reaction in ADP-induced platelet aggregation. J Biol Chem 255:154, 1980.

60. Plow EF, Pierschbacher MD, Ruoslahti E, Marguerie GA, Ginsberg MH. The effect of Arg-Gly-Asp-containing peptides on fibrinogen and von Willebrand factor binding to platelets. Proc Natl Acad Sci USA 82:8057, 1985.

61. Kloczewiak M, Timmons S, Hawiger J. Localization of a site interacting with human platelet receptor on carboxy-terminal segment of human fibrinogen gamma chain. Biochem Biophys Res Commun 107:181, 1982.

62. Kloczewiak M, Timmons S, Lukas TJ, Hawiger J. Platelet receptor recognition site on human fibrinogen. Synthesis and structure-function relationship of peptides corresponding to the carboxy-terminal segment of the gamma chain. Biochemistry 23:1767, 1984.

63. Marguerie GA, Plow EF. Interaction of fibrinogen with its platelet receptor: Kinetics and the effect of pH and temperature. Biochemistry 20:1074, 1981.

64. Poncz M, Eisman R, Heidenreich R. Structure of the platelet membrane glycoprotein IIb: Homology to the alpha subunits of the vitronectin and fibronectin membrane receptors. J Biol Chem 262:8476, 1987.

65. Fitzgerald LA, Steiner B, Rall SC Jr, Lo SS, Phillips DR. Protein sequence of endothelial glycoprotein IIIa derived from a cDNA clone: Identity with platelet glycoprotein IIa and similarity to "integrin." J Biol Chem 262:3936, 1987.

66. Phillips DR, Charo IF, Parisc LV, Fitzgerald LA. The platelet membrane glycoprotein IIb-IIIa complex. Blood 71:831, 1988.

67. Weisel JW, Nagaswami C, Vilaire G, Bennett JS. Examination of the platelet membrane glycoprotein IIb-IIIa complex and its interaction with fibrinogen and other ligands by electron microscopy. J Biol Chem 267:16637, 1992.

68. Plow EF, Pierschbacher MD, Ruoslaht E, Marguerie GA, Ginsberg MH. The effect of Arg-Gly-Asp-containing peptides on fibrinogen and von Willebrand factor binding to platelets. Proc Natl Acad Sci USA 82:8057, 1985.

69. Haverstick DM, Cowan JF, Yamada KM, Santoro SA. Inhibition of platelet adhesion to fibronectin, fibrinogen and von Willebrand factor substrates by a synthetic tetra-peptide derived from the cell-binding domain of fibronectin. Blood 66:946, 1985.

70. Thiagarajan P, Kelley KL. Exposure of binding sites for vitronectin on platelets following stimulation. J Biol Chem 263:3035, 1988.

71. Weiss HJ, Hawiger J, Ruggieri ZM, Turrito VT, Thiagarajon P, Hoffman T. Fibrinogen-independent platelet adhesion and thrombus formation on subendothelium mediated by glycoprotein IIb-IIIa complex at high shear rate. J Clin Invest 83:288, 1989.

72. Ludlam CA, Bolton AE, Moore S, Cash JD. New rapid method for deep venous thrombosis. Lancet 3:259, 1975.

73. Bolton AE, Ludlam CA, Pepper DS, Moore S, Cash JD. A radioimmunoassay for platelet factor 4. Thromb Res 8:51, 1976.

74. Handin RI, McDonough M, Lesch M. Elevation of platelet factor 4 in acute myocardial infarction: Measurement by radioimmunoassay. J Lab Clin Med 91:340, 1978.

75. White GL II, Morouf AA. Platelet factor 4 level in patients with coronary artery disease. J Lab Clin Med 97:369, 1981.

76. Smitherman TC, Milam M, Woo J, Willerson JT, Frenkel EP. Elevated β thromboglobulin in peripheral venous blood of patients with acute myocardial ischemia: Direct evidence for enhanced platelet reactivity in vivo. Am J Cardiol 48:395, 1981.

77. Fisher M, Levine PH, Fullerton AL, Fosberg A, Duffy CP, Hoogasian JJ, Drachman DA. Marker proteins of platelet activation in patients with cerebrovascular disease. Arch Neurol 39:692, 1982.

78. Nossel HL, Wasser J, Kaplan KL, LaGamma KS, Yudelman I, Canfield RE. Sequence of fibrinogen proteolysis and platelet release after intrauterine infusion of hypertonic saline. J Clin Invest 64: 1371, 1979.

79. Niewiorowski S, Holt JC. Biochemistry and physiology of secreted platelet proteins. In Colmon RW, Hirsch J, Marder VJ, Solzman EW (eds). Hemostasis and Thrombosis, Basic Principles and Clinical Practice. Philadelphia: JB Lippincott, 1987:618.

80. Curtis AD, Kerry PJ. Standardization of β thromboglobulin and platelet factor 4: A collaborative study to investigate the sources and extent of variation in the measurement of platelet specific proteins. Thromb Haemost 50:686, 1983.

81. Musial J, Niewarowski S, Edmunds LH Jr, Addonizio VP Jr, Nicolau KC, Colman RW. In vivo release and turnover of secreted platelet antiheparin protein in rhesus monkey (M. mulatta). Blood 56:596, 1980.

82. Kaplan KL, Owen J. Plasma levels of β thromboglobulin and platelet factor 4 as indices of platelet activation in vivo. Blood 57:199, 1981.

83. Nichols AB, Owen J, Kaplan KL, Sciacco RR, Cannon PJ, Nossel HL. Fibrinopeptide A, platelet factor 4 and β-thromboglobulin levels in coronary heart disease. Blood 60:650, 1982.

84. Wu KK. Platelet activation mechanisms and markers in arterial thrombosis. J Intern Med 239:17, 1996.

85. Born GVR. Aggregation of blood platelets by adenosine diphosphate and its reversal. Nature 194:927, 1962.

86. Wu KK, Hoak JC. Spontaneous platelet aggregation in arterial insufficiency: Mechanism and implication. Thromb Haemost 35:702, 1976.

87. Trip MD, Cats VM, von Capelle FJ, Vrecken J. Platelet hyperreactivity and prognosis in survivors of acute myocardial infarction. N Engl J Med 323:1549, 1990.

88. Wu KK, Hoak JC. A new method for the quantitative detection of platelet aggregates in patients with arterial insufficiency. Lancet 11:924, 1974.

89. Dougherty JH, Levy DE, Weksler BB. Platelet activation in acute cerebral ischemia. Lancet 1:821, 1977.

90. Wu KK, Hoak JC. Increased platelet aggregates in patients with transient ischemic attacks. Stroke 6:521, 1975.

91. Preston FE, Ward JD, Marcola BH, Porter NR. Timperley WR. Elevated β thromboglobulin levels and circulating platelet aggregates in diabetic microangiopathy. Lancet 1:238, 1978.

92. Chiang VL, Castleden WM, Leahy MF. Detection of reversible platelet aggregates in the blood of smokers and ex-smokers with peripheral vascular disease. Med J Aust 156:601, 1992.

93. Michelson A. Flow cytometry: A clinical test of platelet function. Blood, 87:4925, 1996.

94. Shattil SJ, Hoxie JA, Cunningham M, Brass LF. Changes in the platelet membrane glycoprotein IIb-IIIa complex during platelet activation. J Biol Chem 260:11107, 1985.

95. Abrams CS, Ellison N, Budzynski AZ, Shattil SJ. Direct detection of activated platelets and platelet-derived microparticles in humans. Blood 75:128, 1990.

96. Zamarron C, Ginsberg MH, Plow EF. Monoclonal antibodies specific for a conformationally altered state of fibrinogen. Thromb Haemost 64:41, 1990.

97. Granick HR, Williams SB, McKeown L, Shafer B, Connaghan GD, Hansmann K, Vail M, Magruder L. Endogenous platelet fibrinogen: Its modulation after surface expression is related to size selective access to and conformational changes in the bound fibrinogen. Br J Haematol 80:347, 1992.

98. Michelson AD, Barnard MR, Hechtman HB, MacGregor H, Connolly RJ, Valeri CR. In vivo tracking of platelets: Circulatory degranulated platelets rapidly lose surface P-selectin but continue to circulate and function (abstr). Blood 84:320, 1994.

99. Michelson AD, Benoit SE, Furman MI, Barnard MR, Nurden P, Nurden AT. The platelet surface expression of glycoprotein V is regulated by two independent mechanisms: Proteolysis and a reversible cytoskeletal-mediated redistribution to the surface-connected canalicular system. Blood 1996, in press.

100. Hourdille P, Heilmann E, Combrie R, Winckler J, Clemetson KJ, Nurden AT. Thrombin induces a rapid redistribution of glycoprotein 1b-IX complexes within the membrane systems of activated human platelets. Blood 76:1503, 1990.

101. Kestin AS, Ellis PA, Barnard MR, Errichetti A, Rosner BA, Michelson AD. The effect of strenuous exercise on platelet activation state and reactivity. Circulation 88:1502, 1993.

102. Becker RC, Tracy RP, Bovill EG, Mann KG, Ault K. The clinical use of flow cytometry for assessing platelet activation in acute coronary syndromes. TIMI-III Thrombosis and Anticoagulation Group. Cor Art Dis 5:339, 1994.

103. Furman MI, Benoit SE, Becker RC, Borbone M, Weiner BH, Michelson AD. Thrombin receptor mediated platelet reactivity is increased in stable coronary artery disease (abstrt). Circulation 1995.

104. Redl H, Hammerschmidt DE, Schlag G. Augmentation by platelets of granulocyte aggregation in response to chemotaxins: Studies utilizing an improved cell preparation technique. Blood 61:125, 1983.

105. Boogaerts MA, Vercellotti G, Roelant C, Malbrain S, Verwilghen RL, Jacob HS. Platelets augment granulocyte aggregation and cytotoxicity: Undercovering of their effects by improved cell separation techniques using Percoll gradients. Scand J Haemotol 37:229, 1986.

106. De Gaetano G, Evangelista V, Ratjar G, Del Moshio A, Cerletti C. Activated polymorphonuclear leukocytes stimulate platelet function. Thromb Res 11:25, 1990.

107. Oda M, Satouchi K, Yasunage K, Saito K. Polymorphonuclear leukocyte-platelet interactions: Acetylglycerol ether phosphocholine-induced platelet activation under stimulation with chemotactic peptide. J Biochem 100:1117, 1986.

108. Coeffier E, Joseph D, Prevost MC, Vargaftig BB. Platelet-leukocyte interaction: Activation of rabbit platelets by FMLP-stimulated neutrophils. Br J Pharmacol 92:393, 1987.

109. Del Muschio A, Evangelista V, Ratjar G, Chen ZM, Cerletti C, De Gaetano G. Platelet activation by polymorphonuclear leukocytes exposed to chemotactic agents. Am J Physiol 258:870, 1990.

110. Dinerman J, Mehta J, Lawson D, Mehta P. Enhancement of human neutrophil function by platelets: Effects of indomethacin. Thromb Res 15:509, 1988.

111. Del Moschio A, Corvazier E, Maillet F, Kazatchkine MD, MacLouf J. Platelet dependent induction and amplification of polymorphonuclear leukocytes lysosomal enzyme release. Br J Haematol 72:329, 1989.

112. Coeffier F, Delautier D, Le-Couedic JP, Chignard M, Denizot Y, Benveniste J. Cooperation between platelets and neutrophils for paf-acether (platelet-activation factor) formation. J Leukoc Biol 47:234, 1990.

113. Palmantier R, Borgeat P. Throbmin-activated platelets promote leukotriene B$_4$ synthesis in polymorphonuclear leukocytes stimulated by physiological agonists. Br J Pharmacol 103:1909, 1991.

114. Spanguolo PJ, Ellner JJ, Hussiel A. Thromboxane A$_2$ mediates augmented polymorphonuclear leukocyte adhesiveness. J Clin Invest 66:406, 1980.

115. Goldman G, Welbourn R, Klausner JM, Valeri CR, Shepro D, Hechtman HB. Thromboxane mediates diapedesis after ischemia by activation of neutrophil adhesion receptor interactions with basally expressed intercellular adhesion molecule-1. Circ Res 68:1013, 1991.

116. Mügge A, Heistad DD, Densen P, Piegors DJ, Armstrong ML, Pudgett RC, Lopez JA. Activation of leukocytes with complement C5a is associated with prostanoid-dependent constriction of large arteries in atherosclerotic monkeys in vivo. Atherosclerosis 95:211, 1992.

117. Padgett RC, Heistad DD, Mügge A, Armstrong ML, Piegros DL, Lopez JA. Vascular responses to activated leukocytes after regression of atherosclerosis. Circ Res 70:423, 1992.

118. Mullane KM, Fornabaio D. Thromboxane synthetase inhibitors reduce infarct size by a platelet-dependent, aspirin-sensitive mechanism. Circ Res 62:668, 1988.

119. Wargovich TJ, Mehta J, Nichols W, Ward MB, Lawson D, Franzini D, Conti CR. Reduction in myocardial neutrophil accumulation and infarct size following administration of thromboxane inhibitor U-63, 577A. Am Heart J 114:1078, 1987.

120. Huddleston CB, Lupinetti FM, Laws KH, Collins JC, Clanton?? JA, Hawiger JJ, Oates JA, Hammon JW Jr. The effects of RO-22-4679, a thromboxane synthetase inhibitor on ventricular fibrillation induced by coronary occlusion in conscious dogs. Circ Res 52:608, 1983.

121. Toki Y, Hieda N, Okumura K, Hashimoto H, Ho T, Ogawa K, Satake T, Ozawa T. Myocardial salvage by a novel thromboxane A$_2$ synthetase inhibitor in a canine coronary occlusion-reperfusion model. Arzneim-Forsch/Drug Res 38:224, 1988.

122. Grover GJ, Schumacher WA. Effect of the thromboxane receptor antagonist SQ 29.548 on myocardial infarct size in dogs. J Cardiovasc Pharmacol 11:29, 1988.

123. Smith EF III, Griswold DE, Egan JW, Hillegass LM, DiMartino MJ. Reduction of myocardial damage and polymorphonuclear leukocyte accumulation following coronary artery occlusion and reperfusion by the thromboxane receptor antagonist BM13.505. J Cardiovasc Pharmacol 13:715, 1989.

124. Deuel TF, Huang JS. Platelet derived growth factor: Structure, function and roles in normal and transformed cells. J Clin Invest 74:669, 1984.

125. Deuel TF, Senior RM, Huang JS. Chemotaxis of monocytes and neutrophils to platelet derived growth factor. J Clin Invest 69:1046, 1982.

126. Tahara A, Yasuda M, Itagane H, et al. Plasma levels of platelet-derived growth factor in normal subjects and patients with ischemic heart disease. Am Heart J 122:986, 1991.

127. Deuel TF, Senior KM, Chang D, Griffin GL, Heinrichson RL, Kaiser ET. Platelet factor 4 is chemotactic for neutrophils and monocytes. Proc Natl Acad Sci USA 78:4584, 1981.

128. Lonky SA, Wohl H. Stimulation of human leukocyte elastase by platelet factor 4. Physiologic, morphologic, and biochemical effects of hamster lungs in vitro. J Clin Invest 67:817, 1981.

129. Goetzl EJ, Woods JM, Gorman RR. Stimulation of human eosinophil and neutrophil. PMN leukocyte chmotaxis and random migration by 12-L-hydroxy-5,8,10,14 elcosatetraenoic acid (HETE). J Clin Invest 59:179, 1977.

130. Maclouf J, Lados BF, Borgeat P. Stimulation of leukotriene biosynthesis in human blood leukocytes by platelet derived 12-hydroperoxy-eicosatetraneoic acid. Proc Natl Acad Sci USA 79:6042, 1982.

131. Rhee BG, Hall ER, McIntire LV. Platelet modulation of polymorphonuclear leukocyte shear induced aggregation. Blood 67:240, 1986.

132. Boogaerts MA, Yamada O, Jacob HS, Moldow CF. Enhancement of granulocyte-endothelial adherence and granulocyte-induced cytotoxicity by platelet release products. Proc Natl Acad Sci USA 79:7019, 1982.

133. Goldman G, Welbourn R, Klausner JM, Valeri CR, Shepro D, Hechtman HB. Thromboxane mediates diapedesis after ischemia by activation of neutrophil adhesion receptor interacting with basally expressed intercellular adhesion molecule-1. Circ Res 68:1013, 1991.

134. Siminiak T, Flores NA, Sheridan DJ. Neutrophil interactions with endothelium and platelets: Possible role in the development of cardiovascular injury. Eur Heart J 16:160, 1995.

135. Handin RI, Karabin R, Boxer GJ. Enhancement of platelet function by superoxide anion. J Clin Invest 59:959, 1977.

136. Levine PH, Weinger RS, Simon J, Scoon KL, Krinsky NI. Leukocyte-platelet interaction. Release of hydrogen peroxide by granulocytes as a modulator of platelet reactions. J Clin Invest 57:955, 1976.

137. Weksler BB. Platelets. In Gallin JI, Godstein IM, Synderman R (eds). Inflammation: Basic Principles and Clinical Correlates. New York: Raven Press, 1988:543.

138. Mehta P, Mehta J, Lawson D, Krop I, Letts LG. Leukotrienes potentiate the effects of epinephrine and thrombin on human platelet aggregation. Thromb Res 41:731, 1986.

139. Zhou W, Javors MA, Olson MS. Platelet-activating factor as an intercellular signal in neutrophil-dependent platelet activation. J Immunol 149:1763, 1992.

140. De Gaetano G, Evangelista V, Ratjar G, Del Mashio A, Cerletti C. Activated polymorphonuclear leukocytes stimulate platelet function. Thromb Res 11:25, 1990.

141. Del Maschio A, Evangelista V, Ratjar G, Chen ZM, Cerletti C, De Gaetano G. Platelet activation by

polymorphonuclear leukocytes exposed to chemotactic agents. Am J Physiol 258:870, 1990.

142. Nash GB. Adhesion between neutrophils and platelets: A modulator of thrombotic and inflammatory events. Thromb Res 74:S3, 1994.

143. Field EJ, MacLeod I. Platelet adherence to polymorphs. Br Med J 2:388, 1963.

144. Kjeldsberg C, Swanson J. Platelet satellitism. Blood 43:831, 1974.

145. Skinnider LF, Musclow CE, Kahn W. Platelet satellitism. An ultrastructural study. Am J Hematol 4:179, 1978.

146. Joseph J, Welch KMA, D'Andrea G, Riddle JM. Evidence for the presence of red and white cells within "platelet" aggregates formed in whole blood. Thromb Res 53:485, 1989.

147. Banks DC, Mitchell JRA. Leukocytes and thrombosis. I. A simple test of leukocyte behaviour. Thromb Diasthes Haemorrh (Stuttg.) 30:36, 1973.

148. Rasp FL, Clawson CC, Repine JE. Platelets increase neutrophil adherence in vitro to nylon fiber. J Lab Clin Med 97:812, 1981.

149. Maeda T, Nash GB, Christopher B, Pecsvarady Z, Dormandy JA. Platelet-induced granulocyte aggregation in vitro. Blood Coagul Fibrinolysis 2:699, 1991.

150. Jungi TW, Spycher MO, Nydegger UE, Barandun S. Platelet-leukocyte interaction: Selective binding of thrombin-stimulated platelets to human monocytes, polymorphonuclear leukocytes, and related cell lines. Blood 67:629, 1986.

151. Hamburger SA, McEver RP. GMP-140 mediates adhesion of stimulated platelets to neutrophils. Blood 75:550, 1990.

152. Larsen E, Celi A, Gilbert GE, Furie BC, Erban JK, Bonfanti R, Wagner DD, Furie B. PADGEM protein: A receptor that mediates the interaction of activated platelets with neutrophils and monocytes. Cell 59:305, 1989.

153. McEver RP, Beckstead JH, Moore KL, Marshall-Carlson L, Bainton DF. GMP-140, a platelet alpha-granule membrane protein, is also synthesized by vascular endothelial cells and is localized in Weibel-Palade bodies. J Clin Invest 84:92, 1989.

154. Beckstead JH, Stenberg PE, McEver RP, Shuman MA, Bainton DF. Immunohistochemical localization of membrane and alpha-granule proteins in human megakaryocytes. Blood 67:285, 1986.

155. Rinder HM, Bonan JL, Rinder CS, Ault KA, Smith BR. Activated and unactivated platelet adhesion to monocytes and neutrophils. Blood 78:1760, 1991.

156. Rinder HM, Bonan JL, Rinder CS, Ault KA, Smith BR. Dynamics of leukocyte-platelet adhesion in whole blood. Blood 78:1730, 1991.

157. Larsen E, Palabrica T, Sajer S, Gilbert GE, Wagner DD, Furie BC, Furie B. PADGEM-dependent adhesion of platelets to monocytes and neutrophils is mediated by a lineage-specific carbohydrate, LNF III (CD15). Cell 63:467, 1990.

158. Moore KL, Varki A, McEver RP. GMP-140 binds to a glycoprotein receptor on human neutrophils: Evidence for a lectin-like interaction. J Cell Biol 112:491, 1991.

159. Corral L, Singer MS, Macher BA, Rosen SD. Requirement for sialic acid on neutrophils in a GMP-140 (PADGEM) mediated adhesive interaction with activated platelets. Biochem Biophys Res Commun 172:1349, 1990.

160. Spangenberg P, Redlich H, Bergmann I, Lösche W, Götzrath M, Kehrel B. The platelet glycoprotein IIb/IIIa complex is involved in the adhesion of activated platelets to leukocytes. Thromb Haemost 70:514, 1993.

161. Kroll MH, Schafer AJ. Biochemical mechanisms of platelet activation. Blood 74:1181, 1989.

162. Coller BS. Platelets in cardiovascular thrombosis and thrombolysis. In The Heart and Cardiovascular System. H.A. Fozzard, E. Haber, R. Jennings, A.M. Katz, and H.E. Morgan, editors. Raven Press, Ltd., New York 219.

SECTION III: FIBRINOLYSIS

David C. Stump, M.D.

Maintenance of blood fluidity is essential for normal vasculature to preserve critical function of vital organs. The fibrinolytic system is composed of a number of naturally occurring proteases and their inhibitors. Its activation leads to lysis of obstructing vessel thrombi, and its inhibition results in maintenance of a prothrombotic state. Pharmacologic use of fibrinolytic activators is now an established means of therapy for diseases caused by acute thrombotic vascular occlusion. This section provides an overview of the fibrinolytic system, its components, potential sequelae of its deficiency, and its role as a target for therapeutic antithrombotic strategies.

4. MOLECULAR REGULATION OF FIBRINOLYSIS

H. Roger Lijnen

Introduction

Mammalian blood contains a fibrinolytic system comprised of a proenzyme, plasminogen, that can be converted to the active enzyme, plasmin, by several types of plasminogen activators. Plasmin, in turn, degrades fibrin into soluble fibrin degradation products [1]. Two physiological plasminogen activators have been identified that are immunologically distinct, the tissue-type (t-PA) and the urokinase-type plasminogen activator (u-PA). t-PA–mediated plasminogen activation is mainly involved in the dissolution of fibrin in the circulation [1]. u-PA binds to a specific cellular receptor (u-PAR) and activates cell-bound plasminogen; its main role appears to be in the induction of pericellular proteolysis via the degradation of matrix components or via activation of latent proteases or growth factors. Thus, u-PA may play a role in events such as tissue remodeling and repair, macrophage function, ovulation, embryo implantation, and tumor invasion [2,3]. The recent observation that mice deficient in u-PAR display a virtually normal phenotype has, however, somewhat challenged an important role of the u-PA/u-PAR system in these phenomena [4].

Inhibition of the fibrinolytic system may occur either at the level of t-PA or u-PA, by specific plasminogen activator inhibitors (PAI), or at the level of plasmin, mainly by α_2-antiplasmin. The fibrinolytic system is schematically represented in Figure 4-1, and some of the biochemical properties of its main components are summarized in Table 4-1.

Physiological fibrinolysis is a fibrin-specific process that is regulated by specific molecular interactions between its main components as well as by controlled synthesis and release, presumably primarily from endothelial cells, of plasminogen activators and PAIs. The physiological importance of the fibrinolytic system is demonstrated by the association between abnormal fibrinolysis and a tendency toward bleeding or thrombosis. Impairment of fibrinolysis, due to a de-

fective synthesis and/or release of t-PA from the vessel wall, to a deficiency or functional abnormality in the molecular interactions regulating plasminogen activation, or to increased levels of inhibitors of t-PA or of plasmin, may be associated with thrombosis. Excessive fibrinolysis due to increased levels of t-PA, or to α_2-antiplasmin or PAI-1 deficiency, may result in tendency to bleed [5,6].

Thrombolytic therapy, consisting of intravenous administration of plasminogen activators, has become an important therapeutic approach to the treatment of patients with thromboembolic disease [1]. Plasminogen activators, such as streptokinase, anisoylated plasminogen streptokinase activator complex (APSAC), and two-chain u-PA (tcu-PA), induce extensive systemic activation of the fibrinolytic system and, after saturation of α_2-antiplasmin, excess plasmin may degrade several plasma proteins, including fibrinogen, factor V, and factor VIII. The physiological plasminogen activators, t-PA, and single-chain u-PA (scu-PA), as well as the bacterial plasminogen activator staphylokinase, in contrast, preferentially activate plasminogen at the fibrin surface, albeit via different mechanisms. Once formed, plasmin, associated with the fibrin clot, is protected from rapid inhibition by α_2-antiplasmin and may thus efficiently degrade the fibrin of a thrombus [1]. These molecular interactions are schematically illustrated in Figure 4-2. We discuss the molecular mechanisms involved in the regulation of fibrinolysis, with special emphasis on the role of fibrin in fibrin-specific clot lysis.

Molecular Structure of Plasminogen and Plasminogen Activators

PLASMINOGEN

Human plasminogen is a single-chain glycoprotein of 92 kd with a plasma concentration of $1.5-2 \mu M$. It consists of 791 amino acids and contains seven struc-

TABLE 4-1. Properties of proteins involved in physiological fibrinolysis

	M_r (kd)	No. of amino acids	Plasma concentration (mg/L)	Catalytic triad	Reactive site
Plasminogen	92	791	200	—	—
Plasmin	85	±715	—	$His^{603},Asp^{646},Ser^{741}$	—
α_2-antiplasmin	67	464	70	—	Arg^{376}-Met^{377}
PAI-1	52	379	0.05	—	Arg^{346}-Met^{347}
PAI-2	60	415	<0.005	—	Arg^{380}-Thr^{381}
t-PA	68	527	0.005	$His^{322},Asp^{371},Ser^{478}$	—
u-PA	54	411	0.008	$His^{204},Asp^{255},Ser^{356}$	—

t-PA = tissue-type plasminogen activator; u-PA = urokinase-type plasminogen activator, pro-urokinase; PAI-1 = plasminogen activator inhibitor-1; PAI-2 = plasminogen activator inhibitor-2.

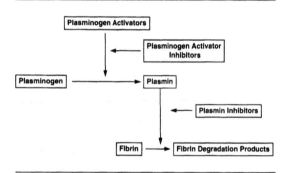

FIGURE 4-1. Schematic representation of the fibrinolytic system. Plasminogen activators convert plasminogen to plasmin, which degrades fibrin to soluble fibrin degradation products. Plasminogen activators can be inhibited by plasminogen activator inhibitors, whereas plasmin can be inhibited by plasmin inhibitors.

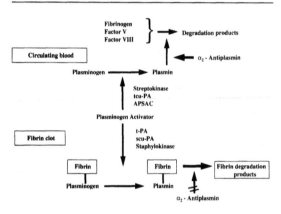

FIGURE 4-2. Molecular interactions involved in the fibrin specificity of plasminogen activation. Non–fibrin-specific plasminogen activators convert plasminogen to plasmin mainly in the circulation, resulting in depletion of α_2-antiplasmin and degradation of several plasma proteins. Fibrin-specific plasminogen activators mainly activate fibrin-bound plasminogen into fibrin-bound plasmin, which is protected from rapid inhibition by α_2-antiplasmin, and efficiently degrades fibrin.

tural domains. Starting from the NH_2 terminus, there are a preactivation peptide (amino acids 1–77), five homologous disulfide-bonded triple-loop structures or "kringles" (about 90 amino acids each), and a proteinase domain (residues 562–791) [7,8]. The kringles contain lysine binding sites and aminohexyl binding sites, which mediate specific binding of plasminogen to fibrin and to cell surfaces, as well as the interaction of plasmin with α_2-antiplasmin, and thereby play a crucial role in the regulation of fibrinolysis. The strongest binding site for lysine and omega amino acids is located on kringle 1, with weaker sites present on kringles 4 and 5. Most of the available structure–function evidence suggests that the kringle regions of plasminogen are independent domains [9]. Nuclear magnetic resonance stud-

ies have suggested that the first kringle is a compact globular structure built around a core of hydrophobic aromatic amino acids, whereas chemical modification studies have revealed that specific arginine residues are involved in fibrin binding [10]. Kringle 4 of plasminogen mediates binding to tetranectin [11].

Native plasminogen, with NH_2-terminal glutamic acid (Glu-plasminogen), may adopt distinct conformations involving two intramolecular interactions, one mediated by regions of the NH_2-terminal peptide and kringle 5, and the other between kringles 3 and 4 [12]. Hydrolysis by plasmin of the Arg^{68}–Met^{69}, Lys^{77}–Lys^{78}, or Lys^{78}–Val^{79} peptide bonds in Glu-plasminogen yields modified forms designated *Lys-plasminogen*, which are more easily activated to plasmin. Plasminogen is converted to plasmin by cleavage of the Arg^{561}–Val^{562} peptide bond by plasminogen activators [13]. Activation of Glu-plasminogen in a buffer milieu yields Lys-plasmin, whereas in human plasma it occurs primarily by direct cleavage of the Arg^{561}–Val^{562} peptide bond, without generation of Lys-plasminogen intermediates [14]. Plasmin is a two-chain trypsin-like serine proteinase, the NH_2-terminal (A-) chain containing the kringles and the COOH-terminal (B-) chain containing the active site (composed of His^{603}, Asp^{646}, and Ser^{741}) of which are connected by two disulfide bonds [7,8]. Digestion of plasminogen with elastase yields three major fragments — kringles 1–3, kringle 4, and low M_r plasminogen (kringle 5 with the proteinase domain) [15]. Low M_r plasminogen lacks lysine-binding sites and does virtually not bind to fibrin. A physiological role for low M_r plasminogen has been suggested in the mediation of intercellular interactions between microglia and neurons [16]. A 38-kd plasminogen fragment comprising the first four kringle structures, called *angiostatin*, was reported to be generated in primary Lewis lung carcinoma and to inhibit angiogenesis and growth in secondary metastasis [17].

TISSUE-TYPE PLASMINOGEN ACTIVATOR

A tissue-type plasminogen activator (t-PA), first identified in tissues and tissue extracts, was purified in the 1970s from several sources, and human t-PA cDNA was cloned and expressed in 1983 [18]. In vivo, t-PA is primarily synthesized and secreted by vascular endothelial cells. The plasma concentration of t-PA antigen is about 5 ng/mL, whereas the concentration of free t-PA is probably less than 1 ng/mL. These levels are highly variable under physiological and pathophysiological conditions. Human t-PA is a single-chain serine proteinase of about 70 kd, consisting of 527 amino acids, with Ser as the NH_2-terminal amino acid [18]. It was later shown that native t-PA contains an NH_2-terminal extension of three amino acids, but, in general, the initial numbering system has been maintained.

Limited plasmic hydrolysis of the Arg^{275}–Ile^{276} peptide bond converts t-PA to a two-chain molecule held together by one interchain disulfide bond. In contrast to the single-chain precursor form of most serine proteinases, single-chain t-PA is enzymatically active. On the basis of conformational similarities between single-chain and two-chain t-PA, it was postulated that the activity of single-chain t-PA would involve an equilibrium between an active and a zymogenic conformation, which would be shifted to the active conformation on substrate binding [19]. Alternatively, the high activity of single-chain t-PA has been ascribed to the absence of a *zymogen triad* in the proteinase domain [20]. The t-PA molecule contains four domains: (1) an NH_2-terminal region of 47 residues (residues 4–50; F domain), which is homologous to the finger domains mediating the fibrin affinity of fibronectin; (2) residues 50–87 (E domain), which are homologous to epidermal growth factor; (3) two regions comprised of residues 87–176 and 176–262 (K_1 and K_2 domains), which share a high degree of homology to the five kringles of plasminogen; and (4) a serine proteinase domain (P, residues 276–527) with the active site residues His^{322}, Asp^{371}, and Ser^{478} [18]. Physicochemical characterization of t-PA suggested that the individual domains are folded within the molecule, yielding a globular structure, which is stabilized by strong interactions between the proteinase domain and the F and/or E domains [21]. Nuclear magnetic resonance studies on the solution structure of the finger domain of t-PA support this model [22]. The t-PA molecule has of three potential N-glycosylation sites, at Asn^{117} (K_1), Asn^{184} (K_2), and Asn^{448} (P). t-PA preparations usually contain a mixture of variant I (with all three glycosylation sites) and variant II (lacking carbohydrate at Asn^{184}) [18]. Classical O-linked carbohydrate chains have not been found in t-PA, but it has been shown that fucose is glycosidically linked to Thr^{61} in the E domain [23] (see Chapters 19 and 20).

SINGLE-CHAIN UROKINASE-TYPE PLASMINOGEN ACTIVATOR

Urokinase-type plasminogen activator (u-PA) was first found in urine at relatively high concentrations (200–300 ng/mL) and was later identified in human plasma at a level of about 3–5 ng/mL. Its cDNA has been cloned and expressed in 1985 [24]. u-PA is comprised of 411 amino acids in a single polypeptide chain (scu-PA) and contains the serine proteinase active site triad His^{204}, Asp^{255}, and Ser^{356}. The molecule contains an NH_2-terminal growth factor domain and one kringle structure homologous to the five kringles found in plasminogen and the two kringles in t-PA. Conversion of scu-PA to two-chain u-PA (tcu-PA) occurs after proteolytic cleavage at position Lys^{158}–Ile^{159} by plasmin [25], kallikrein [26], trypsin [26], cathepsin B [27], human T-cell–associated serine proteinase-1 [28], and thermolysin [29]. A fully active tcu-PA derivative is obtained after additional proteolysis by plasmin at position Lys^{135}–Lys^{136}. In addition, a low molecular weight form of scu-PA (32 kd) can be obtained by selective cleavage at position Glu^{143}–Leu^{144} [30]; this cleavage can be obtained with the matrix metalloproteinase Pump-1 [31]. In contrast, scu-PA is converted to an inactive two-chain molecule by thrombin after proteolytic cleavage at position Arg^{156}–Phe^{157} [26]. This inactivation is strongly enhanced in the presence of thrombomodulin and is dependent on the O-linked glucosaminoglycan of thrombomodulin [32]. The cofactor effect of thrombomodulin on the inactivation of scu-PA by thrombin was demonstrated in a perfused rabbit heart model [33]. u-PA contains only one N-glycosylation site (at Asn^{302}) and contains a fucosylated threonine residue at position 18 [34] (see Chapter 17).

STAPHYLOKINASE

Natural staphylokinase has been purified from *Staphylococcus aureus* strains that were transformed with bacteriophages containing the staphylokinase gene or that had undergone lysogenic conversion to staphylokinase production [35]. It was shown in the 1940s to have profibrinolytic activity [36]. More recently, the staphylokinase gene has been cloned from bacteriophages as well as from the genomic DNA of a lysogenic *Staphylococcus aureus* strain and has been expressed in bacterial systems [37].

Mature staphylokinase consists of 136 amino acids in a single polypeptide chain without disulfide bridges [37]. The solution structure of staphylokinase has been analyzed by x-ray scattering, dynamic light scattering, ultracentrifugation, and ultraviolet circular dichroism spectroscopy. The physical parameters obtained in these studies indicate that the molecule is very elongated and consists of two folded domains of similar size, the mutual positions of which are variable [38].

Several molecular forms of staphylokinase have been purified with slightly different M_r (16.5–18 kd) and isoelectric points. Lower M_r derivatives of mature staphylokinase were obtained lacking the 6 (Sak-Δ6) or the 10 (Sak-Δ10) NH_2-terminal amino acids. On interaction with plasmin(ogen) in a buffer milieu, mature staphylokinase (NH_2-terminal Ser-Ser-Ser-) is rapidly and quantitatively converted to Sak-Δ10 (NH_2-terminal Lys-Gly-Asp-). Mature staphylokinase and Sak-Δ10 have the same fibrinolytic activity and a comparable plasminogen activating and fibrinolytic potential in human plasma in vitro [39].

The amino acid at position 26 appears to be of crucial importance for the activation of plasminogen by staphylokinase. Indeed, substitution of the unique Met residue in position 26 dramatically influenced its potency, depending on the nature of the exchanged amino acid [40]. A "clustered charge-to-alanine scan," in which the 45 charged amino acids of the protein were substituted with Ala in clusters of two or three residues, revealed that mutagenesis in three regions of the protein (amino acids 11–14, 46–50, and 65–69) resulted in impairment of the interaction with plasminogen [41] (see Chapter 18).

Molecular Structure of Inhibitors of Fibrinolysis

α_2-ANTIPLASMIN

α_2-Antiplasmin is the main physiological plasmin inhibitor in human plasma, whereas plasmin formed in excess of α_2-antiplasmin may be neutralized by α_2-macroglobulin. α_2-Antiplasmin is a 67-kd single-chain glycoprotein containing 13% N-linked carbohydrate; it is synthesized in the liver and its plasma concentration is about $1\,\mu M$. Two forms of α_2-antiplasmin were detected in about equal amounts in purified preparations of the inhibitor [42]: a native 464 residue long inhibitor with NH_2-terminal methionine (Met^1–α_2-antiplasmin) and a form that is 12 residues shorter with NH_2-terminal asparagine (Asn^{13}–α_2-antiplasmin). Previously it was reported that native α_2-antiplasmin contains only 452 amino acids (Asn^{13}–α_2-antiplasmin) [43], with reactive site peptide bond Arg^{364}–Met^{365} (Arg^{376}–Met^{377} for Met^1–α_2-antiplasmin). It is not known whether Asn^{13}–α_2-antiplasmin is present in the circulating blood or whether it is generated in vitro. α_2-Antiplasmin is unique among serpins (serine proteinase imhibitors) in having a COOH-terminal extension of 51 amino acid residues [43], which contains a secondary binding site that reacts with the lysine-binding sites of plasminogen and plasmin [44]. The plasminogen-binding form of α_2-antiplasmin becomes partly (about 30% of the total) converted in the circulating blood to a non–plasminogen-binding, less reactive form [45], which lacks the 26 COOH-terminal residues [44]. The NH_2-terminal Gln^{14} residue of $Met^{1-}$$\alpha_2$–antiplasmin can crosslink to Aα chains of fibrin in a process that requires Ca^{2+} and is catalyzed by activated coagulation factor XIII [46]; this crosslinking is more efficient for Asn^{13}–α_2-antiplasmin [47].

PLASMINOGEN ACTIVATOR INHIBITOR-1

Rapid inhibition of both t-PA and u-PA in normal human plasma occurs primarily by plasminogen activator inhibitor-1 (PAI-1) [48]. PAI-1 was first identified in conditioned media of cultured human endothelial cells and subsequently in plasma, platelets, placenta, and conditioned media of fibrosarcoma cells and hepatocytes [49]. In healthy individuals, highly variable plasma levels of both PAI activity and PAI-1 antigen have been observed. PAI activity ranges from 0.5 to 47 U/mL (t-PA neutralizing units; 1 mg active PAI-1 corresponds to 700,000 units), with 80% of the values below 6 U/mL. PAI-1 antigen ranges between 6 and 85 ng/mL (geometric mean: 24 ng/mL) but is strongly elevated in several thromboembolic disease states [50]. The serpin PAI-1 is a single-chain glycoprotein of 52 kd consisting of 379 amino acids without disulfide bonds. Three potential N-glycosylation sites are present at Asn^{209}, Asn^{265}, and Asn^{329}. Its reactive-site peptide bond consists of Arg^{346}–Met^{347}; a basic amino acid is required at P1 for significant inhibitory activity, whereas all substitutions, except Pro, are tolerated at P'1 [51].

PAI-1 occurs in different structural forms. It is synthesized as an active inhibitory form that spontaneously converts to a latent non-inhibitory form with a half-life of 2 hours in a purified system and of 4 hours in plasma. Latent PAI-1 can be partially reactivated by treatment with denaturing agents followed by renaturation of the unfolded molecule [52]. In the circulation in vivo, some reactivation of PAI-1 may occur by interaction with negatively charged phospholipids on the membrane of endothelial cells [53]. The structural basis of the latency in PAI-1 has been resolved by determination of its structure by single-crystal x-ray diffraction. Part of the reactive center loop is inserted into the major β-sheet of PAI-1 and is therefore not accessible to the target enzyme (locked conformation). Reactivation of latent PAI-1 by denaturants results in partial elimination of this insertion [54]. Another molecular form of intact PAI-1 has been isolated that does not form stable complexes with t-PA but is cleaved at the P1–P1' peptide bond (*substrate PAI-1*) [55]. PAI-1 could be converted from an inhibitor to a substrate by point mutations in the reactive site loop [56]. Thus, inhibitory PAI-1 may not only convert to latent PAI-1, which can be reactivated, but also to substrate PAI-1, which is irreversibly degraded by its target proteinases.

PAI-1 is stabilized by binding to a plasminogen activator inhibitor binding protein identified as S-protein or vitronectin [57], which may contribute to its longer half-life in vivo than in vitro. Vitronectin binds active PAI-1 with high affinity ($K_d = 0.3$ nM) and does not bind latent PAI-1 [58]. The PAI-1 binding site on vitronectin was mapped to the region comprising residues Lys^{348} to Arg^{370} [59]. PAI-1 also binds to heparin through positively charged amino

acids in the region 65–88 [60], but this binding does not stabilize the inhibitor (see Chapter 5).

PLASMINOGEN ACTIVATOR INHIBITOR-2
The serpin plasminogen activator inhibitor-2 (PAI-2) was first demonstrated in human placenta but was later also demonstrated in leukocytes, monocytes, and macrophages. PAI-2 levels in plasma are very low but are drastically elevated during pregnancy [50]. PAI-2 exists in two different forms with comparable inhibitory properties, which are derived from a single mRNA: an intracellular nonglycosylated 47-Kd and pI-5.0 form and a secreted glycosylated 60-kd and pI-4.4 form [49]. The function of intracellular PAI-2 is unclear because its main target enzyme (u-PA) occurs extracellularly. It may constitute a storage pool from which PAI-2 can be secreted on cell injury [61]. The 1.9-kb PAI-1 cDNA encodes a single-chain protein of 415 amino acids with the reactive-site peptide bond Arg^{380}–Thr^{381} and three potential N-glycosylation sites. PAI-2 extracted from placenta is essentially nonglycosylated, whereas circulating PAI-2 observed during pregnancy is glycosylated. Pregnancy plasma also contains a 130-kd form of PAI-2, which may represent a complex or an aggregate [61].

Inhibitory Mechanisms Involved in Fibrinolysis

Serpins inhibit their target proteinases by formation of a 1:1 stoichiometric reversible complex, followed by covalent binding between the hydroxyl group of the active-site serine residue of the proteinase and the carboxyl group of the P1 residue at the reactive center (the *bait region*) of the serpin.

INHIBITION OF PLASMIN BY α_2-ANTIPLASMIN
The inhibition of plasmin (P) by α_2-antiplasmin (A) can be represented by two consecutive reactions: a fast, second-order reaction producing a reversible inactive complex (PA), which is followed by a slower first-order transition resulting in an irreversible complex (PA'). This model can be represented by

$$P + A \underset{k_{-1}}{\overset{k_1}{\rightleftarrows}} PA \xrightarrow{k_2} PA'.$$ The second-order rate constant of the inhibition of plasmin by α_2-antiplasmin is very high ($k_1 = 2-4 \times 10^7 M^{-1} s^{-1}$) [62], but this high inhibition rate is dependent on the presence of a free lysine binding site and active site in the plasmin molecule and on availability of a plasminogen binding site and reactive-site peptide bond in the inhibitor. The plasmin–α_2-antiplasmin complex is schematically represented in Figure 4-3. From

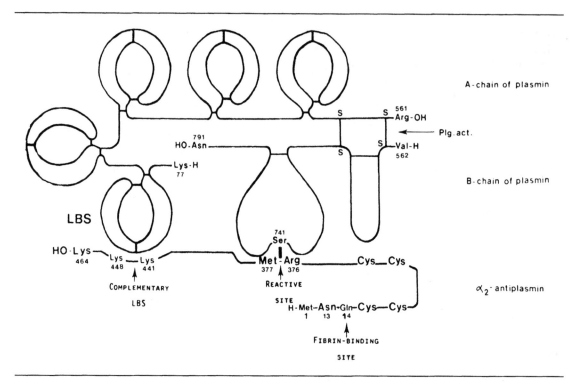

FIGURE 4-3. Schematic representation of the plasmin–α_2-antiplasmin complex. Inhibition of plasmin by α_2-antiplasmin involves a high-affinity interaction between the lysine binding site (LBS) in kringle 1 of plasmin and the complementary plasminogen binding site in the COOH-terminal region of α_2-antiplasmin, and cleavage of the Arg[376]–Met[377] reactive site peptide bond in the inhibitor following interaction with Ser[741] in the active site of plasmin.

kinetic data, the half-life of plasmin molecules on the fibrin surface, which have both their lysine binding sites and active site occupied, is estimated to be two to three orders of magnitude longer than that of free plasmin [62]. Inhibition of plasmin by α_2-antiplasmin is accelerated by Lp(a) in the presence of fibrin or fibrinogen fragments, which may result in impairment of fibrinolysis [63].

INHIBITION OF PLASMINOGEN ACTIVATORS BY PLASMINOGEN ACTIVATOR INHIBITORS

PAI-1 reacts very rapidly with single-chain and two-chain t-PA and with two-chain u-PA, with second-order inhibition rate constants of the order of $10^7 \, M^{-1} \, s^{-1}$. PAI-2 primarily inhibits two-chain u-PA. The inhibition rate of two-chain u-PA, single-chain t-PA, and two-chain t-PA by PAI-2 is about 10, 1200, and 150 times slower, respectively, than that with PAI-1. PAI-1 and PAI-2 do not react with scu-PA [49]. Rapid inhibition of both t-PA and u-PA by PAI-1 involves a reversible high-affinity second-site interaction that does not depend on a functional active site [64]. Modeling based on the assumption that the interaction between t-PA and PAI-1 is similar to that between trypsin and a bovine trypsin inhibitor suggested that sequence 350–355 of PAI-1, which

contains three negatively charged amino acids, interacts with highly positively charged regions in t-PA (residues 296–304) [65] and in u-PA (residues 179–184) [66]. In the presence of fibrin, single-chain t-PA is protected from rapid inhibition by PAI-1 [64]. It has, however, also been reported that PAI-1 binds to fibrin and that fibrin-bound PAI-1 my inhibit t-PA–mediated clot lysis [67,68] (see Chapter 5).

Mechanisms of Fibrin Specificity

TISSUE-TYPE PLASMINOGEN ACTIVATOR

t-PA functions poorly as an enzyme in the absence of fibrin, but the presence of fibrin strikingly enhances the activation rate of plasminogen. Kinetic data support a mechanism in which fibrin provides a surface to which t-PA and plasminogen adsorb in a sequential and ordered manner, yielding a cyclic ternary complex. Formation of this complex is mainly associated with a decrease in the K_m for the t-PA catalyzed activation of plasminogen, leading to an efficient and localized plasminogen activation (a decrease in the K_m from $65\,\mu M$ in the absence of fibrin to $0.16\,\mu M$ in its presence). The maximal stimulation of plasminogen activation by this mechanism is about three orders of magnitude [69]. Plasmin formed on the fibrin surface has both its lysine binding sites and active site occupied, and is thus only slowly inactivated by α_2-antiplasmin (half-life, ~10–100 seconds); in contrast, free plasmin, when formed, is rapidly inhibited by α_2-antiplasmin (half-life, ~0.1 second) [62].

The effector function of fibrin during fibrinolysis is variable because both fibrinogen and fibrin itself are continuously modified by cleavage with thrombin or plasmin, yielding a diversity of reaction products [70]. Thrombin-catalyzed release of fibrinopeptide A from the NH_2-terminal Aα-chain of fibrinogen, yielding the desA-fibrin monomer and some desA-fibrin polymerization, are essential for stimulation of plasminogen activation by t-PA [71]. Optimal stimulation is only obtained after early plasmin cleavage at the COOH terminal Aα-chain and the NH_2-terminal Bβ-chain of fibrin, yielding the fragment X-polymer [70]. Further cleavage of fragment X-polymer by plasmin in the coiled coil region yields the soluble fragments Y and D, and results in abolishment of the stimulatory effect on plasminogen activation. Lysine binding sites and aminohexyl binding sites located in the kringle structures of t-PA and plasminogen, and complementary sites on fibrin (COOH-terminal and internal lysine residues, respectively) play an important role in these interactions.

It was suggested that the initial binding of t-PA to fibrin was mediated via the finger domain, whereas partial fibrin degradation would result in enhanced binding of t-PA via kringle 2. The increase in fibrin stimulation after formation of fibrin X-polymers is indeed associated with an augmented and qualitatively altered binding of t-PA [72] and plasminogen [71]. This increased and altered fibrin binding of enzyme and substrate is mediated in part by COOH-terminal lysines generated by plasmin cleavage of the COOH-terminal α chains of fibrin. Interaction of these COOH-terminal lysines with lysine binding sites on t-PA and plasminogen may permit improved alignment as well as allosteric changes in the t-PA and plasminogen moieties, thus enhancing the rate of plasminogen activation. The physiological relevance of this model for plasminogen activation by t-PA in

the presence of fibrin is supported by cases of dysfibrinogenemia in which decreased binding of either plasminogen (e.g., fibrinogen Dusard [73]) or t-PA (e.g., fibrinogen New York I [74]) to fibrin clots results in defective fibrinolysis and is associated with thrombotic complications.

During fibrin clot lysis, single-chain t-PA is converted to its two-chain form at the fibrin surface; this conversion is probably of little physiological relevance because the activity of single-chain t-PA and two-chain t-PA is comparable in the presence of fibrin [75]. Fibrin-bound single-chain t-PA may adopt a conformation similar to that of two-chain t-PA [76]. Whether conversion of Glu-plasminogen to the more easily activatable Lys-plasminogen contributes significantly to the increased plasminogen activation rate during fibrinolysis is still somewhat controversial.

Binding studies as well as kinetic studies have revealed that Lp(a) competes with plasminogen for binding to fibrin as a result of binding of Lp(a) to fibrin via its lysine-binding domains. With regard to plasminogen, binding of Lp(a) to fibrin is enhanced by partial proteolytic degradation of the fibrin surface. The functional consequence of the competition between Lp(a) and plasminogen for binding to fibrin would be inhibition of the fibrin-dependent enhancement of plasminogen activation by t-PA. Other studies, however, did not find an inhibitory effect of Lp(a) on fibrinolysis, but one study reported an enhancement of fibrin clot lysis by t-PA in the presence of Lp(a) [77]. These discrepancies may be reconciled by the findings that the inhibitory effects of Lp(a) on plasminogen activation are only seen at a low concentration of reactants, whereas at physiological plasminogen concentration Lp(a) stimulates plasminogen activation by t-PA, probably as a result of binding of plasminogen to fibrin-bound Lp(a) [78] (see Chapters 19 and 20).

UROKINASE-TYPE PLASMINOGEN ACTIVATOR

u-PA is a serine proteinase with a high substrate specificity for plasminogen. In contrast to tcu-PA derivatives, scu-PA displays very low activity toward low M_r chromogenic substrates, while conversion to tcu-PA generates full amidolytic activity. scu-PA appears to have some intrinsic plasminogen-activating potential, which represents $\leq 0.5\%$ of the catalytic efficiency of tcu-PA [79,80]. Other investigators, however, have claimed that scu-PA has no measurable intrinsic amidolytic or plasminogen activator activities [81]. The occurrence of a transitional state of scu-PA with a higher catalytic efficiency against native plasminogen than tcu-PA has been postulated [82]. Furthermore, it was reported that fibrin fragment E-2 selectively promotes the activation of plasminogen by scu-PA, mainly by enhancing the catalytic rate constant of the activation [83]. scu-PA, indeed, does not appear to be an efficient activator for plasminogen bound to internal lysine residues on intact fibrin, whereas it develops an activity similar to that of t-PA toward plasminogen bound to newly generated COOH-terminal lysine residues on partially degraded fibrin [84]. Subsequent studies confirmed that the fibrin specificity of scu-PA does not require its conversion to tcu-PA, nor conversion of Glu-plasminogen to Lys-plasminogen, but appears to be mediated by enhanced binding of plasminogen to partially digested fibrin [85].

In plasma, in the absence of fibrin, scu-PA is stable and does not activate plasminogen; in the presence of a fibrin clot, scu-PA, but not tcu-PA, induces fibrin-specific clot lysis [79]. scu-PA does not bind to a significant extent to fibrin, although in the presence of Zn^{2+} ions some binding has been reported [86]. The intrinsic activity of scu-PA towards fibrin-bound plasminogen may contribute to its fibrin specificity. Furthermore, α_2-antiplasmin in plasma prevents conversion of scu-PA to tcu-PA outside the clot and thus preserves fibrin specificity [87] (see Chapter 17).

STAPHYLOKINASE
Like streptokinase, staphylokinase is not an enzyme but forms a complex with plasmin(ogen), which, in turn, activates other plasminogen molecules. The plasminogen–streptokinase complex exposes an active site in the plasminogen moiety without proteolytic cleavage, whereas generation of plasmin is required for exposure of an active site in the plasminogen–staphylokinase complex [88]. Kinetic data support a model in which plasminogen and staphylokinase produce an inactive 1:1 stoichiometric complex. Activation may be initiated by tract amounts of contaminating plasmin, generating an active plasmin–staphylokinase complex that converts excess plasminogen to plasmin and, even more rapidly, inactive plasminogen–staphylokinase to active plasmin–staphylokinase complex [41]. The lysine binding sites in kringles 1–4 of plasminogen are not required for formation of the active complex [89].

Staphylokinase does not bind to fibrin, and fibrin stimulates the initial rate of plasminogen activation by staphylokinase only fourfold [90]. Nevertheless, staphylokinase was found to be an efficient and highly fibrin-specific plasminogen activator in human plasma in vitro and in vivo [37]. The fibrin specificity of staphylokinase in human plasma has been explained by rapid inhibition of the generated plasmin–staphylokinase complex by α_2-antiplasmin [90–92] and by a more than 100-fold reduction of this inhibition rate at the fibrin surface [93], which may allow preferential plasminogen activation at the fibrin clot. However, staphylokinase dissociates in active form from the plasmin–staphylokinase complex following neutralization by α_2-antiplasmin and is recycled to other plasminogen molecules [94]. Thus, extensive systemic plasminogen activation with staphylokinase would be expected in plasma, which clearly contradicts its well-established fibrin specificity.

It was shown that when the plasmin–staphylokinase complex is formed in the absence of fibrin but in the presence of excess α_2-antiplasmin, it is rapidly neutralized and staphylokinase is recycled to other plasminogen molecules. However, conversion of plasminogen–staphylokinase to plasmin–staphylokinase does not occur at a significant rate because it is prevented by α_2-antiplasmin; without the plasmin–staphylokinase complex, no significant plasminogen activation occurs [95]. In the presence of fibrin, generation of the plasmin(ogen)–staphylokinase complex is facilitated and inhibition of plasmin–staphylokinase by α_2-antiplasmin at the clot surface is delayed. Recycling of staphylokinase to fibrin-bound plasminogen, after neutralization of the plasmin–staphylokinase complex, results in more efficient production of the plasmin(ogen)–staphylokinase complex. This mechanism is mediated via the lysine binding sites of plasminogen and results in significantly enhanced plasminogen activation at the fibrin surface [95].

Staphylokinase, in contrast to streptokinase, also induces efficient and fibrin-specific lysis of platelet-rich plasma clots in human plasma [39]. This differential sensitivity might result from alteration of the α_2-antiplasmin to plasminogen ratio in the clot during retraction. Extrusion of non–fibrin-bound plasminogen during platelet-mediated clot retraction may indeed result in an enhanced ratio of α_2-antiplasmin to plasminogen associated with the clot. It was shown previously that retracted blood clots are more sensitive to lysis with fibrin-specific plasminogen activators, probably because enhanced systemic plasminogen activation with non–fibrin-specific agents precludes recruitment of plasminogen from the surrounding plasma, resulting in reduced clot lysis [96]. With the highly fibrin-specific agent staphylokinase, circulating plasminogen levels are not significantly decreased, thus allowing plasminogen supplementation from the plasma to the clot [39] (see Chapter 18).

Conclusions

Plasmin, the proteolytic enzyme responsible for the degradation of fibrin, is generated following activation of the proenzyme plasminogen by plasminogen activators. Inhibition of fibrinolysis may occur at the level of the plasminogen activators by PAIs or at the level of plasmin, mainly by α_2-antiplasmin. Physiological fibrinolysis is a fibrin-specific process resulting from specific molecular interactions between its main components. This implies that the generation of plasmin occurs preferentially at the surface of a fibrin clot and not in the circulation, where it may, after exhaustion of α_2-antiplasmin, degrade several plasma proteins, thus inducing a *lytic state*. In addition to the two physiological plasminogen activators (tissue-type and urokinase-type), staphylokinase, a bacterial plasminogen activator, was also found to display a high fibrin specificity, although via different mechanisms.

References

1. Collen D, Lijnen HR. Basic and clinical aspects of fibrinolysis and thrombolysis. Blood 78:3114, 1991.
2. Blasi F. Urokinase and urokinase receptor: A paracrine/autocrine system regulating cell migration and invasiveness. BioEssays 15:105, 1993.
3. Bachmann F. The plasminogen-plasmin enzyme system. In Colman RW, Hirsch J, Marder VJ, Salzman FW (eds). Hemostasis and Thrombosis: Basic Principles and Clinical Practice, 3rd ed. Philadelphia: JB Lippincott 1993:1592.
4. Bugge TH, Suh TT, Flick MJ, Daugherty CC, Romer J, Solberg H, Ellis V, Danø K, Degen JL. The receptor for urokinase-type plasminogen activator is not essential for mouse development or fertility. J Biol Chem 270:16886, 1995.
5. Lijnen HR, Collen D. Congenital and acquired deficiencies of components of the fibrinolytic system and their relation to bleeding or thrombosis. Fibrinolysis 3:67, 1989.
6. Wiman B, Hamsten A. The fibrinolytic enzyme system and its role in the etiology of thromboembolic disease. Semin Thromb Hemost 16:207, 1990.
7. Sottrup-Jensen L, Petersen TE, Magnusson S. Atlas of Protein Sequence and Structure, Vol. 5, Suppl. 3. Dayhoff MO (ed). Washington DC: National Biomedical Research Foundation 1978:91.
8. Forsgren M, Raden B, Israelsson M, Larsson K, Heden LO. Molecular cloning and characterization of a full-length cDNA clone for human plasminogen. FEBS Lett 213:254, 1987.
9. Menhart N, McCance SG, Sehl LC, Castellino FJ. Functional independence of the kringle 4 and kringle 5 regions of human plasminogen. Biochemistry 32:8799, 1993.
10. Wu TP, Padmanabhan KP, Tulinsky A. The structure of recombinant plasminogen kringle 1 and the fibrin binding site. Blood Coagul Fibrinolysis 5:157, 1994.
11. Berglund L, Petersen TE. The gene structure of tetranectin, a plasminogen binding protein. FEBS left 309:15, 1992.
12. Marshall JM, Brown AJ, Ponting CP. Conformational studies of human plasminogen and plasminogen fragments: Evidence for a novel third conformation of plasminogen. Biochemistry 33:3599, 1994.
13. Robbins KC, Summaria L, Hsieh B, Shah RJ. The peptide chains of human plasmin. Mechanism of activation of human plasminogen to plasmin. J Biol Chem 242:2333, 1967.
14. Holvoet, P, Lijnen HR, Collen D. A monoclonal antibody specific for Lys-plasminogen. Application to the study of the activation pathways of plasminogen in vivo. J Biol Chem 260:12106, 1985.
15. Sottrup-Jensen L, Claeys H, Zajdel M, Petersen TE, Magnusson S. The primary structure of human plasminogen: Isolation of two lysine-binding fragments and one "mini-" plasminogen (MW, 38,000) by elastase-catalyzed-specific limited proteolysis. In Davidson JF, Rowan RM, Samama MM, Desnoyers PC (eds). Progress in Chemical Fibrinolysis and Thrombolysis, 3rd ed. New York: Raven Press 1978:191.
16. Nakajima K, Nagata K, Hamanoue M, Takemoto N, Kohsaka S. Microglia-derived elastase produces a low-molecular-weight plasminogen that enhances neurite outgrowth in rat neocortical explant cultures. J Neurochem 61:2155, 1993.
17. O'Reilly MS, Holmgren L, Shing Y, Chen C, Rosenthal RA, Moses M, Lane WS, Cao Y, Sage EH, Folkman J. Angiostatin: A novel angiogenesis inhibitor that mediates the suppression of metastases by a Lewis lung carcinoma. Cell 79:315, 1994.
18. Pennica D, Holmes WE, Kohr WJ, Harkins RN, Vehar GA, Ward CA, Bennett WF, Yelverton E, Seeburg PH, Heyneker HL, Goeddel DV, Collen D. Cloning and expression of human tissue-type plasminogen activator cDNA in E. coli. Nature 301:214, 1983.
19. Nienaber VL, Young SL, Birktoft JJ, Higgins DL, Berliner LJ. Conformational similarities between one-chain and two-chain tissue plasminogen activator (t-PA): Implications to the activation mechanism on one-chain t-PA. Biochemistry 31:3852, 1992.
20. Madison EL, Kobe A, Gething M-J, Sambrook JF, Goldsmith EJ. Converting tissue plasminogen activator to a zymogen: A regulatory triad of Asp-His-Ser. Science 262:419, 1993.
21. Novokhatny VV, Ingham KC, Medved LV. Domain structure and domain-domain interactions of recombinant tissue plasminogen activator. J Biol Chem 266: 12994, 1991.
22. Downing AK, Driscoll PC, Harvey TS, Dudgeon TJ, Smith BO, Baron M, Campbell ID. Solution structure of the fibrin binding finger domain of tissue-type plas-

minogen activator determined by ^{1}H nuclear magnetic resonance. J Mol Biol 225:821, 1992.

23. Harris RJ, Leonard CK, Guzzetta AW, Spellman MW. Tissue plasminogen activator has an O-linked fucose attached to threonine-61 in the epidermal growth factor domain. Biochemistry 30:2311, 1991.

24. Holmes WE, Pennica D, Blaber M, Rey MW, Günzler WA, Steffens GJ, Heyneker HL. Cloning and expression of the gene for pro-urokinase in *Escherichia coli*. Biotechnology 3:923, 1985.

25. Günzler WA, Steffens GJ, Ötting F, Kim SM, Frankus E, Flohe L. The primary structure of high molecular mass urokinase from human urine. The complete amino acid sequence of the A chain. Hoppe-Seyler's Z Physiol Chem 363:1155, 1982.

26. Ichinose A, Fujikawa K, Suyama T. The activation of pro-urokinase by plasma kallikrein and its inactivation by thrombin. J Biol Chem 261:3486, 1986.

27. Kobayashi H, Schmitt M, Goretzki L, Chucholowski N, Calvete J, Kramer M, Günzler WA, Janicke F, Graeff H. Cathepsin B efficiently activates the soluble and the tumor cell receptor-bound form of the proenzyme urokinase-type plasminogen activator (Pro-uPA). J Biol Chem 266:5147, 1991.

28. Brunner G, Vettel U, Jobstmann S, Kramer MD, Schirrmacher U. A T-cell-related proteinase expressed by T-lymphoma cells activates their endogenous pro-urokinase. Blood 79:2099, 1992.

29. Marcotte PA, Henkin J. Characterization of the activation of pro-urokinase by thermolysin. Biochim Biophys Acta 1160:105, 1993.

30. Stump DC, Lijnen HR. Collen D. Purification and characterization of a novel low molecular weight form of single-chain urokinase-type plasminogen activator. J Biol Chem 261:17120, 1986.

31. Marcotte PA, Kozan IM, Dorwin SA, Ryan JM. The matrix metalloproteinase Pump-1 catalyzes formation of low molecular weight (pro)urokinase in cultures of normal human kidney cells. J Biol Chem 267:13803, 1992.

32. de Munk GA, Parkinson JF, Groeneveld E, Bang NU, Rijken DC. Role of the glycosaminoglycan component of thrombomodulin in its acceleration of the inactivation of single-chain urokinase-type plasminogen activator by thrombin. Biochem J 290:655, 1993.

33. Molinari A, Giorgetti C, Lansen J. Thrombomodulin is a cofactor for thrombin degradation of recombinant single-chain urokinase plasminogen activator "in vitro" and in a perfused rabbit heart model. Thromb Haemost 67:226, 1992.

34. Buko AM, Kentzer EJ, Petros A, Menon G, Zuiderweg ER, Sarin UK. Characterization of a posttranscriptional fucosylation in the growth factor domains of urinary plasminogen activator. Proc Natl Acad Sci USA 88:3992, 1991.

35. Winkler KC, DeWaart J, Grootsen C, Zegers BJM, Tellier NF, Vertegt CD. Lysogenic conversion of staphylococci to loss of beta-toxin. J Gen Microbiol 39:321, 1965.

36. Lack CH. Staphylokinase: An activator of plasma protease. Nature 161:559, 1948.

37. Collen D, Lijnen HR. Staphylokinase, a fibrin-specific plasminogen activator with therapeutic potential? Blood 84:680, 1994.

38. Damaschun G, Damaschun H, Gast K, Misselwitz R, Zirwer D, Gührs KH, Hartmann M, Schlott B, Triebel H, Behnke D. Physical and conformational properties of staphylokinase in solution. Biochim Biophys Acta 1161:244, 1993.

39. Lijnen HR, Van Hoef B, Vandenbossche L, Collen D. Biochemical properties of natural and recombinant staphylokinase. Fibrinolysis 6:214, 1992.

40. Schlott B, Hartmann M, Gührs K-H, Birch-Hirschfeld E, Gase A, Vetterman S, Collen D, Lijnen HR. Functional properties of recombinant staphylokinase variants obtained by site-specific mutagenesis of methionine 26. Biochim Biophys Acta 1204:235, 1994.

41. Silence K, Hartmann M, Gührs K-H, Gase A, Schlott B, Collen D, Lijnen HR. Structure-function relationships in staphylokinase as revealed by "clustered charge-to-alanine" mutagenesis. J Biol Chem, 270:27192, 1995.

42. Bangert K, Johnsen AH, Christensen U, Thorsen S. Different N-terminal forms of α_2-plasmin inhibitor in human plasma. Biochem J 291:623, 1993.

43. Holmes WE, Nelles L, Lijnen HR, Collen D. Primary structure of human α_2-antiplasmin, a serine protease inhibitor (serpin). J Biol Chem 262:1659, 1987.

44. Sugiyama N, Sasaki T, Iwamoto M, Abiko Y. Binding site of α_2-plasmin inhibitor to plasminogen. Biochim Biophys Acta 952:1, 1988.

45. Clemmensen I, Thorsen S, Müllertz S, Petersen LC. Properties of three different molecular forms of α_2-plasmin inhibitor. Eur J Biochem 120:105, 1981.

46. Kimura S, Aoki N. Cross-linking site in fibrinogen for α_2-plasmin inhibitor. J Biol Chem 261:15591, 1986.

47. Sumi Y, Ichikawa Y, Nakamura Y, Miura O, Aoki N. Expression and characterization of pro α_2-plasmin inhibitor. J Biochem (Tokyo) 106:703, 1989.

48. Kruithof EKO, Tran-Thang C, Ransijn A, Bachmann F. Demonstration of a fast-acting inhibitor of plasminogen activators in human plasma. Blood 64:907, 1984.

49. Kruithof EKO. Plasminogen activator inhibitors — a review. Enzyme 40:113, 1988.

50. Kruithof EKO, Gudinchet A, Bachmann F. Plasminogen activator inhibitor 1 and plasminogen activator inhibitor 2 in various disease states. Thromb Haemost 59:7, 1988.

51. Sherman PM, Lawrence DA, Yang AY, Vandenberg ET, Paielli D, Olson ST, Shore JD, Ginsburg D. Saturation mutagenesis of the plasminogen activator inhibitor-1 reactive center. J Biol Chem 267:7588, 1992.

52. Hekman CM, Loskutoff DJ. Endothelial cells produce a latent inhibitor of plasminogen activators that can be activated by denaturants. J Biol Chem 260:11581, 1985.

53. Vaughan DE, Declerck PJ, Van Houtte E, De Mol M, Collen D. Studies of recombinant plasminogen activator inhibitor-1 in rabbits. Circ Res 67:1281, 1990.

54. Mottonen J, Strand A, Symersky J, Sweet RM, Danley DE, Geoghegan KF, Gerard RD, Goldsmith EJ. Structural basis of latency in plasminogen activator inhibitor-1. Nature 355:270, 1992.

55. Declerck PJ, De Mol M, Vaughan DE, Collen D. Identification of a conformationally distinct form of plasminogen activator inhibitor-1, acting as a non-inhibitory substrate for tissue-type plasminogen activator. J Biol Chem 267:11693, 1992.

56. Audenaert A-M, Knockaert I, Collen D, Declerck PJ. Conversion of plasminogen activator inhibitor-1 from inhibitor to substrate by point mutations in the reactive-site loop. J Biol Chem 269:19559, 1994.

57. Declerck PJ, De Mol M, Alessi MC, Baudner S, Paques EP, Preissner KT, Müller-Berghaus G, Collen D. Purification and characterization of a plasminogen activator inhibitor-1 binding protein from human plasma. Identification as a multimeric form of S protein (Vitronectin). J Biol Chem 263:15454, 1988.

58. Seiffert D, Loskutoff DJ. Kinetic analysis of the interaction between type 1 plasminogen activator inhibitor and vitronectin and evidence that the bovine inhibitor binds to a thrombin-derived amino-terminal fragment of bovine vitronectin. Biochim Biophys Acta 1078:23, 1991.

59. Gechtman Z, Sharma R, Kreizman T, Fridkin M, Shaltiel S. Synthetic peptides derived from the sequence around the plasmin cleavage site in vitronectin. Use in mapping the PAI-1 binding site. FEBS lett 315:293, 1993.

60. Ehrlich HJ, Gebbink PK, Keijer J, Pannekoek H. Elucidation of structural requirements on plasminogen activator inhibitor 1 for binding to heparin. J Biol Chem 267:11606, 1992.

61. Booth NA, Reith A, Bennett B. A plasminogen activator inhibitor (PAI-2) circulates in two molecular forms during pregnancy. Thromb Haemost 59:77, 1988.

62. Wiman B, Collen D. On the kinetics of the reaction between human antiplasmin and plasmin. Eur J Biochem 84:573, 1978.

63. Edelberg JM, Pizzo SV. Lipoprotein (a) promotes plasmin inhibition by α_2-antiplasmin. Biochem J 286:79, 1992.

64. Chmielewska J, Ranby M, Wiman B. Kinetics of the inhibition of plasminogen activators by the plasminogen-activator inhibitor. Evidence for "second site" interactions. Biochem J 251:327, 1988.

65. Madison EL, Goldsmith EJ, Gerard RD, Gething MJ, Sambrook JF, Serpin-resistant mutants of human tissue-type plasminogen activator. Nature 339:721, 1989.

66. Adams DS, Griffin LA, Nachajko WR, Reddy VB, Wei CM. A synthetic DNA encoding a modified human urokinase resistant to inhibition by serum plasminogen activator inhibitor. J Biol Chem 266:8476, 1991.

67. Wagner OF, de Vries C, Hohmann C, Veerman H, Pannekoek H. Interaction between plasminogen activator inhibitor type 1 (PAI-1) bound to fibrin and either tissue-type plasminogen activator (t-PA) or urokinase-type plasminogen activator (u-PA). J Clin Invest 84:647, 1989.

68. Reilly CF, Hutzelmann JE. Plasminogen activator inhibitor-1 binds to fibrin and inhibits tissue-type plasminogen activator-mediated fibrin dissolution. J Biol Chem 267:17128, 1992.

69. Hoylaerts M, Rijken DC, Lijnen HR, Collen D. Kinetics of the activation of plasminogen by human tissue plasminogen activator. Role of fibrin. J Biol Chem 257:2912, 1982.

70. Thorsen S. The mechanism of plasminogen activation and the variability of the fibrin effector during tissue-type plasminogen activator-mediated fibrinolysis. Ann N Y Acad Sci 667:52, 1992.

71. Suenson E, Petersen LC. Fibrin and plasminogen structures essential to stimulation of plasmin formation by tissue-type plasminogen activator. Biochim Biophys Acta 870:510, 1986.

72. Higgins DL, Vehar GA. Interaction of one-chain and two-chain tissue plasminogen activator with intact and plasmin-degraded fibrin. Biochemistry 26:7786, 1987.

73. Collet JP, Soria J, Mirshahi M. Dusard syndrome: A new concept of the relationship between fibrin clot architecture and fibrin clot degradability: Hypofibrinolysis related to an abnormal clot structure. Blood 82:2462, 1993.

74. Liu CY, Koehn JA, Morgan FJ. Characterization of fibrinogen New York 1. A dysfunctional fibrinogen with a deletion of Bβ (9–72) corresponding exactly to exon 2 of the gene. J Biol Chem 260:4390, 1985.

75. Andreasen PA, Petersen LC, Danø K. Diversity in catalytic properties of single chain and two chain tissue-type plasminogen activator. Fibrinolysis 5:207, 1991.

76. Loscalzo J. Structural and kinetic comparison of recombinant human single- and two-chain tissue plasminogen activator. J Clin Invest 82:1391, 1988.

77. Harpel PC, Hermann A, Zhang X, Ostfeld I, Borth W. Lipoprotein (a), plasmin modulation, and atherogenesis.Thromb Haemost 74:382, 1995.

78. Liu J, Harpel PC, Gurewich V. Fibrin-bound lipoprotein (a) promotes plasminogen binding but inhibits fibrin degradation by plasmin. Biochemistry 33:2554, 1994.

79. Gurewich V, Pannell R, Louie S, Kelley P, Suddith RL, Greenlee R. Effective and fibrin-specific clot lysis by a zymogen precursor form of urokinase (pro-urokinase). A study in vitro and in two animal species. J Clin Invest 73:1731, 1984.

80. Lijnen HR, Van Hoef B, Nelles L, Collen D. Plasminogen activation with single-chain urokinase-type plasminogen activator (scu-PA). Studies with active site mutagenized plasminogen (Ser^{740} → >Ala) and plas-

min resistant scu-PA (Lys[158] → Glu). J Biol Chem 265:5232, 1990.

81. Husain SS. Single-chain urokinase-type plasminogen activator does not possess measurable intrinsic amidolytic or plasminogen activator activities. Biochemistry 30:5797, 1991.

82. Liu J, Pannell R, Gurewich V. A transitional state of pro-urokinase that has a higher catalytic efficiency against Glu-plasminogen than urokinase. J Biol Chem 267:15289, 1992.

83. Liu J, Gurewich V. Fragment E-2 from fibrin substantially enhances pro-urokinase-induced Glu-plasminogen activation. A kinetic study using the plasmin-resistant mutant pro-urokinase Ala-158-rpro-UK. Biochemistry 31:6311, 1992.

84. Fleury V, Gurewich V, Anglés-Cano E. A study of the activation of fibrin-bound plasminogen by tissue-type plasminogen activator, single chain urokinase and sequential combinations of the activators. Fibrinolysis 7:87, 1993.

85. Fleury V, Lijnen HR, Anglés-Cano E. Mechanism of the enhanced intrinsic activity of single-chain urokinase-type plasminogen activator during ongoing fibrinolysis. J Biol Chem 268:18554, 1993.

86. Husain SS. Fibrin affinity of urokinase-type plasminogen activator. Evidence that Zn^{2+} mediates strong and specific interaction of single-chain urokinase with fibrin. J Biol Chem 268:8574, 1993.

87. Declerck PJ, Lijnen HR, Verstreken M, Collen D. Role of α_2-antiplasmin in fibrin-specific clot lysis with single-chain urokinase-type plasminogen activator in human plasma. Thromb Haemost 65:394, 1991.

88. Collen D, Schlott B, Engelborghs Y, Van Hoef B, Hartmann M, Lijnen HR, Behnke D. On the mecha-

nism of the activation of human plasminogen by recombinant staphylokinase. J Biol Chem 268:8284, 1993.

89. Lijnen HR, Van Hoef B, Collen D. Interaction of staphylokinase with different molecular forms of plasminogen. Eur J Biochem 211:91, 1993.

90. Lijnen HR, Van Hoef B, De Cock F, Okada K, Ueshima S, Matsuo O, Collen D. On the mechanism of fibrin-specific plasminogen activation by staphylokinase. J Biol Chem 266:11826, 1991.

91. Sakai M, Watanuki M, Matsuo O. Mechanism of fibrin-specific fibrinolysis by staphylokinase: Participation of α_2-plasmin inhibitor. Biochem Biophys Res Commun 162:830, 1989.

92. Matsuo O, Okada K, Fukao H, Tomioka Y, Ueshima S, Watanuki M, Sakai M. Thrombolytic properties of staphylokinase. Blood 76:925, 1990.

93. Lijnen HR, Van Hoef B, Matsuo O, Collen D. On the molecular interactions between plasminogen-staphylokinase, α_2-antiplasmin and fibrin. Biochim Biophys Acta 1118:144, 1992.

94. Silence K, Collen D, Lijnen HR. Interaction between staphylokinase, plasmin (ogen) and α_2-antiplasmin. Recycling of staphylokinase after neutralization of the plasmin-staphylokinase complex by α_2-antiplasmin. J Biol Chem 268:9811, 1993.

95. Silence K, Collen D, Lijnen HR. Regulation by α_2-antiplasmin and fibrin of the activation of plasminogen with recombinant staphylokinase in plasma. Blood 82:1175, 1993.

96. Sabovic M, Lijnen HR, Keber D, Collen D. Effect of retraction on the lysis of human clots with fibrin specific and non-fibrin specific plasminogen activators, Thromb Haemost 62:1083, 1989.

5. PLASMINOGEN ACTIVATOR INHIBITOR-1

Daniel T. Eitzman, William P. Fay, and David Ginsburg

General Overview of the Plasminogen Activation System

Fibrinolysis, the dissolution of fibrin clots, is an integral component of the hemostatic system that involves the concerted action of a complex system of zymogens, activators, and inhibitors [1]. Plasmin, the primary protease of the fibrinolytic system, digests fibrin, thereby converting insoluble clot to soluble fibrin degradation products. Plasmin formation is regulated, in large part, by plasminogen activators, which are responsible for converting the zymogen, plasminogen, to plasmin. The two major plasminogen activators in humans are tissue-type plasminogen activator (t-PA) and urokinase-type plasminogen activator (u-PA). Both types of activators are serine proteases that specifically convert plasminogen to the broad-specificity protease, plasmin, by cleaving a single peptide bond (Arg_{560}–Val_{561}) [1]. Plasmin, in turn, appears to participate in a multitude of biological processes, including vascular fibrinolysis [2], ovulation [3], inflammation [4], tumor metastasis [5], angiogenesis [6], and tissue remodeling [7] (Figure 5-1). Regulation of the plasminogen activation system is a complex process that is controlled on many levels. The synthesis and release of plasminogen activators (PAs) is governed by various hormones, growth factors, and cytokines [5,7]. Following secretion, PA activity can be regulated both positively and negatively by a number of specific protein–protein interactions. Activity can be enhanced or concentrated by interactions with fibrin [8], the u-PA and t-PA receptors [9,10], and plasminogen receptors [11]. In contrast, PA activity can be downregulated by the presence of PA inhibitors (PAIs) [12,13], or by direct plasmin inhibition [14]. The overall activity of the PA sytem is determined by the interactions among these various elements, and the balance between the opposing activities of enzymes and inhibitors.

There are at least four immunologically distinct PA inhibitors, that is, PAI-1, PAI-2 [15], activated protein C inhibitor (also known as PAI-3) [16], and protease nexin [17]. However, whereas several inhibitors of plasminogen activation have been demonstrated in vitro, the primary physiologically significant inhibitor of intravascular plasminogen activation is believed to be PAI-1. Accordingly, this chapter focuses on the structure, function, and potential clinical significance of PAI-1 as it relates to intravascular fibrinolysis.

Plasminogen Activator Inhibitor-1

BACKGROUND

In 1983, a rapid inhibitor of u-PA and t-PA was found in plasma and endothelial cells [18,19]. Initially called the endothelial cell PAI, the fast-acting PAI, and the β-migrating PAI, PAI-1 is one of the principal regulators of the plasminogen activation system. PAI-1 is a member of the serpin protease inhibitor superfamily (serpins), as are many of the other protease inhibitors found in blood [20–22]. These serpins share a common tertiary structure and are thought to have evolved from a common ancestral gene [23,24]. Like many other active inhibitory serpins, PAI-1 acts as a suicide inhibitor that reacts irreversibly with its target protease to form sodium dodecyl sulfate (SDS)–stable complexes. PAI-1 is an extremely efficient inhibitor of the single- and two-chain forms of t-PA and u-PA, with second-order rate constants ranging between 0.45 and $3.5 \times 10^7 M^{-1} s^{-1}$ [19]. PAI-1 also inhibits plasmin, trypsin, thrombin, and activated protein C, although these reactions are much less efficient [25–29].

PAI-1 is present in plasma at very low concentrations, with an average of about 20 ng/mL (0.5 nM) [30,31], and has a half-life of approximately 6–7 minutes [32,33]. PAI-1 is also present in platelets, vascular smooth muscle cells, endothelial cells, and a variety of cultured cells [34–36]. The predominant source of PAI-1 in plasma is not known, although in certain pathological states, such as endotoxemia, endothelial cells are a major site of PAI-1 synthesis [37–

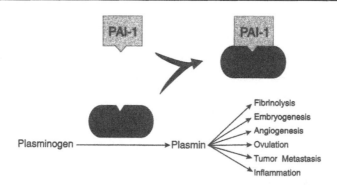

FIGURE 5-1. Plasminogen is converted to plasmin by plasminogen activators (urokinase-type plasminogen activator or tissue-type plasminogen activator), which are both rapidly inhibited by plasminogen activator inhibitor-1. Plasmin appears to participate in a wide variety of physiological and pathological processes. (Adapted from Lawrence and Ginsburg [130], with permission.)

39]. PAI-1 circulates in plasma as a complex with vitronectin [40,41] and is also found to be associated with vitronectin in the extracellular matrix in culture [42]. Although no direct evidence has yet been reported, PAI-1 may also function to regulate fibrinolysis in the extracellular matrix in vivo.

PAI-1 STRUCTURE AND FUNCTION

The gene for human PAI-1 is located on chromosome 7 bands q21.3–22 [43]. It is 12.3 kb in length, composed of 9 exons and 8 introns [44], and encodes a protein of 402 amino acids that includes a typical secretion signal sequence [45]. The gene is highly regulated, with its synthesis and release in cell culture modulated by such agents as endotoxin, serum, transforming growth factor β, basic fibroblast growth factor, interleukin-1, tumor necrosis factor, thrombin, dexamethasone, hydrocortisone, and phorbol esters [36,46].

The PAI-1 protein is a single-chain glycoprotein with a molecular weight of 50 kd [18]. It is unique amongst the serpins in that it exists both in active and latent forms [47] (Figure 5-2). Although the precise mechanism of interaction between serpins and their proteases is controversial, active PAI-1 has been proposed to react with u-PA or t-PA by forming a 1:1 stoichiometric complex, followed by the formation of a covalent bond between the hydroxyl group of the reactive site serine of the protease and the carboxyl group of the P_1 residue at the reactive center of the serpin. This inhibitory function of the serpin is correlated with a conformation in which the reactive-site loop is exposed. On cleavage of PAI-1, the N-terminal end of the reactive center loop (approximately P_1–P_{14}) inserts as an antiparallel strand (s4A) into β-sheet A [48,49]. As with several other serpins, a distinct substrate form of PAI-1 has also been described [50]. While the latent form of PAI-1 does not interact with

plasminogen activators, the substrate form of PAI-1 is cleaved at the $P1$–$P1'$ position by its target proteinase without the formation of a stable stoichiometric complex.

Although controversial, it has been suggested that partial insertion of the reactive-center loop is a prerequisite for serpin inhibitory function, whereas complete insertion of the reactive-center loop leads to the latent form. In support of this theory, synthetic tetradecapeptides corresponding to the reactive-site loops of the serpins antithrombin III [51], α_1-antitrypsin [52], and PAI-1 [53] have been demonstrated to inhibit the activity of serpins toward their cognate protease, presumably by preventing the partial insertion of the native reactive-center loop into the cleft now occupied by the synthetic peptide. Other studies have suggested that partial insertion of the reactive-center loop does not occur prior to interaction with a serpin [54]. The reactive-center loop of PAI-1 may be particularly flexible, accounting for its rapid kinetics of interaction with plasminogen activators and its latent form.

To further support this view of a mobile reactive-center loop determining the functional state of PAI-1, mutant PAI-1 molecules have been engineered to either prevent or reduce the rate of loop insertion into β-sheet A. Mutants that slow the rate of loop insertion lead to an increase in the PAI-1 half-life [55]. A random mutation strategy has produced PAI-1 variants with an even greater prolongation of the PAI-1

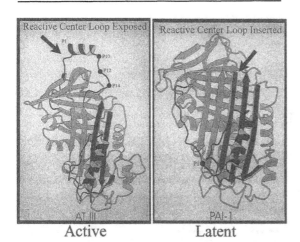

Active   Latent

FIGURE 5-2. Ribbon backbone conformations of the serpins antithrombin III (AT III) and latent PAI-1. The residues corresponding to the reactive-center loop from P_{14} to P_1 are marked by an arrow. The active serpin conformation is demonstrated for antithrombin III, with the reactive-center loop exposed. The latent form of PAI-1 is demonstrated with the reactive-center P_{14}–P_1 residues fully inserted as the central strand in β sheet A. (Adapted from Stein and Carrell [131], with permission.)

half-life [56]. The location of these mutations indicates that other regions of the PAI-1 molecule also play an important role in determining the functional state of PAI-1. The characteristics of these mutations, in comparison with other serpin sequences, suggest that the decreased functional stability and unique latent form of PAI-1 may have resulted from positive evolutionary selection [56]. Although the biological significance of the latent PAI-1 conformation is currently unknown, the lability of the PAI-1 structure may provide a mechanism for sharply restricting the localization of PAI-1 activity.

PAI-1 is secreted by cells in an active conformation [57] but converts spontaneously to the thermodynamically more stable latent conformation [47]. The half-life of active free PAI-1 in solution is 60–90 minutes at 37°C [19], but when bound to vitronectin (kd = 0.3 nM) [58] the active form is stabilized and the half-life is prolonged to 120–180 minutes in solution [40] and to geater than 24 hours on extracellular matrix [42]. The stabilization of PAI-1 by vitronectin has been hypothesized to result from restriction of PAI-1 β-sheet A, thus interfering with the reactive-center loop insertion that is required for PAI-1 conversion to latency [59]. In addition to stabilizing

active PAI-1, vitronectin may act to decrease the rate of PAI-1 clearance from the plasma [60] and also alters the specificity of PAI-1 towards other proteases. Vitronectin-bound PAI-1 has a 270-fold greater second-order rate constant toward thrombin than free PAI-1 [61]. In addition, vitronectin has been shown to stimulate the inhibition of t-PA by PAI-1 [62,63]. PAI-1 also binds to fibrin (kd = 3.8 μM) [64], and when bound retains its capacity to inhibit t-PA and u-PA. Fibrin may serve to localize PAI-1 to sites of forming thrombi [65].

Most of the PAI-1 present in normal, fresh plasma is in the active conformation. Although >90% of the total PAI-1 antigen in blood is localized to the platelet [30,31], this platelet PAI-1 appears to be predominantly latent [30,31]. The physiological relevance of this large platelet PAI-1 pool remains unclear. Platelet PAI-1 may play an important role in thrombolysis resistance. Platelet-mediated resistance to the action of t-PA by a PAI-1–dependent mechanism has been demonstrated using in vitro clot lysis assays [66,67]. Whether or not latent PAI-1 secreted by platelets in the setting of an acute thrombus can be reactivated has not been demonstrated. However, the latent form of PAI-1 can be converted into the active form by treatment with denaturing agents, negatively charged phospholipids, or vitronectin [47,68,69], and evidence for the conversion of latent to active PAI-1 in vivo has been reported when latent PAI-1 was infused into rabbits [33]. Platelets contain significant amounts of vitronectin, suggesting the potential for an interaction between platelet PAI-1 and vitronectin.

CLINICAL SIGNIFICANCE

Genetic Abnormalities of PAI-1 Expression. Human subjects with partial and complete PAI-1 deficiency associated with excessive bleeding have been described [70–72]. In one of these cases, a 9-year-old Amish girl with a moderate bleeding disorder was found to have complete absence of PAI-1 in plasma and platelets [72]. The patient was shown to be homozygous for a two base-pair insertion at the end of exon 4 of the PAI-1 gene. This defect results in a frameshift, leading to an unstable mRNA product and a nonfunctional truncated PAI-1 protein (Figure 5-3A). The deficiency is inherited as an autosomal recessive disorder. Although heterozygous parents and siblings all had plasma PAI-1 activity in the normal range, they were consistently decreased compared with homozygous normal family members (Figure 5-3B).

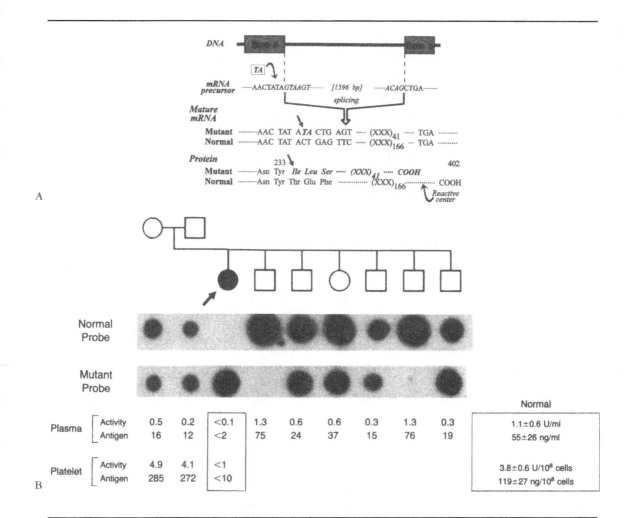

FIGURE 5-3. **A**: TA insertion leading to frameshift and unstable, truncated mRNA. No PAI-1 protein was detected in the patient homozygous for this mutation. **B**: Family pedigree of the PAI-1–deficient patient with the proband indicated by an arrow. Analysis of allele-specific oligonucleotide hybridization of amplified DNA from exon 4 of each individual is shown beneath the pedigree. The proband is homozygous for the TA insertion mutation. The parents and four siblings are heterozygous for the mutation, whereas two siblings are homozygous for the normal sequence. Levels of PAI-1 from plasma or platelets are shown below each individual. (Reprinted from Fay et al. [72], with permission.)

The correlation of complete PAI-1 deficiency with abnormal bleeding clearly demonstrates that PAI-1 is critical for the regulation of hemostasis. Although PAI-1–deficient mice generated by homologous recombination in embryonic stem cells demonstrate enhanced fibrinolytic capacity, significant hemorrhage was not observed [73]. However, it is difficult to compare the hemostatic challenges experienced by human PAI-1–deficient subjects with those used to study this PAI-1–deficient mouse model, and the apparent difference in bleeding tendency may not be significant. Mice with targeted deletions of other components of the PA system have confirmed a critical role of the PA system in fibrin clearance because mice deficient in plasminogen or both plasminogen activators (u-PA and t-PA) exhibit extensive fibrin deposition in multiple tissues [74,75].

Polymorphisms at the PAI-1 genetic locus have been associated with variations in plasma PAI-1 levels. A guanosine insertion/deletion polymorphism was identified 675 base pairs upstream from the start of transcription of the PAI-1 gene, where one allele has a sequence of four guanosines (4G) and the other has five guanosines (5G). Both alleles were shown to bind a putative transcriptional activator, whereas the 5G allele also appears to bind a repressor protein at an overlapping binding site. In vitro assays of promoter activity demonstrated that under conditions of cytokine stimulation, such as are found in the acute phase, the 4G allele had significantly higher activity than the 5G allele [76]. The 4G allele is also associated with higher plasma PAI-1 activity [77]. The prevalence of the 4G allele in one study was significantly higher in patients with myocardial infarction under the age of 45 than in population-based controls [77]. The role of the 4G allele in the predisposition to thrombosis is controversial. Another study (ECTIM) did not find the 4G/5G polymorphism to be a genetic risk factor for myocardial infarction, although it was associated with variations in plasma PAI-1 levels [78].

Vascular Thrombosis. While PAI-1 deficiency is associated with abnormal bleeding, increased levels of PAI-1 in the circulation may be associated with thrombotic disease, including deep venous thrombosis and myocardial infarction [79–84]. Not all studies have demonstrated a positive correlation between plasma PAI-1 and thrombotic events [85]. The conflicting results may reflect the marked variation of PAI-1 levels both between and within individuals, as well as varying methods of sample collection and analysis. In addition, plasma levels of PAI-1 may fail to reflect the potentially potent local effect of PAI-1 in thrombotic processes.

Animal studies have supported a causal role of PAI-1 in thrombotic disease states. In a rabbit model of jugular venous thrombosis, administration of a PAI-1–neutralizing monoclonal antibody enhanced endogenous lysis of thrombus and reduced thrombus growth [67,86]. In addition, PAI-1–deficient mice are able to lyse fibrin thrombi embolized to the lung faster than wild-type littermates and are resistant to the formation of venous thrombosis following footpad endotoxin injection [73]. Conversely, mice that overexpress human PAI-1 experience venous thrombosis [87].

Resistance to Thrombolysis. In acute thrombosis, PAI-1 may contribute to the suboptimal rate of reperfusion observed in patients presenting with acute myocardial infarction who are treated with t-PA. Only 50% of patients presenting with acute myocardial infarction (MI) experience successful reperfusion defined as normal or TIMI grade 3 flow, even though the vast majority of patients with acute

MI are known to have acute thrombus present [88]. This resistance to thrombolysis may be mediated by several factors, including clot retraction [89] and high local concentrations of α_2-antiplasmin [90] or PAI-1 [34]. Evidence favoring PAI-1 as a significant contributor to t-PA resistance was provided in a canine coronary arterial thrombus model [86]. In this model, administration of a PAI-1–neutralizing monoclonal antibody in combination with t-PA significantly reduced time to reperfusion and delayed the occurrence of reocclusion.

In a porcine acute coronary thrombosis model, analysis of extracts derived from acute platelet-rich thrombi has revealed a total PAI-1 antigen concentration of aproximately 100 μg/mL with the active PAI-1 component measuring 30 μg/mL, suggesting the potential of a potent local PAI-1 effect [91]. As plasma concentrations of t-PA reach approximately 1 μg/mL following a therapeutic dose, a local active PAI-1 concentration of approximately 1 μg/mL at the site of thrombosis could neutralize the effect of t-PA on a platelet-rich thrombus. It is also possible that vascular cells at the site of arterial injury, either endothelial or subendothelial, secrete significant amounts of active PAI-1 into the forming thrombus, as has been demonstrated in vitro [92].

Human and animal studies have suggested that it is the platelet-rich *white thrombi* that are more resistant to the lytic effects of t-PA than are platelet-poor *red thrombi*, suggesting that the platelets may be the source of resistance [93]. Using a model that mimics the formation of arterial thrombi in vivo (the *Chandler loop*) and that can be manipulated in terms of rheological parameters and composition of blood cells, Stringer et al. have demonstrated that resistance toward t-PA–mediated thrombolysis parallels the presence of platelets that are fully activated in this system [94]. PAI-1 released by alpha granules was preferentially retained within the thrombus, and the concentration of PAI-1 antigen was higher in the platelet-rich head than the red blood cell–rich tail of the thrombus. Furthermore, the relative thrombolysis resistance of the heads of the Chandler thrombi was largely abolished with an anti–PAI-1 antibody.

Thus, it appears that PAI-1 plays an important role in the resistance of thrombi to lysis with t-PA and that the major source of the PAI-1 in arterial thrombi is the platelet. To further address the clinical relevance of PAI-1 as a contributing factor to t-PA resistance, a human clinical trial is currently underway comparing the efficacy of standard recombinant t-PA versus a mutant form of t-PA that has resistance to PAI-1 inhibition as one of its properties.

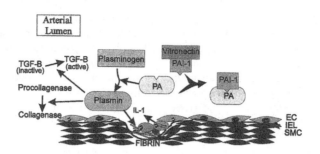

Atherosclerosis. In addition to associations of elevated PAI-1 in young survivors of MI [80] and recurrent myocardial infarction [95], elevations of PAI-1 have also been associated with atherosclerotic burden, and markedly increased PAI-1 expression is found at the site of atherosclerotic plaque [38]. Whether PAI-1 plays a causal role in this chronic disease process or is merely a marker of damaged endothelium remains to be established. Preliminary studies with a novel PAI-1 inhibitor, nicanartine [96], favor a causal role of PAI-1 in atherosclerosis. In rabbits with aortic atherosclerosis induced by hypercholesterolemia and implantation of indwelling plastic tubing, oral administration of nicanartine for 8 weeks attenuated the increase in plasma PAI-1 activity induced by vascular injury, reduced aortic PAI-1 mRNA expression, and inhibited the development of atherosclerotic lesions without affecting the lipid profile. As a regulator of fibrinolysis, PAI-1 may affect the development of atherosclerosis by determining the rate of local fibrin clearance (Figure 5-4).

In addition to the space fibrin occupies as a component of atherothrombi, local deposition of fibrin may serve as a scaffold upon which monocyte/macrophages invade, in addition to inducing the elaboration of inflammatory cytokines by monocyte/macrophages [97]. Fibrin deposition may also cause endothelial dysfunction and may facilitate the migration of vascular smooth muscle cells [98,99]. In addition to affecting fibrin clearance, PAI-1 may protect neovascularized tissue from excessive proteolysis [100] and affect the plasmin-mediated conversion of procollagenase to collagenase [101].

In support of alterations in plasminogen activation influencing human atherosclerosis, a high concentration of serum lipoprotein(a) is a risk factor for atherosclerosis, myocardial infarction, stroke, and restenosis [102]. Lipoprotein(a) consists of low-density lipoprotein with an additional protein compo-

FIGURE 5-4. The potential role of PAI-1 in the development of atherosclerotic lesions. Cross section of artery showing endothelial cells (EC), internal elastic lamina (IEL), and smooth muscle cells (SMC) with early atherosclerotic plaque characterized by a break in the endothelium, fibrin deposition, and the infiltration of monocyte/macrophages (foam cell precursors). Increased expression of PAI-1 could limit the local plasmin concentration, which could decrease the plasmin-mediated activation of transforming growth factor-β (TGF-β) and conversion of procollagenase to collagenase. In addition, PAI-1 inhibition of fibrin clearance might lead to an increased atherothrombotic component of atherosclerotic plaque as well as more scaffolding for cell migration and induction of proinflammatory cytokines (i.e., IL-1) from monocytes.

nent, apoliprotein (a), which is a plasminogen homologue and appears to inhibit plasminogen activation [103]. Transgenic mice that overexpress only the apoliprotein (a) component of lipoprotein (a) develop vascular lesions, when fed a high-fat diet, that are similar to the fatty streak lesions seen in early human atherosclerosis [102]. Immunofluorescence labeling of apoliprotein (a) in aortic sections from these

FIGURE 5-5. **A**: Effect of intracheal bleomycin on the development of pulmonary fibrosis in wild-type mice and PAI-1–overexpressing littermates. Lung tissue from mice that overexpressed PAI-1 exhibited greater fibrin deposition as assessed with an anti-murine fibrinogen antibody (arrows indicate material staining positive for fibrin/fibrinogen) and greater fibrosis as assessed by Masson trichrome staining and quantitative hydroxyproline analysis. **B**: Effect of intracheal bleomycin on the development of pulmonary fibrosis in wild-type mice and PAI-1–deficient littermates. Lung tissue from mice that lacked the gene for PAI-1 exhibited less fibrin deposition and less fibrosis as assessed by Masson trichrome staining and quantitative hydroxyproline analysis. (Adapted from Eitzman et al. [117], with permission.)

Wild-type

anti-Fibrin   Trichrome

PAI-1 Overexpression

anti-Fibrin   Trichrome

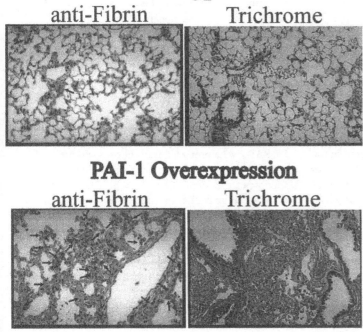

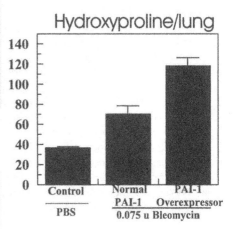

Hydroxyproline/lung

Wild-type

anti-Fibrin   Trichrome

PAI-1 Deficiency

anti-Fibrin   Trichrome

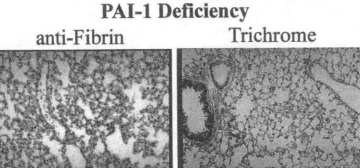

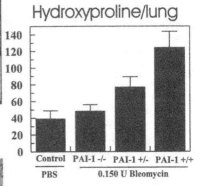

Hydroxyproline/lung

B

transgenic mice shows foci of apoliprotein (a) accumulation near the luminal surface and lesser amounts in the media [102].

The inhibition of plasminogen activation by apoliprotein (a) may contribute to the development of atherosclerosis by inhibiting fibrinolysis or by influencing the activity of TGF-β. Studies of human vascular smooth muscle cells in culture have demonstrated that by inhibiting plasminogen activation, apoliprotein (a) promotes smooth muscle cell proliferation and migration by suppressing the activation of TGF-β [104]. It has also been shown that the activation of TGF-β is inhibited in vivo in the aortic wall and serum of mice expressing apolipoprotein (a), as a consequence of apolipoprotein (a) inhibition of plasminogen activation, effects correlated with vascular smooth muscle cell activation [105]. Thus, there exist several mechanisms by which PAI-1, as a regulator of the plasminogen activation system, may influence the development of atherosclerotic lesions.

Other Disease States

PULMONARY FIBROSIS. PAI-1 also appears to play an important role in other disorders in which fibrin clearance is believed to influence the outcome. In pulmonary fibrosis, plasmin may limit scar formation by dismantling the provisional fibrin matrix on which fibroblasts invade and secrete interstitial collagens. During many acute and chronic inflammatory lung disorders, fibrin accumulates in lung tissue [106, 107]. The fibrinolytic activity in bronchoalveolar lavage fluid from patients with adult respiratory distress syndrome (ARDS) [106,108], idiopathic pulmonary fibrosis [109], sarcoidosis [110], and bronchopulmonary dysplasia [111] has been found to be suppressed. All of these diseases have been associated with the development of pulmonary fibrosis.

PAI-1 has been found to be elevated in BAL fluid from patients with ARDS and has been shown to reduce the fibrinolytic capacity of the fluid [106,108]. Bleomycin administration to animals has been widely used to study the pathogenesis of pulmonary fibrosis [112–115]. When instilled intratracheally into mice, bleomycin causes a pneumonitis that progresses to fibrosis in a dose-dependent manner, with increased collagen content occurring as early as 2 weeks after instillation [113]. Bleomycin treatment suppresses the fibrinolytic activity of BAL fluid in a pattern similar to that seen in human inflammatory lung diseases [112,115]. In mice, Olman et al. have demonstrated that PAI-1 is upregulated following bleomycin administration and that PAI-1 expression

localizes to areas of fibrin-rich fibroproliferative lesions [116].

To determine whether a cause and effect relationship exists between PAI-1 expression and the development of pulmonary fibrosis, intratracheal bleomycin was administered to transgenic mice that either overexpress or are completely deficient in PAI-1 [117]. The results of this study demonstrated a strong relationship between PAI-1 gene dose and the degree of pulmonary fibrosis that follows bleomycin administration. In particular, PAI-1–overexpressing mice experienced greater fibrosis than wild-type mice (Figure 5-5A), whereas mice homozygous deficient for PAI-1 were protected from fibrosis (Figure 5-5B), with heterozygotes showing an intermediate effect. In support of the role of fibrin as a provisional matrix, there was a direct relationship between the amount of fibrin immunostaining, the PAI-1 gene dose, and the degree of collagen deposition, as quantitated by measurement of hydroxyproline. These findings suggest that alterations in the fibrinolytic environment of the alveolar space during inflammatory injury influence the subsequent development of pulmonary fibrosis and that therapeutic interventions designed to enhance fibrinolysis, such as administration of either plasminogen activators or inhibitors of PAI-1, may limit the development of pulmonary fibrosis that occurs as a consequence of acute or chronic inflammatory diseases.

HEMOLYTIC UREMIC SYNDROME. Another disease process characterized by fibrin deposition and subsequent fibrosis is the hemolytic uremic syndrome. Human subjects with this disease experience glomerular fibrin deposition, and end-stage renal failure is not uncommon. A recent human clinical study suggests that PAI-1 is the circulating inhibitor of fibrinolysis in this syndrome and that the duration of elevated PAI-1 activity is strongly correlated with the outcome of the disease. Furthermore, normalization of plasma PAI-1 levels (i.e., by peritoneal dialysis) was correlated with improvement in renal function [118]. Consistent with this human data, elevated PAI-1 expression has also been demonstrated in a model of murine lupus nephritis [119].

METASTATIC MELANOMA. The plasminogen activation system has also been proposed to play an important role in tumor invasion and metastasis. Urokinase is expressed at high levels by a variety of tumors [5,120–122] and is considered critical for the phenotype of metastasizing cells [123–128]. Blockade of the cell surface–associated u-PA in murine B16 melanoma cells with antibodies has been shown to significantly decrease the number of pulmonary metastases after intravenous injection of these cells into mice [121]. Therefore, PAI-1 as a regulator of u-PA activity has been proposed to affect the growth and metastatic potential of this melanoma cell line. To examine the role of host PAI-1 in tumor invasion and metastasis, genetically altered mice that overexpress murine PAI-1 or lack PAI were analyzed in a mouse metastatic melanoma model [129]. In this model, wide variations of host PAI-1 did not significantly affect primary tumor size, metastases, or survival.

Future Directions

Plasminogen activation has been postulated to play a major role in a diverse group of biololgical processes, and PAI-1 many function as a central regulator in many of these systems. The observation of a significant hemorrhagic diathesis in a patient with complete PAI-1 deficiency demonstrates the critical role for PAI-1 in the regulation of vascular fibrinolysis in vivo. The functions of other known PAIs in vivo are currently unknown. With the recent introduction of transgenic mouse technology, many strains of mice with targeted disruptions of genes involved in fibrinolysis have been generated and have provided new insights into the role of plasminogen activation in vivo. Analysis of these powerful animal models should provide further insight into the role of plasminogen activation in diverse disease processes. The development of new pharmacologic inhibitors of PAI-1 may provide novel approaches to therapy for many of these disease processes.

References

1. Francis CW, Marder VJ. Physiologic regulation and pathologic disorders of fibrinolysis. In Colman RW, Hirsh J, Marder VJ, Salzman EW (eds). Hemostasis and Thrombosis. Basic Principles and Clinical Practice, Philadelphia: JB Lippincott, 1987:358.
2. Bachmann F. Fibrinolysis. In Verstraete M, Vermylen J, Lijnen HR, Arnout J (eds). Thrombosis and Haemostasis. Leuven, Belgium: Leuven University Press, 1987:227.
3. Hsueh AJW, Liu YX, Cajander SB, Ny T. Molecular mechanisms in the hormone regulation of plasminogen activator activity in ovarian granulosa cells and cumulus–oocyte complexes. In Haseltine FP, First NL (eds). Meiotic Inhibition: Molecular Control of Meiosis. New York: Liss, 1988:227.
4. Pöllänen J, Stephens RW, Vaheri A. Directed plasminogen activation at the surface of normal and malignant cells. Adv Cancer Res 57:273, 1991.
5. Dano K, Andreasen PA, Grondahl-Hansen J, Kristensen P, Nielsen LS, Skriver L. Plasminogen

6. Moscatelli D, Rifkin DB. Membrane and matrix localization of proteinases: A common theme in tumor cell invasion and angiogenesis. Biochim Biophys Acta 948:67, 1988.
7. Saksela O, Rifkin DB. Cell-associated plasminogen activation: Regulation and physiological functions. Annu Rev Cell Biol 4:93, 1988.
8. Hoylaerts M, Rijken DC, Lijnen HR, Collen D. Kinetics of the activation of plasminogen by human tissue plasminogen activator. J Biol Chem 257:2912, 1982.
9. Ellis V, Dano K. Plasminogen activation by receptor-bound urokinase. Semin Thromb Hemost 17:194, 1991.
10. Hajjar KA, Hamel NM. Identification and characterization of human endothelial cell membrane binding sites for tissue plaminogen activator and urokinase. J Biol Chem 265:2908, 1990.
11. Plow EF, Felez J, Miles LA. Cellular regulation of fibrinolysis. Thromb Haemost 66:32, 1991.
12. Kruithof EKO. Plasminogen activator inhibitors — a review. Enzyme 40:113, 1988.
13. Hart DA, Rehemtulla A. Plasminogen activators and their inhibitors: Regulators of extracellular proteolysis and cell function. Comp Biochem Physiol [B] 90B:691, 1988.
14. Aoki N. Hemostasis associated with abnormalities of fibrinolysis. Blood Rev 3:11, 1989.
15. Astedt B, Lecander I, Ny T. The placental type plasminogen activator PAI-2. Fibrinolysis 1:203, 1987.
16. Meijers JC, Chung DW. Organization of the gene coding for human protein C inhibitor (plasminogen activator inhibitor-3). Assignment of the gene to chromosome 14. J Biol Chem 266:15028, 1991.
17. Scott RW, Bergman BL, Bajpai A, Hersh RT, Rodriguez H, Jones BN, Barreda C, Watts S, Baker JB. Protease nexin. Properties and a modified purification procedure. J Biol Chem 260:7029, 1985.
18. van Mourik JA, Lawrence DA, Loskutoff DJ. Purification of an inhibitor plasminogen activator (antiactivator) synthesized by endothelial cells. J Biol Chem 259:14914, 1984.
19. Lawrence D, Strandberg L, Grundström T, Ny T. Purification of active human plasminogen activator inhibitor 1 from Escherichia coli. Comparison with natural and recombinant forms purified from eucaryotic cells. Eur J Biochem 186:523, 1989.
20. Boswell DR, Carrell RW. Genetic engineering and the SERPINs. Bioessays 8:83, 1988.
21. Huber R, Carrell RW. Implications of the three-dimensional structure of alpha 1-antitrypsin for structure and function of serpins. Biochemistry 28:8951, 1989.
22. Carrell R, Travis J. a_1-Antitrypsin and the serpins: Variation and countervariation. Trends Biochem Sci 10:20, 1985.

activators, tissue degradation, and cancer. Adv Cancer Res 44:139, 1985.

23. Doolittle RF. Angiotensinogen is related to the antitrypsin-antithrombin-ovalbumin family. Science 222:417, 1983.

24. Hunt LT, Dayhoff MO. A surprising new protein superfamily containing ovalbumin, antithrombin III, and alphal-proteinase inhibitor. Biochem Biophys Res Commun 95:864, 1980.

25. Hekman CM, Loskutoff DJ. Bovine plasminogen activator inhibitor 1: Specificity determinations and comparison of the active, latent, and guanidine-activated forms. Biochemistry 27:2911, 1988.

26. Sakata Y, Curriden S, Lawrence D, Griffin JH, Loskutoff DJ. Activated protein C stimulates the fibrinolytic activity of cultured endothelial cells and decreases antiactivator activity. Proc Natl Acad Sci USA 82:1121, 1985.

27. Sakata Y, Loskutoff DJ, Gladson CL, Hekman CM, Griffin JH. Mechanism of protein C-dependent clot lysis: Role of plasminogen activator inhibitor. Blood 68:1218, 1986.

28. Fay WP, Owen WG. Platelet plasminogen activator inhibitor: Purification and characterization of interaction with plasminogen activators and activated protein C. Biochemistry 28:5773, 1989.

29. Ehrlich HJ, Gebbink RK, Keijer J, Linders M, Preissner KT, Pannekoek H. Alteration of serpin specificity by a protein cofactor. J Biol Chem 265:13029, 1990.

30. Declerck PJ, Verstreken M, Kruithof EKO, Juhan-Vague I, Collen D. Measurement of plasminogen activator inhibitor 1 in biologic fluids with a murine monoclonal antibody-based enzyme-linked immunoabsorbent assay. Blood 71:220, 1988.

31. Booth NA, Simpson AJ, Croll A, Bennett B, MacGregor IR. Plasminogen activator inhibitor (PAI-1) in plasma and platelets. Br J Haematol 70:327, 1988.

32. Colucci M, Páramo JA, Collen D. Generation in plasma of a fast-acting inhibitor of plasminogen activator in response to endotoxin stimulation. J Clin Invest 75:818, 1985.

33. Vaughan DE, Declerck PJ, Van Houtte E, De Mol M, Collen D. Studies of recombinant plasminogen activator inhibitor-1 in rabbits. Pharmacokinetics and evidence for reactivation of latent plasminogen activator inhibitor-1 in vivo. Circ Res 67:1281, 1990.

34. Erickson LA, Ginsberg MH, Loskutoff DJ. Detection and partial characterization of an inhibitor of plasminogen activator in human platelets. J Clin Invest 74:1465, 1984.

35. Sawdey MS, Loskutoff DJ. Regulation of murine type 1 plasminogen activator inhibitor gene expression in vivo. Tissue specificity and induction by lipopolysaccharide, tumor necrosis factor-a, and transforming growth factor-b. J Clin Invest 88:1346, 1991.

36. Krishnamurti C, Alving BM. Plasminogen activator inhibitor type 1: Biochemistry and evidence for modulation of fibrinolysis in vivo. Semin Thromb Hemost 18:67, 1992.

37. Pyke C, Kristensen P, Ralfkiaer E, Eriksen J, Dano K. The plasminogen activation system in human colon cancer: Messenger RNA for the inhibitor PAI-1 is located in endothelial cells in the tumor stroma. Cancer Res 51:4067, 1991.

38. Schneiderman J, Sawdey MS, Keeton MR, Bordin GM, Bernstein EF, Dilley RB, Loskutoff DJ. Increased type 1 plasminogen activator inhibitor gene expression in atherosclerotic human arteries. Proc Natl Acad Sci USA 89:6998, 1992.

39. Keeton M, Eguchi Y, Sawdey M, Ahn C, Loskutoff DJ. Cellular localization of type 1 plasminogen activator inhibitor messenger RNA and protein in murine renal tissue. Am J Pathol 142:59, 1993.

40. Declerck PJ, De Mol M, Alessi MC, Baudner S, Pâques E-P, Preissner KT, Müller-Berghaus G, Collen D. Purification and characterization of a plasminogen activator inhibitor 1 binding protein from human plasma. J Biol Chem 263:15454, 1988.

41. Wiman B, Almquist Å, Sigurdardottir O, Lindahl T. Plasminogen activator inhibitor 1 (PAI) is bound to vitronectin in plasma. FEBS Lett 242:125, 1988.

42. Mimuro J, Schleef RR, Loskutoff DJ. Extracellular matrix of cultured bovine aortic endothelial cells contains functionally active type I plasminogen activator inhibitor. Blood 70:721, 1987.

43. Klinger KW, Winqvist R, Riccio A, Andreasen PA, Sartorio R, Nielsen LS, Stuart N, Stanislovitis P, Watkins P, Douglas R, Grzeschik K-H, Alitalo K, Blasi F, Dano K. Plasminogen activator inhibitor type 1 gene is located at region q21.3–q22 of chromosome 7 and genetically linked with cystic fibrosis. Proc Natl Acad Sci USA 84:8548, 1987.

44. Loskutoff DJ, Linders M, Keijer J, Veerman H, van Heerikhuizen H, Pannekoek H. Structure of the human plasminogen activator inhibitor 1 gene: Nonrandom distribution of introns. Biochemistry 26:3763, 1987.

45. Ginsburg D, Zeheb R, Yang AY, Rafferty UM, Andreasen PA, Nielsen L, Dano K, Lebo RV, Gelehrter TD. cDNA cloning of human plasminogen activator-inhibitor from endothelial cells. J Clin Invest 78:1673, 1986.

46. Loskutoff DJ, Sawdey M, Mimuro J. Type 1 plasminogen activator inhibitor. Prog Hemost Thromb 9:87, 1989.

47. Hekman CM, Loskutoff DJ. Endothelial cells produce a latent inhibitor of plasminogen activators that can be activated by denaturants. J Biol Chem 260:11581, 1985.

48. Stein P, Chothia C. Serpin tertiary structure transformation. Mol Biol 221:615, 1991.

49. Loebermann H, Tokuoka R, Deisenhofer J, Huber R. Human a₁-proteinase inhibitor. Crystal structure analysis of two crystal modifications, molecular model and preliminary analysis of the implications for function. J Mol Biol 177:531, 1984.

50. Declerck PJ, De Mol M, Vaughan DE, Collen D. Identification of a conformationally distinct form of

plasminogen activtor inhibitor-1, acting as a non-inhibitory substrate for tissue-type plasminogen activator. J Biol Chem 267:11693, 1992.

51. Björk I, Ylinenjärvi K, Olson ST, Bock PE. Conversion of antithrombin from an inhibitor of thrombin to a substrate with reduced heparin affinity and enhanced conformational stability by binding of a tetradecapeptide corresponding to the P_1 to P_{14} region of the putative reactive bond loop of the inhibitor. J Biol Chem 267:1976, 1992.

52. Schulze AJ, Baumann U, Knof S, Jaeger E, Huber R, Laurell C. Structural transition of a_1-antitrypsin by a peptide sequentially similar to b-strand s4A. Eur J Biochem 194:51, 1990.

53. Eitzman DT, Fay WP, Lawrence DA, Francis-Chmura AM, Shore JD, Olson ST, Ginsburg D. Peptide-mediated inactivation of recombinant and platelet plasminogen activator inhibitor-1 in vitro. J Clin Invest 95:2416, 1995.

54. Lawrence DA, Ginsburg D, Day DE, Berkenpas MB, Verhamme IM, Kvassman J-O, Shore JD. Serpin-protease complexes are trapped as stable acyl-enzyme intermediates. J Biol Chem 270:25309, 1995.

55. Sherman PM, Lawrence D, Paielli D, Olson S, Shore JD, Ginsburg D. Structure-function analysis of the plasminogen activator inhibitor-1 reactive center by site-directed mutagenesis (abstr). Fibrinolysis 4:267, 1990.

56. Berkenpas MB, Lawrence DA, Ginsburg D. Molecular evolution of plasminogen activator inhibitor-1 functional stability. EMBO J 14:2969, 1995.

57. Levin EG, Santell L. Conversion of the active to latent plasminogen activator inhibitor from human endothelial cells. Blood 70:1090, 1987.

58. Seiffert D, Loskutoff DJ. Kinetic analysis of the interaction between type 1 plasminogen activator inhibitor and vitronectin and evidence that the bovine inhibitor binds to a thrombin-derived amino-terminal fragment of bovine vitronectin. Biochim Biophys Acta 1078:23, 1991.

59. Lawrence DA, Berkenpas MB, Palaniappan S, Ginsburg D. Localization of vitronectin binding domain in plasminogen activator inhibitor-1. J Biol Chem 269:15223, 1994.

60. Zheng X, Saunders TL, Camper SA, Samuelson LC, Ginsburg D. Vitronectin is not essential for normal mammalian development and fertility. Proc Natl Acad Sci USA 92:12426, 1995.

61. Naski MC, Lawrence DA, Mosher DF, Podor TJ, Ginsburg D. Kinetics of inactivation of a-thrombin by plasminogen activator inhibitor-1. J Biol Chem 268:12367, 1993.

62. Keijer J, Linders M, Wegman JJ, Ehrlich HJ, Mertens K, Pannekoek H. On the target specificity of plasminogen activator inhibitor 1: The role of heparin, vitronectin, and the reactive site. Blood 78:1254, 1991.

63. Edelberg JM, Reilly CF, Pizzo SV. The inhibition of tissue type plasminogen activator by plasmi-

nogen activator inhibitor-1. J Biol Chem 266:7488, 1991.

64. Keijer J, Linders M, van Zonneveld A-J, Ehrlich HJ, de Boer J-P, Pannekoek H. The interaction of plasminogen activator inhibitor 1 with plasminogen activators (tissue-type and urokinase-type) and fibrin: Localization of interaction sites and physiologic relevance. Blood 78:401, 1991.

65. Stringer HAR, Pannekoek H. The significance of fibrin binding by plasminogen activator inhibitor 1 for the mechanism of tissue-type plasminogen activator-mediated fibrinolysis. J Biol Chem 270:11205, 1995.

66. Fay WP, Eitzman DT, Shaprio AD, Madison EL, Ginsburg D. Platelets inhibit fibrinolysis in vitro by both plasminogen activator inhibitor-1 dependent and independent mechanisms. Blood 83:351, 1994.

67. Levi M, Biemond BJ, van Zonneveld A-J, Wouter Ten Cate J, Pannekoek H. Inhibition of plasminogen activator inhibitor-1 activity results in promotion of endogenous thrombolysis and inhibition of thrombus extension in models of experimental thrombosis. Circulation 85:305, 1992.

68. Lambers JW, Cammenga M, Konig BW, Mertens K, Pannekoek H, van Mourik JA. Activation of human endothelial cell-type plasminogen activator inhibitor (PAI-1) by negatively charged phospholipids. J Biol Chem 262:17492, 1987.

69. Wun T-C, Palmier MO, Siegel NR, Smith CE. Affinity purification of active plasminogen activator inhibitor-1 (PAI-1) using immobilized anhydrourokinase. J Biol Chem 264:7862, 1989.

70. Schleef RR, Higgins DL, Pillemer E, Levitt LJ. Bleeding diathesis due to decreased functional activity of Type 1 plasminogen activator inhibitor. J Clin Invest 83:1747, 1989.

71. Diéval J, Nguyen G, Gross S, Delobel J, Kruithof EKO. A lifelong bleeding disorder associated with a deficiency of plasminogen activator inhibitor type I. Blood 77:528, 1991.

72. Fay WP, Shapiro AD, Shih JL, Schleef RR, Ginsburg D. Complete deficiency of plasminogen-activator inhibitor type 1 due to a frame-shift mutation. N Engl J Med 327:1729, 1992.

73. Carmeliet P, Stassen JM, Schoonjans L, Ream B, van den Oord JJ, De Mol M, Mulligan RC, Collen D. Plasminogen activator inhibitor-1 gene-deficient mice. II. Effects on hemostasis, thrombosis, and thrombolysis. J Clin Invest 92:2756, 1993.

74. Carmeliet P, Schoonjans L, Kieckens L, Ream B, Degen JL, Bronson R, De Vos R, van den Oord JJ, Collen D, Mulligan RC. Physiological consequences of loss of plasminogen activator gene function in mice. Nature 368:419, 1994.

75. Ploplis VA, Carmeliet P, Vazirzadeh S, Van Vlaenderen I, Moons L, Plow EF, Colleen D. Effects of disruption of the plasminogen gene on thrombosis, growth, and health in mice. Circulation 92:2585, 1995.

76. Dawson SJ, Wiman B, Hamsten A, Geen F, Humphries S, Henney AM. The two allele sequences of a common polymorphism in the promoter of the plasminogen activator inhibitor-1 (PAI-1) gene respond differently to interleukin-1 in HepG2 cells. J Biol Chem 268:10739, 1993.

77. Eriksson P, Kallin B, Van't Hooft FM, Båvenholm P, Hamsten A. Allele-specific increase in basal transcription of the plasminogen-activator inhibitor 1 gene is associated with myocardial infarction. Proc Natl Acad Sci USA 92:1851, 1995.

78. Ye S, Green FR, Scarabin PY, Nicaud V, Bara L, Dawson SJ, Humphries SE, Evans A, Luc G, Cambou JP, Arveiler D, Henney AM, Cambien F. The 4G/5G genetic polymorphism in the promoter of the plasminogen activator inhibitor-1 (PAI-1) gene is associated with differences in plasma PAI-1 activity but not with risk of myocardial infarction in the ECTIM study. Thromb Haemost 74:837, 1995.

79. Vague-Juhan I, Moerman B, DeCock F, Aillaud MF, Collen D. Plasma levels of a specific inhibitor of tissue-type plasminogen activator (and urokinase) in normal and pathological conditions. Thromb Res 33:523, 1984.

80. Hamsten A, Wiman B, de Faire U, Blombäck M. Increased plasma levels of a rapid inhibitor of tissue plasminogen activator in young survivors of myocardial infarction. N Engl J Med 313:1557, 1985.

81. Wiman B, Ljungberg B, Chmielewska J, Urden G, Blombäck M, Johnsson H. The role of the fibrinolytic system in deep vein thrombosis. J Lab Clin Med 105:265, 1985.

82. Paramo JA, Colucci M, Collen D, van de Werf F. Plasminogen activator inhibitor in the blood of patients with coronary artery disease. Br Med J (Clin Res Ed) 291:573, 1985.

83. Aznar J, Estelles A, Tormo G, Sapena P, Tormo V, Blanch S, Espana F. Plasminogen activator inhibitor activity and other fibrinolytic variables in patients with coronary artery disease. Br Heart J 59:535, 1988.

84. Angles-Cano E, Gris JC, Loyau S, Schved JF. Familial association of high levels of histidine-rich glycoprotein and plasminogen activator inhibitor-1 with venous thromboembolism. J Lab Clin Med 121:646, 1993.

85. Ridker PM, Vaughan DE, Stampfer MJ, Manson JE, Shen C, Newcomer LM, Goldhaber SZ, Hennekens CH. Baseline fibrinolytic state and the risk of future venous thrombosis: A prospective study of endogenous tissue-type plasminogen activator and plasminogen activator inhibitor. Circulation 85:1822, 1992.

86. Biemond BJ, Levi M, Coronel R, Janse MJ, ten Cate JW, Pannekoek H. Thrombolysis and reocclusion in experimental jugular vein and coronary artery thrombosis: Effects of a plasminogen activator inhibitor type 1-neutralizing monoclonal antibody. Circulation 91:1175, 1995.

87. Erickson LA, Fici GJ, Lund JE, Polites HG, Marotti KR. Transgenic mice expressing plasminogen activator inhibitor-1 develop thrombotic vascular occlusions (abstr). Unknown 583a, 1989.

88. Lincoff AM, Topol EJ. Illusion of reperfusion. Does anyone achieve optimal reperfusion during acute myocardial infarction? Circulation 88:1361, 1993.

89. Kunitada S, Fitzgerald GA, Fitzgerald DJ. Inhibition of clot lysis and decreased binding of tissue-type plasminogen activator as a consequence of clot retraction. Blood 79:1420, 1992.

90. Robbie LA, Booth NA, Croll AM, Bennett B. The roles of a$_2$-antiplasmin and plasminogen activator inhibitor 1 (PAI-1) in the inhibition of clot lysis. Thromb Haemost 70:301, 1993.

91. McEver RP. Selectins: Novel receptors that mediate leukocyte adhesion during inflammation. Thromb Haemost 65:223, 1991.

92. Handt S, Jerome WG, Braaten JV, Lewis JC, Kirkpatrick CJ, Hantgan RR. PAI-1 released from cultured human endothelial cells delays fibrinolysis and is incorporated into the developing fibrin clot. Fibrinolysis 8:104, 1994.

93. Jang I-K, Gold HK, Ziskind AA, Fallon JT, Holt RE, Leinbach RC, May JW, Collen D. Differential sensitivity of erythrocyte-rich and platelet-rich arterial thrombi to lysis with recombinant tissue-type plasminogen activator. Circulation 79:920, 1989.

94. Stringer HAR, Van Swieten P, Heijnen HFG, Sixma JJ, Pannekoek H. Plasminogen activator inhibitor-1 released from activated platelets plays a key role in thrombolysis resistance: Studies with thrombi generated in the Chandler loop. Arterioscler Thromb 14:1452, 1994.

95. Hamsten A, de Faire U, Walldius G, Dahlen G, Szamosi A, Landou C, Blombäck M, Wiman B. Plasminogen activator inhibitor in plasma: Risk factor for recurrent myocardial infarction. Lancet 2:3, 1987.

96. Adamson IY, bowden DH. The pathogenesis of bleomycin-induced pulmonary fibrosis. Am J Pathol 77:185, 1974.

97. Perez RL, Roman J. Fibrin enhances the expression of IL-1b by human peripheral blood mononuclear cells. Implications in pulmonary inflammation. J Immunol 154:1879, 1995.

98. Schwartz CJ, Valente AJ, Kelley JL, Sprague EA, Edwards EH. Thrombosis and the development of atherosclerosis: Rokitansky revisited. Semin Thromb Hemost 14:189, 1988.

99. Thompson WD, Smith EB. Atherosclerosis and the coagulation system. J Pathol 159:97, 1989.

100. Bacharach E, Itin A, Keshet E. In vivo patterns of expression of urokinase and its inhibitor PAI-1 suggest a concerted role in regulating physiological angiogenesis. Proc Natl Acad Sci USA 89:10686, 1992.

101. Werb Z, Mainardi CL, Vater CA, Harris ED. Endogenous activation of latent collagenase by synovial

cells: Evidence for a role for plasminogen activator. N Engl J Med 296:1017, 1977.

102. Lawn RM, Wade DP, Hammer RE, Chiesa G, Verstuyft JG, Rubin EM. Atherogenesis in transgenic mice expressing human apolipoprotein (a). Nature 360:670, 1992.

103. Palabrica TM, Liu AC, Aronovitz MJ, Furie B, Lawn RM, Furie BC. Antifibrinolytic activity of apolipoprotein(a) in vivo: Human apolipoprotein(a) transgenic mice are resistant to tissue plasminogen activator-mediated thrombolysis. Nature Med 1:256, 1995.

104. Grainger DJ, Kirschenlohr HL, Metcalfe JC, Weissberg PL, Wade DP, Lawn RM. Proliferation of human smooth muscle cells promoted by lipoprotein(a). Science 260:1655, 1993.

105. Grainger DJ, Kemp PR, Liu AC, Lawn RM, Metcalfe JC. Activation of transforming growth factor-b is inhibited in transgenic apolipoprotien(a) mice. Nature 370:460, 1994.

106. Bertozzi P, Astedt B, Zenzius L, Lynch K, LeMaire F, Zapol W, Chapman HJ. Depressed bronchoalveolar urokinase activity in patients with adult respiratory distress syndrome. N Engl J Med 322:890, 1990.

107. Fukuda Y, Ishizaki M, Masuda Y, Kimura G, Kawanami O, Masugi Y. 5768. Am J Pathol 126:171, 1987.

108. Idell S, James KK, Levin EG, Schwartz BS, Manchanda N, Maunder RJ, Martin TR, McLarty J, Fair DS. Local abnormalities in coagulation and fibrinolytic pathways predispose to alveolar fibrin deposition in the adult respiratory distress syndrome. J Clin Invest 84:695, 1989.

109. Chapman HA, Allen CL, Stone OL. Abnormalities in pathways of alveolar fibrin turnover among ptients with interstitial lung disease. Am Rev Respir Dis 133:437, 1986.

110. Hasday JL, Bachwich PR, Lynch JP, Sitrin RG. Procoagulant and plasminogen activator activities of bronchoalveolar fluid in patients with pulmonary sarcoidosis. Exp Lung Res 14:261, 1988.

111. Viscardi RM, Broderick K, Sun CC, Yale LA, Hessamfar A, Taciak V, Burke KC, Koenig KB, Idell S. Disordered pathways of fibrin turnover in lung lavage of premature infants with respiratory distress syndrome. Am Rev Respir Dis 146:492, 1992.

112. Idell S, James KK, Gillies C, Fair DS, Thrall RS. Abnormalities of pathways of fibrin turnover in lung lavage of rats with oleic acid and bleomycin-induced lung injury support alveolar fibrin deposition. Am J Pathol 135:387, 1989.

113. Schrier DJ, Phan SH, McGarry BM. The effects of the nude (nu/nu) mutation of bleomycin-induced pulmonary fibrosis. A biochemical evaluation. Am Rev Respir Dis 127:614, 1983.

114. Idell S, Gonzales KK, MacArthur CK, Gillies C, Walsh PN, McLarty J, Thrall RS. Bronchoalveolar lavage procoagulant activity in bleomycin-induced lung injury in marmosets. Characterization and rela-

tionship to fibrin deposition and fibrosis. Am Rev Respir Dis 136:124, 1987.

115. Wuelfroth P, Okada H, Vinogradsky B, Bell SP, Fujii S. A novel inhibitor of plasminogen activator inhibitor-1 in vitro modulates development of atherosclerosis in vivo in rabbits (abstr). Circulation 92:I-303, 1995.

116. Olman MA, Mackman N, Gladson CL, Moser KM, Loskutoff DJ. Changes in procoagulant and fibrinolytic gene expression during bleomycin-induced lung injury in the mouse. J Clin Invest 96:1621, 1995.

117. Eitzman DT, McCoy RD, Zheng X, Fay WP, Shen T, Ginsburg D. Bleomycin-induced pulmonary fibrosis in transgenic mice that either lack or overexpress the murine plasminogen activator inhibitor-1 gene. J Clin Invest 97:232, 1996.

118. Bergstein JM, Riley M, Bang NU. Role of plasmino-gen-activator inhibitor type 1 in the pathogenesis and outcome of the hemolytic uremic syndrome. N Engl J Med 327:755, 1992.

119. Keeton M, Ahn C, Eguchi Y, Burlingame R, Loskutoff DJ. Expression of type 1 plasminogen activator inhibitor in renal tissue in murine lupus nephritis. Kidney Int 47:148, 1995.

120. Cajot JF, Kruithof EK, Schleuning WD, Sordat B, Bachmann F. Plasminogen activators, plasminogen activator inhibitors and procoagulant analyzed in twenty human tumor cell lines. Int J Cancer 38:719, 1986.

121. Hearing VJ, Law LW, Corti A, Appella E, Blasi F. Modulation of metastatic potential by cell surface urokinase of murine melanoma cells. Cancer Res 48:1270, 1988.

122. Pyke C, Kristensen P, Ralfkiaer E, Grondahl-Hansen J, Eriksen J, Blasi F, Dano K, Grndahl-Hansen J, Dan K. Urokinase-type plasminogen activator is expressed in stromal cells and its receptor in cancer cells at invasive foci in human colon adenocarcinomas. Am J Pathol 138:1059, 1991.

123. Mignatti P, Robbins E, Rifkin DB. Tumor invasion through the human amniotic membrane: Require-ment for a proteinase cascade. Cell 47:487, 1986.

124. Ossowski L. In vivo invasion of modified chorioallan-toic membrane by tumor cells: The role of cell surface-bound urokinase. J Cell Biol 107:2437, 1988.

125. Crowley CW, Cohen RL, Lucas BK, Liu G, Shuman MA, Levinson AD. Prevention of metastasis by inhibition of the urokinase receptor. Proc Natl Acad Sci USA 90:5021, 1993.

126. Sordat B, Reiter L, Cajot J-F. Modulation of the ma-lignant phenotype with the urokinase-type plasmino-gen activator and the type 1 plasminogen activator inhibitor. Cell Different Dev 32:277, 1990.

127. Ossowski L, Reich E. Antibodies to plasminogen activator inhibit human tumor metastasis. Cell 35:611, 1983.

128. Ossowski L. Plasminogen activator dependent path-
     ways in the dissemination of human tumor cells in
     the chick embryo. Cell 52:321, 1988.
129. Eitzman DT, Krauss JC, Shen T, Cui J, Ginsburg D.
     Lack of plasminogen activator inhibitor-1 effect in a
     transgenic mouse model of metastatic melanoma.
     1995, unpublished.

130. Lawrence DA, Ginsburg D. Plasminogen activator
     inhibitors. In High KA, Roberts HR (eds). Molecular
     Basis of Thrombosis and Hemostasis, New York:
     Marcel Dekker, 1995:517.
131. Stein PE, Carrell RW. What do dysfunctional serpins
     tell us about molecular mobility and disease? Struct
     Biol 2:96, 1995.

6. BIOLOGICAL EFFECTS OF TARGETED GENE INACTIVATION AND GENE TRANSFER OF THE COAGULATION AND FIBRINOLYTIC SYSTEMS IN MICE

Peter Carmeliet and Désiré Collen

Coagulation System

Preservation of vascular integrity following traumatic or infectious challenges is essential for the survival of multicellular organisms. A major defense mechanism involves the formation of hemostatic plugs by activation of platelets and polymerization of fibrin. Initiation of the plasma coagulation system on exposure of blood to nonvascular cells is triggered by tissue factor (TF), which is expressed by a variety of cells surrounding the vasculature as a hemostatic envelope and which functions as a cellular receptor and cofactor for activation of the serine proteinase factor VII to VIIa [1]. This complex activates factor X directly or indirectly via activation of factor IX, resulting in the generation of thrombin-mediated conversion of fibrinogen to fibrin [2,3]. Thrombin and factor Xa produce a positive feedback stimulation of coagulation by activating factors VIII and V, which serve as membrane-bound receptors/cofactors for the proteolytic enzymes factors IXa and Xa, respectively [2,3].

In contrast, thrombin, when bound to its cellular receptor thrombomodulin, also functions as an anticoagulant by activating the protein C anticoagulant system [4,5]. Activated protein C in the presence of its cofactor protein S inactivates factors Va and VIIIa, thereby reducing thrombin generation [4,5]. Anticoagulation is further provided by antithrombin III, which binds to and inactivates thrombin, factor IXa, and factor Xa in a reaction that is greatly enhanced by heparin [6]. Anticoagulation is further secured by tissue factor pathway inhibitor, which directly inhibits factor Xa and, in a factor Xa–dependent manner, produces feedback inhibition of the factor VIIa–tissue factor catalytic complex [7].

A revised hypothesis of coagulation has been suggested in which factor VIIa–TF is responsible for the initiation of coagulation but, owing to tissue factor pathway inhibitor–mediated feedback inhibition, amplification of the procoagulant response through the actions of factor VIII, IX, and XI is required for sustained hemostasis [7]. Deficiencies of anticoagulant factors or aberrant expression of procoagulant factors have been implicated in hemostasis during inflammation, sepsis, atherosclerosis, and cancer [1,6], whereas deficiencies of procoagulant factors have been related to increased bleeding tendencies [8,9]. Evidence has been provided that the coagulation system may also be involved in other functions beyond coagulation, including cellular migration and proliferation, immune response, angiogenesis, embryonic development, cancer, and brain function [1,10,11]. Its precise role and relevance in these processes in vivo remains, however, largely unknown.

Plasminogen System

The plasminogen system is composed of an inactive proenzyme plasminogen (Plg) that can be converted to plasmin by either of two plasminogen activators (PA), tissue-type PA (t-PA) or urokinase-type PA (u-PA) [12–14]. This system is controlled at the level of plasminogen activators by plasminogen activator inhibitors (PAIs), of which PAI-1 is believed to be physiologically the most important [15–17], and at the level of plasmin by α_2-antiplasmin [13]. Vitronectin stabilizes PAI-1 in its active conformation and may also localize PAI-1 to specific sites in

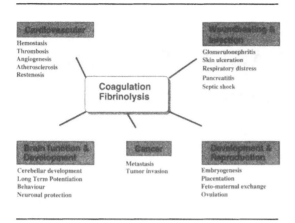

FIGURE 6-1. Schematic overview of the in vivo role of the coagulation and fibrinolytic system as revealed from targeting studies.

the extracellular matrix [17]. Other inhibitors include PAI-2, PAI-3, proteinase nexin-1, and α_2-macroglobulin [13,18]. Due to its fibrin specificity, t-PA is primarily involved in clot dissolution, although it has also been involved in ovulation, bone remodeling, and brain function [14,19]. Cellular receptors for t-PA and Plg have been identified that might localize plasmin proteolysis to the cell surface [20,21].

u-PA also binds a cellular receptor, the urokinase receptor (u-PAR), and has been implicated in pericellular proteolysis during cell migration and tissue remodeling in a variety of normal and pathological processes, including ovulation, trophoblast invasion, angiogenesis, keratinocyte migration, inflammation, wound healing, and cancer [22–24]. u-PAR and PAI-1 interact with vitronectin, suggesting a role in coordinating cell adhesion [25]. As discussed later, it is presently unclear whether or in which conditions binding of u-PA to u-PAR is required in vivo. Plasmin can degrade fibrin and extracellular matrix proteins but can also activate or liberate growth factors from the extracellular matrix (including latent transforming growth factor, basic fibroblast growth factor, and vascular endothelial growth factor), and can activate other matrix-degrading proteinases (such as the metalloproteinases) [26]. Cell-specific clearance of plasminogen activators or of complexes with their inhibitors by low-densitiy lipoprotein receptor-related protein (LRP) or gp330 may modulate pericellular plasmin proteolysis [27]. Figure 6-1 schematically represents the in vivo role of the coagulation and fibrinolytic system, as revealed by the gene targeting and transfer studies described later.

Targeted Manipulation and Adenovirus-Mediated Transfer of Genes in Mice

Novel gene technologies that were developed over the last decade have allowed manipulation of the genetic balance of candidate molecules in mice in a controllable manner. Targeting of genes via homologous recombination in embryonic stem cells allows the study of the consequences of deficiencies, mutations, conditional, or tissue-specific expression of gene products in transgenic mice [28,29]. Using a novel embryonic stem cell technology (aggregation of embryonic stem cells with tetraploid embryos), it has become possible to generate completely embryonic stem cell–derived embryos in a single step. In addition, the technology allows us to bypass conventional germline transmission, to separate extra- from intra-embryonic phenotypes, and to study homozygous deficient phenotypes of genes that cause embryonic lethality when heterozygous deficient [30,31].

Viral gene transfer can also be used to manipulate the expression of genes, for example, via implantation of retrovirally transduced cells [32] or via adenoviral-mediated gene transfer in vivo [33]. In fact, intravenous administration of a recombinant adenovirus results in expression of target genes to plasma levels above $10\,\mu g/mL$ [34]. Such studies allow one to generate and to rescue disease models, and to evaluate possible gene-transfer therapies. Table 6-1 summarizes the phenotypes associated with genetic alterations in the fibrinolytic or coagulation system that result from targeted inactivation in mice compared with those that occur spontaneously in humans.

Embryonic Development and Reproduction

COAGULATION SYSTEM

Only limited information is available on the expression of coagulation factors during embryonic development. Tissue factor expression has been identified in embryonic epithelia, the heart, the nervous system, and the visceral endoderm of the yolk sac, whereas expression of the thrombin receptor has been localized in the heart, blood vessels, and the brain [35,36]. Thrombomodulin expression was observed in the endoderm of the parietal yolk sac at 7.5 days postcoitum, in the aortic arch of 9.5-day postcoitum embryos, and in the blood vessels, heart, lung buds, and central nervous system in 10.5-day postcoitum embryos [37]. It is intriguing that expression of prothrombin and factor VII was undetectable in the early embryo, raising the question of whether these mol-

TABLE 6-1. Phenotypes resulting from the targeted gene deletions in mice and spontaneous mutations in humans

Deficiency	Mouse	Human
Coagulation system		
Tissue factor (TF)	Embryonic lethality due to defective blood vessel formation	Unknown
Thrombomodulin (TM)	Embronic lethality due to defective feto-maternal interaction	Unknown
Factor V (fV)	Postnatal lethality due to severe spontaneous bleeding	Bleeding
Fibrinogen (Fbg)	Bleeding associated with trauma	Bleeding
	Abnormal wound healing	
	Abortion due to maternal bleeding	
Factor VIII (fVIII)	Bleeding	Bleeding
Fibrinolytic system		
Tissue-type plasminogen activator (t-PA)	Increased thrombotic susceptibility	Unknown
	Mild glomerulonephritis	
	Reduced neurotoxicity	
	Abnormal long-term potentiation	
	Impaired neuronal migration	
Urokinase-type plasminogen activator (u-PA)	Increased thrombotic susceptibility	Unknown
	Impaired neointima formation	
	Mild glomerulonephritis	
	Impaired macrophage function	
	Reduced decidual vascularization	
	Reduced trophoblast invasion	
	Reduced platelet activation and trapping	
	Reduced tumor invasion	
t-PA:u-PA	Severe spontaneous thrombosis	Unknown
	Impaired neointima formation	
	Reduced ovulation and fertility	
	Cachexia and shorter survival	
	Severe glomerulonephritis	
	Abnormal tissue remodeling	
Urokinase receptor (u-PAR)	Normal	Unknown
t-PA:u-PAR	Normal	Unknown
Plasminogen (Plg)	Severe spontaneous thrombosis	Thrombosis
	Reduced ovulation and fertility	
	Cachexia and shorter survival	
	Severe glomerulonephritis	
	Reduced neurotoxicity	
	Impaired skin healing	
	Reduced macrophage and keratinocyte migration	
Plasminogen activator inhibitor-1 (PAI-1)	Reduced thrombotic incidence	Bleeding
	No bleeding	
	Accelerated neointima formation	
	Reduced lung inflammation	
	Reduced atherosclerosis	
Plasminogen activator inhibitor-2 (PAI-2)	Normal[a]	Unknown
Vitronectin (VN)	Normal[a]	Unknown
α-Macrogobulin	Reduced lung inflammation	Unknown
	Severe pancreatitis	
	Increased resistance to endotoxin shock	
Proteinase nexin-1 (PN-1)	Reduced fertility	Unknown
LDL receptor-related protein (LRP)	Embryonic lethality due to bleeding	Unknown

Only those genetic deficiencies in humans that correspond to published genetic deficiencies in mice are summarized. The table displays only the abnormal phenotypes, which are described in more detail in the text. The possible lack of a phenotype is discussed in the text.
[a] Initial phenotypic analysis has not revealed any major abnormalities thus far.

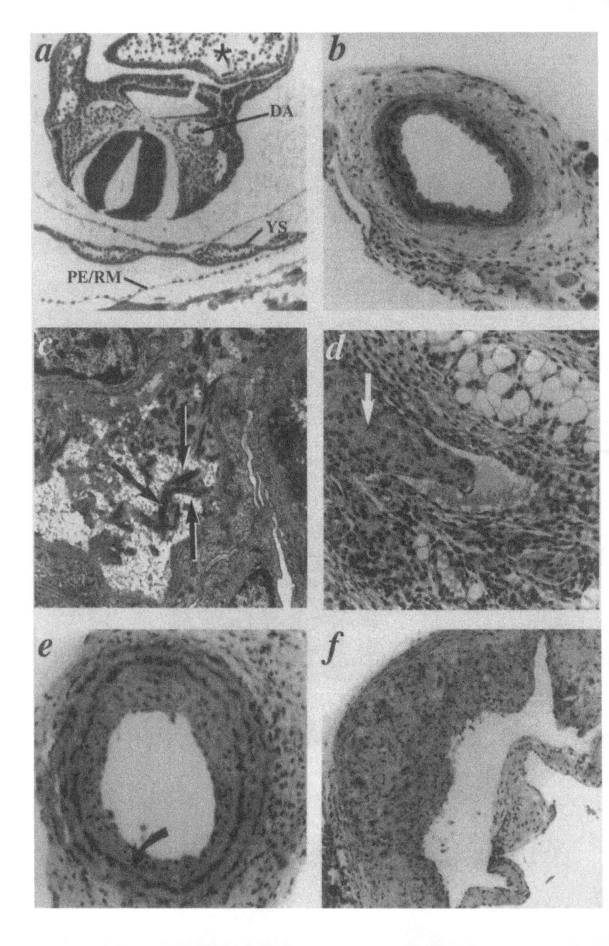

ecules might act independently of their currently known ligands [35,36].

The gene inactivation studies of the coagulation factors that have thus far been performed have yielded an unanticipated involvement in embryogenesis. Indeed, thrombomodulin deficiency resulted in overall growth retardation and embryonic death at around 9.5 days postcoitum [38]. Notably, removal of thrombomodulin-deficient embryos from the maternal decidua rescued the arrested organogenesis, suggesting that defective feto-maternal interactions might compromise the development of the embryo proper [38]. Increased fibrin deposition proteolysis did not seem to affect the barrier function of Reichert's membrane or the parietal endoderm [38]. Figure 6-2A shows Reichert's membrane and the parietal endoderm in a normal postimplantation embryo.

Another surprising finding is that tissue-factor deficiency resulted in embryonic death around 10.5 days postcoitum, most likely due to insufficient vitello-embryonic blood circulation as a result of abnormal vessel formation in the yolk sac [39]. Figure 6-2A illustrates the vessels in the visceral yolk sac in a normal embryo. In particular, loss of tissue factor appeared to result in impaired periendothelial cell recruitment, thereby causing abnormal vessel fragility and rucpture. How tissue factor exerts its role in vessel formation is unclear. Tissue factor could be involved in the formation of fibrin (which might act as a scaffold and chemotactic stimulus for endothelial cell; [40] or of downstream signaling factors such as factor Xa [10] or thrombin [11].

Alternatively, tissue factor may induce the expression of angiogenic or other factors such as vascular endothelial growth factor (VEGF) [41]. In this respect, it is interesting to note that the abnormal vessel development in the yolk sac of tissue factor–deficient embryos resembled that in embryos lacking a single VEGF allele [34], possibly suggesting a link between tissue factor and VEGF. An intriguing but unresolved question is whether the role of tissue factor in embryonic development is mediated by factor VII, the only currently known ligand of tissue factor.

These targeting studies extend the recently documented role of tissue factor in tumor-associated angiogenesis [42] and warrant further study of its involvement in other processes of normal and pathological vessel formation.

Ovulation, embryo implantation, and placentation involve tissue remodeling and breeching of intact vessels, requiring proper hemostasis. Somewhat surprisingly, intraovarian bleeding did not occur following ovulation in fibrinogen-deficient mice [43]. However, fibrinogen deficiency significantly affected embryogenesis [43]. Indeed, development of fibrinogen-deficient embryos in homozygous fibrinogen-deficient females was arrested at 9–10 days postcoitum due to severe intrauterine bleeding. There was no evidence of bleeding within developing embryos or their amniotic or yolk sacs as long as the placentas were intact. Rather, the location, volume, and absence of nucleated (embryonic) red blood cells within the hemorraghic areas suggest that hemorrhaging was from a maternal source. It is possible that bleeding was caused by the invasion of embryonic trophoblasts into and disruption of maternal vasculature within the placenta. Abortion was not observed in heterozygous fibrinogen-deficient females mated to heterozygous or homozygous fibrinogen-deficient males, indicating the importance of the maternal fibrinogen during gestation [43].

FIBRINOLYTIC SYSTEM

The plasminogen system has been claimed to be involved in ovulation, spermatocyte migration, fertilization, embryo implantation, and embryogenesis, and in the associated remodeling of the ovary, prostate, and mammary gland [12,14]. Because homozygous deficiencies of several fibrinolytic system components, including t-PA and u-PA, have not been observed, it was anticipated that inactivation of these genes might cause embryonic lethality. However, transgenic mice overexpressing PAI-1 [44,45], u-PA [46], or the amino-terminal fragment of u-PA [47] and mice with single or combined deficiencies of t-PA and/or u-PA [48,49], t-PA and u-PAR [50], PAI-1 [51,52], u-PAR [53,54], plasminogen [55,56], PAI-

FIGURE 6-2. Formation and pathology of blood vessels in the mouse. A: Section through a 9.0-day postcoitum wild-type embryo revealing the heart (asterisk), dorsal aorta (DA), yolk sac vessels (arrowheads), vitello-embryonic vessels (arrows), parietal endoderm (PE), and Reichert's membrane (RM). B: Section through a normal femoral artery revealing two to three layers of smooth muscle cells in the media and a single layer of endothelial cells in the intima. C: Section through a capillary from a combined t-PA:u-PA–deficient mouse revealing intraluminal fibrin deposits (arrows) indicative of severe thrombosis (electron microscopy). D: Section through a vein from a wild-type mouse 3 days after endotoxin injection in the footpad, revealing an organized thrombus (arrow). E: Section through a femoral artery from a wild-type mouse 3 weeks after electric injury, revealing a smooth muscle cell–rich neointima. F: Section through the aorta from an apolipoprotein E–deficient mouse after 15 weeks on a cholesterol-rich diet, revealing an atherosclerotic plaque.

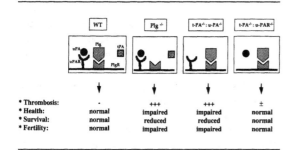

	WT	Plg⁻/⁻	t-PA⁻/⁻:u-PA⁻/⁻	t-PA⁻/⁻:u-PAR⁻/⁻
* Thrombosis:	-	+++	+++	±
* Health:	normal	impaired	impaired	normal
* Survival:	normal	reduced	reduced	normal
* Fertility:	normal	impaired	impaired	normal

FIGURE 6-3. u-PA is biologically active in the absence of u-PAR. Mice with a single deficiency of plasminogen or a combined deficiency of t-PA and u-PA, but not of t-PA and u-PAR, suffered severe thrombosis, impaired health and fertility, and shorter survival, suggesting that sufficient u-PA—mediated pericellular plasmin proteolysis can occur in the absence of u-PAR.

2 [57], vitronectin [58], or α_2-macroglobulin [59] survived embryonic development and were viable at birth. Thus far, u-PA deficiency has only been found to reduce the rate of trophoblast migration during early embryogenesis and the formation of blood lacunae in late pregnancies, possibly due do impaired endothelial cell function (Teesalu, Blasi, and Tallerico, personal communication).

Inactivation of the LRP gene resulted in embryonic lethality at midgestation, secondary to abdominal bleeding [60]. It is presently unclear to what extent lethality in these mice is caused by abnormal plasmin proteolysis because LRP is a multifunctional clearance receptor, not only for fibrinolytic system components but also for other unrelated molecules [27]. Another interesting but unresolved question is why homozygous but not heterozygous proteinase nexin-1—deficient mice are unable to sire offspring (Botteri and Vander Putten, personal communication).

Mice with a single deficiency of t-PA or u-PA [48,49], u-PAR [53,54], PAI-1 [51,52], vitronectin [58], or α_2-macroglobulin [59] are fertile. Normal fertility was also observed in a transgenic mouse strain expressing an antisense t-PA mRNA, with reduction of t-PA activity in the oocytes by more than 50% [61]. Both plasminogen activators appeared, however, to cooperate, because Plg-deficient and combined t-PA:u-PA—deficient mice were less fertile than wild-type mice or mice with a single deficiency of t-PA or u-PA [48,55]. In part, this could be due to poor general health and fibrin deposits in the gonads once they became sick and cachectic. However, gonadotropin-induced ovulation was also signifi-

cantly reduced in healthy 25-day-old female mice lacking both plasminogen activators [62] and plasminogen (Ny et al., personal communication). The observation that combined t-PA:u-PAR–deficient mice are fertile [50] suggests that u-PA can still mediate sufficient pericellular proteolysis in the absence of u-PAR to rescue the defective ovulation of combined t-PA:u-PA–deficient mice (Figure 6-3) [48]. Thus, ovulation can occur in the absence of t-PA, u-PA, u-PAR, PAI-1, or α_2-macroglobulin, but is reduced in mice with Plg deficiency or combined t-PA and u-PA deficiency.

Health and Survival

COAGULATION SYSTEM

Deficiencies of the procoagulant factors V, VIII, and fibrinogen significantly affect the survival of mutant mice due to bleeding complications. Within 2 days after birth, approximately 30% of the fibrinogen-deficient offspring developed overt intra-abdominal bleeding, but surprisingly only 10% of these neonates died [43]. A second period of increased risk of developing fatal intra-abdominal bleeding occurred between 30 and 60 days, resulting in a 50–60% survival rate. Survival of fibrinogen-deficient mice was highly dependent on the genetic background, possibly due to differences in general activity level [43]. Factor V–deficient mice also revealed intra-abdominal bleeding, resulting in early postnatal death [63]. In contrast, factor VIII–deficient mice did not bleed spontaneously but displayed life-threatening bleeding when challenged with trauma during tail cutting [64].

FIBRINOLYTIC SYSTEM

No effects on health and survival were observed in t-PA-, u-PAR-, PAI-1-, vitronectin-, or α_2-macroglobulin–deficient mice [48–59]. A small percentage of u-PA–deficient mice developed chronic (nonhealing) ulcerations and rectal prolapse, but without an effect on survival [48]. Plg-deficient [55,56] and combined t-PA:u-PA–deficient [48], but not combined t-PA:u-PAR–deficient [50] mice, developed chronic ulcerations and rectal prolapse, suggesting that sufficient u-PA–mediated plasmin proteolysis can occur in the absence of u-PAR (Figure 6-3). In addition, these mice suffered significant growth retardation, developed a wasting syndrome with anemia, dyspnea, lethargia, and cachexia, and had a significantly shorter lifespan. Generalized thrombosis in the gastrointestinal tract, the lungs,

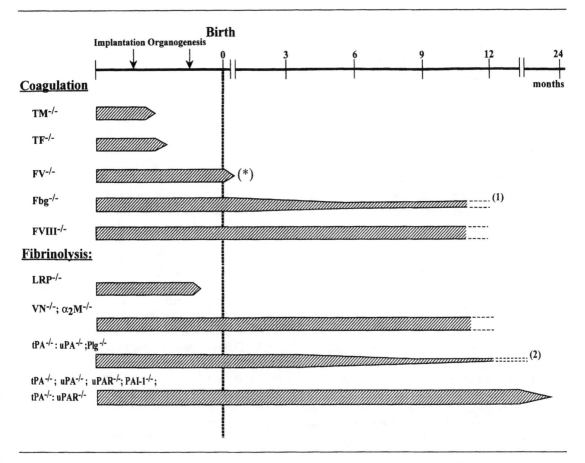

FIGURE 6-4. Relative survival of mice with inactivation of components of the coagulation or fibrinolytic systems. The thickness of the bars denotes the percent of mice surviving for the indicated time period. Interrupted bars indicate that the studies are still ongoing [1]Approximately 10% of the fibrinogen deficient mice die shortly after birth and another 40% around 1–2 months after birth due to bleeding. [2]Plg-deficient and combined t-PA:u-PA–deficient mice start to die after 3 months of age such that less than 30% of these mice survive after 1 year. TM-/- = thrombomodulin deficient; TF-/- = tissue factor deficient; FV-/- = factor V deficient; FVIII-/- = factor VIII deficient; LRP-/- = LDL-related protein deficient; VN-/- = vitronectin deficient; α_2-M-/- = α_2-macroglobulin deficient. Other abbreviations as in the text. (*): preliminary analysis

and other organs (including the gonads, liver, and kidney) might, at least in part, explain their increased morbidity and mortality. Figure 6-4 depicts, on an arbitrary time scale, the viability and survival of these different knock-out strains.

Hemostasis

COAGULATION SYSTEM
Deficiency of fibrinogen resulted in overt intra-abdominal, subcutaneous, joint, and/or periumbilical bleeding in the neonatal period [43]. These are the common sites of spontaneous bleeding events in humans with acquired or congenital coagulation disorders [65]. The bleeding manifestations in adult fibrinogen-deficient mice (e.g., hemoperitoneum, epistaxis, and hepatic, renal, intraintestinal, intrathoracic, and soft tissue hematomas) are generally comparable with those observed in the rare human congenital disorder afibrinogenemia and probably resulted from coincidental mechanical trauma [66]. Although afibrinogenemic murine blood was totally unclottable and platelets failed to aggregate, bleeding was not consistently life threatening [43]. Bleeding was possibly somewhat controlled by the residual thrombin generation and platelet activation. Whether other platelet receptors beyond the GPIIb/IIIa receptor or ligands other than fibrinogen (including vitronectin, fibronectin, or von

Willebrand factor) might rescue deficient platelet interactions remains to be determined.

Initial analysis indicats that Factor V–deficient mice appeared to suffer from a more severe bleeding phenotype (resulting in early postnatal death), suggesting critical hemostatic functions of thrombin activation beyond fibrin generation [63]. The more severe phenotype of factor V deficiency in mice than in humans is consistent with the detection of residual factor V activities in most patients [67].

Factor VIII deficiency (hemophilia A) in humans predisposes to spontaneous and trauma-induced bleeding in the joints and soft tissues [2]. Mice deficient in factor VIII suffered life-threatening bleeding in association with tail injury but did not appear to bleed spontaneously [64]. Factor VIII–deficient mice may provide useful models for studying the immune response that limits recombinant factor VIII substitution in hemophiliac patients as well as for designing possible gene therapy strategies.

FIBRINOLYTIC SYSTEM

Hemostasis involves platelet deposition and coagulation to stabilize hemostatic plugs. Failure to stabilize the clot, for example, as a result of hyperfibrinolytic activity, might result in delayed rebleeding. A hemorrhagic tendency has indeed been observed in patients with increased plasma t-PA or reduced plasma α_2-antiplasmin or PAI-1 activity levels [68,69]. Delayed rebleeding might also explain the hemorrhagic tendency in transgenic mice, expressing high levels of plasma u-PA [46] and in transgenic mice overexpressing granulocyte-macrophage–colony-stimulating factor (GM-CSF), in which increased production of u-PA by peritoneal macrophages occurs [70]. Contrary to patients with low or absent plasma PAI-1 levels, PAI-1–deficient mice did not reveal spontaneous or delayed rebleeding, even after trauma [52]. Lower plasma PAI-1 levels and the occurrence of alternative PAIs in murine plasma (unpublished data) might explain the less pronounced hyperfibrinolytic phenotype and the species-specific difference in the control of plasmin proteolysis.

Thrombosis and Thrombolysis

COAGULATION SYSTEM

Coagulation inhibitor deficiencies in humans predisposes them to an increased risk for thrombosis [6]. Heterozygous thrombomodulin-deficient mice were viable and did not appear to develop spontaneous thrombosis, possibly indicating that the mice need to be challenged either genetically (by crossbreeding them with other thrombosis-prone transgenic mice) or physiologically (by administration of proinflammatory reagents, injury, etc). The recently generated mutant factor V mice [63] engineered to have a similar activated protein C-resistance phenotype as humans [5] might be valuable for examining the role of this anticoagulant protein in vivo.

FIBRINOLYTIC SYSTEM

t-PA is believed to be primarily responsible for removal of fibrin from the vascular tree via clot-restricted plasminogen activation [13]. The role of u-PA in thrombolysis is less well defined. It lacks affinity for fibrin and probably requires conversion from a single-chain precursor to a catalytically active two-chain derivative [13]. The conditions under which u-PA might participate in fibrin clot dissolution in vivo remain to be identified. Other plasminogen activation pathways, such as the intrinsic pathway (involving blood coagulation factor XII, high molecular weight kininogen, prekallikrein, and possibly u-PA) [71], as well as plasminogen-independent mechanisms [72], have been proposed to contribute to clot lysis, but their role in vivo remains to be defined.

Deficient fibrinolytic activity, for example, resulting from increased plasma PAI-1 levels or reduced plasma t-PA or plasminogen levels, might participate in the development of thrombotic events [69]. Elevated plasma PAI-1 levels have indeed been correlated with a higher risk of deep venous thrombosis and of thrombosis during the hemolytic uremic syndrome, disseminated intravascular coagulation, sepsis, surgery, and trauma [15,16]. PAI-1 plasma levels have also been elevated in patients with ischemic heart disease, angina pectoris, and recurrent myocardial infarction [73]. However, the acute-phase reactant behavior of PAI-1 does not allow us to deduce whether increased PAI-1 levels are a cause or consequence of thrombosis. To date, abnormal fibrin clot surveillance resulting from genetic deficiencies in t-PA or u-PA has not been reported in humans, but quantitative and qualitative deficiencies of plasminogen have been associated with an increased tendency to thrombosis [69,74]. Table 6-2 summarizes the consequences of targeted gene manipulation of the fibrinolytic system on fibrin surveillance.

Fibrin Deposits and Pulmonary Plasma Clot Lysis in Transgenic Mice. Microscopic analysis of tissues from u-PA–deficient mice revealed occasional minor fibrin deposits in liver and intestines and excessive fibrin deposition in chronic nonhealing skin ulcerations,

TABLE 6-2. Effects of targeted gene-inactivation and adenovirus-mediated gene transfer of the plasminogen system on vascular wound healing and fibrin surveillance

Mice	Neointima formation	Fibrin deposition		Fibrin degradation	
		Spontaneous	Induced	Plasma clot lysis	Matrix breakdown
Wild type	++	−	++	+++	++++
t-PA−/−	++	−	++++	+	++++
Ad.t-PA in t-PA−/−	N.D.	N.D.	N.D.	++++	N.D.
u-PA−/−	−[a]	+	++++	+++[c]	−
TU−/−	−[b]	++++	++++	−[d]	−
u-PAR−/−	++	−	++	+++	+++[e]
TR−/−	N.D.	+	N.D.	N.D.	N.D.
PAI-1−/−	++++[b]	−	−	++++	++++
Ad.PAI-1 in PAI−/−	−[(1)]	N.D.	N.D.	−	N.D.
Plg−/−	−[(1)]	++++	++++	−[d]	N.D.

Overview of the consequences of targeted gene inactivation or rescue by adenovirus-mediated gene transfer on neointima formation, fibrin deposition (thrombosis), and fibrin degradation (thrombolysis) semiquantitatively expressed on a scale from "−" (very little to absent response) to "++++" (maximal response). Intra- and extra-vascular fibrin deposition was examined in knock-out mice without (spontaneous) or with (induced) endotoxin challenge, locally injected in the footpad, as described in Carmeliet et al. [48,52]. Fibrin degradation was evaluated by monitoring lysis of a ^{125}I-labeled fibrin pulmonary plasma clot or degradation of a ^{125}I-labeled fibrin matrix, as described in Carmeliet et al. [48,52].
[a] Neointima formation in these mice was reduced but not absent [88].
[b] Neointima formation was accelerated in PAI-1–deficient mice [88].
[c] The apparent lack of an effect by u-PA on pulmonary plasma clot lysis might be related to the residual presence of t-PA, which because of its high fibrin specificity is able to rapidly degrade the fibrin-rich platelet-poor plasma clots.
[d] Spontaneous lysis in these knock-out mice occurred at a very slow rate and became significant only after 72 hours [48,55].
[e] Degradation by u-PAR+ macrophages occurred at a somewhat slower initial rate but was similar after 8 hours [53,88].
t-PA−/− = t-PA deficient; u-PA−/− = u-PA deficient; u-PAR−/− = u-PAR deficient; PAI-1−/− = PAI-1 deficient; TU−/− = combined t-PA and u-PA deficient; TR−/− = combined t-PA and u-PAR deficient; Plg−/− = plasminogen deficient; Ad.t-PA in t-PA−/− = intravenous injection of recombinant adenovirus expressing human t-PA in t-PA deficient mice; Ad.PAI-1 in PAI-1−/− = intravenous injection of recombinant adenovirus expressing human PAI-1 in PAI-1 deficient mice; N.D. = not done.

whereas in t-PA–deficient mice, no spontaneous fibrin deposits were observed [48]. Mice with a single deficiency of plasminogen (Plg) or a combined deficiency of t-PA and u-PA, however, had extensive fibrin deposits in several organs (including the liver, lung, gastrointestinal tract, reproductive organs, etc.) associated with ischemic necrosis, possibly resulting from thrombotic occlusions (Figure 6-2C) [48,55,56]. Fibrin deposits were observed at the same sites and around the same age in Plg-deficient as in combined t-PA:u-PA–deficient mice, suggesting that t-PA and u-PA are the only physiologically significant plasminogen activators in vivo. Interestingly, mice with a combined deficiency of t-PA and u-PAR did not display such excessive fibrin deposits, suggesting that sufficient plasmin proteolysis can occur in the absence of u-PA binding to u-PAR (Figure 6-3) [50].

Transgenic mice overexpressing human PAI-1 under the control of the metallothionin promoter displayed cell-, fibrin-, and platelet-rich venous occlusions in the tail and hindlegs [44], whereas mice overexpressing murine PAI-1 under the control of the cytomegaleous virus promoter did not suffer such complications [45] (Ginsburg et al., personal communication). The reason for this discrepancy is at present unclear. Mice with a single deficiency of t-PA or u-PA were significantly more susceptible to the development of venous thrombosis following local injection of proinflammatory endotoxin in the footpad (Figure 6-2D) [48].

Hypoxia also induced ^{125}I-labeled fibrin deposition in t-PA– or u-PA–deficient mice, but not in wild-type or PAI-1–deficient mice (Pinsky et al., personal communication). The increased susceptibility of t-PA–deficient mice to endotoxin and the severe spontaneous thrombotic phenotype of combined t-PA:u-PA– or Plg–deficient mice could be explained by their significantly reduced rate of spontaneous lysis of ^{125}I-fibrin–labeled plasma clots, injected via the jugular vein and embolized into the pulmonary arteries [48,55]. On the contrary, PAI-1–deficient mice were virtually protected against the development of venous thrombosis following the injection of endotoxin, consistent with their ability to lyse ^{125}I-fibrin–labeled plasma clots at a significantly higher rate than wild-type mice [52]. The increased susceptibility of u-PA–deficient mice to thrombosis associated with inflammation or injury might be due to their impaired macrophage function. Indeed, thioglycolate-stimulated macrophages (which are known to express cell-associated u-PA), isolated from u-PA–deficient mice, lacked plasminogen-dependent breakdown of ^{125}I-labeled fibrin (fibrinolysis) or of ^{3}H-labeled subendothelial matrix (mostly collagenolysis), whereas macrophages from t-PA–deficient or PAI-1–deficient mice did not [48,49].

Lipoprotein (a) contains the lipid and protein components of low-density lipoprotein plus apolipoprotein (a) [75]. Extensive homology of apolipoprotein (a) to plasminogen has prompted the proposal that apolipoprotein (a) forms a link between thrombosis and atherosclerosis, but in vitro studies have not yielded conclusive evidence. Transgenic mice overexpressing apolipoprotein (a) displayed reduced thrombolytic potential, but only after administration of pharmacological doses of recombinant t-PA, suggesting a mild hypofibrinolytic condition [76]. Studies using transgenic mice overexpressing lipoprotein (a) extended these findings and revealed that spontaneous lysis of ^{125}I-fibrin–labeled pulmonary plasma clots (and thus, not lysis induced by exogenous administration of recombinant t-PA) was also reduced (Carmeliet et al., unpublished observations).

Adenovirus-Mediated Transfer of t-PA or PAI-1. More recently, we have used adenoviral-mediated transfer of fibrinolytic system components in these knock-out mice in an attempt to revert their phenotypes. Intravenous injection of adenoviruses, expressing a recombinant PAI-1–resistant human t-PA (*rt-PA*) gene, in t-PA–deficient mice increased plasma rt-PA levels 100- to 1000-fold above normal and restored their impaired thrombolytic potential in a dose-related manner [34]. Notably, adenoviral t-PA gene transfer increased thrombolysis to significant levels by 4 hours and was sustained for more than a week, suggesting that it might be useful for restoring deficient thrombolysis in subacute conditions. Conversely, adenovirus-mediated transfer of recombinant human PAI-1 in PAI-1–deficient mice resulted in 100- to 1000-fold increased plasma PAI-1 levels above normal and efficiently reduced the increased thrombolytic potential of PAI-1–deficient mice (Carmeliet et al., unpublished observations).

Collectively, these gene targeting and gene transfer studies confirm the importance of the plasminogen system in maintaining vascular patency and indicate that t-PA and u-PA are the only physiologically significant plasminogen activators in vivo that appear to cooperate significantly in fibrin surveillance. Interestingly, u-PA appears to play a more significant role than previously anticipated in the prevention of fibrin deposition during conditions of inflammation or injury, possibly through cell-associated plasmin proteolysis. A surprising finding, however, is that u-PA can still exert its biological role (pericellular proteolysis) in the absence of u-PAR. Whether the marginal role of u-PAR is related to the ability of u-PA to become *localized around* but not *bound to* the cell surface via interaction with other macromolecules, such as fibrin, plasminogen, vitronectin, or proteoglycans, remains to be determined.

Neointima Formation

Vascular interventions for the treatment of atherothrombosis, such as bypass surgery, percutaneous transluminal balloon angioplasty, atherectomy, or the in situ application of vascular stents, restore blood flow and improve tissue oxygenation but induce restenosis of the vessel within 3–6 months in 30–50% of treated patients [77]. This may result from remodeling of the vessel wall and/or accumulation of cells and extracellular matrix in the intimal or adventitial layer. Several mechanisms are believed to participate in intimal thickening as part of a hyperactive wound healing response, including thrombosis, proliferation, apoptosis, and migration of smooth muscle cells [78,79]. Proteinases participate in the degradation of the extracellular basement membrane surrounding the smooth muscle cells, allowing them to migrate to distant sites. Two proteinase systems have been implicated, the plasminogen (or fibrinolytic) system and the metalloproteinase system, which in concert can degrade most extracellular matrix proteins.

In contrast to the constitutive expression of t-PA by quiescent endothelial cells [13] and of PAI-1 by uninjured vascular smooth muscle cells [80], u-PA and t-PA activity in the vessel wall are significantly increased after injury, at the time of smooth muscle cell proliferation and migration [81–83]. This increase in plasmin proteolysis is counterbalanced by increased expression of PAI-1 in injured smooth muscle and endothelial cells, and by its release from accumulating platelets [84]. Expression of components of the fibrinolytic system is also induced in cultured endothelial cells, smooth muscle cells, and macrophages as a result of wounding or treatment with growth factors and cytokines that are released after injury [22,85]. t-PA has been proposed to act as an autocrine mitogen after injury [86]. The precise

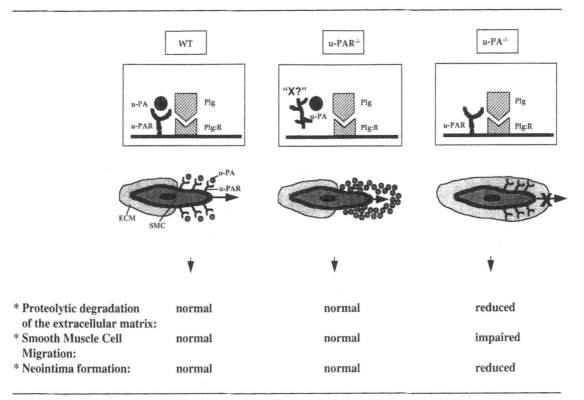

FIGURE 6-5. Hypothetical model of the role of receptor-independent u-PA–mediated plasminogen activation in neointima formation. The smooth muscle cell (SMC) is surrounded by an extracellular matrix (ECM) that needs to be proteolytically degraded to allow cellular migration. In the wild-type (WT) smooth muscle cells, u-PA is bound to u-PAR, mediating plasminogen activation and plasmic degradation of the extracellular matrix such that the cell can migrate. In the u-PAR–deficient smooth muscle cells, u-PA becomes localized to the cell surface, possibly via interaction with other matrix molecules (denoted as "X?"), allowing sufficient pericellular plasmin proteolysis for the cells to migrate. u-PA might also accumulate to increased levels due to deficient u-PAR–mediated clearance [54]. In contrast, smooth muscle cells that lack u-PA have reduced pericellular plasmin proteolysis and fail to migrate efficiently, resulting in reduced neointima formation. The proposed impairment of smooth muscle cell migration in mice lacking u-PA–mediated plasminogen activation is indirectly suggested by the observations that proliferation of u-PA–deficient cells was to that in wild-type cells and that smooth muscle cells migrated over a shorter distance in the Plg-deficient than in wild-type arteries.

and causative role of the plasminogen system in matrix remodeling, passivation of the injured luminal vessel surface, migration, or proliferation of vascular cells remains to be determined.

We have used an experimental model based on the use of an electric current to examine the molecular mechanisms of neointima formation in mice deficient in fibrinolytic system components (Figure 6-2E) [87]. The electric current injury model differs from mechanical injury models in that it induces a more severe injury accross the vessel wall, resulting in necrosis of all smooth muscle cells. This necessitates that wound healing is initiated from the adjacent uninjured borders and progresses into the central necrotic region. Microscopic and morphometric analysis

revealed that the rate and degree of neointima formation and neointimal cell accumulation after injury was similar in wild-type, t-PA–deficient, and u-PAR–deficient arteries [88]. However, neointima formation in PAI-1–deficient arteries occurred at earlier times postinjury [88]. In contrast, both the degree and rate of arterial neointima formation in u-PA–deficient, Plg-deficient, and combined t-PA:u-PA–deficient arteries was significantly reduced until 6 weeks postinjury [88,89]. Evaluation of the mechanisms responsible for these genotype-specific differences in neointima formation revealed that proliferation of medial and neointimal smooth muscle cells differed only marginally between the genotypes [88,89]. Impaired migration of smooth muscle cells could be a significant cause of reduced neointima formation in mice lacking u-PA–mediated plasmin proteolysis because smooth muscle cells migrated over a shorter distance from the uninjured border into the central injured region in Plg-deficient than in wild-type arteries [89]. Table 6-2 summarizes the consequences of the gene deletions on neointima formation in these gene-inactivated mice.

A surprising observation was that deficiency of u-PA, but not of u-PAR, reduced neointima formation in vivo. Because u-PAR is expressed by smooth muscle [88] and endothelial cells [22] and u-PAR is the only currently known receptor for u-PA [22–24], binding of u-PA to its cellular receptor appears to be more neglible for the role of u-PA than anticipated. Such a conclusion is supported by previous observations that an increase in soluble (not membrane-bound) human u-PA in murine tumor cells enhances their invasiveness [90] and that scavenging of soluble u-PA by a truncated (non–membrane-anchored) u-PAR impairs cellular invasion [91]. Furthermore, a membrane-anchored form of u-PA catalyzes plasminogen activation on the cell surface with characteristics comparable with those of u-PAR–bound u-PA [92], suggesting that *cell surface localization* rather than *binding to* u-PAR is important. Possibly, the kinetic advantage resulting from u-PAR–accelerated plasminogen activation may be irrelevant for certain u-PA-dependent phenomena that develop over long time periods, or may be compensated by the increased extracellular accumulation of u-PA in u-PAR–deficient mice (probably resulting from defective clearance of u-PA) [54]. Alternatively, u-PA may be localized to the cell surface via binding to other molecules, such as fibrin, plasminogen, extracellular matrix, or cell adhesion molecules [21,25,93].

Our results also suggest that pericellular proteolysis can still occur in the absence of u-PAR. This is confirmed by the observation that degradation of ^{125}I-labeled fibrin or subendothelial matrix over 8 hours is only transiently affected by u-PAR deficiency [53,88] and that thrombosis, sterility, and organ dysfunction in combined t-PA:u-PAR–deficient mice is significantly less severe than in combined t-PA:u-PA–deficient mice [48,50]. Figure 6-5 schematically represents a hypothetical model of smooth muscle cell function and neointima formation in the absence of u-PA or u-PAR. It should be noted, however, that the lack of an appreciable effect on neointima formation in u-PAR knock-out mice does not exclude a role for this receptor in other biological processes (e.g., cancer), because the relevance of u-PAR may depend on the amount and the cell-specific, temporal, and spatial expression of u-PAR. Whether, to what extent,

and under what conditions u-PAR may be more important in other u-PA–dependent phenomena, such as cancer or angiogenesis, remains to be determined.

Inhibition of Neointima Formation by Adenovirus-Mediated PAI-1 Gene Transfer. The involvement of plasmin proteolysis in neointima formation was supported by intravenous injection in PAI-1–deficient mice of a replication-defective adenovirus that expresses human PAI-1, which resulted in more than 1000-fold increased plasma PAI-1 levels and in a similar degree of inhibition of neointima formation as observed in u-PA–deficient mice [88]. Proteinase-inhibitors have been suggested as anti-restenosis drugs. Our studies suggest that strategies aimed at reducing u-PA–mediated plasmin proteolysis may be beneficial for reduction or prevention of restenosis. However, antifibrinolytic strategies should be targeted at inhibiting plasmin proteolysis and not at preventing the interaction of u-PA with its receptor.

Atherosclerosis

Epidemiologic, genetic, and molecular evidence suggests that impaired fibrinolysis resulting from increased PAI-1 or reduced t-PA expression, or from inhibition of plasminogen activation, may contribute to the development and/or progression of atherosclerosis [16,94–96], presumably by promoting thrombosis or matrix deposition. A possible role for increased plasmin proteolysis in atherosclerosis is, however, suggested by the enhanced expression of t-PA and u-PA in plaques [97–98]. Plasmin proteolysis might indeed participate in plaque neovascularization, induction of plaque rupture, or ulceration and the formation of aneurysms [97,98]. However, a causative role of the plasminogen system in these processes has not been conclusively demonstrated.

In an initial analysis of atherosclerosis in mice deficient in apolipoprotein E (apoE) and t-PA, u-PA, or PAI-1, and fed a cholesterol-rich diet for 10–25 weeks, a significant reduction of plaque development was observed in apoE:PAI-1–deficient mice after 10 and 15 weeks (Figure 6-2F). In contrast, plaques in apoE:u-PA–deficient arteries were devoid of media destruction and aneurysm formation. Further study will be required to unravel these molecular defects in more detail (Carmeliet et al., unpublished observations).

Lipoprotein (a) has been proposed to reduce plasminogen activation and to predispose to atherosclerosis by reducing clot lysis [75]. Alternatively, reduced plasmin proteolysis could diminish activation of latent transforming growth factor-β (TGFβ), thus providing a growth stimulus for smooth muscle cells [99]. A significant correlation between high levels of apolipoprotein (a) and reduced in situ plasmin activity was observed in atherosclerotic vessels of transgenic mice overexpressing apolipoprotein (a) [99]. Ongoing experiments in mice deficient in t-PA, u-PA, PAI-1, u-PAR, or plasminogen will demonstrate whether plasmin is a significant activator of latent TGFβ in vivo.

Tissue Remodeling Associated with Wound Healing

Impaired fibrinolysis, resulting from reduced u-PA or increased PAI-1 activity, has been implicated in the deposition of fibrin and extracellular matrix components in the kidney and lung during inflammation [100,101]. Electron microscopic analysis demonstrated that adult combined t-PA:u-PA–deficient mice developed fibrin deposition not only in the intravascular lumen but also in extravascular compartments, such as in the lung alveoli, kidney mesangium and the subendothelial space of Disse in the liver (Figure 6-2C; Carmeliet et al., unpublished observations). Furthermore, severe tissue remodeling, such as fusion of podocytes in the glomerulus and endothelial cell necrosis in adjacent capillaries, were frequently observed. Notably, extravascular fibrin deposition appeared to precede intravascular thrombosis, possibly suggesting that the triggering event for abnormal fibrin deposition and tissue remodeling is located in the extracellular compartment. These pathological findings are reminiscent of those observed in glomerulonephritis and in acute respiratory distress syndrome in humans [100,101].

Involvement of the plasminogen system in inflammation and wound healing was further extended by observations that plasminogen and combined t-PA:u-PA–deficient mice, and to a lesser extent t-PA–deficient or u-PA–deficient mice, suffered severe experimental glomerulonephritis, characterized by increased formation of fibrin-rich glomerular crescents after challenge with antiglomerular membrane antibodies [102]. In addition, PAI-1–overexpressing mice suffered more severe lung injury and deposition of fibrin and collagen-rich matrix after bleomycin challenge [45] or hyperoxia [102], whereas PAI-1–deficient [45] or α₂-macroglobulin–deficient [59] mice were protected against such a fibrotic reaction. α₂-Macroglobulin deficiency also increased the mortality associated with experimentally induced acute pancreatitis, possibly because of uncontrolled proteolysis [59]. Plg-deficient mice also displayed fibrin-rich gastric ulcerations, in association with infection by pathogenic *Helicobacter* [55,56].

They also suffered delayed and impaired closure of skin wounds [104]. Notably, keratinocyte migration appeared to be reduced, but, surprisingly, the granulation tissue was not qualitatively different from normal, except for the more abundant presence of fibrin(ogen) and fibronectin at the wound edges [104]. In fact, Plg-deficient mice, like their wild-type controls, had an abundant infiltration of macrophages, neutrophilic granulocytes, and fibroblast-like cells, and pronounced neovascularization [100]. Taken together, the plasminogen system appears to play a significant role in tissue remodeling during wound healing, in part mediated by its role in fibrin surveillance. This notion is supported by the observation that fibrinogen-deficient mice had an unusual wound healing response in which the migrating and proliferating cells (primarily fibroblasts) form a thick layer *encapsulating* but not *infiltrating* hematomas [43]. It is thus possible that fibrin provides a critical initial matrix for the movement of cells into sites of injury.

Different degrees of wound healing responses have been reported, depending on environmental conditions and infectious challenges. The most significant phenotype occurred in u-PA–deficient mice after infection with botryomycosis (Shapiro et al., personal communication). In contrast with their wild-type littermates, housed in the same environmental conditions, u-PA–deficient mice developed a suppurative infection of the skin, characterized by the presence of abcesses and granulomas, and containing large numbers of polymorphonuclear leukocytes and histiocytes, which were surrounded by a capsule of fibrous connective tissue. Such destructive tissue remodeling is indeed more severe than observed in combined t-PA:u-PA–deficient or Plg-deficient mice [48,55], indicating that the phenotypes observed in these knock-out mice are importantly determined by the infectious or inflammatory challenge.

Despite a well-documented expression pattern of the fibrinolytic system during certain (patho) biological processes, experimental studies have not always confirmed its relevance in vivo. Biological processes, in which knock-out studies have thus far failed to demonstrate a significant role of the plasminogen system, are corneal wound healing (unpublished data) and bone remodeling. Plasmin proteolysis might facilitate bone resorption via activation of latent collagenases or TGF-β, by freeing insulin-like growth factor-1 from its inhibitory binding proteins, or by promoting osteoclast migration [19].

Nevertheless, bone resorption in cultured fetal metatarsals and calvariae from t-PA– or u-PA–deficient mice did not differ from that in wild-type mice [105]. Bone turnover was slightly increased, but total body calcium content and radiographic examination of the skeleton in young and old t-PA–deficient mice were normal; only a minor degree of cancellous osteopenia (as revealed by dynamic bone histomorphometric analysis of the tibial metaphysis) was observed [106]. In aggregate, although the present results have not revealed an absolute requirement of the plasminogen system for normal bone remodeling or corneal wound healing, a more subtle role of this system remains possible. It should be noted, however, that lack of an obvious phenotype in a knock-out mouse does not exclude a possible role for the target gene during conditions of ectopic or abnormal expression. It is also possible that the knock-out mouse may have adapted to the deficiency of the target gene by alternative mechanisms. However, compensatory upregulation of the residual plasminogen activators has not been observed thus far [48,104].

Infection

The expression of proteinases, and in particular of the u-PA:u-PAR system, by leukocytes is thought to be critical for the ability of cells to degrade matrix proteins and to traverse tissue planes during recruitment to inflammatory sites. u-PA has also been implicated, however, in the modulation of cytokine and growth factor expression. It is required for tumor necrosis factor alpha (TNF-α) expression by mononuclear phagocytes [107], transforms latent transforming growth factor beta (TGF-β) to its active form [26], and may also be involved in the release of interleukin-1 (IL-1) [108]. In addition, serine proteinase inhibitors reduce interleukin-2 (IL-2) expression [109]. u-PA–deficient mice were unable to mount an adequate pulmonary inflammatory response to a challenge with the nonlethal 52D *Cryptococcus neoformans* pathogen [110]. They were unable to recruit sufficient mononuclear phagocytes, neutrophils, and lymphocytes; did not contain the infection to the lung; and could not eliminate the organism, which disseminated widely and ultimately infected the brain, leading to death. This pattern of wide dissemination and death with strain 52D has only been seen in profoundly immunoincompetent mice. Whereas u-PA and u-PAR may promote the recruitment of monocytes and neutrophils by enhancing the degradation of matrix components, u-PA may also play a role in lymphocyte recruitment by modulating the cytokine network. Thus, the absence of u-PA may result in

inadequate signaling via IL-1 or IL-2, significant modulators of lymphocyte cell function.

Treatment of patients with TNF-α frequently induces transient thrombocytopenia. Platelet consumption and trapping within organs was significantly decreased in u-PA–deficient but not in t-PA–deficient mice, consistent with a reduced activation of u-PA–deficient platelets in vitro [111]. Another interesting observation is that α$_2$-macroglobulin–deficient mice were significantly more resistant to lethal doses of endotoxin, possibly related to deficient interaction of cytokines and growth factors [59]. Thus, the role of the plasminogen system in the inflammatory response may extend beyond the proteolytic activities required to allow for the movement of cells, and may participate in the orchestration of cytokine networks that serve to intensify the inflammatory response.

Brain Function

Evidence has been provided that the plasminogen system might be involved in brain function. Fibrinolytic system components are expressed in specialized areas of the brain during development [112] or in adulthood following different forms of brain activity [113,114]. In addition, in vitro studies with cultured neurons revealed that these cells are able to produce and respond to plasminogen activators [115]. Restricted and temporal specific expression of t-PA in the nervous system during development has also been observed in transgenic mice expressing the LacZ marker gene driven by various t-PA promotor constructs [116,117]. Ectopic expression and overexpression of murine u-PA in the brain (e.g., in the hippocampus and limbic system) was associated with impaired learning of tasks in transgenic mice [118] and reduced food intake (Miskin et al., personal communication).

cAMP-dependent de novo synthesis of proteins, including t-PA, has been proposed to participate in long-term potentiation. Deficiency of t-PA, but not u-PA, abolished the late phase of long-term potentiation in both the Schaffer collateral and mossy fiber pathways of the hippocampus that was induced by electrical stimulation or by treatment with dopamine agonists or cAMP analogs [119]. Somewhat surprisingly, a t-PA deficiency did not affect hippocampus-related learning tasks, including spatial memory in the Barnes circular maze and Morris water maze, exploration in a novel environment, and context conditioning [119]. However, t-PA deficiency significantly impaired, active avoidance learning and slightly affected the acquisition learning in the Morris water maze test [119]. Because t-PA is expressed in certain nuclei of the limbic system [114], this impairment might be due to abnormal coping of t-PA–deficient mice with stress. Another study reported that t-PA–deficient mice completely lacked conventional, homosynaptic, late long-term potentiation at the Schaffer collateral–CA1 pyramidal cell synapses and exhibited a different form of (heterosynaptic) long-term potentiation that not only required glutaminergic but also GABA-dependent transmission [120]. This heterosynaptic form of potentiation provided t-PA–deficient mice with an output of CA1 neurons similar to that seen in wild-type mice during conventional late long-term potentiation. Compensation of conventional long-term potentiation by a GABA-dependent potentiation could explain the relative lack of hippocampal-related learning defects [120]. Taken together, these data suggest that t-PA plays a significant role in the late phase of long-term potentiation as a downstream target of cAMP.

Another remarkable observation is that t-PA–deficient and Plg-deficient mice are resistant to neuronal degeneration and are protected against neuroexcitatory induced seizures [121] (Tsirka et al., personal communication). t-PA appears to be produced by microglial cells, the non-neuronal, macrophage-like cells that are transformed from a resting to an activated state on neuronal injury [121]. Activated microglia participate in the phagocytosis of neurons, and microglial proteinases have been involved in neuronal degradation. Thus, the lack of neuronal degeneration in excitotoxin-injected t-PA–deficient mice could be due to a failure of microglial cell activation. The lack of t-PA confers resistance to experimentally induced neuronal degeneration and seizure, suggesting that t-PA activity might contribute to pathologies associated with accelerated neuronal degeneration, such as Alzheimer's disease. Whether the increased plasma t-PA levels during thrombolytic therapy for stroke and brain ischemia might play a similar deleterious effect remains to be determined.

t-PA has been implicated in the migration of granule neurous in the developing cerebellum [122]. Interestingly, there were two to three times more granule neurons in the molecular layer of the developing cerebellum of neonatal t-PA–deficient mice, suggesting that the absence of t-PA leads to retardation in granule neuron migration. This retardation was not observed in wild-type or u-PA–deficient mice (Seeds and Haffke, personal communication).

Trans-section or crush of peripheral motor nerves leads to a retrograde reaction in the neuronal cell bodies, accompanied by the activation of glial cells in the vicinity of the damaged neurons. These microglia extend processes into the synaptic clefts, thus stripping synapses from the motorneuron cell bodies, a process that was proposed to be mediated by plasminogen activators based on induced expression of t-PA, u-PA, and PAI-1 [123,124]. The initial studies suggest that stripping of the synapses from the motorneuron cell bodies still occurs in t-PA–deficient mice (Reddington et al., personal communication). Further studies are required to determine the precise involvement of the plasminogen system in the tissue remodeling accompanying neuronal injury.

Taken together, these findings suggest that improper plasmin proteolytic balance (either due to u-PA overexpression or t-PA deficiency may significantly affect brain functioning. An interesting but unresolved question is whether t-PA and u-PA exert such effects directly or through activation of plasminogen or other related molecules. Indeed, plasminogen levels in the brain have been reported to be low to undertectable [114]. The studies by Tsirka et al. indicate, however, that Plg-deficient mice displayed a reduced susceptibility to excitatory stimuli, similar to t-PA–deficient mice (Tsirka et al., personal communication), suggesting that this phenomenon is dependent on plasmin proteolysis. Whether t-PA binds to a putative (neuronal) receptor [125] and/or processes signaling factors, or proteolytically remodels neuronal tissue, remains to be elucidated.

Malignancy, Macrophage Function, and Neovascularization

Pericellular plasmin proteolysis has been claimed to play a role in tumor invasion and metastasis by facilitating the migration of malignant cells through anatomical barriers via degradation of extracellular matrix constituents [24]. Increased expression of u-PA, u-PAR, and PAI-1 by tumor cells or the surrounding stroma has, indeed, been observed [24]. In addition, administration of synthetic serine proteinase inhibitors or of u-PA–specific antibodies reduced, whereas genetically engineered overexpression of u-PA increased, tumor dissemination [24]. Furthermore, fibrinolytic system components have been used as clinical markers for the prognosis of certain tumors in humans [126].

No significant effect on "spontaneous" pulmonary metastases of the Lewis lung carcinoma (3LL) cells was observed in transgenic mice overexpressing the amino-terminal fragment of u-PA [47]. PAI-1–overexpressing mice, injected intramuscularly with 3LL cells and treated with $ZnSO_4$ (which increased the activity of the metallothionin promoter that directs the human PAI-1 transgene), displayed a signifi-

cant reduction of "spontaneous" pulmonary metastases, with no effect on tumor growth [127]. Furthermore, formation of "artificial" lung nodules
occurred at a reduced frequency in these mice. Because PAI-1 was localized to the endothelial lining
of capillary vessels in the primary tumor and in the
lungs of 3LL-bearing PAI-1 transgenic mice, reduced
lodging of the 3LL tumor cells to the pulmonary
vessels may explain the inhibition of metastatic
spread [127]. Recently, carcinogen-induced me-
lanocytic neoplasms in u-PA–deficient mice were
found to invade the underlying tissues at a reduced
rate (Shapiro et al., personal communication). The use
of knock-out mice and other models, including crossbreeding with a tumor-developing transgenic mouse
strain, may provide means to further examine the role
of the plasminogen system in malignancy.

The plasminogen system has also been implicated
in re-endothelialization, neoangiogenesis, and macrophage invasion. Increased expression of u-PA, u-
PAR, and also of PAI-1 has been observed in
migrating endothelial cells and macrophages in vitro
and in vivo [22–24]. Invasion into the peritoneal
cavity by u-PA–deficient or by u-PAR–deficient
macrophages, 3 d after thioglycolate injection, was
not reduced, despite the absence of plasminogen-
dependent breakdown of the extracellular matrix
[48,49]. Recent studies suggest, however, that migration of plasminogen-deficient macrophages is significantly impaired, possibly suggesting that plasmin
proteolysis needs to be sufficiently reduced [128].

No evidence of abnormal angiogenesis was observed on microscopic examination of tissues from
mice with deficiencies of t-PA, u-PA, PAI-1, u-PAR,
or Plg [48–56], although the degree of decidual vas-
cularization in the late placenta was transiently reduced in u-PA–deficient mice (Teesalu, Blasi, and
Tallerico, personal communication). Wound healing
studies in Plg-deficient mice also revealed no apparent defects in neovascularization of the granulation
tissue [104]. Studies with normal and polyoma virus
middle T (PymT)–transformed endothelial cells suggest that balanced plasmin proteolysis is required
for appropriate formation of capillary tubes [129].
PymT-induced hemangioma formation occurred at a
reduced rate and frequency in mice with single and
combined deficiencies of t-PA and u-PA, (Wagner et
al., personal communication). Collectively, only a
subtle role for plasmin proteolysis has thus far been
documented for the formation of new blood vessels
during development but its role during pathological
neovascularization may be more significant. This
might suggest the involvement of plasminogen-
independent proteinases.

Gene Regulation

Transgenic animals expressing a LacZ reporter gene
have been used for characterization of tissue-specific
regulatory elements in the t-PA and u-PA promoter.
Expression of a LacZ reporter gene by a 3.0-kb fragment of the human t-PA promoter or by a 4.0-kb
fragment of the murine t-PA promoter in transgenic
mice and rats during embryonic development and
adulthood occurred in discrete regions of the central
and peripheral nervous system and in some non-
neuronal sites, but not in the vascular system
[116,117]. The reporter gene was, however, expressed
in the vascular system when a 1.4-kg human t-PA
promoter fragment was used, suggesting that expression of t-PA in the vascular system is regulated by
repressor/silencer elements in more upstream regions
[117]. A 0.5-kg murine t-PA promoter fragment
failed to direct expression of LacZ during embryonic
development, presumably due to the lack of the appropriate regulatory elements [116]. Because expression patterns of LacZ overlapped largely, but not
completely, with the distribution of t-PA mRNA
and enzyme activity, these studies provide evidence
for the involvement of neuronal and cardiovascular
specific regulatory elements in t-PA promoter
activity.

Expression of a reporter gene in peripheral neuronal sites was also observed in transgenic mice,
expressing LacZ under the activity of a 4.7-kb
fragment of the porcine u-PA promoter [130] or
of a 7-kb fragment of the murine u-PA promoter
(Vigo, Blasi, and Karlström, personal communication). The latter promoter fragment directed expression of LacZ to migrating keratinocytes during
wound healing but failed to direct expression in the
urogenital or gastrointestinal system, presumably due
to the lack of the appropriate tissue-specific regulatory elements (Vigo, Blasik, and Kallestrøm, personal
communication).

Monoclonal Antibodies Against
Knocked-Out Murine Proteins

Mice with inactivated t-PA, u-PA, or PAI-1 genes,
which were immunized with the targeted proteins,
produced a significant number of monoclonal antibodies directed against the "knocked-out" proteins
[131]. Monoclonal antibodies against murine u-PA
did not cross-react with human u-PA, confirming
previous observations with polyclonal anti-u-PA antibodies. Monoclonal antibodies against murine t-PA
were largely directed towards epitopes in kringle 1
and 2, and in the catalytic domain. Significantly, 60%

of the antibodies cross-reacted with rat and human t-PA, whereas 15% cross-reacted with human, rat, and vampire-bat t-PA [131], suggesting that production of monoclonal antibodies in gene-inactivated mice might provide a means to generate antibodies against epitopes that are conserved across species, a possibly useful strategy for structure–function analyses of molecules.

Conclusions

Studies with transgenic mice over- or under-expressing components of the coagulation or fibrinolytic system not only confirmed the significant role of these proteinase systems in hemostasis and fibrin clot surveillance but have also revealed novel insights in the precise role and interaction of the individual molecules. The coagulation, and not the fibrinolytic, system appeared to play a more essential role in embryonic development than anticipated. Although life without plasminogen is possible, health and survival are severity compromised. Both systems are involved in infection, inflammation, and wound healing, such as in arterial neointima formation, glomerulonephritis, skin ulcerations, pancreatitis, and lung inflammation.

A novel role for the plasminogen system in the brain has been revealed by gene targeting studies. Unexpectedly, these studies have revealed a more neglible role of the plasminogen system in corneal healing, bone remodeling, and blood vessel development, although this may be due to the type of challenge or analysis used to study these phenotypes. Furthermore, lack of an appreciable effect of a specific gene deletion does not rule out its possible involvement in pathological processes when inappropriately expressed and warrants examination for compensatory mechanisms. These transgenic mice may not only provide suitable models for further elucidatation of the relevance of the plasminogen system in other (patho)physiological processes, such as atherosclerosis or malignancy, but also serve as models for the evaluation of new (gene) therapies.

Acknowledgments

The authors are grateful to the members of the Center for Transgene Technology and Gene Therapy and to Drs. V. Ploplis, E. Plow, and R.C. Mulligan for their contribution to these studies and acknowledge Drs. D. Belin, F. Blasi, F. Botteri, R. Bouillon, M.B. Donati, D. Ginsburg, M. Gyetko, E. Kandel, H.P. Lipp, T. Ny, M. Pepper, D. Rifkin, R. Shapiro, S. Strickland, H. Van der Putten, F. Van Leuven, E. Wagner, and D. Wolffer for sharing unpublished information.

References

1. Edgington TS, Mackman N, Brand K, Ruf W. The structural biology of expression and function of tissue factor. Thromb Haemost 66:67, 1991.
2. Furie B, Furie BC. The molecular basis of blood coagulation. Cell 53:505, 1988.
3. Davie E. Biochemical and molecular aspects of the coagulation cascade. Thromb Haemost 74:1, 1995.
4. Esmon CT. The protein C anticoagulant pathway. Arterioscler Thromb 12:135, 1992.
5. Dahlbäck B. New molecular insights into the genetics of thrombophilia. Resistance to activated protein C caused by Arg506 to Gln mutation in factor Va a pathogenic risk factor for thrombosis. Thromb Haemost 74:139, 1995.
6. Bick RL, Pegram M. Syndromes of hypercoagulability and thrombosis: A review. Semin Thromb Hemost 20:109, 1994.
7. Broze, GJ. Tissue factor pathway inhibitor and the revised hypothesis of blood coagulation. Trends Cardiovasc Med 2:72, 1992.
8. Hoyer LW. Hemophila A. N Engl J Med 330:38, 1996.
9. Bolton-Maggs PHB, Hill FGH. The rarer inherited coagulation disorders: A review. Blood Rev 9:65, 1995.
10. Altieri DC. Xa receptor EPR-1. FASEB J 9:860, 1995.
11. Coughlin SR. Molecular mechanisms of thrombin signaling. Semin Hematol 31:270, 1994.
12. Astrup T. In Davidson JF, Rowan RM, Samama MM, Desnoyers PC (eds). Progress in Chemical Fibrinolysis and Thrombolysis, Vol. 3. New York: Raven Press, 1978:1.
13. Collen D, Lijnen HR. Basic and clinical aspects of fibrinolysis and thrombolysis. Blood 78:3114, 1991.
14. Vassalli JD, Sappino JD, Belin D. The plasminogen activator/plasmin system. J Clin Invest 88:1067, 1991.
15. Schneiderman J, Loskutoff DJ. Plasminogen activator inhibitors. Trends Cardiovasc Med 1:99, 1991.
16. Wiman B. Plasminogen activator inhibitor 1 in plasma: Its role in thrombotic disease. Thromb Haemost 74:71, 1995.
17. Lawrence DA, Ginsburg D. In High KA, Roberts HR (eds). Plasminogen Activator Inhibitors. New York: Dekker, 1995:517.
18. Bachmann F. The engima of PAI-2. Gene expression, evolutionary and functional aspects. Thromb Haemost 74:172, 1995.
19. Martin TJ, Allan EH, Fukumoto S. The plasminogen activator and inhibitor system in bone remodeling. Growth Regul 3:209, 1993.
20. Hajjar KA. Cellular receptors in the regulation of plasmin generation. Thromb Haemost 74:294, 1995.
21. Plow EF, Herren T, Redlitz A, Miles LA, Hoover-Plow JL. The cell biology of the plasminogen system. FASEB J 9:939, 1995.

22. Vassalli JD. The urokinase receptor. Fibrinolysis 8(Suppl 1):172, 1994.
23. Blasi F, Conese M, Moller LB, Pedersen N, Cavallaro U, Cubellis MV, Fazioli F, Hernandez-Marrero L, Limongi P, Munoz-Canoves P, Resnati M, Rüttininen L, Sidenius N, Soravia E, Soria MR, Stoppelli MP, Talarico D, Teesalu T, Valcamonica S. The urokinase receptor: Structure, regulation and inhibitor-mediated internalization. Fibrinolysis 8(Suppl 1):182, 1994.
24. Dano K, Behrendt N, Brünner N, Ellis V, Ploug M, Pyke C. The urokinase-receptor. Protein structure and role in plasminogen activation and cancer invasion. Fibrinolysis 8(Suppl 1):189, 1994.
25. Wei Y, Waltz DA, Rao N, Drummond RJ, Rosenberg S, Chapman HA. Identification of the urokinase receptor as an adhesion receptor for vitronectin. J Biol Chem 269:32380, 1994.
26. Saksela O, Rifkin D. Cell-associated plasminogen activation: Regulation and physiological functions. A Rev Cell Biol 4:93, 1988.
27. Andreasen PA, Sottrup-Jensen LL, et al. Receptor-mediated endocytosis of plasminogen activators and activator/inhibitor complexes. FEBS Lett 338:239, 1994.
28. Capecchi MR. Targeted gene replacement. Sci Amer 1994:34.
29. Nagy A. Engineering the mouse genome. Methods Enzymol, in press.
30. Nagy A, Rossant J. Targeted mutagenesis: Analysis of phenotype without germline transmission. J Clin Invest 6:1360, 1996.
31. Carmeliet P, Ferreira V, Breier G, Pollefeyt S, Kieckens L, Gertsenstein M, Fahrig M, Vandenhoeck A, Harpal K, Eberhardt C, Declercq C, Pawling J, Moons L, Collen D, Risau W, Nagy A. Abnormal blood vessel development and lethality in embryos lacking a single VEGF allele. Nature 380:435, 1996.
32. Mulligan RCM. The basic science of gene therapy. Science 260:926, 1993.
33. Schneider MD, French BA. The advent of adenovirus: Gene therapy for cardiovascular disease. Circulation 88:1937, 1995.
34. Carmeliet P, Stassen JM, Collen D, Meidell R, Gerard R. Adenovirus-mediated gene transfer of rt-PA restores thrombolysis in t-PA deficient mice. Submitted.
35. Soifer SJ, Peters KG, O'Keefe J, Coughlin SR. Disparate temporal expression of the prothrombin and thrombin receptor genes during mouse development. Am J Pathol 144:60, 1994.
36. Luther T, Flössel C, Mackman N, Bierhaus A, Kasper M, Albrecht S, Sage HA, Iruela-Arispe L, Grossman H, Ströhlein A, Zhang Y, Nawroth PP, Carmeliet P, Loskutoff DJ, Müller M. Tissue factor expression during human and mouse development. Am J Pathol 1996, in press.
37. Imada S, Yamaguchi H, Nagumo N, Katyanagi S, Iwasaki H, Imada M. Identification of fetomodulin, a surface marker protein of fetal development as thrombomodulin by gene gene cloning and functional assays. Dev Biol 140:113, 1990.
38. Healy A, Rayburn H, Rosenberg R, Weiler H. Absence of the blood-clotting regulator thrombomodulin causes embryonic lethality in mice before development of a functional cardiovascular system. Proc Natl Acad Sci USA 92:850, 1995.
39. Carmeliet P, Mackman N, Moons L, Wyns S, Van Vlaenderen I, Luther T, Breier G, Lissens A, Rosen E, Müller M, Risau W, Edgington T, Collen D. Role of the cellular receptor tissue factor in embryonic vessel development. Submitted.
40. Dvorak HF, Brown LF, Detmar M, Dvorak AM. Vascular permeability factor/vascular endothelial growth factor, microvascular hyperpermeability and angiogenesis. Am J Pathol 146:1029, 1995.
41. Zhang Y, Deng Y, Luther T, Müller M, Ziegler R, Waldherr R, Stern DM, Nawroth PP. Tissue factor controls the balance of angiogenic and antiangiogenic properties of tumor cells in mice. J Clin Invest 94:1320, 1994.
42. Contrino J, Hair G, Kreutzer DL, Rickles FR. In situ detection of tissue factor in vascular endothelial cells: Correlation with the malignant phenotype of human breast disease. Nature Med 2:209, 1996.
43. Suh TT, Holmbäck K, Jensen NJ, Daugherty CC, Small K, Simon DI, Potter SS, Degen JL. Resolution of spontaneous bleeding events but failure of pregnancy in fibrinogen deficient mice. Genes Dev 9:2020, 1995.
44. Erickson LA, Fici GJ, Lund JE, Boyle TP, Polites HG, Marotti KR. Development of venous occlusions in mice transgenic for the plasminogen activator inhibitor-1 gene. Nature 346:74, 1990.
45. Eitzman DT, McCoy RD, Zheng X, Fay WP, Shen T, Ginsburg D. Bleomycin-induced pulmonary fibrosis in transgenic mice that either lack or overexpress the murine plasminogen activator inhibitor-1 gene. J Clin Invest 97:232, 1996.
46. Heckel JL, Sandgren EP, Degen JL, Palmiter RD, Brinster RL. Neonatal bleeding in transgenic mice expressing urokinase-type plasminogen activator. Cell 62:447, 1990.
47. Sidenius N. Expression of the aminoterminal fragment of urokinase-type plasminogen activator in transgenic mice. PhD thesis, University of Copenhagen, Denmark, 1993.
48. Carmeliet P, Schoonjans L, Kieckens L, Ream B, Degen J, Bronson R, De Vos R, van den Oord JJ, Collen D, Mulligan R. Physiological consequences of loss of plasminogen activator gene function in mice. Nature 368:419, 1994.
49. Carmeliet P, De Clercq C, Janssen S, Pollefeyt S, Bouché A, Wijns S, Mulligan RC, Collen D. Biological effects of disruption of the tissue-type plasminogen activator, urokinase-type plasminogen activator and plasminogen activator inhibitor-1 genes in mice. Ann N Y Acad 748P:367, 1995

50. Bugge TH, Flick MJ, Danton MJ, Daugherty CC, Romer J, Dano K, Carmeliet P, Collen D, Degen JL. Urokinase-type plasminogen activator is effective in fibrin clearance in the absence of its receptor or tissue-type plasminogen activator. Proc Natl Acad Sci USA, in press.

51. Carmeliet P, Kieckens L, Schoonjans L, Ream B, Van Nuffelen A, Prendergast G, Cole M, Bronson R, Collen D, Mulligan RC. Plasminogen activator inhibitor-1 gene deficient mice. I. Generation by homologous recombination and characterization. J Clin Invest 92:2746, 1993.

52. Carmeliet P, Stassen JM, Schoonjans L, Ream B, van den Oord JJ, De Mol M, Mulligan RC, Collen D. Plasminogen activator inhibitor-1 gene deficient mice. II. Effects on hemostasis, thrombosis and thrombolysis. J Clin Invest 92:2756, 1993.

53. Dewerchin M, Van Nuffelen, Wallays G, Bouché A, Moons L, Carmeliet P, Mulligan RCM, Collen D. Generation and characterization of urokinase receptor deficient mice. J Clin Invest 97:870, 1996.

54. Bugge TH, Suh TT, Flick MJ, Daugherty CC, Romer J, Solberg H, Ellis V, Dano K, Degen JL. The receptor for urokinase-type plasminogen activator is not essential for mouse development or fertililty. J Biol Chem 270:16886, 1995.

55. Ploplis V, Carmeliet P, Vazirzadeh S, Van Vlaenderen I, Moons L, Plow E, Collen D. Effects of disruption of the plasminogen gene on thrombosis, growth and health in mice. Circulation 92:2585, 1995.

56. Bugge TH, Flick MJ, Daugherty CC, Degen JL. Plasminogen deficiency causes severe thrombosis but is compatible with development and reproduction. Genes Dev 9:794, 1995.

57. Dougherty K, Yang A, Harris J, Saunders T, Camper S, Ginsburg D. Targeted deletion of the murine plasminogen activator inhibitor-2 gene by homologous recombination. Blood 86(Suppl I):455, 1995.

58. Zheng X, Saunders TL, Camper SA, Samuelson LC, Ginsburg D. Vitronectin is not essential for normal mammalian develoment and fertility. Proc Natl Acad Sci, USA 92:12426, 1995.

59. Umans L, Serneels L, Overbergh L, Lorent K, Van Leuven F, Van den Berghe H. Targeted inactivation of the mouse alpha₂-macroglobulin gene. J Biol Chem 270:19778, 1995.

60. Herz J, Clouthier DE, Hammer RE. LDL receptor-related protein internalizes and degrades uPA:PAI-1 complexes and is essential for embryo implantation. Cell 71:411, 1992.

61. Richards WG, Carroll PM, Kinloch RA, Wassarman PM, Strickland S. Creating matarnal effect mutations in transgenic mice: Antisense inhibition of an oocyte gene product. Dev Biol 160:543, 1993.

62. Leonardsson G, Peng XR, Liu K, Nordström L, Carmeliet P, Mulligan R, Collen D, Ny T. Ovulation efficiency is reduced in mice that lack plasminogen activaor gene function: Functional redundancy among physiological plasminogen activators. Proc Natl Acad Sci USA 92:12446, 1995.

63. Cui J, Saunders TL, Ginsburg D. Analysis of factor V function by gene targeting in embryonic stem cells. Blood 86(Suppl I):449a, 1995.

64. Bi L, Lawler AM, Antonarakis SE, High KA, Gearhart JD, Kazazaian HH Jr. Targeted disruption of the mouse factor VIII gene produces a model of haemophilia A. Nature Genet 10:119, 1995.

65. Montgomery RR, Scott JP. Hemostasis: Diseases of the fluid phases. In Nathan GD, Oski FA (eds). Haematology of Infancy and Childhood. Philadelphia: WB Saunders, 1993:1605.

66. Al-Mondhiry H, Ehmann WC. Congenital afibrinogenemia. Am J Hematol 46:343, 1994.

67. White GC. Coagulation factors V and VIII: Normal function and clinical disorders. In Handin RI, Lux SE, Stossel TP (eds). Blood. Principles & Practice of Hematology. Philadelphia: JB Lippincott, 1995: 1151.

68. Fay WP, Shapiro AD, Shih JL, Schleef RR, Ginsburg D. Complete deficiency of plasminogen-activator inhibitor type 1 due to a frameshift mutation. N Engl J Med 327:1729, 1992.

69. Aoki N. Hemostasis associated with abnormalities of fibrinolysis. Blood Rev 3:11, 1989.

70. Elliott MJ, Faulkner-Jones BE, Stanton H, Hamilton JA, Metcalf D. Plasminogen activator in granulocyte-macrophage-CSF transgenic mice. J Immunol 149: 3687, 1992.

71. Kluft C, Dooijewaard G, Emeis JJ. Role of the contact system in fibrinolysis. Semin Thromb Hemost 13:50, 1987.

72. Plow EF, Edgington TS. An alternative pathway for fibrinolysis. I. The cleavage of fibrinogen by leukocyte proteases at physiologic pH. J Clin Invest 56:30, 1975.

73. Hamsten A, de Faire U, Walldius G, et al. Plasminogen activator inhibitor in plasma: Risk factor for recurrent myocardial infarction. Lancet 2:3, 1987.

74. Robbins KC. Dysplasminogenemias. Enzyme 40:70, 1988.

75. Liu AC, Lawn RM. Lipoprotein(a) and atherogenesis. Trends Cardiovasc Medi 4:40, 1994.

76. Palabrica TM, Liu AC, Aronowitz MJ, Furie B, Lawn RM, Furie BC. Antifibrinolytic activity of apolipoprotein (a) in vivo: Human apolipoprotein (a) transgenic mice are resistant to tissue plasminogen activator-mediated thrombolysis. Nature Med 1:256, 1995.

77. Forrester JS, Fishbein M, Helfant R, Fagin J. A paradigm for restenosis based on cell biology: Clues for the development of new preventive therapies. J Am Coll Cardiol 17:758, 1991.

78. Libby P, Schwartz D, Brogi E, Tanaka H, Clinton SK. A cascade model for restenosis. A special case of atherosclerotic progression. Circulation 86(Suppl III):III47, 1992.

79. Clowes AW, Reidy MA. Prevention of stenosis after

vascular reconstruction: Pharmacologic control of intima hyperplasia — A review. J Vasc Surg 13:885, 1991.

80. Simpson AJ, Booth NA, Moore NR, Bennett B. Distribution of plasminogen activator inhibitor (PAI-1) in tissues. J Clin Pathol 44:139, 1991.

81. Clowes AW, Clowes MM, An YPT, Reidy MA, Belin D. Smooth muscle cells express urokinase during mitogenesis and tissue-type plasminogen activator during migration in injured rat carotid artery. Circ Res 67:61, 1990.

82. Jackson CL, Reidy MA. The role of plasminogen activation in smooth muscle cell migration after arterial injury. Ann N Y Acad Sci 667:141, 1992.

83. Jackson CL, Raines EW, Ross R, Reidy MA. Role of endogenous platelet-derived growth factor in arterial smooth muscle cell migration after balloon catheter injury. Arterioscl Thromb 13:1218, 1993.

84. Sawa H, Fujii S, Sobel BE. Augmented arterial wall expression of type-1 plasminogen activator inhibitor induced by thrombosis. Arterioscler Thromb 12:1507, 1992.

85. Carmeliet P, Collen D. Physiological consequences of over- or under-expression of fibrinolytic system components in transgenic mice. In Vadas M, Harlan J (eds). Vascular Control of Hemostasis; Advances of Vascular Biology, in press.

86. Herbert JM, Lamarche I, Prabonnaud V, Dol F, Gauthier T. Tissue-type plasminogen activator is a potent mitogen for human aortic smooth muscle cells. J Biol Chem 269:3076, 1994.

87. Carmeliet P, Stassen JM, Declercq C, Kockx M, Moons L, Collen D. A model for arterial neointima formation using perivascular electric injury in mice. Submitted.

88. Carmeliet P, Moons L, Dewerchin M, Stassen JM, Declercq C, Gerard R, Collen D. Receptor-independnet role of urokinase-type plasminogen activator in arterial neointima formation in mice. Submitted.

89. Carmeliet P, Moons L, Van Vlaenderen I, Ploplis V, Plow EF, Collen D. Role of plasmin proteolysis in arterial neointima formation in mice. Submitted.

90. Yu HR, Schultz RM. Relationship between secreted urokinase plasminogen activator activity and metastatic potential in murine B16 cells transfected with human urokinase sense and antisense genes. Cancer Res 50:7623, 1990.

91. Wilhelm O, Weidle U, Hohl S, Rettenberger P, Schmitt M, Graeff H. Recombinant soluble urokinase receptor as a scavenger for urokinase-type plasminogen activator. Inhibition of proliferation and invasion of human ovarian cancer cells. FEBS Lett 337:131, 1994.

92. Lee SW, Kahn ML, Dichek DA. Expression of an anchored urokinase in the apical endothelial cell membrane. J Biol Chem 267:13020, 1992.

93. Stephens RW, Bokman AM, Myöhänen HT, Reisberg T, Tapiovaara H, Pedersen N, Grondahl-

Hansen J, Llinas M, Vaheri A. Heparin binding to the urokinase kringle domain. Biochemistry 31:7572, 1992.

94. Hamsten A, Eriksson P. Fibrinolysis and atherosclerosis: An update. Fibrinolysis 8(Suppl 1):253, 1994.

95. Juhan-Vague I, Collen D. On the role of coagulation and fibrinolysis in atherosclerosis. Ann Epidemiol 2:427, 1992.

96. Schneiderman J, Sawdey MS, Keeton MR, Bordin GM, Bernstein EF, Dilley RB, Loskutoff DJ. Increased type 1 plasminogen activator inhibitor gene expression in atherosclerotic human arteries. Proc Natl Acad Sci USA 89:6998, 1992.

97. Schneiderman J, Bordin GM, Engelberg I, Adar R, Seiffert D, Thinnes T, Bernstein EF, Dilley RB, Loskutoff, DJ. Expression of fibrinolytic genes in atherosclerotic abdominal aortic aneurysm wall. A possible mechanism for aneurysm expansion. J Clin Invest 96:639, 1995.

98. Lupu F, Heim DA, Bachmann F, Hurni M, Kakkar VV, Kruithof EKO. Plasminogen activator expression in human atherosclerotic lesions. Arterioscler Thromb Vasc Biol 15:1444, 1995.

99. Grainger DJ, Kemp PR, Liu AC, Lawn RM, Metcalfe JM. Activation of transforming growth factor-β is inhibited in transgenic apolipoprotein (a) mice. Nature 370:460, 1994.

100. Bertozzi P, Astedt B, Zenzius L, Lynch K, LeMaire F, Zapoli W, Chapman HA. Depressed bronchioalveolar urokinase activity in patients with adult respiratory distress syndrome. N Engl J Med 322:890, 1990.

101. Tomooka S, Border WA, Marshall BC, Noble NA. Glomerular matrix accumulation in liked to inhibition of the plasmin protease system. Kidney Int 42:1462, 1992.

102. Kitching R, Carmeliet P, Ploplis V, Collen D, Plow E, Holdsworth ER, Tipping P. Glomerulonephritis in mice with genetic deficiencies of the plasminogen system. XIIIth International Congress on Fibrinolysis and Thrombolysis, Barcelona, June 24–28, 1996. Fibrinolysis Suppl.

103. Barazzone C, Belin D, Huarte J, Vassalli JD, Sappino AP. Deleterious role of plasminogen activator inhibitor-1 in response to hyperoxia in mouse. Presented at 1996 International Conference, New Orleans, Louisiana.

104. Romer J, Bugge TH, Pyke C, Lund LR, Flick MJ, Degen JL, Dano K. Impaired wound healing in mice with a disrupted plasminogen gene. Nature Med 2:287, 1996.

105. Leloup G, Lemoine P, Carmeliet P, Vaes G. Bone resorption and response to parathyroid hormone or 1,25 dihyroxyvitamin D3 in fetal metatarsals and calvariae from transgenic mice devoid of tissue or urokinase type plasminogen activator or of their inhibitor, PAI-1. Twenty-Fourth European Symposium on Calcified Tissues, May 1995, Aarhus, Denmark. Calcified Tissue International (abstract).

106. Bouillon R, Van Herck E, Verhaeghe J, Carmeliet P. Bone metabolism in transgenic mice, deficient in tissue type plasminogen activator (abstr). Xth International Congress on Calcium regulatory hormones, February 1995, Melbourne, Australia. Bone Miner.

107. Sitrin RG, Shollenberger SB, Strieter RM, Gyetko MR. Endogenously produced urokinase activity amplifies tumor necrosis factor-alpha secretion by THP-1 mononuclear phagocytes. J Leukoc Biol, 1996, in press.

108. Matsushima K, Taguchi M, Kovacs EJ, Young HA, Oppenheim JJ. Intracellular localization of human monocytic interleukin-1 (IL-1) activity and release of biologically IL-1 from monocytes by trypsin and plasmin. J Immunol 136:2883, 1986.

109. Auberger P, Sonthonnax S, Peyron JF, Mari B, Fehlmann M. A chymotryptic-type serine proteinase is required for IL-2 production by Jurkat T cells. Immunology 70:547, 1993.

110. Gyetko MR, Chen GH, McDonald RA, Goodman R, Huffnagle GB, Wilkinson CC, Fuller JA, Toews GB. Urokinase is required for the pulmonary inflammatory response to *Crytococcus neoformans*. In press.

111. Tacchini-Cottier F, Vesin C, Philippeaux MM, Belin D, Vassalli P, Piguet PF. Tumor necrosis factor induces platelet activation and consumption in vivo, a process involving urokinase-type plasminogen activator and plasminogen. Abstracts of the Sixth International TNF Congress, May 8–12, 1996, Rhodes, Hellas.

112. Menoud PA, Debrot S, Schowing J. Roux's Arch Dev Biol 198:219, 1989.

113. Qian Z, Gilbert ME, Colicos MA, Kandel ER, Kuhl D. Tissue-type plasminogen activator is induced as an immediate-early gene during seizure, kindling and long-term potentiation. Nature 361:453, 1993.

114. Sappino AP, Madani R, Huarte J, Belin D, Kiss JZ, Wohlwend A, Vassalli JD. Extracellular proteolysis in the adult murine brain. J Clin Invest 92:679, 1993.

115. Krystosek A, Seeds NW Plasminogen activator release at the neuronal growth cone. Science 213:1532, 1981.

116. Carroll PM, Tsirka S, Richards WG, Fronhman MA, Strickland S. Promoter sequences of the tissue-type plasminogen activator gene are able to confer tissue-specific expression of LacZ during mouse development. In press.

117. Theuring F, Aguzzi A, Turner JD, Kropp C, Wohn KD, Hoffmann S, Schleuning WD. Analysis of human tissue-type plasminogen activator gene promotoer activity during embryogenesis of transgenic mice and rats and its induction in the adult mouse brain Submitted.

118. Meiri N, Masos T, Rosenblum K, Miskin R, Dudai Y. Overexpression of urokinase-type plasminogen activator in transgenic mice is correlated with impaired learing. Proc Natl Acad Sci USA 91:3196, 1994.

119. Huang YY, Bach ME, Wolfer DP, Zhuo M, Lipp HP, Hawkins RD, Schoonjans L, Godfraiend JM, Kandel ER, Mulligan RC, Collen D, Carmeliet P. Selective interference with a late stage of both Schaffer collateral and mossy fiber long term potentiation in mice lacking the gene encoding tissue-type plasminogen activator. Submitted.

120. Frey U, Müller M, Kühl D. A different form of long-lasting potentiation revealed in tissue plasminogen activator mutatn mice. J Neurosci 16:2057, 1996.

121. Tsirka SE, Gualandris A, Amaral DG, Strickland S. Excitotoxin-induced neuronal degeneration and seizure are mediated by tissue plasminogen activator. Nature 377:340, 1995.

122. Seeds NW, Haffke S, Christensen K, Schoonmaker J. Cerebellar granule cell migration involves proteolysis. In Lander JM (ed). Molecular Aspects of Development and Aging of the Nervous System. New York: Plenum, 1990:169.

123. Nakajima K, Reddington M, Kohsaka S, Kreutzberg GW. Induction of urokinase-type plasminogen activator in rat facial nucleus by axotomy of the facial nerve. J Neurochem 66, in press.

124. Reddington M, Haas C, Kreutzberg GW. The plasminogen activator system in neurons and glia during motorneuron regeneration. Neuropathol Appl Neurobiol 20:188, 1994.

125. Verral S, Seeds NW. Characterization of ^{125}I-tissue type plasminogen activator binding to cerebellar granule neurons. J Cell Biol 109:265, 1989.

126. Jänicke F, Schmitt M, Graeff H. Clinical relevance of the urokinase-type and tissue-type plasminogen activators and of their type 1 inhibitor in breast cancer. Semin Thromb Hemos 17:303, 1991.

127. Poggi A, Bellelli E, Carmela R, Castelli MP, Salvatore L, Marinacci R, Erickson LA, Benedetta Donati M, Bini A. Reduced pulmonary metastases of Lewis Lung Carcinoma in mice transgenic for the plasminogen activator inhibitor-1 gene. Submitted.

128. Ploplis V, French E, Carmeliet P, Collen D, Plow E. The plasminogen system and cell migration during an inflammatory response. XIIIth International Congress on Fibrinolysis and Thrombolysis, Barcelona, June 24–28, 1996. Fibrinolysis Suppl.

129. Wagner EF. On transferring genes into stem cells and mice. EMBO J 9:3024, 1990.

130 Botteri FM, Van der Putten H, Rajput B, Ballmer-Hofer K, Nagamine Y. Induction of the urokinase-type plasminogen activator gene by cytoskeleton-disrupting agents. In Festoff BW (ed). Serine Proteases and their Serpin Inhibitors in the Nervous System. New York: Plenum Press, 1990:105.

131 Declercq P, Carmeliet P, Verstreken M, Decock F, Collen D. Monoclonal antibodies raised against the targeted proteins in gene-inactivated mice. J Biol Chem 270:8397, 1995.

7. MOLECULAR APPROACHES TO THE DESIGN OF NEW THROMBOLYTIC AGENTS

Bruce A. Keyt and Ted W. Love

Introduction

Tissue plasminogen activator (t-PA) is a glycoprotein that converts plasminogen to plasmin, which cleaves the gel form of fibrin to soluble fibrin degradation products. Recombinant t-PA (Activase® t-PA) is currently used as a thrombolytic agent in the treatment of acute myocardial infarction. Using recombinant DNA technology, the protein sequence can be altered, possibly improving the function of t-PA. Numerous investigators have taken different approaches to the design and evaluation of t-PA variants. Several comprehensive reviews of the literature describe a variety of t-PA mutants and discuss the effects of these mutations on fibrinolytic activity [1,2].

In this chapter we examine different protein design approaches, including the construction of chimeric proteins, substitution and deletion of amino acids, domain deletion, carbohydrate insertion and/or deletion, and a combination of these strategies. These approaches to altering protein structure by mutagenesis are evaluated with respect to maintaining or enhancing t-PA function. Various fibrinolytic functions of t-PA have been modified, including fibrin binding and fibrin specificity, clot lysis activity, interaction with plasma inhibitors, and circulating plasma half-life. The methods used for constructing and evaluating t-PA variants are of crucial importance because these altered molecules may be considered to be clinical candidates with enhanced therapeutic value.

This chapter focuses on functional changes in t-PA that can be achieved by protein engineering and discusses different mutagenic strategies that have been used in attempts to improve t-PA. Most of the improvements in t-PA are actually the result of mutations that decrease selected functional activity. It is this decrease in selected activity that may result in an improved therapeutic profile for a variant of t-PA as compared with the wild-type molecule. Selected examples, especially those variants of t-PA in clinical testing, are described to illustrate certain protein design strategies.

Molecular Interactions of t-PA

Tissue plasminogen activator (t-PA) is a plasma protein that converts plasminogen (an inactive zymogen), to its active form, plasmin (Figure 7-1). Plasmin cleaves the fibrin gel into soluble degradation products. t-PA and plasminogen bind to the fibrin clot, and the rate of plasminogen activation is greater in the presence of fibrin. Hence, fibrin acts as cofactor or template in forming the complex of t-PA and plasminogen. t-PA is *fibrin specific* in that plasminogen activation by t-PA is stimulated by fibrin much more than by fibrinogen [3]. Activities of t-PA and plasmin are regulated by serine protease inhibitors (serpins) present in plasma, such as plasminogen activator inhibitor-type I (PAI-1) and α_2-antiplasmin, respectively. These inhibitors serve to localize the action of t-PA and plasmin to the site of a fibrin clot by rapidly inhibiting the enzymes in circulation, whereas t-PA bound to fibrin is not as rapidly inhibited by PAI-1 [4].

In addition to the interactions of t-PA with its substrate (plasminogen), cofactor (fibrin or fibrinogen), and inhibitor (PAI-1), there is evidence for multiple receptors that rapidly remove t-PA from plasma in vivo [5,6]. The initial half-life of t-PA in the circulation is 4–6 minutes in humans [7]. The relative rates of biosynthesis (by endothelial cells) and clearance (by hepatic cells) result in the relatively low concentration of t-PA observed in normal human plasma (0.1–0.2 nM) compared with plasminogen (1–2 μM) [8,9]. The plasma concentrations of PAI-1 and α_2-antiplasmin are approximately 0.4 nM and 1 μM, respectively, indicating that the concentration of the inhibitors and relevant proteases are of the same order [10,11].

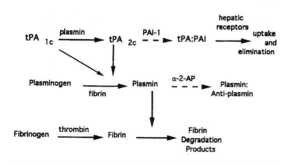

FIGURE 7-1. Schematic diagram of the fibrinolytic system. The proenzyme plasminogen is activated to the enzyme, plasmin, by tissue-type plasminogen activator (t-PA). The activation of plasminogen by t-PA is stimulated in the presence of fibrin. Plasmin can also convert one-chain t-PA to the two-chain species, resulting in feedback activation. Inactivation of t-PA (either the one-chain or two-chain species) occurs by reaction with plasminogen activator inhibitor-type 1 (PAI-1). Fibrin is formed by the action of thrombin on fibrinogen. A fibrin clot is dissolved by active plasmin, which is capable of degrading fibrin to low molecular weight fibrin degradation products. Active plasmin may be inactivated by α_2-antiplasmin (as indicated by the dashed line). t-PA and t-PA–PAI-1 complexes can be bound, internalized, and eliminated by carbohydrate-dependent and -independent hepatic receptors.

With the cloning and sequencing of the cDNA in the early 1980s [12], t-PA was identified as a glycoprotein composed of 527 amino acids that are organized in five distinct modules — finger (F), growth factor (G), two kringle regions (K1,K2), and a serine protease domain (P) — which are homologous with modules found in numerous other plasma proteins (13) (Figure 7-2). Plasmin cleaves t-PA between Arg 275 and Ile 276. The resultant two-chain t-PA is composed of an A chain (amino acids 1–275, containing F, G, K1, and K2 domains) linked to the B chain or protease domain (amino acids 276–527) by a disulfide bond connecting Cys 264 and Cys 395. t-PA has 35 cysteines that form 17 disulfide bonds, with one unpaired cysteine at position 83. Most of the disulfides are intradomain linkages, which have been assigned on the basis of homology with other proteins, such as fibronectin, epidermal growth factor, and plasminogen [12,13]. When the t-PA gene was sequenced in 1984, some of the intron/exon splice junctions were localized to the connecting regions between domains or "modules" of the protein [14]. It has been suggested that the t-PA gene was the result of evolutionary exon shuffling [15] and the domain structures of t-PA could be correlated with individual functions [16].

FIBRIN BINDING: LOCALIZATION OF T-PA ACTIVITY TO THE SITE OF A CLOT

t-PA displays high affinity for fibrin, which targets the enzymatic activity of t-PA to the clot. The domain structures on t-PA that mediate fibrin binding are located predominantly within the A-chain of t-PA. Isolation of A and B chains after mild reduction of two-chain t-PA [17], provided evidence for the targeting function of the A-chain domain, separate from the enzymatic activity of the protease domain [18]. These studies indicated that the isolated A chain bound fibrin, whereas the protease domain did not. Studies with domain deletion variants of t-PA demonstrated that the F and K2 domains of t-PA were involved in fibrin binding [16]. Verheijen et al. also demonstrated the requirement of the F domain for high-affinity fibrin binding [19]. If either the F and/or G domains were deleted, the fibrin affinity of the variant t-PA decreased by 10-fold [20]. Of the t-PA variants with individual domain deletions, the des-K1 t-PA, was the least defective with respect to fibrin binding [21].

Charged to alanine scanning mutagenesis was used to identify the fibrin binding determinants on t-PA [22]. Alanine variants of t-PA were labeled at the active site with ^{125}I YPRck and tested for fibrin binding [23]. Mutations in all domains had major effects on high-affinity fibrin binding, especially mutations located in the K1 domain. Interestingly, mutations in the K2 domain had a minimal effect on fibrin binding. A novel fibrin-binding site localized in t-PA protease was observed [22]. Fibrin binding–deficient variants involving charged residues at positions 403, 432, 434, 460, and 462, co-localized in a "patch" on a three-dimensional model of the t-PA protease. In contrast to the earlier view of autonomous functions for individual domains [24], results with the alanine scan variants indicate that all domains of t-PA are involved in high affinity fibrin binding [22]. No site-specific variants of t-PA have been observed to increase fibrin affinity over that of wild-type single-chain t-PA. Many site-directed variants of t-PA, constructed with a variety of protein engineering strategies, have resulted in decreased fibrin binding. However, high-affinity fibrin binding is a sensitive indicator of overall intact t-PA structure. This contrasts with lysine binding, which is effected by a limited set of mutations localized in one domain. Furthermore, there appears to be little correlation between the lysine binding function (mediated by the

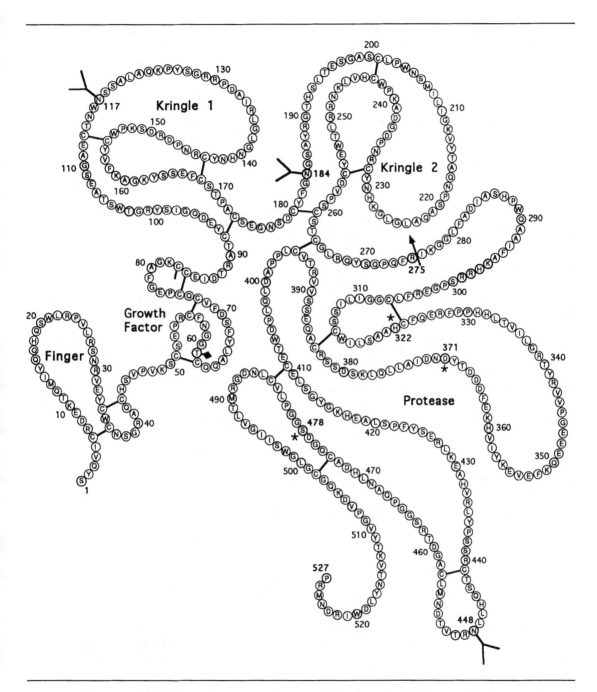

FIGURE 7-2. Diagram of TNK-tPA structure showing domains, disulfides, and glycosylation sites. The primary sequence of this t-PA variant (adapted from refs. 12 and 13) is represented by amino acids abbreviated using the single-letter code. Domains or modules of the protein are described as finger, growth factor, kringle 1, kringle 2, and protease. Disulfide linkages are indicated with black bars between cysteines. N-linked glycosylation sites are represented as black Y-shaped structures at Asn 117, Asn 184, and Asn 448. The active site Ser 478 is noted by an asterisk. The arrow indicates the plasmin cleavage site for conversion of the single-chain to the two-chain form.

K2 domain) and binding to non-degraded, intact fibrin (mediated by multiple domain interactions).

PLASMINOGEN ACTIVATION: FIBRIN STIMULATION

t-PA both binds to fibrin and is stimulated by fibrin. Unlike other plasminogen activators, such as urokinase or streptokinase, t-PA is *fibrin specific* in that its activity is stimulated by fibrin much more than by fibrinogen [3,25,26]. Fibrin stimulation of t-PA activity has been shown to be the result of a large increase in the affinity of the enzyme (t-PA) for the substrate (plasminogen) induced by the cofactor (fibrin). In the absence of fibrin, the K_m of t-PA for Glu-plasminogen is 65 μM. The value for K_m decreases to 0.16 μM in the presence of fibrin, which represents a 400-fold increase in the affinity of t-PA for plasminogen on fibrin [3]. Because the circulating concentration of plasminogen is 2 μM in vivo [9], the role of fibrin serves to regulate and localize the activity of t-PA to the site of the clot. This property of t-PA is important because it restricts the production of plasminogen to sites of fibrin deposition and limits systemic activation of plasminogen, which can lead to a loss of circulating fibrinogen and an increased risk of hemorrhage. The fibrin-specific nature of t-PA is considered to be a significant advantage compared with other fibrinolytic agents for the treatment of thrombotic disorders.

INHIBITION BY PAI-1: REGULATION OF t-PA ACTIVITY

The activity of exogenous t-PA is thought to be primarily localized at the surface of a clot by the fibrin-specific activity of t-PA as well as the affinity of both t-PA and plasminogen for fibrin. The activities of t-PA and plasmin are further regulated and localized by the action of serine protease inhibitors (serpins) in plasma. The most rapid and specific inhibitor of t-PA in plasma is plasminogen activator inhibitor-type I (PAI-1) [27]. PAI-1 rapidly inactivates t-PA by forming a stable, specific 1:1 complex, with a second-order rate constant of approximately $10^7 M^{-1} s^{-1}$ [28,29]. PAI-1 is synthesized by vascular endothelial cells and is released into plasma as a 50-kd protein [30]. In addition to plasma PAI-1, platelet alpha granules also contain high concentrations of PAI-1; however, greater than 90% of platelet PAI-1 is inactive [31].

Although the majority of PAI-1 in platelets is the latent form, the concentration of PAI-1 in platelet-rich clots is orders of magnitude greater than that found in platelet-poor plasma. Thus, the contribution of active PAI-1 from platelets can represent a significant inhibitory activity when localized at the site of a clot. The release of PAI-1 from activated platelets during thrombus formation has led many investigators to suggest that PAI-1 may play a role in stabilizing platelet-rich arterial thrombi, which are known to be resistant to thrombolysis [32,33]. A PAI-1–resistant variant of t-PA may therefore display increased potency as a fibrinolytic agent, especially toward platelet-rich thrombi [34].

BINDING TO HEPATIC RECEPTORS MEDIATES THE PLASMA CLEARANCE OF t-PA

In vivo, t-PA is rapidly removed from circulation by hepatic receptors [35]. Early studies of t-PA pharmacokinetics in rabbits indicated that the liver is the major organ of clearance [36]. The rapid clearance of human t-PA occurs in mice, rats, rabbits, dogs, and rhesus monkeys [37–39]. The pharmacokinetic profile is characterized by a fast alpha phase, which removes most of the circulating t-PA, followed by a slower beta phase of elimination. These and other observations provide evidence for multiple types of hepatic receptors that bind, internalize, and degrade t-PA. There is in vitro and in vivo evidence that implicates at least two types of receptor-mediated clearance: a carbohydrate-dependent and a carbohydrate-independent clearance pathway.

Glycosylation represents the major source of heterogeneity in recombinant t-PA. There is high mannose carbohydrate located at Asn 117 and complex carbohydrate sites at Asn 184 and Asn 448 [40,41] Glycosylation at Asn 184 occurs in approximately 50% of t-PA molecules; hence, the presence or absence of carbohydrate at 184 differentiates t-PA isozymes, known as type I and type II, respectively [42,43]. In addition to the three N-linked glycosylation sites, there is an unusual O-linked glycosylation site, which was identified in the growth factor module of t-PA. Greater than 95% of Thr 61 is modified with a single fucose [44]. The presence of O-linked fucose has also been established in other proteins of fibrinolysis and coagulation, such as urokinase, factor VII, and factor XII [45–47].

The clearance of t-PA has been shown to be mediated, in part, by its glycosylation. In vitro studies have confirmed the binding of wild-type t-PA to the hepatic mannose receptor [5]. Competition binding studies with labeled t-PA incubated with isolated rat hepatocytes in the presence of excess mannosylated ovalbumin showed that much of the t-PA uptake in vitro was mannose dependent [48]. Furthermore, antibodies to the mannose receptor decreased the binding and uptake of t-PA into rat hepatocytes [48]. These studies indicate that the high mannose carbohydrate at Asn 117 contributes to carbohydrate-mediated t-PA clearance via the mannose receptor [5]. Additionally, the presence of exposed terminal galactose residues has also been implicated in t-PA clearance. Lack of complete sialylation of the complex carbohydrate on t-PA leads to accelerated clearance [49] via the hepatic asialoglycoprotein receptor [50]. Complete sialylation (or low levels of exposed galactose) on complex carbohydrate moieties is important for maintaining the circulating lifetime of t-PA.

The recent discovery of fucose on Thr 61 has been considered as another mechanism for hepatic binding of t-PA. Hajjar et al. reported on the binding and uptake of t-PA by the hepatic cell line, Hep-G2 [51]. In these studies, t-PA binding was inhibited by the monosaccharides fucose and galactose, and by fucosylated albumin. Fucosidase was used to remove the O-linked sugar at Thr 61 of t-PA. Hep-G2 cells exhibited 60% reduced binding and uptake of the fucosidase-treated t-PA. These results indicate that O-linked α-fucose may mediate t-PA binding and degradation by Hep-G2 cells, and suggest a potential mechanism for carbohydrate-mediated clearance of t-PA [51].

An additional carbohydrate-independent mechanism for t-PA clearance has been demonstrated by a number of investigators [6,52]. These studies suggest that the low-density lipoprotein receptor–related protein (LRP) [53] can bind and internalize both t-PA and the complex of t-PA plus PAI-1 [54,55]. LRP, also identified as the α_2-macroglobulin receptor [56–58], is a complex of 515-kd and 85-kd proteins present on hepatic parenchymal cells [59,60]. LRP can bind and mediate the endocytosis of a number of unrelated ligands, including t-PA [54], the t-PA–PAI-1 complex [53], the urokinase–PAI-1 complex [61], activated α_2-macroglobulin [57], lipoprotein lipase [62], lactoferrin [63], and apo E–bound very low density lipoprotein (VLDL) [64]. This receptor may be the carbohydrate-independent mechanism for hepatic clearance of t-PA. It is not presently known if there are additional receptors for t-PA.

Approaches to Optimizing Fibrinolytic Function

Can the fibrinolytic properties of t-PA be enhanced by mutagenesis? How can a protein be "improved" that has evolved over millions of years of mammalian development [65]? Presumably natural selection has produced the best possible proteases to dissolve blood clots.

t-PA has been implicated in many cellular processes in which plasminogen activation is involved, such as cell migration, embryogenesis, and neuronal development, as well as fibrinolysis [66–68]. Recent genetic knock-out studies have shown that mice with a t-PA deficiency develop normally, are fertile, and have a normal life span [69]. These mice, whose t-PA gene function has been deleted, do have impaired clot lysis and an increased incidence of endotoxin-induced thrombosis. Because the t-PA–deficient mice are viable and appear to have developed normally, it was suggested that urokinase-type plasminogen activator (u-PA) can effectively serve as an alternative means of generating plasmin in the absence t-PA [69]. With respect to protein engineering of fibrinolytic agents, we must consider that t-PA evolved for various physiological function(s), but not for administration as a therapeutic agent. Compared with wild-type t-PA, variant proteins may exhibit improved properties, which result in more rapid dissolution of large pathologic thrombi.

In designing improved variants of t-PA, one needs to consider what functional changes can be accomplished by altering the protein structure. What are the opportunities for improving t-PA? From a biochemical point of view, there are at least four areas for potential improvement: (1) increasing the fibrin binding of t-PA, (2) increasing the fibrin specificity, (3) decreasing the inhibition of t-PA by plasma inhibitors, and (4) decreasing the plasma clearance rate of t-PA. The feasibility of altering these biochemical parameters can be approached by creating and testing variants of t-PA using in vitro and in vivo experiments. Many assays have been developed to study t-PA function and have been used in the evaluation of t-PA variants. Variants with alterations in specific functions can be used to assess the relative significance of those functional properties to the fibrinolytic activity of t-PA. Protein engineering using site-directed mutagenesis is a integral part in the overall effort of rational drug design. In this chapter, we describe the protein engineering strategies that have been used by different investigators using selected examples of new thrombolytic agents, some of which have been tested in human clinical trials.

INCREASED FIBRIN BINDING

Numerous domain deletion variants were constructed that generally yielded variants having poor fibrin affinity [70,71]. Domain duplication was used with limited success to increase the lysine affinity of t-PA variants. Double K2 variants had increased lysine binding (i.e., FGK2K2P and FGK2K1K2P); however, these molecules displayed no significant increase in fibrin affinity [72,73]. Ikenaka and coworkers attempted to increase fibrin binding by altering the K1 such that both kringles would bind lysine [74].

Mutations were constructed to replicate a portion of the lysine binding sequence of K2 into K1; however, none of these variants displayed greater fibrin affinity; in fact, some were considerably deficient in fibrin binding [74].

The only variants of t-PA observed with increased fibrin affinity are found as naturally occurring isozymes of t-PA. One-chain t-PA has a greater affinity for fibrin than two-chain t-PA [75]. A single-chain variant of t-PA with the plasmin cleavage site deleted (R275E t-PA) exhibits greater fibrin binding than two-chain t-PA [76]. Interestingly, type II t-PA (absence of glycosylation at N184) also has higher fibrin binding than type I t-PA (Keyt and Paoni, unpublished observations). Similarly, deglycosylation variants such as N184Q t-PA (effectively 100% type II t-PA) have increased fibrin affinity compared with wild-type t-PA [77], which is a mixture of approximately equal amounts of type I and type II t-PA [42,43]. The specific activity of type II t-PA was found to be approximately twofold greater than that observed for type I t-PA [78].

Antifibrin Antibody–T-PA Chimeric Molecules. The fibrin specificity of t-PA is mediated by two major mechanisms. First, tPA's catalytic efficiency (k_{cat}/K_m) in converting plasminogen to plasmin is increased by approximately 500- to 1000-fold in the presence of fibrin [3]. Secondly, t-PA binds fibrin and thus increases its local concentration at the site of fibrin clot. In an attempt to enhance this mechanism, Haber and coworkers covalently attached anti-fibrin antibodies to the t-PA molecule [79].

The first step in this approach required a monoclonal antibody that binds to fibrin with high affinity but does not cross-react with fibrinogen. This was accomplished by immunization with a peptide that corresponds to a unique epitope present on fibrin. Exposure of this neo-epitope occurs only after thrombin cleaves fibrinogen to create fibrin [80]. Finally, anti-fibrin antibodies (or fibrin-binding antibody fragments) are attached to t-PA or the catalytic site containing B-chain of t-PA.

Initially, anti-fibrin antibodies were attached to t-PA by means of the disulfide crosslinking reagent N-succinimidyl 3-(2-pyridyldithio)propionate [81,82]. The resulting t-PA–antibody conjugates were 10-fold more potent than t-PA with respect to in vitro fibrinolysis, 3-fold more potent than t-PA in human plasma clot lysis, and 3- to 10-fold more potent than t-PA in vivo [82,83]. The increased fibrinolytic potency was associated with a decrease in the consumption of fibrinogen, plasminogen, and α_2-antiplasmin. Subsequently, recombinant DNA methods were used to make chimeric anti-fibrin antibody–t-PA molecules, proving that it is possible to endow t-PA with enhanced fibrin selectivity through attachment of a fibrin-specific antibody binding site.

ENHANCED FIBRIN SPECIFICITY
The activity of t-PA on plasminogen is unique in its regulation by the physiological cofactors, fibrinogen and/or fibrin. The rate of plasminogen activation is sixfold greater in the presence of fibrinogen versus in its absence [22]. This effect has been called *fibrinogen stimulation*. However, the activity of t-PA on plasminogen is increased 40 times in the presence versus the absence of fibrin [22]. Therefore, the more physiologically relevant cofactor activity is one that measures the *fibrin specificity* of t-PA in plasma, that is, the ratio of t-PA activity on plasminogen in the presence of fibrin (i.e., clotted plasma) over its activity in the presence of fibrinogen (unclotted plasma). This assay evaluates the *clot selectivity* of the plasminogen activator, which is an important function of t-PA that serves to restrict the activation reaction to fibrin clot surfaces rather than in unclotted plasma. Non-specific systemic activation of plasminogen leads to fibrinogen degradation and, in severe instances, can contribute to hemorrhaging [84]. Hence, fibrin specificity or selectivity is a significant attribute to be evaluated in the engineering of t-PA variants.

Vampire Bat Plasminogen Activator. A novel approach to enhancing fibrin selectivity can be observed using diverse animal species as a source of t-PA variants. In the 1970s, it was noticed that the saliva from vampire bats interfered with clot formation in the blood of its host [85]. A plasminogen activator, homologous to human t-PA, was isolated and cloned from the salivary glands of vampire bats (*Desmodus rotundus*) [86,87]. Vampire bat PA is highly homologous (85% identical) with human t-PA, but it lacks kringle 2 and a plasmin cleavage site. The in vitro fibrinolytic activity of vampire bat PA was approximately 65% of wild-type human t-PA on purified human fibrin clots. However, the fibrin specificity of vampire bat PA appeared to be increased by approximately 200-fold compared with wild-type t-PA. Using a soluble form of fibrin, plasminogen activation rates of wild-type t-PA and vampire bat PA were stimulated 205- and 45,000-fold, respectively [86].

The increased fibrin selectivity of the vampire bat PA observed in vitro correlated with increased conservation of circulating fibrinogen, plasminogen, and α_2-antiplasmin in rabbits [88]. Using an equivalent bolus dose of vampire bat PA or wild-type t-PA in a rabbit femoral artery thrombosis model, the levels of these plasma proteins decreased to about 80% or 30% of initial levels, respectively [88]. With a pulmonary embolism model in rats, wild-type t-PA and vampire bat PA were compared in a dosing regimen more appropriate to the intravenous infusion of rapidly cleared thrombolytic agents [89]. Wild-type t-PA decreased fibrinogen, plasminogen, and α_2-antiplasmin by 33%, 38%, and 61%, respectively, whereas bat PA significantly decreased only the α_2-antiplasmin (by 29%). The increased fibrin selectivity exhibited by vampire bat PA is an interesting property to incorporate into a thrombolytic agent such that the conservation of circulating fibrinogen and plasminogen may result in fewer and less severe bleeding complications.

Making t-PA More Fibrin Specific. Increasing the *safety profile* of thrombolytic therapy is at least part of the rationale for making t-PA variants with enhanced fibrin specificity. Early therapeutic regimens used prolonged infusions of t-PA at doses that have been associated with fibrinogen depletion (150 mg per patient), which may put some patients at risk for bleeding [84,90–92]. Increasing the fibrin specificity of t-PA would, in theory, limit the activity of t-PA in the circulation (in the presence of fibrinogen) and localize its lytic action to the site of a fibrin clot. However, the sites or structures on t-PA that confer fibrin stimulation and/or specificity have been considered controversial and were not well characterized. A high-resolution analysis using site-directed mutagenesis allowed the identification of determinants on t-PA that mediate increased plasminogen activation in the presence of fibrin as a cofactor compared with that observed with fibrinogen.

A series of t-PA variants was constructed with point mutations to generate a high-resolution structure-to-function analysis. From one to four charged residues (Arg, Lys, His, Asp, and Glu) in close linear proximity were substituted with alanine, using a scheme called *clustered charged-to-alanine scanning* [93]. Sixty-four alanine variants of t-PA were expressed in cell culture and tested in a variety of assays, including a plasminogen activation assay that compared the relative activity in the presence of fibrin with fibrinogen [22]. A number of mutations in the protease domain significantly decreased plasminogen activation by t-PA in the presence fibrinogen, but not in the presence of fibrin (compared with that observed for wild-type t-PA). The ratio of fibrin- versus fibrinogen-stimulated activity indicated enhanced fibrin specificity for certain t-PA mutants over that of wild-type t-PA. Of particular interest was the 10-fold

increased fibrin specificity ratio for a variant with tetra-alanine substitution: K296A, H297A, R298A, R229A (referred to as the KHRR variant).

Kinetic analyses of the purified KHRR variant and wild-type t-PA were done using fibrinogen and fibrin [94]. In the presence of fibrinogen, wild-type t-PA and the KHRR variant had similar values for the K_m of plasminogen activation. However, in the presene of fibrin the K_m decreased approximately sevenfold and threefold for wild-type t-PA and KHRR t-PA, respectively. The k_{cat} of wild-type t-PA plasminogen activation was virtually unchanged with respect to fibrin or fibrinogen. In contrast, the k_{cat} for the KHRR variant increased 15-fold with fibrin compared with fibrinogen. These data indicated the fibrin specificity of wild-type t-PA is largely due to a reduction in the K_m (for plasminogen) with fibrin instead of fibrinogen. However, the enhanced fibrin specificity of KHRR t-PA was predominantly due to the decreased catalytic efficiency of plasminogen activation in the presence of fibrinogen versus fibrin. Paoni et al. [95] showed that virtually any mutation in the 296–299 region of t-PA generated a variant with the same characteristics of plasminogen activation as the tetra-alanine substitutions. Other sites in the protease domain of t-PA have been described that confer additional fibrin specificity [96,97].

The effect of enhanced fibrin specificity was demonstrated in vitro using a plasma-based assay for fibrinogen conservation [98]. Various concentrations of wild-type or KHRR t-PA were incubated with human plasma for 1 hour at 37°C, after which the amount of clottable fibrinogen was determined. in these studies, approximately 10-fold greater concentrations of KHRR t-PA, compared with wild-type t-PA, were required for consumption of 50% of the fibrinogen. KHRR t-PA was also tested for increased conservation of fibrinogen in vivo and decreased systemic activation of plasminogen. Refino et al. [99] evaluated systemic activation with high doses of wild-type t-PA and KHRR t-PA (2.5 mg/kg intravenous bolus injection) in rabbits by determining the circulating levels of fibrinogen, plasminogen, and α_2-antiplasmin. These plasma proteins, whose levels are sensitive to circulating plasmin, decreased to 20–30% of their initial concentrations 30 minutes after a bolus dose of wild-type t-PA. In contrast, fibrinogen, plasminogen, and α_2-antiplasmin levels were unchanged after administration of KHRR t-PA [99]. Enhanced fibrin specificity and in vitro fibrinogen conservation are correlated with decreased in vivo systemic activation of plasminogen.

The sequence, K296, H297, R298, and R299, is involved in mediating some aspect of the fibrin-

TABLE 7-1. Alignment of the amino-terminal region of selected human serine proteases

	270	280	290	300	310	320
	*	↓ *	*	*	*	*
t-PA	SQPQFRIKGGLFADIASHPWQAAIFA**KHRR**SPGERFLCGGILISSCWILSAAHCF
urokinase	LRPRFKIIGGEFTTIENQPWFAAIY**RRH-R**GGSVTYVCGGSLMSPCWVISATHCF
prothrombin	SYIDGRIVEGSDAEIGMSPWQVMLFR----KSPQELLCGASLISDRWVLTAAHCL
plasminogen	KKCPGRVVGGCVAHPHSWPWQVSLRT-----RFGMHFCGGTLISPEWVLTAAHCL
Factor VII	SKPQGRIVGGKVCPKGECPWQVLLL------VNGAQLCGGTLINTIWVVSAAHCF
Factor IX	FNDFTRVVGGEDAKPGQFPWQVVLN------GKVDAFCGGSIVNEKIVTAAHCV
Factor X	DNNLTRIVGGQECKDGECPWQALLIN-----EENEGFCGGTILSEFYILTAAHCL
trypsin	FDDDDKIVGGYNCEENSVPYQVSLN-------SGYHFCGGSLINEQWVVSAGHCY

These proteases (or protease homologs, such as hepatocyte growth factor) are aligned on the basis of conserved cysteines and the zymogen-activation cleavage site (Arg or Lys followed by Ile or Val), which is indicated by an arrow. The numbering of amino acids is that of human t-PA. The bold residues, including K296, H297, R298, and R299, of t-PA indicate the unique sequence that exists as an apparent insertion in fibrinolytic enzymes (t-PA and u-PA) but not in other related serine proteases.

t-PA = human tissue plasminogen activator [12]; ukn = human urokinase-type plasminogen activator [100]; pro = human prothrombin [149]; plgn = human plasminogen [150]; FVII = human factor VIII [151]; FIX = human factor IX [152]; FX = human factor X [153]; tryp = human trypsin [154].

specific function of t-PA. By inspection of this region from various serine proteases (Table 7-1), this tetrapeptide insertion appears unique to plasminogen activators, t-PA [12] and urokinase [100], both of which have a highly basic series of amino acids in this location (KHRR and RRHR, respectively). By homology with other proteases whose three-dimensional structure is known by x-ray crystallography, this region of t-PA is likely to be an exposed loop near the active-site cleft [22]. Recently, the three-dimensional structure of the catalytic domain of t-PA has been elucidated with 2.3 Å resolution [101]. Lamba and coworkers prepared a nonglycosylated form of two-chain t-PA protease in E. coli, which shows the region Lys 296 to Arg 304 as an exposed, partially disordered loop; therefore, this region is able to adopt different structures during interaction with other proteins, such as plasminogen and PAI-1. It is hypothesized that the fibrin specificity mediated by mutations of the 296–304 sequence occurs by decreasing the strength of the local interaction of t-PA with plasminogen. Although this region does not interact directly with fibrin, the KHRR(296–299)AAAA mutation makes t-PA more dependent on its other interactions with fibrin, namely, the *fibrin binding patch* in the protease [22] and domain interactions of the A-chain. Decreased plasminogen activation in solution (absence of fibrin) is exhibited by molecules such as KHRR t-PA. However, this variant and other fibrin-specific molecules recover normal levels of plasminogen activation (in the presence of fibrin) as a result of the other t-PA structures that serve to co-localize t-PA on fibrin in a productive complex with plasminogen.

RESISTANCE TO PLASMINOGEN ACTIVATOR INHIBITOR-TYPE I

In addition to the presence of fibrin cofactors, the activity of t-PA is also regulated by the action of a fast-acting protease inhibitor in plasma. The most rapid and specific inhibitor of t-PA in plasma is plasminogen activator inhibitor-type I [81]. Because PAI-1 circulates in plasma at a higher concentration than that of t-PA, most of the endogenous t-PA is identified in plasma as an inactive complex with PAI-1 [102]. It is anticipated that a PAI-1–resistant variant of t-PA may display increased potency as a fibrinolytic agent, especially towards platelet-rich thrombi [34,103].

Deletion of Serpin Binding Loop in t-PA. By aligning the sequences of trypsin and t-PA (see Table 7-1), Madison and coworkers noticed a unique heptapeptide region present in t-PA (amino acids 296–303) and urokinase but not in other serine proteases [104]. Furthermore, these investigators reasoned that the interaction of t-PA and PAI-1 would be comparable with that of trypsin and bovine pancreatic trypsin inhibitor (BPTI). Based on analogy with trypsin in its complex with BPTI [105], the loop peptide 296–303 of t-PA was predicted to interact with PAI-1 [104]. A variant of t-PA with residues 296–302 deleted was constructed and tested for PAI-1 resistance [104]. Under conditions in which t-PA was fully inhibited by PAI-1, des (296–302) t-PA was approximately 95% active. This degree of resistance corresponded to a 470-fold decrease in the second-order rate constant for the inhibition of des (296–302) t-PA by PAI-1 [106]. The greatest degree of resistance to PAI-1 was observed with a charge reversal variant (K296E, R298E, R229E t-PA), which displayed a 2800-fold decreased inhibition rate constant. A reversion mutant of PAI-1 (E350R) was constructed that was inhibited by the serpin-resistant mutant, R304E t-PA [107].

Charge Neutralization in T-PA. The determinants involved in mediating the t-PA–PAI-1 interaction were surveyed by analyzing charged-to-alanine t-PA mutants. Sixty-four alanine mutants were incubated with a molar excess of PAI-1, and then were evaluated for residual enzymatic activity. Only a single t-PA mutant, which contained the KHRR(296–299)AAAA substitution, exhibited a significant degree of resistance to PAI-1 [22]. The second-order rate of inhibition for the KHRR variant was decreased 90-fold compared with that of wild-type t-PA [98]. The studies with charged-to-alanine scan variants of t-PA indicated that there appeared a single PAI-1 interaction site on t-PA and that PAI-1 resistance is mediated by a restricted set of positively charged amino acids near the active site of t-PA. It is anticipated that this basic sequence on t-PA interacts with negatively charged amino acids in PAI-1 at the P4' and P5' positions [101] (Table 7-2).

The role of PAI-1 in the lysis of platelet-rich clots has been examined in vitro and in vivo by numerous investigators [31,33,108]. PAI-1 is released from platelets during thrombus formation, binds to fibrin, and contributes to the thrombolytic resistance of platelet-rich clots. Anti–PAI-1 monoclonal antibodies have been used to neutralize the effect of PAI-1 on endogenous thrombolysis in experimental models of thrombosis [33]. Based on these observations, PAI-1–resistant variants were tested in vivo for increased efficacy in thrombolysis of whole-blood clot lysis or platelet-rich clots. The thrombolytic potency in rabbits of the KHRR variant of t-PA was similar to wild-type t-PA on thrombi made from rabbit whole blood [99]. However, this PAI-1–resistant variant was 2.6-fold more potent than wild-type t-PA in the lysis of platelet-enriched thrombi. These results indicate that the PAI-1–resistant variants are more active on platelet-rich clots, suggesting that PAI-1 may contibure to the thrombolytic resistance of platelet-rich clots. In a rabbit model of endotoxin-induced PAI-1 induction, the KHRR mutant of t-PA demonstrated increased in vivo thrombolysis compared with that observed using wild-type t-PA [34].

PROLONGING THE CIRCULATING LIFETIME OF T-PA

Considerable effort has been dedicated to altering the rate of t-PA clearance to create a more convenient therapeutic agent having a longer half-life. Because t-PA is rapidly cleared from circulation, thrombolytic therapy requires a relatively large dose of t-PA (100 mg) administered by continous intravenous infusion to maintain adequate plasma concentrations for lysis. Many slow-clearing variants of t-PA have been constructed, using the techniques of molecular biology, to facilitate the therapeutic use of a single-bolus intravenous administration. Three long half-life variants of t-PA have been studied in clinical trials; the biological properties of selected t-PA variants are summarized in the following sections.

Domain Deletions of t-PA. Single or multiple domain deletion mutants of t-PA have been constructed by numerous investigators [19,24,109], and the resulting proteins have been analyzed for functional differences. Many domain deletion variants exhibited a significantly increased circulating half-life, indicating that major clearance determinants are localized in one or more of the amino-terminal domains (F, G, and K1). Des-finger t-PA (lacking residues 6–50) had a 10-fold decreased clearance in rats and a 20-fold increase in circulating half-life [110] compared with wild-type t-PA. Similar results were observed with the des-growth factor t-PA (des 51–87) in a variety of species; in vivo half-life was extended from 4- to

TABLE 7-2. Sequences near the scissile bonds of the t-PA substrate, plasminogen, and the inhibitor, PAI-1

	P4	P3	P2	P1	↓	P1'	P2'	P3'	P4'	P5'
Plasminogen	Cys	Pro	Gly	Arg		Val	Val	Gly	Gly	Cys
PAI-1	Val	Ser	Ala	Arg		Met	Ala	Pro	Glu	Glu

PAI-1 = plasminogen activator inhibitor-type 1.

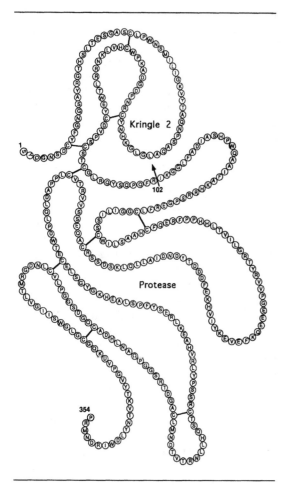

FIGURE 7-3. Diagram of the truncated t-PA variant, r-PA (Reteplase, BM 06.022). This domain deletion form of t-PA is lacking the finger, growth factor, and kringle 1 modules. The amino terminus contains the first three amino acids of t-PA, followed by the kringle 2 and protease sequences. This nonglycosylated protein is expressed in *E. coli.*

Although many domain deletion variants have substantially reduced clearance, the thrombolytic activity of these proteins has been compromised. Specific in vivo thrombolytic potency is a measure of clot lysis in an animal model for a given plasma concentration of lytic agent [114]. For example, the in vivo thrombolytic potency of des-FG t-PA was similar to that of wild-type t-PA, despite a 10-fold increase in plasma concentration [113,114]. Thus, the specific in vivo thrombolytic activity of des-FG t-PA was markedly reduced compared with wild-type t-PA. Numerous domain deletion, insertion, and chimeric variants of t-PA have been constructed with reduced plasma clearance; however, all exhibited reduced in vivo specific thrombolytic activity [114]. Deletion of whole domains appears to be a destructive approach to constructing t-PA mutants with reduced clearance and has resulted in truncated forms of t-PA with less than the full thrombolytic activity.

The first three domains of t-PA were deleted in a variant consisting of the second kringle and the catalytic domain (K2P) (Figure 7-3). This protein, termed *r-PA*, is expressed in *E. coli* as a nonglycosylated variant (Reteplase, Boehringer Mannheim 06.022) with a molecular weight of 39 kd [118]. As expected, r-PA exhibits decreased fibrin binding and increased half-life in rats, rabbits, dogs, and primates [119,120]. In a rabbit model, the effective doses for half-maximal thrombolysis were 0.28 mg/kg and 1.09 mg/kg for r-PA and t-PA, respectively, indicating a 3.9-fold increase in relative potency for r-PA [119]. Plasma clearance for r-PA was 4.3-fold slower than for t-PA in rabbits (4.7 vs. 1.2 ml/min/kg), suggesting that the increased potency of r-PA is due solely to the increased in vivo half-life. An initial half-life of 14–18 minutes was observed with r-PA in healthy human volunteers and in acute myocardial infarct patients [121,122]. In a pilot study with 320 patients, a double bolus of r-PA (10 million units, twice, 30 minutes apart) achieved patency rates that were greater than those observed with front-loaded t-PA [123]. However, in a large-scale randomized trial with 6000 patients, a double bolus of r-PA was equivalent to streptokinase with respect to 30-day mortality [124]. Currently, the double-bolus administration of r-PA is being compared with accelerated infusion of Activase®t-PA in over 10,000 myocardial infarction patients (GUSTO III).

Glycosylation Variants of t-PA. Some of the early site-specific mutants of t-PA altered glycosylation sites. Enzymatically deglycosylating t-PA, using either N-glycanase or α-mannosidase, leads to a two-fold reduction in the clearance rate in rabbits [125].

10-fold in rats, rabbits, and guinea pigs [110–112]. Deletion of both F and G domains (des 6–86 t-PA) resulted in approximately 10-fold reduced clearance in mice and rabbits [110,113–116]. Des-kringle 1 t-PA displayed reduced clearance similar to that of des-G t-PA, whereas des-kringle 2 t-PA was cleared more rapidly than wild-type t-PA [117]. These studies indicate the major clearance determinants of t-PA are located in the F, G, and K1 domains, or possibly that disruption of any of these domains alters other structure(s) of t-PA that directly mediate in vivo clearance.

Site-specific mutagenesis (i.e., N117Q) was employed to delete the glycosylation at position 117, which resulted in 50% reduction in clearance in rabbits [125,126]. Furthermore, a double deglycosylation variant (N117Q, N184Q t-PA) was shown to have a 2.3-fold slower clearance rate than wild-type t-PA [77,127]. Substitution of N184Q or N448Q as single-site mutations did not alter the clearance of t-PA in mice (B. Keyt, unpublished observation). In contrast to many slow-clearing variants that exhibit decreased in vivo specific thrombolytic activity, the deglycosylated variant, N117Q t-PA, yields a modest reduction in clearance (twofold) and exhibits the normal fibrinolytic activity of t-PA [125,126].

Novel Sites of Glycosylation. In 1988, Anderson and Keyt constructed variants of t-PA with additional N-linked glycosylation sites not present in the wild-type protein [128]. Introducing novel glycosylation sites on t-PA in the appropriate location may block or mask a clearance determinant and thus prolong the circulating half-life. Nominal requirements for N-linked glycosylation include the presence of a consensus sequence — Asn-X-Ser or Asn-X-Thr (where X is any amino acid except proline) at a surface-accessible site [129,130]. An appropriate site for extra-glycosylation within the growth factor domain was identified as Tyr 67-Phe 68-Ser 69, a sequence found only in t-PA and urokinase [128]. A variant, prepared with Tyr 67 replaced by Asn, displayed 60% of the clearance rate of wild-type t-PA in rabbits [128]. However, the in vitro fibrin binding and fibrinolytic activities decreased by twofold, such that the in vivo thrombolytic potency was not increased with Y67N t-PA in rabbits (C. Refino, unpublished results). Bassell-Duby et al. also prepared Y67N t-PA and related variants, which were evaluated by hepatocyte binding and clearance in rats [131]. The addition of carbohydrate (Y67N t-PA), and the combination of addition and deletion of carbohydrate (Y67N, S119M t-PA), had twofold and fivefold longer alpha-phase half-lives in rats, respectively.

Additional neo-glycosylation sites in other t-PA domains were evaluated to identify variants that exhibit reduced clearance and normal fibrinolytic activity [128]. The most effective site for addition of carbohydrate, with respect to reducing plasma clearance, was identified by alanine scanning (unpublished observations) as a site in kringle 1 of t-PA. The substitution of Asn for Thr at position 103 was used to design a variant, T103N t-PA, which cleared at a rate 6-fold and 13-fold less in rats and rabbits, respectively [98]. Interestingly, the four sites of N-

linked glycosylation on T103N t-PA are all of the complex carbohydrate type [132]. The addition of carbohydrate at position 103 is associated with the conversion of the high mannose carbohydrate at N117 to the complex glycoform. It is likely that some of the slow-clearing phenotype of the T103N mutation is due to the lack of mannosyl glycoforms and the associated binding to the hepatic mannose receptor.

Combination of Selected Mutations in Tissue Plasminogen Activator

Using recombinant DNA technology, the t-PA protein sequence can be altered, possibly improving its function. Foremost in these efforts to improve t-PA was the identification of variants with a reduced rate of plasma clearance, such that the t-PA variant could effectively be administered by bolus injection. In this chapter we have examined protein design strategies, such as the creation of chimeric molecules, homologous loop "swaps" and/or deletion, charged-to-alanine scanning, charge reversal, domain deletion, and carbohydrate insertion and/or deletion. These approaches to altering protein structure by mutagenesis were evaluated in animal models and, in some instances, in human clinical trials for treatment of acute myocardial infarction.

There is a potential problem that must be addressed when considering bolus administration of a fully active t-PA: When t-PA is given as a bolus (or even as an infusion at high doses), the plasma levels of enzyme increase rapidly and plasminogen becomes activated throughout the circulation as well as on the surface of the clot. This systemic plasmin generation causes decreased levels of circulating plasminogen, fibrinogen, and α_2-antiplasmin. An undesirable consequence of systemic activation is bleeding, which may be related to plasminemia rather than fibrinogen depletion per se; both peripheral and intracranial hemorrhage are associated with systemic activation [84]. One way to reduce systemic activation is to make t-PA even more fibrin specific; that is, to reduce its activity in the absence of clotted plasma. Systematic mutagenesis of t-PA yielded mutations in the protease domain that have this property of increased fibrin specificity [22]; the best characterized example is a tetra-alanine substitution at positions 296–299 [95,96].

In our mutagenesis studies, we found variants that exhibit reduced plasma clearance of t-PA sufficient to provide effective thrombolysis when the agent is administered as a bolus. It was a novel type of mutation, T103N (which has an additional glycosylation site on kringle 1), that produced a variant with the most suitable pharmacokinetic profile. That mutation in combination with the tetra-alanine substitution at positions 296–299 yielded a t-PA variant with the desired clearance rate and enhanced fibrin specificity [98,99]. However, this combination variant still did not yield full in vitro or in vivo fibrinolytic activity when compared with wild-type t-PA. The key factor appears to be maintenance of the fibrin affinity of the molecule, which was achieved by an additional mutation, N117Q [125]. With the appropriate combination of mutations at three distinct sites of t-PA, it is possible to reduce the clearance while retaining full fibrinolytic activity. The resultant variant, TNK-tPA, is substantially more potent than wild-type t-PA [133].

BIOCHEMISTRY AND PHARMACOLOGY OF T103N, N117Q, KHRR(296–299)AAA

The most effective, long half-life tPA variant contained an extra-glycosylation site in kringle 1 created by the substitution of Asn for Thr at 103 (T103N, henceforth T) [98]. In another variant, the high mannose structure at position 117 was removed by a de-glycosylation substitution, N117Q (abbreviated N). This variant exhibited a modest reduction in clearance in rabbits, with minimal perturbation of fibrinolytic activity [125,126]. A combination variant (TN-tPA) was created with extra-glycosylation and de-glycosylation at positions 103 and 117, respectively, which effectively moved the glycosylation site on kringle 1 from position 117 to position 103.

Alanine scanning mutagenesis was used to identify KHRR(296–299)AAAA, a mutation that confers both fibrin specificity and PAI-1 resistance [22,104]. This variant (abbreviated as K) has improved fibrin specificity, because it has eightfold less activity in the absence of fibrin while retaining full activity in the presence of fibrin. The K variant of t-PA was shown to be approximately 90-fold more resistant to the "fast-acting" plasminogen activator inhibitor 1 (PAI-1), as determined by the second-order inhibition rate constants of variant and wild-type t-PA [98]. To create a variant of t-PA with reduced clearance, enhanced fibrin specificity, and PAI-1 resistance, the mutations at three loci were combined in the T103N, N117Q, KHRR(296–299)AAAA variant of tPA (TNK-tPA).

TNK-tPA has been engineered to be more fibrin specific than t-PA. This property is the result of the KHRR(296–299)AAAA mutation (K of TNK-tPA). To determine the effect of increased fibrin specificity on fibrinogen degradation, various concentrations of t-PA or TNK-tPA were incubated in human citrated plasma for 1 hour at 37°C and were subsequently assayed for residual fibrinogen by the Clauss method [134]. The concentration of activator at which 50% of the initial fibrinogen concentration was depleted (EC_{50}) was determined from a four-parameter fit of the fibrinogen versus activator concentration data. These data (Figure 7-4) indicate that the K mutation allows TNK-tPA to be present at approximately 12-fold higher concentrations before significant fibrinogen depletion is observed in human plasma [135].

Pharmacokinetics and Pharmacodynamics of TNK-tPA in Rabbits. The clearance of TNK-tPA and t-PA was compared in rabbits following bolus intravenous injections. The area under the curve was 8.4-fold greater than for wild-type t-PA, which yielded clearance values of 1.9 versus 1.61 mL/min/kg for TNK-tPA and t-PA, respectively [133]. Pharmacokinetic analysis of TNK-tPA indicated alpha- and beta-phase half-lives of approximately 9 and 31 minutes, compared with t-PA, which exhibited alpha, beta, and gamma phases with half-lives of 1.3, 6, and 33 minutes, respectively. The thrombolytic potency of TNK-tPA (by bolus) was compared with that of t-PA (by infusion) in a rabbit arteriovenous shunt model of clot lysis [96]. Clots were made from fresh rabbit whole blood or citrate collected plasma spiked with rabbit platelet-enriched plasma to a platelet concentration of 0.8×10^6 platelets/μL. The extent of lysis after 2 hours was evaluated with doses ranging from 7

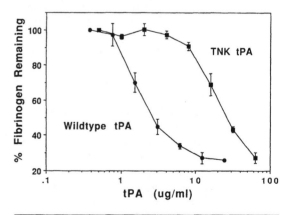

FIGURE 7-4. In vitro fibrinogenolysis in human plasma.

to 180 μg/kg for TNK-tPA, and from 20 to 540 μg/kg for Activase® t-PA. The relative potency of TNK-tPA was determined from the ED_{50} of a fit of the dose–response curves. From this analysis, TNK-tPA was 7.5 and 13.5 times more potent than t-PA in lysing rabbit whole-blood and platelet-enriched clots, respectively [133].

Biological Activity of TNK-tPA in a Rabbit Model of Embolic Stroke. The biological activity of TNK-tPA was also tested in a rabbit model of embolic stroke. In this model, described in detail previously [136,137], a preformed, radiolabeled clot is instilled into the middle cerebral artery via the internal carotid artery. Clot lysis is monitored by gamma scintigraphy. TNK-tPA was shown to be active in this model when given as a single bolus, and the extent of lysis was dose dependent. With an intravenous dose of 0.6 mg/kg, 21 of 34 animals exhibited greater than 75% lysis of the instilled clot 2 hours after treatment [137]. This bolus regimen of TNK-tPA was as effective as an infusion regimen of Activase® (3.3 mg/kg/h).

Biological Activity of TNK-tPA in a Rabbit Model of Electrically Induced Carotid Artery Thrombosis. Thrombolytic properties of TNK-tPA were compared with those of t-PA in a rabbit model of carotid artery occlusion. In this model, a thrombus was formed in a rabbit carotid artery by electrical stimulation, which resulted in disrupted vessel endothelium and 50% occlusion of the artery [for a related canine model, see refs. 138–140]. After 1 hour, TNK-tPA or t-PA was administered intravenously by bolus or front-loaded infusion for 1.5 hours, respectively. Blood flow in the vessel was monitored for 2 hours, during which bleeding was assessed by blood loss from a surgical incision. The following parameters were monitored: incidence of reperfusion, time to reperfusion, duration of patency, residual thrombus weight, and blood loss from the abdominal wall incisional site. In addition, systemic plasminogen activation in vivo was evaluated by measuring the plasma concentration of fibrinogen, plasminogen, and α_2-antiplasmin.

In this model, bolus intravenous administration of TNK-tPA will restore blood flow rapidly in a thrombosed carotid artery without increasing systemic plasmin generation [141]. TNK-tPA was administered as a bolus at doses of 0.38, 0.75, and 1.5 mg/kg. For comparison, t-PA was administered as an infusion at doses of 1.5, 3.0, 6.0, and 9.0 mg/kg. The doses that produced greater than 80% incidence of patency with the longest duration of patency were

1.5 mg/kg for TNK-tPA and 9.0 mg/kg for t-PA. At these doses, the time to reperfusion was significantly less for TNK-tPA (11 ± 2 minutes) when compared with t-PA (23 ± 7 minutes). Similarly, the duration of patency was significantly greater for TNK-tPA (82 ± 9 minutes) when compared with t-PA (51 ± 18 minutes). At the maximal doses tested, the residual thrombus weight of the TNK-tPA–treated animals (4.2 ± 0.4 mg) was significantly less ($P < 0.01$) than saline-treated controls (8.6 ± 0.4 mg) and the t-PA–treated rabbits (8.0 ± 0.7 mg).

The effects of TNK-tPA on fibrinogen, plasminogen, and α_2-antiplasmin levels were modest when compared with those observed with t-PA. At the highest dose of TNK-tPA (1.5 mg/kg), the plasma levels of fibrinogen, plasminogen, or α_2-antiplasmin were significantly greater than the corresponding values for t-PA at either 6.0 mg/kg or 9.0 mg/kg [141]. Blood loss with TNK-tPA–treated animals was significantly less compared with that observed with t-PA–treated rabbits. These studies indicate that a bolus intravenous administration of TNK-tPA, compared with a front-loaded infusion of t-PA, produces rapid and complete recanalization of an occluded carotid artery without increasing systemic plasmin generation or peripheral bleeding. The thrombolytic potency of TNK-tPA was fourfold to sixfold greater than that of t-PA with respect to incidence of reperfusion, duration of patency, and extent of lysis.

Biological Activity of TNK-tPA in a Canine Model of Electrically Induced Coronary Thrombosis. The biological activity of TNK-tPA versus t-PA was tested in a canine model of coronary thrombosis. In this canine model, a thrombus is formed by the disruption of the intimal surface of the coronary artery induced by electrical current [142–146]. The thrombolytic effects of TNK-tPA and t-PA were compared with respect to time of reperfusion, extent of thrombolysis, and the incidence of recurrent rethrombosis. In this model, bolus intravenous administration of TNK-tPA restored blood flow effectively in a thrombosed coronary artery. TNK-tPA (administered as a bolus at 1 mg/kg) achieved 100% patency (n = 9), whereas t-PA (administered intravenously as a 1 mg/kg infusion over 20 minutes) resulted in 67% patency rates (n = 12). The rate of reocclusion was lower in the TNK-tPA group (67%) versus the t-PA group (88%), and the duration of vessel patency was greater with TNK-tPA compared with that observed with t-PA (78 minutes vs 51 minutes, respectively). TNK-tPA–treated animals exhibited a higher incidence of patency, a lower rate of reocclusion, and a greater duration of patency than animals treated with t-PA.

CLINICAL EXPERIENCE WITH TNK-tPA IN TIMI 10A

TNK-tPA has undergone initial clinical evaluation in the treatment of acute myocardial infarction (AMI) in a phase I trial (TIMI 10A) [147]. TIMI 10A was an open-label, dose-ranging, pilot trial of single-bolus, intravenous TNK-tPA in patients with acute myocardial infarction (AMI). Eligible patients were greater than 70 years old, with symptom onset of less than 12 hours duration and electrocardiographic evidence of AMI or new left bundle branch block without contraindications to thrombolytic therapy. All patients received oral aspirin and intravenous heparin therapy titrated to an activated partial thromboplastin time (aPTT) of 55–85 seconds. Endpoints included pharmacokinetic analysis, effect on hemostatic parameters, angiographic assessment by TIMI flow grade and TIMI frame count, and safety evaluation. Doses ranging from 5 mg to 50 mg were studied in a total of 113 patients.

Preliminary results of the TIMI 10A trial were presented at the 68th Annual Scientific Sessions of the American Heart Association [147]. At the 30, 40, and 50 mg doses, patency rates achieved with TNK-tPA were at least as good as, if not superior to, patency rates achieved with accelerated t-PA in the GUSTO I trial. Preliminary pharmacokinetic data from the TIMI 10A trial showed TNK-tPA to have a plasma clearance of approximately one-third that of Activase t-PA (198 ± 42 mL/min) and an elimination half-life of 15–19 minutes. Little effect was observed on coagulation parameters, and negligible fibrinogen or plasminogen consumption was noted. No intracranial (IC) bleeding, anaphylaxis, or antigenicity was observed. Adverse events reported in the TIMI 10A trial, which included escalating bolus doses of TNK-tPA, resulted in a safety profile comparable with that observed in other thrombolytic trials. Due to the limited sample size (113 patients), additional, larger trials are necessary to define the efficacy and safety profile of TNK-tPA.

References

1. Madison EL. Probing structure-function relationships of tissue-type plasminogen activatory by site-specific mutagenesis. Fibrinolysis 8(Suppl. 1):221, 1994.
2. Keyt BA, Paoni NF, Bennett WF. Site-directed mutagenesis of tissue-type plasminogen activator. In Cleland JL, Craik CS (eds). Protein Engineering: Principles and Practice. New York: Wiley-Liss, 435, 1996.
3. Hoylaerts M, Rijken DC, Lijnen HR, Collen D. On the regulation and control of fibrinolysis. J Biol Chem 257:2912, 1982.
4. Wagner OF, de Vries C, Hohmann C, Veerman H, Pannekoek H. Interaction between plasminogen activator inhibitor 1 (PAI-1) bound to fibrin and either tissue-type plasminogen (t-PA) or urokinase-type plasminogen activator (u-PA). J Clin Invest 84:647, 1989.
5. Otter M, Barrett-Bergshoeff MM, Rijken DC. Binding of tissue-type plasminogen activator by the mannose receptor. J Biol Chem 266:13931, 1991.
6. Bu G, Warshawsky I, Schwartz AL. Cellular receptors for the plasminogen activators. Blood 83:3427, 1994.
7. Garabedian HD, Gold HK, Leinbach RC, Johns JA, Yasuda T, Kanuke M, Collen D. Comparative properties of two clinical preparations of recombinant human tissue-type plasminogen activator in patients with acute myocardial infarction. J Am Coll Cardiol 9:599, 1987.
8. Rijken DC, Juhan-Vague I, De Cock F, Collen D. Measurement of human tissue-type plasminogen activator by a two-site immunoradiometric assay. J Lab Clin Med 101:274, 1983.
9. Rabiner SF, Goldfine JD, Hart A, Summaria L, Robbins KC. Radioimmunoassay of human plasminogen and plasmin. J Lab Clin Med 74:265, 1969.
10. Booth, NA, Simpson AJ, Croll A, Bennett B, MacGregor IR. Plasminogen activator inhibitor (PAI-1) in plasma and platelets. Br J Haematol 70:327, 1988.
11. Moroi M, Aoki N. Isolation and characterization of alpha-2-plasmin inhibitor from human plasma. A novel proteinase inhibitor which inhibits activator-induced clot lysis. J Biol Chem 251:5956, 1976.
12. Pennica D, Holmes WE, Kohr WJ, Harkins RN, Vehar GA, Ward CA, Bennett WF, Yelverton E, Seeberg PH, Heyneker HL, Goeddel DV, Collen D. Cloning and expression of human tissue-type plasminogen activator cDNA in E. coli. Nature 301:214, 1983.
13. Banyai L, Varadi A, Patthy L. Common evolutionary origin of the fibrin-binding structures of fibronectin and tissue-type plasminogen activator. FEBS Lett 163:37, 1983.
14. Ny T, Elgh F, Lund B. The structure of the human tissue-type plasminogen activator gene: Correlation of intron and exon structures to functional and structural domains. Proc Natl Acad Sci USA 81:5355, 1984.
15. Patthy L. Evolution of the proteases of blood coagulation and fibrinolysis by assembly from modules. Cell 41:657, 1985.
16. van Zonneveld AJ, Veerman H, Pannekoek HJ. Autonomous functions of structural domains on human tissue-type plasminogen activator. Proc Natl Acad Sci USA 83:4670, 1986.

17. Rijken DC, Groenveld E. Isolation and functional characterization of the heavy and light chains of human tissue-type plasminogen activator. J Biol Chem 261:3098, 1986.

18. Holvoet P, Lijnen HR, Collen D, Characterization of functional domains in human tissue-type plasminogen activator with the use of monoclonal antibodies. Eur J Biochem 158:173, 1986.

19. Verheijen JH, Caspers MPM, Chang GTG, de Munk GAW, Pouwels PH, Enger-Valk BE. Involvement of finger domain and kringle 2 domain of tissue-type plasminogen activator in fibrin binding and stimulation of activity of fibrin. EMBO J 5:3525, 1986.

20. Larsen GR, Hensen K, Blue Y. Variants of human tissue-type plasminogen activator. J Biol Chem 263:1023, 1988.

21. de Vries C, Veerman H, Pannekoek H. Identification of the domains of tissue-type plasminogen activator involved in the augmented binding to fibrin after limited digestion with plasmin. J Biol Chem 264:12604, 1989.

22. Bennett WF, Paoni NF, Keyt BA, Botstein D, Jones AJS, Presta L, Wurm FM, Zoller MJ. High resolution analysis of functional determinants on human tissue-type plasminogen activator. J Biol Chem 266:5191, 1991.

23. Keyt B, Berleau LT, Nguyen H, Bennett WF. Radioiodination of the active site of tissue plasminogen activator: A method for radiolabeling serine proteases with tyrosylprolylarginyl chloromethyl ketone. Anal Biochem 206:73, 1992.

24. van Zonneveld AJ, Veerman H, Pannekoek H. On the interaction of the finger and the kringle-2 domain of tissue-type plasminogen activator with fibrin. J Biol Chem 261:14214, 1986.

25. Rijken DC, Hoylaerts M, Collen D. Fibrinolytic properties of one-chain and two-chain human extrinsic (tissue-type) plasminogen activator. J Biol Chem 257:2920, 1982.

26. Rånby M. Studies on the kinetics of plasminogen activation by tissue plasminogen activator. Biochim Biophys Acta 704:461, 1982.

27. Schneiderman J, Loskutoff DJ. Plasminogen activator inhibitors. Trends Cardiovasc Med 1:99, 1991.

28. Hekman C, Loskutoff DJ. Kinetic analysis of the interactions between plasminogen activator inhibitor 1 and both urokinase and tissue plasminogen activator. Arch Biochem Biophys 262:199, 1988.

29. Chmielewska J, Ranby M, Wiman B. Kinetics of the inhibition of plasminogen activators by the plasminogen-activator inhibitor. Biochem J 251:327, 1988.

30. DeClerck PJ, Alessi M-C, Verstreken M, Kruithof EKO, Juhan-Vague I, Collen D. Measurement of plasminogen activator inhibitor 1 in biologic fluids with a murine monoclonal antibody-based enzyme-linked immunosorbant assay. Blood 71:220, 1988.

31. Booth NA, Robbie LA, Croll AM, Bennett B. Lysis of platelet-rich thrombi: The role of PAI-1. Ann N Y Acad Sci 667:70, 1992.

32. Potter van Loon BJ, Rijken DC, Brommer EJP, van der Maas APC. The amount of plasminogen, t-PA and PAI-1 in human thrombi and the relation to ex-vivo lysibility. Thromb Haemost 67:101, 1992.

33. Levi M, Biemond BJ, van Zonneveld A-J, ten Cate JW, Pannekoek H. Inhibition of plasminogen activator inhibitor-1 activity results in promotion of endogenous thrombolysis and inhibition of thrombus extension in models of experimental thrombosis. Circulation 85:305, 1992.

34. Krishnamurti C, Keyt B, Maglasang P, Alving BM. PAI-1 resistant t-PA: Low doses prevent fibrin deposition in rabbits with increased PAI-1 activity. Blood 87:14, 1996.

35. Krause J. Catabolism of tissue-type plasminogen activator (t-PA), its variants, mutants and hybrids. Fibrinolysis 2:133, 1988.

36. Korninger C, Stassen JM, Collen D. Turnover of human extrinsic (tissue-type) plasminogen activator in rabbits. Thromb Haemost 46:658, 1981.

37. Beebe DP, Aronson DL. Turnover of tissue-type plasminogen activator (t-PA) in rabbits. Thromb Res 43:663, 1986.

38. Einarsson M, Smedrød B, Pertoft H. Uptake and degradation of tissue-type plasminogen activator in rat liver. Thromb Haemost 59:474, 1988.

39. Berleau LT, Refino CJ, Modi N, Bennett WF, Keyt BA. Interspecies scaling of wildtype t-PA and TNK-tPA: Prediction of TNK-tPA clearance in humans. Fibrinolysis 8 (Suppl 1):26, 1994.

40. Pohl G, Kenne L, Nilsson B, Einarsson M. Isolation and characterization of three different carbohydrate chains from melanoma tissue plasminogen activator. Eur J Biochem 170:69, 1987.

41. Spellman MW, Basa LJ, Leonard CK, Chakel JA, O'Connor JV, Wilson S, van Halbeek H. Carbohydrate structures of human tissue plasminogen activator expressed in Chinese hamster ovary cells. J Biol Chem 264:1410, 1989.

42. Bennett WF. Two forms of tissue-type plasminogen activator (t-PA) differ at a single glycosylation site. Thromb Haemost 50:106, 1983.

43. Rånby M, Bergsdorf N, Pohl G, Wallen P. Isolation of two variants of native one-chain tissue plasminogen activator. FEBS Lett 146:289, 1984.

44. Harris RJ, Leonard CK, Guzzetta AW, Spellman MW. Tissue plasminogen activator has 0-linked Fucose attached to Threonine-61 in the epidermal growth factor domain. Biochemistry 30:2311, 1991.

45. Kentzer EJ, Buko A, Menon G, Sarin VK. Carbohydrate composition and presence of a fucose-protein linkage in recombinant human pro-urokinase. Biochem Biophys Res Commun 171:410, 1990.

46. Bjoern S, Foster DC, Thim L, Wiberg FC, Christensen M, Komihyama Y, Pedersen AH, Kisiel W. Human plasma and recombinant factor. VII. Characterization of O-glycosylations at serine resi-

dues 52 and 60 and effects of site-directed mutagenesis of serine 52 to alanine. J Biol Chem 266:11051, 1991.

47. Harris RJ, Ling VT, Spellman MW. O-linked fucose is present in the first epidermal growth factor domain of Factor XII but not protein C. J Biol Chem 267:5102, 1992.

48. Kuiper J, Otter M, Rijken DC, van Berkel TJC. Characterization of the interaction in vivo of tissue-type plasminogen activator with liver cells. J Biol Chem 263:18220, 1988.

49. Cole ES, Nichols EH, Poisson L, Harnois ML, Livingston DJ. In vivo clearance of tissue plasminogen activator: The complex role of sites of glycosylation and level of sialylation. Fibrinolysis 7:15, 1993.

50. Ashwell G, Harford J. Carbohydrate specific receptors of the liver. Ann Rev Biochem 51:531, 1982.

51. Hajjar KA, Reynolds CM. Alpha-fucose-mediated binding and degradation of tissue-type plasminogen activator by HepG2 cells. J Clin Invest 93:703, 1994.

52. Morton PA, Owensby D, Sobel BE, Schwartz AL. Catabolism of tissue-type plasminogen activator by the human hepatoma cell line HepG2. J Biol Chem 264:7228, 1989.

53. Herz J. Surface location and high affinity for calcium of a 500 kd liver membrane protein closely related to the LDL-receptor suggest a physiological role as a lipoprotein receptor. EMBO J 7:4119, 1988.

54. Orth K, Madison EL, Gething M-J, Sambrook JF, Herz J. Complexes of tissue-type plasminogen activator and its serpin inhibitor plasminogen activator inhibitor type I are internalized by means of the low density lipoprotein receptor-related protein/α_2-macroglobulin receptor. Proc Natl Acad Sci USA 89:7422, 1992.

55. Bu G, Williams S, Strickland DK, Schwartz AL. Low density lipoprotein receptor/α_2-macroglobulin receptor is an hepatic receptor for tissue-type plasminogen activator. Proc Natl Acad Sci USA 89:7427, 1992.

56. Gliemann J, Davidsen O. Characterization of receptors for α_2-macroglobulin-trypsin complex in rat hepatocytes. Biochim Biophys Acta 885:49, 1986.

57. Strickland DK, Ashcom JD, Williams S, Burgess WH, Migliorini M, Argraves WS. Sequence identity between the α_2-macroglobulin receptor and low density lipoprotein receptor-related protein suggests that this molecule is a multi-functional receptor. J Biol Chem 265:17401, 1990.

58. Kristensen T, Moestrup SK, Gliemann J, Bendtsen L, Sand O, Sottrup-Jensen L. Evidence that the newly cloned low density lipoprotein receptor-related protein (LRP) is the α_2-macroglobulin receptor. FEBS Lett 276:151, 1990.

59. Bu G, Maksymovitch EA, Schwartz AL. Receptor-mediated endocytosis of tissue-type plasminogen activator by low density lipoprotein receptor-related protein on human hepatoma HEP G2 cells. J Biol Chem 268:13002, 1993.

60. Warshawsky I, Bu G, Schwartz AL. 39 kD protein inhibits tissue-type plasminogen activator clearance in vivo. J Clin Invest 92:937, 1993.

61. Nykaer A, NyKjaer A, Petersen CM, Moller B, Jensen PH, Moestrup SK, Holtet TL, Etzerodt M, Thogersen HC, Munch M, Andreasen P, Gliemann J. Purified α_2-macroglobulin receptor/LDL receptor-related protein binds urokinase: plasminogen activator inhibitor type-1 complex. J Biol Chem 267:14542, 1992.

62. Beiseigel U, Weber W, Ihrke G, Herz J, Stanley KK. The LDL receptor-related protein, LRP, is an apolipoprotein E-binding protein. Nature 341:162, 1989.

63. Willnow TE, Goldstein JL, Orth K, Brown MS, Herz J. Low density receptor-related protein/α_2-macroglobulin receptor and gp330 bind similar ligands, including plasminogen activator-inhibitor complexes and lactoferrin, an inhibitor of chylomicron remnant clearance. J Biol Chem 267:26172, 1992.

64. Kowal RC, Herz J, Goldstein JL, Esser V, Brown MS. Low density lipoprotein receptor-related protein mediates uptake of cholesteryl esters derived from apoprotein E-enriched lipoproteins. Proc Natl Acad Sci USA 86:5810, 1989.

65. Doolittle RF. The evolution of vertebrate blood coagulation: A case of yin and yang. Thromb Haemost 70:24, 1993.

66. Astrup T. Fibrinolysis: An overview. In Davidson JF, Rowan RM, Samama MM, Desnoyers PC (eds). Progress in Chemical Fibrinolysis and Thrombolysis, Vol. 3. New York: Raven Press, 1978:1.

67. Collen D, Lijnen HR. Basic and clinical aspects of fibrinolysis and thrombolysis. Blood 78:3114, 1991.

68. Vassalli JD, Sappino AP, Belin D. The plasminogen activator/plasmin system. J Clin Invest 88:1067, 1991.

69. Carmeliet P, Schoonjans L, Kieckens L, Ream B, Degen J, Bronson R, De Vos R, van den Oord JJ, Collen D, Mulligan RC. Physiological consequences of loss of plasminogen activator gene function in mince. Nature 368:419, 1994.

70. Higgins DH, Bennett WF. Tissue plasminogen activator: The biochemistry and pharmacology of variants produced by mutagenesis. Annu Rev Pharmacol Toxicol 30:91, 1990.

71. Lijnen HR, Collen D. Strategies for the improvement of thrombolytic agents. Thromb Haemost 66:88, 1991.

72. Lijnen HR, Nelles L, Van Hoef B, De Cock F, Collen D. Biochemical and functional characterization of human tissue-type plasminogen activator variants obtained by deletion and/or duplication of structural/functional domains. J Biol Chem 265:5677, 1990.

73. Kalyan NK, Wilhelm J, Lee SG, Dheer SK, Cheng S, Hjorth R, Pierzchala WA, Wiener F, Hung PP. Construction, expression and biochemical characterization of a novel tris-kringle plasminogen activator gene. Fibrinolysis 4:79, 1990.

74. Ikenaka Y, Yajima K, Yahara H, Maruyama H, Matsumoto K, Okada K, Ueshima S, Matsuo O. Characterization of human tissue-type plasminogen activator variants with amino acid mutations in the kringle-1 domain. Blood Coagul Fibrinolysis 3:381, 1992.

75. Higgins DH, Vehar GA. Interaction of one-chain and two-chain tissue plasminogen activator with intact and degraded fibrin. Biochemistry 26:7786, 1987.

76. Tate KM, Higgins DL, Holmes WE, Winkler ME, Heyneker HL, Vehar GA. Functional role of proteolytic cleavage at arginine-275 of human tissue plasminogen activator as assessed by site-directed mutagenesis. Biochemistry 26:338, 1987.

77. Haigwood NL, Mullenbach GT, Moore GK, DesJardin LE, Tabrizi A, Brown-Shimer SL, Stauss H, Stohr HA, Paques E-P. Variants of human tissue-type plasminogen activator substituted at the protease cleavage site and glycosylation sites, and truncated at the N- and C-termini. Protein Eng 2:611, 1989.

78. Wittwer AJ, Howard SC, Carr LS, Harakas NK, Feder J, Parekh RB, Rudd PM, Dwek RA, Rademacher TW. Effects of N-glycosylation on in vitro activity of Bowes melanoma and human colon fibroblast derived tissue plasminogen activator. Biochemistry 28:7662, 1989.

79. Haber E, Quertermous T, Matsueda GR, Runge MS Innovative approaches to plasminogen activator therapy. Science 243:51, 1989.

80. Hui KY, Haber E, Matsueda GR. Monoclonal antibodies to a synthetic fibrin-like peptide bind to human fibrin but not fibrinogen. Science 222:1129, 1983.

81. Bode C, Matsueda GR, Hui KY, Haber E. Antibody-directed urokinase: A specific fibrinolytic agent. Science 229:765, 1985.

82. Runge MS, Bode C, Matsueda GR, Haber E. Conjugation to an anti-fibrin monoclonal antibody enhances the fibrinolytic potency of tissue plasminogen activator in vitro. Biochemistry 27:1153, 1988.

83. Runge MS, Bode C, Matsueda GR, Haber E. Antibody-enhanced thrombolysis: Targeting of tissue plasminogen activator in vivo. Proc Natl Acad Sci USA 84:7659, 1987.

84. Bovill EG, Terrin ML, Stump DC, Berke AD, Frederick M, Collen D, Feit F, Gore JM, Hillis LD, Lambrew CT, Leiboff R, Mann KG, Markis JE, Pratt CM, Sharkey SW, Sopko G, Tracy RP, Chesebro JH. Hemorrhagic events during therapy with recombinant tissue-type plasminogen activator, heparin, and aspirin for acute myocardial infarction. Results of the thrombolysis in myocardial infarction (TIMI), phase II trial. Annu Int Med 115:256, 1991.

85. Cartwright, T. The plasminogen activator of vampire bat saliva. Blood 43:317, 1974.

86. Gardell SJ, Duong LT, Diehl RE, York JD, Hare TR, Register RB, Jacobs JW, Dixon RAF, Friedman PA. Isolation, characterization, and cDNA cloning of a vampire bat salivary plasminogen activator. J Biol Chem 264:17947, 1989.

87. Kratzschmar J, Haendler B, Langer G, Boidol W, Bringmann P, Alagon A, Donner P, Schleuning W-D. The plasminogen activator family from the salivary gland of the vampire bat Desmodus rotundus: Cloning and expression. Gene 105:229, 1991.

88. Gardell SJ, Ramjit DR, Stabilito II, Fujita T, Lynch JJ, Cuca GC, Jain D, Wang S, Tung J, Mark GE, Shebuski RJ. Effective thrombolysis without marked plasminemia after bolus intravenous administration of vampire bat salivary plasminogen activator in rabbits. Circulation 84:244, 1991.

89. Witt W, Baldus B, Bringmann P, Cashion L, Donner P, Schleuning W-D. Thrombolytic properties of Desmodus rotundus (vampire bat) salivary plasminogen activator in experimental pulmonary embolism in rats. Blood 79:1213, 1992.

90. Califf RM, Topol EJ, George BS, Boswick JM, Abbotsmith C, Sigmon KN, Candel R, Masek R, Kereiakes D, O'Neill WW, Stack RS, Stump D, and the TAMI Study Group. Hemorrhagic complications associated with the use of intravenous tissue plasminogen activator in treatment of acute myocardial infarction. Am J Med 85:353, 1988.

91. Rao AK, Pratt C, Berke, A, Jaffe A, Ockene I, Schreiber TL, Bell WR, Knatterud G, Robertson TL, Terrin ML. For the TIMI Investigators Thrombolysis in myocardial infarction (TIMI) trial-phase I: Hemorrhagic manifestations and changes in plasma fibrinogen and the fibrinolytic system in patients treated with recombinant tissue plasminogen activator and streptokinase. J Am Coll Cardiol 11:1, 1988.

92. Stump DC, Califf RM, Topol EJ, Sigmon K, Thornton D, Masek R, Anderson L, Collen D, and the TAMI Study Group. Pharmacodynamics of thrombolysis with recombinant tissue-type plasminogen patients with acute myocardial infarction. Circulation 80:1222, 1989.

93. Cunningham BC, Wells JA. High-resolution epitope mapping of hGH-receptor interactions by alanine-scanning mutagenesis. Science 244:1801, 1989.

94. Eastman D, Wurm FM, van Reis R, Higgins DL. A region of tissue plasminogen activator that affects plasminogen activation differentially with various fibrin(ogen)-related stimulators. Biochemistry 31:419, 1992.

95. Paoni NF, Refino CJ, Brady K, Peña LC, Nguyen HV, Kerr EM, Johnson AC, Wurm FM, van Reis R, Botstein D, Bennett WF. Involvement of residues 296–299 in the enzymatic activity of tissue-type plasminogen activator. Protein Eng 5:259, 1992.

96. Paoni NF, Chow AM, Pena LC, Keyt BA, Zoller MJ, Bennett WF. Making tissue-type plasminogen activator more fibrin specific. Protein Eng 6:529, 1993.

97. Strandberg L, Madison E. Variants of tissue-type plasminogen activator with substantially enhanced response and selectivity toward fibrin co-factors. J Biol Chem 270:23444, 1995.

98. Paoni NF, Keyt BA, Refino CJ, Chow AM, Nguyen H, Berleau LT, Badillo JM, Peña LC, Brady K, Wurm FM, Ogez J, Bennett WF. A slow clearing, fibrin-specific, PAI-1 resistant variant of t-PA (T103N, KHRR296–299AAAA). Thromb Haemost 70:307, 1993.

99. Refino CJ, Paoni NF, Keyt BA, Pater CS, Badillo JM, Wurm FM, Ogez J, Bennett WF. A variant of t-PA (T103N, KHRR 296–299 AAAA) that, by bolus, has increased potency and decreased systemic activation of plasminogen. Thromb Haemost 70:313, 1993.

100. Riccio A, Grimaldi G, Verde P, Sebastio G, Boast S, Blasi F. The human urokinase-plasminogen activator gene and its promoter. Nucleic Acids Res 13:2759, 1985.

101. Lamba D, Bauer M, Huber R, Fischer S, Rudolph R, Kohnert U, Bode W. The 2.3 Å crystal structure of the catalytic domain of recombinant two-chain human tissue-type plasminogen activator. J Mol Biol 258:117, 1996.

102. Lucore CL, Sobel B, Interactions of tissue-type plasminogen activator with plasma inhibitors and their pharmacologic implications. Circulation 77:660, 1988.

103. Shohet RV, Spitzer S, Madison EL, Bassel-Duby R, Gething M-J, Sambrook JF. Inhibitor-resistant tissue-type plasminogen activator: An improved thrombolytic agent in vitro. Thromb Haemost 71:124, 1994.

104. Madison EL, Goldsmith EJ, Gerard RD, Gething M-JH, Sambrook JF. Serpin-resistant mutants of human tissue-type plasminogen activator. Nature 339:721, 1989.

105. Huber R, Kukla D, Bode W, Schwager P, Bartels K, Deisenhofer J, Steigeman W. Structure of the complex formed by bovine trypsin and bovine pancreatic trypsin inhibitor. II. Crystallographic refinement at 1.9 Å resolution. J Mol Biol 89:73, 1974.

106. Madison EL, Goldsmith EJ, Gerard RD, Gething M-JH, Sambrook JF, Bassel-Duby RS. Amino acid residues that affect interaction of tissue-type plasminogen activator with plasminogen activator inhibitor 1. Proc Natl Acad Sci USA 87:3530, 1990.

107. Madison EL, Goldsmith EJ, Gething M-JH, Sambrook JF, Gerard RD. Restoration of serine protease-inhibitor interaction by protein engineering. J Biol Chem 265:21423, 1990.

108. Braaten JV, Handt S, Jerome WG, Kirkpatrick J, Lewis JC, Hantgan RR. Regulation of fibrinolysis by platelet-released plasminogen activator inhibitor 1: Light scattering and ultrastructural examination of lysis of a model platelet-fibrin thrombus. Blood 81:1290, 1993.

109. Gething M-J, Adler B, Boose J-A, Gerard RD, Madison EL, McGookey D, Meidell RS, Roman LM, Sambrook J. Variants of human tissue-type plasminogen activator that lack specific structural domains of the heavy chain. EMBO J 7:2731, 1988.

110. Larsen GR, Metzger M, Hensen K, Blue Y, Horgan P. Pharmacokinetic and distribution analysis of variant forms of tissue-type plasminogen activator with prolonged clearance in rat. Blood 73:1842, 1989.

111. Browne MJ, Carey JE, Chapman CG, Tyrrell WR, Entwisle C, Mark G, Lawrence P, Reavy B, Dodd I, Esmail A, Robinson JH. A tissue-type plasminogen activator mutant with prolonged clearance in vivo. J Biol Chem 263:1599, 1988.

112. Johannessen M, Diness V, Pingel K, Petersen LC, Rao D, Lioubin P, O'Hara P, Mulvihill E. Fibrin affinity and clearance of t-PA deletion and substitution analogues. Thromb Haemost 6:54, 1990.

113. Collen D, Stassen JM, Larsen G. Pharmacokineticsand thrombolytic properties of deletion mutants of human tissue-type plasminogen activator in rabbits. Blood 71:216, 1988.

114. Collen D, Lijnen HR, Vanlinthout I, Kieckens L, Nelles L, Stassen JM. Thrombolytic and pharmacokinetic properties of human tissue-type plasminogen activator variants, obtained by deletion and/or duplication of structural/functional domains, in a hamster pulmonary embolism model. Thromb Haemost 65:174, 1991.

115. Kalyan NK, Lee SG, Wilhelm J, Fu KP, Hum W-T, Rappaport R, Hartzell R, Urbano C, Hung PP. Structure-function analysis with tissue-type plasminogen activator. J Biol Chem 263:3971, 1988.

116. Fu KP, Lee S, Hum WT, Kalyan N, Rappaport R, Hetzel N, Hung PP. Disposition of a novel recombinant tissue plasminogen activator, des 2-89 t-PA, in mice. Thromb Res 50:33, 1988.

117. Browne MJ, Chapman CG, Dodd I, Reavy B, Esmail AF, Robinson JH. The role of tissue-type plasminogen activator A-chain domains in plasma clearance. Fibrinolysis 3:207, 1989.

118. Kohnert U, Rudolph R, Verheijen JH, et al. Biochemical properties of the kringle 2 and protease domains are maintained in the refolded t-PA deletion variant BM 06.022. Protein Eng 5:93, 1992.

119. Martin U, Fischer S, Kohnert U, Opitz U, Rudolph R, Sponer G, Stern A, Strein K. Thrombolysis with an Escherichia coli-produced recombinant plasminogen activator (BM 06.022) in the rabbit model of jugular vein thrombosis. Thromb Haemost 65:560, 1991.

120. Martin U, novel Köhler J, Sponer G, Strein K. Pharmacokinetics of the recombinant plasminogen activator (BM 06.022) in rats, dogs, and non-human primates. Fibrinolysis 6:39, 1992.

121. Martin U, van Möllendorf E, Akpan W, Kientsch-Engel R, Kaufmann B, Neugebauer G. Dose-ranging study of the novel recombinant plasminogen activator BM 06.022 in healthy volunteers. Clin Pharmacol Ther 50:429, 1991.

122. Neuhaus K-L, von Essen R, Vogt A, Tebbe U, Rustige J, Wagner H-J, Appel K-L, Stienen U, König R, Meyer-Sabellek W. Dose-finding with a novel recombinant plasminogen activator (BM

06.022) in patients with acute myocardial infarction: Results of the German recombinant plasminogen activator study. J Am Coll Cardiol 24:55, 1994.

123. Bode C, Smalling RW, Berg G, Burnett C, Lorch G, Kalbfleisch JM, Chernoff R, Christie LG, Feldman RL, Seals AA, Weaver WD. Randomized Comparison of coronary thrombolysis achieved with double-bolus Reteplase and front-loaded, accelerated Alteplase in patients with acute myocardial infarction. Circulation 94:891, 1996.

124. Internation Joint Efficacy Comparison of Thrombolytics. Randomized, double-blind comparison of reteplase double-bolus administration with streptokinase in acute myocardial infarction: Trial to investigate equivalence. Lancet 346:329, 1995.

125. Hotchkiss A, Refino CJ, Leonard CK, O'Connor JV, Crowley C, McCabe J, Tate K, Nakamura G, Powers D, Levinson A, Mohler M, Spellman MW. The influence of carbohydrate structures on the clearance of recombinant tissue-type plasminogen activator. Thromb Haemost 60:255, 1990.

126. Sobel BE, Sarnoff SJ, Nachowiak BA. Augmented and sustained plasma concentrations after intramuscular injections of molecular variants and deglycosylated forms of tissue-type plasminogen activator. Circulation 81:1362, 1990.

127. Paques E-P, Just M, Reiner G, Romisch J. Pharmcological and pharmacokinetic properties of a deglycosylated mutant of the tissue-type plasminogen activator expressed in CHO cells. Fibrinolysis 6:125, 1992.

128. Anderson S, Keyt BA. Variants of Plasminogen Activators and Processes for their Production. International Patent Application WO89/11531, filed May 20, 1988 and published November 30, 1989, U.S. Patent 5,270,198, 1988.

129. Marshall RD. The nature and metabolism of the carbohydrate-peptide linkages of glycoproteins. Biochem Soc Symp 40:17, 1974.

130. Aubert JP, Helbecque N, Loucheux-Lefebvre MH. Circular dichroism studies of synthetic Asn-X-Ser/Thr-containing peptides: Structure-glycosylation relationship. Arch Biochem Biophys 208:20, 1981.

131. Bassell-Duby R, Jiang NY, Bittick T, Madison E, McGookey D, Orth K, Shohet R, Sambrook J, Gething M-J. Tyrosine 67 in the epidermal growth factor-like domain of tissue-type plasminogen activator is important for clearance by a specific hepatic receptor. J Biol Chem 267:9668, 1992.

132. Guzzetta AW, Basa LJ, Hancock WS, Keyt BA, Bennett WF. Identification of carbohydrate structures in glycoprotein peptide maps by the use of LC/MS with selected ion extraction with special reference to tissue plasminogen activator and a glycosylation variant produced by site directed mutagenesis. Anal Chem 65:2953, 1993.

133. Keyt BA, Paoni NF, Refino CJ, Berleau L, Nguyen H, Chow A, Lai J, Peña L, Pater C, Ogez J, Etcheverry T, Botstein D, Bennett WF. A faster-acting and more

potent form of tissue plasminogen activator. Proc Natl Acad Sci USA 91:3670, 1954.

134. Clauss A. Gerinnungsphysiologische schnellmethode zur bestimmung des fibrinogens. Acta Haematol (Basel) 17:237, 1957.

135. Refino CJ, Keyt BA, Paoni NF, Badillo JM, Pater CS, van Peborgh J, Pena L, Berleau LT, Nguyen HV, Bennett WF. A variant of tissue plasminogen activator (T103N, N117Q, KHRR 296-299AAAA) with a decreased plasma clearance rate, is substantially more potent than Activase t-PA in a rabbit thrombolysis model. Thromb Haemost 69:841, 1993.

136. Thomas GR, Thibodeaux H, Bennett WF, Refino CJ, Badillo JM, Errett CJ, Zivin JA. Optimized thrombolysis of cerebral clots with tissue-type plasminogen activator in a rabbit model of embolic stroke. J Pharmacol Exp Ther 264:67, 1993.

137. Thomas GR, Thibodeaux H, Errett CJ, Badillo JM, Keyt BA, Refino CJ, Zivin JA, Bennett WF. A long half-life and fibrin-specific form of tissue plasminogen activator in rabbit models of embolic stroke and peripheral bleeding. Stroke 25:2073, 1994.

138. Benedict CR, Mathew B, Rex KA, Cartwright J Jr, Sordahl LA. Correlation of plasma serotonin changes with platelet aggregation in an in vivo dog model of spontaneous occlusive coronary thrombus formation. Circ Res 7:58, 1986.

139. Benedict CR, Ryan J, Wolitzky B, Gerlach M, Stern D. Active site-blocked factor IXa prevents intravascular thrombus formation in the coronary vasculature without inhibiting extravascular coagulation in a canine thrombosis model. J Clin Invest 88:1760, 1991.

140. Benedict CR, Ryan J, Todd J, Kuwabara K, Tijburg P, Cartwright J Jr, Stern D. Active site-blocked factor Xa prevents intravascular thrombus formation in the coronary vasculature in parallel with inhibition of extravascular coagulation in a canine thrombosis model. Blood 81:2059, 1993.

141. Benedict CR, Refino CJ, Keyt BA, Pakala R, Paoni NF, Thomas GR, Bennett WF. New variant of human tissue plasminogen activator (tPA) with enhanced efficacy and lower incidence of bleeding compared with recombinant human tPA. Circulation 92:3032, 1995.

142. Nicolini FA, Nichols WW, Saldeen TGP, Mehta JL. Cardiovasc Res 25:283, 1991.

143. Nicolini FA, Mehta JL, Nichols WW, Saldeen TGP, Grant M. Prostacyclin analogue Iloprost decreases thrombolytic potential of tissue-type plasminogen activator in canine coronary thrombosis. Circulation 81:1115, 1990.

144. Nicolini FA, Nichols WW, Mehta JL, Schofield R, Ross M, Player D, Pohl G, Mattsson C. J Am Coll Cardiol 20:228, 1992.

145. Romson JL, Haack DW, Lucchesi BR. Thromb Res 17:841, 1980.

146. Nicolini FA, Lee P, Rios G, Kottke-Marchant K, Topol EJ. Combination of platelet fibrinogen receptor antagonist and direct thrombin inhibitor at low doses

markedly improves thrombolysis. Circulation 89:1802, 1994.

147. Cannon CP, McCabe CH, Gibson CM, Ghali M, Sequeira RF, McKendall GR, Breed J, Modi NB, Fox NL, Tracy RP, Love TW, Braunwald E, and the TIMI 10A Investigators. TNK-Tissue Plasminogen Activator in Acute Myocardial Infarction: Results of the Thrombolysis in Myocardial Infarction (TIMI) 10A Dose-Ranging Trial. Circulation 95:351, 1997.

148. The GUSTO Angiographic Investigators. The effect of tissue plasminogen activator, streptokinase, or both on coronary-artery patency, ventricular function, and survival after acute myocardial infarction. N Engl J Med 329:1615, 1993.

149. Dihanich M, Monard D. cDNA sequence of rat prothrombin. Nucleic Acids Res 18:4251, 1990.

150. Sottrup-Jensen L, Claeys H, Zajdel M, Petersen TE, Magnusson S. The primary structure of human plasminogen: Isolation of two lysine-binding fragments and one "mini-" plasminogen (MW 38,000) by elastase-catalyzed-limited proteolysis. In Davidson JF, Rowan RM, Samama MM, Desnoyers PC (eds).

Progress in Chemical Fibrinolysis and Thrombolysis, Vol. 3. New York: Raven Press, 1978:191.

151. Hagen FS, Gray CL, O'Hara PJ, Grant FJ, Saari GG, Woodbury RG, Hart CE, Insley MY, Kisiel W, Kurachi K, Davie EW. Characterization of a cDNA coding for human factor VII. Proc Natl Acad Sci USA 83:2412, 1986.

152. Jaye M, De La Salle H, Schamber F, Balland A, Kohli V, Findeli A, Tolstoshev P, Lecocq JP. Isolation of a human anti-haemophilic factor IX cDNA clone using a unique 52-base synthetic oligonucleotide probe deduced from the amino acid sequence of bovine factor IX. Nucleic Acids Res 11:2325, 1983.

153. Fung MR, Hay CW, McGillivray RTA. Characterization of an almost full-length cDNA coding for human blood coagulation factor X. Proc Natl Acad Sci USA 82:3591, 1985.

154. Emi M, Nakamura Y, Ogawa M, Yamamoto T, Nishide T, Mori T, Matsubara K. Cloning, characterization and nucleotide sequences of two cDNAs encoding human pancreatic trypsinogens. Gene 41:305, 1986.

SECTION IV: VASCULAR BIOLOGY

Joseph Loscalzo

The blood vessel has historically been viewed as a passive conduit within which the blood volume is retained. The contemporary view of the blood vessel is, by contrast, vastly different. Vascular cells, endothelial cells, vascular smooth muscle cells, and fibroblasts comprise a dynamic organ that has important regulatory and homeostatic functions. Under normal conditions, these cells regulate vascular resistance and blood pressure, maintain blood fluidity by inhibiting platelet function and thrombin activation, and limit the adhesion and diapedesis of leukocytes from the blood pool. As a result, tissue perfusion is maintained. With loss of vascular integrity, these cells are poised to staunch the flow of blood and to minimize hemodynamic compromise. In pathophysiologic conditions, however, vascular cells develop phenotypic characteristics that mimic more those of an acutely injured vessel rather than a normal, intact vessel. Thus, endothelial cells from atherosclerotic vessels are less able to inhibit platelet function and vascular smooth muscle migration and proliferation, and readily adhere to leukocytes. This section provides a contemporary view of the normal and abnormal functions of the cells of the vasculature. The dynamic nature of the responses of vascular cells is emphasized, and their roles in physiologic and pathophysiologic states are reviewed.

8. ENDOTHELIAL CELL BIOLOGY

Una S. Ryan

Introduction

The endothelium is a critical component of all organs yet itself represents a complex, unique organ with a vast surface area and an aggregate mass equal to that of the liver. In cross sections of the vessel wall, the endothelium appears as a thin and insignificant layer that belies its importance and significance in homeostasis [1].

In fact, the strategic interposition of the endothelium between the blood and all other tissues in the body, is ideal for subserving its many functions as a regulator of cellular and molecular traffic, both within the circulation and between the vascular lumen and the surrounding tissues. It also provides a dynamic interface for responding to cellular and molecular clues arriving via the blood or from the tissue side [2]. For example, endothelial cells (ECs), particularly those of the pulmonary capillaries, are capable of converting angiotensin I to angiotensin II and of degrading bradykinin [3]. Thus, the endothelium can regulate blood pressure by inactivating a hypotensive substance (bradykinin) and by causing the delivery of a potent hypertensive substance (angiotensin II) directly into the circulation [4]. Both of these effects are achieved by interaction of the circulating substrates with an enzyme, angiotensin converting enzyme, (ACE; kininase II), localized on the surface of endothelial cells in situ and in culture [3]. Localization of ACE on endothelial cells was the first of many studies that led to the recognition of a number of processing, or "metabolic," functions of endothelium [1]. The endothelial disposition of ACE also led to the development of assays useful for the identification of endothelial cells in culture and to the development of antihypertensive drugs that target ACE.

Subsequent studies of EC properties have received much impetus from the development of techniques for the isolation, characterization, and culture of ECs [5]. Endothelial cells from a wide variety of species and vessel origins, including the microvasculature, can now be grown in culture reproducibly. In the quiescent state, the endothelium acts to maintain the blood's fluidity and resists thrombosis, but thrombotic functions take over when the cells are perturbed (Figure 8-1). The endothelium also acts as a selective barrier between the elements in the blood and the extravascular space, and serves to convey signals between the tissues and the circulating elements. During infection or when activated by cytokines or components of the coagulation or complement systems, the endothelium functions to attract leukocytes, allowing their emigration to sites of inflammation. The endothelium also has local regulatory functions, being a key controller of vascular tone as well as an important modulator of vascular remodeling through its influence on the growth of the underlying vascular smooth muscle cells and by secretion of extracellular matrix components. Toward all these functions, the endothelium synthesizes a diverse armament of hormones, mediators, and growth modulators, some of which are expressed constitutively and others of which are only induced in response to various stimuli. It is significant that the same anatomic location that makes the endothelium so unique and diverse in its biologic functions makes it an immediate target of vascular injury and an ideal candidate to initiate events leading both to local and systemic damage.

Endothelial Barrier and Transducing Functions

The interactions between neighboring ECs serve to maintain vascular integrity, to regulate vascular permeability, and to control leukocyte traffic. The junctions between ECs vary in different parts of the circulation and in different organs. In much of the vasculature, where ECs form a continuous monolayer, gap junctions predominate [6]. A decrease in both gap junctions and tight junctions is seen in areas of regenerating endothelium [7]. In contrast, in the brain and retina, where the development of edema can be dangerous, tight (occluding) junctions predominate. While the blood–brain barrier is recognized to

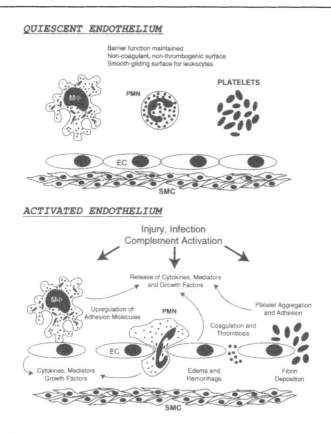

FIGURE 8-1.

be the most highly selective anatomic and physiological barrier that regulates the entry and exit of cerebral nutrients and biologically important substances necessary for the maintenance of cerebral metabolism and neuronal activity, the endothelium of all organs serves to mediate the passage of solutes, nutrients, lipids, and hormones to the interstitium, often involving a complex system of membrane receptors and transporters.

In addition to endothelial–endothelial cell interactions, endothelial smooth-muscle cell interactions occur primarily via gap junctions, where cytoplasmic bridges of smooth muscle cells extend through fenestrations in the internal elastic lamina to contact the endothelium [8]. Gap junctions provide a pathway for the transport of ions and small molecules and could provide a route of entry of mediators from endothelium to smooth muscle and vice versa. In addition, some endothelium-derived factors are freely diffusible and penetrate smooth muscle cells directly, independent of gap junctions. Others bind to receptors on the surface of the smooth muscle cell and elicit responses through second messengers.

The endothelium and smooth muscle cells form an integrated alliance; the close association of these two cell types allows for the efficacy of the most influential of the endothelium-derived vasomodulating factors, endothelium-derived relaxing factor (EDRF/NO), and demonstrates the transducing role of the endothelium: a blood-borne agonist interacting with receptors on the ECs leads to release of a mediator that modulates smooth muscle relaxation (see Endothelial Control of Vascular Wall Function).

Endothelial Hemostatic Functions

Endothelial cells have both thrombotic and thromboresistant properties. In the quiescent state, they are antithrombotic, but they can be induced to become procoagulant (see Figure 8-1). Endothelial cells inhibit thrombus formation by interfering with the coagulation cascade, inhibiting platelet adhesion/aggregation, and activating fibrinolytic pathways. The luminal surface of the EC contains anionic heparin-like glycosaminoglycans, which are synthesized by the ECs and bind thrombin, the key enzyme of blood coagulation, and antithrombin III, a serum protein that binds and inactivates thrombin. In the presence of ECs, thrombin reacts primarily with antithrombin II, resulting in rapid inactivation of the enzyme. Thrombin also interacts with thrombomodulin on the EC surface. Thrombomodulin binds both thrombin and protein C, and the thrombin–thrombomodulin–protein C complex markedly accelerates the activation of protein C [9]. Protein C, with the intermediary protein S, inhibits factor Va and factor XIII in the coagulation cascade [10,11]. Endothelial cells are also thought to produce a lipoprotein-associated inhibitor of coagulation known as tissue factor pathway inhibitor (TFPI) or lipoprotein-associated coagulation inhibitor (LACI) [12]. This factor is a potent inhibitor of factor Xa and the factor VIIa–TF complex [13]. TFPI is primarily synthesized in endothelial cells. A major fraction remains with the endothelium, whereas a small fraction is secreted into the blood [14,15]. It is currently hypothesized that the heparin-releasable form is associated with endothelial glycosaminoglycans [16]. Endothelial cells also synthesize prostacyclin (PGI_2), a potent inhibitor of platelet aggregation [17]. Other products released by ECs that prevent platelet adhesion/aggregation include adenosine and nitric oxide (NO). Moreover, there is clear synergism between the antiaggregatory effect of PGI_2 and the effect of NO at subthreshold levels [18].

Clot dissolution through enhancement of the fibrinolytic system is another EC anticoagulant defense mechanism. Endothelial cells synthesize both tissue-type plasminogen activators (t-PA) as well as urokinase-type plasminogen (u-PA) activators [19]. The synthesis and release of plasminogen activators by ECs is stimulated by thrombin, activated protein C, epinephrine, vasopressin, and bradykinin.

In contrast to the anticoagulant mechanisms described earlier the EC, when perturbed mechanically or exposed to bacterial endotoxin, thrombin, tumor necrosis factor, or interleukin-1, can interact with blood components to promote coagulation [20–22]. The procoagulant activity is the result of increased production of tissue factor (thromboplastin), von Willebrand factor (vWF), plasminogen activator inhibitor, platelet activating factor, and extracellular matrix components. Tissue factor, released by damaged cells, functions with factor VII in activating factor X, initiating the *extrinsic pathway* of coagulation, and potentiates the cleavage of factor IX (activating the *intrinsic pathway* as well). In the presence of vWF, activated factor IX further activates factor X. The activated factor X, formed via either pathway, then converts prothrombin to thrombin in a reaction that requires factor V. Thrombin converts soluble fibrinogen to insoluble fibrin, activates platelets, and inhibits vessel-wall fibrinolytic activity.

The vWF synthesized by ECs is also bound by collagen types I, III, IV, and V, and helps mediate platelet adhesion to the subendothelium through a specific glycoprotein receptor on the platelet surface, glycoprotein IIb/IIIa (which also serves as a receptor for fibrinogen) [23]. The importance of vWF in platelet adhesion to the subendothelium and subsequent thrombosis is evidenced by the fact that in von Willebrand's disease there is a marked decrease in platelet adhesion, which can be reversed by administration of vWF [24]. Endothelial cells also synthesize other proteins that stimulate the coagulation cascade (although this may not be the primary function of these proteins), including thrombospondin, collagens, and fibronectin. Procoagulant activity also involves alterations in fibrinolysis through the regulated expression of t-PA and specific plasminogen activator inhibitors (PAI). In fact, the activity of t-PA in plasma is based on the amount of t-PA released as well as on the level of PAI present [25,26].

Thus, the hemostatic potential of the endothelium results from a complex balance between active factors that have opposing biological actions and between active factors and specific inhibitors. Upset of this balance could lead to conditions predisposing both to local and widespread embolic and thrombotic responses.

Endothelial Control of Vascular Wall Function

Endothelial cells play a key role in modulating vasomotor tone. Many substances produced by ECs affect local vasomotor tone and a complex interaction exists among those elements that control hemostasis, vascular modeling, and vasomotor reactivity. Angiotensin converting enzyme localized on ECs established a role for endothelium in the control of blood pressure [3]. The renin-angiotensin system is now also known to play a role in vascular remodeling [27].

Abluminally released, PGI$_2$ is a potent vasodilator and antiaggregant. PGI$_2$ release by ECs can be stimulated by pulsatile pressure as well as the endogenous mediators thrombin, bradykinin, angiotensin II, histamine, platelet-derived growth factor (PDGF), interlenkin-1 (IL-1), and adenine nucleotides [28–30]. The effects of PGI$_2$ are opposed by thromboxane, a prostanoid produced by activated platelets that induces platelet aggregation and vasoconstriction [31]. Aspirin, an irreversible inhibitor of cyclooxygenase, owes its efficacy to the EC's ability to synthesize cyclooxygenase continuously while the platelet cannot do so. This leads to cumulative inhibition of thromboxane A$_2$ formation while the ECs continue to produce PGI$_2$ [32].

EDRF was first described by Furchgott and Zawadzki, who demonstrated that the relaxation of the rabbit aorta by acetylcholine depended on the presence of an endothelial lining and was the result of a nonprostanoid diffusible substance [33]. Subsequently, it was suggested that EDRF may be NO or a related species [34–37]. A fuller description of NO and its pharmacology will be found in Chapter 10 [38]. NO is synthesized from the amino acid L-arginine by the enzyme NO synthase (NOS), and its actions are mediated by increases in cellular cGMP [39–41]. Arginine analogs (such as L-NG-monomethyl arginine) are potent inhibitors of NO production, and their effects can be reversed by arginine. Blockade of NO synthesis in animals results in marked increases in blood pressure, underlining the importance of NO release in maintaining resting blood pressure [42,43]. Several isozymes of NOS exist. The constitutive enzyme is Ca^{2+}/calmodulin dependent and releases picomolar concentrations of NO. In several cell types, a second form of Ca^{2+}-independent NOS can be induced by inflammatory mediators [44,45]. The inducible NOS produces NO at the nanomolar level, and its induction can be prevented by pretreatment with glucocorticoids. NO, in addition to mediating vasodilation, inhibits platelet adhesion and aggregation as previously described. It also limits smooth muscle cell (SMC) proliferation and inhibits leukocyte–EC interactions. After reperfusion injury, sodium nitrite prevents leukocytes from adhering and infiltrating into the vessel wall [46], perhaps by an effect of NO on EC adhesion molecule expression.

More than 30 substances have been shown to elicit endothelium-dependent relaxations of isolated blood vessels, including acetylcholine, the calcium ionophore A23187, bradykinin, thrombin, and endothelin, indicating the importance of this factor in local autoregulation of vascular tone. Defects in EC production of EDRF/NO have been seen in a number of disease states, including atherosclerosis, hypertension, and diabetes, and may contribute to their pathogenesis [47–49]. There is mounting evidence to suggest that mild trauma to microvessels is sufficient to impair the dilating responses of microvessels temporarily without irreversible injury to the vessels.

In addition to the vasodilators PGI$_2$ and NO, the endothelium also releases vasoconstrictor substances in response to a variety of stimuli [50]. In 1988, Yanagisawa et al. identified endothelin, a linear 21 amino acid peptide secreted by ECs [51]. Endothelin is the most potent vasoconstrictor substance yet discovered, with a potency 10 times that of angiotensin II. Intense vasoconstriction and decreased blood flow have been seen in multiple species in which endothelin-1 (ET-1) has been infused, although it is rapidly removed from the bloodstream, suggesting a local vasoregulatory role [52,53]. Three pharmacologically separate endothelin isopeptides have been identified in mammalian species and are named endothelin-1, endothelin-2, and endothelin-3. ET-1 is the only endothelin known to be made by ECs.

Many substances, including thrombin, epinephrine, transforming growth factor-β, and the Ca^{2+} ionophore A23187, increase preproendothelin mRNA as well as the release of vasoactive ET-1 from ECs [51]. The release of ET-1 is slow, consistent with the fact that it requires new synthesis. The fact that ET-1 is secreted by numerous cell types and that receptors are widely distributed among many tissues, including blood vessels, brain, lungs, kidneys, adrenal glands, spleen, and intestines, suggests that endothelin has multiple roles.

In addition to its long-acting vasoconstrictor and pressor actions, ET-1 has numerous biological activities, including mitogenicity for cultured mesangial cells, Swiss 3T3 cells, capillary ECs, and SMCs. Elevated levels of ET-1 have been detected in patients who have suffered a myocardial infarction as well as in acute renal failure, acute ischemic stroke, and hypertensive states; however, it is unclear whether the elevated ET-1 levels actually contribute to the pathogenesis of these diseases or are the result of concurrent disease processes [54,55]. In a rat model of arterial injury, high levels of ET-1 worsen postangioplasty restenosis and may act through a direct mitogenic effect on the underlying SMCs [56].

Leukocyte/Endothelial Cell Adhesive Interactions

Interaction of leukocytes with the endothelium is a routine physiologic function. Under normal circumstances, over 75% of granulocytes are adherent to the endothelium, where they remain ready for release by specific stimuli to join the circulating pool. Lymphocytes, on the other hand, circulate through the plasma and as part of their normal course emigrate through specialized postcapillary venules in lymphoid tissues, returning to the plasma after a few hours. When this delicate system is upset by an inflammatory process, changes occur on the endothelium that allow not only adhesion but emigration of leukocytes to the site (see Figure 8-1). These interactions of leukocytes with the endothelium are carefully controlled by specific adhesion molecules. At present, three different groups of adhesive receptors/ligands are known to participate in leukocyte adhesion. These include proteins of the integrin family or leukocyte cellular adhesion molecules (LEU-CAMS) [57,58], members of the immunoglobulin-related molecules or intercellular adhesion molecules (ICAMs) [59], and carbohydrate binding proteins called selections or lectin-epidermal growth factor–complement cell adhesion molecules (LEC-CAMs) [60,61].

The most important integrins present on leukocytes belong to the β1 (CD11/CD18) and β2 (VLA-4, CD49d/CD29) subfamilies [6,62]. Although integrins are constitutively expressed on the surface of leukocytes, they are normally in a functionally inactive state. Conversion to the active state is rapid in response to chemotactic factors, cytokines, antigens, or mitogens. The importance of leukocyte integrins to immunologic defense against inflammatory processes is demonstrated by the human disease leukocyte adhesion deficiency (LAD). Neutrophils from patients with LAD lack expression of leukocyte integrins and exhibit defective leukocyte-EC adhesion in in vitro assays correlating with the absence of these cells at sites of inflammation [63].

ECs possess at least three adhesive receptors in the immunoglobulin family, namely, ICAM-1, ICAM-2, and VCAM (INCAM-110), which serve as counter receptors for the leukocyte integrins [64–66]. They are single-chain N-glycosylated polypeptides. ICAM-1 contains five immunoglobulin domains. It is not only present on ECs but is present on a variety of other cells, including leukocytes. Endothelial cells constitutively express ICAM-1 in low amounts, but increased levels are easily induced by a variety of cytokines, including interferon-γ, IL-1, and tumor necrosis factor (TNE)-α [67]. Following stimulation, increased expression can be detected within 4 hours, and expression is maintained for over 24 hours. ICAM-2 is similar to ICAM-1 but contains only two immunoglobulin domains. ICAM-2 is constitutively expressed by ECs and is not increased after cytokine

activation [68]. This may indicate more of a role for ICAM-2 in routine EC–leukocyte interactions, whereas ICAM-1 becomes more important in activated ECs. VCAM-1 is also expressed following endothelial activation by cytokines [69]. VCAM-1 selectively binds mononuclear cells, such as lymphocytes and monocytes, and is the counter-receptor for the β2 integrin VLA-4 [70]. VCAM-1 has been found at sites of chronic inflammation, but its expression is not restricted to ECs. Macrophages and fibroblast-like cells also appear to express VCAM-1 [71].

Three members of the selectin family currently exist: L-selectin (LEC-CAM-1, LAM-1, Leu 8, TQ-1), E-selectin (LEC-CAM-2, ELAM-1, endothelial-leukocyte adhesion molecule), and P-selectin (LEC-CAM-3 PADGEM, platelet-activation-dependent-granulocyte-external-membrane protein, GMP-140, CD62 [72–77]. L-selectin is confined to leukocytes and is involved in leukocyte homing. E-selectin is found on ECs, and P-selectin is found on both ECs and platelets. These molecules are transmembrane glycoproteins that contain an amino-terminal lectin domain, followed by an epidermal growth factor–like domain, and a varying number of complement-like consensus repeats. P- and E-selectin bind sialyated Lewis x (sLe^x) carbohydrates, which are commonly found on glycoproteins and glycolipids of myeloid cells. Although the physiological ligands for the selectins may still not be completely identified, P-selectin glycoprotein ligand (PSGL-1) is a high-affinity ligand that may well represent an important leukocyte counter-receptor for both P- and E-selectins [78–82]. In addition, the E-selectin ligand (ESL-1), a variant of a receptor for fibroblast growth factor, functions as a cell adhesion ligand of E-selectin [83].

E-selectin is an adhesion protein for monocytes and neutrophils, but not lymphocytes. It is expressed on the EC surface 4–6 hours after stimulation by cytokines and is downregulated by 24 hours [84]. It is not contained within the cytoplasm of cells and requires new protein synthesis for expression [73]. E-selectin has been shown to be expressed on microvascular endothelium transiently in certain pathologic settings, particularly acute and chronic inflammatory processes in which cytokine generation is thought to occur [85]. P-selectin is present in both platelets and ECs, although the endothelial protein is primarily found in postcapillary venules [86]. Endothelial P-selectin is expressed constitutively and is located in membranes of Weibel-Palade bodies, the secretory granules of endothelium in which large multimers of vWF are stored [76,87,88]. Following stimulation with agonists such as thrombin or histamine, P-selectin is rapidly distributed to the cell surface, where it binds neutrophils, monocytes, and platelets [89]. In stimulated cultured endothelium, surface expression of P-selectin is rapid, within 10 minutes. Downregulation then occurs over the next 30 minutes. Exposure of ECs to oxidants results in prolonged expression of P-selectin on their surface and thus may provide a direct role for oxygen radicals in neutrophil adhesion [90]. P-selectin is an excellent candidate for directing the initial aherence of unstimulated neutrophils and monocytes to sites of inflammation. Progression of the inflammatory stimulus can then activate other adhesive receptors on both cells, thus stimulating leukocyte emigration to the site of tissue damage [91]. P-selectin's presence on platelets and its localization with vWF also suggest a role for this molecule in hemostasis. Stimulated platelets expressing P-selectin may then recruit neutrophils and monocytes to the thrombus. The activated monocyte with its procoagulant surface could then amplify thrombin generation and clot formation.

The migration of leukocytes throughout the vasculature provides the body with the ability to maintain immune surveillance and to protect tissues from injury caused by foreign antigens. In addition to their participation in host defense, leukocytes may also be involved in the mounting of pathological inflammation in disease states [92]. However, the precise mechanisms of the binding of leukocytes to inflamed endothelium may still not be completely understood. In the current consensus model, leukocytes interact with endothelium through a series of events; initial attachment and "rolling" of leukocytes on endothelium is mediated by selectin molecules. Tethering leads to activation of integrins, which cause strong adhesion of leukocytes to the vessel wall.

Migration of leukocytes into tissues is mediated by chemokines and possibly other cytokines that are secreted by subendothelial tissues or by the endothelium itself [93,94]. The accumulation of leukocytes, often the result of bacterial infection and release of endotoxin, causes injury to the endothelium as a result of the interplay of activated adhesion molecules [92,95] and the release of chemotactic molecules, including TNF-α, interleukins, and chemokines [95–97]. The chemokines comprise a family of chemoattractant cytokines that are classified into two subfamilies based on sequence homology and the sequence around two cystine residues [96–98]. The C-X-C or α chemokine family acts predominantly on neutrophils and nonhematopoietic cells, and the C-C or β cytokine family acts mainly on monocytes as well as on eosinophils and lymphocytes. The recently discovered lymphotactin cytokine has been proposed to belong to a new group of chemokines, designated the *C family* [99].

Chemokines are thought to play an important role in inflammatory cell recruitment and subsequent tissue damage. The TNF-induced expression of the macrophage inflammatory protein 1-α (MIP-1α), a member of the C-C chemokine family, has been shown to mediate neutrophil and macrophage influx, probably by regulating the expression of ICAM-1. Clearly, the identification and characterization of the adhesive molecules that orchestrate the increasingly complex interactions of ECs, platelets, and leukocytes have provided new insights [100], and current investigation has focused on the exploitation of this knowledge to identify pathways for therapeutic intervention.

Endothelial Cells in Ischemia/Reperfusion

Ischemia-reperfusion injury is twofold. The initial insult results in tissue hypoxia, with its associated cellular alterations, whereas the second insult occurs after reperfusion, leading to complement activation, neutrophil recruitment, and the generation of toxic oxygen radicals.

The initial hypoxic episode results in specific alteration in cellular metabolism as the oxygen-deprived cell switches from aerobic metabolism to anaerobic metabolism, decreasing the cellular pH concurrent, with a buildup in metabolites such as lactate. Cells starved of oxygen for too long eventually die; however, a number of cells can survive the initial hypoxic episode quite well. A hypoxic environment is not necessarily toxic to ECs. However, the hypoxic state does induce activation of endothelial cells and multiple reversible changes in endothelial pathology [101], one of which is a switch from the normal anticoagulant state of the EC to one that promotes clot formation. Hypoxia induces thrombomodulin activity on the EC cell surface, resulting in activation of factor X as well as inhibition of EC fibrinolytic activity. Hypoxia also results in inhibition of the barrier function of the endothelium, and because the production of NO requires oxygen, the hypoxia and ischemia result in vasospasm. Clearly, the initial hypoxic insult sets the stage for continued thrombosis and contributes to the pathology seen in ischemic injury. For instance, the loss of barrier function in areas of ischemic vascular injury is a direct result of injury to the endothelium.

Adhesion of neutrophils to vascular endothelium is an early event in their recruitment into acute inflammatory or ischemic regions. It is important to recognize that endothelial–neutrophil adhesive mechanisms occur very rapidly following injury and that the specificity of the reaction resides with the altered endothelium and does not occur randomly, as would be the case if activation of the neutrophils were to activate adhesion. The complement system is known to be involved in inflammatory [102] and ischemic [103] injury. Complement fixation has recently been shown to provide a potent and rapid stimulus for neutrophil adhesion [104].

Restenosis and Longer Term Responses to Endothelial Injury

Percutaneous transluminal coronary angioplasty (PTCA) is a highly successful procedure for increasing the luminal diameter of atherosclerotic coronary arteries in order to improve distal perfusion of the myocardium. However, PTCA induces a series of events following endothelial injury, culminating in vascular remodeling, which becomes life threatening, while apparently not deviating substantially from "appropriate" responses to endothelial injury. Activation of the coagulation and complement cascades, platelet activation and aggregation, thrombus formation, leukocyte adherence, activation of the inflammatory response, vascular smooth muscle (VSM) migration and proliferation, and deposition of extracellular matrix (ECM) [105–111] lead to restenosis (narrowing or blockage of the lumen of the coronary artery) and the necessity for a repeat PTCA or a coronary artery bypass graft (CABG) in up to 50% of patients at 6 months.

PTCA failure within a day or two of the procedure occurs in 10% of patients and is due to acute closure of the arterial lumen by the formation of a platelet and thrombotic plug, blockage caused by separation of the atherosclerotic plaque from the vessel wall, elastic recoil of the stretched coronary artery, vasospasm, or a combination of the these [112]. Efforts are aimed at preventing acute closure center on mechanical devices, such as stents, and the prevention of platelet aggregation and thrombosis. PTCA failure within 6 months of the procedure is due to intimal hyperplasia that causes restenosis of the newly expanded arterial lumen. The high frequency of delayed failure, 30–50% of patients, has provided the impetus for the continued effort to find a therapeutic regimen that will effectively prevent is occurrence [105,106,108].

Restenosis begins with injury to the arterial wall, caused by expansion of the balloon catheter, and progresses through at least three phases [109,110,113]. The first phase, lasting up to 3 days, is largely a normal tissue response to injury, involving the coagulation cascade, platelet activation, and deposition of neutrophils and monocytes. The release of numerous growth factors and cytokines in this phase is believed to initiate the subsequent phases. In the second phase, smooth muscle cells are stimulated to proliferate in the media and begin to migrate to the intima. In the third phase, the smooth muscle cells populate the intima and begin to synthesize ECM, which constitutes the bulk of the restenotic lesion.

In the first phase, inflation of the balloon catheter injures the coromary artery by causing de-endothelialization, disruption, and fracture of the atherosclerotic plaque and internal elastic lamina, and stretching and rupturing of vascular smooth muscle cells and remaining endothelial cells. One of the first events is activation of the coagulation cascade via the extrinsic pathway [114]. Plaque rupture and fissuring exposes tissue factor, expressed by macrophages, to serum coagulation factors, causing their activation. Thrombin is formed, leading to fibrin deposition and contributing to platelet activation. Plaque rupture also exposes collagen, which can directly activate platelets [106]. Platelets adhere to the exposed subendothelial matrix and may also aggregate. Peak platelet deposition occurs within 2 hours of the PTCA procedure [113]. Thromboxane A_2 (TxA$_2$), synthesized and secreted by activated platelets, adenosine diphosphate (ADP) and serotonin, released by degranulation of activated platelets, serve to amplify the platelet response. Together with thrombin, these agents promote the growth of an obstructive thrombus, which may contribute to acute closure in a small but significant percentage of patients. In most patients, natural antithrombotic regulatory elements, such as antithrombin III and activated protein C, as well as flow dilution of the activating agents, limit the growth of the thrombus and platelet aggregate.

Neutrophils, lymphocytes, and monocytes are recruited to the site of injury by chemotactic factors and adhesion molecules that appear on the surface of platelets and endothelial cells following degranulation, and that are upregulated in activated and injured endothelial cells [108,109,114]. A likely chemotactic factor is PDGF, and the adhesion molecules include P-selectin, E-selectin, and ICAM-1. Neutrophils and monocytes are activated by platelet-activating factor (PAF), thrombin, PDGF, C5a, and leukotrienes to release proteases and oxygen free radicals, which may exacerbate the injury, and mitogens to promote smooth muscle cell proliferation [114,115]. A significant, though small, fraction

(1–11%) of the cells in the enlarging lesion are leukocytes, and the particular role of each type of leukocyte remains unclear [106,107].

The proliferation of vascular smooth muscle cells and endothelial cells begins in the first phase, in response to thrombin, basic fibroblast growth factor (bFGF), angiotensin II (AII), insulin-like growth factor-I (IGF-I), epidermal growth factor (EGF), and PDGF [110,114]. Thrombin directly stimulates smooth muscle cell proliferation in vitro and is present in regenerating arteries for days [116]. There is an intracellular pool of bFGF that is released by cell injury, lysis, and death [117]. Angiotensin II is formed by the local renin-angioitensin system. Degranulating platelets release growth factors, including PDGF, IGF-1, and EGF. However, the induction of medial smooth muscle proliferation can occur without platelets, indicating that the release and expression of factors from other sources are sufficient [118].

Activated monocytes also contribute several growth factors and cytokines, including PDGF, bFGF, and interleukin (IL)-1. IL-1 maintains the activated states of endothelial cells, smooth muscle cells, and monocytes, which result in the continued synthesis and release of mitogens. The primary effect of these agents is to induce a phenotypic change in smooth muscle cells from a quiescent, nonsecreting, and contractile phenotype to a proliferative and secretory phenotype [107,113]. This change perpetuates the proliferative response because smooth muscle cells begin to secrete PDGF and bFGF, thus stimulating their own proliferation in an autocrine fashion. However, by the end of the first phase most, but not all, smooth muscle cells return to a quiescent state [116]. The return to a quiescent state is attributed to re-endothelialization of the luminal surface, which may occur within several days [109,114].

The second phase of restenosis, beginning on the first to third day and lasting up to 2 weeks, is characterized by the migration from the media to the intima of the subpopulation of smooth muscle cells that escaped growth inhibition in the first phase [116]. PDGF, in addition to bFGF and AII, are believed to mediate this phase [110]. Smooth muscle cells and endothelial cells begin to synthesize and secrete ECM proteins, including fibronectin, heparan sulfate proteoglycans, tenascin, thrombospondin, and collagen. In addition, transforming growth factor-β (TGF-β), which stimulates the synthesis of ECM proteins, is produced [107,116,119,120].

In the third phase, beginning after about 7 days and continuing for several months, neointimal proliferation is reduced, but deposition of matrix contin-

ues. The bulk of the neointima is composed of newly synthesized ECM proteins [110,111,114,116,120]. The matrix undergoes remodeling and becomes organized. By 6 months all the smooth muscle cells have returned to their contractile phenotype [121]. The issue of the contribution and time course of changes in smooth muscle proliferation is controversial. Recent work has suggested that there is no peak in smooth muscle proliferation; instead, proliferation seems to occur at a steady, but low ($\leq 1\%$ of smooth muscle cells), rate for more than 9 months following PTCA [110].

In patients who do not develop restenosis, the third phase completes the healing process. This desirable outcome of the events following PTCA — re-endothelialization, recovery of vascular tone, clearance of cellular debris, replacement of dead cells by new cells, vascular remodeling, formation of scar tissue, and maintenance of vessel patency — occurs by the processes described earlier. In patients developing restenosis, neointimal proliferation and matrix deposition continues, probably mediated by the presence of mitogens and other mediators. Thus, the progression of events that are a normal response to injury also leads to restenosis. This abnormal response has been called the *fourth phase* or *wave* [110] and leads to the view that restenosis is an exaggerated response to injury.

If this view is correct, then certain mediating factors must have sufficient influence to convert a controlled response to injury, leading to vessel patency, into continued proliferation and matrix deposition, leading to restenosis. These factors may be pre-existing, they may occur as a result of a problematic procedure that causes severe injury, or they may emerge later. Attempts to define the risk factors that are predictive of restenosis have, for the most part, been inconclusive [112]. Several studies have been unable to correlate serum lipoprotein, lipid, and/or cholesterol levels with restenosis [122,123], while others have shown a correlation [124,125]. Some have proposed that the greater the severity of arterial injury, the greater the neointimal thickening and risk of restenosis [109,111]. The goal of therapy to prevent restenosis is therefore not to prevent the response to injury but to control the response such that the benefits of a healed coronary artery are realized without causing restenosis.

Many different strategies have been attempted, and many of these have proven efficacious in various animal models of restenosis. However, human clinical trials have largely been disappointing [105,106,108]. In the belief that inhibition of the early events will prevent progression to restenosis, many therapeutic strategies have targeted coagulation, platelets, inflammation, and the generation of free radicals. Another strategy has been to target classical risk factors of atherosclerosis, based on the argument that mechanisms promoting neointimal hyperplasia in restenosis are similar to those in atherosclerosis. This rationale has supported the testing of lipid-lowering drugs, vasodilators, and antihypertensive drugs.

Recent advances in the development of novel drug delivery technologies and in the understanding of the initiating mechanisms of smooth muscle proliferation have resulted in other approaches [126]. Success in animal models by targeting smooth muscle cell proliferation directly with antisense oligonucleotides targeting cdc2 kinase and proliferating-cell nuclear antigen [127], and the cellular oncogenes c-*myc* or c-*myb* [128,129], have been reported. In a gene therapy approach, balloon-injured porcine iliofemoral arteries were exposed to adenovirus vectors encoding thymidine kinase, and then the animals were treated with ganciclovir [130]. In several rat and rabbit studies, a direct inhibitor of proliferation, angiopeptin, has also proven effective in inhibiting restenosis following balloon injury [131–133].

Endothelial Injury and Complement Activation

Many vascular procedures, including CABG, endarterectomy, PTCA, and thrombolysis, would be expected to lead to immediate complement activation. Numerous types of injuries, including burns [134], pulmonary inflammation [135,136], hyperacute transplant rejection [137,138], and myocardial, skeletal muscle, and hepatic ischemia [119,139–145], are associated with complement activation. When cells and tissues are damaged, complement is activated by the release of subcellular components from injured and ischemic cells, including mitochondrial proteins [119,141], which may be associated with cardiolipin [142], a phospholipid abundant in mitochondrial membranes, or cardiolipin alone [146]. These components bind and activate C1q, the first component of the classical pathway of complement activation. Evidence for complement activation following myocardial ischemia in dogs includes the detection of C1q in cardiac lymph [141,142] and the deposition of C1q in reperfused myocardium [119]. Complement-activating lipid particles, composed of cholesterol, cholesteryl esters, and phospholipids, have also been extracted from human atherosclerotic lesions [147]. In addition, activation of the alternative pathway in ischemia-reperfusion injury of skeletal muscle has been reported [139]. Complement

may also be activated by plasmin through the activation of C1r and C3 [148,149]. Plasmin is formed from plasminogen by the release of t-PA from thrombin-activated endothelial cells, and its generation in animal models of balloon injury is increased [120]. Moreover, plasmin-mediated complement activation occurs in patients undergoing thrombolytic therapy [150,151]. Reperfusion of ischemic myocardium and localized injury to the endothelium and underlying cells by inflation of a balloon catheter and coronary artery recanalization provide ample stimuli for complement activation.

Complement activation results in the formation of the anaphylatoxins, C3a, C4a, and C5a, and the formation and deposition of the membrane attack complex (MAC) on cell membranes. In the setting of PTCA-mediated injury, these proinflammatory products would be expected to contribute to the normal response to injury, but could also exacerbate the normal response and contribute to the development of restenosis. The anaphylatoxins are chemotactic for neutrophils, inducing them to cross the endothelial cell barrier, if it still exists. Moreover, the anaphylatoxins can directly activate neutrophils, causing degranulation and the release of oxygen free radicals and proteolytic enzymes, highly toxic products that may contribute to additional cell injury. This, in turn, causes the release of more subcellular components and continued activation of complement.

The formation and deposition of the MAC, a pore-forming complex of multiple complement components (C5b,6,7,8,9), on cell membranes causes the collapse of the electrochemical gradient, leading to ion and water fluxes that ultimately lead to cell death by lysis. Sublytic deposition of the MAC stimulates mitogenesis on fibroblasts and smooth muscle cells [152], both alone and synergistically with PDGF. The MAC also stimulates the release of bFGF and PDGF from endothelial cells, resulting in smooth muscle cell proliferation [153]. Endothelial cells are also stimulated by the MAC to degranulate, releasing von Willebrand factor and exposing P-selectin, and to assemble the prothrombinase complex, promoting coagulation [154,155]. Support for a role of complement in vascular disease has been obtained by the study of atherosclerotic plaques. C5b-9, CR1, CR3, decay accelerating factor (DAF), CD59, factor H, C3c, C3d, and S-protein have been found in plaques, suggesting a contributory role of complement in the development of atherosclerosis [156–159]. In addition to plaques, complement deposition and depletion of complement regulatory proteins have been reported in infarcted human myocardium [160–163].

Activated complement may exacerbate the response to injury and may lead to restenosis by the following mechanisms: (1) Anaphylatoxins are chemotactic for neutrophils and monocytes, leading to the recruitment of these cell types to the injury site. (2) Anaphylatoxins activate neutrophils and monocytes, causing the release of oxygen free radicals and proteases that contribute to tissue injury, and growth factors and cytokines that may prolong the proliferative response. (3) The formation and deposition of sublytic amounts of the MAC activate cells at the injury site, stimulating proliferation and coagulation via prothrombinase assembly, and depleting complement regulatory proteins.

Soluble complement receptor 1 (sCR1) is a recombinant protein that lacks the cytoplasmic and transmembrane domains of complement receptor 1 (CR1) [140]. CR1 is a naturally occurring membrane-bound inhibitor of C3 and C5 convertases, and a cofactor for the degradation of C3b and C4b by factor I, that is found primarily on erythrocytes and leukocytes. Substantial evidence indicates that sCR1 retains all of the functions of CR1 and suggests that it may counteract many of the initiating and continuing processes that lead to restenosis. In models of myocardial ischemia-reperfusion injury, sCR1 significantly decreased myeloperoxidase activity, a marker for neutrophil accumulation, in infarcted myocardium and reduced infarct size [140,144]. In a model of skeletal ischemia-reperfusion injury, sCR1 prevented leukocyte adherence and increased the number of reperfusing capillaries [164]. In various models of dermal and lung inflammation, sCR1 has demonstrated potent antiinflammatory effects [135,136,165]. In a hyperacute xenograft rejection model, in which complement is rapidly activated by xenoreactive antibodies present on the surface of the endothelium of transplanted hearts, sCR1 prolonged xenograft survival, in part by reducing the number of occlusive platelet thrombi and cellular infiltrates [137,138].

The complex nature of the vascular response to injury has frustrated numerous attempts to inhibit restenosis in human trials. The failure of inhibitors of the early events of restenosis in clinical trials, including antiplatelet drugs, anticoagulants, and antioxidants, suggests either that the most critical early event was not targeted or that combination therapy may ultimately be necessary to prevent restenosis. So far no studies have targeted complement activation. Because the progression of events leading to restenosis is largely comparable with the responses to vascular injury in which complement-mediated responses have been identified and shown to be abrogated by sCR1,

it is tempting to speculate that a new class of therapeutics, complement inhibitory agents, may join the long list of useful drugs based on inhibiting the other blood enzyme cascades.

Concluding Comments

Despite their deceptive thinness in transverse section, ECs are highly active and responsive cells. It is clear from the foregoing discussion that ECs perform a multitude of functions, some of which occur constitutively and some of which are induced following activation. Not all aspects of endothelial activation occur concomitantly; nevertheless, many activation responses share common triggers and common mechanisms of cellular signal transduction.

Many pathological and pathophysiological conditions involve situations that alter the normal interactions of ECs with blood-borne molecules and alter the communication systems between endothelium and other cell types. Thus conditions that do not necessarily involve loss or death of ECs may set the stage for later irreversible endothelial damage. All injuries to endothelial cells result in alterations in vascular function; these alterations may lead to acute inflammatory reactions and subsequently to long-term remodeling of vessels. On one way or another, vascular dysfunction results and almost always involves compromise of hemostatic properties. It may well be that the ability of vessels to sustain local damage, leading to occlusion, may operate to preserve overall vascular function and to subserve the larger goal of homeostasis of the organism. Studies of the mechanisms underlying regulation of EC activation and interaction of ECs with hemostatic, inflammatory, immune, and complement systems should allow improved understanding of modulations of EC structure, function, and behavior during a wide variety of diseases and lead to improved understanding of targets for therapeutic intervention.

Acknowledgments

It is a pleasure to thank Selma Carlson for typing the manuscript and Gayle O'Neil for producing the figure.

References

1. Ryan US. Structural bases for metabolic activity. Ann Rev Physiol 44:223, 1982.
2. Ryan US. Pulmonary endothelium: A dynamic interface. Clin Invest Med 9:124, 1986.
3. Ryan US, Ryan JW, Whitaker C, Chiu A. Localization of angiotensin converting enzyme (kininase II):

Immunocytochemistry and immunofluorescence. Tissue Cell 8:125, 1976.

4. Ryan US. Processing of angiotension and other peptides by the lungs. In Fishman AP (ed). Handbook of Physiology — Section 3: The Respiratory System. Bethesda, MD: American Physiological Society, 351, 1985.

5. Ryan US, Maxwell G. Isolation, culture and subculture of bovine pulmonary artery endothelial cells: Mechanical methods. J Tissue Culture Meth 10:3, 1986.

6. Larson RS, Springer TA. Structure and function of leukocyte integrins. Immunol Rev 114:181, 1990.

7. Spagnoli LG, Pietra GC, Villaschi S, Jones LW. Morphometric analysis of gap junctions in regenerating endothelium. Lab Invest 46:139, 1982.

8. Ryan US, Ryan JW. Vital and functional activities of endothelial cells. In Nossel HL, Vogel HJ, (eds). Pathobiology of the Endothelial Cell. New York: Academic Press, 445, 1982.

9. Esmon NL, Owen WG, Esmon CT. Isolation of a membrane bound cofactor for thrombin-catalyzed activation of protein C. J Biol Chem 257:859, 1982.

10. Walker FJ, Secton PW, Esmon CT. The inhibition of blood coagulation by activated protein C through the selective inactivation of activated factor V. Biochim Biophys Acta 571:333, 1979.

11. Stern DM, Nawroth PP, Harris K, Esmon CT. Cultured bovine aortic endothelial cells promote activated protein C- protein S-mediated inactivation of factor Va. J Biol Chem 261:713, 1986.

12. Broze GJ Jr. The role of tissue factor pathway inhibitor in a revised coagulation cascade. Semin Hematol 29:159, 1992.

13. Broze GJ Jr, Warren LA, Novotny WF, Higuchi DA, Girard JJ, Miletich JP. The lipoprotein-associated coagulation inhibitor that inhibits the factor VII-tissue factor complex also inhibits factor Xa: Insight into its possible mechanism of action. Blood 71:335, 1988.

14. Sabharwal AK, Bajaj SP, Ameri A, Tricomi SM, Hyers TM, Dahms TE, et al. Tissue factor pathway inhibitor and von Willebrand factor antigen levels in adult respiratory distress syndrome and in a primate model of sepsis. Am J Respir Crit Care Med 151:758, 1995.

15. Ameri A, Kuppuswamy MN, Basu S, Bajaj SP. Expression of tissue factor pathway inhibitor by cultured endothelial cells in response to inflammatory mediators. Blood 79:3219, 1992.

16. Sandset PM, Abildgaard U, Larsen ML. Heparin induces release of extrinsic pathway inhibitor. Thromb Res 50:803, 1988.

17. Weksler BB, Marcus AJ, Jaffe EA. Synthesis of prostaglandin I_2 (prostacyclin) by cultured human and bovine endothelial cells. Proc Natl Acad Sci USA 126:365, 1977.

18. Radomski MW, Palmer RM, Moncada S. The anti-aggregating properties of the vascular endothelium: Interactions between prostacyclin and nitric oxide. Br J Pharmacol 82:6539, 1987.

19. Levin E, Loskutoff DJ. Cultured bovine endothelial cells product both urokinase and tissue-type plasminogen activators. J Cell Biol 94:631, 1982.

20. Colucci M, Balcon GI, Lorenzet R, et al. Cultured human endothelial cells generate tissue factor in response to endotoxin. J Clin Invest 71:1893, 1983.

21. Bevilacqua MP, Pober JS, Majeau GR, Fiers W, Cotran RS, Gimbrone MA Jr. Recombinant tumor necrosis factor induces procoagulant activity in cultured human vascular endothelium: Characterization and comparison with the actions of interleukin 1. Proc Natl Acad Sci USA 83:4533, 1986.

22. Nawroth PP, Stern DM. Modulation of endothelial cell hemostatic properties by tumor necrosis factor. J Exp Med 163:740, 1986.

23. Sakariassen KS, Nievelstein PF, Coller BA, Sixma JJ. The role of glycoprotein 1b and 11b-111a in platelet adherence to human artery subendothelium. Br J Haematol 63:681, 1986.

24. Weiss HJ, Baumgartner HR, Tchopp TB, Turitto VT, Cohen D. Correction by factor VIII of the impaired platelet adhesion to subendothelium in von Willebrand's disease. Blood 51:267, 1978.

25. Brommer EJP,Verheijen JH, Chang GTG, Rijken DC. Masking of fibrinolytic response to stimulation by an inhibitor of tissue-type plasminogen activator in plasma. Thromb Haemost 52:154, 1984.

26. Nilsson IM, Ljunger H, Tengborn L. Two different mechanisms in patients with venous thrombosis and defective fibrinolysis: Low concentration of plasminogen activator or increased concentration or plasminogen activator inhibitor. Br Med J 290:1453, 1985.

27. Powell JS, Rouge M, Muller RK, Baumgartner HR, Cilazapril suppresses myointimal proliferation after vascular injury: Effects on growth factor induction in vascular smooth muscle cells. Basic Res Cardoil 86:65, 1991.

28. Bhagyalakshmi A, Frangos JA. Mechanism of shear-induced prostacyclin production in endothelial cells. Biochem Biophys Res Commun 158:31, 1989.

29. Baenziger NL, Fogerty FJ, Mertz LF, Chernuta LF. Regulation of histamine-mediated prostacyclin synthesis in cultured human vascular endothelial cells. Cell 24:915, 1981.

30. Crutchley DJ, Ryan JW, Ryan US, Fischer GH. Bradykinin-induced release of prostacyclin and thromboxanes from bovine pulmonary artery endothelial cells. Biochim Biophys Acta 751:99, 1983.

31. Hamberg M, Svensson J, Samuelson G. Thromboxanes: A new group of biologically active compounds derived from prostaglandin endoperoxides. Proc Natl Acad Sci USA 72:2994, 1975.

32. Fitzgerald GA, Oates JA, Hawiger J, et al. Endogenous biosynthesis of prostacyclin and thromboxane and platelet function during chronic administration of aspirin in man. J Clin Invest 71:676, 1983.

33. Furchgott RF, Zawadzki JV. The obligatory role of endothelial cells in the relaxaation of arterial smooth muscle by acetycholine. Nature 373:299, 1980.

34. Khan MT, Furchgott RF. Similarities of behavior of (NO) and endothelium-derived relaxing factor in perfusion cascade bioassay system. Fed Proc 46:385, 1987.

35. Ignarro LJ, Byrns RE, Buga GM, Wood KS. Endothelium-derived relaxing factor (EDRF) released from artery and vein appears to be nitric oxide (NO) or a closely related radical species. Fed Proc 46:644, 1987.

36. Palmer RM, Ferrige AG, Moncada S. Nitric oxide release accounts for the biological activity of endothelium-derived relaxing factor. Nature 357:524, 1987.

37. Hutchinson PJ, Palmer RM, Moncada S. Comparative pharmacology of EDRF and nitric oxide on vascular strips. Eur J Pharmacol 141:445, 1987.

38. Diaz MN, Cohen R. Coronary Vascalar Pharmacology. In Becker RC (ed). Textbook of Coronary Thrombosis and Thrombolysis Boston: Kluwer Academic 1996.

39. Moncada S, Palmer RMJ, Higgs EA. Biosynthesis and endogenous roles of nitric oxide. Pharmacol Rev 43:109, 1991.

40. Palmer RM, Ashton DS, Moncada S. Vascular endothelial cells synthesize nitric oxide from L-arginine. Nature 333:664, 1988.

41. Rapoport RM, Murad F. Agonist induced endothelium-dependent relaxation in rat thoracic aorta may be mediated through cyclic GMP. Circ Res 52:352, 1983.

42. Rees DD, Palmer RMJ, Moncada S. Role of endothelium-derived nitric oxide in the regulation of blood pressure. Proc Natl Acad Sci USA 86:3375, 1989.

43. Aiska K, Gross SS, Griffith OW, Levi R. NG-Methylarginine, an inhibitor of endothelium-derived nitric oxide synthesis, is a potent pressor agent in the guinea pig: Does nitric oxide regulate blood pressure in vivo? Biochem Biophys Acta 160:881, 1989.

44. Knowles RG, Merrett M, Salter M, Moncada S. Differential induction of brain, lung and liver nitirc oxide synthase by endotoxin in the rat. Biochem J 270:833, 1990.

45. Busse R, Mulch A. Induction of nitric oxide synthaseby cytokines in vascular smooth muscle cells. FEBS Lett 275:87, 1990.

46. Johnson GPS, Tsa D, Malloy D, Leffer AM. Cardioprotective effects of acidified sodium nitrite in myocardial ischemia with reperfusion. J Pharmacol Exp Ther 252:35, 1990.

47. Gryglewski RJ, Botting RM, Vane JR. Mediators produced by the endothelial cell. Hypertension 12:530, 1988.

48. Flavahan NA. Atherosclerosis or lipoprotein-induced endothelial dysfunction. Potential mechanisms underlying reduction in EDRF/nitric oxide activity. Circulation 85:1927, 1992.

49. Venturini CM, Ryan US. Endothelial control of vascular smooth muscle: The importance of nitric oxide.

In Sperelakis N (ed). Physiology and Paraphysiology of the Heart, 3rd ed. Boston: Kluwer Academic, 1994.

50. Rubanyi GM, Vanhoutte PM, Hypoxia releases a vasoconstrictor substance from the canine vascular endothelium. J Physiol 364:45, 1985.

51. Yanagisawa M, Kurihara H, Kimura S, et al. A novel potent vasoconstrictor peptide produced by vascular endothelial cells. Nature 332:411, 1995.

52. Goetz KL, Wang BC, Madwed JB, Zhu JL, Leadley RJ Jr. Cardiovascular, renal, and endocrine responses to intravenous endothelin in conscious dogs. Am J Physiol 255:R1604, 1988.

53. DeNucci G, Thomas R, D'Orleans-Juste P, et al. Pressor effects of circulating endothelin are limited by its removal in the pulmonary circulation and by the release of prostacyclin and endothelium-derived relaxing factor. Proc Natl Acad Sci USA 87:9797, 1988.

54. Miyauchik T, Yangisawa M, Tomizawa T, et al. Increased plasma concentrations of endothelin-1 and big endothelin-1 in acute myocardial infarction [letter]. Lancet 2:53, 1989.

55. Tomita K, Ujiie K, Nakanishi T, et al. Plasma endothelin levels in patients with acute renal failure. N Engl J Med 321:1127, 1989.

56. Trachtenberg JD, Sun S, Rapp NS, Choi ET, Callow AD, Ryan US. The effect of endothelin-1 infusion on the development of intimal hyperplasia after balloon catheter injury. J Cardiovasc Pharmacol 22:S355, 1993.

57. Hynes RO. Integrins: A family of cell surface receptors. Cell 48:549, 1986.

58. Ruoslahi E. Integrins. J Clin Invest 87:1, 1991.

59. Williams AF, Barclay AN. The immunoglobulin superfamily—domains for cell surface recognition. Annu Rev Immunol 6:381, 1988.

60. Brandley BK, Swiedler SJ, Robbins PW. Carbohydrate ligands of the LEC cell adhesion molecules. Cell 63:861, 1990.

61. Springer TA, Lasky LA. Sticky sugars for selectins. Nature 349:196, 1991.

62. Arnout MA. The structure and function of the leukocyte adhesion molecules CD11/CD18. Blood 75:1037, 1990.

63. Kishimoto TK, Larson RS, Corbi AL, Dustin ML, Staunton DE, Springer TA. The leukocyte integrins. Adv Immunol 46:149, 1991.

64. Marlin SD, Springer TA. Purified intercellular adhesion molecule-1 (ICAM-1) is a ligand for lymphocyte function-associated antigen 1 (LFA-1). Cell 51:813, 1987.

65. Gahmberg CG, Nortamo P, Zimmermann D, Ruoslahti E. The human leukocyte-adhesion ligand, intercellular-adhesion molecule 2. Expression and characterizationof the protein. Eur J Biochem 195:197, 1991.

66. Springer TA. Adhesion receptors of the immune system. Nature 346:425, 1990.

67. Dustin ML, Rothlein R, Bhan AK, Dinarello CA, Springer TA. Induction by IL-1 and interferon-gamma: Tissue distribution, biochemistry, and function of a natural adherence molecule (ICAM-1). J Immunol 137:245, 1986.

68. Nortamo P, Li R, Renkonen R, et al. The expression of human leukocyte adhesion molecular intercellular adhesion molecule-2 is refractory to inflammatory cytokines. Eur J Immunol 21:2629, 1991.

69. Carlos TM, Schwartz BR, Kovach NL, et al. Vascular cell adhesion molecule—1 mediates lymphocyte adherence to cytokine-activated cultured human endothelial cells. Blood 76:965, 1990.

70. Elices MJ, Osborn L, Takada Y, et al. VCAM-1 on activated endothelium interacts with the leukocyte integrin VLA4 at a site distinct from the VLA4/fibronectin binding site. Cell 60:577, 1990.

71. Koch AE, Burrows JC, Haines GK, Carlos TM, Harlan JM. Immunolocalization of endothelial and leukocyte adhesion molecules in human rheumatoid and osteoarthritic synovial tissues. Lab Invest 64:313, 1991.

72. Bevilacqua M, Butcher E, Furie B, et al. Selectins: A family of adhesion receptors. Cell 67:233, 1991.

73. Bevilacqua MP, Stengelin S, Gimbrone MA Jr, Seed B. Endothelial leukocyte adhesion molecule 1: An inducible receptor for neutrophils related to complement regulatory proteins and lectins. Science 243:1160, 1989.

74. Kansas GS. Structure and function of L-selectin. APMIS 100:287, 1992.

75. Michl J, Qiu QY, Kuerer HM. Homing receptors and addressins. Curr Opin Immunol 3:373, 1991.

76. McEver RP, Beckstead JH, Moore KL, Marshall-Carlson L, Bainton DF. GMP-140, a platelet alpha-granule membrane protein, is also synthesized by vascular endothelial cells and is localized in Weibel-Palade bodies. J Clin Invest 84:92, 1989.

77. Lasky LA. Lectin cell adhesion molecules (LEC-CAMs): A new family of cell adhesion proteins involved with inflammation. J Cell Biochem 45:139, 1991.

78. Sako D, Chang X, Barone KM, Vachino G, White HM, Shaw G, et al. Expression cloning of a functional glycoprotein ligand for P-selectin. Cell 75:1179, 1993.

79. Moore KL, Patel KD, Bruehl RE, Fugang L, Johnson DA, Lichenstein HS, et al. P-selectin glycoprotein Ligand-1 mediates rolling of human neutrophils on P-selectin. J Cell Biol 128:661, 1995.

80. Asa D, Raycroft L, Ma L, Aeed PA, Kaytes PS, Elhammer AP, et al. The P-selectin glycoprotein ligand functions as a common human leukocyte ligand for P- and E-selectins. J Biol Chem 270:11662, 1995.

81. Vachino G, Chang X, Veldman GM, Kumar R, Sako D, Fouser LA, et al. P-selectin glycoprotein ligand-1 is the major counter-receptor for P-selectin on stimulated T cells and is widely distributed in non-functional form on many lymphocytic cells. J Biol Chem 270:21996, 1995.

82. Wilkins PP, Moore KL, McEver RP, Cummings RD. Tyrosine sulfation of P-selectin glycoprotein ligand-1 is required for high affinity binding to P-selectin. J Biol Chem 270:22677, 1995.

83. Steegmaler M, Levinovitz A, Isenmann S, Borges E, Lenter M, Kocher HP, et al. The E-selectin-ligand ESL-1 is a variant of a receptor for fibroblast growth factor. Nature 373:615, 1995.

84. Pober JS, Bevilacqua MP, Mendrick DL, Lapierre LA, Fiers W, Gimbroine MA Jr. Two distinct monokines, interleukin 1 and tumor necrosis factor, each independently induce biosynthesis and transient expression of the same antigen on the surface of culture human vascular endothelial cells. J Immunol 136:1680, 1986.

85. Cotran RS, Gimbrone MA Jr. Bevilacqua MP, Mendrick DL, Pober JS. Induction and detection of a human endothelial activation antigen in vivo. J Exp Med 164:661, 1986.

86. McEver RP. GMP-140: A receptor for neutrophils and monocytes on activated platelets and endothelium. J Cell Biochem 45:156, 1991.

87. Hattori R, Hamilton KK, Fugate RD, McEver RP, Sims PJ. Stimulated secretion of endothelial von Willebrand factor is accompanied by rapid redistribution to the cell surface of the intracellular granule membrane protein GMP-140. J Biol Chem 264:7768, 1989.

88. Bonfanti R, Furie BC, Furie B, Wagner DD. PADGEM (GMP140) is a component of Weibel-Palade bodies of human endothelial cells. Blood 73:1109, 1989.

89. Geng JG, Bevilacqua MP, Moore KL, et al. Rapid neutrophil adhesion to activated endothelium mediated by GMP-140. Nature 343:575, 1990.

90. Patel KD, Zimmerman GA, Prescott SM, Mclntyre TM. Oxygen radicals induce human endothelial cells to express GMP-140 and bind neutrophils. J Cell Biol 112:749, 1991.

91. Lo SK, VanSeventer GA, Levin SM, Wright SD. Two leukocyte receptors (CD11a/CD18 and CD11b/CD18) mediate transient adhesion to endothelium by binding to different ligands. J Immunol 143:3325, 1989.

92. Albelda SM, Smith CW, Ward PA. Adhesion molecules and inflammatory injury. FASEB J 8:504, 1994.

93. Adams DH, Shaw S. Leucocyte-endothelial interactions and regulation of leucocyte migration. Lancet 343:831, 1994.

94. Mackay C. Lymphocyte migration: A new spin on lymphocyte homing. Curr Biol 5:733, 1995.

95. Springer TA. Traffic signals for lymphocyte recirculation and leukocyte emigration: The multistep paradigm. Cell 76:301, 1994.

96. Oppenheim JJ, Zachariae COC, Mukaida N, Matsushima K. Properties of the novel

proinflammatory supergene "intercrine" cytokine family. Annu Rev Immunol 9:617, 1991.

97. Miller MD, Krangel MS. Biology and biochemistry of the chemokines: A family of chemotactic and inflammatory cytokines. CRC Crit Rev Immunol 14:54, 1992.

98. Kuna P, Reddigari SR, Schall TJ, Rucinski D, Sadick M, Kaplan AP, Characterization of the human basophil response to cytokines, growth factors, and histamine releasing factors of the intercrine/chemokine family. J Immunol 150:1932, 1993.

99. Kelner GS, Kennedy J, Bacon KB, Kleyensteuber S, Largaespada DA, Jenkins NA, et al. Lymphotactin: A cytokine that represents a new class of chemokine. Science 266:1395, 1994.

100. Ryan US, Worthington RE. Cell-cell contact mechanisms. Curr Opin Immunol 4:33, 1992.

101. Ogawa S, Gerlach H, Esposito C, Pasagian-Macaulay A, Brett J, Stern D. Hypoxia modulates the barrier and coagulant function of culture bovine endothelium. J Clin Invest 85:1090, 1990.

102. Mulligan MS, Yeh CG, Rudolph AR, Ward PA. Protective effects of soluble CR1 in complement- and neutrophil-mediated tissue injury. J Immunol 148:1479, 1992.

103. Hill J, Lindsay TD, Oritz F, Yeh CG, Hechtman HB, Moore FD. Soluble complement receptor type 1 ameliorates the local and remote organ injury after intestinal ischemia-reperfusion in the rat. J Immunol 149:1723, 1992.

104. Marks RM, Todd RFI, Ward PA. Rapid induction of neutrophil-endothelial adhesion by endothelial complement fixation. Nature 339:314, 1989.

105. Popma JJ, Califf RM, Topol EJ. Clinical trials of restenosis after coronary angioplasty. Circulation 84:1426, 1991.

106. Ferns GAA, Stewart-Lee AL, Anggard EE. Arterial response to mechanical injury: Balloon catheter de-endothelialization. Atherosclerosis 92:89, 1992.

107. Wilcox JN. Molecular biology: Insight into the causes and prevention of restenosis after arterial intervention. Am J Cardiol 72:88E, 1993.

108. Herrman JR, Hermans WRM, Vos J, Serruys PW. Pharmacological approaches to the prevention of restenosis following angioplasty. The search for the Holy Grail? (Part I). Drugs 46:18, 1993.

109. Schwartz RS, Edwards WD, Huber KC, Antoniades LC, Bailey KR, Camrud AR, et al. Coronary restenosis: Prospects for solution and new perspectives from a porcine model. Mayo Clin Proc 68:54, 1993.

110. O'Brien ER, Schwartz SM. Update on the biology and clinical study of restenosis. Trends Cardiovsc Med 4:169, 1994.

111. Casscells W, Engler D, Wilkerson JT. Mechanisms of restenosis. Tex Heart Inst J 21:68, 1994.

112. Landau C, Lange RA, Hillis LD. Percutaneous transluminal coronary angioplasty. N Engl J Med 330:981, 1994.

113. Currier JW, Haudenschild C, Faxon DP. Pathophysiology of restenosis: Clinical implications. In Anonymous Strategies in Primary and Secondary Prevention of Coronary Artery Disease. New York: W. Zuckschwerdt Verlag GmbH, 1992:181.

114. Shirotani M, Yui Y, Kawai C. Restenosis after coronary angioplasty: Pathogenesis of neointimal thickening initiated by endothelial loss. Endothelium 1:5, 1993.

115. Ricevuti G, Mazzone A, Paotti D, deServi S, Specchia G. Role of granulocytes in endothelial injury in coronary heart disease in humans. Atherosclerosis 91:1, 1991.

116. Majesky MW. Neointima formation after acute vascular injury. Role of counteradhesive extracellular matrix proteins. Tex Heart Inst J 21:78, 1994.

117. Lindner V, Reidy MA. Proliferation of smooth muscle cells after vascular injury is inhibited by an antibody against basic fibroblast growth factor. Proc Natl Acad Sci USA 88:3739, 1991.

118. Fingerle J, Johnson R, Clowes AW, Majesky MW, Reidy MA. Role of platelets in smooth muscle cell proliferation and migration after vascular injury in rat carotid artery. Proc Natl Acad Sci USA 86:8412, 1989.

119. Rossen RD, Swain JL, Michael LH, Weakley S, Giannini E, Entman ML. Selective accumulation of the first component of complement and leukocytes in ischemic canine heart muscle. A possible initiator of an extra myocardial mechanism of ischemic injury. Circ Res 57:119, 1985.

120. Gibbons GH, Dzau VJ. The emerging concept of vascular remodeling. N Engl J Med 330:1431, 1994.

121. Nobuyoshi M, Kimura T, Ohishi H, Horiuchi H, Nosaka H, Hamasaki N, et al. Restenosis after percutaneous transluminal coronary angioplasty: Pathologic observations in 20 patients. J Am Coll Cardiol 17:433, 1991.

122. Califf RM, Ohman EM, Frid DJ, Fortin DF, Mark DB, Hlatky MA, et al. Restenosis: The clinical issues. In Topol EJ (ed). Textbook of Interventional Cardiology. Philadelphia: WB Saunders, 1990:363.

123. Austin GE. Lipids and vascular restenosis. Circulation 85:1613, 1992.

124. Reis GJ, Kuntz RE, Silverman DI, Pasternak RC. Effects of serum lipid levels on restenosis after coronary angioplasty. Am J Cardiol 68:1431, 1991.

125. Shah PK, Amin J. Low high density lipoprotein level is associated with increased restenosis rate after coronary angioplasty. Circ 85:1279, 1992.

126. Herrman JR, Hermans WRM, Vos J, Serruys PW. Pharmacological approaches to the prevention of restenosis following angioplasty. The search for the Holy Grail? (Part II). Drugs 46:249, 1993.

127. Morishita R, Gibbons GH, Ellison KE, Nakajima M, Zhang L, Kaneda Y, et al. Single intraluminal delivery of antisense cdc2 kinase and proliferating-cell nuclear antigen oligonucleotides results in chronic

inhibition of neointimal hyperplasia. Proc Natl Acad Sci USA 90:8474, 1993.

128. Simons M, Edelman ER, DeKeyser J, Langer R, Rosenberg RD. Antisense c-*myb* oligonucleotides inhibit intimal arterial smooth muscle cell accumulation in vivo. Nature 359:67, 1992.

129. Epstein SE, Speir E, Finkel T. Do antisense approaches to the problem of restenosis make sense? Circulation 88:1351, 1993.

130. Ohno T, Gordon D, San H, Pompili VJ, Imperiale MJ, Nabel GJ, et al. Gene therapy for vascular smooth muscle cell proliferation after arterial injury. Science 265:781, 1994.

131. Conte JV, Foegh ML, Calcagno D, Wallace RB, Ramwell PW. Peptide inhibition of proliferation following angioplasty in rabbits. Transplant Proc 21:3686, 1989.

132. Lundergan C, Foegh ML, Vargas R, Eufemio M, Bormes GW, Kot PA, et al. Inhibition of myointimal proliferation of the rat carotid artery by the peptides angiopeptin and BIM 23034. Atherosclerosis 80:49, 1989.

133. Hong MK, Bhatti T, Matthews BJ, Stark KS, Cathaperman S, Foegh ML, et al. The effect of porous infusion balloon-delivered angiopeptin on myointimal hyperplasia after balloon injury in the rabbit. Circulation 88:638, 1993.

134. Gelfand JA, Donelan M, Burke JF. Preferential activation and depletion of the alternative complement pathway by burn injury. Ann Surg 198:58, 1982.

135. Mulligan MS, Warren JS, Smith CW, Anderson DC, Yeh CG, Rudolph AR, et al. Lung injury after deposition of IgA immune complexes. Requirements for CD18 and L-arginine. J Immunol 148:3086, 1992.

136. Mulligan MS, Yeh CG, Rudolph AR, Ward PA. Protective effects of soluble CR1 in complement- and neutrophil-mediated tissue injury. J Immunol 148:1479, 1992.

137. Pruitt SK, Baldwin WMI, Marsh HC, Jr, Lin SS, Yeh CG, Bollinger RR. The effect of soluble complement receptor type 1 on hyperacute xenograft rejection. Transplantation 52:868, 1992.

138. Pruitt SK, Kirk AD, Bollinger RR, Marsh HC, Jr, Collins BH, Levin JL, et al. The effect of soluble complement receptor type 1 on hyperacute rejection of porcine xenografts. Transplantation 57:363, 1994.

139. Rubin BB, Smith A, Liauw S, Isenman D, Romaschin AD, Walker PM. Complement activation and white cell sequestration in postischemic skeletal muscle. Am J Physiol 259:H525, 1990.

140. Weisman HF, Bartow T, Leppo MK, Marsh HC Jr, Carson GR, Concino MF, et al. Soluble human complement receptor type 1: in vivo inhibitor of complement suppressing post-ischemic myocardial inflammation and necrosis. Science 249:146, 1990.

141. Rossen RD, Michael LH, Kagiyama A, Savage HE, Hanson G, Reisberg MA, et al. Mechanism of complement activation after coronary artery occlusion: Evidence that myocardial ischemia in dogs causes release of constitutents of myocardial subcellular origin that complex with human C1q in vivo. Circ Res 62:572, 1988.

142. Rossen RD, Michael LH, Hawkins HK, Youker K, Dreyer WJ, Baughn RE, et al. Cardiolipin-protein complexes and initiation of complement activation after coronary artery occlusion. Circ Res 75:546, 1994.

143. Kagiyama A, Savage HE, Michael LH, Hanson G, Entman ML, Rossen RD. Molecular basis of complement activation in ischemic myocardium: Identification of specific molecules of mitochondrial origin that bind human C1q and fix complement. Circ Res 64:607, 1989.

144. Smith EF III, Griswold DE, Egan JW, Hillegass LM, Smith RAG, Hibbs MJ, et al. Reduction of myocardial reperfusion injury with soluble complement receptor 1 (BRL 55730). Eur J Pharmacol 236:477, 1993.

145. Jaeschke H, Farhood A, Bautista AP, Spolarics Z, Spitzer JJ. Complement activates Kupffer cells and neutrophils during reperfusion after hepatic ischemia. Am J Physiol 264:G801, 1993.

146. Kovacsovics T, Tschopp J, Kress A, Isliker H. Antibody-independent activation of C1, the first component of complement, by cardiolipin. J Immunol 135:2695, 1985.

147. Seifert PS, Hugo F, Tranum-Jensen J, Zahringer U, Muhly M, Bhakdi S. Isolation and characterization of a complement-activating lipid extracted from human atherosclerotic lesions. J Exp Med 172:547, 1990.

148. Ratnoff OD, Naff GB. The conversion of C'1s the C'1 esterase by plasma and trypsin. J Exp Med 125:337, 1967.

149. Ward P. A plasmin-split fragment of C3 as a new chemotactic factor. J Exp Med 126:189, 1967.

150. Frangi D, Gardinali M, Cafaro C, Pozzoni L, Agostoni A. Abrupt complement activation and transient neutropenia in patients with acute myocardial infarction treated with streptokinase. Circulation 89:76, 1994.

151. Ewald GA, Eisenberg PR. Plasmin-mediated activation of contact system in response to pharmacological thrombolysis. Circulation 91:28, 1995.

152. Halperin JA, Taratuska A, Nicholson-Weller A. Terminal complement complex C5b-9 stimulates mitogenesis in 3T3 cells. J Clin Invest 91:1974, 1993.

153. Benzaquen LR, Nicholson-Weller A, Halperin JA. Terminal complement proteins C5b-9 release basic fibroblast growth factor and platelet-derived growth factor from endothelial cells. J Exp Med 179:985, 1994.

154. Hattori R, Hamilton KK, McEver RP, Sims PJ. Complement proteins C5b-9 induce secretion of high molecular weight multimers of endothelial von Willebrand factor and translocation of granule membrane protein GMP-140 to the cell surface. J Biol Chem 264:9053, 1989.

155. Hamilton KK, Hattori R, Esmon CT, Sims PJ. Complement proteins C5b-9 induce vesiculation of the endothelial plasma membrane and expose catalytic surface for assembly of the prothrombinase enzyme complex. J Biol Chem 265:3809, 1990.

156. Niculescu F, Rus HG, Vlaicu R. Immunohistochemical localization of C5b-9, S-protein, C3d and apolipoprotein B in human arterial tissues with atherosclerosis. Atherosclerosis 65:1, 1987.

157. Seifert PS, Hansson GK. Decay-accelerating factor is expressed on vascular smooth muscle cells in human atherosclerotic lesions. J Clin Invest 84:597, 1989.

158. Seifert PS, Hansson GK, Complement receptors and regulatory proteins in human atherosclerotic lesions. Arteriosclerosis 9:802, 1989.

159. Seifert PS, Roth I, Schmiedt W, Oelert H, Okada N, Okada H, et al. CD59 (homologous restriction factor 20), a plasma membrane protein that protects against complement C5b-9 attack, in human atherosclerotic lesions. Atherosclerosis 96:135, 1992.

160. Shafter H, Mathey D, Hugo F, Bhakdi S. Deposition of the terminal C5b-9 complement complex in infarcted areas of human myocardium. J Immunol 137:1945, 1986.

161. Hugo F, Hamdoch T, Mathey D, Schafer H, Bhakdi S. Quantiative measurement of SC5b-9 and C5b-9(m) in infarcted areas of human myocardium. Clin Exp Immunol 81:132, 1990.

162. Zimmermann A, Gerber H, Nussenzweig V, Isliker H. Decay-accelerating factor in the cardiomyocytes of normal individuals and patients with myocardial infarction. Virchows Arch A Pathol Anat 417:299, 1990.

163. Vakeva A, Laurila P, Meri S. Loss of expression of protection (CD59) is associated with complement membrane attack complex deposition in myocardial infarction. Lab Invest 67:608, 1992.

164. Pemberton M, Anderson G, Vetvicka V, Justus DE, Ross GD. Microvascular effects of complement blockade with soluble recombinant CR1 on ischemia/reperfusion injury in skeletal muscle. J Immunol 150:5104, 1993.

165. Rabinovici R, Yeh CG, Hillegass LM, Griswold DC, DiMartino MJ, Vernick J, et al. Role of complement in endotoxin/platelet-activating factor-induced lung injury. J Immunol 149:1744, 1992.

9. PHYSIOLOGY OF VASCULAR HOMEOSTASIS

Harsch Sanchorawala and John F. Keaney, Jr.

Introduction

Over the past 15 years the vasculature has been recognized as more than simply a conduit for the delivery of nutrients and oxygen. The vasculature is an organ composed of endothelial, smooth muscle, and fibroblast cell types with an integrated system of autocrine–paracrine interactions. The vascular system is responsive to changes within both the vascular wall and target organs through the action of local factors that influence its structure and function. In this chapter, we review the anatomic and functional properties of the vasculature, with particular reference to the maintenance of vascular homeostasis.

ANATOMIC CONSIDERATIONS

The arterial vasculature, through a branching system of conduit vessels, carries blood from the heart to the capillaries, where the exchange of nutrients and waste products takes place. In addition to the transport of blood, these conduit vessels maintain arterial pressure and flow during diastole. The conduit vessels terminate in small arteries and arterioles that are the site of greatest hemodynamic resistance and are thus called *resistance vessels*. Resistance vessels, in combination with precapillary sphincters, modulate peripheral resistance, and thus, tissue blood flow. Resistance vessels also provide a reduction in hydrostatic pressure in the capillaries that prevents excessive transudation of plasma. The venous vasculature, in contrast, comprises a series of capacitance vessels that, compared with the arterial system, exhibit a blunted pressure-volume relationship and ultimately transport blood back to the heart from tissues. The venous system also serves as a volume reservoir that maintains relatively constant arterial blood volume over a wide range of changes in total intravascular volume.

As shown in Figure 9-1, the vessel wall consists of three concentric layers: (1) the tunica adventitia, the outermost layer, consisting primarily of fibroblasts and connective tissue on the extralumenal surface of the external elastic lamina; (2) the tunica media, composed of vascular smooth muscle, along with subintimal tissue located between the internal and external elastic laminae; and (3) the tunica intima, consisting of endothelial cells and a thin layer of collagen and elastin fibers located on the lumenal side of the internal elastic lamina.

ADVENTITIA

The adventitia consists of collagen, elastin, and other extracellular matrix interspersed with fibroblasts. The external elastic lamina is the layer of interwoven elastin fibrils between the adventitia and the media. The adventitia, along with the external elastic lamina, contribute to the compliance of a given blood vessel. For example, the aorta has a thick adventitia with a modest elastin content relative to collagen and, thus, is a relatively noncompliant vessel. In contrast, the pulmonary artery also has a thick adventitia, but it contains a higher proportion of elastin relative to collagen and is much more compliant. The anatomic layer inside the adventitia, the media, is also an important determinant of vascular compliance.

MEDIA

The media is composed of vascular smooth muscle cells enmeshed in collagen and elastin, and this layer is separated from the intima by the internal elastic lamina. This collagen and elastin extracellular matrix forms a scaffold for the vascular smooth muscle cells and greatly contributes to the strength and compliance of the blood vessel wall. Using the example cited earlier the aorta has many layers of smooth muscle in the intima, with a great abundance of collagen and elastin in order to withstand arterial pressure. The pulmonary artery, in contrast, has fewer layers of smooth muscle with relatively more elastin, making it suitable for large changes in volume without much change in pressure.

Blood Vessel Cross-Section

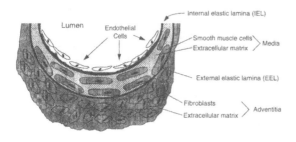

FIGURE 9-1. Cross-section of a blood vessel. The lumenal surface is lined with endothelium and subendothelial connective tissue. The tunica intima is bordered by the lumen and the internal elastic lamina, whereas the internal and external elastic laminae define the tunica media. The abluminal portion of the vessel outside the external elastic lamina defines the tunica adventitia.

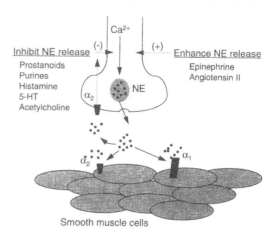

FIGURE 9-2. Adrenergic neural transmission in the blood vessel wall. Neural stimulation results in action potential propagation and an icrease in intracellular Ca^{2+}, which facilitates norepinephrine (NE) release into the synaptic cleft. Nitric oxide release is augmented by epineprine and angiotensin II, whereas prostanoids, purines, histamine, 5-hydroxytryptamine (5-HT), and acetylcholine impair NE release. Norepinephrine interaction with postsynaptic α_1 adrenergic receptors leads to smooth muscle cell contraction. In contrast, prejunctional stimulation of α_2 receptors results in feedback inhibition of NE release. (Adapted from Marlar et al. [87], with permission.)

Vascular smooth muscle cells are connected with tight junctions, providing close mechanical coupling of cells for vascular contraction. In addition, smooth muscle cells have pathways of low electrical resistance via gap junctions in order to facilitate cellular communication and to propagate electrical stimuli for contraction. The arterial vascular smooth muscle maintains a basal level of active tension (i.e., tone), and the control of vessel diameter is achieved through modulation of this tension in response to neural, hormonal, or pharmacologic stimulation. Contraction of resistance vessels (50–100 microns in diameter) modulates tissue blood flow and peripheral vascular resistance. In addition to the control of vascular tone, vascular smooth muscle cells also play an important role in vascular remodeling after arterial injury [1].

INTIMA

The intima is the anatomic layer of the vascular wall between the internal elastic lamina and the vessel lumen space. It is composed of endothelial cells in a single layer embedded in connective tissue. This connective tissue provides mechanical strength, modulates the function of endothelial cells, and participates in maintaining local homeostasis. Collagen is a major component of intimal connective tissue, and types I and III are the major types of collagen in the intima. In addition to providing mechanical strength, collagen plays an important role in hemostasis at sites of vascular injury.

The third component of the intimal connective tissue are the *amorphous ground substances*. This term refers to glycoproteins and glycosaminoglycans that are contained in the subendothelial space. These substances provide a number of important functions. Fibronectin represents the most well-characterized glycoprotein and is an important component of the extracellular matrix. Fibronectin binds to fibrin, collagen, and vascular cells, thus promoting cellular adhesion to the connective tissue. Fibronectin appears particularly important for cellular migration in the arterial wall [2]. Laminin is another glycoprotein in the extracellular matrix that binds endothelial cells, providing an anchor to the basement membrane.

Glycosaminoglycans are the major macromolecular elements of the amorphous ground substance and consist of long unbranched chains of carbohydrate polymers with recurrent disaccharide units. Glycosaminoglycans bind to specific core proteins, forming complexes called *proteoglycans*. Common proteoglycans in the vascular wall include chondroitin sulfate, dermatan sulfate, heparin, and heparan sulfate. These proteoglycans are involved in vascular homeostasis, modulating local thrombin activity and smooth muscle cell proliferation.

TABLE 9-1. Adrenergic influences on vascular smooth muscle

Receptor	Ligand preference	Location	Physiologic effect
α_1-adrenergic	NE > Epi	Postjunctional	Increased release and influx of Ca^{2+} and decreased intracellular cAMP
α_2-adrenergic	NE > Epi	Postjunctional	Same as α_2 receptor
		Prejunctional	Reduces NE release in response to neuronal stimulation
β-adrenergic	Epi > NE	Postjunctional	Increased cAMP and reduced intracellular Ca^{2+}

NE = norepinephrine; Epi = epinephrine; cAMP = cyclic 3',5'-adenosine monophosphate.

Thus, the extracellular matrix is responsible for a number of structural and regulatory functions in the vessel wall. These functions are also complemented by the actions of vascular smooth muscle and endothelial cells, such as control of blood flow, vascular tone, thrombosis, fibrinolysis, and the modulation of vessel geometry.

Control of Blood Flow

The cardiovascular system ensures appropriate perfusion of tissues and organs of the body during rest as well as in conditions of stress. This requires a complex interplay between neural, humoral, and local factors that affect the heart and vascular tone. At the precapillary level, active changes in vessel diameter that occur in response to vasoactive influences regulate blood flow to specific tissues. These changes in vessel diameter are determined by the balance of vasoconstrictive and vasodilatory influences on vascular smooth muscle cells.

NEURAL CONTROL OF VASCULAR TONE

The vessel wall is innervated by sympathetic neurons that utilize norepinephrine as a neurotransmitter to act on α- and β-adrenergic receptors (Table 9-1). The sympathetic outflow to peripheral blood vessels originates in the reticular formation of the brainstem. In most blood vessels, α-adrenergic receptors predominate, and they are characterized by two subtypes, α_1 and α_2. The α_1 receptors are predominantly postjunctional and are present on vascular smooth muscle cells of most large arteries. In contrast, α_2 receptors are predominantly prejunctional and, in response to activation, limit the prejunctional response, thus exerting a negative feedback. Postjunctional α_1-adrenergic stimulation leads to smooth muscle cell contraction and vasoconstriction.

In the coronary arteries, β-adrenergic receptors are the predominant adrenergic receptors. The β receptors are also subdivided into β_1 and β_2 subtypes. β_1 receptors predominate in the coronary smooth muscle, whereas β_2 receptors are more prevalent in the systemic vasculature. The postjunctional stimulation of β receptors leads to vasodilation. Under normal physiologic conditions, neurally released norepinephrine predominantly stimulates postjunctional α-adrenergic receptors on blood vessels, causing vasoconstriction in the systemic circulation and activation of β-adrenergic receptors in the coronary circulation, resulting in vasodilation [3–5]. The systemic vasoconstriction mediated by adrenergic release of norepinephrine is attenuated by the stimulation of prejunctional α_1-adrenergic receptors. There is also evidence that α and β (specifically β_1) stimulation may lead to the generation of prostacyclin by endothelial cells in cardiovascular tissue that may, in part, modulate the vascular effects of adrenergic stimulation [6]. Adrenergic neural transmission is outlined schematically in Figure 9-2.

The vessel wall is also innervated by parasympathetic nerves that utilize acetylcholine as a neurotransmitter to activate muscarinic receptors. In general, the activation of muscarinic receptors has the opposite effect of adrenergic stimulation, namely, vasodilation and a reduction of the heart rate. Activation of cholinergic neurons results in vasodilation through two distinct mechanisms. The first, and most direct, mechanism of cholinergic vasodilation appears to be dependent on the endothelium [5,7]. In experiments conducted in dogs, coronary vasodilation due to vagal stimulation was attenuated by inhibition of endothelial nitric oxide (NO) synthesis [8] (see later for further details). The second mechanism for cholinergic vasodilation is related to modulation of sympathetic tone. Some cholinergic nerves terminate in the prejunctional region of adrenergic neurons. Stimulation of these cholinergic nerves inhibits the release of norepinephrine and limits the extent of α-adrenergic stimulation [9], thus reducing vasoconstriction and promoting vasodilation.

HUMORAL CONTROL OF VASCULAR TONE

Circulating catecholamines and vasoactive peptides impact on the contractile state of vascular smooth muscle cells and, thus, vascular tone. The influence of circulating catecholamines on vascular tone is primarily a consequence of epinephrine generated in the adrenal medulla. Because physiologic levels of epinephrine primarily result in stimulation of peripheral β-adrenergic receptors, the overall effect of circulating epinephrine is vasodilation, which results from an increase in smooth muscle cell cyclic 3′,5′-adenosine monophosphate (cAMP).

Circulating atrial natriuretic peptide, as the name suggests, is derived primarily from atrial myocytes and is released in response to elevations of atrial pressure. This peptide mediates vasodilation and decreases blood pressure by activation of particulate guanylyl cyclase [10] in vascular smooth muscle cells. In addition, atrial natriuretic peptide produces an increase in glomerular filtration rate and renal blood flow, resulting in a natriuresis that counters any increase in atrial pressure. Other circulating peptides that influence vascular tone include glucagon and insulin. These peptides are derived from the pancreas, and their primary function is the regulation of glucose metabolism. In addition to their effect on glucose metabolism, both hormones produce vasodilation. Insulin induces vasodilation both by stimulation of endothelial NO production [11] and direct activation of smooth muscle cell β-adrenergic receptors [12]. Glucagon produces vasodilation through an increase in smooth muscle cell cAMP that is not mediated by β-adrenergic receptors [13].

The humoral control of vascular tone also involves circulating facotors that mediate vasoconstriction, such as catecholamines and peptides, including angiotensin II, arginine vasopressin, and endothelin. As stated earlier, the primary circulating catecholamine is epinephrine, which at normal circulating levels mediates vasodilation. Under conditions of stress, such as shock or vigorous exercise, however, plasma levels of norepinephrine increase and may produce peripheral vasoconstriction through stimulation of α-adrenergic receptors.

The renin-angiotensin system is an important humoral mediator of vascular tone through the action of angiotensin II, an octapeptide. Control of circulating angiotensin II levels begins in the kidney with the release of renin, an enzyme that catalyzes the conversion of plasma angiotensinogen to angiotensin I, a decapeptide with limited biologic activity. Circulating angiotensin I is then cleaved to the more active angiotensin II through the action of angiotensin converting enzyme in the pulmonary and, perhaps, peripheral circulation. The rate-limiting step in this process is renin-mediated production of angiotensin I.

Angiotensin II is among the most potent vasoconstrictors and acts on all manner of vascular smooth muscle, including conduit arteries, arterioles, and some veins. Angiotensin II also stimulates adrenal aldosterone production, resulting in renal sodium reabsorption and an expansion in plasma volume that serves to increase arterial pressure. Thus, circulating angiotensin II regulates vascular tone and arterial pressure, both through direct and indirect mechanisms. The important of circulating angiotensin II in the control of arterial pressure is underscored by the widespread use of angiotensin converting enzyme inhibitors as antihypertensive agents.

Arginine vasopressin is a peptide released by the posterior pitutary gland in response to volume depletion or stimulation of low-pressure baroreceptors in the atrium and pulmonary vessels. The systemic response to vasopressin is dependent on the target circulation. In the cerebral circulation vasopressin produces vasodilation, whereas in the peripheral circulation the response to vasopressin is vasoconstriction. The effects of vasopressin are mediated by two classes of vasopressinergic receptors, V_1 and V_2. The V_1 subtype is located in the vascular wall in vascular smooth muscle cells and mediates peripheral vasoconstriction through a direct increase in cellular Ca^{2+} and augmentation of postjunctional adrenergic responses. The V_2 receptors are principally responsible for water reabsorption in the distal nephron and, thus, indirectly modulate arterial pressure. In contrast to peripheral responses, the cerebral response to vasopressin is an endothelium-dependent process [14], resulting in NO-mediated vasorelaxation. The neurohumoral control of vascular tone is summarized in Table 9-2.

LOCAL CONTROL OF VASCULAR TONE

A variety of factors are produced and released by the endothelium to modulate vascular tone (Table 9-3). The important mediators in endothelial control of vascular tone include arachidonic acid derived cyclooxygenase and lipoxygenase products, endothelium-derived NO, endothelin, and angiotensin II.

TABLE 9-2. Neural and humoral control of vascular tone

Influence	Mediator	Effect
Neural		
Sympathetic	Norepinephrine	Vasoconstriction
Parasympathetic	Acetylcholine	Vasodilation; attenuate alpha-adrenergic effect
Humoral		
Catecholamine	Epinephrine	Vasoconstriction of skin and viscera vasculature (predominant alpha receptors); vasodilation of skeletal muscle vasculature (predominant beta receptors)
	Norepinephrine	Vasoconstriction
Peptide	Atrial natriuretic peptide	Vasodilation by guanylyl cyclase
	Vasoactive intestinal peptide	Vasodilation via stimulation of adenylyl cyclase
	Glucagon	Vasodilation by a cAMP-dependent mechanism
	Insulin	Vasodilator
	Angiotensin II	Vasoconstrictor; growth stimulatory properties; potentiates adrenergic influences
	Arginine vasopressin	Vasoconstriction; endothelium-dependent vasodilation in cerebral vasculature

TABLE 9-3. Endothelial mediators of vascular tone

Agent	Precursor	Secondary messenger	Effects	Comments
Arachidonic acid products				
Prostacyclin	PGH_2	cAMP	Vasodilation and inhibition of platelet aggregation/adhesion	Effects are additive effects with EDNO and antagonized by TxA_2
Leukotrienes (LTC_4, LTD_4, LTE_4)	Leukotriene A_4		Conductance and resistance vessel vasoconstriction	Effects impair the responses to EDNO
EDRF/NO	L-arginine	cGMP, K^+ channels	Vasodilation; inhibition of platelet aggregation/ adhesion	Additive effects with prostacyclin
Endothelin-1	Preproendothelin	IP_3, Ca^{2+} channels	Vasoconstriction	Effects are antagonized by NO
Angiotensin II	Angiotensinogen	IP_3	Potent vasoconstriction	potentiates adrenergic influences

EDRF = endothelium-derived relaxation factor; NO = nitric oxide; cGMP = cyclic 3′,5′-guanosine monophosphate; cAMP = cyclic 3′,5′-adenosine monophosphate; TxA_2 = thromboxane A_2; IP_3 = inositol triphosphate; PGH_2 = prostaglandin endoperoxide; EDNO = endothelium-derived nitric oxide.

Arachidonic Acid Derivatives. A number of arachidonic acid–derived lipid mediators play an important role in the regulation of vascular tone. The initial step in the generation of these vasoactive substances is the release of arachidonic acid from membrane phospholipids. This process begins by activation of receptors on the cell surface, followed by G-protein–coupled stimulation of phospholipase C, an enzyme located on the internal surface of the plasma membrane.

Phospholipase C catalyzes the hydrolysis of membrane-bound phosphatidylinositol-2,4-biphosphate (PIP_2) and results in the formation of inositol 1,4,5-triphosphate (IP_3) and diacylglycerol. Calcium is released from intracellular storage sites, notably the sarcoplasmic reticulum, through the action of IP_3. In association with this increase in intracellular Ca^{2+}, diacylglycerol stimulates translocation and activation of protein kinase C (PKC). Increased Ca^{2+} also activates phospholipase A_2, releasing arachidonic acid from membrane phospholipids, and this represents the major source for arachidonic acid. The other source of arachidonic acid is diacylglycerol through the action of diacylglycerol lipase [15,16].

Cyclooxygenase System. Increased arachidonic acid serves as a substrate for cyclooxygenase, an enzyme that converts arachidonic acid into cyclic endoperoxides, key precursor molecules for the formation of prostacyclin (PGI_2), a potent vasodilator; thromboxane (TxA_2), a potent vasoconstrictor; and the other prostaglandins (PGE_2, $PGF_{2\alpha}$, and PGD_2). Arachidonic acid is initially converted into prostaglandin G_2, which is then converted into prostaglandin H_2, via the peroxidase activity of the cyclooxygenase enzyme [16]. Prostaglandin H_2 then serves as the precursor for the above-mentioned active compounds. Prostacyclin is the most important product of this system in the vessel wall and is generated from prostaglandin H_2 in vascular smooth muscle cells and endothelial cells by the action of an enzyme, prostacyclin synthase. Thromboxane synthesis is principally important in the action of platelets [16].

Endothelial cells are the most important site of prostacyclin formation. The production of prostacyclin is stimulated by a number of physiologically relevant stimuli, including increased shear stress in the vessel wall [17], hypoxia [18], and neurohumoral mediators, such as thrombin and acetylcholine [16] (Figure 9-3). Prostacyclin exerts its physiologic effect by receptor-mediated stimulation of adenylyl cyclase in vascular smooth muscle cells and, thus, increased intracellular cAMP levels. Increased cAMP stimulates intracellular sequestration of calcium, producing a decrease in the intracellular Ca^{2+} levels. These effects are mediated by cAMP-dependent protein kinase and probably cGMP-dependent protein kinase [19]. In smooth muscle cells, a decrease in Ca^{2+} levels leads to relaxation and thus vasodilation. There is also evidence to suggest that prostacyclin may cause relaxation of coronary vasculature by opening outward-rectifying K^+ channels, leading to hyperpolarization and relaxation [20].

Lipoxygenase System. Arachidonic acid is also subject to oxidation via the lipoxygenase system, and the products of this reaction, the leukotrienes, play a role in regulation of vascular tone. The initial step in the generation of these vasoactive substances is the release of arachidonic acid from membrane phospholipids in response to appropriate agonists as described earlier. Under appropriate stimulatory conditions, including the presence of Ca^{2+} and adenosine triphosphate,

lipoxygenase converts free arachidonic acid into the unstable epoxide, leukotriene A_4. This compound is then converted into leukotriene B_4 and leukotriene C_4.

Leukotriene C_4 and its metabolites, leukotrienes D_4 and E_4, increase vascular permeability and contract vascular smooth muscle in both large [21] and resistance [22] coronary arteries. Leukotriene B_4 is a potent chemoattractant for neutrophils and stimulates adherence of neutrophils to the endothelial surface [23]. Other lipoxygenase derivatives may play a role in modulation of vascular tone in pathologic states. For example, isolated aortas of diabetic rabbits contain an increased level of the lipoxygenase product, 15-hydroxyeicosatetraenoic acid, and this compound impairs endothelium-dependent vasodilation and may, in part, explain the endothelial dysfunction associated with diabetes mellitus [24]. The precise role of lipoxygenase products in the modulation of basal vascular tone, however, is not known.

Endothelium-Derived Nitric Oxide. In 1980, Furchgott and Zawadzki noted that acetylcholine treatment of isolated vessels with intact endothelium leads to vasodilation, whereas de-endothelialized vessels respons with vasoconstriction [25]. These investigators hypothesized that endothelial cells produce a relaxing factor they termed *endothelium-deived relaxing factor.* Endothelium-derived relaxing factor has now been identified as NO or a closely related redox form of NO [26,27], which is synthesized constitutively by endothelial cells through the action of NO synthase [28]. Its release is stimulated by a variety of agents, including shear stress, aggregating platelets, thrombin, serotonin, acetylcholine, substance P, α_2-adrenergic agonists, and bradykinin, all of which act via specific endothelial cell membrane receptors [29] (see Figure 9-3).

Nitric oxide is synthesized from L-arginine by the action of a family of enzymes, the NO synthases [30]. Three distinct subtypes of NO synthase have been described, and they differ in subcellular location, regulation, and, thus, functional roles. For the purposes of this discussion, the endothelial NO synthase, known as eNOS, is the most relevant. This enzyme is constitutively active and has a N-myristoylation site, which results in its localization in the cell membrane [31]. Agonist activation of endothelial cell membrane receptors leads to a transient increase in intracellular Ca^{2+}. The Ca^{2+} facilitates calmodulin association with eNOS to allow electron transfer from NADPH, via flavin groups (flavin mononucleotide and flavin adenine dinucleotide) within NO synthase, to the active site on the enzyme [32]. This activation

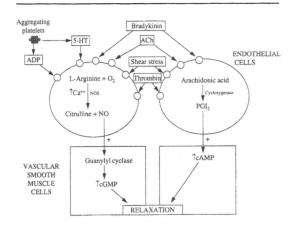

FIGURE 9-3. Receptor-mediated control of vascular tone. In response to a number of physiologically relevant stimuli, endothelial cells produce both arachidonic acid and L-arginine derivatives that modulate vascular tone. The secondary messengers for these signals in smooth muscle cells are distinct and thus act synergistically to limit inappropriate vasospasm.

leads to the production of NO in the presence of cofactors such as tetrahydrobiopterin and glutathione [33].

Nitric oxide activates soluble guanylyl cyclase through an interaction with the heme component of this enzyme, leading to the generation of cyclic $3',5'$-guanosine monophosphate (cGMP) in vascular smooth muscle cells. The cGMP stimulates cAMP phosphodiesterase, causing hydrolysis of cAMP. In addition, cGMP stimulates cGMP-dependent protein kinase, leading to phophorylation of Ca^{2+} transport proteins, with the net result being a decrease in the intracellular Ca^{2+}. This decrease in the intracellular Ca^{2+} results in relaxation and, thus, vasodilation. In this manner, cGMP serves as a secondary messenger for NO. There is also evidence that NO may also exert its effects through the stimulation of potassium channels [34].

The importance of endothelium-derived NO in maintaining vascular tone is illustrated by the response of the blood vessels to aggregating platelets. Vasoconstriction in response to aggregating platelets in isolated blood vessel preparations has been demonstrated and is due to platelet release of serotonin and adenine nucleotides as well as the generation of thrombin. This effect is markedly attenuated in the presence of intact endothelium [35]. In fact, the process of platelet aggregation actually stimulates endothelial cell generation of NO as part of a feedback

mechanism to prevent excessive vasoconstriction. This effect is mediated by serotonergic and purinergic receptors on the endothelial surface that are stimulated in response to serotonin [36] and adenine nucleotides [37], respectively. Thus, the endothelium is important in preventing excess vasospasm in response to aggregating platelets.

Endothelin. Endothelin is a potent vasoconstrictor peptide released from endothelial cells [38]. Three subtypes of endothelins have been recognized that are encoded by three distinct genes [39], although endothelin-1 is secreted from endothelial cells. Endothelin-1 is first synthesized as preproendothelin, a 203 amino acid peptide that is converted to big endothelin-1 (proendothelin) by an endopeptidase. Proendothelin is then subject to hydrolysis in the vascular wall by endothelin converting enzyme into endothelin-1. Endothelin-1 is continuously secreted by cultured endothelial cells, and its expression is enhanced when endothelial cells are stimulated by hyperglycemia, hypoxia, thrombin, epinephrine, and mediators of inflammation such as interleukin-1 [15]. In vascular smooth muscle cells, endothelin-mediated constriction is initiated by binding of endothelin-1 to endothelin receptors on vascular smooth muscle cells that activate phospholipase C. This, in turn, leads to an increase in inositol phosphates and diacylglycerol, causing increased intracellular Ca^{2+} via mobilization from intracellular stores [40]. Endothelin also activates voltage-dependent Ca^{2+} channels in vascular smooth muscle as a second mechanism of increasing intracellular Ca^{2+} [41]. Vasoconstriction caused by endothelin is reversed with endothelium-derived vasodilators such as NO [42] and prostacyclin, as well as exogenous nitrates [42]. This functional antagonism between endothelin and endothelium-derived NO plays an important role in local regulation of vascular tone.

Renin-Angiotensin System. Renin catalyzes the conversion of angiotensinogen to angiotensin I, which is then converted into angiotensin II through the action of angiotensin converting enzyme. There is growing evidence that angiotensin II is produced in the heart and blood vessels, in part through the action of local angiotensin converting enzyme activity [43,44]. This observation is based on evidence that both the renin and angiotensinogen genes are actively transcribed in peripheral tissue. In addition, angiotensin converting enzyme activity has been demonstrated in peripheral tissue by enzyme activity assay, immunostaining, and autoradiographic studies [45]. With respect to blood vessels, angiotensin converting enzyme is found in

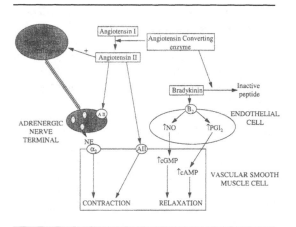

FIGURE 9-4. The renin-angiotensin system and the control of vascular tone. Angiotensin converting enzyme acts both to produce angiotensin II (AII), and inactivate bradykinin. The former action results in vasoconstriction via AII receptors on the smooth muscle cell surface and an effective increase in norepinephrine (NE) through enhancement of both local and central sympathetic activity. The inactivation of bradykinin further promotes vasoconstriction through a reduction in endothelial cell production of nitric oxide (NO) and prostacyclin (PGI$_2$).

endothelial cells [44] and, to a lesser degree, in the adventitia [43]. The wide-ranging effects of angiotensin II in blood vessels are depicted in Figure 9-4.

The vasoconstrictive effects of angiotensin II are mediated through multiple mechanisms. In vascular smooth muscle cells, angiotensin II stimulates voltage-sensitive Ca^{2+} channels, leading to a rise in the intracellular calcium and, thus, vasoconstriction [46]. Angiotensin II also enhances sympathetic activity by stimulation of prejunctional angiotensin II receptors on adrenergic nerve endings, leading to augmented local release of norepinephrine in response to adrenergic stimulation [47]. In addition, angiotensin II inhibits neuronal reuptake of norepinephrine, thus increasing its half-life at the neuromuscular interface and enhancing the effect of central nervous system sympathetic outflow.

In addition to the generation of angiotensin II, angiotensin converting enzyme is the main pathway for degradation of bradykinin, a peptide that is formed from the kininogens. Because bradykinin is a potent stimulus for the generation of endothelium-derived NO, inhibition of the angiotensin converting enzyme may indirectly increase the local concentration of NO [48]. Thus, inhibition of angiotensin

converting enzyme would not only inhibit the direct effects of angiotensin II (i.e., vasoconstriction, cellular proliferation), but may also promote the formation of endothelium-derived NO, resulting in vasodilation. In this manner, local vascular angiotensin converting enzyme activity may exert a dual effect on vascular homeostasis.

Control of Arterial Patency

The endothelium and underlying intimal connective tissue play a pivotal role in maintaining normal blood fluidity and preventing imappropriate thrombus formation. Endothelial cells constitutively produce autocrine and paracrine factors that inhibit platelet adhesion and thrombus formation, and modulate fibrinolysis. In addition, many components of the extracellular matrix that are produced by the endothelium also contribute to the regulation of thrombosis. Under both normal and pathologic conditions, endothelial denudation and turnover occurs. In response, platelet adhesion and thrombin generation leads to the formation of a fibrin plug that maintains vascular integrity. In the following section we discuss the major mediators of arterial patency.

NEURAL CONTROL OF ARTERIAL PATENCY
As discussed earlier, blood vessels are innervated by sympathetic and parasympathetic neurons. Parasympathetic stimulation leads to vasodilation, which appears to be dependent on the endothelium, likely as consequence of NO generation. These observations raise the possibility that parasympathetic stimulation may exert a beneficial effect on platelet adhesion. In contrast, sympathetic stimulation causes postjunctional α-adrenergic stimulation, which may, in theory, increase the local concentration of norepinephrine and reduce the threshold for platelet aggregation. The precise role of neural input in modulating local control of platelet adhesion and thrombus formation, however, is not known.

HUMORAL CONTROL OF ARTERIAL PATENCY
There is considerable evidence to indicate that circulating humoral factors have an influence on platelet "tone" and, thus, the propensity towards adhesion and aggregation. The fact that epinephrine stimulates platelet aggregation has been known for some time [49], and infusion of epinephrine results in platelet activation in vivo [50]. These findings have prompted speculation that circulating catecholamines may modulate the platelet propensity for aggregation. Support for this hypothesis is derived from observations that epinephrine release from the adrenal

medulla follows a circadian pattern and has been implicated in the timing of myocardial infarction [51].

There is also evidence that resistance vessels may influence systemic platelet tone. For example, Yao and colleagues found that inhibition of constitutive nitric oxide synthesis with N^G-monomethyl-L-arginine (L-NMMA) induced platelet adhesion and aggregation to injured segments of dog coronary artery [52]. These injured arterial segments were devoid of endothelium and, thus, unable to produce NO [25], suggesting that systemic NO production by the endothelium, in part, modulates platelet function. Thus, circulating humoral substances may impact on platelet adhesion and aggregability, and play a role in vascular homeostasis.

LOCAL CONTROL OF ARTERIAL PATENCY

Arachidonic Acid Products. A number of arachidonic acid derivatives are important in the modulation of hemostasis. As discussed earlier, release of arachidonic acid from the cell membrane leads to enzymatic oxidation of the arachidonic acid by cyclooxygenase and lipoxygenase to generate bioactive mediators of vascular function. As we discuss later, these arachidonic acid derivatives also modulate local platelet function.

Cyclooxygenase System. Prostacyclin is produced in endothelial cells by the action of cyclooxygenase and prostacylcin synthase, as described earlier. In addition to its effects on vascular smooth muscle, prostacyclin in also a potent inhibitor of platelet aggregation. As with vascular smooth muscle cells, prostacyclin activates platelet adenylyl cyclase, leading to the generation of cAMP. This increase in cAMP activates cAMP-dependent protein kinase and blunts the Ca^{2+} rise associated with platelet stimulation and, thus, inhibits platelet aggregation [53]. Thus, endothelial cell production of prostacyclin contributes to the maintainence of vessel patency through both vasodilation and inhibition of platelet aggregation.

The fate of arachidonic acid is cell specific. For example, unlike endothelial cells, arachidonic acid oxidation in platelets by cyclooxygenase ultimately leads to the formation of thromboxane A_2, a potent stimulant of vasoconstriction and platelet aggregation. Platelet stimulation leads to phospholipase C–mediated liberation of arachidonic acid, which is oxidized to prostaglandin H_2, as discussed earlier. Platelets, however, contain no prostacyclin synthase. Instead, thromboxane synthase is freely available in platelets and catalyzes the formation of thromboxane

A_2 from prostaglandin H_2. Thus, in the blood vessel wall arachidonic acid release generates prostacyclin, whereas in platelets it generates thromboxane A_2.

Lipoxygenase System. Platelet-derived arachidonic acid is a substrate for both cyclooxygenase and lipoxygenase in the platelet [54]. The precise role of lipoxygenase in the local control of platelet function is not well defined. Inhibition of lipoxygenase enhances the aggregation response to arachidonic acid, perhaps by making more substrate available for cyclooxygenase-mediated thromboxane formation [55]. Lipoxygenase products, such as the hydroperoxyeicosatetraenoic acids (HpETEs), also sensitize platelets to arachidonate-mediated aggregation [55]. Recent data by Freedman and colleagues [56], have shed light on the mechanism for this observation. These investigators found that HpETEs impair NO-mediated platelet *inhibition*, and this effect is reversed by glutathione peroxidase. Because platelets are known to produce NO during aggregation [57], it is possible that lipoxygenase products, such as HpETEs, impair the feedback regulation of platelet aggregation by NO.

Endothelium-Derived Nitric Oxide. Platelet adhesion and aggregation are inhibited by NO via mechanism(s) similiar to that for vasodilation [58,59]. Nitric oxide leads to an increase in the platelet cGMP, blunts the calcium rise in the platelets in response to agonists of platelet aggregation, and reduces fibrinogen binding to platelets [60]. The clinical relevance of these observations in human vascular disease is emphasized by observations that atherosclerotic vessels demonstrate a defect in the effective release of endothelium-derived NO [61]. Given that clinical manifestations of atherosclerosis, such as unstable angina [62] and myocardial infarction [63], involve platelet activation and thrombus formation, it is attractive to speculate that impaired action of endothelium-derived NO plays some role in this process.

LOCAL CONTROL OF THROMBOSIS/FIBRINOLYSIS

The fibrinolytic system is responsible for feedback regulation of clot formation and clot dissolution. Plasminogen activators are principal components of the fibrinolytic system and catalyze the conversion of plasminogen to plasmin, a serine protease that catalyzes fibrin degradation [64]. Tissue-type plasminogen activator (t-PA) and single-chain urokinase-type plasminogen activator are the two main endogenous plasminogen activators, and they are constitutively synthesized by endothelial cells [65]. In tissue culture, physiologic stimuli associated with clot formation (i.e., thrombin, activated protein C, and histamine) stimulate endothelial cell tissue-type plasminogen activator production [66,67].

Endothelial cells also exert another level of control over the fibrinolytic system through the secretion of plasminogen activator inhibitors [68]. Plasminogen activator inhibitor is a glycoprotein serine protease inhibitor and the primary inhibitor of plasminogen activators in vivo. Like tissue-type plasminogen activator, the synthesis of plasminogen activator inhibitor-1 (PAI-1) is regulated by a number of relevant stimuli, including thrombin [69], inflammatory cytokines, endotoxin, and angiotensin II [70]. High PAI-1 activity and low t-PA activity have been demonstrated in patients with coronary artery disease [71,72] and diabetes [73], suggesting that altered endothelial control of fibrinolysis may be important in the clinical expression of coronary artery disease.

Renin-Angiotensin System and Fibrinolysis. Clinical studies of angiotensin converting enzyme inhibitors in patients with left ventricular systolic dysfunction following a myocardial infarction demonstrate a significant decrease in recurrent myocardial infarction and ischemic events [74]. Furthermore, hypertensive patients with high plasma renin levels, and presumably high angiotensin II activity, have a higher risk of a myocardial infarction than hypertensive with a normal plasma renin level [75]. These clinical observations led to speculation that there was a link between the renin-angiotensin system and fibrinolytic system. Vaughan and colleagues shed light on these speculations by demonstrating that angiotensin II induced the release of PAI-1 from cultured endothelial cells [70]. In addition, increased circulating levels of PAI-1 are observed following infusion of angiotensin II [76]. Thus, it appears that local angiotensin II production can cause the generation of PAI-1, increasing the plaminogen activator inhibitor to plasminogen activator ratio, creating a thrombogenic local environment. Furthermore, angiotensin converting enzyme catalyzes the degradation of bradykinin, a stimulant for endothelial expression of prostacyclin and endothelium-derived NO. These findings lend credence to the hypothesis that local angiotensin converting enzyme activity may contribute to the development of coronary pathology.

Thrombomodulin. Thrombomodulin is a cell-surface protein that is abundantly present on endothelial cells

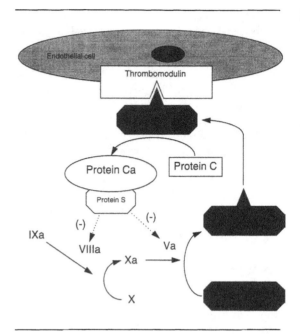

FIGURE 9-5. The interaction of thrombomodulin and thrombin on the endothelial cell surface. In response to activation, thrombin binds to thrombomodulin on the endothelal cell surface, producing a dual effect. The first is to catalyze the activation of protein C, ultimately producing inactivation of activated clotting factors VIII and V, and thus, feedback inhibition of thrombin formation. The second effect is to facilitate thrombin inactivation by endothelial cell endocytosis.

and is important for endothelial cell control of thrombin activity (Figure 9-5). Activation of the coagulation cascade leads to the formation of thrombin, which binds to thrombomodulin, accounting for 50–60% of thrombin binding sites on endothelial cells. The thrombin–thrombomodulin complex is internalized into the cell by endocytosis, leading to degradation of thrombin [77]. The free thrombomodulin then returns to the cell surface and is available for binding. In addition, the thrombin–thrombomodulin complex activates protein C, a naturally occuring vitamin K–dependent anticoagulant [78]. Activated protein C, in the presence of activated protein S, rapidly degrades activated factors VIII and V [78–80]. Thus, thrombomodulin serves as an endothelium-dependent physiologic anticoagulant by removing thrombin from the circulation and by activating protein C. Activated protein C also exerts an anticoagulant effect by inhibition of plasminogen activator inhibitor [81], thus further promoting local fibrinolysis.

EXTRACELLULAR MATRIX

As discussed earlier, extracellular matrix provides structural integrity to the vessel wall. In addition, the extracellular matrix of subintimal tissue plays an important role in the control of arterial patency. Glycosaminoglycans and proteins present in the subintimal tissue serve as cofactors for important antithrombotic influences as well as key molecules for primary hemostasis, and these are discussed later.

Glycosaminoglycans. Heparan sulfate and dermatan sulfate are glycosaminoglycans present in the extracellular matrix and subendothelial connective tissue, and play an important role in the maintenance of blood fluidity. Heparan sulfate and heparin-like proteoglycans are ubiquitous in the vasculature and are most abundant in the microvasculature, where they are tightly bound to endothelial cells [82]. Antithrombin III is a serine protease inhibitor that circulates in plasma, and its physiologic action is to neutralize thrombin. Antithrombin III inactivates thrombin at a slow rate; however, this inactivation is markedly enhanced by binding of antithrombin-III to heparin or heparan sulfate on the endothelial cell surface [82]. In addition to its effect on thrombin, antithrombin III inactivates the activated coagulation factors XII, XI, X, and IX.

Dermatan sulfate is present primarily in subintimal connective tissue and exerts an antithrombotic effect through heparin cofactor II. Heparin cofactor II is a glycoprotein present in plasma that is also a specific inhibitor of thrombin. Heparin cofactor II neutralizes thrombin at a rate that approaches that of the antithrombin III saturated with heparin [83]. Dermatan sulfate catalyzes the formation of a heparin cofactor II–thrombin complex, which enhances the heparin cofactor II–mediated inhibiton of thrombin approximately 1000-fold. Thus glycaosaminoglycans in the intimal and subintimal connective tissue exert antithrombotic properties that contri-bute importantly to the maintenance of vascular homeostasis.

Proteins. Proteins located in the subintimal tissue, such as vitronectin, von Williebrand factor (vWF), and collagen, also contribute to the maintainence of blood fluidity and the response to endothelial injury. Vitronectin is a single-chain glycoprotein found in plasma and platelet granules, and bound to the subintimal connective tissue. Plasminogen activator inhibitor-1 binds to and is stabilized by vitronectin in plasma and subintimal connective tissue within the vessel wall. Because plasminogen activator inhibitor-

1 inhibits the action of plasmin, tissue-type plasminogen activator, and activated protein C, vitronectin indirectly modulates fibrinolysis within the vascular wall [64].

Von Williebrand factor is another protein that is synthesized and expressed by endothelial cells [84]. The presence of vWF in plasma and subendothelial tissue is important for the initial response to vascular injury associated with the loss of endothelium. In this respect, vWF has two important function: (1) vWF is necessary for platelet adhesion to the denuded vascular wall, particularly in high shear stress conditions; and (2) vWF serves as a carrier of factor VIII, a cofactor for activation of factor X. With vascular injury and loss of the endothelium, collagen-bound vWF is exposed to the circulation, and plasma vWF binds to the exposed collagen. This layer of vWF facilitates platelet adhesion to the injured vessel surface, which is mediated by the glycoprotein Ib receptor on platelets. Adherent platelets become activated and release preformed storage granules, which result in platelet aggregation and the formation of a platelet plug.

Vascular Remodeling

Endothelial injury is an obligate byproduct of both normal and pathologic events, such as shear stress, elevated blood cholesterol, and mechanical factors. Despite the fact that endothelial injury results from a variety of stimuli, the blood vessel response to this injury is, in many ways, uniform. The loss of endothelium from an arterial segment initiates a cascade of events that begins with the accumulation of platelets at the site of injury and ultimately leads to a focal accumulation and proliferation of smooth muscle cells and their extracellular matrix. In the following section, the arterial response to injury is reviewed, with particular reference to its implications for hemostasis and the control of vascular tone.

The response to acute vascular injury can be divided into three stages. In the first stage, platelets adhere to the de-endothelialized surface of the vessel and become activated. As a consequence, growth and chemotactic factors are released and initiate the recruitment and activation of smooth muscle cells and mononuclear cells as the second stage of the injury response. In the final stage, these activated cells produce a number of cytokines and growth factors that result in smooth muscle cell proliferation and matrix production, leaving the arterial segment with a proportionally larger intima than a normal artery.

PLATELET ADHESION AND THE INITIAL RESPONSE TO INJURY

Removal of the endothelium exposes the intimal connective tissue and extracellular matrix to the circulation. The presence of vWF in the subendothelial connective tissue facilitates platelet adhesion to the de-endothelialized vessel segment. Platelet adhesion is followed by platelet aggregation, resulting in the release of serotonin, adenosine triphosphate, and fibrinogen at the site of injury. These platelet products lead to continued platelet adhesion and aggregation and the formation of a platelet plug. Among other platelet contents released during this response is platelet-derived growth factor (PDGF). The primary function of this peptide is the induction of smooth muscle cell migration from the arterial media to the intimal space. Other factors released by the platelet include transforming growth factor-β (TGF-β), basic fibroblast growth factor (bFGF), and platelet-derived endothelial cell growth factor (PD-ECGF).

Platelet products released at the site of arterial injury also impair the endogenous homeostatic functions of the vascular wall. For example, platelets also release an endoglycosidase that cleaves heparin proteoglycan from the surface of remaining endothelial cells and adjacent smooth muscle cells. Because heparins in the vessel wall inhibit smooth muscle cell proliferation, the removal of these proteoglycans by endoglycosidase activity renders smooth muscle cells more receptive to growth factors. The loss of heparins from the vessel wall also facilitates activation of the coagulation cascade because the formation of thrombin–antithrombin III complexes is reduced.

SMOOTH MUSCLE CELL ACTIVATION

In response to PDGF, smooth muscle cells leave the media and migrate to the intimal space, where they become activated and assume a "secretory" phenotype. This migration of smooth muscle cells is associated with profound alterations in functional characteristics of both vascular smooth muscle cells and endothelial cells. Smooth muscle cell migration in response to PDGF involves the local generation of plasmin and an increase in the fibrinolytic activity of the vascular wall. Specifically, activation of plasmin by t-PA in the blood vessel wall is associated with extracellular matrix degradation [85]. Recent evidence has implicated T-cell production of interleukin-4 and gamma-interferon as important mediators of smooth muscle cell migration.

As discussed previously, heparin and heparin-like proteoglycans in the blood vessel wall usually limit smooth muscle cell migration and proliferation. In the setting of vascular injury, however, endothelial cells are temporarily unavailable for proteoglycan synthesis. In addition, smooth muscle cell migration and proliferation are also facilitated by the removal of heparins in the vascular wall by the endoglycosidase activity derived from platelets. Thus, vascular injury is associated with an impaired function of the heparin-like glucosaminoglycan components of the vascular wall.

During the migration and proliferation of intimal smooth muscle cells, the endothelium begins to migrate from be border zone of the injured segment. The absence of endothelium is an important component of the proliferative response. Normally, the endothelium produces NO, which may act to limit smooth muscle cell migration, proliferation and, thus, intimal thickening. In fact, treatment of injured rabbit vessels with an NO donor prevents smooth muscle cell migration and intimal proliferation [86]. Without an overlying endothelium, the contribution of NO to vascular homeostasis is lost. In addition, when the endothelium does regenerate, it is dysfunctional and, thus, may further contribute to persistent smooth muscle cell matrix production late in the response to injury.

MATRIX PRODUCTION AND REMODELING

With the recovery of the endothelium and the arrival of smooth muscle cells in the intima, the production of extracellular matrix continues. The major extracellular matrix component, fibronectin, becomes replaed with proteoglycan. The intimal fibroblasts and smooth muscle cells synthesize chondroitin sulfate and dermatan sulfate, principally in response to TGF-β. Both of these proteoglycans promote cell migration and proliferation, in effect further stimulating the proliferation of intimal components and encroaching upon the vessel lumen. Eventually, endothelial cell production of heparin leads to the slowing of smooth muscle cell proliferation, although proteoglycan synthesis is not necessarily curtailed. The recovery of endothelial integrity is accompanied by an increase retention of proteoglycan in the intimal space and further intimal hyperplasia. Complete restoration of vascular homeostasis requires up to 6 months.

Conclusions

In conclusion, blood vessels are structuraly composed of endothelium, vascular smooth muscle cells, and extracellular matrix. In addition to being conduits for blood, the vessel wall plays a critical role in the maintainence of vascular homeostasis. These include control of vascular tone and blood flow, control of arterial patency through modulation of the hemo-static and fibrinolytic systems, and modulation of growth factors. The control and modulation of these physiologically important functions is the sum total of the checks and balances of neural influences mediated by the autonomic nervous system, humoral influences mediated by circulating mediators, and local factors generated in the vessel wall.

Acknowledgments

Dr. Keaney is supported by a Clinical Investigator Development Award from the NIH and grants from the American Heart Association, Massachusetts Affiliate and The Council for Tobacco Research-USA.

References

1. Gibbons GH, Dzau VJ. The emerging concept of vascular remodeling. N Engl J Med 330:1431, 1994.
2. Skinner MP, Raines EW, Ross R. Dynamic expression of alpha 1 beta 1 and alpha 2 beta 1 integrin receptors by human vascular smooth muscle cells. Alpha 2 beta 1 integrin is required for chemotaxis across type I collagen-coated membranes. Am J Pathol 145:1071, 1994.
3. Young MA, Vatner SF. Regulation of large coronary arteries. Circ Res 59:579, 1985.
4. Vatner S. Regulation of coronary resistance vessels and large coronary arteries. Am J Cardiol 56:16E, 1985.
5. Young MA, Knight DR, Vatner SF. Autonomic control of large coronary arteries and resistance vessels. Prog Cardiovasc Dis 30:211, 1987.
6. Malik KU. Interaction of arachidonic acid metablites and adrenergic nervous system. Am J Med Sci 295:280, 1988.
7. Shen W, Ochoa M, Xu X, Wang J, Hintze TH. Role of EDRF/NO in parasympathetic coronary vasodilation following carotid chemoreflex activation in conscious dogs. Am J Physiol 267:H605, 1994.
8. Broten SP, Miyashiro JK, Moncada S, Feigl EO. Role of endothelium-derived relaxing facotr in parasympathetic coronary vasodilation. Am J Physiol 262:H1579, 1992.
9. Vanhoutte PM, Levy MN. Prejunctional cholinergic modulation of adrenergic neurotransmission in the cardiovascular system. Am J Physiol 238:H275, 1990.
10. Ohlstein EH, Berkowitz BA. Vasodilation: Vascular smooth muscle, peptides, autonomic nerves, and endothelium. New York: Raven Press, 1988:113.
11. Scherrer U, Randin D, Vollenweider P, Vollenweider L, Nicod P. Nitrix oxide release accounts for insulin's vascular effects in humans. J Clin Invest 94:2511, 1994.
12. Creager MA, Liang CS, Coffman JD. Beta adrenergic-mediated vasodilator response to insulin in the human forearm. J Pharmacol Exp Ther 235:709, 1985.
13. Gagnon G, Regoli D, Rioux F. A new bioassay for glucagon. Br J Pharmacol 64:99, 1978.
14. Consentino F, Sill JC, Katusic ZS. Endothelial L-arginine pathway and relaxations to vasopressin in canine basilar artery. Am J Physiol 264:H413, 1993.
15. Vane JR, Anggard EE, Botting RM. Regulatory functions of the vascular endothelium. N Engl J Med 323:27, 1990.
16. Schror K. The effect of prostaglandins and thromboxane A2 on coronary vessel tone — mechanisms of action and therapeutic implications. Eur Heart J 14(Suppl. 1):34, 1993.
17. Francos JA, Eskin SG, McIntire LV, Ives LV. Flow effects on prostacyclin production by cultured human endothelial cells. Science 227:1477, 1985.
18. Rubanyi GM, Vanhoutte PM. Hypoxia releases a vasoconstrictor substance from the canine vascular endothelium. J Physiol 364:45, 1985.
19. Lincoln TM, Cornwell TL, Taylor AE. cGMP-dependent protein kinase mediates the reduction of Ca^+ by cAMP in vascular smooth muscle cells. Am J Physiol 258:C399, 1990.
20. Luscher TF, Vanhoutte PM (eds). The Endothelium: Modulator of Cardiovascular Function, 1st ed. Boca Raton, FL: CRC Press, 1990.
21. Roth DM, Lefer AM. Studies on the mechanism leukotriene induced coronary artery constriction. Prostaglandins 26:573, 1983.
22. Tomoike H, Egashira K, Yamada A, Hayashi Y, Nakamura M. Leukotriene C_4 and D_4-induced diffuse peripheral contstriction of swine coronary artery accompanied by ST elevation on the electrocardiogram. Circulation 76:480, 1987.
23. Mayatepek E, Hoffman GF. Leukotrienes: Biosynthesis, metabolism, and pathophysiologic significance. Pediatr Res 37:1, 1995.
24. Tesfamariam B, Brown ML, Cohen RA. 15-Hydroxyeicosatetraenoic acid and diabetic endothelial dysfunction in rabbit aorta. J Cardiovasc Pharmacol 25:748, 1995.
25. Furchgott RF, Zawadzki JV. The obligatory role of endothelial cells in the relaxation of arterial smooth muscle by acetylcholine. Nature 288:373, 1980.
26. Ignarro LJ, Buga GM, Wood KS, Byrns RE, Chaudhuri G. Endothelium-derived relaxing factor produced and released from artery and vein is nitric oxide. Proc Natl Acad Sci USA 84:9265, 1987.
27. Stamler JS, Singel DJ, Loscalzo J. Biochemistry of nitric oxide and its redox-activated forms. Science 258:1898, 1992.
28. Furchgott R. Role of endothelium in responses of vascular smooth muscle. Circ Res 35:557, 1983.
29. Vita JA, Keaney JF Jr, Loscalzo J. Endothelial dysfunction in vascular disease. In Loscalzo J, Creager MA, Dzau VJ (eds). Vascular Medicine, 2nd ed. Boston: Little Brown, 1996:245.
30. Palmer RM, Ashton DS, Moncada S. Vascular endothelial cells synthesize nitric oxide from L-arginine. Nature 333:664, 1988.
31. Sessa WC, Barber CM, Lynch KR. Mutation of N-myristoylation site converts endothelial nitric oxide

synthase from a membrane to a cytosolic protein. Circ Res 72:921, 1993.

32. Lopez-Jaramillo P, Gonzalez MC, Palmer RMJ, Moncada S. The crucial role of physiological Ca^{2+} concentrations in the production of endothelial nitric oxide and the control of vascular tone. Br J Pharmacol 101:489, 1990.

33. Stuehr DJ, Kwon NS, Nathan CF. FAD and GSH participate in macrophage synthesis of nitric oxide. Biochem Biophys Res Commun 168:558, 1990.

34. Bolotina VM, Najibi S, Palacino JJ, Pagano PJ, Cohen RA. Nitric oxide directly activates calcium-dependent potassium channels in vascular smooth muscle. Nature 368:850, 1994.

35. Cohen RA, Shepherd JT, Vanhoutte PM. The inhibitory role of the endothelium in the response of isolated coronary arteries to platelets. Science 221:273, 1983.

36. Vanhoutte PM. Platelet-derived serotonin, the endothelium, and cardiovascular disease. J Cardiovasc Pharmacol 17(Suppl. 5):S6, 1991.

37. Vanhoutte PM. Hypercholesterolaemia, atherosclerosis and release of endothelium-derived relaxing factor by aggregating platelets. Eur Heart J 12(Suppl. E):25, 1991.

38. Yanagisawa M, Kurihara H, Kimura S, Tomobe Y, Kobayashi M, Mitsui Y, Yazaki Y, Goto K, Masaki T. A novel potent vasoconstrictor peptide produced by vascular endothelial cells. Nature 332:411, 1988.

39. Inoue S, Yanagisawa M, Kimura S, Kasuya Y, Miyauchi T, Goto K, Masaki T. The human endothelin family: Three structurally and pharmacologically distinct isopeptides predicted by three separate genes. Proc Natl Acad Sci USA 86:2863, 1989.

40. Resink TJ, Scott-Burden T, Buhler FR. Endothelin stimulates phsospholipase C in cultured vascular smooth muscle cells. Biochem Biophy Res Commun 157:1360, 1988.

41. Goto K, Kasuya Y, Matsuki N, Takuwa Y, Kurihara H, Ishikawa T, Kimura S, Yanagisawa M, Masaki T. Endothelin activates the dihydropyridine-sensitive, voltage-dependent Ca^{2+} channel in vascular smooth muscle. Proc Natl Acad Sci USA 86:3915, 1989.

42. Boulanger C, Luscher TF. Release of endothelin from the porcine aorta. Inhibition by endothelium-derived nitric oxide. J Clin Invest 85:587, 1990.

43. Falkenhahn M, Golhlke P, Paul M, Stoll M, Unger T. The renin-angiotensin system in the heart and vascular wall: New therapeutic aspects. J Cardiovasc Pharmacol 24(Suppl. 2):S6, 1994.

44. Dzau V. Circulating versus local renin-angiotensin system in cardiovascular homeostasis. Circulation 77(Suppl. 1):4, 1988.

45. Rogerson F, Chai S, Schlawe I, Murray W, Marley PH, Mendelsohn F. Presence of angiotensin converting enzyme in the adventitia of large blood vessels. J Hypertens 10:615, 1992.

46. Ullian ME, Linas SL. Angiotensin II surgace receptor coupling to inositol triphosphate formation in vascular smooth muscle cells. J Biol Chem 265:195, 1990.

47. Szabo B, Hedler L, Schurr C, Starke K. Periperal presynaptic facilitatory effect of angiotensin II on noradrenaline release in anesthetized rabbits. J Cardiovasc Pharmacol 15:968, 1990.

48. Vanhoutte PM, Boulanger CM, Illiano SC, Nagao T, Vidal M, Mombouli JV. Endothelium-dependent effects of converting-enzyme inhibitors. J Cardiovasc Pharmacol 22(Suppl. 5):S10, 1993.

49. Marthel W, Markwardt F. Aggregation of blood platelets by adrenaline and its uptake. Biochem Pharmacol 24:1903, 1975.

50. Folts JD. An in vivo model of experimental arterial stenosis, intimal damage, and periodic thrombosis. Circulation 83(Suppl. IV):IV3, 1991.

51. Muller JE, Tofler GH, Verrier RL. Sympathetic activity as the cause of the morning increase incardiac events. A likely culprit, but the evidence remains controversial. Circulation 91:2508, 1995.

52. Yao S-K, Ober JC, Krishnaswami A, Ferguson JJ, Anderson HV, Golino P, Buja LM, Willerson JT. Endogenous nitric oxide protects against platelet aggregation and cyclic flow variations in stenosed and endothelium-injured arteries. Circulation 86:1302, 1992.

53. Booyse FM, Marr J, Yang DC, Guiliani D, Rafelson ME Jr. Mechanism of cyclic adenosine 3',5'-monophosphate regulation of platelet membrane phosphorylation-dephosphorylation, Ca binding, and aggregation. In Lutin ON (ed). Platelets. Amsterdam: Exerpta Medica, 1975:84.

54. Chevy F, Wolf C, Colard O. A unique pool of free arachidonate serves as substrate for both cyclooxygenase and lipoxygenase in platelets. Lipids 26:1080, 1991.

55. Hill TD, Thite JG, Rao GH. Platelet hypersinsitivity induced by 1-chloro-2, 4-dinitrobenzene, hydroperoxides, and inhibition of lipoxygenase. Thromb Res 53:447, 1989.

56. Freedman JE, Frei B, Welch GN, Loscalzo J. Glutathrove peroxidase potentiates the inhibition of platelet function by 5-nitrosothiols. J Clin Invest 96:394, 1995.

57. Malinski T, Radomski MW, Taha Z, Moncada S. Direct electrochemical measurement of nitric oxide released from human platelets. Biochem Biophys Res Commun 194:960, 1993.

58. Azuma H, Ishikawa M, Sekizaki S. Endothelium-dependent inhibition of platelet aggregation. Br J Pharmacol 88:411, 1986.

59. Radomski MW, Palmer RMJ, Moncada S. The role of nitric oxide and cGMP in platelet adhesion to the vascular endothelium. Biochem Biophys Res Commun 148:1482, 1987.

60. Mendelsohn ME, O'Neill S, George D, Loscalzo J. Inhibition of fibrinogen binding to human platelets by S-nitroso-N-acetylcysteine. J Biol Chem 265:19028, 1990.

61. Ludmer PL, Selwyn AP, Shook TL, Wayne RR, Mudge GH, Alexander RW, Ganz P. Paradoxical vasoconstriction induced by acetylcholine in atherosclerotic coronary arteries. N Engl J Med 315:1046, 1986.

62. Mizuno K, Satomura K, Miyamoto A, Arakawa K, Shibuya T, Arai T, Kurita A, Nakamura H, Ambrose JA. Angioscopic evaluation of coronary-artery thrombi in acute coronary syndromes. N Engl J Med 326:287, 1992.

63. DeWood MA, Spores J, Notske R, Mouser LT, Burroughs R, Golden MS, Lang HT. Prevalence of total coronary occlusion during the early hours of transmural myocardial infarction. N Engl J Med 303:897, 1980.

64. Keaney JF Jr, Loscalzo J. The pharmacology of thrombolytic agents. In Loscalzo J, Schaefer AI (eds). Thrombosis and Hemorrhage. Boston: Blackwell Scientific, 1173, 1991.

65. Loskutoff DJ, Edgington DS. Synthesis of a fibrinolytic activator and inhibitor by endothelial cells. Proc Natl Acad Sci USA 74:3903, 1977.

66. Levin EG, Marzec U, Anderson J, Harker LA. Thrombin stimulates tissue plasminogen activator release from cultured human endothelial cells. J Clin Invest 74:1988, 1984.

67. Hanss M, Collen D. Secretion of tissue-type plasminogen activator and plasminogen activator inhibitor by cultured human endothelial cells: Modulation by thrombin, endotoxin and histamine. J Lab Clin Med 109:97, 1987.

68. Hekman CM, Loskutoff DJ. Fibrinolytic pathways and the endothelium. Semin Thromb Haemost 13:514, 1987.

69. Gelehrter TD, Szneyeer-Laszuk R. Thrombin induction of plasminogen activator inhibitor in cultured human endothelial cells. J Clin Invest 77:165, 1986.

70. Vaughan DE, Lazos SA, Tong K. Angiotensin II regulates the expression of plasminogen activator inhibitor-1 in cultured endothelial cells. A potential link between the renin angiotensin system and thrombosis. J Clin Invest 95:995, 1995.

71. Aznar J, Estelles A, Tormo G, Sapena P, Tormo V, Blanch S, Espana F. Plasminogen activator inhibitor activity and other fibrinolytic variables in patients with coronary artery disease. Br Heart J 59:535, 1988.

72. Paramo JA, Colucci M, Collen D, van de Werf F. Plasminogen activator inhibitor in the blood of patients with coronary artery disease. Br Med J 291:573, 1985.

73. Auwerx J, Bouillon R, Collen D, Gaboers J. Tissue-type plasminogen activator antigen and plasminogen activator inhibitor in diabetes mellitus. Arteriosclerosis 8:68, 1988.

74. Pfeffer MA, Braunwald E, Moye LA, Basta L, Brown EJ Jr, Cuddy TE, Davis BR, Geltman EM, Goldman S, Flaker GC, et al. Effect of captopril on mortality and morbidity in patients with left ventricular dysfunction after myocardial infarction. N Engl J Med 327:676, 1992.

75. Alderman MH, Madhavan S, Ooi WL, Cohen H, Sealey JE, Laragh JH. Association of the renin-sodium profile with the risk of myocardial infarction in patients with hypertension. N Engl J Med 324:1098, 1991.

76. Ridker PM, Gaboury CL, Conlin PR, Seely EW, Williams GH, Vaughan DE. Stimulation of plasminogen activator inhibitor in vivo by infusion of angiotensin II. Evidence of a potential interaction between the renin-angiotensin system and fibrinolytic function. Circulation 87:1969, 1993.

77. Horvat R, Palade GE. Thrombomodulin and thrombin localization on the vascular endothelium; their internalization and transcytosis by plasmalemmal vesicles. Eur J Cell Biol 61:299, 1993.

78. Esmon CT. The roles of protein C and thrombomodulin in the regulation of blood coagulation. J Biol Chem 264:4743, 1989.

79. Stern DM, Nawroth PP, Harris K, Esmon CT. Cultured bovine aortic endothelial cells promote activated protein C-protein S-mediated inactivation of factor Va. J Biol Chem 261:713, 1986.

80. Marlar RA, Kleiss AJ, Griffin JH. Mechanism of activation of human activated protein C, a thrombin-dependent anticoagulant enzyme. Blood 59:1067, 1982.

81. De Fouw NJ, van Hinsbergh VW, de Jong YF, Haverkate F, Bertina RM. The interaction of activated protein C and thrombin with the plasminogen activator inhibitor released from human endothelial cells. Thromb Haemost 57:176, 1987.

82. Marcum JA, Mckinney JB, Rosenberg RD. Acceleration of thrombin-antithrombin complex formation in rat hindquarters via heparinlike molecules bound to the endothelium. J Clin Invest 74:341, 1984.

83. Tollefsen DM, Petska CA, Nibafi WJ. Activation of heparin cofactor II by dermatan sulfate. J Biol Chem 258:6713, 1983.

84. Jaffe EA, Hoyer LW, Nachman RL. Synthesis of von Williebrand factor by cultured human endothelial cells. Proc Natl Acad Sci USA 71:1906, 1974.

85. Reuning U, Bang NU. Regulation of the urokinase-type plasminogen activator receptor on vascular smooth muscle cells is under the control of thrombin and other mitogens. Arterioscler Thromb 12:1161, 1992.

86. Marks DS, Vita JA, Folts JD, Keaney JF Jr, Welch GN, Loscalzo J. Inhibition of neointimal proliferation in rabbits after vascular injury by a single treatment with a protein adduct of nitric oxide. J Clin Invest 95:2630, 1995.

87. O'Rourke ST, Vanhoutte PM. Vascular pharmacology. In Loscalzo J, Creager MA, Dzao VJ (eds). Vascular Medicine, 1st ed. Boston: Little Brown, 1992:133.

10. CORONARY VASCULAR PHARMACOLOGY

Marco N. Diaz and Richard A. Cohen

Introduction

This chapter reviews a basic understanding of coronary artery physiology and pharmacology. Mechanisms of physiological control of coronary blood flow are discussed first. This serves as a basis for a discussion of the major classes of drugs used clinically which affect coronary blood flow including nitrates, angiotension converting enzyme inhibitors, calcium channel blockers, and alpha- and beta-adrenergic antagonists. The mechanism of action of each drug class, the evidence for its effects on coronary blood flow, and its clinical use in myocardial infarction, and acute and chronic myocardial ischemia are reviewed.

Physiologic Regulation of Coronary Blood Flow

Coronary blood flow is normally regulated directly in response to cardiac work. Although metabolic rate is the primary determinant of coronary blood flow, extravascular compressive forces, and local factors, including autoregulation, neurotransmitters, and endothelial factors, play a significant role (Figures 10-1 and 10-2). Cardiac work is determined primarily by contractility, tension of the myocardium, and heart rate.

METABOLIC REGULATION

Normally, coronary blood flow increases linearly as myocardial oxygen demand increases, primarily related to coronary vasodilatation as a result of the accumulation of several metabolic mediators [1]. Metabolic autoregulation of coronary blood flow has been attributed to changes in oxygen or carbon dioxide tension, vasodilator metabolites such as adenosine or lactate, or changes in hydrogen or potassium ions that accumulate in the underperfused myocardium and reduce coronary vascular resistance [2]. Adenosine, a strong coronary vasodilator, is formed during states when ATP utilization exceeds the capacity of myocardial cells to synthesize high-energy phosphates, resulting in accumulation of AMP [1]. Local accumulation of potassium, hydrogen, and calcium ions and increased osmolality also appear to be involved in coronary vasodilatation during increased metabolic demand [2]. Other potential metabolic mediators of coronary blood flow include other nucleotides, prostaglandins, and kinins [2].

AUTOREGULATION

The phenomenon of autoregulation refers to the nonlinear relationship between blood pressure and blood flow. Autoregulation in the coronary vascular bed maintains blood flow relatively constant over a range of blood pressure between 60 and 130 mmHg [2]. Autoregulation may, in part, be secondary to changes in coronary vascular tone occurring as a result of myogenic responses of the smooth muscle cells to the varying stretch exerted by coronary perfusion pressure [1]. In this way, increased coronary perfusion pressure stimulates vascular smooth muscle contraction, resulting in increased coronary vascular resistance and maintenance of stable coronary flow [1]. Several other mechanisms have been implicated in autoregulation, including metabolic factors, release of vasoactive substances from the endothelium (see later), and extravascular compressive forces.

PHYSICAL FACTORS REGULATING CORONARY BLOOD FLOW

The arterial pressure gradient between the aorta and the left ventricle during diastole plays a significant role in determining coronary blood flow. Normally if the diastolic pressure is elevated, no change in coronary blood flow occurs due to autoregulation. However, as the diastolic pressure drops to very low levels, the coronary bed is maximally dilated and coronary blood flow is then linearly correlated with perfusion pressure [1]. Because coronary blood flow occurs primarily during diastole, the time spent in diastole

155

correlates in a linear fashion with coronary blood flow. Thus, as the heart rate increases, coronary blood flow per cardiac cycle declines. In addition to affecting the diastolic filling period, an increase in heart rate results in increases in coronary blood flow, owing to increased myocardial oxygen demand and changes in autoregulation. Systemic arterial pressure also contributes to the regulation of coronary blood flow by influencing myocardial wall tension and myocardial oxygen demand [2]. Myocardial contractility in-

creases myocardial oxygen consumption as well. Thus, several factors that increase myocardial oxygen consumption mediate increases in coronary blood flow.

Once blood has entered the epicardial conductance coronary vessels, there is little resistance to flow until reaching the intramural vessels and coronary arterioles [2]. The dense capillary network of resistance vessels possesses sphincters that regulate flow, depending on the needs of the myocardium. This capillary density is reduced in left ventricular hypertrophy. Collateral vessels, which are anastomotic connections without intervening capillary beds between the same or different coronary arteries, also influence coronary blood flow. These vessels develop under conditions of repeated ischemia or occlusion of coronary arteries, and can be influenced by the same metabolic, autoregulatory, and humoral influences as the noncollateral coronary circulation, but to different degrees [2].

Determinants of Coronary Artery Resistance

Supply ⟷	Demand
Coronary Blood Flow:	**Cardiac Work:**
Metabolism	Contractility
Extravascular Compression	Heart rate
Autoregulation	Wall tension
Humoral factors	
Neurotransmitters	
Endothelium-derived factors	

FIGURE 10-1. Determinants of coronary artery resistance.

HUMORAL REGULATION

Large coronary vessels have $alpha_1$, $alpha_2$, $beta_1$, and $beta_2$ receptors, while small vessels have predominantly $beta_2$ receptors [1]. Circulating catecholamines, norepinephrine, and epinephrine can cause coronary constriction by stimulating alpha-adrenoreceptors of conductance vessels and coronary resistance vessels, although coronary smooth muscle also possesses beta-adrenoreceptors, which mediate counteracting vasodilatation [1]. The direct action of

Determinants of Coronary Artery Blood Flow

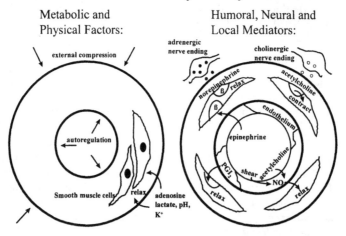

FIGURE 10-2. Determinants of coronary artery blood flow.

catecholamines on coronary smooth muscle may be overwhelmed by their indirect effect on myocardial metabolism by increasing afterload, heart rate, and contractility, resulting in coronary vasodilatation. Similarly, angiotensin II produces coronary vasoconstriction, which is partially offset by increases in myocardial oxygen demand secondary to increased systemic pressure, left ventricular wall stress, heart rate, and contractility [1]. In addition, angiotensin II may also mediate the release of prostaglandins E_2 and I_2, which produce coronary vasodilatation [1]. Several circulating substances mediate coronary vasodilatation by increasing myocardial oxygen demand, including thyroid hormone, glucagon, and histamine [1].

NEURAL REGULATION OF CORONARY BLOOD FLOW
Coronary vessels are innervated by both adrenergic and parasympathetic nerve fibers. Stimulation of cardiac sympathetic nerves causes coronary vasoconstriction via stimulation of alpha-adrenoceptors when the inotropic and chronotropic effects on the myocardium and the direct beta-adrenoceptor effects are blocked [1]. As with the humoral effects of catecholamines, the many neural vasoconstrictor effects are overwhelmed by the vasodilatory effects produced by enhanced myocardial metabolism [1].

Stimulation of the parasympathetic nerves produce both coronary vasodilatation and vasoconstriction in experimental animal models. The cholinergic neurotransmitter, acetylcholine, can cause direct coronary smooth muscle contraction, or vasodilatation via stimulation of endothelial cells. In intact animals stimulation of the vagus nerve results in bradycardia and a reduction in contractility, resulting in a decline in myocardial oxygen demand and secondary coronary vasoconstriction [1]. In summary, the direct effects of both vagal and sympathetic neural input on coronary vascular tone are modulated, to a large degree, by the indirect effects of neural input on myocardial oxygen demand and subsequent metabolic regulation.

ENDOTHELIAL REGULATION OF CORONARY BLOOD FLOW
The coronary endothelium produces several vasoactive substances that play a crucial role in the regulation of coronary blood flow. Nitric oxide is synthesized by the endothelium via metabolism of the amino acid L-arginine [2], and this free radical is released from endothelial cells through the activation of multiple receptors, including muscarinic, thrombin, histamine, vasopressin, alpha-adrenoceptors, and

serotonergic receptors [2]. Nitric oxide release can be stimulated by acetylcholine, thrombin, bradykinin, thromboxane A_2, histamine, platelet aggregation, and catecholamines stimulating alpha$_2$ receptors [2]. This endothelial product acts on smooth muscle cell guanylyl cyclase to increase intracellular cyclic guanosine monophosphate (cyclic GMP), which subsequently inhibits calcium release from the sarcoplasmic reticulum and entry via calcium channels, resulting in vascular smooth muscle relaxation [2]. In addition, nitric oxide causes hyperpolarization of the smooth muscle cell membrane, which mediates smooth muscle relaxation [2]. The continuous basal release of nitric oxide contributes to normal resting vascular tone [2], and its basal formation is regulated by shear forces on endothelial cells, enabling autoregulation of coronary artery diameter via changes in blood flow. A number of substances produced by endothelial cells, including endothelin, serotonin, and prostaglandins, may produce opposing vasoconstriction [2]. Prostacyclin, another prostaglandin produced by endothelial cells, causes coronary artery vasodilatation by increasing smooth muscle intracellular cAMP [2].

Nitrates

MECHANISM OF ACTION
The family of compounds containing -ONO_2 groups, such as nitroglycerin, isosorbide dinitrate, and isosorbide-5-mononitrate, shares a potent vasodilatory effect. On a biochemical level, nitrates interact with sulfhydryl groups at the level of the plasma membrane to form nitric oxide or S-nitrosothiols [3]. These compounds then activate guanylyl cyclase to produce cyclic GMP [3]. As previously outlined, this results in protein kinase G activation, protein phosphorylation, a decrease in free intracellular calcium, and vascular smooth muscle relaxation. Sulfhydryl groups are required for both the formation of nitric oxide and for the stimulation of guanylyl cyclase. Nitroglycerin-induced vasodilatation can be enhanced by administration of N-acetyl-L-cysteine, a compound that increases the availability of sulphydryl groups [4].

The vasodilatory effect of nitrates occurs in both the venous and arterial circulation, but their hemodynamic effects are due predominantly to their effect on the venous circulation. The decrease in venous tone results in sequestration of blood in the venous capacitance bed, particularly in the limbs, and in splanchnic and mesenteric circulations [5]. The decline in blood return to the heart reduces preload, right and left ventricular volume, and wall tension. In addition to venodilation, the reduction in arterial tone caused by nitrates results in a modest reduction in afterload. Taken together, these hemodynamic effects of nitrates lead to a decline in systolic and diastolic ventricular wall tension and a resultant reduction in myocardial oxygen demand [5]. The vasodilation due to these metabolic effects of nitrates reinforces their direct effects on coronary smooth muscle.

EFFECTS ON CORONARY CIRCULATION

The effect of nitrates on coronary blood flow in patients with atherosclerotic coronary artery disease involves a complex interaction between its effect on myocardial metabolism, hemodynamics, the endothelium, and vascular smooth muscle. It has been demonstrated by angiographic quantitative analysis that nitrates dilate the larger conductance coronary arteries, particularly at the site of epicardial coronary stenosis [6]. Elliptical or eccentric coronary artery stenotic lesions contain vascular smooth muscle in the wall, which retains its ability to vasodilate in response to nitroglycerin. While the magnitude of dilatation after nitroglycerin treatment may be small in terms of increased luminal diameter, it is substantial in terms of the reduction in stenosis resistance [6]. While some studies have demonstrated that this reduced stenotic resistance results in increased coronary blood flow [7], other studies have not substantiated this effect [8,9].

Despite this controversy, several studies have demonstrated improved regional or ischemic zone blood flow in the setting of coronary atherosclerosis after nitroglycerin [10–12]. Cohn and colleagues demonstrated that nitroglycerin equally reduced the blood pressure–heart rate product in both patients with angiographic coronary artery stenosis and in those with normal coronary arteries [12]. In addition, using a xenon-133 washout technique, it was shown that nitroglycerin increased coronary vascular resistance and decreased myocardial blood flow in patients with either normal or diseased coronary arteries. It is hypothesized that this occurs secondary to autoregulation of coronary resistance vessels in response to reduced myocardial oxygen demand. Despite this reduction in overall coronary blood flow, ischemic zone blood flow increased in those patients with angiographic collateral vessels, but not in those without collaterals. This study suggests that improved ischemic zone blood flow in response to nitroglycerin in patients with atherosclerosis may be secondary to increased collateral circulation blood flow.

In addition to it effects in chronic atherosclerosis, nitrates also enhance coronary blood flow in patients

with vasospastic (Prinztmetal's) angina by reducing coronary vasospasm [13,14]. Nitrates also reverse or prevent the abnormal vasoconstrictor responses observed after administration of intracoronary acetylcholine and serotonin in patients with atherosclerosis [15,16]. It is hypothesized that nitroglycerin may replace the endothelium-derived relaxing factor (EDRF) in the diseased coronary bed where EDRF release is impaired [5]. In summary, improvement in coronary blood flow after nitrate therapy may be due to hemodynamic effects (i.e., decline in ventricular diastolic pressure, leading to reduced subendocardial compression of coronary arteries), dilatation of epicardial coronary arteries and stenotic segments, and increased collateral blood flow. In addition, nitroglycerin can improve blood flow in the specific settings of coronary spasm and endothelial dysfunction.

MYOCARDIAL INFARCTION

In 1972 cardiologists at Johns Hopkins Hospital were the first to study the use of intravenous nitroglycerin in acute myocardial infarction [17]. In the 12 patients studied, an average 7 mmHg reduction in blood pressure, a significant lowering of left ventricular filling pressure, and a reduction in the sum of the precordial ST-segment voltages were observed. In subsequent studies, with higher infusion rates (15–30 mmHg reduction in mean arterial pressure), antiischemic effects as assessed by precordial ST-segment mapping were observed [18]. At lower infusion rates, nitroglycerin acts primarily as a venodilator, lowering left ventricular pressure by a mean of 10 mmHg (45%), with little effect on mean arterial pressure. At higher doses, a similar (52%) lowering of left ventricular filling pressure is observed, but an arterial dilating effect is also noted (20% lowering of mean arterial pressure) [18]. The effect of nitroglycerin on left ventricular filling pressures varies according to the degree of left ventricular failure. Those patients with acute myocardial infarction without congestive failure demonstrate a decrease in both stroke volume and left ventricular filling pressure, reflecting a predominant lowering of preload secondary to venodilation. In contrast, patients with severe heart failure demonstrate a decrease in left ventricular filling pressure, but in addition they experience an increase in stroke volume, suggesting a reduction in both preload and afterload [18]. Review of several trials shows that the cardiac output in acute myocardial infarction increases or remains the same with nitroglycerin therapy [19]. Thus, short-term infusion of nitroglycerin in acute myocardial infarction results in a reduction in electrocardiographic evidence of ischemia and improved hemodynamics, particularly in patients with congestive heart failure.

Several clinical trails have assessed the role of nitrates on outcome following acute myocardial infarction. Flaherty and colleagues treated 102 patients presenting with acute myocardial infarction with 48 hours of intravenous nitroglycerin followed by nitropaste or placebo for a 7-day period [20]. In this study a statistically insignificant reduction in mortality was observed; however, a significant reduction in the combined endpoints of in-hospital death, infarct extension, or new congestive heart failure was noted, as well as a significant increase in ejection fraction at 10 hours. In a study of 310 patients presenting with transmural myocardial infarction, Jugdutt and Warnica demonstrated a reduced 30-day mortality (14% vs. 26%, $P < 0.01$), reduced echocardiographic evidence of infarct expansion, and reduced infarct size as assessed by creatine kinase release [21]. A meta-analysis of pooled results of 10 studies demonstrated that intravenous nitrates reduce mortality by 10–30% in myocardial infarction [22]. Others studies have demonstrated reduction of ventricular remodeling after myocardial infarction with nitrate therapy [19].

It must be noted that these studies were performed prior to the use of thrombolytic therapy. More recently, two large trials have examined the role of nitrate therapy in patients receiving thrombolytic therapy. In the GISSI-3 trial, patients receiving thrombolytic therapy for acute myocardial infarction did not have a significant reduction in mortality or reduction in the combined endpoints of mortality and ventricular dysfunction with transdermal nitrate therapy [23]. A significant reduction in the incidence of cardiogenic shock and a trend toward a reduction in postinfarction angina was observed in this trial. Similarly, in the ISIS-4 study no mortality benefit was observed with oral nitrate therapy in patients receiving thrombolytic therapy [24]. Based on these large trials, nitrate therapy appears to be safe in acute myocardial infarction, but its indiscriminant use is associated with an increased frequency of episodes of hypotension [23,24].

UNSTABLE ANGINA
The pathogenesis of unstable angina involves a complex interaction between atherosclerotic plaque rupture, local platelet activation, thrombosis, coronary endothelial dysfunction, and vasomotion. Nitrates may be of benefit by reducing myocardial oxygen demand via reduction in preload and reduced peripheral resistance [5], dilating epicardial coronary arteries [25], preventing coronary vasoconstriction

[15,16], and inhibiting platelet function [26]. Given the perceived benefits of nitrates in coronary artery syndromes, no studies have analyzed the effects of nitrates compared with placebo in the unstable angina population. Curfman and colleagues randomized 40 patients to receive either intravenous nitroglycerin or isosorbide dinitrate/transdermal ointment and found no significant difference in clinical outcomes when comparing the two strategies [27].

Nitrate tolerance can occur in the setting of unstable angina and may be important with regard to both the hemodynamic and antiplatelet effects of nitrates [28]. Because of the need to maintain nitrate efficacy in patients prone to ischemia over a 24-hour period, prevention of tolerance is important in unstable angina. One approach to the problem of tolerance is to infuse N-acetyl-L-cysteine (NAC), a sulfhydryl antioxidant known to potentiate the hemodynamic response to nitroglycerin, and to reverse or prevent tolerance [28]. In a study of 46 patients with unstable angina, Horowitz and colleagues reported a lower incidence of myocardial infarction in patients randomized to receive nitroglycerin/NAC compared with those receiving nitroglycerin alone [29]. However, the NAC/nitroglycerin-treated patients had a higher incidence of symptomatic hypotension [29].

CHRONIC ANGINA PECTORIS
Nitrates were first administered to patients with angina pectoris in 1879 by Murrell [30]. Since that time sublingual nitroglycerin has been used extensively for the treatment and prevention of anginal attacks. Nitrates have been shown to reduce exercise-induced angina and electrocardiographic ischemia in patients with established coronary artery disease [31]. In addition, when taken prophylactically in the sublingual, buccal, or oral forms, nitrates can reduce the incidence of ischemic episodes and prolong exercise tolerance in patients with coronary artery disease [32]. While nitrates are quite effective for short-term therapy, long-term administration is influenced by tolerance to both hemodynamic and anti-ischemic effects [32]. Tolerance develops with four times daily administration of isosorbide dinitrate and continuous therapy with nitroglycerin patches [32]. Use of a twice-daily or three-times-daily drug schedule promotes a sustained drug effect without significant attenuation of efficacy [33]. Alternatively, use of once-daily sustained-release formulations of isosorbide dinitrate or isosorbide 5-mononitrate can eliminate drug tolerance [33].

Angiotensin-Converting Enzyme Inhibitors

Angiotensin-converting enzyme inhibitors (ACEI) prevent the conversion of angiotensin I to angiotensin II by inhibiting the converting enzyme peptidyl dipeptidase [34]. This enzyme also inactivates brady-kinin, a potent vasodilator, and ACEI thereby promote accumulation of bradykinin. Converting enzyme inhibitors have in common a 2-methyl propranolol-L-proline moiety, which is critical for blocking the active site of the converting enzyme [35].

The physiologic actions of ACEI are, in large part, related to the lowering of angiotensin II levels. Angiotensin II is a potent peripheral and coronary vasoconstrictor, and also increases myocardial contractility by raising cytosolic calcium [36]. In addition to the systemic effects of angiotensin II, local tissue renin-angiotensin systems exist in blood vessels and many organs, including the heart [37]. In fact, local generation of angiotensin II in the myocardium may participate in the processes of left ventricular hypertrophy and left ventricular remodeling [37]. By promoting the release of norepinephrine and interfering with its neuronal reuptake, angiotensin II enhances sympathetic nervous system activity [38]. Angiotensin II also inhibits both central and peripheral vagal activity. The increase in myocardial contractility, autonomic effects, and vasoconstrictive effects of angiotensin II result in increased myocardial oxygen demand.

By inhibiting the formation of angiotensin II, ACEIs promote arterial vasodilation and reduce both preload and afterload [36]. These hemodynamic effects lead to decreased left ventricular wall stress and myocardial oxygen demand [36]. ACEIs also reduce sympathetic tone and increase parasympathetic tone due to inhibition of the renin-angiotensin system and sympathetic nervous activity. These neural effects may underlie the lack of reflex tachycardia after administration of ACEIs.

EFFECTS ON CORONARY CIRCULATION

Several studies have demonstrated that ACEIs block angiotensin II–mediated coronary vasoconstriction and thus increase coronary blood flow in both humans and animals [36]. In addition to a direct effect, coronary vasodilatation after ACEI treatment is also mediated by accumulation of bradykinin and prostaglandins [39]. Karsch and colleagues showed that intravenous captopril increased coronary artery diameter at the site of existing atherosclerotic lesions (but not in normal segments), both at rest and with

pacing-induced ischemia, in patients with chronic angina [40]. In the study, despite an increase in coronary artery luminal diameter, reduced left ventricular end-diastolic pressure, and peripheral arterial vasodilatation, a significant reduction in anginal symptoms during pacing was not observed after ACEI therapy. In contrast, Ikram and colleagues showed that intravenous captopril reduced the time to angina, increased the paced heart rate for the development of angina, and showed a trend toward increased coronary blood flow [41]. Thus, while ACEIs have been shown to have coronary vasodilatory effects, the ability of ACEI to reduce pacing-induced ischemia remains controversial.

MYOCARDIAL INFARCTION

A role for the renin-angiotensin system in the pathogenesis of acute coronary syndromes has been suggested from epidemiological evidence linking elevated plasma renin levels with risk of myocardial infarction [36]. Three recent large randomized trials in patients with depressed left ventricular function have provided data regarding ACEI treatment and the risk of acute coronary syndromes [42–44]. The SOLVD (Studies Of Left Ventricular Dysfunction) trial, which consisted of patients with ejection fractions of less than 35% who had symptomatic heart failure (treatment trial) [45] or who were asymptomatic (prevention trial) [43], demonstrated a reduction in ischemic events (unstable angina, myocardial infarction) over an average 40-month follow-up period in enalapril-treated patients compared with placebo [46]. Similarly, the SAVE (Survival and Ventricular Enlargement) trial, which randomized patients within 3–16 days after myocardial infarction to captopril or placebo, also showed a reduction in risk of myocardial infarction [44]. Combining the results of the SAVE and SOLVD trials, the risk reduction in secondary myocardial infarction rates was 23% (95% CI, 12–33%); $P < 0.001$ [36].

The reduction in the risk of myocardial infarction observed in the SAVE and SOLVD trials did not become apparent until 6 months after initiation of treatment. Likewise, the reduction in unstable angina observed in the SOLVD trials displayed a similar time course. This delay in the reduction of ischemic events suggests that the mechanism is unlikely to be related solely to the hemodynamic effects of ACE inhibition but may reflect antiatherogenic effects, improved endothelial function, stabilization of atherosclerotic plaques [36], or reduced plasminogen activator inhibitor-1 [47].

In addition to their role in the prevention of myocardial infarction, ACEIs improve on mortality in patients with acute myocardial infarction. Several trials have examined the role of ACE inhibition in patients with evidence of cardiac dysfunction after myocardial infarction. The SAVE trial, a large, randomized placebo-controlled trial (2231 patients), treated patients 3–16 days after myocardial infarction with ejection fractions less than 40% without symptomatic heart failure with captopril [44]. A 19% mortality reduction, a 37% decrease in the development of severe heart failure, and a 22% reduction in admissions for congestive failure were observed over a mean 42-month follow-up. Similarly, in the AIRE (Acute Infarction Ramipril Efficacy) study, patients with symptomatic heart failure after myocardial infarction were treated with ramipril and a 27% mortality reduction over a mean 15-month period was observed [42].

ACEIs also improve outcome in patients without evidence of left ventricular dysfunction with acute myocardial infarction. The ISIS-4 study (58,050 patients) demonstrated that captopril given for 1 month after acute myocardial infarction reduced overall mortality by 7% after 5 weeks and showed a trend toward a 12-month mortality reduction [24]. Similarly, in the GISSI-3 study (19,394 patients), lisinopril therapy reduced 6-week mortality by 11% and decreased the incidence of severe ventricular dysfunction in patients presenting with acute myocardial infarction [23]. It is important to note that the use of thrombolytic therapy varied in these trials (SAVE trial, 33%; ISIS-4, 70%; and GISSI-3, 71%), suggesting that the benefits of ACEI are present irrespective of the use of fibrinolysis. The CONSENSUS II trial was terminated early owing to excessive hypotension and lack of mortality benefit in patients given intravenous enalapril within the first 24 hours after myocardial infarction [48]. Thus some caution must be exercised with ACEI therapy in the early hours after myocardial infarction. In summary, ACEI therapy reduce mortality and the development of heart failure in patients presenting with acute myocardial, regardless of the presence or absence of congestive heart failure. The mechanism of the mortality reduction observed with ACEI therapy after myocardial infarction may involve inhibition of neurohumoral activation [44], reduced ventricular remodeling [49], improvement in endothelial dysfunction [50], antiatherogenic effects [36], or improved plaque stability [36].

CHRONIC ANGINA
By blocking both circulating and tissue renin-angiotensin systems, ACEIs exert a multitude of theoretically cardioprotective effects in patients with chronic coronary artery disease. The vascular effects outlined earlier result in a reduction in ventricular wall stress and improved coronary blood flow. In addition, reduced sympathetic stimulation would also be expected to reduce myocardial oxygen demand in patients with chronic angina. ACEIs also reduce left ventricular mass, which has been shown to be an independent predictor of coronary heart disease and cardiac mortality [36]. In animal models, ACEIs have been shown to have a direct antiatherogenic effect [51,52]. ACEIs also have antiplatelet effects, improve endothelial function, and may increase atherosclerotic plaque stability [36].

Despite the many potential mechanisms for reduction in atherogenesis and myocardial ischemia with ACEI therapy, several small trials in patients with chronic stable angina have reported variable clinical benefit. Some trials have shown no impact on the frequency of angina [53,54], exercise-induced ST depression [55,56], or ambulatory ECG ischemia [54,56] with ACEI therapy, while others have demonstrated improvement in these indices [57,58]. Several large ongoing trials have been designed to better examine the antiischemic effects of ACEI in patients with coronary artery disease (Heart Outcomes Prevention Evaluation [HOPE], Study to Evaluate Carotid Ultrasound Changes with Ramapril and Vitamin E [SECURE], The Quinapril Ischemic Event Trial [QUIET], Simvastatin and Enalapril Coronary Atherosclerosis Trial [SCAT], and the Prevention of Atherosclerosis with Ramapril Therapy [PART] trial) [36].

Calcium Channel Blockers

The calcium channel blockers are a heterogeneous group of compounds sharing in common the ability to interfere with calcium entry into cardiac and smooth muscle myocytes. These agents can be classified chemically into the dihydropyridine (e.g., nifedipine), phenylalkylamine (e.g., verapamil), and benzothiazepine (e.g., diltiazem) derivatives [59]. Calcium can enter cells by three main mechanisms: voltage-dependent calcium channels, receptor-operated channels, and sodium–calcium exchange. All three classes of calcium channel blockers inhibit calcium entry, primarily by blocking the voltage-dependent calcium channels. Diltiazem and verapamil slow the rate of opening of voltage-dependent calcium channels, while nifedipine reduces the number of these ion channels that are opening [60]. Verapamil also blocks alpha-adrenergic receptors and reduces calcium entry via this mechanism [59].

Vascular smooth muscle cells are dependent on transmembrane calcium influx for normal resting tone and contractile responses [34]. By inhibiting calcium entry in vascular smooth muscle cells, calcium channel blockers cause vascular relaxation, resulting in a decrease in total peripheral resistance [61]. Force generation during cardiac muscle contraction also depends on calcium influx during membrane depolarization [62]. Thus, antagonism of calcium entry in the myocardium can result in a negative inotropic effect. Calcium influx also plays an integral role in spontaneous depolarization of cardiac pacemaker cells in the sinoatrial node and conduction in the atrioventricular (AV) node. Calcium channel blockade results in reduced sinus node activity and slowed conduction in the AV node [60].

The physiologic effects of calcium channel blockers are, to some extent, determined by chemical class. For example, dihydropyridine calcium channel blockers have a more prominent vasodilator effect than negative inotropic effect [60]. Diltiazem has less prominent peripheral vascular effects and more negative inotropic effects [4]. Verapamil has a more evenly balanced effect on the myocardium and peripheral vascular bed [4]. The chronotropic and dromotropic effects are greater with verapamil than diltiazem [34], and the dihydropyridines have little negative chronotropic effect, owing to peripheral vasodilatation and baroreceptor-mediated augmentation of sympathetic tone [63]. The so-called second-generation dihydrophyridine calcium channel blockers (amlodipine, felodipine, isradipine, nicardipine, and nimodipine) have longer half-lives and even greater vascular selectivity than nifedipine [4].

EFFECTS ON CORONARY BLOOD FLOW
All three classes of calcium channel blockers can produce epicardial coronary artery vasodilatation [64,65]. In addition, calcium channel blockers have been shown to prevent the effects of various stimuli that can induce abnormal coronary vasoconstriction. Brown and colleagues showed that diltiazem treatment reduced handgrip-induced coronary vasoconstriction as measured by quantitative coronary angiography [25]. The presumed mechanism of this effect is attenuation of receptor-activated adrenergic coronary vasoconstriction, which requires calcium entry into smooth muscle cells. In contrast to isometric hand-grip exercise, exercise causes an increase in the diameter of normal coronary segments mediated by the increased metabolic demand [66]. Coronary vasodilatation during exercise overwhelms the modest increase in sympathetic tone observed with this type of exercise [65]. Coronary vasoconstriction occurs in diseased coronary segments in response to bicycle exercise [66], possibly as a result of increased neurogenic tone or impaired endothelial vasodilator function. Either nitroglycerin or diltiazem prevents the exercise-induced decrease in stenotic cross-sectional area during exercise [66,67].

In addition to acting on epicardial coronary arteries, calcium channel blockers also dilate coronary resistance vessels, resulting in increased coronary blood flow [65]. The effect of calcium channel blockers on collateral blood flow during acute coronary occlusion remains controversial, with some studies showing improved flow and others showing no benefit [65]. In chronic coronary occlusion animal models, diltiazem (but not nifedipine) appears to increase coronary collateral blood flow [65].

ACUTE MYOCARDIAL INFARCTION
Considering the basic mechanisms of action of calcium channel blockers, it might be expected that these agents would have several beneficial effects in acute myocardial infarction. Indeed, animal experimental models of myocardial infarction have shown that calcium channel blockers reduce infarct size, increase endocardial perfusion, reduce the extent of myocardial stunning, reduce the incidence of arrhythmia [68], and counteract the deleterious effects of intracellular calcium overload [69]. Despite these beneficial effects in animals, clinical trials of calcium blockers in acute myocardial infarction have shown only variable benefit. This variability, in part, correlates with the heterogeneous effects of these agents on heart rate and the inotropic state of the myocardium.

Three large trials have examined the effect of nifedipine in acute myocardial infarction [70–72]. None of these trials demonstrated a reduction in mortality or reinfarction, and two of the three trials were halted in progress due to neutral or adverse outcomes. Pooling the data on 4731 patients studied in these trials, 7.7% died in the nifedipine group compared with 7% in the placebo group [73]. In addition, there was a trend toward a higher reinfarction rate in the nifedipine-treated patients (3.4 vs. 3.0%) [73].

The Multicenter Diltiazem Postinfarction Trial was a randomized placebo-controlled trial examining the role of diltiazem treatment in myocardial infarction [74]. In this large trial of patients with both Q-wave myocardial infarction (n = 1757) and non–Q-wave myocardial infarction (n = 634), there was no overall mortality benefit in the diltiazem-treated group. Prospectively planned subgroup analysis revealed an excess mortality in patients with left ventricular dysfunction and pulmonary congestion (20% of total population) treated with diltiazem. In the remaining 80% of patients, diltiazem treatment was associated with a 27% reduction in nonfatal reinfarction and death. In the subgroup of patients with non–Q-wave infarction, diltiazem was associated with a significant reduction in death and reinfarction over long-term follow-up (43% at 1 year and 34% at 4.5 years) [75]. Thus, treatment with diltiazem appears to be beneficial in patients with myocardial infarction who have intact left ventricular function and/or non–Q-wave events.

The two large Danish Verapamil Infarction Trials have provided insight into the role of verapamil in myocardial infarction. The DAVIT-I trial (3500 patients) compared verapamil with placebo early after myocardial infarction and demonstrated no survival difference after 6 months follow-up [76]. In contrast, the DAVIT-II trial (1800 patients) treated patients 1–3 weeks after the acute event and noted a significant mortality reduction (11% vs. 13% with placebo) after 16 months [77]. Thus, verapamil appears to be safe in myocardial infarction and may provide a modest mortality reduction. In summary, there may be a role for rate-slowing calcium blockers in the setting of acute myocardial infarction. Patients must be screened carefully for evidence of left ventricular dysfunction when considering diltiazem. Nifedipine appears to have no role in the treatment of acute myocardial infarction.

UNSTABLE ANGINA

Several studies have demonstrated the effectiveness of calcium channel blockers in controlling anginal symptoms in patients with unstable angina [78–80]. However, Held and Yusuf pooled data from all randomized trials utilizing calcium channel blockers in unstable angina and found no reduction in mortality or myocardial infarction [73]. In addition, some classes of calcium channel blockers may be harmful in the setting of unstable angina. For example, the Holland Interuniversity Nifedipine/Metoprolol Trial (HINT) was a large, double-blind, placebo-controlled study comparing the use of nifedipine alone, metoprolol alone, or the combination in the management of unstable angina [80]. The study was halted prematurely owing to a greater incidence of nonfatal myocardial infarction in the first 48 hours among patients treated with nifedipine alone compared with those treated with metoprolol or the combination of nifedipine and metoprolol. While monotherapy with nifedipine may be deleterious in unstable angina, adding nifedipine to nitrates or beta-adrenoceptor blockers reduced the incidence of myocardial in-

farction, death, or the need for emergency bypass surgery in one study [79]. In this study, the patients with presumed vasospastic angina associated with transient electrocardiographic ST-segment elevation obtained the most benefit from the addition of nifedipine to beta blockers and nitrates [79].

STABLE ANGINA

Several controlled trials have demonstrated that all three classes of calcium channel blockers are effective in reducing anginal attacks, the need for nitroglycerin, and improving exercise treadmill time in patients with stable angina pectoris [60]. The potential mechanisms for reduction of angina by calcium channel blockers include improved coronary blood flow, a reduction in heart rate, reduced arterial resistance and contractility, and prevention of coronary vasospasm [60]. The degree to which any one of these mechanisms predominates depends on the class of agent and the dosage utilized. When the three agents were compared in one nonrandomized trial, diltiazem and verapamil were more effective than nifedipine when used as single agents [81].

Adrenergic Blockers

BETA-ADRENORECEPTOR BLOCKERS

In 1948 Ahlquist hypothesized that the effects of catecholamines were mediated by activation of distinct alpha and beta receptors [82]. By the late 1950s, Sir James Black and colleagues synthesized propranolol, the first competitive inhibitor of the beta-receptor [83]. Numerous additional beta-adrenoceptor antagonists have since been synthesized and can be distinguished by the following properties: relative affinity for $beta_1$ and $beta_2$ receptors, intrinsic sympathomimetic activity, additional blockade of alpha-adrenergic receptor, differences in lipid solubility, and pharmacokinetics [83]. Propranolol has equal affinity for $beta_1$ and $beta_2$ receptors, whereas metoprolol and atenolol are more selective for the $beta_1$-adrenoreceptor than for the $beta_2$-adrenoreceptor [83]. Unlike propranolol, pindolol is a beta blocker that has intrinsic sympathomimetic activity, implying the ability to activate partially beta receptors in the absence of catecholamine stimulation [83]. Labetalol is an example of a beta-blocking agent with alpha-adrenoreceptor blocking properties [83].

The pharmacological effects of beta-adrenoreceptor blockers are determined by their ability to blunt the effects of catecholamines on effector tissues (the heart, arteries, arterioles of the skeletal system, and bronchi). Catecholamines normally increase cardiac contractility and heart rate by stimulating the $beta_1$ receptor and cause peripheral vasodilatation and bronchial relaxation via stimulation of the $beta_2$ receptor [83]. Accordingly, $beta_1$-adrenoreceptor antagonists slow the heart rate and decrease myocardial contractility [83]. The effects of $beta_1$-adrenoreceptor blockade on contractility and heart rate are proportional to the degree of sympathetic stimulation [83]. For example, when the sympathetic system is activated during stress or exercise, beta blockers greatly attenuate the expected rise in heart rate, while at rest the effect of these agents on heart rate is quite modest. Short-term administration of beta-adrenoreceptor blockers increases peripheral resistance as a result of blockade of vascular $beta_2$ receptors and compensatory sympathetic reflexes that activate vascular alpha-adrenoreceptors [83]. In contrast, long-term use of beta-adrenoreceptor blockers is associated with a return of the peripheral resistance to baseline values [83]. In hypertensive, but not nonhypertensive, individuals, beta blockers may lower blood pressure by attenuating the sympathetically stimulated release of renin from the juxtaglomerular apparatus in the kidney [38,44]. Interestingly, chronic exposure to beta-adrenoreceptor antagonists can result in an increase in the number of available beta-adrenoreceptors. Thus, upon withdrawal of the drug, tissues may be supersensitive to adrenergic stimuli owing to this upregulation of receptors [83].

Coronary Blood Flow. The effects of beta-adrenoceptor blocking drugs on coronary blood flow are varied. Heart rate slowing with beta blockers can enhance coronary blood flow by allowing more time in diastole for coronary blood flow to occur [84]. In addition, some investigators have demonstrated that beta-blocking agents can improve myocardial oxygen supply by improving coronary collateral blood flow [85,86]. Other investigators have not supported these findings [68]. In some patients who are prone to coronary spasm, beta blockers may increase myocardial ischemia and symptoms of angina [84], an effect that may occur secondary to unopposed alpha-adrenoceptor stimulation [87].

Myocardial Infarction. Beta blockers may improve outcome in myocardial infarction by lowering myocardial oxygen demand (decreasing heart rate, blood pressure, and myocardial contractility) during periods of reduced coronary perfusion. Early administration of beta-blockers in the setting of myocardial infarction reduces infarct size [88], lowers the incidence of ventricular fibrillation [89], and reduces overall mortality at 7 days (4.3% placebo vs. 3.7% atenolol treated;

ISIS-1) [90]. The benefits of early beta-blockade in acute myocardial infarction have subsequently been shown to extend to patients receiving thrombolytic therapy (TIMI IIB) [91]. In the TIMI trial a subgroup of patients were randomly assigned to receive intravenous metoprolol followed by oral metoprolol or oral metoprolol alone started on day 6. Although early beta blockade offered no benefit over late administration in improving left ventricular function or reducing mortality, patients receiving early intravenous metoprolol had fewer nonfatal infarctions and less recurrent ischemic events at 6 days.

The long-term use of beta blockers after myocardial infarction has been supported by two large clinical trials. In the Norwegian Multicenter trial in 1884 patients, there was a significant reduction in mortality (16% placebo and 10.4% timolol) and reinfarction (14% placebo and 10% timolol) in patients treated with timolol for an average of 17 months after myocardial infarction [92]. Similarly, the Beta Blocker Heart Attack Trial (BHAT) showed a mortality reduction (9.8% placebo vs. 7.2% propranolol) and a reduction in reinfarction (5% placebo vs. 4% propranolol) after approximately 2 years of follow-up [93]. In summary, in patients with acute myocardial infarction, early initiation and subsequent continuation of beta-blocker therapy reduces mortality, infarct size, and recurrent ischemia. Thus, beta blockers should be given to all patients after myocardial infarction without contraindications (bradycardia or atrioventricular block, clinical congestive heart failure, hypotension, or bronchospasm).

Unstable Angina. In unstable angina, a combination of coronary plaque rupture, thrombosis, and coronary spasm leads to reduced myocardial blood flow. It would be expected that the negative chronotropic and negative inotropic properties of beta blockers would reduce myocardial ischemia in this setting. However, unlike calcium channel blockers, which improve coronary vasospasm, beta blockers may, in theory, worsen coronary spasm. For these reasons, several studies have compared beta blockers with calcium channel blockers in the treatment of unstable angina pectoris. The Holland Interuniversity Nifedipine/Metoprolol Trial compared nifedipine and metoprolol in preventing recurrence of ischemia or infarction in 515 patients presenting with unstable angina. In this study, metoprolol alone or in combination with nifedipine resulted in a reduction in anginal symptoms and recurrent ischemic events [80]. Theroux and colleagues randomized 100 patients with unstable angina to receive propranolol or diltiazem, and found that both drugs were equally effective in reducing the number of chest pain episodes without any difference in long-term cardiac event rates [78]. A third study demonstrated that the addition of propranolol to nifedipine in unstable angina reduced the frequency of both symptomatic and silent ischemic episodes [94]. Thus, it appears that beta blockers are effective in the treatment of unstable angina when used alone or in combination with nitrates and calcium channel blockers.

Stable Angina Pectoris. Angina pectoris occurs when oxygen demand exceeds supply and is often precipitated by conditions that increase sympathetic tone [95]. This concept led to several clinical trials with beta-adrenergic blocking agents in patients with chronic angina pectoris. Numerous studies have demonstrated that beta-blocking agents reduce anginal frequency, nitroglycerin consumption, heart rate, systolic blood pressure, and electrocardiographic ST-segment deviation, and improve exercise tolerance in patients with angina [95]. There are no data confirming an improvement in long-term outcome in patients taking beta-blocking agents for chronic angina; however, one study showed a trend toward a reduction in cardiac events [96].

ALPHA BLOCKERS

Two distinct alpha-adrenoreceptors have been identified in vascular tissue: alpha$_1$ and alpha$_2$ adrenoreceptors. The alpha$_1$ adrenoreceptor exists on postjunctional synapses of smooth cells and mediates vasoconstriction. In contrast, the alpha$_2$ adrenoreceptor (of which there are two subtypes, a and b) is located on sympathetic nerve endings, where it modulates norepinephrine release by a negative-feedback mechanism. Some blood vessels also possess postjunctional alpha$_2$ adrenoreceptors [87].

Activation of both postjunctional alpha adrenoreceptors results in an increase in intracellular ionized calcium [87]. Alpha$_2$ adrenoreceptor activation limits the availability of ionized calcium for release of norepinephrine, possibly through regulation of neural cyclic AMP [87]. In coronary as well as noncoronary vessels, selective blockade of alpha$_1$ adrenoreceptors with prazosin results in inhibition of sympathetically mediated vasoconstriction [97]. In contrast, phentolamine, a nonselective alpha-adrenoreceptor blocker, inhibits alpha$_1$ and alpha$_2$ receptors, resulting in inhibition of vasoconstriction and enhanced release of norepinephrine, which may act on beta adrenoreceptors to enhance further vasodilatation [97]. Alpha-blocking agents have been widely used as antihypertensive agents because of the vasodilating effect [87]. In addition, prazosin has been shown to be useful in refractory coronary artery spasm in humans [98]. Because alpha blockers reduce afterload, they may reduce myocardial oxygen demand in ischemic states [87]. However, alpha blockers have not been utilized as primary agents for the treatment of myocardial ischemia as yet.

References

1. Schlant RC, Sonnenblick EH. Normal physiology of the cardiovascular system. In Schlant RC, Alexander RW (eds). The Heart. New York: McGraw-Hill, 1994:113.
2. Braunwald E, Sobel BE. Coronary blood flow and myocardial ischemia. In Braunwald E. (ed). Heart Disease. Philadelphia: WB Saunders, 1992:1161.
3. Fung HL, Chung SJ, Bauer JA, Chong S, Kowaluk EA. Biochemical mechanism of organic nitrate action. Am J Cardiol 70:4B, 1992.
4. Rutherford JD, Braunwald E. Chronic Ischemic Heart Disease. In Braunwald E (ed). Heart Disease. Philadelphia: WB Saunders, 1992:1292.
5. Abrams J. Mechanisms of action of the organic nitrates in the treatment of myocardial ischemia. Am J Cardiol 70:30B, 1992.
6. Brown BG, Bolson E, Petersen RB, Pierce CD, Dodge HT. The mechanisms of nitroglycerin action: Stenosis vasodilatation as a major component of the drug response. Circulation 64:1089, 1981.
7. Cowan C, Duran PVM, Corsini G. The effects of nitroglycerin on myocardial blood flow in man. Measured by coincidence counting and bolus injections of [84]rubidium. Am J Cardiol 24:154, 1969.
8. Parker JO, West RO, Di Giorgi S. The effect of nitroglycerin on coronary bood flow and the hemodynamic response to exercise in coronary artery disease. Am J Cardiol 27:59, 1971.
9. Ganz W, Marcus HS. Failure of intracoronary nitroglycerin to alleviate pacing-induced angina. Circulation 46:880, 1972.
10. Fam WM, McGregor M. Effect of coronary vasodilator drugs on retrograde flow in areas of chronic myocardial ischemia. Circ Res 15:355, 1964.
11. Cohen MV, Downey JM, Sonnenblick EH. The effects of nitroglycerin on coronary collaterals and myocardial contractility. J Clin Invest 52:2836, 1973.
12. Cohn PF, Maddox D, Holman BL, Markis JE, Adams DF, See JR. Effect of sublingually administered nitroglycerin on regional myocardial blood flow in patients with coronary artery disease. Am J Cardiol 39:672, 1977.
13. Hill JA, Feldman RL, Pepine CJ, Conti CR. Randomized double-blind comparison of nifedipine and isosorbide dinitrate in patients with coronary arterial spasm. Am J Cardiol 49:431, 1982.
14. Ginsburg R, Lamb I, Schroeder JS, Hu M, Harrison DC. Randomized double-blind comparison of nifedipine and isosorbide dinitrate therapy in variant

angina pectoris due to coronary arterial spasm. Am Heart J 103:44, 1982.

15. Ludmer PL, Selwyn AP, Shook TL, Wayne RR, Mudge GH, Alexander RW, Ganz P. Paradoxical vasoconstriction induced by acetylcholine atherosclerotic arteries. N Engl J Med 315:1046, 1986.

16. Golino P, Piccione F, Willerson JT. Divergent effects of serotonin on coronary artery dimensions and blood flow in patients with coronary atherosclerosis and control patients. N Engl J Med 324:641, 1986.

17. Flaherty JT, Come PC, Baird MG, Kelly DT. Intravenous nitroglycerin in acute myocardial infarction. Circulation 51:132, 1975.

18. Flaherty JT. Role of nitrates in acute myocardial infarction. Am J Cardiol 70:73B, 1992.

19. Jugdutt BI. Role of nitrates after acute myocardial infarction. Am J Cardiol 70:82B, 1992.

20. Flaherty JT, Becker LC, Bulkley BH, Weiss JL, Gerstenblith G, Kallman CH, Silverman KJ, Wei JY, Pitt B, Weisbeldt ML. A randomized prospective trial of intravenous nitroglycerin in patients with acute myocardial infarction. Circulation 68:576, 1983.

21. Jugdutt BI, Warnica JW. Intravenous nitroglycerin therapy to limit myocardial infarct size, expansion and complications. Effect of timing, dosage and infarct location. Circulation 78:906, 1988.

22. Yusuf S, Collins R, MacMahon S, Peto S. Effect of intravenous nitrates on mortality in acute myocardial infarction: An overview of the randomized trials. Lancet 1:1088, 1988.

23. Gruppo Italiano per lo Studio della Soprawivenza nell'infarto Miocardico. GISSI-3: Effects of lisinopril and transdermal glyceryl trinitrate singly and together on 6-week mortality and ventricular function after acute myocardial infarction. Lancet 343:1115, 1994.

24. ISIS-4. A randomised factorial trial assessing early oral captopril, oral mononitrate, and intravenous magnesium sulphate in 58,050 patients with suspected acute myocardial infarction. Lancet 345:669, 1995.

25. Brown BG, Lee AB, Bolson EL, Dodge HT. Reflex constriction of significant coronary stenosis as a direct mechanism contributing to ischemic left ventricular dysfunction during isometric exercise. Circulation 70:18, 1984.

26. Loscalzo J. Antiplatelet and antithrombotic effects of organic nitrates. Am J Cardiol 70:18B, 1992.

27. Curfman GD, Heinsimes JA, Lozner EC, Fung HL. Intravenous nitroglycerin in the treatment of spontaneous angina pectoris: A prospective randomized trial. Circulation 67:286, 1983.

28. Horowitz JD. Role of nitrates in unstable angina pectoris. Am J Cardiol 70:64B, 1992.

29. Horowiitz JD, Henry CA, Syrjanen ML. Combined use of nitroglycerine and N-acetylcysteine in the management of unstable angina pectoris. Circulation 77:787, 1988.

30. Murrell W. Nitro-glycerine as a remedy for angina pectoris. Lancet I:80, 1879.

31. Detry JMR, Bruce RA. Effects of nitroglycerin on "maximal" oxygen intake and exercise electrocardiogram in coronary artery disease. Circulation 43:629, 1971.

32. Thadani U. Role of nitrates in angina pectoris. Am J Cardiol 70:43B, 1992.

33. Abrams J. New concepts on using nitrates in angina pectoris. Contemp Intern Med 1991:92.

34. Banowitz NC, Bourne HR. Antihypertensive Agents. In Katzung, BG (ed). Basic and Clinical Pharmacology. Appleton and Lang, 1987:105.

35. Williams GH. Converting-enzyme inhibitors in the treatment of hypertension. N Engl J Med 319:1517, 1988.

36. Lonn EM, Yusuf S, Jha P, Doris CI, Sabine MJ, Dzavik V, Hutchison K, Riley WA, Tucker J, Pogue J, Taylor W. Emerging role of angiotensin-converting enzyme inhibitors in cardiac and vascular protection. Circulation 90:2056, 1994.

37. Kelly RA, Smith TW. Pharmacologic treatment of heart failure. In Hardman J, Limbird L, Molinoff P, Ruddon RW, Gilman AG, Goodman LS (eds). The Pharmacologic Basis of Therapeutics. New York: McGraw Hill, 1996.

38. Davies MK. Effects of ACE inhibitors on coronary haemodynamics and angina pectoris. Br Heart J 72:S52, 1994.

39. Van Gilst WH, Van Wigorgaarden J, Scholters E, de Grueff PA, deLarger CDJ, Wesseling H. Captopril-induced increase in coronary flow: An SH-dependent effect on arachidonic acid metabolism? J Cardiovasc Pharmacol 9:S31, 1987.

40. Karsch KR, Voelker W, Mauser M. Myocardial and coronary effects of captopril during pacing-induced ischaemia in patients with coronary artery disease. Eur Heart J 11:157, 1990.

41. Ikram H, Low CJ, Shirlaw T, Webb CM, Richards AM, Crozier IG. Antianginal, hemodynamic and coronary vascular effects of catopril in stable angina pectoris. Am J Cardiol 66:164, 1990.

42. AIRE Study Investigators. Effect of ramipril on mortality and morbidity of survivors of acute myocardial infarction with clinical evidence of heart failure. Lancet 342:821, 1993.

43. The SOLVD Investigators. Effect of enalapril on mortality and the development of heart failure in asymptomatic patients with reduced left ventricular ejection fractions. N Engl J Med 327:685, 1992.

44. Pfeffer MA, Braunwald E, Moye LA, Basta L, Brown EJ Jr., Cuddy TE, Davis BR, Geltman EM, Goldman S, Flaker GC, Klein M, Lamas GA, Packer M, Rouleau J, Rouleau JL, Rutherford J, Wertheimer JH, Hawkins CM. Effect of captopril on mortality and morbidity in patients with left ventricular dysfunction after myocardial infarction; Results of the survival and ventricular enlargement trial. N Engl J Med 327:669, 1992.

45. The SOLVD Investigators.Effect of enalapril on survival in patients with reduced left ventricular ejection fractions and congestive heart failure. N Engl J Med 325:293, 1991.

46. Yusuf S, Collins R, Peto R, Furberg C, Stampfer MJ, Goldhaber SZ, Hennekens CH. Intravenous and intracoronary fibrinolytic therapy in acute myocardial infarction: Overview of results on mortality, reinfarction and side-effects from 33 randomized controlled trials. Eur Heart J 6:556, 1985.

47. Vaughan DE, Lazos SA, Tong K. Angiotensin II regulates the expression of plasminogen activator inhibitor-1 in cultured endothelial cells. A potential link between the renin-angiotensin system and thrombosis. J Clin Invest 95:995, 1995.

48. Swedberg K, Held P, Kjekshus J, Rasmussen K, Ryden L, Wedel H. Effects of the early administration of enalapril on mortality in patients with acute myocardial infarction; Results of the cooperative New Scandinavian Enalapri Survival Study II (Consensus II). N Engl J Med 327:678, 1992.

49. Pfeffer MA, Lamas GA, Vaughan DE, Parisi AF, Braunwald E. Effect of captopril on progressive ventricular dilatation after anterior myocardial infarction. N Engl J Med 319:80, 1988.

50. Greenwald L, Becker RC. Expanding the paradigm of the renin-angiotensin system and angiotensin-converting enzyme inhibitors. Am Heart J 128:997, 1994.

51. Chobanian AV. The effects of ACE inhibitors and other antihypertensive drugs on cardiovascular risk factors and atherogenesis. Clin Cardiol 13:VII43, 1990.

52. Rolland PH, Charpiot P, Friggi A, Piquet P, Barlatier A, Scalbert E, Bodard H, Tranier P, Mercier C, Luccioni R, Garcon D. Effects of angiotensin-converting enzyme inhibition with perindolol on hemodynamics, arterial structure, and wall rheology in the hindquarters of atherosclerotic mini-pigs. Am J Cardiol 71:22e, 1993.

53. Gibbs JS, Crean PA, Mockus L, Wright C, Sutton GC, Fox KM. The variable effects of angiotensin converting enzyme inhibition on myocardial ischaemia in chronic stable angina. Br Heart J 62:112, 1989.

54. Thurmann P, Odenthal HJ, Rietbrock N. Converting enzyme inhibition in coronary artery disease: A randomised, placebo-controlled trial with benazepril. J Cardiovasc Pharmacol 17:718, 1991.

55. Klein WW, Khurmi NS, Eber B, Dusleag J. Effects of benazepril and metoprolol OROS alone and in combination on myocardial ischemia in patients with chronic stable angina. J Am Coll Cardiol 16:948, 1990.

56. Ikram H, Low CJ, Shirlaw T. Angiotensin converting enzyme inhibition in chronic stable angina: Effects on myocardial ischaemia and comparison with nifedipine. Br Heart J 71:30, 1994.

57. Stompe KO, Overlack A. A new trial of the efficacy, tolerability, and safety of angiotensin converting enzyme inhibition in mild systemic hypertension with concomitant disease and therapies. Am J Cardiol 71:32E, 1993.

58. Akhras F, Jackson G. The role of captopril as single therapy in hypertension and angina pectoris. Int J Cardiol 33:259, 1991.

59. Wood AJJ. Calcium antagonists. Circulation 80:IV84, 1989.

60. Weiner DW, Klein MD. Calcium Antagonist for the Treatment of Angina Pectoris. In Weiner DW, Frishman WH (eds). Therapy of Angina Pectoris. New York: Marcel Dekker, 1986:145.

61. Frohlich ED. Calcium antagonists as cardioprotective agents. Am J Cardiol 70:7I, 1992.

62. Frishman WH. Current status of calcium channel blockers. Curr Probl Cardiol 19:637, 1994.

63. Epstein M. Calcium antagonists should continue to be used for first-line treatment of hypertension. Arch Intern Med 155:2150, 1995.

64. Vatner SF, Hintze TH. Effects of a calcium-channel antagonist on large and small coronary arteries in conscious dogs. Circulation 66:579, 1982.

65. Bache RJ. Effects of calcium entry blockade on myocardial blood flow. Circulation 80:IV40, 1989.

66. Gage JE, Hess OM, Murakami T, Ritter M, Grimm J, Krayenbuehl HP. Vasoconstriction of stenotic coronary arteries during dynamic exercise in patients with classic angina pectoris: Reversibility by nitroglycerin. Circulation 73:865, 1986.

67. Nonogi H, Hess OM, Ritter M, Bortone A, Corin WJ, Grimm J, Krayenbuehl HP. Prevention of coronary vasoconstriction by diltiazem during dynamic exercise in patients with coronary artery disease. J Am Coll Cardiol 12:892, 1988.

68. Kloner RA, Reimer K, Jennings R. Distribution of coronary collateral flow in acute myocardial ischemic injury. Cardiovasc Res 10:81, 1976.

69. Nayler WG, Ferrari R, Williams A. Protective effect of pretreatment with verapamil, nifedipine and propranolol on mitochondrial function in the ischemic and reperfused myocardium. Am J Cardiol 46:242, 1980.

70. The Israeli SPRINT Study Group. Secondary Prevention Reinfarction Israeli Nifedipine Trial (SPRINT). A randomized intervention trial of nifedipine in patients with acute myocardial infarction. Eur Heart J 9:354, 1988.

71. SPRINT Study Group. The Secondary Prevention Reinfarction Israeli Nifedipine Trial (SPRINT) II. Design, methods and results. Eur Heart J 9:350A, 1988.

72. Wilcox RG, Hampton JR, Banks DC. Trial of nifedipine in acute myocardial infarction: The TRENT Study. Br Med J 293:1204, 1986.

73. Held PH, Yusuf S. Effects of -blockers and calcium channel blockers in acute myocardial infarction. Eur Heart J 14(Suppl F):18, 1993.

74. Multicenter Diltiazem Postinfarction Trial Research Group. The effect of diltiazem on mortality and reinfarction after myocardial infarction. N Engl J Med 319:385, 1988.

75. Gibson RS, Boden WE, Theroux P. Diltiazem and reinfarction in patients with non-Q-wave myocardial infarction. N Engl J Med 315:423, 1986.

76. Danish Study Group on Verapamil in Myocardial

Infarction. Verapamil in acute myocardial infarction. Eur Heart J 5:516, 1984.

77. The Danish Study Group on Verapamil in Myocardial Infarction. Effect of verapamil on mortality and major events after acute myocardial infarction. Am J Cardiol 66:779, 1990.

78. Theroux P, Taeymans Y, Morissette D, Bosch X, Pelletier GB, Waters DD. A randomized study comparing propranolol and diltiazem in the treatment of unstable angina. J Am Coll Cardiol 5:717, 1995.

79. Gerstenblith G, Ouyang P, Achuff SC, Bulkley BH, Becker LC, Mellits ED, Baughman KL, Weiss JL, Flaherty JT, Kallman CH, Llewellyn M, Weisfeldt ML. Nifedipine in unstable angina. N Engl J Med 306:885, 1982.

80. Holland Interuniversity Nifedipine/Metoprolol Trial Research Group. Early treatment of unstable angina in the coronary care unit: A randomized, double-blind, placebo controlled comparison of recurrent ischemia in patients treated with nifedipine or metoprolol or both. Br Heart J 56:400, 1986.

81. Bala Subnamanian V, Khurmi NS, Bowles MJ, O'Hara M, Ratery FB. Objective evaluation of three dose levels of diltiazem in patients with chronic stable angina. J Am Coll Cardiol 1:1144, 1983.

82. Ahlquist RP. A study of the adrenotropic receptors. Am J Physiol 153:586, 1948.

83. Hoffman BB. Catecholamines, sympathomimetic druys and adrenergic receptor antagonist. In Hardman JE, Lindbery CF, Mclinitt K, Ruddon RW (eds). The Pharmacological Basis of Therpeutics. New York: McGraw Hill, 1995.

84. Frishman WH. Multifactorial actions of beta-adrenergic blocking drugs in ischemic heart disease: Current concepts. Circulation 67:I-11, 1983.

85. Becker LC, Fortuin NJ, Pitt B. Effect of ischemia and antianginal drugs on the distribution of radioactive microspheres in the canine left ventricle. Circ Res 28:263, 1971.

86. Vatner SF, Baig H, Manders WT, Ochs H. Effects of propranolol on regional myocardial function, electrograms, and blood flow in conscious dogs with myocardial ischemia. J Clin Invest 60:353, 1977.

87. Graham RM. Selective alpha-adrenergic antagonists: Therapeutically relevant antihypertensive agents. Am

J Cardiol 16A, 1984.

88. The International Collaborative Study Group. Reduction of infarct size with the early use of timolol in aorta myocardial infarction. N Engl J Med 310:9, 1984.

89. Singh BN. Advantages of beta-blockers versus anti-arrhythmic agents and calcium antagonists in secondary prevention after myocardial infarction. Am J Cardiol 66:9C, 1990.

90. ISIS-1 Collaborative Group. Randomised trial of intravenous atenolol among 16,027 cases of suspected acute myocardial infarction. Lancet 2:57, 1986.

91. The TIM1 Study Group. Comparison of invasive and conservative strategies after treatment with intravenous tissue plasminogen activator in acute myocardial infarction: Results of the thrombolysis in myocardial infarction. N Engl J Med 6320:618, 1989.

92. The Norwegian Multicenter Study Group. Timolol-induced reduction in mortality and reinfarction in patients surviving acute myocardial infarction. N Engl J Med 304:801, 1981.

93. Beta Blocker Heart Attack Trial Research Group. A randomized trial oif propranolol in patients with acute myocardial infarction: 1. Mortality results. JAMA 247:1701, 1982.

94. Gottlieb SO, Weisfeldt ML, Ouyang P, Achuff SC, Baughman KL, Traill TA, Brinker JA, Shapiro EP, Chandra NC, Mellits ED, Townsend SN, Gerstenblith G. Effect of the addition of propranolol to therapy with nifedipine for unstable angina pectoris: A randomized, double-blind, placebo-controlled trial. Circulation 73:331, 1986.

95. Frishman WH. Beta adrenergic blockade for treatment of angina pectoris. In Weiner DA, Frishman WH (ed). Therapy of Angina Pectoris. Marcel Dekker, New York: 1986:83.

96. Fox KM, Mulcahy D, Purcell H. Unstable and stable angina. Eur Heart J 14:15, 1993.

97. Cohen RA, Shepherd JT, Vanhoutte PM. Effects of the adrenergic transmitter on epicardial coronary arteries. Fed Proc 43:2862, 1984.

98. Tzivoni D, Keren A, Benhorin J. Prazosin therapy for refractory variant angina. Am Heart J 105:262, 1983.

SECTION V: EXPERIMENTAL MODELS OF PLAQUE RUPTURE, THROMBOSIS, AND THROMBOLYSIS

Richard C. Becker

Coronary arteriosclerosis, a common disease process in westernized societies, varies widely in its natural history, rate of development, and clinical expression. Although advanced stages of coronary atherosclerosis can remain silent, the clinical signs and symptoms of disease are, in general, closely correlated with pathologic features of the vessel wall. Acute coronary syndromes, including unstable angina and myocardial infarction, coincide with unique features of the atherosclerotic plaque and are the end result of disruption within thin fibrous caps that overlie a prominent lipid core. This event is followed by platelet deposition and either a partially or totally occlusive thrombus. A clear understanding of the pathobiology underlying coronary atherosclerosis, and the events predisposing to plaque rupture and intraluminal thrombosis, through scientific investigation in vital to both the prevention and treatment of this common disease entity.

11. EXPERIMENTAL MODELS OF CORONARY ARTERIAL RESISTANCE AND BLOOD FLOW

William P. Santamore

Introduction

In this chapter, experimental preparations that have been used to examine facets of coronary artery resistance and its effects on blood flow are reviewed. Before discussing the experimental models, the characteristics of human coronary vessel – the characteristics that we are trying to model in our experimental studies – are reviewed. Also, because most clinical problems involve restriction of blood flow through the large epicardial coronary vessels, the focus is on these large coronary arteries and not on small-vessel disease models. Remember that there are no perfect experimental models; they all have shortcomings. The biggest shortcoming is using models to address questions the models were not designed to answer.

Characteristics of Human Stenoses

Morphologically, most human coronary lesions have some normal wall segments and, thus, may exhibit dynamic characteristics. In a postmortem study, Vlodaver and Edwards observed that 70% of atherosclerotic lesions are eccentric with some normal wall segment [1]. Freudenberg and Lichtlen examined 384 stenotic coronary segments postmortem and observed that 74% of all obstructions showed a normal wall segment [2]. Thus, based on these studies, 70–74% of human coronary lesions are eccentrically shaped with normal wall sections. In another study from Edwards' laboratory, the mean disease-free wall are length measured between 17% and 23% of the total vessel circumference in eccentric coronary artery lesions, but the amount of normal arterial wall is variable (Figure 11-1) [3]. For example, for an 80% stenosis one postmortem case had only a 2% disease-free wall segment,

whereas another case had 38% of the wall disease free. These large variations in the proportion of normal wall present at the stenotic site might help to explain the clinically observed variations in stenotic vasomotion.

Consistent with these morphological observations, many clinical studies have shown vasomotion within an arterial stenosis. Brown et al., who pioneered quantitative coronary angiography, observed exaggerated stenotic vasomotion in response to isometric exercise and to isosorbide dinitrate [4]. Tousoulis et al. infused serotonin directly into the coronary arteries [5]. One hundred percent of complicated stenosis and 50% of concentric stenoses constricted by over 20%. However, the magnitude of constriction was greater at eccentric stenoses than concentric stenoses, and was greater in complicated stenoses than in eccentric stenoses. Gage et al. studied patients with classic angina pectoris who performed symptom-limited supine bicycle exercise during cardiac catheterization [6]. During exercise, the luminal area of the normal coronary segment increased, while, in contrast, stenotic luminal area decreased [6,7].

Nabel et al. studied the response to the cold pressor test using quantitative angiography and Doppler flow velocity measurements [8]. In patients with angiographically normal coronary arteries, the cold pressor test produced vasodilation and increased flow by 65%. In patients with mild coronary artery disease, the cold pressor test dilated normal segments but constricted irregular segments, which resulted in an attenuated flow increase of only 15%. In patients with severe coronary artery disease, the cold pressor test constricted irregular arterial segments and reduced flow by 39%, but still dilated normal arterial segments. Thus, catheterization studies have proven that coronary stenoses can exhibit vasomotion and that different segments of the coronary artery can have opposite responses to the same stimulus.

Vasomotion is an important component in many cases of angina pectoris, as demonstrated by variable thresholds for ischemia, ischemia unrelated to work load, and variant angina [9–13]. In patients with chronic stable angina, Deanfield et al. found that an increase in heart rate was uncommon prior to the onset of myocardial ischemia [9]. Rocco et al. found that the increased frequency of early morning electrocardiogram (ECG) ST depression was not explained by increases in activity, mental stress, or heart rate [12]. Chiechia et al. found that, prior to ischemic episodes, the heart rate, left ventricular pressure, peak dP/dt, aortic mean and systolic pressure, and pressure–rate product were unchanged in patients with rest angina [11]. Benhorin et al. observed a second prominent peak in ischemia between 6 and 9 p.m. [14]. This peak had a low threshold, suggesting that the mechanism of ischemia is probably reduced coronary flow due to increased coronary tone.

Not only can coronary artery stenoses constrict, but they are capable of exaggerated constriction as compared with normal arteries or normal arterial segments. In 18 patients with resting and exertional angina, Reiber et al. observed that mean minimal diameters of 20 stenotic lesions decreased to 1.0 mm after 0.4 mg ergometrine, and then increased to 2.7 mm after 3 mg isosorbide dinitrate [15]. In patients with positive ergonovine tests, Freedman et al. found that the normal arterial segments constricted by 15% (SD), whereas the stenotic segments constricted by 83% [17]. Kaski et al. observed that during spontaneous coronary spasm or ergonovine challenge, the degree of vasoconstriction observed in the spastic segments far exceeded that in the normal arterial segments [16]. During intravenous ergonovine, the luminal diameter of spastic segments was reduced by 92%, while the luminal diameter of nonspastic proximal segments was only reduced by 18%. Thus, exaggerated diameter shortening occurs within many arterial stenoses. Reiber et al., Freedman et al., and Kaski et al. observed diameter reductions of 63–92% within the arterial stenosis, while in the nonstenotic segments, vasoconstriction reduced the diameter by 15–20% [15–17]. In comparison, the maximal vasoconstriction-induced diameter shortening that occurs in nonstenotic coronary arteries, even under conditions that increased the sensitivity of the artery to vasoconstrictors (e.g., endothelial denudation) ranged 20–30% [18]. This value is far less than the observed diameter reductions that can occur within coronary artery stenoses.

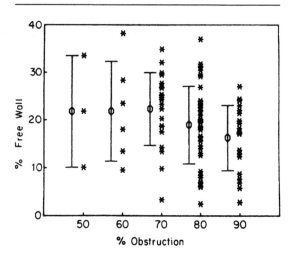

FIGURE 11-1. Ratio of disease-free wall arc length to total vessel circumference compared with the severity of obstruction of the coronary lumen. *Single values. Mean value ± SD in 100 cross sections of eccentric coronary artery atherosclerosis. % free wall = percent of the uninvolved wall of total vessel circumference. (From Saner et al. [3], with permission.)

In summary, the literature shows that most human coronary artery stenoses are capable of vasomotion, cardiac catheterization studies have demonstrated vasomotion, many cases of angina pectoris have a vasomotion component, and exaggerated constriction can occur with a stenosis. The experimental models described here represent an attempt to examine these aspects of coronary arteries, generally in acute experimental preparations.

Theoretical Models

Theoretical analysis can examine wide ranges in values, difficult experimental situations, and pathological conditions. As an author of several theoretical analyses, it is my personal view that theoretical analysis should never be viewed as proof. Rather, theoretical analysis should test possibilities, provide insight, and aid in the design of experimental and clinical studies [19–21].

With these limitations in mind, we modeled the coronary circulation as two resistors in series: proximal resistance offered by the proximal coronary artery stenosis, and flow resistance offered by the coronary circulation distal to the stenosis. Standard hemodynamic equations were used to express the pressure and flow relations across the coronary stenosis. Our unique contribution was that we expressed the cross-sectional area in terms of the vessel circumference [19]. By using this approach, we could incorporate arterial wall characteristics into the stenotic model. As in most human stenoses, the vessel wall within the stenosis was composed of both normal and rigid sections.

This theoretical analysis suggested that intra-luminal pressure changes within the stenosis significantly affected the hemodynamic responses. Decreasing aortic pressure or decreasing distal coronary arterial resistance decreased pressure within the stenosis. In turn, this reduction in stenotic pressure caused a decrease in the luminal area and increased the sensitivity to vasoconstriction [19]. In other words, to increase the hemodynamic resistance and decrease flow through a vessel, the luminal area must be decreased. The ability of a vasoconstrictor to shorten the smooth muscle is inversely related to the afterload — the intraluminal pressure. Interventions that decrease the intraluminal pressure theoretically would increase the effective strength of a vasoconstrictor.

In another study, we wanted to determine how much plaque rupture with subsequent thrombus formation was needed to occlude a coronary artery and how much was needed to cause a myocardial infarction [20]. For a dynamic stenosis, this analysis assumed that plaque rupture would induce proximal coronary artery vasoconstriction and that autoregulation would occur. This model suggested that a stenosis capable of vasomotion needed significantly less thrombus formation for total vessel occlusion as compared with a geometrically fixed stenosis.

In Vitro Models

ARTERIAL RING PREPARATIONS

This relatively simple preparation has been and will continue to be a mainstay of pharmological examination of arteries. A big advantage of this preparation is that tissue can be obtained from many sources. The tissue can be obtained from slaughterhouses, from normal experimental animals, and from experimental animals that have been preconditioned, undergone hypertrophy, high cholesterol diets, etc. Because we are primarily interested in human responses, the arteries can also be obtained from discarded human tissue: umbilical arteries and veins, excess segments of arteries and veins obtained during bypass operations, and from transplant operations. A good friend and

colleague, Dr. Bob Ginsburg, obtained the recipients' heart during heart transplantation and then went to his laboratory in the basement of the Standford Medical Center to study human coronary artery responses [22].

While the exact methods vary, most arterial ring preparations use the following approach. This is depicted in Figure 11-2 for human arterial graft specimens. Attention and care is given to maintaining and not disrupting the integrity of the endothelium. The vessels are immediately placed in an oxygenated physiological salt solution maintained at 4°C and then transferred to the laboratory. The artery segments are then cut into 2–3 mm long ring segments, or helical strips, and mounted on wire hooks passed through the lumen. The tissues are immersed in water-jacketted organ baths containing Krebs solution (34–37°C).

After setting the initial resting tension, drugs are added to the baths in a cumulative fashion, and changes in isometric tension are measured with a force-displacement transducer. Two measurements quantified arterial ring segment reactivity to different vasoactive drugs: maximum developed tension and sensitivity (EC_{50}). This easy preparation and these measurements have provided us with a wealth of information on the vasculature.

The limitations of ring preparations are that they do not simulate or measure hemodynamic responses. Most vascular smooth muscle studies use isolated arterial ring or strip preparations, studied under isometric or isotonic contractions. These studies implicitly assume that the observed responses and contractions will be similar to human arteries. In large conduit arteries, the primary force opposing constriction is systemic pressure. Localized contractions in large arteries do not alter systemic pressure. Thus, this contraction is probably similar to isotonic contractions. In stenotic coronary arteries, however, small changes in cross-sectional area cause large decreases in stenotic distending pressure. This decrease in afterload further increases shortening, with a further decrease in cross-sectional area and (stenotic) pressure [23]. Thus, unlike rings or normal arteries, contraction within an arterial stenosis is neither isometric nor isotonic; nor is the contraction a combination of isometric and isotonic contractions. Rather, the contraction is shortening with decreasing load (heterotonic), a unique contraction present only in stenotic arteries [24,25]. Because of this unique contraction, arterial ring preparations cannot predict responses to very basic interventions, such as vasoconstriction, vasodilation, and endothelial denudation [18].

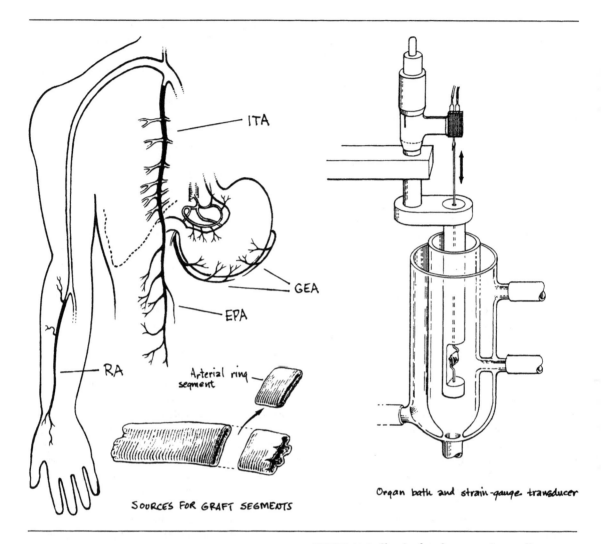

ITA

GEA

EPA

RA

Arterial ring segment

SOURCES FOR GRAFT SEGMENTS

Organ bath and strain-gauge transducer

FIGURE 11-2. Sketch of study to examine small segments of human arteries in an arterial ring preparation. ITA = internal thoracic artery; GEA = gastroepipoic artery; EPA = epigastric artery; RA = radial artery.

PERFUSED ARTERIAL SEGMENTS

For the perfused arterial segments, the arteries are handled similar to the in-vitro arterial ring preparation. The perfusion apparatus consist of a reservoir and an arterial bath, both containing physiological salt solutions. The proximal part of the artery is cannulated and attached to the perfusion system. The arteries are perfused at either a constant flow rate or at a constant perfusion pressure.

The perfused arterial segment preparations have all of the advantages of the isolated arterial ring preparations and most of the same disadvantages. However, the arteries are studied under hemodynamic conditions. Note that for large-conduit arteries, the cross-sectional area must be decreased by over 85% to reduce the lumen sufficiently to cause either a pres-

sure gradient along the length of the vessel or to cause a decrease in flow. Thus, at least for large coronary conduit vessels, vasoconstriction does not reduce the lumen sufficiently to cause either a pressure gradient along the length of the vessel or to cause a decrease in flow.

Figure 11-3 shows the typical effects of norepinephrine on carotid artery hemodynamic in a non-stenotic vessel. In this experiment, the vessel was subjected to endothelial denudation. With maximal vasoconstriction, norepinephrine decreased the diameter and cross sectional area. However, without a

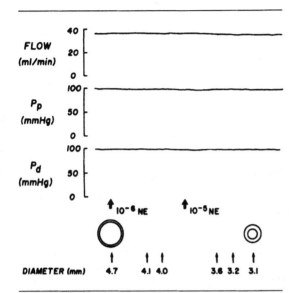

FIGURE 11-3. Hemodynamic effects of increasing concentration of norepinephrine in a nonstenotic, endothelial denuded carotid artery. Proximal pressure and distal pressure are shown. (From Tulenko et al. [24], with permission.)

stenosis, even in a denuded vessel, maximal vasoconstriction had negligible effects on the pressure gradient across or the flow through the vessel, despite the reduction in arterial diameter. In all of my experience, I have never been able, nor do I know of, any other studies in which vasoconstriction within a large-conduit artery has reduced flow through the artery. No vasoconstrictor (thromboxane, endothelin, calcium), concentration, combination of vasoconstriction, and endothelial dysfunction can induce enough smooth muscle shortening to cause a sufficient decrease in luminal area to result in a pressure gradient or flow decrease.

Thus, for the constant-flow experiments, the distal segment remains unattached to the perfusion system. The arterial responses are recorded as changes in the proximal perfusion pressure [26]. While this makes for easy measurement, the physiological relevance of the resulting vascular constriction is questionable. The proximal part of the artery is constricting against an increasing load, while the distal portion is constricting against a decreasing load. For this reason, the author would not recommend this preparation. For the constant perfusion pressure experiments, the arterial response is generally recorded as some change in arterial dimensions. Earlier experiments used strain gauges to assess dimensional changes [27]. More recent studies have used ultrasonic crystals or video detection to directly measure arterial dimensions.

In Vivo Preparations

ACUTE APPROACHES

In the normal coronary circulation, changes in blood flow are usually caused by changes in small-vessel resistance. Thus, measuring coronary blood flow by itself does not provide information about large epicardial coronary-artery responses. To circumvent this problem, the initial studies also measured the pressure in a distal portion of the coronary artery. In a typical protocol, coronary blood flow was measured by an electromagnetic flow probe; pressure transducers were inserted into the arch of the aorta and into a distal apical branch of the left anterior descending coronary artery to measure aortic pressure (coronary perfusion pressure) and peripheral coronary pressure, respectively. Large coronary artery end-diastolic resistance and small coronary end-diastolic resistance were computed from end-diastolic coronary blood flow and the coronary artery pressure gradient [28].

Using this approach, differences in large proximal and smaller distal coronary arteries responding to pharmacologic agents were observed. For instance, at normal perfusion pressure, nitroglycerin injected directly into the coronary artery caused a transient fall in small-vessel resistance and a prolonged decrease in large-vessel resistance. During ischemia, when small vessels autoregulated and small-vessel resistance was minimal, nitroglycerin lowered only large-vessel resistance [29,30].

In later studies, large coronary artery reactivity was directly assessed by measuring arterial diameters with ultrasound crystals (Triton, San Diego, CA). For example, Vatner and colleagues implanted ultrasonic dimensional crystals on the circumflex artery in calves [31–33]. Proximal to the dimensional crystals, a Silastic catheter was implanted in the coronary artery. For pressure measurements, catheters were implanted in the descending aorta and left atrium, and a solid-state pressure transducer was placed in the left ventricle. The experiments were conducted 2–4 weeks after the operation in conscious calves. Using this approach, Vatner and colleagues investigated the regulation of coronary resistance vessels and large coronary arteries [33]. The major advantage of this preparation is the observations on vascular responses can be made in conscious animals. The disadvantages are the difficulty in the experimental preparation and that only normal arteries are studied.

STENOTIC MODELS

External Constrictors. The most commonly used acute model of an arterial stenosis is an external constrictor. Although the exact details vary, the methods are as follows: The left anterior descending or circumflex coronary artery is exposed, and a flow probe is placed on the proximal part of the artery. The circumflex artery tends to be easier to prepare because the proximal artery is embedded in a fat pad with few side branches. The left anterior descending coronary artery has many side branches, the septal branches of which are the most difficult to occluder and sever. Distal to the flow probe, an external occluder is placed on the artery. The occluder can be a balloon type (In Vivo Metric, Healdsburg, CA), a plastic constrictor, or just a snare (suture, wire, or umbilical tape).

Establishing the amount of constriction and doing it reproducibly can be difficult. The relationship between the percent stenosis and flow is very steep [34]. An 85% or greater reduction in cross-sectional luminal area is needed before resting blood flow begins to decrease. Anyone who has tried to use an external constrictor develops an appreciation for this steep relationship between percent stenosis and flow. The artery is constricted more and more, with no effect on flow. Then, a slight further constriction leads to an almost total cessation of flow.

In most experiments, the goal is establish an 85–95% stenosis. Because this is not directly measured, a variety of approaches have been used. The most common approach is to constrict the artery until reactive hyperemia is abolished. Another easy approach is to place a tube with the desired cross-sectional area on the artery, tie the artery and tube, and then remove the tube. Personally, I prefer to measure the pressure distal to the obstruction [35]. As the coronary artery is constricted, the distal coronary vasculature dilates to maintain resting coronary blood flow. The flow is maintained, but this is at the cost of the coronary pressure. Thus, the pressure falls before the coronary blood flow decreases; the pressure measurement is more sensitive than the flow measurement.

Vasoreactivity of External Constrictors. The above-mentioned models show the *consequences* of an arterial stenosis on the distal coronary circulation. In other words, these models tell us how the effects of a vasodilator or vasoconstrict on the *distal coronary circulation* is attenuated by the proximal upstream stenosis. Thus, for example, we can study how the vasodilation effects of dipyridamole are attenuated, as the severity of the proximal upstream stenosis increase.

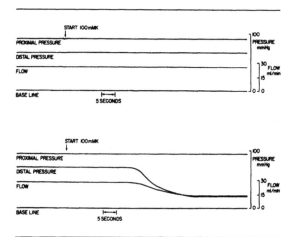

FIGURE 11-4. Typical stenotic hemodynamic response to coronary artery vasoconstriction with an external circumferential snare (top) and with an intraluminal obstructional (bottom). (From Santamore et al. [35], with permission.)

However, this tells us nothing about large-vessel reactivity itself; about how, for example, dipyridamole affects the stenosis. In fact, *all external constrictors* (plastic occluder, snare, or external balloon occluder) *are completely nonresponsive* to proximal coronary artery vasodilation and/or vasoconstriction [36]. Figure 11-4 (top panel) shows the vasoconstriction response when an external snare is used to create a stenosis [35]. In this example, a coronary artery was perfused in vitro. An external constrictor created a pressure gradient across the artery. To induce vasoconstriction, the perfusate was switched from a normal physiological salt solution to a high-potassium salt solution. The artery was totally nonresponsive to vasoconstriction, and neither distal pressure nor flow decreased.

In the author's experience, no vasoconstrictor or combination of vasoconstrictors has resulted in a decrease in distal pressure or flow when an external constrictor is used. Conceivably, the external snare shortens the circumferential vessel fibers to a maximal degree, so that no further shortening is possible by vasoconstriction. This observation may be relevant to the clinical situation in which, although two patients may have a similar degree of stenosis, only one patient exhibits coronary artery spasm. Thus, all external constriction devices are nonresponsive to vasoconstriction. This limitation needs to be kept in mind when using external constrictors. Given the fact that human coronary artery stenoses are capable of vasomotion, this is a very severe limitation of external constrictor stenotic models. Further, most of these models have little, if any, interaction with the blood elements. The noteable exception is the model developed by John Folts.

Folts Model. With this model, the mechanisms of platelet interaction with endothelial and medial damaged stenosed arteries can be reproducibily studied [36,37]. The key elements in the Folts model are vessel injury, a long length of stenosis, and severe stenosis. The artery is compressed with a vascular clamp to produce endothelial and medial injury. Then, an encircling plastic cylinder (4 mm or longer in length) is placed around the outside of the injured artery, producing a "critical stenosis." Acute platelet thrombus formation begins to occur in the stenosed lumen. This causes the coronary flow to decline and reach zero (or near zero) flow. Then, the thrombus is embolized into the distal circulation and flow is restored. This occurs repeatedly, causing cyclic flow reductions. These cyclic flow reductions can be made larger and made to occur more frequently by increasing in vivo platelet activity.

The Folts model is a *very good model to study platelet interactions* and has been used extensively for this purpose. As for the exact relationship of this model to the pathophysiology of angina, the author has a few reservations. The model is totally nonresponsive to vasoconstriction. The platelet plugging occurs only in very severe stenoses (greater than 95% area reduction) with extensive endothelial and vascular damage [38,39]. Thus, it is unclear whether subsequent platelet activation is due to the hemodynamic conditions present in the arterial stenosis or the clotting cascade caused by the arterial damage.

Intraluminal Obstructions. Simialr to human stenoses, we developed a stenotic model that responds to vasoconstriction and pressure changes [36,40,41]. To achieve this, we created an intraluminal stenosis by inserting either a rubber plug (Figure 11-5) or a partially inflated angioplasty balloon catheter into the coronary artery [24,42,43]. Like the external constriction, the intraluminal obstruction decreased flow and caused a pressure gardient across the vessel.

Using the same artery as illustrated in the top panel of Figure 11-4, the bottom panel shows the vasoconstriction response when the artery was partially obstructed by an intraluminal stenosis. The initial stenotic resistance, flow, and distal pressure were almost identical for stenoses created by either an external snare (top panel) or an intraluminal obstruction (bottom panel). Yet the intraluminal obstruction was responsive to vasoconstriction: Switching to the

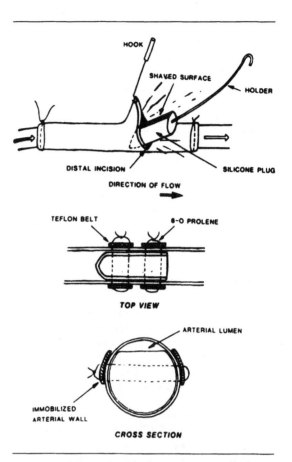

FIGURE 11-5. Insertion of silicone plug into arterial segment top. **Top:** A transverse incision was made in the distal end of artery. The plug was inserted and advanced retrogradely into the vessel. This procedure was done while the artery was perfused under pressure to minimize collapse of the vessel during the insertion procedure. Longitudinal (**middle**) and cross-sectional (**bottom**) views of the stenotic plug sutured in place are shown. (From Tulenko et al. [24], with permission.)

high-potassium solution caused a large decrease in distal pressure and flow.

This is the only animal model in which proximal coronary artery constriction alone (vasoconstriction along the first 3 cm of the coronary artery) has been able to reduce flow through the vessel. This intraluminal stenosis has both qualitative and quantitative responses similar to human arterial stenoses [44]. The major disadvantages of these preparations are that they are more difficult to use than an external constrictor and that the artifical surface makes blood element–flow interactions irrelevant to study.

UNIQUE CONTRACTION WITHIN A STENOSIS

Using this intraluminal stenotic model, we have determined that a unique type of constriction occurs within a stenotic artery, information that would be unobtainable with an arterial ring preparation or with an external constrictor. Figure 11-6 shows the pattern of constriction that we believe occurs within normal and stenotic coronary arteries. Figure 11-6 presents the pressure–diameter relation for a dilated and constricted coronary artery [27]. The force opposing arterial constriction is the intraluminal pressure. In normal (nonstenotic) arteries, this pressure is the systemic arterial pressure, which is relatively constant. Localized contraction does not change systemic pressure, and therefore does not change the afterload for the vascular smooth muscle. Vasoshortening occurs along isopressure lines.

Within a stenosis, the pressure is initially less than systemic pressure, which by itself results in greater shortening for any given amount of agonist [27]. More importantly, local vasoconstriction further decreases this pressure [45]. Thus, in a stenotic artery, as the artery begins to shorten, the stenotic pressure opposing vasoconstriction decreases dramatically (see Figure 11-6). This decrease in stenotic pressure leads to further diameter shortening, with a resulting decrease in cross-sectional area and stenotic pressure — a positive feedback mechanism. Thus, within a stenosis a unique type of constriction occurs. When the artery contracts, it is able to change its own afterload — a phenonemon that does not happen in other large conduit arteries.

Using this model, we observed that in a stenotic artery, the entire response or the vast majority of the response occurs at one incremental dose of the agonist. As increasing doses of vasoconstrictor are administered, one dose is reached at which flow rapidly and abruptly decreased to near or total occlusion (all or none) [25,46]. We measured an increased vasoshortening within the stenoses. This increased shortening occurred when the stenotic arterial distending pressure decreased [23]. We observed that nitroglycerin was much more effective when given before, rather than after, vasoconstriction. After vasospasm, greater concentrations of nitroglycerin were required to reestablish flow compared with the concentration required to prevent spasm [23]. Lastly, with endothelial denudation we observed apparent changes in the sensitivity to vasoconstrictors, even without real changes in sensitivity of the arterial smooth muscle [24]. None of these response patterns occurred in isometrically or isotonically contracted vascular tissue.

Our studies showed the inability of isometric arterial rings, normal conduit arterial contractions, or

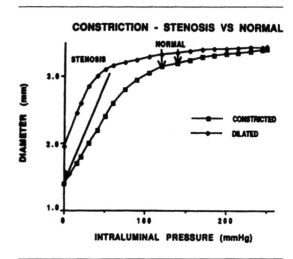

FIGURE 11-6. Graph of the decrease in initial intraluminal pressure due to the effects of atherosclerotic plaque in a stenotic artery. This initial decrease in intraluminal pressure makes constriction more effective. Further, localized vasoconstriction decreases the intraluminal pressure. As the vessel constricts, the pressure decrease leads to further vessel shortening. Thus, the constriction is along a decreasing pressure line. The combination of an initial decrease in intraluminal pressure together with pressure decreases as the vessel constricts causes exaggerated constriction within the stenosis. (From Ghods et al. [25], with permission.)

external snares to predict stenotic arterial responses to basic interventions, such as vasoconstriction, vasodilation, and denudation [46]. As stated at the beginning of this chapter, the limitations of each method must be kept in mind. Using an arterial ring preparation to examine hemodynamic response can be very misleading.

Chronic Models

Other chapters cover the pros and cons of the many atherosclerotic models. Thus, the rabbit and miniature pig models are discussed only briefly here. In the rabbit model, the endothelium is damaged generally by rubbing an inflated balloon catheter against the endothelium in the iliac artery. The rabbit is then placed on a high-cholesterol diet and develops atherosclerotic lesions within 2–3 weeks. While this model has many disadvantages, the technique is relatively simple and reproducible. For the hemodynamic point of view, the lesions that are produced can partially obstruct the arterial lumen and can respond to pressure and vasoconstriction. In this respect, the lesions are similar to human stenoses. A major limitation is the size of the arteries. Even the iliac arteries are significantly smaller than human coronary arteries.

Using this model, we have observed not only quantitatively, but also qualitatively, different responses between arterial rings and whole artery responses [46]. In arterial rings, (1) normal and hypercholesterolemic arterial rings developed more isometric tension and were more sensitive to norepinephrine than stenotic arterial rings, (2) all arterial rings vasodilated in response to nitroglycerin, and (3) changes in isometric tensions occurred over a 1000-fold change in norepinephrine, serotonin, and nitroglycerin concentrations. In perfused normal and hypercholesterolemic arteries, (1) flow was unaltered, even at the highest norepinephrine or serotonin concentration; (2) in stenotic arteries, norepinephrine and serotonin decreased distal pressure and flow; (3) nitroglycerin did not always successfully dilate stenotic arteries and thereby re-establish flow; and (4) in stenotic arteries, most of the hemodynamic response occurred at one incremental dose of vasoconstrictor or vasodilator.

The above-reported results demonstrate that the choice of experimental models can influence conclusions. If one just examined arterial rings, the conclusions would be very different than perfused artery results. Selection of the experimental model influences the conclusions. Limitations need to be considered when selecting an experimental model and when making conclusions.

MINIATURE PIG MODEL

From the hemodynamic point of view, the best animal model, in the author's opinion, is the miniature pig, as developed by Nakamura and coworkers [47]. In their model, Göttingen miniature pigs were subjected to cholesterol feeding, balloon-induced coronary arterial denudation, and x-ray irradiation. Five months later, coronary spasm was induced. Nakamura and colleagues have used this model to examine the mechanisms for coronary artery spasm, agents that induce spasm, endothelial function, and how the mode of onset and the duration of coronary spasm influence the progression of organic coronary stenosis and acute myocardial infarction [48–51].

The fact that the coronary arterial lesions are similar in size to human arteries is an important strength of this model. Further, with this model large coronary artery vasoreactivity, interactions between the stenosis and blood elements, and interactions between vasoreactivity and blood elements are all possible.

The major problems with this model are that it is difficult to create and expensive.

Human Model

In a chapter devoted to experimental models, it might seem strange to mention the human model. But, given the cost and time needed to develop a quality large-animal research laboratory, the support system already in place in human cardiac catheterization laboratories, and recent technological advancements, more direct observations on humans are to be expected. The major limitation in human studies is that interventions that are potentially dangerous cannot be performed. Sometimes examining things that are detrimental can provide insight into the disease and potential treatment. Lastly, keep in mind that to fully characterize large-vessel hemodynamics three variables are needed: flow through the vessel, the pressure drop across the vessel, and the luminal area.

As mentioned earlier, Greg Brown pioneered quantitative coronary angiography. Thus, dimensional measurements have been available for many years, and recent advances may make this analysis possible in semi-real time [52]. Another technique to measure coronary dimensions is intravascular ultrasound, which has been used to study epicardial coronary vasomotor tone in cardiac transplant recipients and to assess coronary vasomotion and endothelial function in patients with mild atherosclerosis [53,54]. For coronary imaging, a 4.3F ultrasound catheter is positioned within a coronary artery segment, with imaging provided by a 30-MHz transducer. Ultrasound allows continuous determinations of vessel size and morphological characteristics. Given the size of the catheter, however, the ultrasound approach cannot be used to assess vasomotion in severely, or even mildly, stenosed arteries. In other words, given that a 85–90% reduction in luminal area is needed before resting blood flow is affected, a 4.3F ultrasound catheter will reduce flow through a minimally stenotic vessel and may even occlude the vessel.

Advancements in Doppler flow velocity systems make the measurement of coronary blood flow possible in most cardiac catheterization patients. The Doppler flow system consist of a 0.014- to 0.018-in. diameter flexible, steerable guide wire with a 12-MHz piezoelectric ultrasound transducer integrated into the tip [55]. Investigators have used the Doppler flow velocity system to make clinical descisions, such as whether to defer angioplasty in patients with angiographically intermediate lesions [56].

The last vital measurement is pressure. Several studies have measured translesional pressure gradients [56–58]. After recording the translesional flow velocity data, a 2.2F infusion catheter (Ttracker 18, Target Therapeutics) was advanced over a guide wire beyond the stenosis into the distal portion of the coronary artery. The guide wire was removed, and phasic and mean pressures in the distal arterial segment were recorded using fluid-filled tubing and standard transducers.

In some very impressive studies, Morton Kern and colleagues have combined dimensional data with flow and pressure measurements. While these investigators and their efforts to measure translesional pressure should be commended, the limitations must be kept in mind. To measure distal coronary artery pressure, the catheter must be placed through the stenotic segment, that is, the catheter partially occludes the artery. Even a very small 1-mm diameter catheter obstructs over 10% of a normal coronary artery lumen. Given that a 75–80% reduction in luminal area is needed before a pressure gradient develops across a stenosis, the pressure catheter will further obstruct the lumen and thereby affect the resulting pressure measurement. This artifact is hard to remove because the translesional pressure gradient is not constant but is related to the square of the flow rate. This problem is compounded by the inability to simultaneously measure pressure and flow. These two factors can lead to very erroneous measurements. Until advancements in pressure measuring techniques are made, this author would highly recommend not making this measurement. A pressure measuring catheter needs to be 0.5 mm in diameter or less, the size of the Doppler flow wire.

References

1. Vlodaver Z, Edwards JE. Pathology of cornary atherosclerosis. Prog Cardiovasc Dis 14:256, 1971.
2. Freudenberg H, Lichtlen PR. Z. The normal wall segment in coronary stenosis. A postmortem study. Cardiology 70:863, 1981.
3. Saner HE, Gobel FL, Salomonowitz E, Erlien DA, Edwards JE. The disease-free wall in coronary atherosclerosis: Its relation to degree of obstruction. J Am Coll Cardiol 6:1096, 1985.
4. Brown BG, Josephson MA, Petersen RB, Pierce CD, Wong M, Hecht HS, Bolson E, Dodge HT. Intravenous dipyridamole combined with isometric handgrip for near maximal acute increase in coronary flow in patients with coronary artery disease. Am J Cardiol 48:1077, 1982.
5. Tousoulis D, Davies G, McFadden E, Clarke J, Kaski JC, Maseri A. Coronary vasomotor effects of serotonin in patients with angina. Circulation 88:1518, 1993.
6. Gage JE, Hess OE, Murakami T, Ritter M, Grimm J, Krayenbuehl HP. Vasoconstriction of stenotic coronary arteries during dynamic exercise in patients with clasic anginapectoris: Reversibility by nitroglycerin. Circulation 73:865, 1986.
7. Suter TM, Buechi M, Hess OM, Haemmerli-Saner C, Gaglione A, Krayenbuehl HP. Normalization of coronary vasomotion after percutaneous transluminal coronary angioplasty? Circulation 85:86, 1992.
8. Nabel EG, Ganz P, Gordon JB, Alexander RW, Selwyn AP. Dilation of normal and constriction of atherosclerotic coronary arteries caused by the cold pressor test. Circulation 77:43, 1988.
9. Deanfield JE, Maseri A, Selwin AP, Ribeiro P, Chierchia S, Krikler S, Morgan M. Myocardial ischemia during daily life in patients with stable angina: Its relation to symptoms and heart rate changes. Lancet 2:753, 1983.
10. Banai S, Moriel M, Benhorin J, Gavish A, Stern S, Tzivoni D. Changes in myocardial ischemic threshold during daily activities. Am J Cardiol 66:1403, 1990.
11. Chiechia S, Brunelli C, Simonetti I, Lazzari M, Maseri A. Sequence of events in angina at rest: Primary reduction in coronary flow. Circulation 61:759, 1980.
12. Rocco MB, Barry J, Campbell S, Naber E, Cook EF, Goldman L, Selwyn AP. Circadian variation of transient myocardial ischemia in patients with coronary artery disease. Circulation 75:395, 1987.
13. Kishida H, Fukuma N, Saito T. Circadian variation of ischemic threshold in patients with chronic sable angina. Int J Cardiol 35:65, 1992.
14. Benhorin J, Banai S, Moriel M, Gavish A, Keren A, Stern S, Tzivoni D. Circadian variations in ischemic threshold and their relation to the occurrence of ischemic episodes. Circulation 87:808, 1993.
15. Reiber JHC, Serruys PW, Slager CJ. The role of vascular wall thickening during changes in coronary artery tone. In Reiber JHC, Serruys PW, Slager CJ (eds). Quantitative Coronary and Left Ventricular Cineangiography. Martinus Nijhoff, 1986:373.
16. Kaski JC, Maseri A, Vejar M, Crea F, Hackett D. Spontaneous coronary artery spasm in variant angina is caused by a local hyperreactivity to a generalized constrictor stimulus. J Am Coll Cardiol 14:1456, 1989.
17. Freedman B, Richmond DR, Kelly DT. Pathophysiology of coronary artery spasm. Circulation 66:705, 1982.
18. Santamore WP, Tulenko TN, Bove AA. The importance of endothelial function on stenotic hemodynamic responses. Cardiovasc Res 25:988, 1991.
19. Santamore WP, Bove AA. A theoretical model of a compliant arterial stenosis. Am J Physiol 248:H274, 1985.
20. Santamore WP, Yelton B, Ogilby D. Dynamics of coronary occlusion in the pathogenesis of myocardial infarction J Am Coll Cardiol 18:1397, 1991.
21. Barnea O, Santamore WP. Coronary autoregulation

and optimal myocardial oxygen utilization. Basic Res Cardiol 87:290, 1992.

22. Ginsburg R, Bristow MR, Davis K, Dibiase A, Billingham ME. Quantitative pharmacologic responses of normal and atherosclerotic isolated human epicardial coronary arteries. Circulation 69:30, 1984.

23. Li K, Santamore WP, Morley DL, Tulenko TN. Stenosis as an amplifier of stenotic hemodynamic response. Am J Physiol 256:H1044, 1989.

24. Tulenko TN, Constantinescu D, Kikuchi T, Santamore WP, Cox RH. Mutual interaction of vasoconstriction and endothelial damage in stenotic arteries. Am J Physiol Heart Circ 256:H881, 1989.

25. Ghods M, Mangal R, Iskandrian A, Santamore WP. Importance of intraluminal pressure on hemodynamic and vasoconstriction responses of stenotic arteries. Circulation 85:708, 1992.

26. Ogletree ML, Smith JB, Lefer AM. Actions of prostaglandins on isolated perfused cat coronary arteries. Am J Physiol 235:400, 1978.

27. Cox RH. Mechanical aspects of larger coronary arteries. In Santamore WP, Bova AA (eds). Coronary Artery Disease: Etiology, Hemodynamic Consequences, Drug Therapy and Clinical Implications, Baltimore: Urban & Schwarzenberg, 1982:19.

28. Malindzak GS Jr, Kosinski EJ, Green HD, Yarborough GW. The effects of adrenergic stimulation on conductive and resistive segments of the coronary vascular bed. J Pharmacol Exp Ther 206:248, 1978.

29. Cohen MV, Kirk ES. Differential response of large and small coronary arteries to nitroglycerin and angiotensin. Autoregulation and tachyphylaxis. Circ Res 33:445, 1973.

30. Winbury MM, Howe BB, Hefner MA. Effects of nitrates and other coronary dilators on large and small coronary vessels. Hypothesis for the mechanism of action of nitrates. J Pharmacol Exp Ther 168:70, 1969.

31. Vatner SE. Regulation of coronary resistance vessels and large coronary arteries. Am J Cardiol 56:16E, 1985.

32. Vatner SE, Pasipoularides A, Mirsky I. Measurement of arterial pressure dimension relationships in conscious animals. Ann Biomed Eng 12:521, 1984.

33. Young MA, Vatner DE, Knight DR, Graham RM, Homcy CJ, Vatner SE. α-Adrenergic vasoconstriction and receptor subtypes in large coronary arteries of calves. Am J Physiol 255:H1452, 1988.

34. May AG, Van der Berg L, DeWeese JA, Rob CC. Critical arterial stenosis. Surgery 54:250, 1963.

35. Santamore WP, Walinsky P, Bove AA, Cox RH, Carey RA, Spann JF. The effects of vasoconstriction on experimental coronary artery stenosis. Am Heart J 100:852, 1980.

36. Folts JD, Crowell ED, Row GG. Platelet aggregation in partially obstructed vessels and its elimination with aspirin. Circulation 54:365, 1976.

37. Folts J. An in vivo model of experimental arterial stenosis, intimal damage, and periodic thrombosis. Circulation 83(Suppl. IV):IV3, 1991.

38. Gallagher KP, Folts JD, Rowe CG. Comparison of coronary arteriograms with direct measurements of stenosed coronary arteries in dogs. Am Heart J 95:338, 1978.

39. April P, Schmitz JM, Campbell WW, Tilton G, Ashton J, Raheja S, Buja M, Willerson JT. Cyclic blood flow variations induced by platelet-activating factor in stenosed canine coronary arteries despite inhibition of thromboxane synthetase, serotonin receptors, and ALPHA-adrenergic receptors. Circulation 72:397, 1985.

40. Santamore WP, Bove AA, Carey R, Walinsky P, Spann JF. Synergist relation between vasoconstriction and fixed epicardial vessel stenosis in coronary artery disease. Am Heart J 101:428, 1981.

41. Santamore WP, Bove AA, Carey RA. Tachycardia induced reduction in coronary blood flow distal to stenosis. Int J Cardiol 2:23, 1982.

42. Bove AA, Santamore WP, Carey RA. Reduced myocardial blood flow resulting from dynamic changes in coronary artery stenosis. Int J Cardiol 4:301, 1983.

43. Santamore WP, Kent RL, Carey RA, Bove AA. Synergistic effects of pressure, distal resistance and vasoconstriction on stenosis. Am J Physiol 243:H236, 1982.

44. Higgins DR, Santamore WP, Bove AA, Nemir J Jr. Mechanisms for dynamic changes in stenotic severity. Am J Physiol 249:H293, 1985.

45. Higgins DR, Santamore WP, Walinsky P, Nemir J Jr. Hemodynamic of human arterial stenosis. Int J Cardiol 8:177, 1985.

46. Santamore WP, Li KS. Disassociation of intrinsic and haemodynamic responses in stenotic ateries. Cardiovasc Res 27:2058, 1992.

47. Kuga T, Tagawa H, Tomike H, Mitsuoka W, Egashira S, Ohara YI, Takeshita A, Nakamura M. Role of coronary artery spasm in progression of organic coronary stenosis and acute myocardial infection in a swine model. Importance of mode of onset and duration of coronary artery spasm. Circulation 87:573, 1993.

48. Shimokawa H, Tomike H, Nabeyama S, Yamato H, Nakamura M. Histamine induced spasm not significantly modulated by prostanoids in a swine model of coronary artery spasm. J Am Coll Cardiol 6:321, 1985.

49. Shimokawa H, Tomike H, Nabeyama S, Yamamoto H, Ishii Y, Tanaka K, Nakamura M. Coronary artery spasm induced in minature swine: Angiographic evidence and relation to coronary atherosclerosis. Am Heart J 110:300, 1985.

50. Yamamoto Y, Tomike H, Egashira K, Nakamur M. Attenuation of endothelium related relaxation and enhanced responsiveness of vascular smooth muscle to histamine in spastic coronary arterial segments from minature pigs. Circ Res 61:772, 1987.

51. Yamamoto Y, Tomike H, Egashira K, Dobayashi T, Kawasaki T, Nakamura M. Pathogenesis of coronary artery spasm in miniature swine with regional intimal thickening after balloon denudation. Circ Res 60:113, 1987.

52. Gronenschild E, Janssen J, Tijdens F. CSSA II: A second generation system for off-line and on-line quantitative coronary angiography. Cathet Cardiovasc Diagn 33:61, 1994.

53. Pinto FJ, St Goar F, Fischell TA, Stadius ML, Valantine HA, Alderman EL, Popp RL. Nitroglycerin-induced coronary vasoldilation in cardiac transplant recipients. Evaluation with in vivo intracoronary ultrasound. Circulation 85:69, 1992.

54. Dupouy P, Geschwind HJ, Pelle G, Gallot D, Dubois-Randé. Assessment of coronary vasomotion by intracoronary ultrasound. Am Heart J 126:76, 1993.

55. Doucette JW, Corl PD, Payne HM, Flynn AE, Goto M, Nassi M, Segal J. Validation of a Doppler guidewire for intravascular measurements of coronary artery flow velocity. Circulation 85:1899, 1992.

56. Kern MJ, Donohue TJ, Aguirre FV, Bach RG, Caracciolo EA, Wolford T, Mechem CJ, Flynn MS, Chaitman B. Clinical outcome of deferring angioplasty in patients with normal translesional pressure-flow velocity measurements. J Am Coll Cardiol 25:178, 1995.

57. Kern MJ, Aguirre FV, Bach RG, Caracciolo EA, Donohue TJ. Translesional pressure-flow velocity assessment in patients: Part I. Cathet Cardiovasc Diagn 31:49, 1994.

58. Tron C, Kern MJ, Donohue TJ, Back RG, Aguirre FV, Caracciolo EA, Moore JA. Comparison of quantitative angiographically derived and measured translesion pressure and flow velocity in coronary artery disease. Am J Cardiol 75:111, 1995.

12. PATHOGENESIS OF THE ACUTE CORONARY SYNDROMES: HYPOTHESES GENERATED FROM CLINICAL EXPERIENCE

Narinder P. Bhalla and John A. Ambrose

Introduction

The acute coronary syndromes include unstable angina, myocardial infarction (both non–Q-wave and Q-wave), and sudden ischemic death. Common to all these syndromes, in a majority of cases, is the event of plaque disruption. Thrombus generated as a result of plaque disruption is clinically manifested as one of the acute coronary syndromes. Hence, there is considerable overlap amongst the syndromes, and the distinction may simply be the amount of thrombus generated and the presence of collateral circulation. Though many theories have been advanced to elucidate the events leading to plaque rupture, the temporal determinants of the final event remain a mystery. In this chapter we discuss the various hypotheses regarding the events of plaque rupture, the clinical data regarding the acute coronary syndromes, and how these relate to our current understanding of the pathogenesis of the acute coronary syndromes.

Although the event of plaque rupture is sudden in nature, the platform on which it occurs, the atherosclerotic plaque, has been present for a long time. In the United States atherosclerotic lesions have been found in 90% of people who are over 30 years of age [1]. Hence, prior to discussing plaque rupture it is important to briefly discuss the process of atherosclerosis.

Formation of the Atherosclerotic Plaque

The process of atherosclerosis involves an interaction amongst the cellular blood elements and the injured vascular wall. Resulting from these interactions are various pathologic phenomena, such as inflammation, proliferation, necrosis, and calcification/ossification. Thrombus formation may be important in the early stages of the atherosclerotic process, but a flow-limiting thrombus usually occurs only with mature atherosclerosis [2]. The early stages of atherosclerosis occur over a prolonged period of time, during which the patient is without symptoms related to these processes [3]. Indeed, slow progression of coronary disease can result in symptoms, late in its course, once the luminal diameter becomes flow limiting. In these cases the initial symptoms tend to be related to exertion, when there is an imbalance between myocardial blood supply and demand.

The earliest visible lesion of atherosclerosis is the fatty streak. On gross examination, this appears as an area of yellowish discoloration. Microscopically, this relates to the presence of foam cells, which are lipid-laden macrophages/monocytes or smooth muscle cells. The lipid within these cells is mostly in the form of cholesterol and cholesteryl ester (primarily oxidized LDL). Fatty streaks are found at points of turbulence and disturbed flow patterns in the coronary arteries, particularly at bifurcations. Fatty streaks are apparent on walls opposite flow dividers in the coronary tree, and also at bifurcations of the carotid and brachiocephalic circulations [4–6]. These are the regions that are subjected to significant hydrodynamic stresses. Taken together, these stresses constitute the rheology of the flowing blood.

The further progression of the coronary atherosclerotic plaque is variable and is dependent on the coronary risk factors. The fatty streaks may progress to the more advanced lesions of atherosclerosis, known variably as fibrous plaques, atheromas, fibroatheromas,

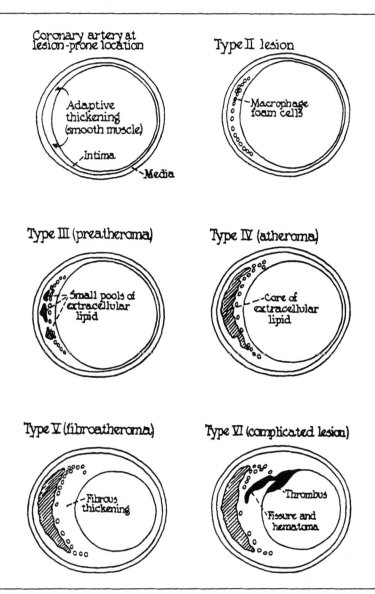

FIGURE 12-1. Schematic showing cross sections from an identical area in the proximal left anterior descending artery (LAD). The morphology of the intima ranges from adaptive intimal thickening to a type VI lesion in advanced atherosclerosis. (Used with permission of the American Heart Association; from Stary et al. [11].)

and/or complicated lesions [7]. The progression is accelerated in individuals with coronary risk factors, such as tobacco use, hypertension, hyperlipidemia, and a family history of early atherosclerosis [4]. Recently, a scheme to type the advanced lesions of atherosclerosis has been proposed, based on the histology of the plaque [8]. The lesions are considered advanced when the accumulation of lipids and cellular components leads to structural disorganization, intimal thickening, and distortion of the arterial wall. These lesions may not necessarily result in a critical narrowing. The clinical importance of these

lesions relates to the fact that while these lesions can be clinically silent, complications can develop suddenly. The initial, fatty streak, and intermediate lesions have been typed as I, II, and III, and the advanced lesions are classified as types IV, V, and VI [9] (Figure 12-1).

TYPE IV LESION

In these lesions there is a significant accumulation of extracellular lipid, which occupies an extensive, but well-defined region of the intima. This lipid accumulation is termed the *lipid core*. Fibrosis is not a prominent characteristic, and surface disruption with thrombosis is not present. The type IV lesion is also known as an *atheroma*. Even though the lipid core thickens the artery wall, the atheroma usually does not cause significant luminal narrowing because there is a compensatory increase in the external boundary of the arterial wall [10]. The region between the lipid core and the intimal surface is mostly composed of proteoglycans, and macrophage foam cells. Because there are few fibromuscular elements in this region, it is susceptible to the formation of fissures and conversion of the lesion to a more advanced form. Furthermore, the periphery of the type IV lesion is vulnerable to rupture because there is a great concentration of macrophages in this area.

TYPE V LESION

These lesions are characterized by an increase in fibrous tissue. When this increase in fibrous tissue is combined with a lipid core, the lesion is called a *fibroatheroma*. The fibroatheroma contains the activated smooth muscle cells that have adopted the proliferative phenotype [5]. This is the characteristic lesion of atherosclerosis. These cells are also capable of ingesting cholesterol and becoming foam cells, hence serving to continue the atherosclerotic process. A fibrous cap covers the fibroatheroma and is composed of smooth muscle cells and connective tissue. The type V lesion can be further classified depending on the amount of lipid and calcification [8]. These lesions result in a greater degree of luminal narrowing, and this is in part due to the size of lipid core and in part due to the amount of reparative connective tissue that forms in response to the obliteration of the normal architecture. These lesions may also develop fissures, hematoma, and/or thrombus. They may be clinically significant, even without these secondary features.

TYPE VI

When type IV and V lesions become ulcerated and disrupted, and develop a hematoma or hemorrhage, they are termed *type VI* or *complicated lesions*. The type VI lesions are further subdivided based on the superimposed features. Needless to say, these lesions are the final common pathway for the pathogenesis of the acute coronary syndromes.

Unstable Plaque

Unstable plaque is a term describing the vulnerable plaques that are susceptible to the process of plaque disruption. These unstable, "vulnerable" plaques often possess four characteristics: a large lipid core, a decrease in fibrous cap thickness, increased inflammatory cell content, and mild to moderate stenosis. Vulnerable plaques rupture when exposed to different stresses. These stresses are related to plaque size or configuration.

Early theories regarding intraluminal thrombus formation hypothesized damage to the vasa vasorum as the cause of plaque rupture. Intraplaque hemorrhage leading to thrombus formation was felt to be the major event. More recent data have indicated that this is an uncommon cause of intraluminal thrombus formation. In most situations the inciting event is the disruption of the fibrous cap [11]. Exposure of the underlying elements to the flowing blood is a potent thrombogenic stimulus. The collagen fibers contained in the fibrous cap, when exposed to blood, stimulate platelet aggregation [12]. The soft material in the plaque, the lipid-rich *gruel*, when exposed to the blood elements is also extremely thrombogenic [2]. An acute increase in shear forces, which can occur during plaque disruption, further magnifies the extent of platelet aggregation [13]. Mechanisms of platelet activation, triggered by the above-mentioned chain of events, include adenosine diphosphate, thromboxane, and thrombin/collagen pathways, leading to exposure of the glycoprotein IIb/IIIa receptor [14]. Activation of the coagulation system results in thrombin formation, and the red cells and fibrin attach to the mass of platelets. Typically, the arterial thrombi consist mostly of platelets at the proximal end, and fibrin and red cells at the distal end. Occlusion of the lumen is related to the fibrin tail of the thrombus.

MILDLY TO MODERATELY STENOTIC PLAQUE

As mentioned earlier, although the events of plaque disruption are well understood, the temporal triggers that result in the event are not well described. Plaque rupture is not a random event in that not every plaque has the same risk of rupture. Retrospective studies by Ambrose et al. and Little et al. have shown that lesions that gave rise to new myocardial infarctions were noted to be only mildly or moderately stenosed on previous angiograms [15,16]. These data were later confirmed in other studies by Giroud et al. and Noboyushi et al. Giroud et al. appropriately pointed out, though, that this may simply have been due to the fact that in their study moderate stenoses outnumbered the more severe stenoses by a factor of 14.

Hence, the relative risk of a severe stenosis leading to acute occlusion or myocardial infarction was five times that of any other segment in their study [17,18].

Prospective data from the CASS study analyzed 2938 coronary artery segments (n = 298 patients), none of which were bypassed during the study. Repeat angiography was performed 5 years after entrance into the study, and factors associated with disease progression were evaluated. Only 89 segments (3%) had an 81–95% stenosis at baseline. Twenty-four percent (n = 21 segments) of these became occluded during the 5-year follow-up, as opposed to 13% (n = 370 segments) of the segments that had a less than 80% stenosis at baseline. In this study the less severely diseased segments outnumbered the severely diseased segments by a factor of 32, and thereby gave rise to a greater number of occlusions [19]. Hence, whether moderate lesions possess characteristics that make them inherently more likely to rupture remains debatable.

It is clear that the more stenosed a vessel, the more likely it is to go onto total occlusion in the future. These events, however, tend to be clinically silent due to the presence of collateral circulation. Conversely, it is the absence of collaterals that makes a total occlusion resulting from a previously moderate stenosis a clinically significant event, that is, a myocardial infarction. Furthermore, angiography seems to be a poor predictor of the site of future plaque rupture, because many total occlusions arise from vessels that on prior angiography had no apparent stenotic lesion. In assessing the significance of these angiographic data, one must realize that angiography underestimates the degree of atherosclerosis compared with pathology and intravascular ultrasound. The fact that a plaque is not significantly stenotic does not mean that it is not a large plaque. However, one has to consider plaque composition rather than plaque size, as determined by angiography, to explain further the propensity of certain plaques to rupture. There are certain features of a plaque that have been found to be associated with increased incidence of rupture.

LIPID CORE
The degree of lipid present in a coronary plaque is extremely variable. Stenotic plaques contain a larger amount of fibrous tissue than soft gruel; however, pathologic studies have shown that culprit lesions in acute coronary syndromes have a greater percentage of lipid within the atheromatous core than non-culprit lesions [20]. Postmortem examination on patients with coronary disease revealed much larger

atheromatous cores in coronary segments with plaque disruption than in those with an intact surface [21]. Davies et al. studied aortic plaques and identified a critical threshold; a plaque with an atheromatous core occupying greater than 40% of the plaque area at its midpoint was much more susceptible to rupture [22]. In ulcerated (disrupted) plaques, the size of the lipid pool exceeded 40% in 91% of cases compared with 11% of intact plaques.

The lipid core consists of extracellular lipids, particularly cholesterol and cholesteryl esters [23,24]. It appears to develop from the confluence of small isolated pools of extracellular lipids that are found in the early lesions of atherosclerosis [11]. The increase in the amount of lipid probably occurs due to a continuous movement of lipid from the plasma into the atheromatous core.

Plaque lipid content is an important determinant of plaque rupture. This is supported by two sources of data. Animal studies have shown a decrease in the plaque lipid content, in addition to other chemical changes, while being maintained on hypolipidemic therapy [25,26]. Decreasing serum lipids, either by hypolipidemic therapy or by other mechanisms, in humans has been shown to decrease the number of acute coronary events [27–31]. Brown et al. performed angiographic follow-up as a part of a lipid regression trial and showed that, even though there was a significant decrease in clinical events, there was only a small change in the angiographic stenosis. Once again, the emphasizes that plaque composition, rather than size, may be a determinant of plaque rupture [32]. It has been hypothesized that with lipid-lowering therapy the liquid cholesterol content of the plaque decreases, hence raising the relative concentration of crystalline cholesterol. The increase in the crystalline cholesterol concentration increases the stiffness of the lipid pool, allowing for better plaque stabilization, and makes the plaque less likely to rupture [24].

FIBROUS CAP
The content and thickness of the fibrous cap is a feature to consider when discussing plaque disruption.

Fibrous Cap and Inflammatory Cell Content. Collagen fibers provide tensile strength to the cap and are an important component of stable plaques. Ruptured aortic plaques, however, have been found to have significantly fewer collagen fibers, and hence smooth muscle cells [22,33]. The reasons for this lack of smooth muscle cells, however, have not been adequately explained. T lymphocytes, which are also found in abundance at sites of plaque disruption, may contribute to the absence of the collagen fibers, through the elaboration of gamma interferon, a cytokine that has been shown to markedly decrease the ability of human smooth muscle cells to express the interstitial collagen genes in both the quiescent and the activated states [34,35].

As discussed earlier, foam cells are an important constituent of any atherosclerotic plaque. The thinnest area of the plaque is usually at the interface of the fibrous cap with the normal arterial wall, which is often the site of disruption. This is also the area of greatest macrophage infiltration [36]. The macrophages at this site are activated, suggesting ongoing inflammation [37]. Multiple studies have reviewed the histopathology of ruptured plaques layered with thrombus (postmortem data) and plaques from patients with acute coronary syndromes (atherectomy samples). A majority of these plaques rupture at these so-called shoulder sites, where the cap meets the normal wall, and show a significant infiltration of foam cells [2,36–38].

Macrophages may play a role in plaque rupture through expression and secretion of metalloproteinases. One of the metalloproteinases is a collagenase and may be involved in plaque destabilization. Recent studies have shown the presence of metalloproteinases in human coronary plaques, and increased monocyte tissue factor expression has been demonstrated in coronary artery disease [39–44]. Furthermore, mast cells have also been identified at the shoulder regions, and the greatest numbers are found in the advanced atheroma [45]. In vitro, the tryptase produced by the mast cells has been shown to activate prostromelysin, a metalloproteinase produced by macrophages in atherosclerotic plaques [41,46]. When activated, prostromelysin can degrade the extracellular matrix [47]. Moreover, activated stromelysin can also activate procollagenase, a precursor of collagenase [48]. Chymase, another proteolytic enzyme produced by mast cells in some atheromas, can further cleave and activate procollagenase [49]. Hence, both tryptase and chymase produced by the mast cells may initiate a set of events that leads to degradation of the extracellular matrix, thereby destabilizing the shoulder region. Tissue factor expressed by macrophages may initiate thrombus formation, through the formation of a complex with factor VII, which activates factor X or factor IX, intrinsic and extrinsic coagulation pathways, leading to thrombin generation and fibrin formation.

Cap Thickness and Plaque Stress. The thickness and stiffness of the cap are key determinants of the amount and distribution of the stress experienced by the plaque. Wall tension in the blood vessel is related to the radius and the luminal pressure, as stated in Laplace's law. Circumferential wall stress is equal to the product of the radius and the pressure divided by the cap thickness. For an equal outer vessel diameter, plaques with mild to moderate stenoses will experience a greater overall wall tension, because of a larger inner lumen, when compared with more severely stenosed vessels under similar conditions of blood pressure and cap thickness [2]. The plaque components are responsible for bearing the imposed stresses, a property that is influenced by cap thickness and plaque contents. The stresses are redistributed to other areas if the components within the wall (the lipid core) are unable to bear the load. These adjacent areas include the shoulder regions, where the plaque meets the normal wall [36]. Hence, the stiffness of the gruel, within the plaque wall, is an important determinant of the response to the imposed stress. The stiffer the lipid core, the more stress it is able to bear, and the less is redistributed to the shoulder regions [26].

Computer-simulated models of plaques have shown that the areas of peak stress are usually concentrated in the shoulder regions when significant amount of soft lipid is present in the plaque. These findings have correlated well with pathological studies, which then identified the site of plaque rupture [36]. Cheng et al., using an elegant computer model, demonstrated that a significant number of plaques (58%) indeed rupture at points of peak circumferential stress [50]. The thickness of the cap is then also important in determining the circumferential tension. The thicker the cap, the less the peak circumferential stress [51]. The stiffness of the plaque lipid pools (gruel) is determined in part by the amount of cholesterol monohydrate crystals. As mentioned earlier, the amount of cholesterol monohydrate crystals increase relatively during the early phase of regression, making the plaque stiffer; this ability to bear stress makes the plaque more stable [26].

However, plaques may rupture at sites other than those predicted by the computed models. This may occur because of the presence of inflammatory cells within the unstable plaque [36,50]. Inflammatory responses within the unstable plaque may serve to weaken certain areas of the cap, making it more susceptible to rupture. It has also been suggested that plaque disruption may also be related to the cyclic stretching, compression, bending, flexion, shear, and pressure fluctuations that occur in the coronary artery [52]. This type of load, when applied repeatedly, may serve to weaken the plaque and may ultimately lead to sudden fracture of the plaque due to cap fatigue, a situation similar to the repetitive bending of a paper clip that weakens it until it suddenly breaks. If fatigue does play a role in plaque disruption, then reducing the frequency (by reducing the heart rate) and magnitude (flow and pressure related) of loading should result in less plaque disruption [53].

OTHER PATHOGENETIC MECHANISMS IN UNSTABLE ANGINA

Inflammation. Though most cases of unstable angina appear to result from plaque rupture and subsequent thrombosis, recent evidence suggests an additional role for inflammatory cell reaction as a pathogenetic mechanism. Activation of leukocytes has been described in patients with unstable angina [54–58]. Increased levels of C-reactive protein were noted by Berk et al. in patients with unstable angina [56]. Liuzzo et al. described elevated levels of C-reactive protein in patients with unstable angina, but without evidence of myocardial necrosis. Patients with elevated C-reactive protein also had worse in hospital outcomes than those with normal levels [57]. A significant increase in the expression of neutrophil and monocyte adhesion molecule CD11b/CD18 was noted by Mazzone et al. in the coronary sinus blood of patients with unstable angina compared with patients with stable angina [58]. Dinerman et al. have found increased levels of neutrophil elastase in patients with unstable angina compared with controls [55].

Histopathologic specimens also show an inflammatory cell reaction in patients with unstable angina. Areas of plaque disruption are usually found to be infiltrated with inflammatory cells [37]. Patients with unstable angina and non–Q-wave myocardial infarction more frequently have macrophage-rich sclerotic tissue and macrophage-rich atherosclerotic material in atherectomy samples [38]. We feel, however, that there is an interrelationship between thrombosis and inflammation. It is very difficult to separate thrombosis and inflammation. Inflammation in unstable angina may lead to plaque disruption and thrombus formation, as outlined earlier, or it may be secondary to thrombosis. Furthermore, prolonged ischemia may lead to activation of white blood cells, as recently shown by de Mazzone et al. [58].

Smooth Muscle Cell Proliferation. Flugelman et al. evaluated atherectomy samples to assess if mechanisms other than plaque rupture were operative in the conversion of stable angina to unstable angina [59]. They reviewed the histopathology and immunocytochemistry of plaques retrieved from patients whose lesions did not show any thrombus on angiography. Thrombus was retrieved in only 34% of patients with unstable angina, and a smooth muscle predominance index was only slightly lower than patients with restenosis (1.4 vs. 1.7). The expression of acidic FGF and basic FGF was noted in 80–100% of unstable angina and restenosis specimens. Hence, they proposed that in a subset of patients with unstable angina, smooth muscle cell proliferation may lead to gradual luminal narrowing through plaque expansion and give rise to unstable symptoms.

Anatomic-Pathophysiologic Correlates of the Acute Coronary Syndromes

Having discussed the features of the atherosclerotic plaque that may make it vulnerable to rupture, we now turn our attention to the clinical correlates of the acute coronary syndromes. The particular syndrome that develops depends on the amount of ischemia and/or necrosis produced by the obstruction. The factors that determine the degree of ischemia and/or necrosis produced include the degree of obstruction present after plaque rupture, the relative acuteness of the obstruction, the duration of the total occlusion, and the ability to recruit collaterals. Over the years much clinical data have been accumulated regarding the acute coronary syndromes. These data have come in the form of therapeutic trials, angiographic and angioscopic, and biochemical studies. In the remaining portion of this chapter we review these data and develop a cohesive approach to understanding the pathogenesis of the acute coronary syndromes. We discuss each syndrome individually and present the currently available data on it.

UNSTABLE ANGINA

The term *unstable angina* usually incorporates all the following clinical scenarios: new-onset angina, angina at rest, or any increase in the anginal pattern. Unstable angina may also occur soon after a myocardial infarction. For new-onset angina to be classified as unstable, it should be present on mild exertion or at rest. The very name of the syndrome, *unstable angina*, implies an instability or a changing anginal pattern, possibly leading to myocardial infarction. On the level of the plaque, unstable angina can result from two scenarios. Plaque rupture can occur, and a new lesion or a transient total occlusion gives rise to symptoms, or plaque growth, which has been occurring chronically and can progress to the point of critical stenosis. In either situation when the demand increases, the supply is limited and angina occurs; this scenario probably also accounts for a significant num-

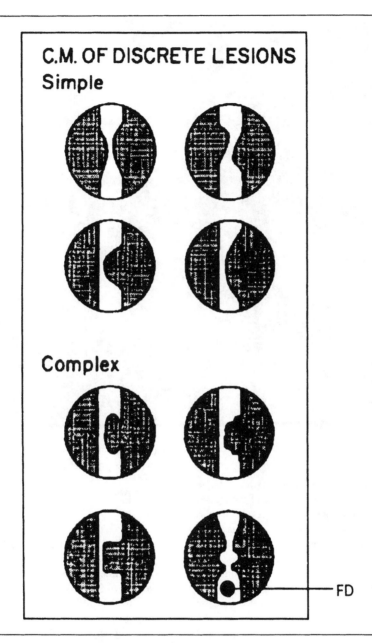

FIGURE 12-2. Diagrammed on the top are the most common lesion morphologies (C.M.) seen in patients presenting with unstable angina. The simple discrete lesions are distinguished from the complex lesions. A filling defect (FD) may be seen proximal or distal to any leison. When a FD is noted in a lesion with simple morphology, it is automatically classified as complex. (Used with permission from Futura Publishing.)

ber of patients with new-onset exertional angina. Interestingly, narrowing by plaque alone was similar on pathological analyses from patients with unstable angina, myocardial infarction, and sudden ischemic death; however, patients with unstable angina had a higher frequency of more severe narrowings [60]. The remainder of the discussion on unstable angina concentrates on rest angina and crescendo angina.

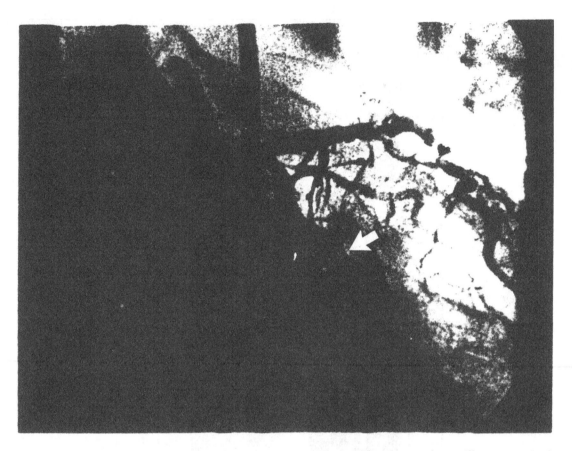

FIGURE 12-3. The photograph top illustrates a simple lesion in the proximal left circumflex artery in the RAO caudal projection. The arrow points to a severe, but concentric, narrowing.

Angiographic Correlates of Unstable Angina. Plaque disruption with thrombosis is the cause of most cases of unstable angina presenting either as rest pain or as an acute change in previously stable angina [61]. Angiography in these patients reveals a stenosis that is greater than 70% but less than 100%; only 10–20% are found to have a total occlusion. The first systematic evaluation of coronary morphology in patients with unstable angina was performed by Ambrose et al. in 1985 [62]. They reviewed the morphology of coronary stenoses in 110 patients with either stable or unstable angina. In patients with unstable angina, an asymmetric or eccentric narrowing with irregular borders and/or a narrow neck was noted in 54% of lesions, as compared with 7% of lesions in patients with stable angina. When ventriculographic and clinical criteria were used to identify the vessel responsible for the ischemic syndrome, this morphology was present in 71% of the culprit or angina-producing lesions. This lesion morphology was classified as type II eccentric, to distinguish it from the smooth eccentric (type I eccentric) or concentric morphology found in patients with

stable angina. Various other studies have confirmed these findings, although different terms have been used to define the lesions, now collectively termed *complex lesions* [63,64] (Figures 12-2 to 12-4).

Intraluminal thrombus has also been demonstrated on angiography in patients with unstable angina [65–68]. The reported prevalence varies from 1% to 75%. This wide variation results from various factors, including the use of heparin, the definition of unstable angina, the duration of the syndrome, the timing of the angiogram from the last episode of pain, and the definition of angiographic thrombus itself (particularly in vessels that are less than 100% occluded). Unfortunately, there is no standard definition for a diagnosis of intracoronary thrombus, and there has been great overlap in the definitions of intracoronary thrombus and complex lesions.

The timing of the angiogram from the last episode of pain is a critical factor in defining the incidence of

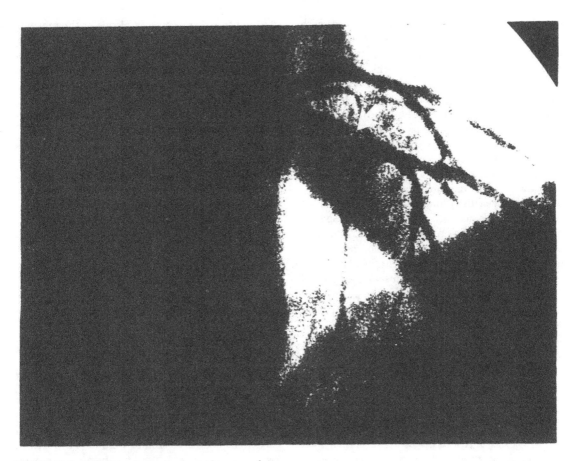

FIGURE 12-4. A complex lesion in the midportion of the left anterior descending coronary artery as seen in the RAO cranial projection. The arrow points to an overhanging edge on the proximal portion of the lesion.

intracoronary thrombus on angiography. Freeman et al. evaluated 80 patients with unstable angina and randomized them to either early angiography (within 24 hours of hospital admission) or later angiography (within 1 week of hospitalization). Patients with on-going chest pain crossed over to a late urgent group. Thrombus was detected in 43% of the patients in the early angiographic group, 75% of the patients in the late urgent group, and 21% of the patients in the late elective group [69]. This study emphasizes the dynamic nature of thrombi in the coronary circulation of patients with unstable angina, and helps partly explain the mixed responses to thrombolytic therapy in patients with unstable angina (see later).

Furthermore, this study also showed that the presence of intracoronary thrombus and complex coronary morphology were strongly associated with in-hospital cardiac events (death, myocardial infarction, and urgent revascularization). Such cardiac events occurred in 73% of the group with intracoronary thrombus and in 55% of the group with complex coronary morphology. Multivessel disease was present in 58% of the patients having cardiac events. Only 17% of patients without any of these angiographic features had cardiac events.

Multiple regression analysis indicated intracoronary thrombus to be the best predictor of cardiac events. Left main coronary artery disease, which is found in 5–10% of unstable angina patients in most angiographic studies but was as high as 25% in one study, were excluded from this analysis [70]. In another study relating prognosis to morphology, Bugardini et al. reported that patients having in-hospital events were at least twice as likely to have complex coronary morphology when compared with patients with a favorable outcome (94% vs. 45%, respectively).

The association between coronary morphology and in-hospital outcome was even more significant when complex coronary morphology was coupled with ischemia on 24-hour continuous electrocardiographic monitoring [71]. A more recent retrospective analysis of the patients in the Unstable Angina Study Using Eminase (UNASEM) study group, however, failed to correlate the presence of thrombus or complex lesion morphology with clinical outcome, even though cardiac events occurred in 63% of the total group [72]. This study included a selected group of patients, and the primary goal was to look at efficacy of thrombolytics in unstable angina, and not to correlate angiography with clinical outcome.

Dissolution of the thrombus and stabilization of the complex plaque then become key therapeutic maneuvers in treating unstable angina. Ongoing chest pain and ischemia after admission on therapy probably represent a group of patients in whom transient episodes of decreased perfusion precipitated by ongoing thrombus formation, due to a persistent hypercoagulable state, and/or increased vasomotion occur at or distal to the lesion site. Merlini et al. prospectively evaluated the degree of coagulation system activity, as measured by F_{1+2} and FPA assays, in a population with unstable angina or myocardial infarction [73]. They found elevated levels of both compounds in the early stages of acute myocardial infarction and in unstable angina; persistent elevation of F_{1+2} was also noted for up to 6 months after the event, whereas FPA levels returned to normal soon after the acute events. The persistent elevation of F_{1+2}, a compound found earlier in the coagulation cascade, indicated that the abnormalities of the hemostatic mechanism were present long after clinical stabilization in patients with acute coronary syndromes. This persistent hypercoagulable state was independent of coronary artery atherosclerosis or drug ingestion. This study also raised the interesting issue of whether a hypercoagulable state could predate the onset of the acute coronary syndromes. This is currently under investigation in the Northwick Park Heart Study II.

Angioscopic Correlations in Acute Coronary Syndromes. Although coronary angiography is quite specific for detecting intracoronary thrombus, its sensitivity is not as good. This has been shown in various studies comparing angioscopy with angiography [74–77]. Moreover, recent studies comparing angioscopy with intracoronary ultrasound continue to show the superiority of angioscopy in defining lesion characteristics [78]. Sherman et al. performed intracoronary angioscopy during coronary artery bypass surgery in patients with unstable and stable angina [79]. None of the 17 arteries in patients with stable coronary

disease had either a complex plaque or thrombus. In the culprit vessels of patients with unstable angina, the three patients with accelerated angina had complex lesions, while all seven with angina at rest had thrombi. Coronary angiography correctly identified the absence of complex plaque and thrombus in 22 vessels but detected only one of four complex plaques and one of seven thrombi.

Mizuno et al. performed angioscopy during coronary arteriography to elucidate the types of lesions found in the various acute coronary syndromes [80]. They studied 10 patients with unstable angina, and thrombi were observed in 9 of the 10 patients. Mural, non-occlusive thrombi were noted in 80% of the patients with unstable angina, as compared with 21% of patients with myocardial infarction. Conversely, occlusive thrombi were noted in only 10% of patients with unstable angina as opposed to 79% of patients with acute myocardial infarction. These data are similar to those reported in various pathological studies.

In another study Mizuno et al. performed angioscopy in patients with unstable angina and acute myocardial infarction in order to define the character of the intracoronary thrombi [81]. The procedure was performed within 48 hours after an episode of rest pain in patients with unstable angina and within 8 hours of onset in those with acute myocardial infarction. Coronary thrombi were found in all but two patients, one in each group. Seventy-one percent of patients with unstable angina had grayish-white thrombi, as compared with none in the group with acute myocardial infarction. Reddish thrombi were found in all the patients with acute myocardial infarction, as opposed to 28% of the patients with unstable angina and thrombi. These differences in the appearance of thrombi relate to the different composition of the thrombi found in these two acute coronary syndromes. On pathological analyses, Kragel et al. found the grayish-white nonocclusive thrombi of unstable angina to consist mostly of platelets, and the reddish occlusive thrombi of acute myocardial infarction to consist mostly of fibrin [82].

More recently, Silva et al. used angioscopy to distinguish unstable lesion characteristics in diabetic and nondiabetic patients [83]. They found a much greater percentage of ulcerated plaques and thrombi, 94% of each, in diabetic patients with unstable angina than in nondiabetic patients with unstable angina (60% ulcerated plaques and 55% thrombi). This finding is consistent with the disproportionately higher incidence of acute coronary events seen in the diabetic population [84,85].

Progression of Coronary Artery Disease in Unstable Angina. A major angiographic feature present in patients with unstable angina is the angiographic progression of coronary disease. In one study by Moise et al., 76% of patients with a new diagnosis of unstable angina had progression of coronary artery disease on a second angiogram compared with 33% of control patients with stable angina. Thirty-eight percent of unstable patients demonstrated progression to obstructive coronary lesions from previously healthy lesions [86].

Ambrose et al. also noted angiographic progression of stenosis severity in a group of patients with new unstable angina who had undergone prior angiography [87]. Disease progression was noted in 75% of patients, and the culprit lesion was less than 50% on a previous angiogram in 72%. In patients with unstable angina who clinically stabilized and were awaiting "elective" coronary intervention, Chen et al. noted significant disease progression, particularly of complex lesions over an 8-month period. Progression was frequently associated with a coronary event and, angiographically, with development of a new total occlusion [88].

TREATMENT STRATEGIES IN UNSTABLE
ANGINA: A PATHOPHYSIOLOGIC APPROACH
Based on the pathogenesis of unstable angina, let us examine the various therapeutic options that have been used in the treatment of unstable angina.

Thrombolysis in Unstable Angina. Thrombolytic therapy has been well established as an effective treatment for myocardial infarction. Because plaque disruption with thrombus formation is the most frequent pathophysiologic mechanism in unstable angina, treatment of this syndrome with thrombolytics would also seem a logical approach. Various trials have looked at the effect of thrombolytics on the unstable plaque, and although variable clinical and angiographic results have been observed, little overall benefit has been demonstrated [68,88–93]. Even though some clinical benefit was demonstrated in some patients, it was often unrelated to the angiographic percentage change in the stenosis [94]. Trials that included totally occluded vessels, such as UNASEM, which randomized to anistreplase (APSAC) or placebo, did demonstrate a significant improvement in the angiographic appearance of the lesion; this improvement was entirely due to the inclusion of the totally occluded vessels [95]. Other studies have shown similar results when totally or subtotally occluded vessels were included in the analysis [94]. However, trials using quantitative

techniques before and after thrombolysis showed no significant angiographic improvement. Ambrose et al. and Topol et al. found no significant differences in percentage stenosis after thrombolysis [89,90].

The controversy regarding the effect of thrombolytics in unstable angina and non–Q-wave myocardial infarction was essentially settled in the Thrombolysis in Myocardial Infarction III (TIMI III) study. In TIMI IIIA, 306 patients were randomized to receive intravenous r-tPA or placebo, and coronary angiography was performed before and after therapy [96]. A substantial improvement was noted on the morphology of the culprit lesion in 15% or the group receiving r-tPA and in 5% of the group receiving placebo. The clinical relevance of this finding failed to be demonstrated in the larger TIMI IIIB trial, a study that examined the potential benefit of r-tPA compared with placebo, as well as an early invasive strategy versus a conservative strategy in 1473 patients [97]. No benefit for r-tPA was demonstrated for the combined endpoint of death, myocardial infarction, or failure of initial therapy at 6 weeks. Interestingly, fatal and nonfatal myocardial infarction after randomization occurred more frequently in the r-tPA group, along with an increased number of intracranial hemorrhages.

The investigators, therefore, concluded that the addition of r-tPA to the treatment regimen of unstable angina and non–Q-wave myocardial infarction was of no benefit, and may even be harmful. Other studies have shown that thrombolytics administered concurrently with heparin in unstable angina resulted in an increased number of myocardial infarctions [98]. It is likely that the main reason for this lack of efficacy is related to the fact that a thrombus, if present, is platelet rich with little fibrin and is thus resistant to the effects of thrombolytics.

Antiplatelet/Antithrombotic Therapy in Unstable Angina. Antiplatelet and antithrombotic therapy remain the mainstay of treatment of unstable angina and non–Q-wave myocardial infarction. The clinical benefits of these therapies are well established, with the first randomized studies being published in 1983 [99–102]. The two agents that formed the cornerstone of this approach were aspirin and heparin. More recently, however, there has been a growing interest in other agents. This interest has been stimulated for various reasons:

1. An increase in thrombin generation and activity is common in acute coronary syndromes [73].
2. Thrombin is involved in both platelet aggregation and the clotting cascade [103].

3. Heparin is unable to bind clot-bound thrombin, and it has its primary effect on circulating thrombin [104].
4. Heparin is also susceptible to neutralization by activated platelets [105,106].
5. Neither aspirin nor heparin is completely able to eliminate the risk of death, nonfatal myocardial infarction, and recurrent ischemic pain in patients with unstable angina [97]. The protection afforded by these agents is not complete, and refractory angina occurs in 10–15% of the patients despite the use of these agents.
6. Heparin therapy is erratic and cumbersome, requiring frequent monitoring of the coagulation profile and frequent boluses, and rare cases can be complicated by heparin-induced thrombocytopenia.

A new class of agents, called *direct antithrombins*, have recently been studied and show promise as additional agents for the treatment of unstable angina. These agents provide a more controlled prolongation of the partial thromboplastin time (PTT), without the peaks and troughs noted with heparin therapy. Most of the preliminary data regarding the efficacy of these agents are from trials looking at clinical endpoints, and there has been little angiographic correlation. However, hirudin was compared with heparin in an angiographic trial conducted by Topol et al. [107]. Patients presenting with ischemic pain and electrocardiographic changes at rest who had angiographic thrombus were eligible for the study. Two different heparin doses were compared with four different hirudin doses. The average cross-sectional area of the culprit lesion improved more in the hirudin-treated group.

Other indices of lesion improvement, such as minimal luminal diameter, and changes in the minimal cross-sectional area were also noted to be better in the hirudin-treated patients. A slightly greater number of patients demonstrated TIMI perfusion grade III flow in the hirudin group as compared with heparin (25% vs 19%) on the day-5 angiogram. Furthermore, even though the study was not designed to assess clinical endpoints, the composite endpoint of death, myocardial infarction, or recurrent angina occurred in 24.0% of heparin-treated patients and in 14.6% of hirudin-treated patients. The incidence of postrandomization myocardial infarction was also lower in the hirudin-treated group.

These data taken together indicate that resolution of intracoronary thrombus, as judged by improved lesion severity, is associated with clinical benefits in patients with unstable angina and non–Q-wave myo-

cardial infarction [108]. Other trials, such as GUSTO II, are examining the clinical benefits of hirudin in patients with unstable angina [109,110].

The effects of antiplatelet therapy in unstable angina may, in part, be due to the inhibition of thrombin generation that has been reported to be increased in patients with unstable angina [111,112]. Aspirin DL-lysine was found to decrease thrombin generation, as measured by a decrease in the levels of thrombin–antithrombin III complexes [113]. Thrombin-induced platelet aggregation may be a key factor in disease progression in patients with unstable angina. Lam et al. found increased disease progression over a 2-year period in patients found to have platelet hyperaggregability [114].

More recently, there has been an increasing interest in another category of antiplatelet agents, the GPIIb/IIIa receptor antagonists. The various compounds in this group include monoclonal antibodies, cyclic peptides, and peptido-mimetic agents [115]. The use of c7E3 Fab (abciximab), a monoclonal antibody in patients with refractory unstable angina, significantly reduced the number of ischemic episodes compared with heparin. Angiographic improvements seen with the abciximab, however, were not significant and may have been a factor of the small numbers studied [116]. Various other trials, some published and some in progress, are evaluating the use of these agents in acute coronary syndromes. Most of these trials are directing attention towards clinical endpoints, or the use of these agents as adjunts to percutaneous coronary intervention [115]. Most of the published data thus far include only trials evaluating the potential role of these agents as adjuncts to percutaneous coronary intervention, such as the EPIC and the recently terminated EPILOG trials of c7E3 Fab [117]. However, preliminary data from other trials show great promise for the use of these agents in acute coronary syndromes [118,119].

NON–Q-WAVE MYOCARDIAL INFARCTION

Non–Q-wave myocardial infarction is a syndrome that pathogenetically lies between unstable angina and Q-wave myocardial infarction. The hallmark of non–Q-wave myocardial infarction, as implied by its name, is the absence of Q waves on a 12-lead electrocardiogram in the presence of myocardial necrosis. Pathologically, this does not necessarily imply a nontransmural infarction. The amount of myocardial necrosis, however, is less than Q-wave myocardial infarction, but the ischemic episode is of longer duration than in unstable angina [120]. Non–Q-wave myocardial infarction usually evolves from one of three conditions:

1. There may be a new persistent total occlusion of an artery, usually with recruitable collaterals that limit myocardial necrosis.
2. Transient total occlusion may occur with spontaneous recanalization, thereby limiting the amount of necrosis.
3. Multiple episodes of occlusion and reperfusion followed by a prolonged episode of occlusion (ischemic preconditioning) are present [121].
4. In the setting of significant multivessel disease, transient hypotension could result in areas of subendocardial necrosis, because myocardial demand may outstrip supply.

As most infarct-related arteries are patent in this setting (see later), a shorter duration of total coronary occlusion followed by spontaneous reperfusion distinguishes this entity from Q-wave myocardial infarction in a majority of cases.

Angiographic Correlates of Non–Q-Wave Myocardial Infarction. Because non–Q-wave myocardial infarction as a clinical syndrome is intermediate between unstable angina and Q-wave myocardial infarction, it is little surprise, then, that the angiographic findings fall somewhere between unstable angina and Q-wave myocardial infarction. The number of culprit vessels is similar in unstable angina and Q-wave myocardial infarction [122]. Total occlusion is seen more frequently than unstable angina, but less frequently than Q-wave myocardial infarction; 60–80% of the vessels are patent on angiography in non–Q-wave myocardial infarction [123,124]. In patients with patent infarct-related arteries, the angiographic morphology is similar to that seen in unstable angina [123]. In approximately 65% of the infarct-related arteries, a complex lesion is present (type II eccentric plaque). The major difference from unstable angina is the presence of more intracoronary thrombus (appearing as filling defects) in non–Q-wave myocardial infarction [125].

Serial studies in patients with non–Q-wave myocardial infarction have shown significant progression in lesion severity when compared with previous angiograms. Little et al. found that progression often occurred from lesions that angiographically had less than a 50% reduction in diameter [16]. However, in another smaller series by Ambrose et al., more severe lesions were also present [15]. Klein et al. compared preinfarct and postinfarct angiograms in a group of patients with Q-wave and non–Q-wave myocardial infarctions. Patients with non–Q-wave myocardial infarction had pre-existing stenoses that were either severe, mild (less than 20%), or absent on the preinfarct angiogram. This variability is explained by the different mechanisms (see earlier discussion) that result in non–Q-wave myocardial infarction.

Q-WAVE MYOCARDIAL INFARCTION

Q-wave myocardial infarction results from sudden total occlusion of a coronary artery, resulting in a sudden cessation of myocardial blood flow without a major change in myocardial oxygen demand. The result is myocardial necrosis, the degree of which is a function of recruitable collaterals, the duration of total occlusion, and the size of the coronary bed being perfused by the culprit vessel. The ability to acutely recruit collaterals is usually less, and the duration of total occlusion is usually longer in patients with Q-wave myocardial infarction than in patients with non–Q-wave myocardial infarction. The net result is a larger amount of myocardial necrosis in the patients with Q-wave myocardial infarction. On pathologic analyses from patients dying with major coronary thromboses, a disrupted atherosclerotic plaque is found in 75% of the patients, while superficial intimal injury is noted in the remaining 25% [126]. The extent of lysable thrombus is greater in Q-wave myocardial infarction than unstable angina, and the importance of this is evident from the results of the various trials showing the benefit of thrombolytic therapy in acute myocardial infarction [127,128]. As mentioned previously, thrombus found at sites of arterial injury (as in unstable angina) is platelet rich, while thrombus extending distally from the site of plaque disruption and occluding the lumen is red cell and fibrin rich. The appearance of these thrombi compared with those found in other acute coronary syndromes has been previously discussed in this chapter.

Perturbations in the blood coagulation system and blood flow play an important role in the pathogenesis of myocardial infarction, in addition to vascular injury. Elevated fibrinogen and factor VII levels correlate with a risk of subsequent myocardial infarction [129,130]. Tobacco smoking, which can increase fibrinogen levels and increase platelet aggregation, is a well-known risk factor for acute myocardial infarction [131]. The role of platelet aggregation as a risk factor for acute myocardial infarction is further supported by the demonstration that aspirin can reduce this risk [132]. Furthermore, acute myocardial infarctions tend to have a peak in the morning hours, when an upright posture may result in increased platelet aggregability [133]. Overall, a large thrombus burden is not necessary for an acute myocardial infarction to occur. Vascular injury can result in the formation of a platelet thrombus and local vasoconstriction. Increased vasomotion at this site can then lead to stasis, and formation of a fibrin-rich thrombus, which subsequently grows and becomes occlusive. Hence, in the initial stages only a small amount of thrombus may be necessary for an acute myocardial infarction to occur in the presence of a dynamic stenosis [134].

Angiographic Correlates of Q-Wave Myocardial Infarction. Total coronary occlusion remains the overwhelming angiographic finding in the early hours after the onset of an evolving Q-wave myocardial infarction. De Wood et al. found that 84% of their patients had total occlusion of the infarct-related coronary artery within 6 hours of the onset of infarction. This frequency decreased to 63% when angiography was performed 12–24 hours after the onset of the event [135]. Needless to say, intracoronary thrombus is nearly universally demonstrated on angiography in this patient group [136–140]. Reperfusion or patency rates with the various thrombolytic agents vary from 60% to 80% when these agents are given either intravenously or directly into the coronary artery. These rates are dependent on several factors, including fibrin selectivity, with the nonselective agents having a lower recanalization rate, and the timing of therapy since the onset of symptoms; recanalization rates diminish as the time from symptom onset increases [141]. In addition to recanalization rates, the flow grade distal to the lesion at 90 minutes after the administration of the thrombolytic is becoming increasingly important in predicting short-term prognosis. TIMI III flow grade (normal antegrade flow and normal washout in the culprit vessel) was only achieved in 54% of the patients receiving rt-PA and intravenous heparin in the GUSTO I trial [142]. A critical finding in this study was the relationship between TIMI III flow and 30-day mortality and left ventricular function. Irrespective of the thrombolytic agent used, the 30-day mortality was 4.4% in the TIMI III group compared with 8.9% in the group with either TIMI 0 or TIMI I flow (TIMI 0, totally occluded vessel with no antegrade flow; TIMI I, slow antegrade flow with incomplete filling, and persistence of dye in the vessel as other vessels wash out). TIMI II flow (slow but complete antegrade flow) did not portend a significantly improved prognosis over TIMI 0 and TIMI I flow.

The coronary artery morphology in patients undergoing successful thrombolysis, and in patients with acute or recent myocardial infarction with patent infarct-related arteries, is usually complex, with irregular and/or ulcerated plaques in the majority of

cases [143]. Wilson et al. studied culprit lesions in a group of patients with recent myocardial infarction and with patent infarct-related arteries. An irregularity noted in the lesion was felt to suggest a role for ulceration or plaque disruption as a cause for the infarction. An ulceration index was defined for these lesions. Lesions responsible for myocardial infarction were noted to have a significantly different ulceration index compared with those found in patients with stable angina [144].

Brown et al., using videodensitometric techniques, found a distinct translucency overlying a less translucent plaque in patients with patent infarct-related arteries after thrombolysis. This translucency was felt to be nonlysed thrombus on top of the ruptured plaque [145]. The residual thrombus and the irregular morphology seen in the early hours after thrombolysis undergoes significant remodeling over the ensuing few days. Davies et al. compared lesion morphology on day 1 and day 8 in a group of patients who had received intravenous thrombolysis. They found eccentric lesions as well as a globular and linear filling defect on day 1. Using Wilson's ulceration index, restudy at day 8 revealed a significant decrease in the ulceration index, and in the number of filling defects if the patients had been maintained on heparin therapy [146].

In the Antithrombotics in The Prevention of Reocclusion in Coronary Thrombolysis (APRICOT) study, nearly half of the initially complex lesions became smooth, with an increase in the luminal diameter, within 3 months [147]. The ulceration index has also been found to be predictive of clinical instability in the days following myocardial infarction. The patients with a higher ulceration index required more frequent and urgent medical intervention, including bypass grafting, or angioplasty, while those with a lower index stabilized on medical therapy [148]. Lesions felt to be thrombotic and complex on angiography have been repeatedly confirmed on angioscopy [128,149].

Angiographic Progression of Coronary Artery Disease and Myocardial Infarction. As mentioned toward the beginning of this chapter, various studies have indicated that the degree of stenosis as detected by angiography that precedes a myocardial infarction is usually mild to moderate. Similar data have been seen in the thrombolytic era. Brown et al. demonstrated that the underlying stenosis in 32% of patients receiving thrombolytics was less than 50%, and in 66% it was less than 60% [145]. In the TIMI and TAMI (Thrombolysis After Myocardial Infarction) trials, however, approximately 10–15% of patients were found to have a less than 50% stenosis within 48 hours after successful thrombolysis [150,151].

It is important to understand, as mentioned earlier, that the finding of a mild or moderate stenotic lesion at the site of an index infarction may simply be a reflection of the greater number of such lesions in the population, as opposed to an inherent characteristic of mild and moderate plaques. Nevertheless, it is clear that patients with previously severe stenoses who go on to total occlusion often do not infarct but occlude asymptomatically [152]. In these patients recruitable and/or already active collaterals, because of the underlying severe stenosis, prevent or limit the size of the infarction. While it is extremely difficult to be sure how often a mild to moderate stenosis leads to a myocardial infarction, suffice it to say that in a majority of cases of large infarctions, the underlying lesion is less than severe. Because these lesions are not hemodynamically significant, no collaterals are formed or recruited, and the abrupt plaque disruption with thrombotic occlusion results in sizable infarction of the unprotected bed.

MEDICAL TREATMENT STRATEGIES IN Q-WAVE MYOCARDIAL INFARCTION

It is no surprise, given the pathophysiology of Q-wave myocardial infarction and the anatomic correlates of this syndrome, that thrombolytics are the mainstay of medical therapy in these patients. In contrast to unstable angina, thrombolytics have shown great benefit in treating acute myocardial infarction when total coronary occlusion is present [127,128,153,154]. The two main agents currently being used are streptokinase and rt-PA. At least for rt-PA, intravenous heparin is required for the first 24–48 hours. Aspirin should be given acutely to all patients with myocardial infarction.

The superiority of rt-PA over streptokinase was shown in GUSTO I, in which this agent was administered in an accelerated fashion over 90 minutes [155]. This trial showed a higher 90-minute patency rate and a small, but statistically significant, decrease in mortality for rt-PA compared with streptokinase. As mentioned earlier, the 90-minute patency with TIMI grade 3 flow is a good marker of mortality. Hence, efforts are now being directed toward increasing the 90-minute patency with TIMI 3 flow for rt-PA and streptokinase.

To this end, newer investigations are focusing on using these agents concurrently with newer antithrombotic and antiplatelet agents. In TIMI 5 hirudin or heparin was given with rt-PA [156]. At 90 minutes there was a nonsignificant trend favoring infarct artery patency of hirudin versus heparin (65%

vs. 57%). At 18–36 hours, however, there was a clear benefit for hirudin — 62% versus 49% for heparin-treated patients. Death or reinfarction occurred in 16.7% of heparin-treated patients and in 6.9% of hirudin-treated patients. Major hemorrhage occurred in 23% of the heparin-treated patients and in 17% of hirudin-treated patients.

The HIT study looked at three different doses of hirudin in conjunction with rt-PA and aspirin [157]. There was no heparin comparison arm. Sixty-one percent of patients in the highest hirudin dose group achieved TIMI 3 flow at 90 minutes. Major spontaneous hemorrhage was noted in 2.4% of patients in the highest dose group.

TIMI 6 studied three different doses of hirudin with streptokinase and aspirin, compared with heparin, aspirin, and streptokinase [158]. The trial was not powered to detect differences in efficacy, but favorable trends were observed for hirudin. Death, reinfarction, congestive heart failure, and cardiogenic shock occurred in 11.6% of the hirudin patients receiving the highest dose, compared with 17.6% of heparin-treated patients. Major hemorrhage rates were similar — 5.7% for hirudin versus 5.6% for heparin.

Given the data from the above-mentioned phase II trials, hirudin was subsequently investigated in large scale phase III trials. These included TIMI 9A, GUSTO IIA, and HIT III [159–161]. Intracranial hemorrhage in TIMI 9A was similar for hirudin and heparin (1.8% vs. 1.9%). Major spontaneous hemorrhage, however, was 8.9% for hirudin and 4.9% for heparin. In GUSTO IIA, intracranial bleeding occurred in 2.2% of hirudin-treated patients and in 1.5% of heparin-treated patients (P = NS). Similar increased bleeding rates were observed in HIT III. This resulted in major protocol changes, which urged for lower doses of heparin and hirudin when administered with thrombolytics. Hence, even though the newer regimens show greater patency rates, their overall efficacy maybe limited by the bleeding risk.

Various other trials are ongoing looking at the concurrent use of GPIIb/IIIa inhibitors with thrombolytics. These include TAMI 8 with Abciximab (phase I/II), IMPACT AMI with Integrelin (phase II), PARADIGM with Lamifiban (phase II), and PARAGON Pilot with Lamifiban (phase I/II) [115]. We eagerly await the data from these studies.

Sudden Ischemic Death

Sudden death in the coronary disease patient occurs via two mechanisms. The first is due to poor left ventricular function and scar, often from previous myocardial infarction. In this setting, the scar provides the arrhythmogenic substrate in the form of a reentrant loop, which when activated results in malignant ventricular arrhythmias. Coronary ischemia is usually not an important factor in this group of patients. The second mechanism involves the sudden occlusion of a coronary artery by a thrombus. In this group, sudden coronary ischemia is an important factor, hence the term *sudden ischemic death*. On pathologic analysis there is an overlap between patients dying from sudden death and those dying after a myocardial infarction. Furthermore, approximately one third of patients who survive an episode of sudden death, from either mechanism, are found to have a concurrent myocardial infarction [162].

In sudden ischemic death, the finding of intraluminal thrombus is variable. Some studies have found it infrequently, while Davies et al. found an intraluminal thrombus in 74% of patients [163–165]. A more recent study by Farb et al. examined the frequency of active coronary lesions, inactive coronary lesions, and myocardial infarction in patients who died from sudden cardiac death [64]. They found active coronary lesions (defined as disrupted plaques, luminal fibrin/platelet thrombus, or both) in 57% of the cohort. Most of the patients (94%) with active coronary lesions had thrombus present, either alone or with disrupted plaque. In another study, patients with sudden ischemic death and intracoronary thrombus were more likely to have single-vessel disease, acute myocardial infarction, and a recent history of clinical ischemia [166]. This group is distinct from the group with scarred left ventricles, who tend to have multivessel disease and a longer history of ischemia/myocardial infarction.

ANGIOGRAPHIC CORRELATES OF
SUDDEN ISCHEMIC DEATH
There are two major drawbacks in analyzing angiograms in patients with sudden death. First, the angiograms are performed in survivors, a group that, by surviving the event, is in a different prognostic category than nonsurvivors. Inherent in this may be a more "benign coronary morphology." Second, many of the studies combine all surviving patients with sudden death, regardless of the mechanism. Though not absolutely perfect, there may be a way to tease out the group of patients who survive sudden death caused by sudden thrombotic occlusion. This group of patients tends not to have inducible ventricular tachycardia on electrophysiologic study, whereas patients with sudden death from scar tend to be inducible. When these former patients are studied

angiographically, approximately 50–65% have complex lesions that are either irregular or eccentric irregular, compared with only 19–25% of patients in the latter group [60,167].

Conclusions

The clinical presentation of the acute coronary syndromes spans a spectrum that includes unstable angina, non–Q-wave myocardial infarction, Q-wave myocardial infarction, and sudden ischemic death. All syndromes share, in most cases, a common pathophysiologic mechanism of plaque disruption and thrombus formation. The differences in the clinical presentation of the different syndromes is determined by the suddenness of the occlusion, the degree of occlusion, the duration of the occlusion, and the ability to recruit collaterals. These differences are important because they determine the response to therapy.

The clinical experience with these syndromes has not only been important in treating the disease process but has also been critical in understanding the disease process. Early pathologic studies found evidence of thrombus on autopsies of patients who died from myocardial infarctions. In these cases, thrombus was felt to be a result of the postmortem changes, rather than a cause of the infarction. It was not until angiography was performed during ongoing infarctions that the hypothesis changed and thrombus formation took center stage as the cause of myocardial infarction. These findings were further corroborated by angioscopy.

Similar findings were then noted in the other acute coronary syndromes, and thrombus formation became the common thread that bound together all the syndromes. Pathologic studies at the cellular level showed a disrupted vessel architecture, with plaque and thrombus, establishing the importance of plaque disruption and thrombus formation. Other studies suggested the importance of the lipid content of the plaque as an important determinant of plaque disruption.

Armed with these data, investigators around the world designed the various therapeutic trials we have discussed in this chapter. For the most part, the trials have been successful, further supporting the hypotheses generated from earlier clinical experiences. When the trials were not successful, reasons were sought and the subtle differences amongst the acute coronary syndromes were elucidated. The field of acute ischemic coronary disease has moved forward rapidly in the last 15 years. The ability to arrive at a hypothesis and be able to test it in the angiography suite, or in a large patient population, has been extremely important in the advancement of this field.

In the clinical arena, the emphasis will remain on two major aspects of the disease: prevention and treatment. Acute coronary events remain the largest cause of death in the United States. The importance of risk factor control in preventing acute coronary events has been shown in many trials and stresses the importance of aggressive risk-factor modification in the population at risk for coronary events. Newer therapeutic agents and strategies are constantly being developed and tested, and the cardiac catheterization laboratory and the coronary care units are taking on an increasing role in evaluating these strategies. The clinical experience gained in this disease will remain an important teaching tool for the generations of physicians to come.

References

1. Berenson G. Epidemiology and prevention. ACCSAP 1995 1.3.
2. Falk E, Shah PK, Fuster V. Coronary plaque disruption. Circulation 92:657, 1995.
3. Ambrose JA. Coronary angiographic findings in the acute coronary syndromes. In Bleifeld W, Braunwald WE, Hamm C (eds). Unstable Angina. Berlin/Heidelberg: Springer Verlag, 1990:112.
4. Fox B, James K, Morgan B, Seed A. Distribution of fatty and fibrous plaques in young human coronary arteries. Arteriosclerosis 48:139, 1983.
5. Kjaernes M, Svindland A, Walloe L, Willie SO. Location of early atherosclerotic lesions in an arterial bifurcation in humans. Acta Pathol Microbiol Immunol Second Sect 89:35, 1981.
6. Zairns CK, Giddens DP, Bhardavaj BK, et al. Carotid bifurcation atherosclerosis. Quantitative correlation of plaque locationwith flow velocity profiles and wall shear stress. Circ Res 53:502, 1983.
7. Fuster V. Pathogenesis of atherosclerosis. In Spittell JA Jr (ed). Clinical Medicine. Philadelphia: Harper & Row 1981:1.
8. Stary HC, Chandler AB, Dinsmore RE, et al. A definition of advanced types of atherosclerotic lesions and a histological classification of atherosclerosis. Circulation 92:1355, 1995.
9. Stary HC, Chandler AB, Glagov S, et al. A definition of initial, fatty streak, and intermediate lesions of atherosclerosis. Arterioscler Thromb 14:840, 1994.
10. Glagov S, Weisenberg E, Zarins CK, et al. Compensatory enlargement of human atherosclerotic coronary arteries. N Engl J Med 316:1371, 1987.
11. Stary HC. Evolution and progression of atherosclerotic lesions in coronary arteries of children and young adults. Arteriosclerosis 9(Suppl. 1):119, 1989.
12. Fuster V, Kottke BA. Atherosclerosis. A. Pathogenesis, pathology, and presentation of atherosclerosis. In Brandenburg RO (ed). Cardiology: Fundamentals and Practice. Year Book Medical, 1987:951.
13. Ross R. The pathogenesis of atherosclerosis — an update. N Engl J Med 314:488, 1986.
14. Chapman I. Morphogenesis of occluding coronary artery thrombosis. Arch Pathol 80:256, 1965.
15. Ambrose JA, Tannenbaum MA, Alexopoulos D, et al. Angiographic progression of coronary artery disease and the development of myocardial infarction. J Am Coll Cardiol 12:56, 1988.
16. Little WC, Constantinescu M, Applegate RJ, et al. Can coronary angiography predict the site of a subsequent myocardial infarction in patients with mild to moderate coronary artery disease? Circulation 78:1157, 1988.
17. Giroud D, Li JM, Urban P, et al. Relation of the site of acute myocardial infarction to the most severe coronary arterial stenosis at prior angiography. Am J Cardiol 69:729, 1993.
18. Nobuyoshi M, Tanaka M, Nosaka H, et al. Progression of coronary atherosclerosis: Is coronary spasm related to progression? J Am Coll Cardiol 18:904, 1991.
19. Alderman EL, Corley SD, Fisher LD, et al. Five year angiographic follow-up of factors associated with progression of coronary artery disease in the Coronary Artery Surgery Study (CASS). J Am Coll Cardiol 22:1141, 1993.
20. Falk E. Morphologic features of unstable ather-thrombotic plaques underlying acute coronary syndromes. Am J Cardiol 63(Suppl. E):114E, 1989.
21. Gertz SD, Roberts WC. Hemodynamic shear force in rupture of coronary arterial athersclerotic plaques. Am J Cardiol 66:1368, 1990.
22. Davies MJ, Richardson PD, Woolf N, et al. Risk of thrombosis in human atherosclerotic plaques: Role of extracellular lipid, macrophage, and smooth muscle cell content. Br Heart J 69:377, 1993.
23. Lundberg B. Chemical composition and physical state of lipid deposits in ahterosclerosis. Athersclerosis 56:93, 1985.
24. Small DM. Progression and regression of atherosclerotic lesions: Insights from lipid physical biochemistry. Arteriosclerosis 8:103, 1988.
25. Wagner WD, St Clair RW, Clarkson TB, Connor JR. A study of atherosclerosis regression in Macaca mulatta, III: Chemical changes in arteries from animals with atherosclerosis induced for 19 months and regressed for 48 months at plasma cholesterol levels of 300 or 200 mg/dl. Am J Pathol 100:633, 1980.
26. Loree HM, Tobias BJ, Gibson LJ, et al. Mechanical properties of model atherosclerotic lesion lipid pools. Arterioscler Thrmob 14:230, 1994.
27. Buchwald H, Vargo RL, Matts JP, et al. Effect of partial ileal bypass surgery on mortality and morbidity from coronary heart disease in patients with hypercholesterolemia: Report of the Program on the

Surgical Control of the Hyperlipidemias (POSCH). N Engl J Med 323:946, 1990.

28. Watts GF, Lewis B, Brunt JNH, et al. Effects on coronary artery disease of lipid lowering diet plus cholestyramine, in the St Thomas' Athersclerosis Regression Study (STARS). Lancet 339:563, 1992.

29. Blankenhorn DH, Azen SP, Dieter KM, et al. Coronary angiographic changes with Lovastatin therapy: The Monitored Atherosclerosis Regression Study (MARS). Ann Intern Med 119:969, 1993.

30. Scandanavian Simvastatin Survival Group. Randomised trial of cholesterol lowering in 4444 patients with coronary heart disease: The Scandanavian Simvastatin Survival Study (4S). Lancet 344:1383, 1994.

31. Shepherd J, Cobbe SM, Ford I, et al. Prevention of coronary heart disease with pravastatin in men with hypercholesterolemia. N Engl J Med 333:1301, 1995.

32. Brown G, Albers JJ, Fisher LD, et al. Regression of coronary artery disease as a result of intensive lipid lowering therapy in men with high levels of apolipoprotein B. N Engl J Med 323:1289, 1990.

33. Burleigh MC, Briggs AD, Lendon CL, et al. Collagen types I and III, collagen content, GAGs and mechanical strength of human atherosclerotic plaque caps: Span-wise variations. Atherosclerosis 96:71, 1992.

34. Libby P. Molecular bases of the acute coronary syndromes. Circulation 91:2844, 1995.

35. Amento EP, Palmer H, Libby P. Cytokines positively and negatively regulate interstitial collagen gene expression in human vascular smooth muscle cells. Arterioscler Thromb 11:1223, 1991.

36. Richardson PD, Davies MJ, Born GVR. Influence of plaque configuration and stress distribution on fissuring of coronary atherosclerotic plaques. Lancet 2:941, 1989.

37. van der Wal AC, Becker AE, van der Loos CM, Das PK. Site of intimal rupture or erosion of thrombosed coronary atherosclerotic plaques is characterized by an inflammatory process irrespective of the dominant plaque morphology. Circulation 89:36, 1994.

38. Moreno PR, Falk E, Palacios IF, et al. Macrophage infiltration in acute coronary syndromes: Implications for plaque rupture. Circulation 90:775, 1994.

39. Shah PK, Falk E, Badimon JJ, et al. Human monocyte-derived macrophages express collagenase and induce collagen breakdown in atherosclerotic fibrous caps: Implications for plaque rupture (abstr). Circulation 88(Suppl. I):I-254, 1993.

40. Shah PK, Falk E, Badimon JJ, et al. Human monocyte-derived macrophages induce collagen breakdown in fibrous caps of atherosclerotic plaques: Potential role of matrix degrading metalloproteinases and implications for plaque rupture. Circulation 92:1565, 1995.

41. Henney AM, Wakeley PR, Davies MJ, et al. Localiza-tion of stromelysin gene expression in atherosclerotic plaques by in situ hybridization. Proc Natl Acad Sci USA 88:8154, 1991.

42. Galis ZS, Sukhova GK, Lark MW, Libby P. Increased expression of matrix-metalloproteinases and matrix degrading activity in vulnerable regions of human atherosclerotic plaques. J Clin Invest 94:2493, 1994.

43. Brown DL, Hibbs MS, Kearny M, et al. Identification of 92-kD gelatinase in human coronary atherosclerotic lesions: Association of active enzyme synthesis with unstable angina. Circulation 91:2125, 1995.

44. Neri Serneri GG, Gensini GF, Poggesi L, et al. The role of extraplatelet thromboxane A_2 in unstable angina investigated with a dual thromboxane A_2 inhibitor: Importance of activated monocytes. Cor Art Dis 5:137, 1994.

45. Kaartinen M, Penttilä A, Kovanen PT. Accumulation of activated mast cells in the shoulder region of human coronary atheroma, the predilection site of atheromatous rupture. Circulation 90:1669, 1994.

46. Gruber BL, Marchese MJ, Suzuki K, et al. Synovial procollagenase activation by human mast cell tryptase: Dependence upon matrix metalloproteinase 3 activation. J Clin Invest 84:1657, 1989.

47. Matrisian LM. Metalloproteinases and their inhibitors in matrix remodeling. Trends Genet 6:121, 1990.

48. Shapiro SD, Campbell EJ, Kobayashi DK, Welgus HG. Immune modulation of metalloproteinase production in human macrophages: Selective pretranslational suppression of interstial collagenase and stromelysin biosynthesis by interferon-γ. J Clin Invest 86:1204, 1991.

49. Saarinen J, Kalkkinen N, Welgus HG, Kovanen PT. Activation of human interstitial procollagenase through direct cleavage of the Leu^{83}-Thr^{84} bond by mast cell chymase. J Biol Chem 269:181340, 1994.

50. Cheng GC, Loree HM, Kamm RD, et al. Distribution of circumferential stress in ruptured and stable atherosclerotic lesions: A structural analysis with histopathological correlation. Circulation 87:1179, 1993.

51. Loree HM, Kamm RD, Stringfellow RG, Lee RT. Effects of fibrous cap thickness on peak circumferential stress in model atherosclerotic vessels. Circ Res 71:850, 1992.

52. MacIsaac AI, Thomas JD, Topol EJ. Toward the quiescent coronary plaque. J Am Coll Cardiol 22:1228, 1993.

53. Fitzgerald JD. By what means might beta blockers prolong life after acute myocardial infarction? Eur Heart J 8:945, 1987.

54. Neri Serneri G, Abbate R, Gori AM, et al. Transient intermittent lymphocyte activation is responsible for the instability of unstable angina. Circulation 86:790, 1992.

55. Dinerman J, Mehta J, Saldeen T, et al. Increased neutrophil elastase in unstable angina and acute myocardial infarction. Am J Cardiol 15:1559, 1990.

56. Berk B, Weintraub W, Alexander R. Elevation of C-reactive proteinin "active" coronary artery disease. Am J Cardiol 65:168, 1990.

57. Liuzzo A, Biasucci LM, Gallimore JR, et al. The prognostic value of C-reactive protein and serum amyloid "a" protein in severe unstable angina. N Engl J Med 331:417, 1994.

58. Mazzone A, De Servi, Ricevuti G, et al. Increased expression of neutrophil and monocyte adhesion molecules in unstable coronary artery disease. Circulation 22:358, 1993.

59. Flugelman MY, Virmani R, Correa R, et al. Smooth muscle cell abundance and fibroblast growth factors in coronary lesions of patients with nonfatal unstable angina: A clue to the mechanism of transformation from stable to the unstable clinical state. Circulation 88:2493, 1993.

60. Roberts WC, Kragel AH, Gertz SD, Roberts CS. Coronary arteries in unstable angina pectoris, acute myocardial infarction, and sudden coronary death. Am Heart J 127:1588, 1994.

61. Ambrose JA. Coronary arteriographic analysis and angiographic morphology. J Am Coll Cardiol 13:1492, 1989.

62. Ambrose JA, Winters SL, Stern A, et al. Angiographic morphology and the pathogenesis of unstable angina pectoris. J Am Coll Cardiol 5:609, 1985.

63. Haft JI, Goldstein JE, Niemiera ML. Coronary arteriographic lesion of unstable angina. Chest 92:609, 1987.

64. Williams AE, Freeman MR, Chisolm RJ, et al. Angiographic morphology in unstable angina pectoris. Am J Cardiol 62:1024, 1988.

65. Bresnahan DR, Davis DR, Holmes DR Jr, Smith HC. Angiographic occurrence and clinical correlates of intraluminal coronary artery thrombus: Role of unstable angina. J Am Coll Cardiol 6:285, 1985.

66. Vetrovec GW, Cowley MJ, Overton H, Richardson DW. Intracoronary thrombus in syndromes of unstable myocardial ischemia. Am Heart J 102:1202, 1981.

67. Capone G, Wolf NM, Meyer B, Meister SG. Frequency of intracoronary filling defects by angiography in angina pectoris at rest. Am J Cardiol 56:403, 1985.

68. Mandlekorn JB, Wolf NM, Singh S, et al. Intracoronary thrombus in nontransmural myocardial infarction and unstable angina pectoris. Am J Cardiol 52:1, 1983.

69. Freeman MR, Williams AE, Chisolm RJ, Armstrong PW. Intracoronary and thrombus and complex morphology in unstable angina. Relation to timing of angiography and in-hospital cardiac events. Circulation 80:17, 1989.

70. Plotnick GD, Greene HI, Carliner NH, et al.Clinical indicators of left main coronary artery disease in unstable angina. Ann Intern Med 91:149, 1979.

71. Bugiardini R, Pozzati A, Borghi A, et al. Angiographic morphology in unstable angina and its relation to transient myocardial ischemia and hospital outcome. Am J Cardiol 67:460, 1991.

72. Bar FW, Raynaud P, Renkin JP, et al. Coronary angiographic findings do not predict clinical outcome in patients with unstable angina. J Am Coll Cardiol 24:1453, 1994.

73. Merlini PA, Bauer KA, Oltrona L, et al. Persistent activation of coagulation mechanism in unstable angina and myocardial infarction. Circulation 90:61, 1994.

74. Lee G, Garcia JM, Corso PJ, et al. Correlation of coronary angioscopic to angiographic findings in coronary artery disease. Am J Cardiol 58:238, 1986.

75. Spears JR, Spokojny AM, Marais HJ. Coronary angioscopy during cardiac catheterization. J Am Coll Cardiol 6:93, 1985.

76. Uchida Y, Tomaru T, Nakamura F, et al. Percutaneous coronary angioscopy in patients with ischemic heart disease. Am Heart J 114:1216, 1987.

77. White CJ, Ramee SR, Collins TJ, et al. Percutaneous coronary angioscopy of saphenous vein coronary bypass grafts. J Am Coll Cardiol 21:1181, 1993.

78. de Feyter PJ, Ozaki Y, Baptista J, et al. Ischemia related lesion characteristics in patients with stable or unstable angina: A study with intracoronary angioscopy and ultrasound. Circulation 92:1408, 1995.

79. Sherman TC, Litvack F, Grundfest W, et al. Coronary angioscopy in patients with unstable angina pectoris. N Engl J Med 315:913, 1986.

80. Mizuno K, Miyamoto A, Satomura K, et al. Angioscopic coronary macromorphology in patients with acute coronary disorders. Lancet 337:809, 1991.

81. Mizuno K, Satomura K, Miyamoto A, et al. Angioscopic evaluation of coronary artery thrombi in acute coronary artery syndromes. N Engl J Med 326:287, 1992.

82. Kragel AH, Reddy SG, Wittes JT, Roberts WC. Morphologic comparison of frequency and types of acute lesions in the major epicardial coronary arteries in unstable angina pectoris, sudden coronary death, and acute myocardial infarction. J Am Coll Cardiol 18:801, 1991.

83. Silva JA, Escobar A, Tyrone J, et al. A comparison of angioscopic findings between diabetic and nondiabetic patients. Circulation 92:1731, 1995.

84. Fein F. Heart disease in diabetes. Cardiovasc Rev Rep 3:877, 1982.

85. Barrett-Connor E, Orchard T. Insulin dependent diabetes mellitus and ischemic heart disease. Diabetes Care 8:65, 1985.

86. Moise A, Theroux P, Taigmans Y, et al. Unstable angina and progression of coronary atherosclerosis. N Engl J Med 309:685, 1983.

87. Ambrose JA, Winters SL, Arora RR, et al. Angiographic evolution of coronary artery morphol-

ogy in unstable angina. J Am Coll Cardiol 7:472, 1986.

88. Chen L, Chester MR, Redwood S, et al. Angiographic stenosis progression and coronary events in patients with "stabilized" unstable angina. Circulation 91:2319, 1995.

89. Ambrose JA, Hjemdahl-Monsen C, Borrico S, et al. Quantitative and qualitative effects of intracoronary steptokinase in unstable angina and non-Q wave myocardial infarction. J Am Coll Cardiol 9:1156, 1987.

90. Topol EJ, Nicklas JM, Kander NH, et al. Coronary revascularization after intravenous tissue plasminogen activator for unstable angina pectoris: Results of a randomized, double blind, placebo controlled trial. Am J Cardiol 62:368, 1988.

91. DeZwaan C, Bar FW, Janssen JHA, et al. Effects of thrombolytic therapy in unstable angina: Clinical and angiographic results. J Am Coll Cardiol 12:301, 1988.

92. Gold HK, Johns JA, Leinbach RC, et al. A randomized, blinded, placebo-controlled trial of recombinant human tissue-type plasminogen activator in patients with unstable angina pectoris. Circulation 75:1192, 1987.

93. Vetrovec GW, Leinbach RC, Gold HK, Cowley MJ. Intracoronary thrombolysis in syndromes of unstable ischemia: Angiographic and clinical results. Am Heart J 104:946, 1982.

94. Gotoh K, Minamino R, Katoh O, et al. The role of intracoronary thrombus in unstable angina: Angiographic assessment and thrombolytic therapy during ongoing angina attacks. Circulation 77:526, 1988.

95. Bar FW, Verheugt FW, Col J, et al. Thrombolysis in patients with unstable angina improves the angiographic but not the clinical outcome: Results of UNASEM, a multicenter, randomized, placebo-controlled, clinical trial with anistreplase. Circulation 86:131, 1992.

96. The TIMI III Investigators. Early effects of tissue-type plasminogen activator added to conventional therapy on the culprit coronary lesion in patients presenting with ischemic cardiac pain at rest. Results of the Thrombolysis in Myocardial Ischemia (TIMI IIIA) Trial. Circulation 87:38, 1993.

97. The TIMI III Investigators. Effects of tissue plasminogen activator and a comparison of early invasive and conservative strategies in unstable angina and non-Q wave myocardial infarction. Results of the TIMI IIIB Trial. Thromobolysis in Myocardial Ischemia. Circulation 89:1545, 1994.

98. Waters D, Lam JY. Is thrombolytic therapy striking out in unstable angina? Circulation 86:1642, 1992.

99. Ouimet TP, McCans J. Aspirin, heparin, or both to treat acute unstable angina. N Engl J Med 319:1105, 1988.

100. Lewis HD, Davis JW, Archibald DG. Protective effects of aspirin against acute myocardial infarction and death in men with unstable angina: Results of a Veterans Administration cooperative study. N Engl J Med 309:396, 1983.

101. Cairns JA, Gent M, Senger J. Aspirin, sulfinpyrazone, or both in unstable angina: Results of a Canadian multicenter trial. N Engl J Med 1985:1369.

102. Telford AM, Wilson C. Trial of heparin versus atenolol in prevention of myocardial infarction in intermediate coronary syndrome. Lancet 1:1225, 1981.

103. Willerson JT, Casscells W. Thrombin inhibitors in unstable angina: Rebound or continuation of angina after argatroban withdrawal? J Am Coll Cardiol 21:1048, 1993.

104. Weitz JI, Hudoba M, Massel D, et al. Clot-bound thrombin is protected from inhibition by heparin-antithrombin III but is susceptible to inactivation by antithrombin III-independent inhibitors. J Clin Invest 86:385, 1990.

105. Hirsh J. Heparin. N Engl J Med 324:1565, 1991.

106. Maraganore JM, Bourdon P, Adelman B, et al. Heparin variability and resistance: Comparisons with a direct thrombin inhibitor. Circulation 86(Suppl. I):I386, 1992.

107. Topol EJ, Fuster V, Harrington RA, et al. Recombinant hirudin for unstable angina pectoris. A multicenter, randomized angiographic trial. Circulation 89:1557, 1994.

108. Cannon CP, Braunwald E. Hirudin: Initial results in acute myocardial infarction, unstable angina and angioplasty. J Am Coll Cardiol 25(Suppl.):30S, 1995.

109. The Global Use of Strategies to Open Occluded Coronary Arteries (GUSTO IIA) Investigators. A randomized trial of intravenous heparin versus recombinant hirudin for acute coronary syndromes. Circulation 90:1631, 1994.

110. Fuchs J, Cannon CP, The TIMI 7 Investigators. Hirulog in the treatment of unstable angina: Results of the Thrombin Inhibition in Myocardial Ischemia (TIMI) 7 Trial. Circulation 92:727, 1995.

111. Neri Serneri GG, Gensini GF, Cinobali M, et al. Association between time of increased fibrinopeptide A levels in plasma and episodes of spontaneous angina: A controlled prospective study. Am Heart J 113:672, 1987.

112. Theroux P, Latour JG, Leger-Gauthier C, Lara JD. Fibrinopeptide A and platelet factor levels in unstable angina pectoris. Circulation 75:156, 1987.

113. Yasu T, Oshima S, Imanishi M, et al. Effects of aspirin DL-lysine on thrombin generation in unstable angina pectoris. Am J Cardiol 71:1164, 1993.

114. Lam JYT, Latour JG, Lesperance J, Waters D. Plate-

let aggregation, coronary artery disease progression and future coronary artery events. Am J Cardiol 73:333, 1994.

115. Coller BS, Anderson KM, Weisman HF. Inhibitors of platelet aggregation: GP IIb/IIIa antagonists. In Braunwald E (ed). Heart Disease (Update). Philadelphia: WB, Saunders, 1995:4.

116. Simoons ML, Jan de Boer M, van den Brand MJBM. Randomized trial of a GPIIb/IIIa platelet receptor blocker in refractory unstable angina. Circulation 89:596, 1994.

117. The EPIC Investigators. Use of a monoclonal antibody directed against the platelet glycoprotein Iib/IIIa receptor in high risk coronary angioplasty. N Engl J Med 330:956, 1994.

118. Topol EJ, Califf RM, Weisman HF, et al. for the EPIC Investigators. Randomized trial of coronary intervention with antibody against platelet IIb/IIIa integrin for reduction of restenosis results at six months. Lancet 343:881, 1994.

119. Tcheng JE, Ellis SG, Kleiman NS, et al. Outcome of patients treated with GPIIb/IIIa inhibitor integrelin during coronary angioplasty: Results of the IMPACT study. Circulation 88(Suppl. II):II595, 1993.

120. Gibson RS. Clinical, functional and angiographic distinctions between Q wave and non-Q wave myocardial infarction: Evidence of spontaneous reperfusion and implications for intervention trials. Circulation 75(Suppl. V):V128, 1987.

121. Braunwald E. Acute myocardial infarction — The value of being prepared. N Engl J Med 34:51, 1996.

122. Huey BL, Gheorghiade M, Crampton RS, et al. Acute non-Q wave myocardial infarction associated with early ST segment elevation: Evidence for spontaneous coronary reperfusion and implications for thrombolytic trials. J Am Coll Cardiol 9:18, 1987.

123. Ambrose JA, Hjemdahl-Monsen CE, Borrico S, et al. Angiographic demonstration of a common link between unstable angina pectoris and non-Q wave acute myocardial infarction. Am J Cardiol 61:244, 1988.

124. DeWood MA, Stifter WF, Simpson CS, et al. Coronary arteriographic findings soon after non-Q wave myocardial infarction. N Engl J Med 315:417, 1986.

125. Rivera W, Sharaf BL, Miele NJ, et al. Coronary anatomy in patients who present with non-Q wave myocardial infarction differs from unstable angina pectoris: A report from TIMI 3B. Circulation 90: I-438, 1994.

126. Davies MJ. Thrombosis and coronary atherosclerosis. In Julian D, Kubler W, Norris RM, Swan HJC, Collen D, Verstraete M (eds). Thrombolysis in Cardiovascular Disease. New York: Marcel Dekker, 1989:25.

127. GISSI (Gruppo Italiano per lo Studio della Streptochinasi nell' Infarcto Miocardico): Effectiveness of intravenous thrombolytic treatment in acute myocardial infarction. Lancet 1:397, 1986.

128. ISIS-2 (Second International Study of Infarct Survival) Collaborative Group: Randomised trial on intravenous streptokinase, oral aspirin, both, or neither among 17,187 cases of suspected acute myocardial infarction: ISIS-2. Lancet 2:349, 1988.

129. Wilhelmsen L, Svarsudd K, Korsan-Bengsten K, et al. Fibrinogen as a risk factor for stroke and myocardial infarction. N Engl J Med 311:501, 1984.

130. Meade TW, Mellows S, Brozovic M, et al. Haemostatic function and ischemic heart disease: Principal results of the Northwick Park Heart Study. Lancet 2:533, 1986.

131. Hawkins R. Smoking, platelets and thrombosis. Nature 236:450, 1972.

132. Ridker PM, Manson JE, Buring JE, et al. Circadian variation of acute myocardial infarction and the effect of low-dose aspirin in a randomized trial of physicians. Circulation 82:897, 1990.

133. Brexinski DA, Tofler GA, Muller JE, et al. Morning increase in platelet aggregability: Association with the assumption of the upright posture. Circulation 78:35, 1988.

134. Santamore WP, Yelton BW, Ogilby JD. Dynamics of coronary occlusion in the pathogenesis of myocardial infarction. J Am Coll Cardiol 18:1397, 1991.

135. DeWood MA, Spores J, Notske RN, et al. Prevalence of total coronary occlusion during the early hours of transmural myocardial infarction. N Engl J Med 303:897, 1980.

136. Verstraete M, Bory M, Collen D, et al. Randomized trial of intravenous recombinant tissue-type plasminogen activator versus intavenous streptokinase in acute myocardial infarction. Lancet 1:842, 1985.

137. The TIMI Study Group. The thrombolysis in myocardial infarction (TIMI) trial. N Engl J Med 312:932, 1985.

138. Neuhaus KL for the GAUS Study Group. Intarvenous recombinant tissue plasminogen activator (rt-PA) and urokinase in acute myocardial infarction: Results of the German Activator Urokinase Study (GAUS). J Am Coll Cardiol 12:581, 1988.

139. Bonnier HJRM, Visser RF, Klomps HC, Hoffmann HJML, Dutch Invasive Reperfusion Study Group. Comparison of intravenous anisoylated plasminogen streptokinase activator complex and intracoronary streptokinase in acute myocardial infarction. Am J Cardiol 62:25, 1988.

140. Rentrop P, Blanke H, Karsch KR, et al. Selective intracoronary thrombolysis in acute myocardial infarction and unstable angina pectoris. Circulation 63:307, 1981.

141. Topol EJ. Thrombolysis. In Topol EJ (ed). Textbook of Interventional Cardiology. Philadelphia: WB Saunders, 1990:77.

142. The GUSTO Angiographic Investigators. The effects of tissue plasminogen activator, streptokinase, or both on coronary artery patency, ventricular function, and survival after acute myocardial infarction. N Engl J Med 329:1615, 1993.

143. Ambrose JA, Winters SL, Arora RR, et al. Coronary angiographic morphology in myocardial infarction: A link between the pathogenesis of unstable angina and myocardial infarction. J Am Coll Cardiol 6:1233, 1985.

144. Wilson RF, Holida MD, White CW. Quantitative angiographic morphology of coronary stenosis leading to myocardial infarction or unstable angina. Circulation 73:286, 1986.

145. Brown BG, Gallery CA, Badger RS, et al. Incomplete lysis of thrombus in the moderate underlying atherosclerotic lesion during intracoronary infusion of streptokinase for acute myocardial infarction: Quantitative angiographic observations. Circulation 73:653, 1986.

146. Davies SW, Marchant B, Lyons JP, et al. Coronary lesion morphology in acute myocardial infarction: Demonstration of early remodeling after streptokinase treatment. J Am Coll Cardiol 16:1079, 1990.

147. Veen G, Meijer A, Werter CJPJ, et al. Dynamic changes of culprit lesion morphology and severity after successful thrombolysis for acute myocardial infarction: An angiographic follow-up study. J Am Coll Cardiol 23:147A, 1994.

148. Davies SW, Marchant B, Lyons JP, et al. Irregular coronary lesion morphology after thrombolysis predicts early clinical instability. J Am Coll Cardiol 18:669, 1991.

149. Forrester JS, Litvack F, Grundfest W, Hickey A. A perspective of coronary disease seen through the arteries of living man. Circulation 75:505, 1987.

150. The TIMI Study Group. Comparison of invasive and conservative strategies following intravenous tissue plasminogen activator in acute myocardial infarction: Results of the thrombolysis in myocardial infarction (TIMI) II trial. N Engl J Med 320:618, 1989.

151. Topol EJ, Califf RM, George BS, et al. A randomized trial of immediate versus delayed elective angioplasty after intravenous tissue plasminogen activator in acute myocardial infarction. N Engl J Med 317:581, 1987.

152. Webster MWI, Cheseboro JH, Smith HC, et al. Myocardial infarction and coronary artery occlusion: A prospective 5-year angiographic study. J Am Coll Cardiol 15:218A, 1990.

153. Laffel GL, Braunwald E. Thrombolytic therapy. A new strategy for treatment of acute myocardial infarction. N Engl J Med 311:710, 1984.

154. Gruppo Italiano Per Lo Studio Della Sopravvivenza Nell Infarcto Miocardico: GISSI-2: A factorial randomized trial of alteplase versus streptokinase and heparin versus no heparin among 12,490 patients with acute myocardial infarction. Lancet 336:65, 1990.

155. The GUSTO Investigators: An international randomized trial comparing four thrombolytic strategies for acute myocardial infarction. N Engl J Med 329:673, 1993.

156. Cannon CP, McCabe CH, Henry TD, et al. A pilot trial of recombinant disulfatohirudin compared with heparin in conjunction with tissue-type plasminogen activator and aspirin for acute myocardial infarction: Results of the Thrombolysis in Myocardial Infarction (TIMI) 5 trial. J Am Coll Cardiol 23:993, 1994.

157. Neuhaus K-L, Niederer W, Wagner J, et al. HIT (Hirdin for the Improvement of Thrombolysis): Results of a dose escalation study (abstr). Circulation 88:I-292, 1993.

158. Lee LV, for the TIMI 6 Investigators. Initial experience with hirudin and streptokinase in acute myocardial infarction: Results of the TIMI 6 trial. Am J Cardiol 75:7, 1995.

159. Antman EM, for the TIMI 9A Investigators. Hirudin in acute myocardial infarction: Safety report from the Thrombolysis and Thrombin Inhibition in Myocardial Infarction (TIMI) 9A trial. Circulation 90:1624, 1994.

160. The Global Use of Strategies to Open Occluded Coronary Arteries (GUSTO) IIa Investigators. A randomized trial of intravenous heparin versus recombinant hirudin for acute coronary syndromes. Circulation 90:1631, 1994.

161. Neuhaus K-L, von Essen R, Tebbe U, et al. Safety observations from the pilot phase of a randomized trial: r-Hirudin for Improvement of Thrombolysis (HIT-III) Study. A study of the Arbeitsgemein-schaft Leitender, Kardiologischer Koinkenhausarzte (ALKK). Circulation 90:1638, 1994.

162. Langer A, Freeman MR, Armstrong PW. ST segment shift in unstable angina: Pathophysiology and association with coronary anatomy and hospital outcome. J Am Coll Cardiol 13:1495, 1989.

163. Davies MJ, Thomas A. Thrombosis and acute coronary lesions in sudden cardiac ischemic death. N Engl J Med 310:1137, 1984.

164. Warnes CA, Roberts WC. Sudden coronary death: Relation of amount and distribution of coronary narrowing at necropsy to previous symptoms of myocardial ischemia, left ventricular scarring and heart weight. Am J Cardiol 54:65, 1984.

165. Baroldi G, Falzi G, Mariani F. Sudden coronary death: A postmortem study in 208 selected cases compared to 97 "control" subjects. Am Heart J 98:20, 1979.

166. Davies MJ, Bland JM, Hangartner JRW, et al. Factors influencing the presence or absence of acute coro-

nary artery thrombi in sudden ischaemic death. Eur Heart J 10:203, 1989.

167. Roberts WC. Qualitative and quantitative comparison of amounts of narrowing by atherosclerotic plaques in the major epicardial coronary arteries at necropsy in sudden death, transmural acute myocardial infarction, transmural healed myocardial infarction and unstable angina pectoris. Am J Cardiol 64:324, 1989.

13. PLAQUE DISRUPTION AND THROMBOSIS: MODELS TO EVALUATE ACUTE CARDIOVASCULAR EVENTS

George S. Abela and Joel D. Eisenberg

Introduction

BACKGROUND

Although the concept of plaque disruption leading to arterial thrombosis is not novel, it was not accepted as a critical pathophysiologic event for many years. In fact, early publications suggested plaque disruption and thrombosis to be the mechanism underlying acute cardiovascular events [1–4]. A historical report in 1912 provides an example of acute plaque disruption and thrombosis that was demonstrated by an autopsy performed immediately after sudden death [1,5]. A subsequent report by Herrick of that event described an ulcerated atheromatous plaque extruding into the arterial lumen and a plugged coronary artery. Two decades ago, similar observations were made by DeWood et al. in patients undergoing coronary artery bypass surgery for acute myocardial infraction [6]. Subsequently, similar observations of intracoronary thrombi were made during cardiac catheterization of patients with acute myocardial infarction [7]. The advent of interventional diagnostic procedures allowed in vivo detection of the pathological processes. Coronary angioscopy could detect intra-arterial thrombi, and intravascular ultrasound (IVUS) could define arterial wall morphology [8–11].

MORPHOLOGIC EVIDENCE OF PLAQUE DISRUPTION AND THROMBOSIS IN HUMANS

In the early 1960s, Constantinides demonstrated in an autopsy study that the majority of plaques beneath a fresh thrombus were fissured and disrupted [12]. This report was not popularized because the teaching at that time did not emphasize the role of thrombosis in acute myocardial events. Subsequent work by Davies et al. has shown that the composition of plaques at increased risk for disruption had three distinct characteristics [13]. These included lipid accumulation in both the extracellular matrix and within the macrophages, a relatively low smooth muscle cell count, and an increase in the number of macrophages in lesions that had undergone disruption. Also, a thin collagenous caps was considered an important feature of vulnerable plaques. The common site of plaque disruption is often at the corners of the lesion, where inflammatory cells seem to aggregate [12,14–16].

Other mechanisms of plaque disruption and thrombosis have been proposed. These include the triggering by arterial vasospasm and intraplaque hemorrhage. In the presence of an eccentric plaque, vasospasm can cause asymmetric contraction of the arterial arterial wall. This can result in the building of stresses at the plaque–normal arterial wall interface, resulting in tears and/or the squeezing out of atheromatous material in an eruptive fashion. This has been compared to a "volcanic eruption," in which the plaque cap is torn and the gruel material is extruded into the arterial lumen [17,18].

The mechanism, proposed by Barger, suggests that hemorrhage from the vasa vasora into the plaque increases the intraplaque pressure, leading to disruption [19]. This is supported by evidence of increased numbers of vasa vasora in the vicinity of plaques. These vasa vasora are very fragile and often penetrate from the adventitia into the media of the arterial wall. While evidence from autopsy studies supports this finding of hemorrhage into the plaque, it is often a less common occurrence compared with those that appear to have only a tear without hemorrhage or an underlying inflammatory process.

It is likely that more than one mechanism or a combination thereof is responsible for plaque disruption and thrombosis. Epidemiologic data reveal a clustering of acute myocardial events in the early morning hours. Thus, a circadian rhythm for acute events may be related to sympathetic discharge and/or elevation in blood pressure [20]. Other triggers of acute myocardial events may be contributing to plaque disruption and thrombosis. At present, it is only possible to account for an associated trigger in less than 20% of acute events. Therefore, in order to understand the pathophysiology of plaque disruption and thrombosis, models could be a highly valuable source of information.

Bench Models of Plaque Disruption

The law of Laplace describes the basic physiologic conditions that determine stress (σ) on the arterial wall. This is derived from the product of arterial lumen radius (r in cm) and pressure (p in dynes/cm^2) divided by wall thickness (h in cm) as follows:

$$\sigma = \frac{p \cdot r}{h}.$$

Thus, a stenosis that reduces lumen radius and increases wall thickness paradoxically enhances arterial plaque stability [21].

To evaluate this scenario specifically for arteries with atherosclerotic plaque, Loree et al. used finite element analysis by computer modeling to demonstrate that plaque cap thickness and the underlying intramural lipid pool size can influence the stress developed at that site [22]. This was performed using two-dimensional cross sections of diseased vessels that were used to evaluate plaque morphology. The analysis compared biomechanical parameters from normal and diseased vessels and determined the stress distribution within the plaque at a mean lumen internal pressure of 110 mmHg.

Results demonstrated that if luminal area reduction was 70%, the maximum circumferencial stress normalized to 110 mmHg (σ_{max}/P) increased from 6.0 to 24.8 as the thickness of the lipid pool was increased from 38% to 54% of the plaque thickness. When the lipid pool thickness was constant, increasing the stenosis severity from 70% to 91% by increasing the fibrous cap thickness decreased the σ_{max}/P from 24.8 to 4.7. When no lipid pool was present and the stenosis severity was increased from 70% to 99%, σ_{max}/P decreased from 5.3 to 4.7. Thus, reducing the fibrous cap thickness dramatically increased peak circumferential stress in the plaque, whereas increasing the stenosis severity decreased peak stress in the plaque. Examples of the method are shown in the atherosclerotic rabbit arteries used as a model for disruption and thrombosis described later (Figure 13-1).

In another study Richardson et al. used computer modeling to demonstrate that the common sites of plaque disruption were the attachment sites of the plaque cap to the normal arterial wall. These sites were shown to constitute areas of high stress. This was especially the case in the presence of calcium or other stiff materials that produced a great local tensile stress differential with adjacent softer tissues [23].

However, to implicate blood pressure elevation as a trigger of plaque disruption in humans using these data required over a 10-fold elevation in the normal blood pressure levels. Thus, the likelihood for plaque disruption to be related only to mechanical stress is not great under normal or even abnormal physiologic

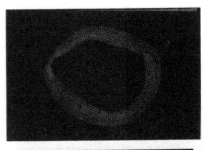

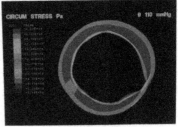

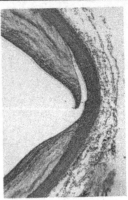

FIGURE 13-1. Finite element mesh of cross-sectional arterial specimen from atherosclerotic plaque in a rabbit aorta. **Top:** Diagram of the geometry of the arterial wall and plaque. Plane-strain elements are shown for the arterial wall and plaque. **Middle:** Contour map of the circumferential stress model (in Pascals). Maximum circumferential stress normalized by luminal pressure (σ_{max}/P) was greatest at 4 o'clock, as shown by the red markings of the circumferential stress key. **Bottom:** Corresponding cross section of atherosclerotic aorta stained with hematoxylin and eosin (Magnification ×40). (Reprinted courtesy of G. Abela.)

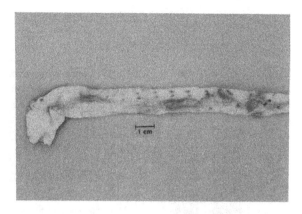

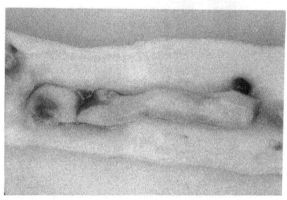

FIGURE 13-2. **Top:** Gross image of an atherosclerotic aorta with exposed intimal surface demonstrating four large platelet-rich thrombi. **Bottom:** Higher magnification of the platelet thrombi shown at the top. (Reprinted courtesy of G. Abela.)

blood pressure. Subsequent studies have demonstrated that degeneration of the fibrous plaque cap by enzymatic lysis may contribute to its mechanical instability. This was demonstrated by the higher concentration of inflammatory cells present at the disrupted sites [12,14,15]. Expression of metallothionen proteins and collagenases by macrophages may result in the lysis of the plaque cap [24]. Also, plaques that were disrupted often had fewer smooth muscle cells [25,26]. These data indicate that the plaque composition and metabolism may also contribute to its stability or vulnerability to disruption and thrombosis.

Animal Models of Plaque Disruption

RABBIT MODEL OF PLAQUE DISRUPTION AND THROMBOSIS

Constantinides and Chakravarti developed an atherosclerotic rabbit model to demonstrate the role of plaque disruption in the development of a platelet-rich thrombus [27–29]. Their hypothesis was that two basic elements, vasospasm and a prothrombotic state, would be necessary to induce plaque disruption and thrombosis. They pulse-fed rabbits with an atherogenic diet alternating with periods of normal chow. The rationale was that the artery would heal and scar to form a fibrous cap over a lipid pool, resembling the human lesions. Another advantage of the pulsed diet was that the rabbits seemed to survive longer because a large load of continuous lipid feeding resulted in fatty infiltration of the liver and death from hepatitis and starvation. Thus, rabbits that lived longer developed more advanced atherosclerotic lesions that were similar to those seen in humans. Similar results have been achieved using a low cholesterol content in rabbit feed for up to 5 years or more [30].

PHARMACOLOGIC TRIGGER

The trigger used to induce plaque disruption was a cocktail of pharmacological agents that simulated the conditions known to be associated with unstable syndromes in humans. The trigger was composed of

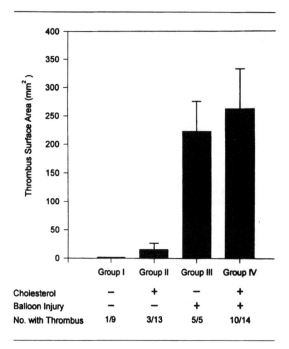

Cholesterol   −   +   −   +
Balloon Injury −   −   +   +
No. with Thrombus 1/9   3/13   5/5   10/14

FIGURE 13-3. Bar graph showing the percentage of arterial surface area covered by white thrombus. The greatest amount of thrombus was present in samples from groups III and IV, and the least in those from group I (error bars indicate SEM). (Reproduced with permission from the American Heart Association and the author.)

an injection of histamine, which induces vasoconstriction in rabbits [31]. The other agent was Russell's viper venom (RVV), which in the doses used has no direct platelet effects; however, it does act as a procoagulant, activating factor X and V [32]. In his model, Constantinides also injected calciferol in an attempt to enhance calcification and endothelial

injury, but this was subsequently discontinued. Constantinides tried several vasoconstrictor agents, including norepinephrine and vasopressin, with often less effective results [27]. Russell's viper venom and a vasoconstrictor agent used alone were not very effective in causing plaque disruption and thrombosis.

In order to develop a model of plaque disruption and thrombosis, Abela et al. [33] re-evaluated the atherosclerotic rabbit model. However, because the model required a long preparation time (over 1 year) and had a low yield of disruption and thrombosis (less than 50%), modifications were introduced to improve the outcome. This was evaluated by inducing different types of plaque in the rabbit. Thus, plaques were induced primarily in the thoracic and abdominal aorta (1) by a high cholesterol diet alone, (2) by mechanical balloon injury of the artery alone, or (3) by a combination of a high-cholesterol diet and balloon injury. Triggering was attempted by injection of RVV and histamine. This resulted in platelet-rich thrombi superimposed on focal plaque disruption (Figure 13-2).

A total of 41 New Zealand White (NZW) rabbits were exposed to one of four preparatory regimens; Group I (n = 9) was fed a regular diet for 8 months; group II (n = 13) was fed a diet of 1% cholesterol for 2 months, alternating with 2 months of a regular diet for a total of 8 months; group III (n = 5) underwent balloon-induced arterial wall injury, followed by a regular diet for 8 months; and group IV (n = 14) underwent balloon-induced arterial wall injury, and then received a diet of 1% cholesterol for 2 months, followed by a regular diet for 2 months, for a total of 4 months. Group IV was maintained for half the time (4 months) when compared with the other groups (8 months) in order to demonstrate that the modified rabbit model is more efficient and less costly.

TABLE 13-1.

Predominant group	Diet	Endothelial debridement	with thrombus/ no. triggered	Surface area (mm²) (mean ± SD)		Histology type[c]
				Thrombus	Plaque	
I	Reg[a]	No	1/9	2	0	0
II	Chol[b]	No	3/13	15 ± 19	1969 ± 699	1
III	Reg	Yes	5/5	223 ± 119	2209 ± 262	2
IV	Chol	Yes	10/14	263 ± 222	2366 ± 464	3

[a] Regular.
[b] 1% cholesterol.
[c] Histology types: 0 = normal artery; 1 = foamy plaque; 2 = fibromuscular plaque; 3 = mixed foamy and fibrous. (Reproduced with permission from the American Heart Association and the author)

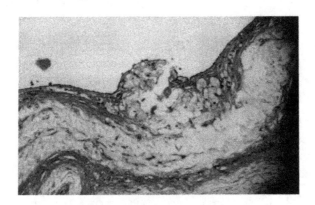

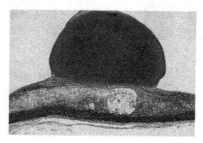

FIGURE 13-4. **Top:** Light micrograph from thoracic aorta of a rabbit in group II. An accumulation of macrophages forms a subintimal lesion. The foam cells appear to have a very thin cap, bulging into the lumen of the vessel (azocarmine-aniline blue, magnification ×50). **Bottom:** Light micrograph of large thrombus attached to the luminal surface of the thoracic aorta in rabbit from group IV. A cavitation is seen below the thrombus, and the intimal surface is markedly thinned (Masson's trichrome, magnification ×16). (Reproduced with permission from the American Heart Association and the author.)

After completion of the preparatory regimen, triggering of plaque disruption and thrombosis was attempted by injection of RVV (0.15 mg/kg, IP) and histamine (0.02 mg/kg, IV). In group I, normal control rabbits without atherosclerosis, only one small thrombus was noted in one of nine rabbits. In group II, cholesterol-fed rabbits, thrombosis occurred in 3 of 13 rabbits. Thrombus occurred in all rabbits in group III (5 of 5) and in 10 of 14 rabbits in group IV. Although the frequency of thrombosis was not significantly different between groups I and II, possibly due to a small sample size, it was significantly different among all four groups ($P < 0.001$). Also, the amount of thrombus formation was significantly different among all four groups ($P < 0.001$). Rabbits with atheromatous plaques (those in groups II and IV) demonstrated plaque disruption and an overlying platelet-rich thrombus formation similar to that observed in patients with acute coronary syndromes. The surface area covered by thrombus was 2 mm^2 in group I, 15.3 ± 19.2 mm^2 in group II, 223 ± 119 mm^2 in group III, and 263 ± 222 mm^2 in group IV. Rabbits in groups III and IV had the greatest amount of thrombus, and this amount was significantly greater than in rabbits in groups I and II ($P < 0.001$ and $P < 0.03$, respectively; Figure 13-3).

Histologic analysis using light microscopy of plaque from the various groups demonstrated the following: normal vascular morphology in group I, predominance of foam cells in the intima in group II, fibromuscular plaque in group III, and muscular with predominantly foam cell infiltration in group IV (Table 13-1; Figure 13-4).

The distribution of plaque for each group is shown in Figure 13-5. Individual comparisons showed a larger amount of plaque in rabbits from groups III and IV than in those in group II ($P = 0.04$ and $P = 0.001$, respectively). Also, the total cholesterol content in the aortic tissue in group IV (16 ± 7.2 mg/g) was significantly greater than in group II (2.8 ± 1.6 mg/g; $P < 0.0001$). A significant but not high correlation ($r = 0.54$; $P < 0.05$) was found between the amount of cholesterol in the arterial tissue and the amount of thrombosis that developed in the two

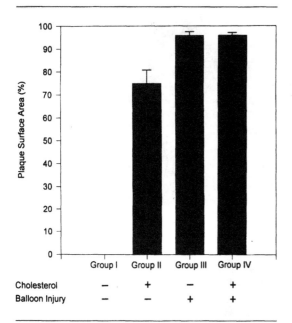

FIGURE 13-5. Bar graph shows percent of surface area of abdominal aorta and iliac arteries covered by plaque as determined by video planimetry. Rabbits in group I had total absence of plaque, those in group II had an intermediate amount, and those in group II and IV had the greatest amount of plaque (error bars indicate SEM). (Reproduced with permission from the American Heart Association and the author.)

groups. Also, coronary occlusions occurred in the majority of rabbits. These were induced by platelet-rich thrombi in intermediate-size arteries (10–20 μm in diameter; Figure 13-6). Other organ systems, including the kidney and lung, were examined for infarction and vascular thrombosis, but these were not detected.

Endothelial dysfunction was shown to occur in rabbits during triggering of plaque disruption (Abela and Myiamoto, unpublished). The role of endothelial function and integrity is currently being assessed in the setting of acute myocardial infarction in humans. Evaluation of endothelial function was tested after administration of RVV intraperitoneally at 24 and 48 hours prior to sacrifice in 5 NZW rabbits. Carotid, iliac, and femoral arteries isolated from rabbits with and without RVV were mounted in a perfusion chamber with constant flow at 60 mmHg. Vascular responses to norepinephrine (NE, 1–3 μM), acetylcholine (AC, 5 μM), and nitroprusside (SN, 5 μM) were monitored and measured using a video-computerized system. Vasoreactivity to NE and SN was not significantly different between both arteries

exposed to RVV and untreated controls. However, vasodilatation to AC varied with the arterial site. RVV significantly impaired the endothelial function of iliac and femoral arteries. (Figure 13-7). Thus, endothelial function in arteries overlying atherosclerotic plaque could become severely impaired by RVV and enhance the potential for plaque disruption and thrombosis.

Studies to Prevent Plaque Disruption and Thrombosis

EFFECT OF ANTIOXIDANTS
In a preliminary study, 16 rabbits were prepared by feeding a 1% cholesterol diet and balloon endothelial injury. After 4 months, eight rabbits received β-carotene (30m/kg IV) 1 week prior to the pharmacological trigger described in the earlier study. The remaining eight did not receive β-carotene. Although, the mean surface area of thrombus (78.6 ± 38.9 vs. 50.3 ± 25.9) and the number of thrombi (5.0 ± 4.3 vs. 2.3 ± 1.3) were less in the β-carotene treated rabbits, these did not achieve statistically significance (Abela and Ma, unpublished). However, since there are variations between antioxidants in their effect on the atherosclerotic process, further investigations in this area may be warranted.

EFFECT OF ASPIRIN, A BETA BLOCKER, AND EPINEPHRINE
Other investigations were conducted using this model to evaluate the effects of aspirin, a beta blocker, and chronic administration of epinephrine on plaque disruption and thrombosis (Abela and Picon, unpublished). None of these interventions appeared to have an effect on plaque disruption. Aspirin and a beta blocker (esmolol) given prior to triggering did not result in a reduction of thrombi formed. Also, chronic administration of epinephrine given intravenously daily for 1 week prior to triggering did not influence the disruption event rate. These data suggest that vasoreactivity of the arterial wall may be the predominant factor in the model. The intravenous use of epinephrine may have a transient constrictor response, but in the absence of RVV would not lead to an event, as had already been shown by earlier work of Constantinides [25,26].

Other Models

The Folts model has been invaluable in assessing enhanced platelet deposition in dog and pig coronary

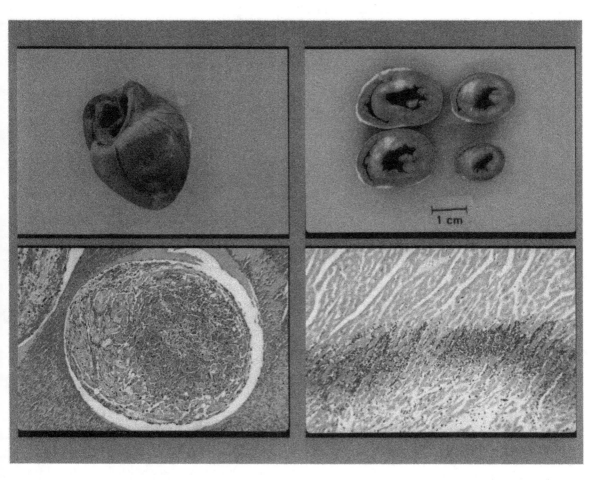

FIGURE 13-6. **Upper panels:** Gross image of heart with antero-apical and septal myocardial infarction 48 hours following triggering with RVV and histamine (triphenyltetrazolium chloride staining for viable myocardium). **Lower left:** Coronary artery (20 μm in diameter) with organizing platelet-rich occlusive thrombus (Masson's Trichrome stain; magnification 50×). **Lower Right:** Micrograph of infarct zone demonstrating early inflammatory cellular infiltration (dense blue line) following myocardial necrosis (hematoxylin and eosin; magnification 50×). (Courtesy of G. Abela.)

arteries; however, it requires both endothelial injury and the production of a high-grade stenosis [34]. The model provides a means of evaluating the interaction between platelets and the damaged arterial wall. The procedure is performed on the circumflex coronary artery in an anesthetized open-chest dog or pig. The artery is dissected and a flow probe is placed on it. Arterial injury is induced by a clamp distal to the flow probe. An encircling plastic cylinder is placed around the injured part of the artery to produce a high-grade stenois. Following this procedure, the flow in the vessel becomes cyclical due to the formation and immobilization of platelet thrombi in the injured and stenosed portion of the artery. Using various drugs that influence platelet activity, the cyclical flow can be improved (i.e., with aspirin) or worsened (i.e., with catecholamines). Thus, the model provides an method of evaluating and studying mechanisms that enhance or inhibit arterial thrombosis in injured or dysfunctional endothelium overlying stenosed arteries.

Badimon et al. developed a flow chamber to evaluate platelet deposition on activated arterial surfaces [35]. This system was used to study the influence of flow and shear stress on platelet deposition on selected biological surfaces. This was accomplished using an ex-vivo perfusion chamber system in which de-endothelialized pig aorta and collagen type I bundles from Achilles tendon were exposed to either

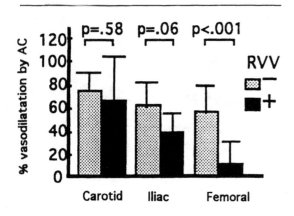

FIGURE 13-7. Bar graph displaying vasomotor response to acetylcholine in rabbit carotid arteries (n = 7 RVV, n = 6 control), iliac arteries (n = 6 RVV, n = 4 control), and femoral arteries (n = 8 RVV, n = 8 control). Shaded bars indicate the mean ± SD of control arteries, while black bars indicate arteries from rabbits treated with RVV. Results demonstrate that RVV significantly impairs vasomotor relaxation to acetylcholine in the iliac and femoral arteries. (Reprinted courtesy of G. Abela.)

native or heparinized pig blood. Flow rates were adjusted to provide shear rates of 106–3380/s. On de-endothelialized vessel wall, platelet deposition increased with exposure time and shear rate. At high shear rates and long exposures (over 10 minutes), platelet deposition decreased from maximal values, indicating embolization of platelets. Collagen from tendon continued to have progressive accumulation of platelet deposition. Deep arterial injury involving the media of the artery resulted in greater platelet deposition compared with more superficial injury limited to the intimal layer. This model provides a useful tool but has some limitations by being ex vivo.

Methods to Detect Vulnerable Plaques

ANGIOGRAPHY

The detection of vulnerable plaques could provide a means of testing and implementing a preventive management. Angiography, which is the most commonly used diagnostic technique to define coronary artery anatomy, cannot predict which atheroslcerotic lesions are most likely to undergo disruption and thrombosis [7,36]. Reports have demonstrated that vascular stenosis is not correlated with a predilection to develop a myocardial infarction. In fact, over 50%

of lesions that were angiographically measured as ≤50% stenosis were the ones that developed total vascular occlusion and myocardial infarction [18,36]. Thus, it is clear from these investigations that other diagnostic technologies were necessary to identify plaques that were vulnerable to disruption and thrombosis.

INTRAVASCULAR ULTRASOUND

Intravascular ultrasound (IVUS) provides imaging of the arterial wall morphology in vivo. Thus plaques with thin fibrous caps may be detected. The lesion morphology is displayed in cross-sectional views showing the fibrous caps overlying a lipid-rich core. IVUS has several advantages. It can be performed rapidly and safely in a blood-filled medium. The disadvantages of IVUS are its invasive nature and the limited resolution with a beam pulse width of 300 μm, which makes it difficult to detect plaques with thinner caps [37]. This could be important, given that the lesions with plaque cap thickness less than 300 μm are mechanically unstable [22].

ANGIOSCOPY

Angioscopy of the coronary arteries provides high-resolution images of the intimal surface of the arterial lumen. One important observation made recently was that plaques associated with unstable cardiovascular syndromes had a yellow color [9,38]. This led to a study by Myiamoto et al., which demonstrated that the yellow color was due to the reflection of yellow color of the lipid core of the plaque through a thin fibrous cap [39]. The hypothesis was that the plaque color was yellow because a thin cap was transparent to the yellow core of the lesion. In both an artificial model of plaque and subsequently in human plaque, a high correlation could be shown between the fibrous plaque thickness and yellow color saturation. This relationship was present if plaques caps were ≤300 μm (Figure 13-8). Greater plaque cap thickness had a white color. Coincidentally, a study by Loree et al. demonstrated that at a cap thickness of 300 μm biomechanical tests demonstrated that plaque cap fragility became markedly increased [22].

The advantages of angioscopy is that it provides a means of direct assessment of the pathological process. However, the disadvantage is its invasive nature, which also adds more time to the interventional procedure. Also, angioscopy involves interruption of blood flow and displacement of the blood column in the artery in order to visualize the plaque. This can intensify the ischemia and may induce ventricular arrhythmias.

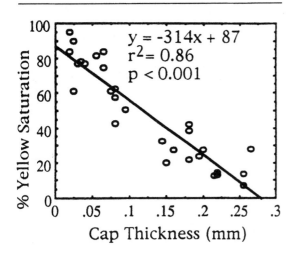

$$y = -314x + 87$$
$$r^2 = 0.86$$
$$p < 0.001$$

FIGURE 13-8. The relationship between the cap thickness and the percent yellow saturation of plaques is shown for plaques with caps $\leq 300\,\mu$m. There is a strong inverse correlation between these two variables. $r^2 = 0.86$; $y = -313X + 87$; $P = 0.0001$. (Reproduced with permission of SPIE and author.)

OTHER DIAGNOSTIC TECHNIQUES

Other techniques are being investigated for purposes of detecting vulnerable plaque. These include magnetic resonance, radiolabeled low-density lipoproteins (LDL), infrared, and fluorescence of plaque with a high lipid content. All of these approaches are currently investigational.

Magnetic resonance imaging (MRI), as a "biochemical imaging" tool, offers the potential to combine anatomic information in conjunction with plaque composition. Cholesterol-rich plaques exhibit a very short T2 (relaxation time of transverse magnetism) as compared with the triglyceride-rich adventitia. This was elegantly demonstrated by Toussaint et al. utilizing ex-vivo arterial segments [40]. These were imaged in a high field-strength (9.4 Tesla) magnet utilizing a fast spin echo technique to maximize the contrast between the cholesterol-rich pool and other arterial wall components.

The non-invasive nature of MRI lends itself to serial studies. Skinner and colleagues have demonstrated serial changes in the rabbit aorta, with fine detail [41,42]. Measurement of the thickness of the fibrous cap, combined with the area of the lipid pool, might afford an index of vulnerability. The limitation

of MRI, at present, is the field strength of the magnets now available at most centers (1.5 Tesla). Anatomic detail in adults, particularly in the coronary circulation, requires further improvements in resolution. However, surface coils with a higher field strength could be utilized in the carotid and peripheral circulations.

The concept of a radiolabeled accumulation of cholesterol and cholesterol esters preceding plaque disruption has led to an interest in measuring LDL flux in and out of lesions. The labeling of LDL with I-123 and performing subsequent scintigraphy to quantitate this flux offers the promise of noninvasive follow-up and monitoring of drug intervention [43].

Attention to inflammation as the final common pathway to plaque disruption has led to the potential of detecting differences in temperature within the plaque, as an index of increasing macrophage activity. Basic work with surgically explanted carotid lesions has confirmed this concept [44].

Ye and Abela used the same atherosclerotic rabbit model described earlier to demonstrate that β-carotene can be used to attenuate normal arterial wall fluorescence and to identify lipid-laden plaques. β-carotene, which is highly lipophilic, is preferentially absorbed into the plaque when compared with the normal surrounding intima [45]. This was demonstrated by a 17-fold attenuation of laser-induced fluorescence by plaque with β-carotene when compared with the surrounding normal artery. Also, in another study conducted in atherosclerotic plaque from human aorta, plaque with fissures had a significantly greater attenuation of fluorescence when compared with plaque with smooth, thick collagen caps [46].

In a preliminary study, an SERP-1 viral serine proteinase inhibitor with anti-inflammatory activity was used to reduce acute macrophage infiltration and plaque growth after balloon injury to the aortic wall in the rabbit model [47]. Laser-induced fluorescence (LIF) was used to detect early changes in the aortic wall after SERP-1 and balloon injury combined with a high-cholesterol diet. LIF spectra were recorded during 308-nm excitation. A significant decrease in normalized LIF emission intensity was detected in SERP-1–treated aorta. This was correlated with the fatty plaque content in the aorta. Thus LIF may be useful in the assessment of the arterial wall for detection of macrophage-rich atherosclerotic plaques.

Future improvements in technology will allow for improved imaging of the anatomic detail of atherosclerotic plaques with intracoronary ultrasound and MRI. Thus, data on plaque morphology, complimented by biochemical information from radiolabeled techniques, fluorescence, and/or MRI, could provide us with more clues about the behavior of atherosclerotic plaques.

References

1. Herrick JB. Clinical features of sudden obstruction of the coronary arteries. JAMA 59:2015, 1912.
2. Chapman I. Morphogenesis of occluding coronary artery thrombosis. Arch Pathol 80:256, 1965.
3. Friedman M, van den Bovenkamp GJ. The pathogenesis of a coronary thrombus. Am J Pathol 80:19, 1966.
4. Constantinides P. Plaque fissures in human coronary thrombosis. J Atheroscler Res 6:1, 1966.
5. Falk E. Why do plaques rupture? Circulation 86(Suppl. III):III30, 1992.
6. Dewood MA, Spores J, Notske R, Lowell T, et al. Prevalence of total coronary occlusion during the early hours of transmural myocardial infarction. N Engl J Med 303:897, 1980.
7. Ambrose JA, Winters SL, Arora RR, Eng A, et al. Angiographic evolution of coronary artery morphology in unstable angina. J Am Coll Cardiol 7:472, 1986.
8. Seeger JM, Abela GS. Angioscopy as an adjunct to arterial reconstructive surgery J Vasc Surg 4:315, 1986.
9. Mizuno K, Miyamoto A, Satomura K. Angioscopic coronary macromorphology in patients with acute coronary disorders. Lancet 337:809, 1991.
10. Sherman CT, Litvack F, Grundfest W, et al. Coronary angioscopy in patients with unstable angina pectoris. N Engl J Med 315:912, 1986.
11. Nissen SE, Gurley JC, Booth DC, et al. Differences in intravascular ultrasound plaque morphology in stable in and unstable patients (abstr). Circulation 84(Suppl. II):II436, 1991.
12. Constantinides P. Plaque fissures in human coronary thrombosis J Atheroscler Res 6:1, 1966.
13. Davies MJ, Richardson PD, Woolf N, Katz DR, et al. Risk of thrombosis in human atherosclerotic plaques: Role of extracellular lipid, macrophage, and smooth muscle cell count. Br Heart J 69:377, 1993.
14. Johannson L, Holm J, Skalli O, Bondjers G, Hansson GK. Regional accumulation of T cells, macrophages and smooth muscle cells in the human atherosclerotic plaque. Arteriosclerosis 6:131, 1986.
15. van der Wal A, Becker AE, Van der Loos C, Das PK. Site of intimal rupture or erosion of thrombosed coronary atherosclerotic plaques is characterized by an inflammatory process irrespective of the dominant plaque morphology. Circulation 89:36, 1994.
16. Li H, Cybulsky MI, Gimbrone MA, Libby P. An atherogenic diet rapidly induces VCAM-1, a cytokine-regulatable mononuclear leukocyte adhesion molecule, in rabbit aortic endothelium. Arterioscler Thromb 13:197, 1993.
17. Lin CS, Penha PD, Zak FG, Lin JC. Morphodynamic interpretation of acute coronary thrombosis, with special reference to volcano-like eruption of atheromatous plaque caused by coronary artery spasm. Angiology 39:535, 1988.
18. Nobuyoshi M, Tanaka M, Nosaka H, Kimura T, et al. Progression of coronary atherosclerosis: Is coronary spasm related to progression? J Am Coll Card 18:904, 1991.
19. Barger AC, Beeuwkes R III, Lainey LL, Silverman KJ. Hypothesis: Vasa vasorum and neovascularization of human coronary arteries. A possible role in the pathophysiology of atherosclerosis. N Engl J Med 310:175, 1984.
20. Muller JE, Tofler GH, Stone PH. Circadian variation and triggers of onset of acute cardiovascular disease. Circulation 79:733, 1989.
21. MacIssacs AI, Thomas JD, Topol EJ. Toward the quiescent coronary plaque. J Am Coll Cardiol 22:1228, 1993.
22. Loree HM, Kamm RD, Stringfellow RG, Lee RT. Effects of fibrous cap thickness on peak circumferential stress in model atherosclerotic vessels. Circ Res 71:850, 1992.
23. Richardson PD, Davies MJ, Born GVR. Influence of plaque configuration and stress distribution on fissuring of coronary atherosclerotic plaques. Lancet 2:941, 1989.
24. Childers JW, Stricklin GP. Increased immunostaining of collagenase and TIMP in eruptive xanthoma. Am J Med Sci 298:172, 1989.
25. Davies MJ, Wolf N, Katz DR. The role of endothelial denudation injury, plaque fissuring, and thrombosis in the progression of human atherosclerosis. In Weber PC, Leaf A (eds). Atherosclerosis: Its Pathogenesis and the Role of Cholesterol. New York: Raven Press, 1991:105.
26. Henney AM, Wakeley PR, Davies MJ, Foster K, et al. Localization of stromelysin gene expression in atherosclerotic plaques by in situ hybridization. Proc Natl Acad Sci USA 88:8154, 1991.
27. Constantinides P, Chakravarti RN. Rabbit arterial thrombosis production by systemic procedures. Arch Pathol 72:197, 1961.
28. Constantinides P. Experimental Atherosclerosis. New York Elsevier, 1965:25.
29. Constantinides P, Booth J, Carlson G. Production of advanced cholesterol atherosclerosis in the rabbit. Arch Pathol 70:80, 1960.
30. Wilson RB, Miller RA, Middleton CC, Kinden D. Atherosclerosis in rabbits fed a low cholesterol diet for five years. Arteriosclerosis 2:228, 1982.
31. Awano K, Mitsuhiro Y, Fukuzaki H. Role of serotonin, histamine and thromboxane A_2 in platelet-induced contractions of coronary arteries and aortae from rabbits. J Cardiovasc Pharm 13:781, 1989.
32. Warn-Cramer BJ, Rapaport SI. Studies of Factor Xa/phospholipid-induced intravascular coagulation in rabbits: Effects of immunodepletion of tissue factor

pathway inhibitor. Atheroscler Thromb 13:1551, 1993.

33. Abela GS, Picon PD, Friedl SE, Gebara O, et al. Triggering of plaque disruption and arterial thrombosis in an atherosclerotic rabbit model. Circulation 91:776, 1995.

34. Folts JD, Crowell EB, Bowe GG. Platelet aggregation in partially obstructed vessels and their elimination with aspirin. Circulation 54:365, 1976.

35. Badimon L, Badimon JJ, Galvez A, Chesebro JH, Fuster V. Influence of arterial damage and wall shear rate on platelet deposition: Ex vivo study in a swine model. Arteriosclerosis 6:312, 1986.

36. Little WC, Constantinescu M, Applegate RJ, Kutcher MA, et al. Can coronary angiography predict the site of a subsequent myocardial infarction in patients with mild-to-moderate coronary artery disease? Circulation 78:1157, 1988.

37. Nissen SE, Gurley JC, Booth DC, DeMaria AN. Intravascular ultrasound of the coronary arteries: Current applications and future directions. Am J Cardiol 69:18H, 1992.

38. Nesto RW, Sassower MA, Manzo KS, Byrnes CM. Angioscopic differentiation of culprit lesions in unstable versus stable coronary artery disease (abstr). J Am Coll Cardiol 21:195, 1993.

39. Miyamoto A, Friedl SE, Lin FC, Nesto RW, Abela GS. Plaque cap thickness can be detected by quantitative color analysis of angioscopic images in a plaque model, diagnostic and therapeutic cardiovascular interventions V (abstr). SPIE (Int Soc Optical Eng), 429:2395, 1995.

40. Tousaint J-F, Southern JF, Fuster V, Kantor HL. T2-weighted contrast for NMR charcterization of human atherosclerosis. Atheroscler Thromb Vasc Biol 15:1533, 1995.

41. Skinner MP, Yuan C, Mitsumori L, et al. Serial magnetic resonance imaging of experimental atherosclerosis detects lesion fine structure, progression and complications in vivo. Nature Med 1:69, 1995.

42. Yuan C, Skinner MP, Kareko E, et al. Magnetic resonance imaging to study lesions of atherosclerosis in the hyperlipidemic rabbit. Magn Reson Imaging 4:93, 1996.

43. Pirich C, Sinzinger H. ^{123}I-LDL scintigraphy in rabbits and humans. Ann N Y Acad Sci 748:613, 1995.

44. Casscells W, Hathorn B, David M, Krabach T, et al. Thermal detection of cellular infiltrates in living atherosclerotic plaques: Possible implications for plaque rupture and thrombosis. Lancet 347:1447, 1996.

45. Ye B, Abela GS. β-carotene enhances plaque detection by fluorescence attenuation in an atherosclerotic rabbit model. Lasers Surg Med 13:393, 1993.

46. Ye B, Abela GS. Beta carotene decreases total fluorescence from human arteries. Optic Eng 32:326, 1993.

47. Luu H, Dai E, Mah M, Liu L Laser-induced fluorescence (LIP): Detection of changes in atherosclerotic plaque after anti-inflammatory therapy in rabbits (abstr). Lasers Surg Med, (Suppl 9), 39:10, 1997.

14. DEVELOPING ANTITHROMBOTIC AND THROMBOLYTIC AGENTS: THE ROLE OF EXPERIMENTAL MODELS

Richard C. Becker

Introduction

Thrombosis is a common and unifying phenomenon among persons with atherosclerotic coronary artery disease and occurs typically at discrete sites of vascular injury, defined pathobiologically as foci of endothelial cell disruption or dysfunction and overt atheromatous plaque rupture. Over a century ago, Rudolf Virchow suggested the now classical triad of associated factors leading to pathological thrombosis: (1) stasis of blood flow, (2) abnormalities of the blood vessel wall, and (3) a procoagulant state. Accordingly, researchers and scientists over the years have developed experimental methods that apply one or more of these sacred tenants. Models have also been developed that can be used in the study of treatments for vascular thrombosis. The recent focus has been on antithrombotic and thrombolytic agents.

To study vascular thrombosis experimentally, it is essential that the thrombi produced are consistent and reproducible. Evaluation of experimental, preventive, and therapeutic measures also depends strongly on this methodological requirement. Furthermore, the reliability of each method and the conclusions drawn are influenced directly by the procedure used and in strictest terms, should be applied solely to thrombi produced by similar methods. This chapter covers an assemblage of experimental methods that have been used in the study and the development of antithrombotic and thrombolytic agents as they apply to vascular thrombosis in general and coronary arterial thrombosis in particular.

Venous Thrombosis Models

Early venous thrombosis models were based on Wessler's principle that combined stasis of blood flow with activation of the clotting system. The latter was

direct and included the injection of serum or serum products. The original Wessler model was as follows [1]: Dogs 18–23 kg in weight were anesthetized with Nembutal®, (pentobarbital). A segment of jugular vein 3–6 cm in length was freed from its surrounding structures and its tributaries were ligated. Canine serum from another animal (~100 cc) was infused through a distant antecubital vein. One minute later, the isolated jugular vein segment was clamped. A large red clot typically formed within 60 seconds.

More recent animal models have combined vascular injury as a physiologic activator of thrombosis with blood stasis; however, modifications of the original Wessler model still utilize injectable thrombogenic challenges, including thromboplastin, activated prothrombin complex concentrate, Russell's viper venom, and factor Xa [2]. The resulting thrombus is fibrin rich and can be graded visually on a scale of 0 to 4+ (4+ representing full thrombus formation without free erythrocytes).

Inferior Vena Cava Ligation Model

The inferior vena cava thrombosis model was developed for use in small animals and combined vascular injury and stasis [3]. Female Wistar rats (180–220 g) are anesthetized. Intravenous hypotonic saline (0.225% NaCl), 2 mL/200 g is then given via a femoral vein (right or left) to produce mild vascular injury. Approximately 1 minute later, the inferior vena cava, exposed through a midline abdominal incision, is isolated and a tight ligature is placed below the left renal vein. The abdominal cavity is closed, reopened 10 minutes latter, and the inferior vena cava is ligated 2 cm below the original ligature. After ligating major side branches, the isolated venous segment is resected and opened longitudinally in a Petri dish. The thrombus is removed with forceps and placed in a wet chamber/Petri dish containing saline-soaked filter paper. The thrombus is weighed 2 hours later.

The inferior vena cava thrombosis model has been used to investigate anticoagulants, thrombolytics, and antiplatelets agents. The test agent is typically administered intravenously through a cannulated femoral vein approximately 5 minutes before vascular injury is produced. Although an uncomplicated procedure, several potential limitations with this model have been recognized: (1) There is profound stimulation of coagulation when the peritoneal cavity is entered, (2) accessibility (of test drugs) to the thrombus is limited, (3) quantitation of antithrombotic and thrombolytic effects is difficult, and, (4) hypotonic saline-induced vascular injury is inconsistent.

Jugular Vein Thrombosis Model

Further developments and variations of the original Wessler model have yielded a simple, quantitative, and reproducible model that can be used to investigate thrombolytics and anticoagulants. Minimal surgical intervention is required, and the technical failure rate is less than 10% [4]. In most instances rabbits are used; however, models using other animals have been developed [5].

An external jugular vein from a New Zealand white rabbit (2–3 kg) is exposed through a 5-cm paramedical incision in the neck. The vein is then cleared over a distance of 4 cm up to the main bifurcation of the external jugular vein and the facial vein. Small venous side branches are ligated and the facial vein is cannulated with 10-cm tubing connected to a syringe. A woolen thread is then introduced in the jugular vein lumen over a distance of 4 cm with an ordinary needle. After bleeding has ceased, the vein is clamped proximally and distally to isolate a segment, which is then emptied of blood by gentle suction. The volume of the segment is measured by injection of saline from a volumetric syringe until the vessel is fully distended (Figure 14-1).

The procedure to form a venous clot is as follows: Approximately 10–20 μL of ^{125}I-labeled human fibrinogen (containing ~500,000 CMP) is aspirated in a 1.0-mL syringe followed by a volume of blood corresponding to the measured volume of the isolated vein segment. The jugular vein segment is then emptied by withdrawal of saline through the facial vein catheter and 0.1 thrombin (100 NIH units/mL) is quickly injected, followed immediately by the volume of blood containing the labeled fibrinogen. A thrombus usually forms quickly and is allowed to age for 30 minutes before both vessel clamps are removed.

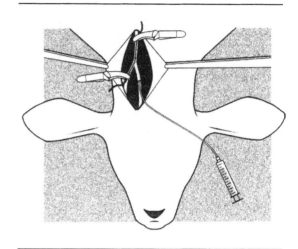

FIGURE 14-1. Jugular vein thrombosis model. The external jugular vein is exposed and the facial vein is cannulated. A woolen thread is introduced into the jugular vein lumen to serve as a nidus for clot formation. The vessel is then ligated proximally and distally. Thrombin is injected to initiate thrombosis (see the text).

Cotton swabs are generally placed over the vessel to absorb blood leaking from the vein segment.

A blood sample is drawn immediately after clamp removal to measure the radioactivity of blood. The cotton swabs are removed for isotope counting, and the amount of radioactivity delivered to the clot is calculated by subtracting the swab loses, the radioactivity remaining in the syringe, and the total blood radioactivity from the original amount of radioactivity in the syringe.

When thrombolytics are studied, an infusion is given through a 21-gauge butterfly needle placed in the contralateral marginal ear vein. After completion of the infusion, the thrombosed jugular vein segment is removed after careful suturing at both ends. The extent of thrombolysis is then calculated as the difference between the radioactivity originally incorporated in the clot and the radioactivity in the vein segment, expressed as a percentage of the original radioactivity.

Platelet-Rich Venous Thrombosis Model

A venous model that produces platelet-rich thrombosis has been described [6]. Male Wistar rats (150–250 g) are anesthestized with an intraperitoneal injection of pentobarbital (50 mg/kg). A longitudinal incision is made from the lower abdomen to the knees bilaterally, and the femoral arteries and veins are dissected from the surrounding tissues. A modified Acland vessel clamp is brought above the vessel and aligned parallel to the long axis of the femoral vein. The adventitia is grasped with microsurgical forceps, and the anterior wall is brought between the jaws of the clamp. The movable tip is rotated five times through 360° (90° clockwise, 180° counterclockwise, and 90° clockwise again, thereby rubbing the opposing endothelial surfaces of the vein against one another). A platelet-rich mural (nonobstructive) thrombus forms in the traumatized area that persists for 35 minutes. The platelet-rich venous thrombosis model can be used to investigate antiplatelet therapies as a prophylactic modality.

Pulmonary Embolism Model

Hamsters 6–8 weeks of age (body weight 80–100 g) are anesthetized with an intraperitoneal injection of 0.3 mL nembutal diluted to 20 mg/mL in saline. Atropine is given intravenously (50 µL of 0.25 mg/mL solution) to reduce oral secretions. A 3F femoral vein sheath is placed for blood sampling.

To create the pulmonary embolism, 6000 µL of fresh-frozen plasma (human), 10 µL of ^{125}I-labeled fibrinogen (human), and 100 µL of a mixture consisting of bovine thrombin (10 NIH units/mL) and 0.5 M $CaCl_2$ are aspirated into an 8F catheter and incubated for 30 minutes at 37°C. The plasma clot is dislodged, washed for 30 minutes in saline, and cut into 1-cm segments (total volume 50 µL), and the radioisotope content is measured (~0.1 µC per thrombus).

The radiolabeled clot is aspirated into a 6F catheter for injection. A jugular vein is exposed and the catheter containing the clot is introduced and advanced for 1 cm into the brachiocephalic vein, where it is injected. In approximately 85% of cases, the clot quickly embolizes to the lungs. The 6F catheter is then replaced with a 3F catheter through which 0.1 mL of sodium iodide solution (20 mg/mL) is injected, followed by a bolus of heparin (1000 U/kg).

Following thrombolytic or anticoagulant experiments, the animal is killed and the heart and lungs are removed for isotope counting. The extent of clot lysis is considered the difference between the radioactivity incorporated in the clot and the sum of residual activity in the heart and lungs. The pulmonary embolism model has several advantages: (1) There is a low failure rate, (2) it is reproducible, (3) limited surgical skill is required, (4) a small amount of drug (and other material) is used per experiment, and (5) up to 10 experiments can be performed daily.

Venous thrombosis models in general, and the rabbit jugular vein model in particular, are well suited for studying thrombolytics and anticoagulants because of the fibrin-rich thrombus that is produced. Both class of drugs have a fairly predictable dose–response to fibrin, erythrocyte-rich whole-blood clots.

Arterial Thrombosis Models

Arterial thrombosis has several unique features, particularly when it occurs in the coronary circulation. Typically, there is endothelial cell injury and dysfunction that significantly alter physiologic thromboresistance. In addition, alterations in blood flow velocity and shearing forces occur, increasing the interaction of circulating cellular components (predominantly platelets) with the vessel wall. The resulting thrombus is characterized by a high density of platelets and fibrin (with the former predominating). Accordingly, experimental models of arterial thrombosis have been developed in an attempt to reproduce, as closely as possible, the unique anatomical, topographic, and physiologic findings of human atherosclerotic vascular disease. They have been valuable in the investigation and development of pharmacologic agents, particularly thrombolytics and adjunctive anticoagulants and platelets antagonists designed to improve thrombolytic efficacy and/or prevent arterial reocclusion.

There are several criteria for an arterial thrombosis model: (1) the technique should produce a fixed amount of coronary stenosis that can either be increased or decreased under controlled conditions, (2) the technique should produce a consistent amount or degree of intimal/medial damage, and (3) the rate and size of the developing thrombus should be predictable and quantitatible.

Endothelial Injury

Endothelial injury and cellular dysfunction are important components contributing greatly to the thrombotic process. Several experimental techniques that cause endothelial cell injury have been described, including external blunt trauma and internal mechanical trauma with foreign materials, laser, and balloon stretching. Unfortunately, none are capable of simulating the human condition perfectly and therein lies a recognized limitation of experimental animal models [7,8].

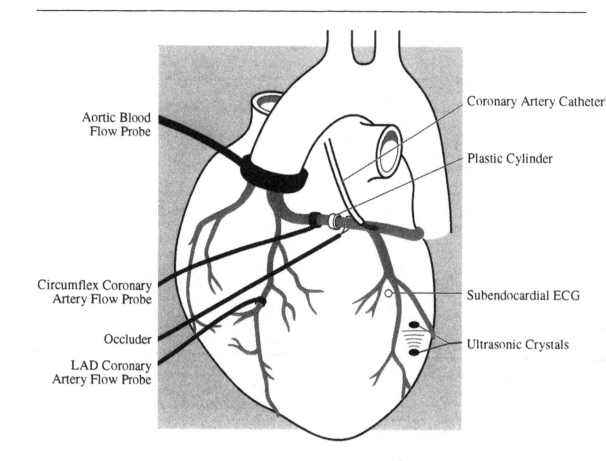

Aortic Blood
Flow Probe

Circumflex Coronary
Artery Flow Probe

Occluder

LAD Coronary
Artery Flow Probe

Coronary Artery Catheter

Plastic Cylinder

Subendocardial ECG

Ultrasonic Crystals

FIGURE 14-2. Coronary thrombosis with high-grade stenosis model. After isolating the coronary arteries (LAD and/or LCX), a plastic cylinder is placed around the vessel to produce a 60–70% internal diameter stenosis. Controlled intimal damage is achieved with surgical clamps. Typically blood flow declines rapidly and can be measured with a coronary artery flow probe. Electrical injury to the intima can be used in place of external trauma (see the text). LAD = left anterior descending coronary artery; LCX = left circumflex coronary artery.

Metallic Coil Arterial Thrombosis Model

More than two decades ago, Blair et al. [9] demonstrated that spiral wires constructed of aluminum-magnesium alloy inserted in the coronary circulation of dogs produced occlusive thrombosis. Several variations and modifications of the original description have since been used experimentally [10,11]. In brief, a thrombogenic coil is advanced via the left common carotid artery into a coronary artery with the aid of a hollow guide catheter or wire. An occlusive thrombus occurs within several minutes and is confirmed both electrocardiographically (injury pattern) and angiographically. Morphologically, the clots are fibrin rich and can be used to study thrombolytic agents [12–14] and anticoagulants [15]. A greater proportion of platelets can be achieved using a copper coil than aluminum-magnesium alloy, permitting investigation of adjunctive therapy and the prevention of reocclusion [16]. Unfortunately, death from ventricular fibrillation occurs in up to 20% of animals. A modification of the copper-coil model makes use of the femoral artery. In general, the thrombus forms more gradually (over 10–20 minutes) and is associated with fewer technical failures than the coronary artery model.

Coronary Thrombosis with High-Grade Stenosis Model

In 1974 Folts [17,18] described a model of repetitive thrombus formation in stenosed coronary arteries of

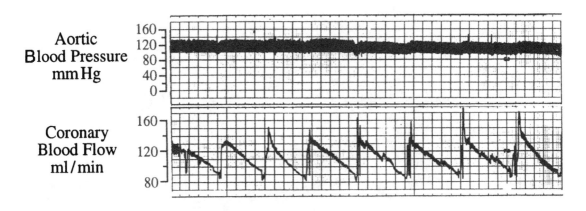

FIGURE 14-3. Simultaneous aortic blood pressure and coronary blood flow measurements. Cyclic flow reductions represent transient decreases in coronary blood flow from periodic platelet thrombus formation.

open-chest, anesthetized dogs. Rheological conditions required to produce turbulent flow and stasis on vessel narrowing dictated that the lumenal diameter be reduced by at least 50%.

The original model is as follows [19]: Adult mongrel dogs are premedicated with morphine sulfate (3 mg/kg) and anesthetized with sodium pentobarbital (20 mg/kg). Respirations are maintained with a positive pressure ventilator. The heart is exposed through a left thoracotomy in the fifth intercostal space and placed in a pericardial cradle. The left anterior descending (LAD) and/or left circumflex (LCX) coronary arteries are dissected out for 2–3 cm, and small side branches are ligated (septal branches of the LAD should be left intact).

An electromagnetic or ultrasonic flow meter probe of appropriate size is placed on the proximal coronary artery for measuring volume flow (mL/min) or flow velocity (cm/s). A controlled amount of intimal damage is produced with vascular clamps (typically 2–3 times over 4–5 seconds for each). A plastic cylinder (constrictor) 2–3 mm in length made from lexan rods, with a diameter that produces a 60–70% internal diameter stenosis of the coronary artery (the point where reactive hyperemia is abolished), is then placed just beyond the site of vessel injury (Figure 14-2).

After damaging and stenosing the coronary artery, blood flow declines rapidly, typically within 5–10 minutes. Blood flow can be restored by "flicking" the constrictor or by sliding the constrictor up and down the vessel to mechanically dislodge the thrombus. The cyclic blood flow seen is the result of intermittent

occlusive thrombus formation followed by restoration of flow as the thrombus is embolized (Figure 14-3). Typically the thrombus is platelet rich.

A variation of the Folt's model employs electrical injury rather than external trauma. Introduced by Salazar [20], a stimulation electrode is constructed from a 25- to 26-gauge stainless-steel hypodermic needle tip attached to a 30-gauge Teflon-insulated, silver-coated copper wire. Anodal current is delivered to the electrode via a 9-volt cadmium battery connected in series to a 250,000-ohm potentiometer. The cathode is placed in a subcutaneous site. The current is adjusted to deliver 50–200 µA, which causes focal endothelial cell disruption and a platelet-rich fibrin thrombus [21]. Thrombolytics, anticoagulants, and antiplatelet therapies can be studied [22–25]. As with other coronary arterial thrombosis models, infarct size and other related phenomena (e.g., reperfusion injury) can be investigated [26,27]. A major limiting factor associated with electrical injury is the potential for vasospasm [28].

The coronary stenosis and intimal damage procedures in other animals are similar to those described in dogs; however, pig coronary arteries are fragile, requiring a technical modification to produce high-grade stenosis. After the coronary artery has been dissected out, an oversized plastic cylinder is selected that decreases the vessel diameter by 20–30%. A conventional 2- to 2.5-mm angioplasty balloon on the end of a catheter is placed between the outside wall of the artery and the inside wall of the plastic cylinder. The balloon is gradually inflated to produce a 70–80% stenosis and to abolish reactive hyperemia (i.e., a critical stenosis; Figure 14-4). The carotid and femoral arteries of rabbits, cynomolgus monkeys, and rats can be used to produce intermittent platelet-rich

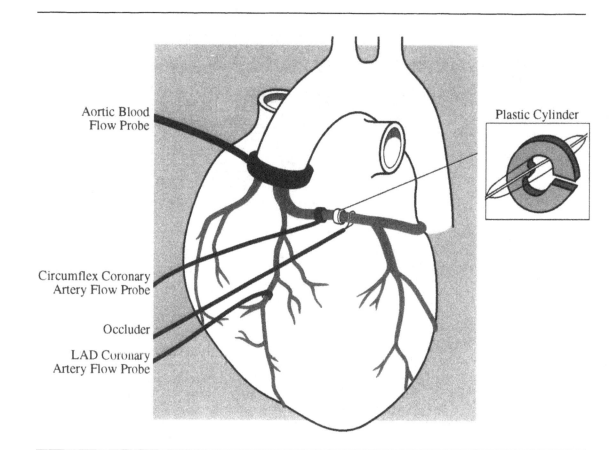

Aortic Blood
Flow Probe

Plastic Cylinder

Circumflex Coronary
Artery Flow Probe

Occluder

LAD Coronary
Artery Flow Probe

FIGURE 14-4. A variation of the Folt's model can be applied to swine. Because the coronary arteries are particularly fragile, an angioplasty balloon is placed between the vessel and the plastic cylinder. The degree of stenosis can be varied by inflating the balloon (see the text).

thrombotic occlusions and cyclic flow variations [29].

Overall, the Folts model is best suited for studying platelet antagonists [17,18,30–33], serotonin blocking agents [34], and possibly glycoprotein IIb/IIIa inhibitors. It has little use in the investigation of thrombolytics and anticoagulants. Its major advantage is the ability to reliably produce platelet-rich thrombi that intermittently recur over a 60-minute period, allowing dose-response studies and reasonable quantitation.

Canine Thrombosis with Endothelial Damage and High-Grade Stenosis

Adult mongrel dogs (10–25 kg) are anesthetized with pentobarbital (30 mg/kg IV), intubated, and placed on a respirator with tidal volumes between 10 and 15 mg/kg. Procainamide (1.5 g IM) and lidocaine (75 mg bolus, continuous infusion 1 mg/min IVs) are given to prevent lethal ventricular arrhythmias (ventricular fibrillation). The left carotid artery is exposed through a paramedial neck incision and is cannulated with a 7F modified amplatz coronary artery catheter, which is then guided into the ascending aorta.

The thorax is entered through the left fifth intercostal space, and the pericardium is opened to create a pericardial cradle. The left anterior descending coronary artery (LAD) is dissected out, and a 2.5-cm segment is isolated distal to the first diagonal branch. An ultrasonic flow probe is placed on the proximal LAD for continuous blood flow monitoring. Selective angiography is performed and 1 mL of blood is withdrawn for thrombus formation. The animal is given heparin 4000 U in an IV bolus, followed by 1000 U at 1-hour intervals. A 2-mm wide plastic wire tie is progressively constricted around the LAD, just distal to the proposed site of thrombus formation, to limit blood flow to 40 ± 10% of baseline.

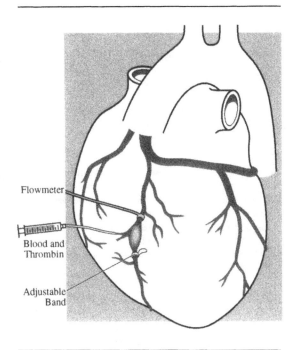

FIGURE 14-5. Coronary thrombosis with endothelial damage and high-grade stenosis. The isolated left anterior descending coronary artery (LAD) is traumatized by external compressions using blunt forceps. A whole blood–thrombin mixture is injected after both proximal and distal occlusion of the vessel. Beyond the site of endothelial damage, a high-grade stenosis is produced using an adjustable band (see the text).

The isolated LAD segment is traumatized by four consecutive external compressions using blunt forceps. Snare occlusions are made distal to the flow probe and proximal to the constriction site (Figure 14-5). Thrombin (0.1 mL of 100 U/mL) is mixed with 0.3 mL blood and injected through an LAD side branch after the LAD is emptied of blood by gentle aspiration. After 5 minutes, the proximal snare is released; 2 minutes later the distal snare is released. Selective angiography is performed 30 minutes later to confirm a stable occlusive thrombus.

When thrombolytic agents are studied, an intravenous infusion (via a femoral vein) is given followed by continuous flow probe monitoring and intermittent angiography over the subsequent 2 hours. Reperfusion is confirmed by a return of blood flow to >25% above baseline (at the time of occlusion) and complete angiographic filling of the vessel to the apex with rapid clearance of dye in less than four heart beats. Reocclusion is considered when flow is

reduced to <25%, with dye clearance requiring greater than five cycles. This model is particularly useful for studying thrombolytic and adjunctive therapies designed to prevent reocclusion [35,36]. The limiting features include the large amount of material and the technical skill required to complete each experiment.

Femoral Artery Thrombosis with Distal Stenosis

New Zealand white rabbits (2.2–4.0 kg) are anesthetized with pentobarbital (35 mg/kg, IV followed by 10 mg at 30- to 60-minute intervals) given through a cannulated marginal ear vein or femoral vein. The left femoral artery and vein are exposed under a surgical microscope. The left superficial epigastric artery is cannulated with a 23-gauge intracath, as is the right brachial artery (for continuous blood pressure monitoring). Blood flow in the left femoral artery is monitored continuously by an ultrasonic flow probe. A constriction (stenosis) is produced proximal to the flow probe using two 3.0 vicryl sutures. A 1-cm segment on the femoral artery is isolated using clamps placed proximal and distal to the superficial epigastric artery (Figure 14-6). The isolated segment is then emptied of blood by gentle suction. Endothelial injury is produced by blunt trauma using external compressions.

Bovine thrombin (0.05 mL Thrombinar, 5000 U per vial) and fresh blood (0.1 mL) taken from the femoral vein are mixed in a syringe and injected into the isolated segment. Approximately 10 minutes later, the proximal and distal clamps are released. An absence of flow is confirmed for 10 minutes. The femoral artery model produces a fibrin-rich thrombus that is useful for studying thrombolytics and anticoagulants.

Coronary Arterial Eversion Graft with Distal High-Grade Stenosis

Mongrel dogs are anesthetized with intravenous pentobarbital, intubated, and artificial ventilated. A left thoracotomy is performed and the left internal mammary artery is cannulated for continuous blood pressure monitoring. Procainamide (1.5 g IM) and lidocaine (75 mg IV bolus, 1 mg/min infusion) are given to prevent arrhythmic death. Heparin (4000 U IV bolus, 1000 U at hourly intervals) is infused via a cannulated femoral vein. An ultrasonic blood flow meter is placed around the left circumflex coronary artery proximal to the site of the eversion graft. A stenosis is then produced with a 2-mm wide plastic

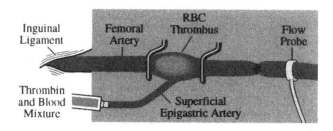

FIGURE 14-6. The femoral artery of small animals (example illustrated is a rabbit) can be used to produce an erythrocyte-rich clot. An isolated segment of artery is evacuated of blood, which is then mixed with thrombin and reinjected. A distal stenosis is produced using a ligature (see the text).

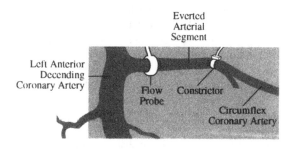

FIGURE 14-7. Platelet-rich thrombus model. An isolated segment of the left circumflex coronary artery (LCX) is surgically removed, everted "inside-out," and reinserted by end-to-end anastomosis. A constriction is placed distal to the reinserted vessel segment to produce a high-grade stenosis. The thrombus that forms after the reinitiation of blood flow is predominantly platelet rich (see the text).

reperfusion or adjunctively in the prevention of reocclusion [37,38]. In general, the thrombus is more platelet rich than those produced in standard blunt trauma/stenosis models and may, therefore, more closely simulate an environment similar to atherosclerotic plaque rupture. Accordingly, thrombolytic resistance and early reocclusion are common. Considerable effort, technical skill, and material are required with the coronary eversion model.

Femoral Artery Eversion Graft

A New Zealand white rabbit (2.2–3.4 kg) is anesthetized with pentobarbital (35 mg/kg IM, followed by 10-mg IV via the marginal ear vein or femoral vein at 30- to 60-minute intervals). The right brachial artery is cannulated with a 23-gauge intracath for continuous blood pressure monitoring. A groin incision is made to expose the femoral artery between the inguinal ligament and distal bifurcation. Small side branches are cauterized. The superficial epigastric artery is cannulated with Silastic tubing (0.012 in. i.d.) for intra-arterial infusion of study drug.

A 5-mm segment of the right femoral artery is excised between two ligatures, stripped of excessive adventitial tissue, everted inside out, and sutured "end-to-end" using 10–12 uninterrupted sutures (10–0 nylon). (The everted segment can also be anastomosed to the contralateral femoral artery.) The proximal and distal microvascular clamps are then released.

Coronary blood flow is monitored continuously by a flow probe placed on the proximal portion of the

wire tie placed around the coronary artery distal to the eversion graft and constricted to reduce blood flow to 40 ± 10% of baseline (typically >90% reduction in luminal diameter is required) (Figure 14-7).

The circumflex coronary artery is dissected from the epicardium. A 1-cm segment is excised between two microvascular clamps, stripped of excessive adventitial tissue, everted inside-out, and reinserted by end-to-end anastomosis using 8–12 interrupted sutures (7–0 nylon). The clamps are then released. Complete occlusion occurs 80% of the time within 5 minutes (decrease of blood flow to <0.5 mL/min, confirmed by angiography). Typically, a 30-minute period is required to document a stable clot before study drug administration.

The eversion graft produces a platelet-rich thrombus that can be used to investigate antiplatelet therapy and thrombolytics in the context of primary

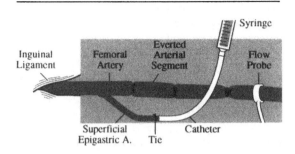

Syringe

Inguinal Ligament

Femoral Artery

Everted Arterial Segment

Flow Probe

Superficial Epigastric A.   Tie   Catheter

FIGURE 14-8. Platelet-rich thrombus can be produced using an everted arterial segment in the femoral artery. This model is particularly applicable in small animals, including rabbits (see the text).

vessel (Figure 14-8). The flow has decreased to <0.5 mL/min once occlusive thrombus is present. Approximately 70% of animals develop an occlusive thrombus within 15 minutes. If flow persists beyond this point, the vessel can be traumatized with blunt forceps. The study drug is typically given after the thrombus has remained stable for 20 minutes. The thrombus is platelet-rich, providing experimental conditions for investigating thrombolytics and antiplatelet strategies. Less technical skill and material are required for the rabbit femoral artery model when compared with canine coronary artery or femoral artery [39] models.

Rat Arteriovenous Shunt Model

Male Wistar rats (300–350 g) are anesthetized, and the trachea is cannulated to allow spontaneous breathing. The right jugular vein and left carotid artery are exposed and cannulated with polypropylene catheters (siliconized) 12 cm in length. A shunt is created by connecting the two catheters to a 3-cm piece of silicon tubing (i.d. 3 mm) containing a length of preweighted cotton thread. All tubes are filled with 3.8% trisodium citrate prior to establishing the circuit.

Once the loop has been created, the clamps on the two catheters are released and blood is allowed to flow. After 10 minutes, the vessel is clamped and the thrombus is removed and weighed. The catheters are flushed with 3.8% tri-sodium citrate to prevent clotting in the lines. A second thrombus can be produced by connecting the catheters to a newly placed silicon tube and allowing blood to flow for 10 minutes.

Thus, it is possible to form one control thrombus and another after study drug administration (by intravenous or subcutaneous administration). The thrombus produced is predominantly platelet rich but does contain an element of fibrin as well. This characteristic permits the experimental evaluation of antiplatelet agents and anticoagulants [40–42].

Nonhuman Primates

There are potential advantages to nonhuman primate models in the study of vascular disease. The baboon vascular anatomy has similarities to that of humans, and it is technically easier to work with than smaller animals. Platelet structure, concentration, kinetics, and function are also similar to humans, as are coagulation, fibrinolytic, and inhibitor proteins in plasma.

The vast experience with baboons is in the study of hemostasis [43–47], blood–vascular surface interactions [48–53], arteriovenous (AV) shunts [45,46], vascular grafts [49–53], and thrombosis. With the latter, exteriorized chronic AV shunts containing thrombogenic segments have been investigated most widely. Collagen-coated tubing, endarterectomized vessels, and prosthetic materials can be inserted to produce a thrombogenic nidus (Figure 14-9).

Juvenile male baboons (8–12 kg) are used for a majority of experiments. An AV shunt is placed surgically between the femoral artery and vein. The permanent shunt system consists of two 5-cm lengths of silicone rubber tubing (3.0 mm i.d.). Blood flow is established by connecting the two shunt segments and ranges from 150 to 250 mL/min. In general the shunt is useful for producing acute occlusive thrombosis that is resistant to heparin and aspirin (resistant thrombosis). The extent of thrombus is measured with scintillation camera imaging of autologous ^{111}In-labeled platelets or by measuring [121]I-labeled fibrinogen incorporated into the thrombus.

Endarterectomized Vascular Segments

Endarterectomized aortic segments are prepared from homologous baboon aorta that is flushed immediately with saline upon removal and divided into 3-cm lengths. Each segment is inverted and the intima is removed over a 1-cm length. It is then reverted back to a normal configuration, and each end is attached to flanged Teflon tubing. The entire vessel segment is encased with tubing before being placed in the externalized AV shunt system.

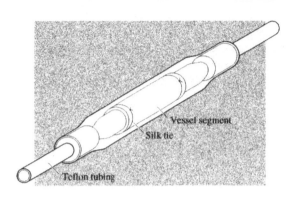

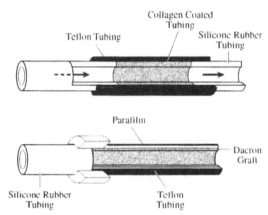

FIGURE 14-9. An exteriorized arteriovenous (AV) shunt containing various thrombogenic materials has been employed in primates to investigate thrombosis and its prevention and treatment. As illustrated, the vessel segment is cannulated at each end by Teflon tubing and secured with silk ties. Silicone rubber tubing can also be used (middle panel) to produce a smooth flow transition. The primate AV shunt model has been used to investigate the thrombogenic properties of Dacron grafts (lower panel). (From Schneider et al. J Vasc Surgery 11:365, 1990, with permission.)

Collagen-Coated Segments

Collagen-coated tubular segments are prepared using soluble type I collagen that is immobilized by crosslinking with glutaraldehyde. Before being placed in the externalized AV shunt, 2-cm segments of collagen-coated tubing are coated with silicone rubber as a butt joint using heat-shrink Teflon casing [54–56].

Dacron Graft Segments

The segments are prepared from externally supported uncrimped knitted Dacron, 5 cm long with a 4-mm internal diameter. Before placement in the AV shunt system, the grafts are rendered impervious to blood leakage by an external wrapping of Parafilm and are placed inside a 5-cm length of 5.3-mm i.d. heat-shrink Teflon tubing.

Biomaterial Tubular Segments

Several smooth-walled biomaterials, including polyurethane and acrylic or methacrylic polymers and copolymers, can be used in the externalized AV shunt system to induce platelet thrombus formation [45,46].

Thrombogenic Arteriovenous Flow Device

This model was developed to study the mechanisms of complex thrombus formation and to compare the relative effects of anticoagulants and antiplatelet agents [56]. A collagen-coated tube is connected to two expansion chambers exhibiting disturbed flow patterns. The proximal tubular segment (2 cm long × 4 mm i.d.) consists of knitted Dacron followed by a distal segment of expanded diameter composed of poly-tetrafluoroethylene tubing (2 cm long × 9.3 mm i.d.). The device is incorporated for 1 hour into an externalized AV shunt system under controlled blood flow (20 mL/min), maintained by a pump placed distal to the device. Collagen thrombi are platelet rich, while the thrombus within the chambers consists predominantly of fibrin and erythrocytes. This combination is reminiscent of thrombi developing at sites of plaque rupture platelet-rich preceded (head) and followed (tail) by erythrocyte-rich zones [57].

Carotid Endarterectomy Model

This model of vascular injury frequently results in reproducible platelet-rich occlusive thrombosis [58]. A midline incision is made exposing the common carotid artery, which is then dissected from surrounding tissues from the aortic arch to the bifurcation. After an intravenous heparin bolus (100 U/kg), the common carotid artery is occluded with vascular clamps and divided 1 cm proximal to the distal clamps. The proximal segment is everted to expose the luminal surface, which is then removed with microvascular forceps. The vessel is restored to its normal configuration, and an end-to-end anastomosis is performed. The clamps are removed and platelet deposition is measured continuously over 90 minutes with ^{111}In-labeled platelet imaging.

Femoral Arterial Injury with Stenosis

This model is based on the original Folt's model [19]; however, in baboons the superficial femoral artery is used because it is easily isolated and of appropriate size (3 mm i.d.). After focal injury is produced by vascular clamps, a stenosis is created at the injury site by placement of a 1-cm long silicone rubber cuff that reduces the luminal diameter to 60–80%. Mean flow rates are recorded continuously by a Doppler probe placed proximal to the stenosis. Predictable cyclic flow variations occur within several minutes [59,60].

Arterial Mural Thrombosis

Mural thrombosis can be studied in baboons with a surgically created iliac artery aneurysm [61]. A preclotted blind-end segment of Dacron vascular graft is anastomosed end-to-side with the right common iliac artery by surgical arteriotomy. Autologous ^{111}In-labeled platelet deposition is measured by serial scintillation camera imaging.

Flow Chambers

Over the past 10 years, it has been recognized that the complex events operating in arterial thrombogenesis are influenced by fluid flow. It is now also clear that the sequence of events involved with protein and cellular interactions with the vessel's surface influence changes in local flow conditions. An increased awareness and understanding of these relationships has fostered the development of flow chambers for experimental use. Flow chambers can be divided into two categories: (1) those in which the local effects are controlled at the solid–liquid interface (e.g., parallel plates, tubular systems, and annular chambers) and (2) those in which the entire fluid phase is subjected to uniform forces (e.g., viscometers of varying configuration).

Constant Shear Systems

Consider a fluid between two large, flat plates places parallel to one another and separated by a small distance. If the upper plate is set in motion (at constant velocity) while the lower plate is held stationary, a steady-state velocity gradient develops within the fluid. Knowing the velocity in the upper plate and the distance between the plates, one can calculate shear rate, shear stress, and fluid velocity.

Because the fluid between parallel plates is exposed to a uniform shear stress, the system is well suited for examining shear and effects on bulk fluid properties.

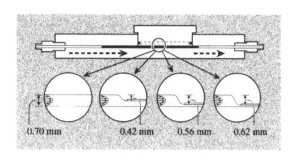

FIGURE 14-10. A parallel-plate perfusion chamber with eccentric stenosis model can be used to investigate thrombogenicity under high shear conditions. Longitudinal sections through the perfusion chamber are shown. The degree of stenosis and the blood flow rate determine the wall shear rates (see the text). (From Barstad et al. Arterioscler Thromb 14:1984, 1994, with permission.)

The same principles apply to cells or proteins suspended in the fluid, and, therefore, the system can also be used to investigate the effects of shear on physical characteristics or biologic functions. The constant-shear system has been particularly useful in understanding shear-induced platelet aggregation [62–68].

A parallel-plate perfusion system with an eccentric stenosis has also been described. The stenosis is introduced as an 18-mm long planar surface with a 0.5-mm cosine-shaped "step" on a coverslip holder that fits into the recess of the perfusion chamber. The extent of stenosis (reduction of cross-sectional area of the blood flow channel) can vary from 0% to nearly 90%. The depths of protrusion vary from 0.42 mm to 0.62 mm, corresponding to stenoses of 60% and 89%, respectively. This model is intended to simulate flow conditions in coronary arteries with advanced eccentric stenoses with a long axial dimension. The coverslip itself may contain collagen, endothelial cells, or extracellular matrix (Figure 14-10).

Variable Shear Devices

In a parallel system flow is produced by moving one plate while the other is kept stationary. In a variable shear system, the lateral ends of the plates are enclosed and flow is pressure driven in the axial direction (either by a pressure drop or a constant displacement pump). The variable shear system is useful for studying the effects of shear on mass exchange with a surface. It has been used extensively to study shear-rate–dependent platelet deposition on various materials and surfaces [69–72]. Variations of the

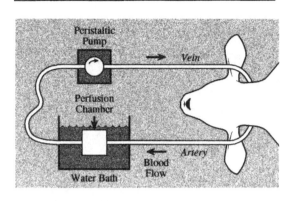

FIGURE 14-11. Schematic representation of a tubular flow chamber with recirculation. Substrate placed within the Plexiglas chamber is perfused continuously using a peristaltic pump. Platelet deposition and thrombus formation can be determined (see the text).

axial flow system, including cylindrical flow chambers and annular flow chambers, have been used extensively in the investigation of platelet and fibrin deposition on surfaces [73–75], the effect of shear on protein–cell interactions with endothelial surfaces, signal transduction, coagulation, and fibrinolysis [76–79].

Annular Flow Chamber

The experimental use of an annular flow chamber in an animal model is described [80]. New Zealand white rabbits (3–4 kg) are anesthetized with sodium pentobarbital (33 mg/kg IV). The right carotid and right femoral arteries, as well as the jugular veins, are dissected and cannulated using silicon eleastomer catheters. The perfusion experiments are started typically 5 minutes after the intravenous administration of study drug.

Native blood is circulated for 5–30 minutes from a carotid artery via silicone elastomer tubing through annular space formed by the outer cylinder of a perfusion chamber and a segment of de-endothelialized rabbit aorta mounted on a small plastic rod [81]. Blood is then returned to the circulation through tubing inserted in the jugular vein. Variable flow rates and chamber dimensions can be used to mimic venous and arterial blood flow conditions. The desired flow rate is controlled by a roller pump [82–84].

Immediately after the perfusion experiment, the vascular segmented (still mounted on the rod) is rinsed with phosphate-buffered saline and fixed with 2.5% glutaraldehyde. The rod with the segment is then removed from the chamber, postfixed with glutaraldehyde, and embedded in epoxy resin. Platelet and fibrin interactions are then quantitated using standard morphometry and computer-assisted morphometry.

Badimon Chamber

The Badimon perfusion chamber consists of a Plexiglas block (1.9 cm wide by 1.1 cm deep) through which a cylindrical hole (0.2 cm) is placed in the center. The upper face of the plastic block, parallel to the axis of the cylinder hole, is milled to create a trough (1.3 cm wide and 3 cm in length). Materials, either biologic (e.g., plaque components) or prosthetic, can be placed in the trough for study.

This model has typically utilized pigs because of their hematologic similarity to humans. A cannulated carotid artery is connected to the input of the perfusion chamber (maintained in a 37°C water bath), and the output is connected to a variable-speed perisystolic pump and finally to a cannulated jugular vein (Figure 14-11). Blood is allowed to pass through the chamber and over the test surface at a preselected flow rate and time. At the experiment's completion, buffer is perfused through the chamber for 30 seconds. Platelet deposition, fibrin formation, and thrombus characteristics can be assessed [85,86]. Variations of the Badimon perfusion chamber have been developed to include stenoses, allowing further (and potentially more physiologic) investigation of platelet adherence and aggregation [87].

Human Ex Vivo Perfusion System

Flow (of unanticoagulated blood) through a perfusion chamber can be directed from a cannulated antecubital vein by a pump placed distal to the chamber [88]. The venipuncture is performed with a #19 butterfly infusion set. The blood flows directly into the chamber at a constant rate (10 mL/min) and ultimately to a collecting chamber. The blood is not recirculated. Each experiment lasts 5 minutes, and the specimens are evaluated morphometrically. Perfusion chambers with differing geometric dimensions of the blood flow channel can be used to vary shear rates at the blood–surface interface.

The human ex vivo perfusion chamber permits experimentation using non-anticoagulated human blood. Human atherosclerotic materials can also be used, thereby avoiding the potential pitfalls of including materials from varying animals or species.

Plasma Systems

Although animal models and perfusion chambers have been developed to simulate physiologic events in humans, the activation of platelets, coagulation, and fibrinolysis in these experimental systems may alter the response to pharmacologic agents. In this regard, plasma systems can be useful. They may also permit the environment to be "controlled," allowing specific drug properties and effects to be investigated. The thrombus itself can be tailored to a variety of specifications, once again permitting specific hypothesis to be tested. Lastly, cost, materials, and technical skills are not a limiting feature, and many experiments can be performed in a brief period of time. An example follows [89].

To make fibrin clots, blood is collected into plastic syringes prefilled with 1/10 volume of 3.8% trisodium citrate. After thorough mixing, the red blood cells are sedimented by centrifugation at $1700 \times g$ for 15 minutes at $4°C$. The harvested plasma is supplemented with ^{125}I-labeled fibrinogen (approximately 100,000 cPM/ML), and 500 µL aliquots are transferred to polypropylene Eppendorf tubes. Labeled fibrin clots form around wire hooks by the addition of CaC_{12} (final concentration 225 mM). The clots are then aged for 60 minutes at $37°C$ and then washed three times with 1 mL aliquots of 0.1 M NaCl buffered with 0.05 m Tris-HCI (pH 7.4) over the course of 30 minutes. The washed clots are then counted for radioactivity over 1 minute.

In thrombolytic experiments, ^{125}I-labeled fibrin clots are incubated in aliquots containing a carefully chosen concentration of drug in fresh citrated plasma. The extent of thrombolysis can be calculated (quantitated) by measuring the radioactivity in residual clots after a set incubation period.

Acknowledgment

The author acknowledges the technical assistance of Clinton F. Becker in preparing this chapter.

References

1. Wessler S, Ward K, Ho C. Studies in intravascular coagulation III. The pathogenesis of serum-induced venous thrombosis. J Clin Invest 34:647, 1955.
2. Walenga LM, Petitou M, Lormeau JC, Samama M, Fareed J, Choay J. Antithrombotic activity of a synthetic heparin pentasaccharide in a rabbit stasis thrombosis model using different thrombogenic challenges. Thromb Res 46:187, 1987.
3. Hladovec J. A sensitive model of venous thrombosis in rats. Thromb Res 43:539, 1986.
4. Collen D, Stassen JM, Verstraete M. Thrombolysis with human extrinsic (tissue-type) plasminogen activator in rabbits with experimental jugular vein thrombosis. J Clin Invest 71:368, 1983.
5. Schaub RG, Simmons CA, Koets MH, Romano PJ, II, Stewart GJ. Early events in the formation of a venous thrombus following local trauma and stasis. Lab Invest 51:218, 1984.
6. Stockmans F, Deckmyn H, Gruwez J, Vermylen J, Acland R. Continuous quantitative monitoring of mural, platelet-dependent, thrombus kinetics in the crushed rat femoral vein. Haemostas Thromb 425, 1991.
7. Baumgartner HR. The role of blood flow in platelet adhesion, fibrin deposition, and formation of mural thrombi. Microvasc Res 5:167, 1973.
8. Weichert W, Breddin HK, Staubesand J. Application of a laser-induced endothelial injury model in the screening of antithrombotic drugs. Semin Thromb Hemost 14(Suppl.):106, 1988.
9. Blair E, Nygren E, Cowley RA. A spiral wire technique for producing gradually occlusive coronary thrombosis. J Thorac Cardiovasc Surgery 48:476, 1964.
10. Kordenat RK, Kezdi P. Experimental intracoronary thrombosis and selective in situ lysis by catheter technique. Am Heart J 83:360, 1972.
11. Bergmann SR, Fox KAA, Ter-Pogossian MM, Sobel BE, Collen D. Clot-selective coronary thrombolysis with tissue-type plasminogen activator. Science 220:1181, 1983.
12. Golino P, Ashton JH, Glas-Greenwalt P, McNatt J, Buja LM, Willerson JT. Mediation of reocclusion by thromboxane A_2 and serotonin after thrombolysis with tissue-type plasminogen activator in a canine preparation of coronary thrombosis. Circulation 77:678, 1988.
13. Bergmann SR, Lerch RA, Ludbrook PA, Welch MJ, Ter-Pogossian MM, Sobel BE. Temporal dependence of beneficial effects of coronary thrombolysis characterized by positron tomography. Am J Med 73:573, 1982.
14. Van der Werf F, Jang IK, Collen D. Thrombolysis with recombinant human single chain urokinase-type plasminogen activator (rscu-PA): Dose-response in dogs with coronary artery thrombosis. J Cardiovasc Pharmacol 9:91, 1987.
15. Cercek B, Lew AS, Hod H, Yano J, Reddy J, Reddy NKN, Ganz W. Enhancement of thrombolysis with tissue-type plasminogen activator by pretreatment with heparin. Am J Heart 74:583, 1986.
16. Shebuski RJ, Storer BL, Fujita T. Effect of thromboxane synthase inhibition on the thrombolytic action of tissue-type plasminogen activator in a rabbit model of peripheral arterial thrombosis. Thromb Res 52:381, 1988.
17. Folts JD, Crowell EB, Rowe GG. Platelet aggregation in partially obstructed coronary arteries and their inhibition with aspirin. Clin Res 22:595A, 1974.
18. Folt JD, Rowe GG. Cyclical reductions in coronary blood flow in coronary arteries with fixed partial obstruction and their inhibition with aspirin. Fed Proc 33:413, 1974.

19. Folts JD, Crowell EB, Rowe GG. Platelet aggregation in partially obstructed vessels and its elimination with aspirin. Circulation 54:365, 1976.
20. Salazar AE. Experimental myocardial infarction, induction of coronary thrombosis in the intact closed-chest dog. Circ Res 9:135, 1961.
21. Bush LR, Shebuski RJ. In vivo models of arterial thrombosis and thrombolysis. FASEB J 4:3087, 1990.
22. Shea MJ, Driscoll EM, Romson JL, Pitt B, Lucchesi BR. Effects of OKY 1581, a thromboxane synthetase inhibitor, on coronary thrombosis in the conscious dog. Eur J Pharmacol 105:285, 1984.
23. Simpson PJ, Smith JB Jr, Rosenthal G, Lucchesi BR. Reduction in the incidence of thrombosis by the thromboxane synthetase inhibitor CGS 13080 in a canine model of coronary artery injury. J Pharmacol Exp Ther 238:497, 1986.
24. Hook BG, Schumacher WA, Lee DL, Jolly SR, Lucchesi BR. Experimental coronary artery thrombosis in the absence of thromboxane A_2 synthesis: Evidence for alternate pathways for coronary thrombosis. J Cardiovasc Pharmacol 7:174, 1985.
25. Schumacher WA, Lucchesi BR. Effect of the thrmboxane synthetase inhibitor UK 37,248 (Dazoxiben) upon platelet aggregation, coronary artery thrombosis and vascular reactivity. J Pharmacol Exp Ther 227:790, 1983.
26. Haskel EJ, Prager NA, Sobel BE, Abendschein DR. Relative efficacy of antithrombin compaed with antiplatelet agents in accelerating coronary thrombolysis and preventing early reocclusion. Circulation 83:1048, 1991.
27. Fitzgerald DJ, Fitzgerald GA. Role of thrombin and thromboxane A_2 in reocclusion following coronary thrombolysis with tissue-type plasminogen activator. Proc Natl Acas Sci USA 86:7585, 1989.
28. Van der Giessen WJ, Harmsen E, de Tombe PP, Hugenholtz PG, Verdouw PD. Coronary thrombolysis with and without nifedipine in pigs. Basic Res Cardiol 83:258, 1988.
29. Bagdy D, Szabö G, Barabás É, Bajusz S. Inhibition of D-MePhe-Pro-Arg-H (GYKI-14766) of thrombus growth in experimental models of thrombosis. Thromb Haemost 68:125, 1992.
30. Folts JD. Experimental arterial platelet thrombosis, platelet inhibitors, and their possible clinical relevance: An update. Cardiovasc Res 6:10, 1990.
31. Folts JD, Hansing CE, Afonso S, Rowe GG. The systemic and coronary hemodynamic effects of ketamine in dogs. Br J Anaesth 47:686, 1975.
32. Folts JD. Inhibition of acute in vivo platelet thrombus formation with U-63557A, a thromboxane A_2 synthase inhibitor, but with renewal of thrombus formation with IV epinephrine. Circulation 74:II355, 1986.
33. Ashton JH, Golino P, McNatt JM, Buja LM, Willerson JT. Serotonin S_2 and thromboxane A_2-prostaglandin H_2 receptor blockades provide protection against epinephrine-induced cyclic flow variations in severely narrowed canine coronary arteries. J Am Coll Cardiol 13:755, 1989.
34. Torr S, Noble MIM, Folts JD. Inhibition of acute platelet thrombosis in stenosed canine coronary arteries by the specific serotonin S_2 receptor antagonist retanserin. Cardiovasc Res 26:465, 1990.
35. Yasuda T, Gold HK, Fallon JT, Leinbach RC, Garabedian HD, Guerrero JL, Collen D. A canine model of coronary artery thrombosis with superimposed high grade stenosis for the investigation of rethrombosis after thrombolysis. J Am Coll Cardiol 13:1409, 1989.
36. Eidt JF, Allison P, Noble S, Ashton J, Golino P, McNatt J, Buja LM, Willerson JT. Thrombin is an important mediator of platelet aggregation in stenosed canine coronary arteries with endothelial injury. J Clin Invest 84:18, 1989.
37. Yasuda T, Gold HK, Fallon JT, Leinbach RC, Guerrero JL, Scudder LE, Kanke M, Shealy D, Ross MJ, Collen D, Coller BS. Monoclonal antibody against the platelet glycoprotein (GP) IIb/IIIa receptor prevents coronary artery reocclusion after reperfusion with recombinant tissue-type plasminogen activator in dogs. J Clin Invest 81:1284, 1988.
38. Gold HK, Coller BS, Yasuda T, Saito T, Fallon JT, Guerrero JL, Leinbach RC, Ziskind AA, Collen D. Rapid and sustained coronary artery recanalization with combined bolus injection of recombinant tissue-type plasminogen activator and monoclonal antiplatelet GP IIb/IIIa antibody in a canine preparation. Circulation 77:670, 1988.
39. Collen D, Rong Lu H, Stassen J-M, Vreys I, Yasuda T, Bunting S, Gold HK. Antithrombotic effects and bleeding time prolongation with synthetic platelet GPIIb/IIIa inhibitors in animal models of platelet-mediated thrombosis. Thromb Haemost 71:95, 1994.
40. Tapparelli C, Metternich R, Gfeller P, Gafner B, Powling M. Antithrombotic activity in vivo of SDZ 217-766, a low-molecular weight thrombin inhibitor in comparison to heparin. Thromb Haemost 73:641, 1995.
41. Ardlie NG, Packham MA, Mustard JF. Adenosine diphosphate-induced platelet aggregation in suspension of washed rabbit platelets. Br J Pharmacol 19:7, 1970.
42. Peters RF, Lees CM, Mitchell KA, Tweed MF, Talbot MD, Wallis RB. The characterization of thrombus development in an improved model of arteriovenous shunt thrombosis in the rat and the effects of recombinant desulphatohirudin (CGP 39393), heparin, and iloprost. Thromb Haemost 65:268, 1991.
43. Hampton JW, Matthews C. Similarities between baboon and human blood clotting. J Appl Physiol 21:1713, 1966.
44. Todd ME, McDevitt EL, Goldsmith EI. Blood-clotting mechanisms of nonhuman primates: Choice of the baboon model to simulate man. J Med Primatol 1:132, 1972.
45. Harker LA, Hanson Sr. Experimental arterial throm-

boembolism in baboons: Mechanism, quantitation and pharmacologic prevention. J Clin Invest 64:559, 1979.

46. Hanson SR, Harker LA, Ratner BD, Hoffman AS. In vivo evaluation of artificial surfaces with a nonhuman primate model of arterial thrombosis. J Lab Clin Med 95:289, 1980.

47. Hanson SR, Reidy MA, Hattori A, Harker LA. Pharmacologic modification of acute vascular graft thrombosis. Scanning Electron Microsc 2:773, 1982.

48. Malpass TW, Hanson Sr, Savage B, Hessel EA II, Harker LA. Prevention of acquired transient plug formation? Blood 57:736, 1981.

49. Hanson SR, Kotze HF, Savage B, Harker LA. Platelet interactions with Dacron Vascular grafts. Arteriosclerosis 5:595, 1985.

50. Callow AD, Ledig CB, O'Donnell TF, Kelly JJ, Rosenthal D, Korwin S, Hatte C, Kahn PC, Vecchione JJ, Valeri CR. A primate model for the study of the interaction of ^{111}In-labeled baboon platelets with Dacron arterial prostheses. Ann Surg 191:363, 1980.

51. Clowes AW, Gown AM, Hanson SR, Reidy MA. Mechanisms of arterial graft failure: Role of cellular proliferation in early healing of PTFE prostheses. Am J Pathol 118:43, 1985.

52. Reidy MA, Chao SS, Kirman TR, Clowes AW. Endothelial regeneration: Chronic nondenuding injury in baboon vascular grafts. Am J Pathol 123:432, 1986.

53. Clowes AW, Kirman TR, Reidy MA. Mechanisms of arterial graft healing: Rapid transmural capillary ingrowth provides a source of intimal endothelium and smooth muscle in porous PTFE prostheses. Am J Pathol 123:220, 1986.

54. Kelly AB, Marzec UM, Krupski W, Bass A, Cadroy Y, Hanson SR, Harker LA. Hirudin interruption of heparin-resistant arterial thrombus formation in baboons. Blood 77:1006, 1991.

55. Schneider PA, Hanson SR, Price TM, Harker LA. Confluent durable endothelialization of endarterectomized baboon aorta by early attachment of cultured endothelial cells. J Vasc Surg 11:365, 1990.

56. Cadroy Y, Horrbett TA, Hanson SR. Discrimination between platelet-mediated and coagulation-mediated mechanisms in a model of complex thrombus formation in vivo. J Lab Clin Med 113:436, 1989.

57. Yokoyama T, Kelly AB, Marzec UM, Hanson SR, Kunitada S, Harker LA. Antithrombotic effects of orally active synthetic antagonist of activated factor X in nonhuman primates. Circulation 92:485, 1995.

58. Torem S, Schneider PA, Paxton LD, Yasuda H, Hanson SR. Factors' Influencing Acute Thrombsis Formation on carotid artery vascular ceragts. Trans Am Soc Artif Intern Organs 34:916, 1988.

59. Hanson SR, Pareti FI, Ruggeri ZM, Kunicki TJ, Montgomery RR, Zimmerman TS, Harker LA. Effects of monoclonal antibodies against the platelet glycoprotein IIb/IIIa complex on thrombosis and hemostasis in the baboon. J Clin Invest 81:149, 1988.

60. Hanson SR, Harker LA. Vascular graft thrombus formation. Ann N Y Acad Sci 516:653, 1987.

61. Hanson SR, Paxton LD, Harker LA. Iliac artery mural thrombus formation: Effect of antiplatelet therapy on ^{111}In-platelet deposition in baboons. Arteriosclerosis 6:511, 1986.

62. Moake JL, Turner NA, Stathopoulos NA, Nolasco LH, Hellums JD. Involvement of large plasma von Willebrand factor (vWF) multimers and unusually large vWF forms derived from endothelial cells in shear stress-induced platelet aggregation. J Clin Invest 78:1456, 1986.

63. Peterson DM, Stathopoulos NA, Giorgio TD, Hellums JD, Moake JL. Shear-induced platelet aggregation requires von Willebrand factor and platelet membrane glycoproteins Ib and IIb–IIIa. Blood 69:625, 1987.

64. Moake JL, Turner NA, Stathopoulos NA, Nolasco LH, Hellums JD. Shear-induced platelet aggregation can be mediated by vWF released by platelets, as well as exogenous large or unusually large vWF multimers, requires adenosine diphosphate, and is resistant to aspirin. Blood 71:1366, 1988.

65. Ikeda Y, Murata M, Araki Y, Watanabe K, Ando Y, Itagaki I, Mori Y, Ichitani M, Sakai K. Importance of fibrinogen and platelet membrane glycoprotein IIb/IIa in shear-induced platelet aggregation. Thromb Res 51:157, 1988.

66. O'Brien JR. Shear-induced platelet aggregation. Lancet 335:711, 1990.

67. Ikeda Y, Handa M, Kawano K, Kamata T, Murata M, Araki Y, Anbo H, Kawai Y, Watanabe K, Itagaki I, Sakai K, Ruggeri Z. The role of von Willebrand factor and fibrinogen in platelet aggregation under varying shear stress. J Clin Invest 87:1234, 1991.

68. Chow TW, Hellums JD, Moake JL, Kroll MH. Shear stress-induced von Willebrand factor binding to platelet glycoprotein Ib initiates calcium influx associated with aggregation. Blood 80:113, 1992.

69. Grabowski EF, Herther KK, Didisheim P. Human vs. dog platelet adhesion to Cuprophane under controlled conditions of whole blood flow. J Lab Clin Med 88:368, 1976.

70. Muggli R, Baumgartner HR, Tschopp TB, Keller H. Automated microdensitometry and protein assays as a measure for platelet adhesion and aggregation on collagen-coated slides under controlled flow conditions. J Lab Clin Med 95:195, 1980.

71. Sakariassen KS, Aarts PAMM, de Groot PG, Houdijk WPM, Sixma JJ. A perfusion chamber developed to investigate platelet interaction in flowing blood with human vessel wall cells, their extracellular matrix and purified components. J Lab Clin Med 102:522, 1983.

72. Sakariassen KS, Muggli R, Baumgartner HR. Growth and stability of thrombi in flowing citrated blood: Assessment of platelet surface interaction with computer-assisted morphometry. Thromb Haemost 60:392, 1988.

73. Turitto VT, Baumgartner HR. Platelet interaction with subendothelium in a perfusion system: Physical role of red blood cells. Microvasc Res 9:335, 1975.

74. Turitto VT, Baumgartner HR. Platelet interaction

with subendothelium in flowing rabbit blood: Effect of blood shear rate. Microvasc Res 17:38, 1979.

75. Turitto VT, Weiss HJ, Baumgartner HR. The effect of shear rate on platelet interaction with subendothelium exposed to citrated blood. Microvasc Res 19:352, 1980.

76. Badimon L, Badimon JJ. Mechanisms of arterial thrombosis in nonparallel streamlines: Platelet thrombi grow on the apex of stenotic severely injured vessel wall. J Clin Invest 84:1134, 1989.

77. Lassila R, Badimon JJ, Vallabhajosula S, Badimon L. Dynamic monitoring of platelet deposition on severely damaged vessel wall in flowing blood. Arteriosclerosis 10:306, 1990.

78. Barstad RM, Roald HE, Turitto VT, Cui W, Sakariassen KS. A novel perfusion chamber for the study of thrombus formation in flowing native human blood at the apex of artificially made stenoses. Submitted.

79. Schoephoerster RT, Oynes F, Nunez G, Kapadvanjwala M, Dewanjee MK. Effects of local geometry and fluid dynamics on regional platelet deposition on artificial surfaces. Arterioscler Thromb 13:1806, 1993.

80. Gast A, Tschopp TB, Baumgartner HR. Thrombin plays a key role in late platelet thrombus growth and/or stability. Effect of a specific thrombin inhibitor on thrombogenesis induced by aortic subendothelium exposed to flowing rabbit blood. Arterioscler Thromb 14:1466, 1994.

81. Baumgartner HR, Muggli R. Adhesion and aggregation: Morphological demonstration and quantification in vivo and in vitro. In Gordon JL (ed). Platelets in Biology and Pathology. Amsterdam: Elsevier/North Holland, 1976:23.

82. Weiss HJ, Turitto VT, Baumgartner HR. Effect of shear rate on platelet interaction with subendothelium in citrated and native blood, I: Shear dependent decrease of adhesion in von Willebrand's disease and the Bernard-Soulier syndrome. J Lab Clin Med 92:750, 1978.

83. Aarts PAMM, Van Broek JATM, Kulken GDC, Sixma JJ, Heethaar RM. Velocity profiles in annular perfusion chamber measured by laser-Doppler velocimetry. J Biomech 9:203, 1984.

84. Turitto VT, Baumgartner HR. Platelet-surface interactions. In Colman RW, Hirsh J, Marder VJ, Salzman EW (eds). Hemostasis and Thrombosis: Basic Principles and Clinical Practice, 2nd ed. Philadelphia: JB Lippincott, 1987:555.

85. Badimon L, Turitto V, Rosemark JA, Badimon JJ, Fuster V. Characterization of a tubular flow chamber for studying platelet interaction with biologic and prosthetic materials: Deposition of indium 111-labeled platelets on collagen, subendothelium, and expanded polytetrafluoroethylene. J Lab Clin Med 110:706, 1987.

86. Badimon L, Badimon JJ. Mechanisms of arterial thrombosis in nonparallel streamlines: Platelet thrombi grow on the apex of stenotic severely injured vessel wall. Experimental study in the pig model. J Clin Invest 84:1134, 1989.

87. Sakariassen KS, Aarts PAMM, de Groot PG, Houdijk WPM, Sixma JJ. A perfusion chamber developed to investigate platelet interaction in flowing blood with human vessel wall cells, their extracellular matrix, and purified components. J Lab Clin Med 1983:522.

88. Barstad RM, Roald HE, Cui Y, Turitto VT, Sakariassen KS. A perfusion chamber developed to investigate thrombus formation and shear profiles in flowing native human blood at the apex of well-defined stenoses. Arterioscler Thromb 14:1984, 1994.

89. Weitz JI, Kuint J, Leslie B, Hirsh J. Standard and low molecular weight heparin have no effect on tissue plasminogen activator induced plasma clot lysis or fibrinogenolysis. Thromb Haemost 65:541, 1991.

PART B: CLINICAL APPLICATION OF SCIENTIFIC PRINCIPLES

SECTION VI: THROMBOLYTIC AGENTS

Felicita Andreotti

Platelet and blood cells in thrombi are held together by a network of fibrin and fibrinogen molecules. Proteolysis of the fibrin/fibrinogen network leads to thrombus fragmentation and dissolution. Human blood contains enzyme systems that can dissolve fibrin: tissue-type and urinary-type plasminogen activators secreted in blood by endothelial cells convert plasminogen to the active fibrin/fibrinogen-digesting enzyme plasmin. These plasminogen activators represent a natural defense against thrombosis and have been developed by the pharmaceutical industry into the thrombolytic drugs alteplase and urokinase.

For most patients with heart attacks, alteplase and urokinase are effective in restoring complete coronary perfusion within 90 minutes of their administration. These drugs, however, can be neutralized by plasminogen activator inhibitors in the thrombus, are cleared from plasma in a few minutes, require continued intravenous administration, and are expensive.

The bacterial fibrinolytic enzymes, streptokinase and staphylokinase, have roughly similar efficacy compared with the human proteins, but may induce allergic reactions.

Chemical engineering has modified streptokinase into the acylated plasminogen-streptokinase complex APSAC, while genetic engineering of alteplase has produced the mutants reteplase and TNK-PA. Because these three substances have longer plasma half-lives than their bacterial or human ancestors, they can be administered as rapid intravenous injections. Recently, powerful fibrin-selective plasminogen activators have been isolated from the saliva of blood-feeding bats. Initial testing of bat-PA in patients is underway.

This Section comprehensively reviews the structure, function, and applications of thrombolytic agents in current use or under clinical investigation.

15. STREPTOKINASE: BIOCHEMISTRY AND PHAMACOKINETICS

H. Joost Kruik, Willemien J. Kollöffel, and Freek W.A. Verheugt

Introduction

Streptokinase, one of the first thrombolytic agents to be discovered, has now been used in many hundreds of thousands of patients with acute myocardial infarction. The drug was first discovered in 1933 by William Tillet, who called it *fibrolysin* [1], but only in 1947 were the first tests done on humans to lyse chronic thoracic empyemas, with considerable success. The intravenous administration of streptokinase was delayed because of difficulties in purifying the protein. In the 1960s, Behringwerke AG and Kabi Pharmacia made the drug available for widespread therapeutic use. The first trials using streptokinase in patients with acute myocardial infarction, published between 1978 and 1988, showed a significant survival benefit compared with conservative treatment or placebo [2–4].

Chemistry

Streptokinase is a bacterial protein produced by β-hemolytic streptococci (Lancefield type C). The 47,000–50,000 d protein consists of a single chain of 414 amino acids. It acts as a relatively non–fibrin-specific activator of endogenous plasminogen, although the protein itself has no intrinsic enzymatic activity [5]. It is commercially supplied as a lyophilized powder (Streptase®, Kabikinase®) for reconstitution in water, with a pH between 6.8 and 7.5. It is also available in complex with its target, plasminogen, in the form of anisoylated (lys) plasminogen-streptokinase activator complex (APSAC, anistreplase, Eminase®, discussed Chapter 16).

Dynamics

Streptokinase activates the fibrinolytic system indirectly, that is, only after binding to circulating plasminogen [6]. The complex formed has plasminogen activating properties. In a three-step mechanism, streptokinase first forms a noncovalent complex with plasminogen. After a transition within the complex,

it acquires plasminogen-activator activity [5]. In the presence of fibrin, a streptokinase–plasmin complex is rapidly formed, thereby causing lysis in the vicinity of the clot. However, in the absence of fibrin (i.e., in plasma), active complexes are also formed, although to a lesser degree, thereby causing a systemic *fibrinolytic state* [7]. The different rate of formation of the active complex in the presence or absence of fibrin, a property known as *fibrin specificity*, is the subject of some controversy.

When the fibrinolytic state occurs, blood viscosity tends to decrease, possibly because of depletion of plasma fibrinogen [7]. This effect may be advantageous in patients with acute myocardial infarction, even if coronary reperfusion has not been achieved. Because streptokinase is a bacterial protein, it is antigenic for the human body and elicits the production of antibodies that recognize, and therefore can inactivate, the drug when administered a second time.

Kinetics

The precise definition of the pharmacokinetics of streptokinase is difficult because different and not always suitable assays have been employed.

ABSORPTION

Streptokinase is given parenterally, for example, intravenously or by the intracoronary route. After oral or rectal administration in 30 patients, no evidence of absorption nor of increased fibrinolytic activity in plasma was found [8]. The intrapleural administration of streptokinase has been used for its local effects.

DISTRIBUTION

After infusion, streptokinase is rapidly distributed in plasma, like other proteins. The measured distribution volumes vary extensively among studies, mostly because of differences in the assays used. Grierson and Bjornsson [5] calculated the distribution volume to be as small as 1.1 L by measuring the activity of an amidolytic activator complex. This assay, however, does not distinguish between active and inactive fragments. In contrast, Gemmill et al. [9] found a larger volume of distribution, 5.7 L, comparable with that of plasma proteins. They used a functional assay that measures fibrinolytic activity on human fibrin plates and is probably more relevant to the clinical situation.

ELIMINATION

Using radiolabeled streptokinase, the plasma clearance of the drug is biphasic. The first phase, with a half-life of 11–17 minutes, is believed to be the result of clearance by antibodies. The second phase, with a half-life of approximately 85 minutes, is thought to be determined by a non–antibody-related mechanism, probably clearance by the reticuloendothelial system [10]. It is useful to point out that radiolabeling is a quantitative method that does not take into account the degradation of streptokinase into active and inactive fragments. Gemmill et al. [9] demonstrated an overall half-life of 37 minutes, based on a functional human fibrin plate lysis assay. In comparison, APSAC has a longer half-life of 67 minutes, probably related to the rate-limiting deacetylation step before it becomes active. The overall clearance of streptokinase is 7.1 L/h.

DOSAGE

Ideally, the dose and regimen of streptokinase should ensure a high early plasma concentration of the drug in order to overcome neutralizing antibodies and to achieve high initial fibrinolytic activity [9]. The elimination phase should be slow, allowing the maintenance of adequate concentrations for an appropriate length of time, thus minimizing early reocclusion of recanalized vessels. The current recommended dose of streptokinase in patients with acute myocardial infarction is 1.5 million units infused intravenously over 30–60 minutes.

Only few dose-finding studies have been carried out. The initial dose to overcome the neutralization by antibodies ranges from 25,000 to 1,500,000 units; a dose of 1,250,000 units is reported to be sufficient to neutralize antibodies in 97% of patients [11]. Dose-finding studies based on efficacy are rare. Six et al. [12] reported no significant difference in coronary reperfusion rates between doses of 750,000 units and 1,500,000 units. A possible advantage was shown with a dose of 3,000,000 units.

Efficacy in Patients with Acute Myocardial Infarction

The intravenous administration of streptokinase in patients with acute myocardial infarction has been tested in large randomized trials such as ISAM, GISSI-1, and ISIS-2. These studies have shown significant preservation of left ventricular function and significant survival benefit with streptokinase compared with placebo or conservative treatment [3,4,13].

In the ISAM trial, infarct size, as measured by serum creatinine kinase levels, was smaller, and left ventricular function, as assessed by angiographic ventricular ejection fraction, was better after streptokinase compared with placebo [13]. The GISSI-1 trial showed an overall 18% reduction in 21-day mortality when streptokinase was administered within 12 hours from the onset of symptoms: 10.7 deaths occurred per 100 streptokinase recipients versus 13 deaths per 100 controls [3]. If treatment was started earlier, the survival benefit was greater; for example, within 1 hour from the onset of symptoms, 8.2% of streptokinase-treated patients had died by 21 days versus 15.4% of controls [3]. The combination of streptokinase with aspirin, as used in the ISIS-2 trial, resulted in an even greater mortality reduction, with about 50 lives saved during the first 5 weeks per 1000 patients treated with streptokinase plus aspirin, versus about 30 lives saved by streptokinase alone, compared with placebo. The significant benefit of streptokinase and aspirin was maintained up to 1 year after treatment [4].

The angiographic arm of the GUSTO trial showed that patients receiving streptokinase, aspirin, and intravenous heparin had a 90-minute coronary patency rate of 60% (TIMI grade 2 or 3) and a 1-week reocclusion rate of 5.5% (from TIMI grade 2 or 3 at 90 minutes to grade 0 or 1 at follow-up) [14]. The corresponding values for patients allocated to the accelerated tissue plasminogen activator (t-PA) regimen were 81% and 5.9% [14]. Studies using intracoronary administrations of streptokinase have shown somewhat higher reperfusion rates compared with the intravenous route [15], but this advantage is hampered by the limited availability of emergency coronary angiography and by the delay of intracoronary access.

Adverse Events

The main adverse event with streptokinase use is the increased risk of bleeding from the cerebral or gastrointestinal circulation and at puncture sites. Other adverse events consist of allergic or anaphylactic reactions, for example, urticaria, bronchospasm, or shock. The incidence of allergic reactions is reported to be between 1.7% and 18% [16]. Serum-sickness–like reactions, such as Henoch-Schönlein purpura and transient proteinuria, have also been described [17]. Transient hypotension and occasional bradycardia, probably caused by bradykinins, have been reported. A lower infusion rate can overcome this reaction [7].

Another major drawback to the widespread use of streptokinase is that it is antigenic. Both previous administration of streptokinase and prior common streptococcal infections can lead to the formation of antibodies, which may neutralize the effects of the drug. Readministration of streptokinase is considered inappropriate between 5 days and 1 year after the initial treatment. A longer interval, of up to 4.5 years, has been reported for the prolonged presence of antibodies [18]. One possible solution would be to measure antibody titers before deciding whether to give streptokinase or another thrombolytic agent, such as alteplase, but this would be time consuming. The administration of corticosteroids does not prevent the appearance of antibodies or the previously mentioned allergic reactions [18].

Concomitant Antithrombotic Medications

Adjunctive therapies can have important effects on thrombolysis with streptokinase. ISIS-2 showed a marked survival benefit when aspirin was added to streptokinase: The odds reduction in vascular death at 35 days was about 20% with streptokinase and about 40% with the combination of streptokinase plus aspirin, compared with neither drug [4]. Therefore, aspirin is now a standard part of thrombolytic therapy. The addition of heparin is still under discussion because studies using adjunctive heparin in the presence of aspirin have shown a small positive effect on death and reinfarction rates, but also a significant increase in bleeding complications [19–21]. Compared with intravenous heparin, the addition of the specific antithrombin agent hirudin to streptokinase has shown unacceptable bleeding complications at higher doses [22] and no significant benefit for 30-day survival at lower doses [23,24]. An aggressive regimen, such as the combination of streptokinase with alteplase, investigated in the GUSTO-I study, failed to show improved short-term or 1-year survivals, or greater thrombolytic efficacy, compared with either t-PA or streptokinase [14,25].

References

1. Tillett WS, Garner RL. The fibrinolytic activity of streptococci. J Exp Med 58:485, 1933.
2. European Cooperative Study Group for Streptokinase Treatment in Acute Myocardial Infarction. Streptokinase in acute myocardial infarction. N Engl J Med 301:797, 1979.
3. Gruppo Italiano per lo Studio della Streptochinasi nell'Infarto miocardico (GISSI). Effectiveness of intravenous thrombolytic treatment in acute myocardial infarction. Lancet 1:397, 1986.
4. ISIS-2 (Second International Study of Infarct Survival) Collaborative Group. Randomised trial of intravenous streptokinase, oral aspirin, both, or neither among 17,187 cases of suspected acute myocardial infarction: ISIS-2. Lancet 2:349, 1988.
5. Grierson DS, Bjornsson TD. Pharmacokinetics of streptokinase in patients based on amidolytic activator complex activity. Clin Pharmacol Ther 41:304, 1987.
6. Peuhkurinen KJ, Risteli L, Melkko JT, Linnaluoto M, Jounela A, Risteli J. Thrombolytic therapy with streptokinase stimulates collagen breakdown. Circulation 83:1969, 1991.
7. Goa KL, Henwood JM, Stolz JF, Langley MS, Clissold SP. Intravenous streptokinase. A reappraisal of its therapeutic use in acute myocardial infarction. Drugs 39:693, 1990.
8. Oliven A, Gidron E. Orally and rectally administered streptokinase. Investigation of its absorption and activity. Pharmacology 22:135, 1981.
9. Gemmill JD, Hogg KJ, Burns JMA, Rae AP, Dunn FG, Fears R, et al. A comparison of the pharmacokinetic properties of streptokinase and anistreplase in acute myocardial infarction. Br J Clin Pharmacol 31:143, 1991.
10. Fletcher AP, Alkjaersig N, Sherry S. The clearance of heterologous protein from the circulation of normal and immunized man. J Clin Invest 37:1306, 1958.
11. Verstraete M, Vermylen J, Amery A, Vermylen C. Thrombolytic therapy with streptokinase using a standard dosage scheme. Br Med J 5485:454, 1966.
12. Six AJ, Louwerenburg HW, Braams R, Mechelse K, Mosterd WL, Bredero AC, et al. A double-blind randomized trial of intravenous streptokinase in acute myocardial infarction. Am J Cardiol 65:119, 1990.
13. The ISAM Study Group. A prospective trial of intravenous streptokinase in acute myocardial infarction (I.S.A.M.). Mortality, morbidity and infarct size at 21 days. N Engl J Med 314:1465, 1986.
14. The GUSTO Angiographic Investigators. The effects of tissue plasminogen activator, streptokinase, or both on coronary-artery patency, ventricular function, and survival after acute myocardial infarction. N Engl J Med 329:1615, 1993.
15. Rogers WJ, Mantle JA, Hood WP Jr, Baxley WA, Whitlow PL, Reeves RC, et al. Prospective randomized trial of intravenous and intracoronary streptokinase in acute myocardial infarction. Circulation 68:1051, 1983.
16. McGrath KG, Zeffren B, Alexander J, Kaplan K, Patterson R. Allergic reactions to streptokinase consistent with anaphylactic or antigen antibody complex mediated damage. J Allergy Clin Immunol 76:453, 1984.

17. Payne ST, Hosker HSR, Allen MB, Bradbury H, Page RL. Transient impairment of renal function after streptokinase treatment. Lancet 2:1398, 1989.

18. Lee HS, Cross S, Davidson R, Reid T, Jennings K. Raised levels of antistreptokinase antibody and neutralization titres from 4 days to 54 months after administration of streptokinase or anistreplase. Eur Heart J 14:84, 1993.

19. Gruppo Italiano per lo Studio della Streptochinasi nell'Infarto Miocardico. GISSI-2: Randomised trial of intravenous alteplase versus intravenous streptokinase in acute myocardial infarction. Lancet 336:65, 1990.

20. ISIS-3: A randomised comparison of streptokinase vs. tissue plasminogen activator vs. anistreplase and aspirin plus heparin vs. aspirin alone among 41,299 cases of suspected acute myocardial infarction. Lancet 339: 753, 1992.

21. Collins R, MacMahon S, Flather M, Baigent C, Remvig L, Mortensen S, et al. Clinical effects of anticoagulant therapy in suspected acute myocardial infarction: Systematic overview of randomised trials. Br Med J 313:652, 1996.

22. Antman EM, for the TIMI 9A Investigators. Hirudin in acute myocardial infarction: Safety report from the Thrombolysis and Thrombin Inhibition in Myocardial Infarction (TIMI)9A trial. Circulation 90:1624, 1994.

23. The Global Use of Strategies to Open Occluded Coronary Arteries (GUSTO) IIb Investigators. A comparison of recombinant hirudin with heparin for the treatment of acute coronary syndromes. N Engl J Med 335:775, 1996.

24. Andreotti F. The TIMI 9B and GUSTO IIb trials and the "thrombin hypothesis." J Thromb Thrombolys 1997, in press.

25. Califf RM, White HD, Van de Werf F, Sadowski Z, Armstrong PW, Vahanian A, et al. One-year results form the Global Utilization of Streptokinase and TPA for Occluded Coronary Arteries (GUSTO-I) trial. Circulation 94:1233, 1996.

16. ANISTREPLASE (ANISOYLATED PLASMINOGEN STREPTOKINASE ACTIVATOR COMPLEX, APSAC) IN CORONARY THROMBOLYSIS

David P. de Bono

Introduction

Anistreplase was introduced and developed as a thrombolytic agent for two reasons: first, the hope that it would act as a fibrin-selective agent and reduce the risks of hemorrhage associated with streptokinase; second, its pharmacokinetic properties, which allow it to be given as a single injection rather than an infusion. The first aspiration has not been fulfilled. The second property has, however, been very useful, particularly for prehospital fibrinolysis.

Pharmacology and Pharmacokinetics

The rationale for the design of anistreplase was the observation that streptokinase, when mixed with plasma, rapidly forms a noncovalent activation complex with plasminogen. The resulting conformational change facilitates plasminogen activation; at the same time, the complex is able to bind to fibrin, because of the kringle motifs in the plasminogen moiety. In anistreplase, the plasmin catalytic site is protected by acylation with an anisoyl group with a deacylation half-life, in vitro, of 105 minutes. The concept is that after injection in vivo, anistreplase will bind to fibrin in thrombi and only then will be activated by hydrolysis, leading to the formation of plasmin, which will activate other plasminogen molecules by cleavage of the $Arg^{561}-Val^{562}$ bond as well as cleavage of fibrin [1,2]. In vitro, anistreplase is more clot slective than streptokinase, but less so than tissue plasminogen activator (t-PA, alteplase).

After intravenous injection in humans, anistreplase is cleared from plasma with a half-life of approximately 90 minutes (compared with 20 minutes for streptokinase and 5 minutes for alteplase). Bolus ad-ministration of 10–30 units causes mild vasodilatation and hypotension, with a nadir at 5 minutes after administration [3]. These mild circulatory effects, together with the relatively long half-life, make it practice to administer the agent clinically as a slow intravenous injection over 4–5 minutes. Anistreplase is presented as a lyophilized powder that is dissolved in water for injection.

Clinical Studies

Virtually all clinical studies with anistreplase have been in the context of acute coronary thrombosis, although there have been anecdotal reports of use in other conditions, such as pulmonary embolism. Early clinical studies [3–6] evaluated anistreplase given by intracoronary or intravenous injection using angiographic coronary patency as the endpoint. On the basis of rather limited dose-ranging studies, a dose of 30 units (equivalent to 30mg or approximately 1.25×10^6 units of streptokinase) was identified for use in clinical outcome trials. This dose causes a similar decrease in plasma fibrinogen concentration, both in magnitude and time course, as that caused by 1.5×10^6 units of streptokinase. Coronary reperfusion rates of 51–62% were obtained in these early studies, but the confidence intervals were wide because of the small numbers.

The AIMS (APSAC Intervention Mortality Study) study [7,8] was a randomized, placebo-controlled trial of anistreplase, 30 units IV, in a relatively high-risk (presentation within 6 hours of marked ST changes) group of 1004 patients with myocardial infarction. Concomitant aspirin was not used, but patients received adjusted-dose intravenous heparin followed by warfarin. There was a marked reduction in 30-day mortality (12.1% with placebo, 6.4% with APSAC), and the trial was discontinued prematurely on the advice of the safety committee. One-year mortality was 17.8% with placebo and 11.4% with APSAC ($P = 0.0007$).

The ISIS-3 (Third International Study of Infarct Survival) Collaborative Group study [9] was a double-blind, mortality-endpoint, 3×2 factorial study in 41,299 patients, comparing streptokinase 1.5×10^6 units, anistreplase 30 units, and tissue plasminogen activator (duteplase) 0.6 MU/kg. All patients received aspirin; half were randomly allocated to receive subcutaneous calcium heparin, 12,500 units twice daily for 7 days or until prior discharge. Patients were eligible if they were thought to be within 24 hours of the onset of acute myocardial infarction. There were no significant differences in survival at 35 days with any of the six possible treatment combinations. Treatment with anistreplase (compared with streptokinase) was associated with significantly more "allergic" reactions (5.1% vs. 3.6%), more minor noncerebral bleeds (5.4% vs. 4.5%), and a slight excess of stroke (1.26% vs. 1.04%). The stroke excess was principally of early stroke due to cerebral hemorrhage. In comparison, duteplase was less likely than streptokinase to cause allergic reactions (0.8% vs. 3.6%), but more likely to cause stroke (1.39% vs. 1.04%).

The European Myocardial Infarction Project (EMIP) Group study [10] was a multicenter double-blind study in which 5469 patients with a clinical and electrocardiographic diagnosis of acute myocardial infarction were randomized within 6 hours of symptom onset to receive either anistreplase before admission followed by placebo in hospital, or vice versa. There was a nonsignificant trend toward reduced overall 30-day mortality (9.7% vs. 11.1%) in patients given anistreplase prior to hospital admission.

The GREAT (Grampian Region Early Anistreplase Trial) study [11,12] was also a randomized trial comparing the effects of domiciliary administration of anistreplase, followed by placebo after hospital admission, with domiciliary placebo followed by anistreplase in hospital. Three hundred and eleven patients with symptoms of infarction seen at home within 4 hours of symptom onset were randomized. By 3 months after trial entry, the relative reduction in risk of all-cause mortality in patients given anistreplase at home was 49% (difference, −7.6%; 95% CI, −14.7% to −0.4%; $P = 0.04$), and there was also a reduction in full-thickness Q-wave infarction. The difference in outcome between EMIP and GREAT may reflect the much greater difference in

time to thrombolysis between the two treatment arms in GREAT (approximately 140 minutes) compared with EMIP (55 minutes). Two angiographic endpoint studies [13,14] have compared coronary patency after anistreplase with that after "front-loaded" alteplase. In both cases alteplase appeared to give better early patency.

Adjunctive Therapy

For historical reasons, early clinical studies such as AIMS used anistreplase followed by intravenous heparin and then warfarin. In the Duke University Clinical Cardiology Study (DUCCS), 250 patients with acute myocardial infarction were treated with 30 units of anistreplase and were randomized to receive either 325 mg aspirin daily alone or aspirin plus heparin 15 IU/kg body weight per hour [15]. Clinical ischemic events and bleeding were monitored; angiography was performed after 5 days. Clinical and angiographic outcomes were similar, but the group randomized to heparin had more bleeding complications (32% vs. 17.2%; $P = 0.006$). In the Anticoagulation Following Thrombolysis with Eminase (AFTER) study of over 1000 patients, there was no clinical outcome difference in patients randomized to aspirin compared with those maintained on warfarin [16].

Safety

The safety profile of anistreplase is broadly similar to that of streptokinase. Overall bleeding complications in trials have been rather more frequent with anistreplase, but this partly reflects the more frequent use of heparin. In the ISIS-3 study (see earlier), in which the agents were used under comparable conditions, safety profiles were very similar.

Appraisal

Anistreplase is an effective agent for coronary thrombolysis. The direct comparison of different thrombolytics inevitably gives an arbitrary weighting to different criteria: Anistreplase is perceived as showing no advantage over streptokinase in terms of survival on the basis of the ISIS-3 study, which took no account of the particular suitability of anistreplase for very early, out-of-hospital administration. This was well demonstrated in the GREAT study, and even the underpowered EMIP trial showed a trend that, had it been confirmed in a trial of appropriate size, would have been comparable with the differences between agents shown in much larger trials such as GUSTO.

It is some consolation to those who have worked on anistreplase to know that a hemodynamically benign, long half-life agent that can be given as a single-bolus injection is now well recognized as a desirable aim in the design of third-generation thrombolytics [17,18].

References

1. Smith RAG, Dupe RJ, English PD, Green J. Thrombolysis with acyl enzymes: A new approach to thrombolytic therapy. Nature (Lond) 290:505, 1981.

2. Been M, de Bono DP, Muir AL, Boulton FE, Hillis WS, Hornung R. Coronary thrombolysis with intravenous anisoylated plasminogen streptokinase activator complex BRL 26921. Br Heart J 53:253, 1985.

3. Been M, de Bono DP, Muir AL, Boulton FE, Fears R, Standring R, Ferres H. Clinical effects and pharmacokinetics of intravenous APSAC (anisoylated plasminogen streptokinase activator complex, BRL26921) in acute myocardial infarction. Int J Cardiol 11:53, 1986.

4. Anderson JL, Rothbard RL, Hackworthy RA, et al. Multicenter reperfusion trial of intravenous anisoylated plasminogen streptokinase activator complex (APSAC) in acute myocardial infarction. Controlled comparison with intracoronary streptokinase. J Am Coll Cardiol 11:1153, 1988.

5. Bonnier HJRM, Visser RF, Klomps HC, Hoffman HJML, and the Dutch Invasive Reperfusion Study Group. Comparison of intravenous anisoylated plasminogen streptokinase activator complex and intracoronary streptokinase in acute myocardial infarction. Am J Cardiol 2:25, 1988.

6. Hogg KJ, Gemmill JD, Burns JMA, et al. Angiographic patency study of anistreplase versus streptokinase in acute myocardial infarction. Lancet 335:254, 1990.

7. AIMS Trial Study Group. Effects of intravenous APSAC on mortality after acute myocardial infarction. Preliminary report of a placebo-controlled clinical trial. Lancet 2:545, 1988.

8. AIMS Trial Study Group. Long term effects of intravenous anistreplase in acute myocardial infarction. Final report of the AIMS study. Lancet 2:427, 1990.

9. ISIS-3 (Third International Study of Infarct Survival) Collaborative Group. ISIS-3: A randomised comparison of streptokinase vs. tissue plasminogen activator vs. anistreplase and of aspirin plus heparin vs. aspirin alone among 41,299 cases of suspected acute myocardial infarction. Lancet 39:753, 1992.

10. The European Myocardial Infarction Project Group. Prehospital thrombolytic therapy in patients with suspected acute myocardial infarction. N Engl J Med 329:383, 1993.

11. GREAT Group. Feasibility, safety and efficacy of domiciliary thrombolysis by general practitioners: Grampian region early anistreplase trial. Br Med J 305:548, 1992.

12. Rawles J, on behalf of the GREAT group. Halving of mortality at one year by domiciliary thrombolysis in the Grampian Region Early Anistreplase Trial (GREAT). J Am Coll Cardiol 23:1, 1994.

13. Cannon CP, McCabe CH, Diver DJ, et al. Comparison of front-loaded tissue-type plasminogen activator, anistreplase and combination thrombolytic therapy in acute myocardial infarction: Results of the thrombolysis in myocardial infarction (TIMI) 4 trial. J Am Coll Cardiol 24:1602, 1994.

14. Neuhaus KL, von Essen R, Tebbe U, et al. Improved thrombolysis in acute myocardial infarction with front loaded administration of alteplase: Result of the rt-PA-APSAC patency study (TAPS). J Am Coll Cardiol 19:885, 1992.

15. O'Connor CM, Meese R, Carney R, et al. A randomized trial of intravenous heparin in conjunction with anistreplase (anisoylated plasminogen streptokinase activator complex) in acute myocardial infarction: The Duke University Clinical Cardiology Study (DUCCS) 1. J Am Coll Cardiol 23:11, 1994.

16. Julian DG. Aspirin or anticoagulants after thrombolysis with anistreplase: Preliminary data from the AFTER study. Eur Heart J 13 (Abstract Suppl.): 307, 1992.

17. Vanderscheuren S, Barrios L, Kerdsinchai P, Van der Heuvel P, Hermans L, Vrolix M, et al. A randomised trial of recombinant staphylokinase versus alteplase for coronary artery patency in myocardial infarction. Circulation 92:2044, 1995.

18. Collen D. Fibrin selective thrombolytic therapy for myocardial infarction. Circulation 93:857, 1996.

17. BIOCHEMISTRY, PHARMACOKINETICS, AND DYNAMICS OF SINGLE- AND TWO-CHAIN UROKINASE

Kurt Huber

Introduction

Enzymes in urine capable of digesting fibrin were described as early as 1885 [1], but the name *urokinase* was first used by Sobel et al. about 45 years ago [2].

Biochemical and Biological Properties of Urokinase

Urokinase (u-PA) is a serine protease with an uncertain physiological role for intravascular fibrin degradation because the latter is believed to be promoted mainly by tissue-plasminogen activator (t-PA) [3,4]. However, u-PA is involved in other physiological and pathological mechanisms, for example, inflammation [5,6], tissue proliferation, tumor invasion and metastasis [7–11], as well as angiogenesis [12,13] and atherosclerosis [14]. u-PA is produced basally and in response to inflammatory stimulation by different cell types, including endothelial cells [15] and monocytes/macrophages [16,17], and has also been detected in platelets [18]. The human u-PA gene is 6.4 kb long and is located on chromosome 10 [19]. In human plasma of healthy volunteers, u-PA antigen concentrations range between 2 and 7 ng/mL (40–150 pmol/L), irrespective of gender [20].

u-PA is not a single molecular species; a number of different forms exist. The major forms are schematically shown in Figure 17-1. Single-chain u-PA (scu-PA, pro-urokinase) is a glycoprotein with a molecular weight (MW) of 54,000 and contains 411 amino acids. A number of proteases are able to convert scu-PA to the high molecular weight two-chain form (tcu-PA, HMW-tcu-PA) by cleavage of the Lys^{158}–Ile^{159} bond. These proteases include plasmin, kallikrein, and, to a minor extent, factor XIIa in plasma [21,22], and cathepsin B and L in tissues [23,24].

A low molecular weight form of tcu-PA (LMW-tcu-PA with a MW of 33,000) can be generated by hydrolysis of the Lys^{135}–Lys^{136} bond by plasmin [25]. Some cultured tumor cell lines contain a low molecular weight scu-PA (MW 32,000) cleaved by a metalloproteinase between Glu^{143} and Leu^{144} [26,27], with similar protelytic activities as the high molecular weight scu-PA [28]. Thrombin converts scu-PA to an inactive two-chain derivative by cleavage of the Arg^{156}–Phe^{157} bond [21,29]. On the basis of homology with other serine proteases, three distinct domains exist in the A-chain [30]: (1) the epidermal growth factor domain (residues 1–45), which interacts with the u-PA receptor (u-PAR) on cell membranes [31]; (2) the single kringle region (residues 45–134); and (3) the proteinase domain (residues 159–411), which contains the active center (composed of His^{204}, Asp^{255}, and Ser^{356}) (Figure 17-2).

Single-Chain Urokinase-Type Plasminogen Activator

CHARACTERISTICS

Single-chain urokinase-type plasminogen activator (scu-PA) appears to be a true zymogen with very low reactivity toward low molecular weight substrates or active-site inhibitors as compared with tcu-PA [32,33]. In contrast with tcu-PA, scu-PA has significant fibrin specificity [34]. The presence of fibrin in a purified system enhances plasminogen activation by scu-PA by about 10-fold [35,36]. Several hypothetical mechanisms for this fibrin specificity have been proposed: (1) scu-PA is inactive towards circulating native Glu-plasminogen, but active towards Lys-plasminogen bound to partially digested fibrin [37]. Whether the increased binding of scu-PA to partially digested fibrin [38] is direct or mediated exclusively via its binding to plasminogen [39] remains uncertain. This model would explain the lag phase that is characteristic of scu-PA–induced thrombolysis [28]. (2) A second possibility is that scu-PA is a genuine proenzyme with negligible activity toward plasminogen [40,41]. Therefore, fibrinolysis with scu-PA would entirely depend on the generation of tcu-PA [42] by, for instance, plasmin generated, in turn, by fibrin-bound tissue-type plasminogen activator (t-PA). However, only about 28% of scu-PA is converted to tcu-PA during thrombolytic therapy in acute myocardial infarction [43]. (3) A third hypothesis is that scu-PA has some intrinsic plasminogen activating potential, which is counteracted by a competitive inhibitory mechanism in plasma, but is reversed by fibrin.

In vitro studies in human plasma have suggested that conversion of scu-PA to tcu-PA during clot lysis represents a primary positive-feedback mechanism, whereas binding of plasminogen to fibrin or predigestion of fibrin by plasmin results in relatively minor additional acceleration of fibrinolysis [44]. The observation that plasmin-resistant mutants of scu-PA have only a three- to fivefold lower thrombolytic potency in vivo as compared with wild-type scu-PA suggests that, for in vivo thrombolysis, conversion of scu-PA to tcu-PA may play a less important role than postulated [45]. The thrombolytic effect of scu-PA is enhanced by kallikrein generated during the contact activation of blood coagulation [22,46] and by glycosaminoglycans [47], and is decreased by lipoprotein (a) [47] or thrombomodulin [48].

For clinical use, scu-PA is produced by recombinant technology in mammalian cells or E. coli [30]. As compared with wild-type scu-PA (MW 54,000; specific activity 170,000 latent urokinase units/mg protein), the substance produced in E. coli (Saruplase) is not glycosylated and has a specific activity of only 135,000 latent urokinase units/mg protein [49,50] and a MW of 47,000. Scu-PA is rapidly metabolized in the liver [51] and exhibits a dominant half-life of about 7–8 minutes [49,52]. For a summary of the biochemical characteristics of scu-PA, see Table 17-1.

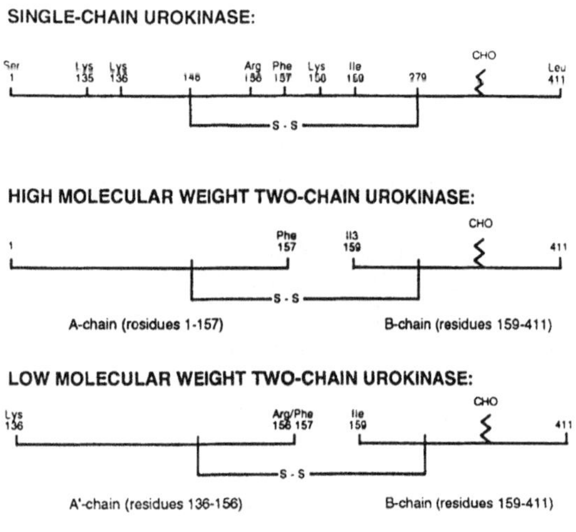

Scu-PA IN ACUTE MYOCARDIAL INFARCTION

For use in acute myocardial infarction, scu-PA has either been preactivated with low doses of recombinant t-PA [53–56] or tcu-PA [57–59], or has been used as a high-dose standard regimen without preactivation (Table 17-2) [60–62]. Preactivation of scu-PA seems to have no additional benefit compared with high-dose regimens of scu-PA [59,63]. Both

FIGURE 17-1. Schematic representation of different forms of urokinase. (Adapted from Gaffney and Heath [84], with permission.)

TABLE 17-1. Biochemical characteristics of scu-PA and tcu-PA

	scu-PA (pro-urokinase)	tcu-PA (urokinase)
Molecular weight	54,000 & 47,000	54,000 & 33,000
Plasminogen activation	Direct	Direct
Half-life (min)	7–8	7–18
kcat/km (−) fibrin	10×10^{-3}	$2–3 \times 10^{-2}$
kcat/km (+) fibrin	50	$2–3 \times 10^{-2}$
Source	E. coli, recombinant	Human urine Fetal kidney

TABLE 17-2. Clinical
characteristics of scu-PA and tcu-PA

	scu-PA	tcu-PA
Generic name	Saruplase	Urokinase
Fibrin specificity	Yes	No
Antigenicity	No	No
Recommended total Dose	80 mg/h	3×10^6 U/h
Intravenous bolus	20 mg	1.5×10^6 U
Infusion	60 mg/h	1.5 ± 10^6 U/h
Coronary patency rate at 90 minutes (TIMI grades 2 and 3)	70–78%	66–70%

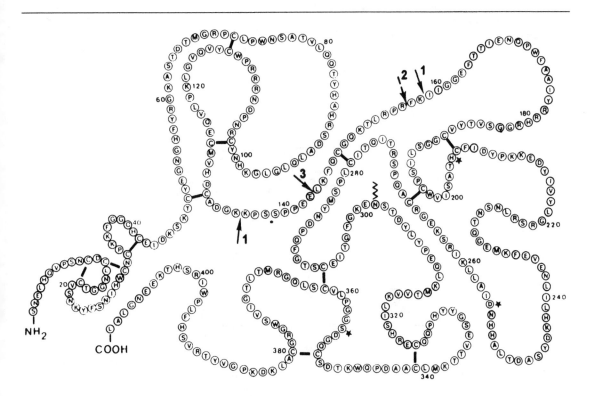

FIGURE 17-2. Schematic representation of the primary structure of scu-PA. The black bars indicate disulphide bonds, based on homology with other serine proteases and kringles. The active site residues His^{204}, Asp^{255}, and Ser^{356} are marked with stars. The arrows indicate the cleavage sites for conversion of the 54,000 MW scu-PA to the 54,000 MW tcu-PA and of the 54,000 MW tcu-PA to the 33,000 MW tcu-PA by plasmin (arrows labeled 1); conversion of the 54,000 MW tcu-PA to inactive tcu-PA by thrombin (arrow labeled 2); and conversion to the 32,000 MW scu-PA by a still unidentified protease (arrow 3). The zigzag line at Asn^{302} indicates the unique glycosylation site. (Adapted from Holmes et al. [29], with permission.)

treatment strategies need the concomitant infusion of high doses of heparin to be highly efficient [62,64]. With both strategies, substantial amounts of scu-PA are converted to active tcu-PA [65] and fibrinogen breakdown occurs [54,58,59]. The rate of fibrinogen breakdown during and following thrombolytic treatment with scu-PA for acute myocardial infarction is related to early vessel patency and bleeding complications [66]. Comparative trials using high-dose scu-PA versus streptokinase, tcu-PA, or rt-PA have achieved comparable coronary patency rates of about 70% (Thrombolysis in Myocardial Infarction [TIMI] grades 2 and 3 [67]) and a comparable outcome with respect to preservation of left ventricular function and in-hospital mortality for all thrombolytic agents used [60,68–71]. The use of an intravenous heparin bolus [5000 IU) before initiation of thrombolytic therapy increased early patency rates (TIMI grades 2 and 3) to 78% [62].

Two-Chain Urokinase-Type Plasminogen Activator

CHARACTERISTICS

As indicated earlier two-chain urokinase-type plasminogen activator (tcu-PA) exists in two distinct molecular entities: a HMW-tcu-PA form, with 411 amino acids, and a LMW-tcu-PA, consisting of 276 amino acids. HMW-tcu-PA is converted to LMW-tcu-PA by limited proteolysis (see Figures 17-1 and 17-2). tcu-PA for clinical use has been isolated from human urine [72,73] and from embryonic human kidney cells [74]. Commercially available preparations predominantly consist of HMW-tcu-PA and only minor amounts of LMW-tcu-PA. During the thrombolytic process, however, HMW-tcu-PA is continuously converted to LMW-tcu-PA, while Glu-plasminogen is continuously converted to Lys-

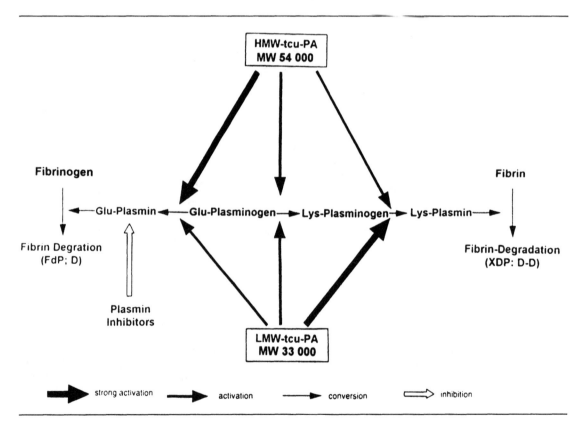

FIGURE 17-3. Schematic representation of the relative fibrin specificity of tcu-PA. Degration = degradation. (Adapted from Gulba et al. [64], with permission.)

plasminogen (Figure 17-3) [25,30]. While HMW-tcu-PA predominantly activates Glu-plasminogen, the catalytic activity of LMW-tcu-PA is predominantly directed toward Lys-plasminogen, which is accumulated at the Lys-binding sites of crosslinked fibrin [74]. The increased binding of LMW-tcu-PA to new Lys-binding sites on the fibrin clot explains the *relative fibrin specificity* of tcu-PA compared with other non-fibrin-specific thrombolytic agents, for example, streptokinase or acylated plasminogen streptokinase complex (see Figure 17-3) [76–79]. The dominant half-life of tcu-PA ranges between 7 and 18 minutes [52–79]. Due to rapid inactivation and clearance, its thrombolytic efficacy ceases rapidly after discontinuation of the infusion. For a summary of the biochemical characteristics of tcu-PA, see Table 17-1.

TCU-PA IN ACUTE MYOCARDIAL INFARCTION
AND UNSTABLE ANGINA
tcu-PA is one of the oldest classical fibrin-nonspecific thrombolytic agents used in the treatment of acute thrombotic occlusions at different sites [80]. Despite its long use in the treatment of acute myocardial infarction, data are available on only a small number of patients [77,81], and with no systematic testing in trials including mortality as an endpoint. In the United States, tcu-PA is not formally approved by the Food and Drug Administration for thrombolytic treatment of acute myocardial infarction [82]. In Europe, the average use of tcu-PA as a thrombolytic agent in acute myocardial infarction ranges at present between 5% and 10% of all thrombolytic procedures. Angiography performed 90 minutes after initiation of thrombolytic therapy with tcu-PA shows patency of the infarct-related artery (TIMI grades 2 and 3) of 65.8% in all patients and 70% in patients treated within 3 hours from the onset of symptoms [77].

The clinical characteristics and recommended doses of tcu-PA are given in Table 17-2. tcu-PA has also been used in a limited number of patients receiving combination therapy with recombinant tissue-plasminogen activator (rt-PA). These data revealed lower in-hospital clinical events and reocclusion rates with the combination therapy as compared with rt-PA or tcu-PA alone [83]. An advantage of combination thrombolytic therapy using a fibrin-specific (rt-PA) and a fibrin-nonspecific agent (tcu-PA) might be the possible reduction of total doses of each fibrinolytic substance [83]. Furthermore, recent data have demonstrated that long-term intermittent tcu-PA therapy in doses of $3 \times 500,000$ IU/wk represents an effective anti-ischemic and antianginal approach for patients with refractory angina and end-stage coro-

nary artery disease, because of its antithrombotic properties and improved blood rheology [84].

Conclusions

Both scu-PA and tcu-PA are highly effective fibrinolytic agents for the treatment of acute myocardial infarction, with a similar safety profile as streptokinase and rt-PA. However, at present only a few studies have been published using these agents in a limited number of patients. To further prove the value of scu-PA and tcu-PA as fibrinolytic substances and to increase their clinical use, well-planned prospective thrombolytic trials comparing these agents with established fibrinolytic drugs have to be performed, using mortality as the endpoint.

References

1. Sahli W. Ueber das Vorkommen von Pepsin und Trypsin im normalen menschlichen Harn. Pflügers Arch Physiol 36:209, 1885.
2. Sobel GW, Mohler SR, Jones NW, Dowdy ABC, Guest MM. Urokinase: An activator of plasma profibrinolysin extracted from human urine. Am J Physiol 171:768, 1952.
3. Astedt B. No crossreaction between circulating plasminogen activator and urokinase. Thromb Res 14:535, 1979.
4. Kok P. Separation of plasminogen activators from human plasma and a comparison with activators from human uterine tissue and urine. Thromb Haemost 41:734, 1979.
5. De Bruin PAF, Crama-Bohbouth G, Verspaget HW, Verheijen JH, Dooijewaard G, Weterman IT, Lamers CBHW. Plasminogen activators in the intestine of patients with inflammatory bowel disease. Thromb Haemost 60:262, 1988.
6. Grondahl-Hansen J, Kirkeby L, Ralfkiaer E, Kristensen P, Lund LR, Dano K. Urokinase-type plasminogen activator in endothelial cells during acute inflammation of the pancreas. Am J Pathol 135:631, 1989.
7. Kirchheimer JC, Köller A, Binder BR. Isolation and characterization of plasminogen activators from hyperplastic and malignant prostate tissue. Biochim Biophys Acta 797:256, 1984.
8. Layer GT, Cederholm-Williams SA, Gaffney PJ, Houlbrook S, Mahmoud M, Pattison M, Burnand KG. Urokinase — the enzyme responsible for invasion and metastasis in human breast carcinoma? Fibrinolysis 1:237, 1987.
9. Markus G. The relevance of plasminogen activators to neoplastic growth: A review of recent literature. Enzyme (Basel) 40:158, 1988.
10. Huber K, Kirchheimer JC, Ermler D, Bell C, Binder BR. Determination of plasma urokinase-type plasmi-

nogen activator antigen in patients with primary liver cancer — characterization as tumor-associated antigen and comparison with alpha-fetoprotein. Cancer Res 52:1717, 1992.

11. Huber K, Kirchheimer JC, Sedlmayr A, Bell C, Ermler D, Binder BR. Clinical value of determination of urokinase-type plasminogen activator antigen in plasma for detection of colorectal cancer: Comparison with circulating tumor-associated antigens CA 19-9 and carcinoembryonic antigen. Cancer Res 53:1788, 1993.

12. Saskela O, Montesano F. Cell-associated plasminogen activation: Regulation and physiological functions. Ann Rev Cell Biol 4:93, 1988.

13. Pepper MS, Montesano F. Proteolytic balance and capillary morphogenesis. Cell Differ Dev 32:319, 1991.

14. Lupu F, Heim DA, Bachmann F, Hurni M, Kakkar VV, Kruithof EKO. Plasminogen activator expression in human advanced atherosclerotic lesions. Arterioscler Thromb Vasc Biol 15:1444, 1995.

15. Van Hinsberg VWM. Regulation of the synthesis and secretion of plasminogen activators by endothelial cells. Haemostasis 18:307, 1988.

16. Vasalli JD, Dayer JM, Wohlwend A, Belin D. Concomitant secretion of prourokinase and of plasminogen activator-specific inhibitor by cultured human monocytes-macrophages. Exp Med 159:1653, 1984.

17. Hart PH, Burgess DR, Vitti GF, Hamilton JA. Interleukin-4 stimulates human monocytes to produce tissue-type plasminogen activator. Blood 74:1222, 1989.

18. Park S, Karker LA, Marzec UM, Levin EG. Demonstration of single chain urokinase-type plasminogen activator on human platelet membrane. Blood 73:1421, 1989.

19. Bachmann F. Fibrinolysis. In Verstraete M, Vermylen J, Lijnen R, Arnout J (eds). Thrombosis and Haemostasis 1987. Leuven University Press 1987:227.

20. Kirchheimer JC, Binder BR. Urokinase antigen in plasma: Age and sex dependent variations. Thromb Res 36:643, 1984.

21. Ichinose A, Fujikawa K, Suyama T. The activation of pro-urokinase by plasma kallikrein and its inactivation by thrombin. J Biol Chem 261:3484, 1984.

22. Hauert J, Nicoloso G, Schleunig WD, Bachmann F, Schapira M. Plasminogen activators in dextran sulfate-activated euglobulin fractions: A molecular analysis for factor XII- and prekallikrein-dependent fibrinolysis. Blood 73:994, 1989.

23. Kobayashi H, Schmitt M, Goretzki L, Chucholowski N, Calvete J, Kramer M, Gunzler WA, Janicke F, Graeff H. Cathepsin B efficiently activates the soluble and the tumor-cell receptor-bound form of the proenzyme urokinase-type plasminogen activator (Pro-uPA). J Biol Chem 266:5147, 1991.

24. Goretzki L, Schmitt M, Mann K, Calvete J, Chucholowski N, Kramer M, Gunzler WA, Janicke F, Graeff H. Effective activation of the proenzyme form of

the urokinase-type plasminogen activator (pro-uPA) by the cysteine protease cathepsin L. FEBS Lett 297:112, 1992.

25. Günzler WA, Steffens GJ, otting F, Buse G, Flohe L. Structural relationship between human high and low molecular mass urokinase. Hoppe-Seyler's Z Physiol Chem 363:133, 1982.

26. Stump DC, Lijnen HR, Collen D. Purification and characterization of a novel low molecular weight form of single-chain urokinase-type plasminogen activator. J Biol Chem 261:17120, 1986.

27. Marcotte PA, Dudlak D, Leski ML, Ryan J, Henkin J. Characterization of a metalloproteinase which cleaves with high site-specificity the glu(143)-leu(144) bond of urokinase. Fibrinolysis 6:57, 1992.

28. Collen D, Zamarron C, Lijnen HR, Hoylaerts M. Activation of plasminogen by pro-urokinase. II. Kinetics. J Biol Chem 261:1259, 1986.

29. Gurewich V, Pannel R. Inactivation of single-chain urokinase (pro-urokinase) by thrombin and thrombin-like enzymes: Relevance of the findings to the interpretation of fibrin-binding experiments. Blood 69:769, 1987.

30. Holmes WE, Pennica D, Blaber M, Rey MW, Guenzler WA, Steffens GJ, Heyneker HL. Cloning and expression of the gene for pro-urokinase in Escherichia coli. Biotechnology 3:923, 1985.

31. Blasi F. Surface receptors for urokinase plasminogen activator. Fibrinolysis 2:73, 1988.

32. Gurewich V, Pannell R, Louie S, Kelley P, Suddith L, Greenlee R. Effective and fibrin-specific clot-lysis by a zymogen precursor form of urokinase (pro-urokinase): A study in vitro and in two animal species. J Clin Invest 73:1731, 1984.

33. Booyse FM, Lin PH, Traylor M, Bruce R. Purification and properties of a single-chain urokinase-type plasminogen activator form produced by subcultured human umbilical vein endothelial cells. J Biol Chem 263:15139, 1988.

34. Gurewich V. Fibrinolytic properties of single-chain urokinase plasminogen activator and how they complement those of tissue plasminogen activator. In Haber E, Braunwald E (eds). Thrombolysis. Basic Contributions and Clinical Progress. St. Louis, MO; Mosby Year Book, 1991:51.

35. Takada A, Sugawara Y, Takada Y. Enhancement of the activation of Glu-plasminogen by urokinase in the simultaneous presence of tranexamic acid or fibrin. Haemostasis 1:26, 1989.

36. Liu J, Gurewich V. A comparative study of the promotion of tissue plasminogen activator and pro-urokinase-induced plasminogen activation by fragments D and E-2 of fibrin. J Clin Invest 88:2012, 1991.

37. Pannell R, Gurewich V. Activation of plasminogen by single-chain urokinase or by two-chain urokinase — a demonstration that single-chain urokinase has a low catalytic activity (pro-urokinase). Blood 69:22, 1987.

38. Lenich C, Pannell R, Gurewich V. The effect of the carboxy-terminal lysine of urokinase on the catalysis of plasminogen activation. Thromb Res 64:69, 1991.

39. Longstaff C, Clough AM, Gaffney PJ. Kinetics of plasmin activation of single chain urinary-type plasminogen activator (scu-PA) and demonstration of a high affinity interaction between scu-PA and plasminogen. J Biol Chem 267:173, 1992.

40. Ellis V, Scully MF, Kakkar VV. Plasminogen activation by single-chain urokinase in functional isolation. J Biol Chem 262:14998, 1987.

41. Petersen LC, Lund LR, Nielsen LS, Dano K, Skriver L. One-chain urokinase-type plasminogen activator from human sarcoma cells is a proenzyme with little or no intrinsic activity. J Biol Chem 263:11189, 1988.

42. Giorgetti C, Molinari A, Bonomini L, Lansen J, Gurewich V. The role of urokinase generation during clot lysis by pro-urokinase in a plasma milieu. Fibrinolysis 7:183, 1993.

43. Koster RW, Cohen AF, Hopkins GR, Beier H, Gunzler WA, van der Wouw PA. Pharmacokinetics and pharmacodynamics of saruplase, an unglycosylated single-chain urokinase-type plasminogen activator, in patients with acute myocardial infarction. Thromb Haemost 72:740, 1994.

44. Lijnen HR, Van Hoef B, De Cock F, Collen D. The mechanism of plasminogen activation and fibrin dissolution by single-chain urokinase-type plasminogen activator in a plasma milieu in vitro. Blood 73:1864, 1989.

45. Lijnen HR, Nelles L, Van Hoef B, Demarsin E, Collen D. Structural and functional characterization of mutants of recombinant single-chain urokinase-type plasminogen activator obtained by site-specific mutagenesis of Lys158, Ile159 and Ile160. Eur J Biochem 177:575, 1988.

46. Loza J, Gurewich V, Johnstone M, Pannell R. Platelet-bound prekallikrein promotes pro-urokinase-induced clot lysis: A mechanism for targeting the factor XII dependent intrinsic pathway of fibrinolysis. Thromb Haemost 71:347, 1994.

47. Edelberg JM, Weissler M, Pizzo SV. Kinetic analysis of the effects of glycosaminoglycans and lipoproteins on urokinase-mediated plasminogen activation. Biochem J 276:785, 1991.

48. de Munk GAW, Groeneveld E, Rijken DC. Acceleration of the thrombin inactivation of single chain urokinase-type plasminogen activator (pro-urokinase) by thrombomodulin. J Clin Invest 88:1680, 1991.

49. van de Werf F, Vanhaecke J, de Geest H, Verstraete M, Collen D. Coronary thrombolysis with recombinant single-chain urokinase-type plasminogen activator in patients with acute myocardial infarction. Circulation 74:1066, 1986.

50. Gulba DC, Fischer K, Barthels M, Polensky U, Reil G-H, Daniel WG, Welzel D, Lichtlen PR. Low dose urokinase preactivated natural pro-urokinase for thrombolysis in acute myocardial infarction. Am J Cardiol 63:1025, 1989.

51. Collen D, De Cock F, Lijnen HR. Biological and thrombolytic properties of proenzyme and active forms of human urokinase. II. Turnover of natural and recombinant urokinase in rabbits and squirrel monkeys. Thromb Haemost 52:24, 1984.

52. Kohler M, Sen S, Miyashita C, Hermes R, Pindur G, Heiden M, Berg G, Morsdorf S, Leipnitz G, Zeppezauer M, Schieffer H, Wenzel E, Schonberger A, Hollemeyer K. Half-life of single-chain urokinase-type plasminogen activator (scu-PA) and two-chain urokinase-type plasminogen activator (tcu-PA) in patients with acute myocardial infarction. Thromb Res 62:75, 1991.

53. Kasper W, Hohnloser SH, Engler H, Meinertz T, Wilkens J, Roth E, Lang K, Limbourg P, Just H. Coronary reperfusion studies with pro-urokinase in acute myocardial infarction: Evidence for synergism of low dose urokinase. J Am Coll Cardiol 16:733, 1990.

54. Bode C, Schuler G, Nordt T, Schönermark S, Baumann H, Richardt G, Dietz R, Gurewich V, Kübler W. Intravenous thrombolytic therapy with a combination of single-chain urokinase-type plasminogen activator and recombinant tissue-type activator in acute myocardial infarction. Circulation 81:907, 1990.

55. Kirshenbaum JM, Bahr RD, Flaherty JT, Gurewich V, Levine HJ, Loscalzo J, Schumacher RR, Topol EJ, Wahr D, Braunwald E. Clot-selective coronary thrombolysis with low-dose synergistic combinations of single-chain urokinase-type plasminogen activator and recombinant tissue-type plasminogen activator. The Pro-Urokinase for Myocardial Infarction Study Group. Am J Cardiol 68:1564, 1991.

56. Zarich SW, Kowalchuk GJ, Weaver WD, Loscalzo J, Sasower M, Manzo K, Byrnes C, Muller JE, Gurewich V for the PATENT Study Group. Sequential combination thrombolytic therapy for acute myocardial infarction: Results of the Pro-urokinase and t-PA enhancement of thrombolysis (PATENT) trial. J Am Coll Cardiol 26:374, 1995.

57. Bode C, Schönermark S, Schuler G, Zimmermann R, Schwarz F, Kübler W. Efficacy of intravenous pro-urokinase and a combination of pro-urokinase and urokinase in acute myocardial infarction. Am J Cardiol 61:971–974, 1988.

58. Loscalzo J, Wharton T, Kirshenbaum JM, Levine HJ, Flaherty JT, Topol EJ, Ramaswamy K, Kosowsky BD, Salem DN, Ganz P, Brinker JA, Gurewich V, Muller JE, and the Pro-Urokinase for Myocardial Infarction Study Group. Clot-selective coronary thrombolysis with pro-urokinase. Circulation 79:776, 1989.

59. Gulba DC, Bode C, Sen S, Topp J, Fischer K, Wolf H, Hecker H and the German Preactivated Pro-Urokinase Study Group. Multicenter dose-finding trial for thrombolysis with urokinase preactivated pro-urokinase (TCL 598) in acute myocardial infarction. Cathet Cardiovasc Diagn 26:177, 1992.

60. PRIMI Trial Study Group. Randomized double-blind trial of recombinant pro-urokinase against streptokinase in acute myocardial infarction. Lancet 1:863, 1989.

61. Diefenbach C, Erbel R, Pop T, Mathey D, Schofer J, Hamm C, Ostermann H, Schmitz-Hübner U, Bleifeld W, Meyer J. Recombinant single-chain urokinase-type plasminogen activator during acute myocardial infarction. Am J Cardiol 61:966, 1988.

62. Tebbe U, Windeler J, Boesel I, Hoffmann H, Wojcik J, Ashmawy M, Schwarz ER, von Loewis of Menar P, Roesmeyer P, Hopkins G, Barth H, on behalf of the LIMITS Study Group. Thrombolysis with recombinant unglycosylated single-chain urokinase-type plasminogen activator (Saruplase) in acute myocardial infarction: Influence of heparin on early patency rate (LIMITS Study). J Am Coll Cardiol 26:365, 1995.

63. Weaver WD, Hartmann JR, Anderson JL, Reddy PS, Sobolski JC, Sasahara AA. New recombinant glycosylated prourokinase for treatment of patients with acute myocardial infarction. Prourokinase Study Group. J Am Coll Cardiol 24:1242, 1994.

64. Gulba DC, Fischer K, Barthels M, Jost S, Moller W, Frombach R, Reil G-H, Daniel WG, Lichtlen PR. Potentiative effect of heparin in thrombolytic therapy of evolving myocardial infarction with natural pro-urokinase. Fibrinolysis 3:165, 1989.

65. Gulba DC, Bode C, Runge MS, Huber K. Thrombolytic agents — an overview. Ann Haematol 73:S9, 1996.

66. Ostermann H, U. S-H, Windeler J, Bar F, Meyer J, van de Loo J. Rate of fibrinogen breakdown related to coronary patency and bleeding complications in patients with thrombolysis in acute myocardial infarction — results from the PRIMI trial. Eur Heart J 13:1225, 1992.

67. TIMI Study Group. The thrombolysis in myocardial infarction (TIMI) trial: Phase I findings. N Engl J Med 312:932, 1985.

68. Kambara H, Kawai C, Kajiwara N, Nitani H, Sasayama S, Kanmatsuse K, Kodama K, Sato H, Nobuyoshi M, Nakashima M, Matsuo O, Matsuda T. Randomized, double-blinded multicenter study: Comparison of intracoronary single-chain urokinase-type plasminogen activator, pro-urokinase (GE-0943), and intracoronary urokinase in patients with acute myocardial infarction. Circulation 78:899, 1988.

69. Pindur G, Koehler M, Sen S, Hermes R, Miyashita C, Wenzel E, Schieffer H. Fibrinolytic effects of pro-urokinase combined with low-dose urokinase compared to high-dose urokinase in patients with acute myocardial infarction. Thromb Res 67:191, 1992.

70. Schofer J, Lins M, Mathey DG, Sheehan FH. Time course of left ventricular function and coronary patency after saruplase vs. streptokinase in acute myocardial infarction. The PRIMI Trial Study Group. Eur Heart J 14:958, 1993.

71. Vogt A, von Essen R, Tebbe U, Feuerer W, Appel KF, Neuhaus KL. Impact of early perfusion status of the infarct-related artery on short-term mortality after thrombolysis for acute myocardial infarction: Retrospective analysis of four German multicenter studies. J Am Coll Cardiol 21:1391, 1993.

72. Huber K, Kirchheimer JC, Binder BR. Rapid isolation of high molecular weight urokinase from native human urine. Thromb Haemost 47:197, 1982.

73. Husain SS, Gurewich V, Lipinski B. Purification and partial characterization of a single-chain-high-molecular-weight form of urokinase from human urine. Arch Biochem Biophys 220:31, 1982.

74. Barlow GH, Lazer L, Rueter A, Tribby I. Production of plasminogen activators by culture cell techniques. In Paoletti R, Sherry S (eds). New York: Academic Press, 1977:758.

75. Harpel PC, Chang T-S, Verderber E. Tissue-plasminogen activator and urokinase mediate the binding of glu-plasminogen to plasma fibrin. I. Evidence for new binding sites in plasma-degraded fibrin. J Biol Chem 260:4432, 1985.

76. van de Loo JCW, Kriessmann A, Trübestein G, Knoch K, de Swart CAM, Asbeck F, Marbert GA, Schmitt HE, Sewell AF, Duckert F, Theiss W, Ritz R. Controlled multicenter pilot study of urokinase-heparin and streptokinase in deep vein thrombosis. Thromb Haemost 50:660, 1983.

77. Neuhaus KL, Tebbe U, Gottwik M, Weber MAJ, Feuerer W, Niederer W, Haerer W, Praetorius F, Grosser K-D, Huhmann W, Hoepp H-W, Alber G, Sheikhzadeh A, Schneider B. Intravenous recombinant tissue plasminogen activator (rt-PA) and urokinase in acute myocardial infarction: Results of the German activator urokinase study (GAUS). J Am Coll Cardiol 12:581, 1988.

78. Goldhaber SZ, Kessler CM, Heit J, Markis J, Sharma GVRK, Dawley D, Nagel JS, Meyerovitz M, Kim D, Vaughan DE, Parker JA, Tumeh SS, Drum D, Loscalzo J, Reagan K, Selwyn AP, Anderson J, Braunwald E. Randomized controlled trial of recombinant tissue plasminogen activator versus urokinase in the treatment of acute pulmonary embolism. Lancet 2:293, 1988.

79. Fletcher AP, Alkjaersig N, Sherry S, Genton E, Hirsh J, Bachmann F. The development of urokinase as a thrombolytic agent: Maintenance of a sustained thrombolytic state in man by its intravenous infusion. J Lab Clin Med 65:713, 1965.

80. Gulba DC, Lichtlen PR. Urokinasetherapie bei thromboembolischen Erkrankungen. In Kirchhof B, Kienast J (eds). Thrombolysetherapie: Daten und Argumente fur verschiedenen Verfahren und Substanzen. Emmendingen: Kesselring, 1988:45.

81. Mathey DG, Schofer H, Sheehan FH, Becher H, Tilsner V, Dodge HT. Intravenous urokinase in acute myocardial infarction. Am J Cardiol 55:878, 1985.

82. Lincoff AM, Topol EJ. Thrombolytic therapy. In Fuster V, Ross R, Topol EJ (eds). Atherosclerosis and Coronary Artery Disease. Philadelphia: Lippincott-Raven, 1996:955.

83. Popma JJ, Califf RM, Ellis SG, George BS, Kereiakes DJ, Samaha JK, Worley SJ, Anderson JL, Stump D, Woodlief L, Sigmon K, Wall TC, Topol EJ. Mechanism of benefit of combination thrombolytic therapy for acute myocardial infarction: A quantitative angiographic and hematologic study. J Am Coll Cardiol 20:1305, 1992.

84. Leschke M, Schoebel F-C, Mecklenbeck W, Stein D, Jax TW, Müller-Gärtner H-W, Strauer B-E. Long-term intermittent urokinase therapy in patients with end-stage coronary artery disease and refractory angina pectoris: A randomized dose-response trial. J Am Coll Cardiol 27:575, 1996.

85. Gaffney PJ, Heath AB. A collaborative study to establish a standard for high molecular weight urinary-type plasminogen activator (HMW/u-PA). Thromb Haemost 64:398, 1990.

18. STAPHYLOKINASE: BIOCHEMISTRY AND PHARMACODYNAMICS

Steven Vanderschueren and Désiré Collen

Structure and Production of Staphylokinase

Although the existence of staphylokinase (Sak) has been known since at least 1908 [1], detailed biochemical evaluation and clinical testing of Sak have only recently been initiated. Staphylokinase is a 136 amino acid protein, made of a single polypeptide chain without disulfide bridges (Figure 18-1), secreted by *Staphylococcus aureus* strains after transformation with bacteriophages or after lysogenic conversion. The production of Sak by *S. aureus* is believed to play a role in tissue penetration and in invasion by the bacteria [2]. The structure of Sak shows no homology with that of other plasminogen activators. Three natural variants that have been characterized (SakSTAR, Sak42D, and SakφC) [3–5] differ at amino acid positions 34, 36, and 43 (Table 18-1), and have a similar plasminogen-activating potential but different thermostability [6].

The purification of Sak from selected *S. aureus* strains for in vivo use has been disappointing because of low expression and concomitant secretion of potent exotoxins. Recently, large quantities of two variants of wild-type Sak (variants SakSTAR and Sak42D) have become available by introducing recombinant plasmids in *Escherichia coli* that subsequently produce intracellular Sak in quantities of up to 10–15% of the total cell protein [7]. This material, after purification, has allowed extended preclinical and early clinical evaluation.

Mechanisms of Action and of Fibrin Specificity

The mechanisms of action and of fibrin specificity of Sak have recently been elucidated [8,9]. Staphylokinase, like streptokinase, is not an enzyme and does not directly convert plasminogen to plasmin, but rather forms a 1:1 stoichiometric complex with plasminogen, which then activates other plasminogen molecules. In contrast to streptokinase, exposure of an active site in the complex of Sak with plasminogen requires conversion to plasmin. The plasmin–Sak complex, unlike the plasmin(ogen)–streptokinase complex, is rapidly neutralized by α_2-antiplasmin in plasma in the absence of fibrin, thus avoiding systemic plasminogen activation and fibrinogen degradation. After inhibition by α_2-antiplasmin, Sak dissociates from the complex and is recycled to other plasminogen molecules. In the presence of fibrin, however, the inhibition by α_2-antiplasmin is delayed >100-fold, allowing preferential plasminogen activation at the fibrin surface.

These molecular interactions between Sak, α_2-antiplasmin, and fibrin endow the Sak molecule with a unique mechanism of fibrin selectivity in the plasma milieu. In the absence of fibrin, no activation of plasminogen by Sak occurs, presumably because α_2-antiplasmin prevents the generation of active plasmin–Sak complex. At the fibrin surface, traces of plasmin are present that form active plasmin-Sak complex that is bound to fibrin via the lysine binding sites of the plasmin molecule and is protected from rapid inhibition by α_2-antiplasmin. After digestion of the fibrin clot, the plasmin–Sak complex is released and inhibited, and further plasminogen activation is interrupted. Thus, the differential neutralization by α_2-antiplasmin of circulating as opposed to fibrin-associated plasmin–Sak complex and the local generation and surface assembly of active plasmin–Sak complex at the fibrin surface form the basis of the fibrin specificity of Sak.

Properties of Staphylokinase Extrapolated from Preclinical Experiments

In vitro and laboratory animal experiments [10–12] demonstrated that in most species studied Sak is a

TABLE 18-1. Amino acid differences
among the three natural staphylokinase variants

	NH₂-Ser	..34......	..36......	..43.......	Lys-COOH
SakSTAR		Ser	Gly	His	
Sak42D		Gly	Arg	Arg	
SakøC		Gly	Gly	His	

1													14
Ser	Ser	Ser	Phe	Asp	Lys	Gly	Lys	Tyr	Lys	Lys	Gly	Asp	Asp
15													28
Ala	Ser	Tyr	Phe	Glu	Pro	Thr	Gly	Pro	Tyr	Leu	Met	Val	Asn
29													42
Val	Thr	Gly	Val	Asp	Ser	**Lys**	Gly	Asn	**Glu**	Leu	Leu	Ser	Pro
						└─────	3	─────┘					
43													56
His	Tyr	Val	Glu	Phe	Pro	Ile	Lys	Pro	Gly	Thr	Thr	Leu	Thr
57													70
Lys	Glu	Lys	Ile	Glu	Tyr	Tyr	Val	Glu	Trp	Ala	Leu	Asp	Ala
71													84
Thr	Ala	Tyr	**Lys**	**Glu**	Phe	**Arg**	Val	Val	**Glu**	Leu	**Asp**	Pro	Ser
			└───────	──┘		└───			└──		──┘		
85			8						9				98
Ala	Lys	Ile	Glu	Val	Thr	Tyr	Tyr	Asp	Lys	Asn	Lys	Lys	Lys
99													112
Glu	Glu	Thr	Lys	Ser	Phe	Pro	Ile	Thr	Glu	Lys	Gly	Phe	Val
113													126
Val	Pro	Asp	Leu	Ser	Glu	His	Ile	Lys	Asn	Pro	Gly	Phe	Asn
127										136			
Leu	Ile	Thr	Lys	Val	Val	Ile	Glu	Lys	Lys				

FIGURE 18-1. Amino acid sequence of SakSTAR with bolds indicating the charged amino acid clusters that are changed to alanine in the mutants SakSTAR.M38 (clusters 3 and 8) and SakSTAR.M89 (clusters 8 and 9). The numbers appear underneath the clusters. The amino acid sequence (1–136) is indicated at the top.

potent and rapidly acting plasminogen activator. In human plasma, Sak, unlike streptokinase, was found to be very fibrin specific. On a theoretical basis, fibrin specificity may improve the efficacy and safety of thrombolytic therapy. Avoidance of the "plasminogen steal" phenomenon and of plasminemia-induced paradoxical prothrombotic effects may ameliorate efficacy. Reduction of the "systemic plasminolytic state" and the resulting hemostatic perturbations may improve safety. Also, the ease of administration may improve because a high affinity for fibrin prolongs the biological half-life beyond the plasma half-life and may thus allow bolus administration, notwithstanding a relatively short circulatory half-life. Of course, these postulated advantages of fibrin specificity await thorough clinical validation.

In contrast with streptokinase, Sak efficiently lysed platelet-rich, contracted, as well as mechanically compressed plasma clots [11]. This differential lysability may be explained by the extrusion of clot-associated plasminogen following retraction or compression. In contrast with non–fibrin-specific plasminogen activators, fibrin-specific agents such as Sak spare circulating plasminogen that can be recruited into the thrombus and activated in loco [12]. Therapeutic doses of Sak did not affect platelet function [12].

In rabbits, Sak, in contrast with rt-PA, did not prolong surface bleeding times unless aspirin and heparin were added [13]. In the cuticle bleeding time model, the lower hemorrhagic tendency of Sak could be attributed to its fibrinogen-sparing potential. In a hamster pulmonary embolism model, streptokinase and Sak were equally sensitive to inhibition with aprotinin, while Sak was significantly more sensitive to the antifibrinolytic effects of tranexamic acid [14]. The higher antifibrinolytic potency of tranexamic acid (which prevents binding of plasminogen to fibrin) toward Sak than toward streptokinase is most likely to be related to the requirement of fibrin-bound plasminogen for efficient fibrinolysis with Sak.

The immunogenicity of streptokinase and Sak (SakSTAR variant) was compared in a dog [15] and baboon [16] extracorporeal thrombosis model. Serial administration of streptokinase induced rapidly increasing IgG-related streptokinase-neutralizing activities in plasma and a progressive resistance to clot lysis in both species, and severe hypotensive reactions, especially in baboons. With Sak, induction of Sak-neutralizing activities was less consistent and thrombolytic potency was relatively maintained, while no acute hypotension occurred.

Promising properties of Sak, deduced from in vitro and laboratory animal experiments, included high thrombolytic efficacy, even toward platelet-rich and retracted thrombi, rapid onset of action, remarkable fibrin specificity, low bleeding risk, sensitivity to inhibition by antifibrinolytic agents, and reduced antigenicity and allergenicity relative to streptokinase. These attractive features prompted the clinical evaluation of Sak.

Initial Clinical Experience with Recombinant Staphylokinase

ACUTE MYOCARDIAL INFARCTION

To study the fibrin specificity and potency of Sak for coronary thrombolysis, pilot-phase angiographic trials were conducted. Conjunctive therapy consisted of aspirin and intravenous heparin. In the first pilot recanalization study, 10 patients with angiographically confirmed infarct-related artery occlusion (TIMI grade 0 flow) were treated with 10 mg intravenous Sak (variant SakSTAR) over 30 minutes [7,17]. Within 40 minutes all but one of the occluded coronary arteries were recanalized (TIMI grade 3 flow in eight patients and TIMI grade 2 flow in one patient). The mean (± SEM) time delay to reperfusion in recanalized arteries, 20 ± 4.0 minutes, compared favorably with $\geq$45-minute delays reported for rt-PA and streptokinase [18].

A subsequent multicenter randomized trial compared the effects of Sak with the present standard regimen, accelerated and weight-adjusted rt-PA, on early coronary artery patency in 100 patients with acute myocardial infarction [19]. Patients randomized to intravenous Sak were given 10 mg over 30 minutes in the first half of the study and, following a prospectively planned interim analysis, 20 mg over 30 minutes in the second half. TIMI perfusion grade 3 rates of the infarct-related artery at 90 minutes were 58% in patients treated with rt-PA (n = 52) and 62% in patients treated with Sak (n = 48; 50% after 10 mg Sak, n = 25; and 74% after 20 mg Sak, n = 23).

The feasibility of bolus Sak administration was first studied in 12 patients with evolving transmural myocardial infarction [20]. At baseline, 20 mg of Sak was given over 5 minutes. Patients with TIMI perfusion grade 0, 1, or 2 at 60 minutes received a second bolus of 10 mg of Sak over 5 minutes. TIMI grade 3 flow was obtained in 7 patients (58%) at 60 minutes and, after addition of the second Sak bolus in the 5 others, in a total of 10 patients (83%) at 90 minutes. Following this small trial, a multicenter randomized study in 102 patients further investigated the bolus administration of Sak, comparing a double bolus of 15 mg of Sak each, given 30 minutes apart, with accelerated rt-PA [21]. At 90 minutes, TIMI grade 3 flow of the culprit artery was achieved in 68% of patients treated with double-bolus Sak (n = 50) versus 57% of patients treated with rt-PA (n = 52).

Sak proved to be highly fibrin specific, preserving plasma fibrinogen and plasminogen, after infusion of up to 40 mg of Sak [19–21]. From a cumulative dose of 30 mg onwards, a slight but statistically significant decline (to 91% of baseline at 90 minutes) of α_2-antiplasmin levels, a sensitive marker of systemic plasmin generation, occurred [21]. rt-PA, in contrast, caused a substantial drop of fibrinogen (mean decrease vs. pretreatment of 30% at 90 minutes) and of plasminogen and α_2-antiplasmin (mean decreases of 60% at 90 minutes) [19].

Pooled data from both randomized trials of Sak versus rt-PA (encompassing a total of 202 patients) demonstrated an excess of in-hospital mortality, mainly due to cardiogenic shock, after rt-PA (6 deaths vs. none after Sak, $P = 0.03$) and more bleeding requiring transfusion after rt-PA (9 vs. 2 after Sak, $P = 0.06$) [19,21]. No study drug–associated allergic reactions occurred. Although these initial data are encouraging, larger studies with clinical endpoints are required to substantiate these differences.

From these studies it is concluded that intravenous Sak, combined with heparin and aspirin, is a potent, rapidly acting, and highly fibrin-specific thrombolytic agent in patients with acute myocardial infarction. Its fibrin specificity, safety, and efficacy in coronary thrombolysis appear to compare well with those of the best available treatment, namely, accelerated rt-PA. More studies are needed to establish the optimal dose and mode of Sak administration and its life-saving potential relative to established thrombolytic agents.

PERIPHERAL ARTERIAL OCCLUSION

Thirty patients (37–86 years of age) with limb ischemia or incapacitating claudication of <120 day duration and with angiographically documented thromboembolic peripheral arterial occlusion, mostly due to in situ thrombosis of native femoropopliteal arteries, were treated in a pilot study [22]. Intra-arterial, catheter-directed Sak was given as a bolus of 1 mg, followed by a continuous infusion of 0.5 mg/h in 20 patients and as a bolus of 2 mg, followed by an infusion of 1 mg/h in 10 patients, together with heparin. After 7.0 ± 0.7 mg of Sak were infused over 8.7 ± 1.0 hours, recanalization was complete in 25 patients (83%), partial in 2, and absent in 3. Poor prognostic signs (including poor distal runoff, long duration, and distal localization of occlusion) characterized the three patients without macroscopic clot lysis. The majority of patients underwent complementary surgical or endovascular procedures, mainly percutaneous transluminal angioplasty, to treat culprit lesions and to promote long-term vessel patency. Major amputations were limited to two patients in whom thrombolysis failed. Three patients developed a reocclusion within 1 month; two major hemorrhagic complications occurred, both in elderly women, including a fatal hemorrhagic stroke. Intra-arterial Sak did not produce a systemic lytic state nor a prolongation of template bleeding times. Staphylokinase thus appeared to be a valuable adjunct to endovascular and surgical revascularization techniques, with rapid and efficient restoration of vessel patency and limb viability in the great majority of patients with acute or subacute peripheral arterial occlusion.

Antigenicity of Staphylokinase and Engineered Variants

The rather low-grade antigenicity of Sak, as suggested by early dog and baboon experiments, unfortunately could not be extended to patients: the vast majority of patients with either myocardial infarction [19–21] or peripheral arterial occlusion [22] developed neutralizing antibodies to Sak after a prolonged lag phase of 10–12 days, which remained elevated well above pretreatment levels for several months after administration [23]. However, the titers of preformed anti-Sak antibodies in the general population appeared to be lower than those of antistreptokinase antibodies, and even systemic *S. aureus* infections failed to induce Sak-neutralizing antibodies in most patients, possibly reflecting the low proportion of *S. aureus* strains that produce Sak [24]. The current clinical experience suggests that major allergic reactions to Sak are rare, but is too limited to allow definite conclusions. The boost of neutralizing antibody titers upon infusion of Sak would predict therapeutic refractoriness on repeated administration. Therefore, restriction to a single use probably applies to both streptokinase and Sak. The absence of cross-reactivity to streptokinase of antibodies elicited by Sak, and vice versa, suggests that the use of both plasminogen activators is not mutually exclusive.

Wild-type Sak (variant SakSTAR) was found to contain three nonoverlapping immunodominant epitopes, at least two of which could be eliminated, albeit with partial inactivation of the molecule, by site-directed mutagenesis of selected clusters of two or three charged amino acids to alanine [25]. The recombinant combination mutants SakSTAR.M38 (with Lys^{35}, Glu^{38}, Lys^{74}, Glu^{75}, and Arg^{77} replaced by Ala) and SakSTAR.M89 (with Lys^{74}, Glu^{75}, Arg^{77}, Glu^{80}, and Asp^{82} replaced by Ala) (see Figure 18-1) had reduced immunoreactivity toward a panel of murine monoclonal anti-SakSTAR antibodies and toward antibodies elicited in patients by treatment with SakSTAR. Relative to wild-type SakSTAR, SakSTAR.M38 and SakSTAR.M89 induced less circulating neutralizing activity and less resistance to thrombolysis on repeated infusion, following intensive immunization of rabbits [26] or baboons [27]. In a comparative study in 16 patients with peripheral arterial occlusion, SakSTAR.M38 and SakSTAR.M89 proved to be equally fibrin specific and thrombolytically effective, but significantly less antigenic than wild-type SakSTAR [26]. Systematic reversal of the substituted amino acids to the wild-type residues suggested that, in humans, lysine at position 74 is involved in the humoral immune response [28,29]. These studies illustrate that genetic engineering of a heterologous protein with therapeutic potential can reduce its antigenicity. Ongoing research is aimed at gaining more mechanistic insight into the humoral and cellular immune response to Sak and at optimizing the ratio of specific activity to antigenicity of Sak mutants.

Pharmacokinetics of Staphylokinase in Patients

In five patients with acute myocardial infarction treated with an intravenous infusion of 10 mg Sak over 30 minutes, the postinfusion disappearance of Sak-related antigen from plasma occurred in a biphasic manner with a $t_{1/2}\alpha$ of 6.3 minutes and a $t_{1/2}\beta$ of 37 minutes, corresponding to a plasma clearance of 270 mL/min [18]. Staphylokinase antigen levels in myocardial infarction patients at 25 and 90 minutes were $0.56 \pm 0.06 \mu g/mL$ and $0.16 \pm 0.04 \mu g/mL$ after 10 mg over 30 minutes (n = 25), $1.9 \pm 0.22 \mu g/mL$ and $0.42 \pm 0.06 \mu g/mL$ after 20 mg over 30 minutes (n = 23), $3.4 \pm 0.45 \mu g/mL$ and $1.3 \pm 0.30 \mu g/mL$ after 40 mg over 30 minutes (n = 5), and $1.6 \pm 0.19 \mu g/mL$ and $0.44 \pm 0.07 \mu g/mL$ after a double 15 mg bolus, 30 minutes apart (n = 50), respectively [20,22].

Conclusions

Staphylokinase, a 136 amino acid protein produced by *S. aureus* and now readily available by recombinant DNA technology, is an indirect plasminogen activator with a unique structure, mechanism of action, and fibrin specificity. Staphylokinase induces efficient and rapid recanalization in patients with arterial thrombosis. Its fibrin specificity at clinically effective doses exceeds that of other available plasminogen activators. Likewise, its speed and rate of clot lysis compare favorably with established agents, but definition of the relative benefits, especially in terms of reduction of mortality and morbidity, awaits larger comparative trials. The optimal dose and rate of infusion in patients with coronary and peripheral arterial thrombosis and a possible role for Sak in other thromboembolic disorders (comprising deep venous thrombosis, pulmonary embolism, and ischemic stroke) remain to be establised. Notwithstanding its rather short circulatory half-life, bolus coronary thrombolysis with Sak appears to be feasible. The antigenicity of wild-type Sak argues against repeated administration, but initial experience with selected recombinant mutants indicates that the immunoreactivity and antigenicity of this bacterial protein can at least be attenuated while preserving fibrinolytic activity and fibrin specificity.

Acknowledgments

S. Vanderschueren is a research assistant of the National Fund for Scientific Research (N.F.W.O.), Belgium.

References

1. Much H. Über eine Vorstufe des Fibrinfermentes in Kulturen von Staphylokokkus aureus. Biochemische Zeitschrift 14:143, 1908.
2. Mölkänen T, Kuikka T, Kuusela P. Production of staphylokinase by staphylococcus strains isolated from bacteremic patients (abstr). Fibrinolysis 10(Suppl. 3):138, 1996.
3. Sako T, Tsuchida N. Nucleotide sequence of the staphylokinase gene from *Staphylococcus aureus*. Nucleic Acids Res 11:7679, 1983.
4. Behnke D, Gerlach D. Cloning and expression in *Escherichia coli*, *Bacillus subtilis* and *Streptococcus sanguis* of a gene for staphylokinase: A bacterial plasminogen activator. Mol Gen Genet 210:528, 1987.
5. Collen D, Zhao ZA, Holvoet P, Marynen P. Primary structure and gene structure of staphylokinase. Fibrinolysis 6:226, 1992.
6. Gase A, Birch-Hirschfeld E, Gührs KH, Hartmann M, Vetterman S, Damaschun G, Damaschun H, Gast K, Misselwitz R, Zirwer D, Collen D, Schlott B. The thermostability of natural variants of bacterial plasminogen-activator staphylokinase. Eur J Biochem 223:303, 1994.
7. Schlott B, Hartmann M, Gührs KH, Birsch-Hirschfeld E, Pohl D, Vanderschueren S, Van de Werf F, Michoel A, Collen D, Behnke D. High yield production and purification of recombinant staphylokinase for thrombolytic therapy. Biotechnology 12:185, 1994.
8. Collen D, Lijnen HR. Staphylokinase, a fibrin-specific plasminogen activator with therapeutic potential? Blood 84:680, 1994.
9. Lijnen HR. Staphylokinase. In Handbook of Experimental Pharmacology. Fibrinolytics and Antifibrinolytics. Heidelberg: Springer Verlag, in press.
10. Vanderschueren SMF, Lijnen HR, Collen D. Properties of staphylokinase and its potential as a thrombolytic agent. Fibrinolysis (Suppl. 1):87, 1995.
11. Lijnen HR, Van Hoef B, Vandenbossche L, Collen D. Biochemical properties of natural and recombinant staphylokinase. Fibrinolysis 6:214, 1992.
12. Lijnen HR, Van Hoef B, Collen D. Interactions of staphylokinase with human platelets. Thromb Haemost 73:472, 1995.
13. Vanderschueren S, Collen D. Comparative effects of staphylokinase and alteplase in rabbit bleeding time models. Thromb Haemost 75:816, 1996.
14. Lijnen HR, Stassen JM, Collen D. Differential inhibition with antifibrinolytic agents of staphylokinase and streptokinase induced clot lysis. Thromb Haemost 73:845, 1995.
15. Collen D, De Cock F, Van Linthout J, Declerck PJ, Lijnen HR, Stassen JM. Comparative thrombolytic and immunogenic properties of staphylokinase and streptokinase. Fibrinolysis 6:232, 1992.
16. Collen D, De Cock F, Stassen JM. Comparative immunogenicity and thrombolytic properties toward arterial and venous thrombi of streptokinase and recombinant

staphylokinase in baboons. Circulation 87:996, 1993.

17. Collen D, Van de Werf F. Coronary thrombolysis with recombinant staphylokinase in patients with evolving myocardial infarction. Circulation 87:1850, 1993.

18. Collen DC, Gold HK. New developments in thrombolytic therapy. Adv Exp Med Biol. 281:333, 1990.

19. Vanderschueren S, Barrios L, Kerdsinchai P, Van den Heuvel P, Hermans L, Vrolix M, De Man F, Benit E, Muyldermans L, Collen D, Van de Werf F. A randomized trial of recombinant staphylokinase versus alteplase for coronary artery patency in acute myocardial infarction. Circulation 92:2044, 1995.

20. Vanderschueren S, Collen D, Van de Werf F. A pilot study on bolus administration of recombinant staphylokinase for coronary artery thrombolysis. Thromb Haemost 76:541, 1996.

21. Vanderschueren S, Dens J, Kerdsinchai P, Desmet W, Vrolix M, De Man F, Van den Heuvel P, Hermans L, Collen D, Van de Werf F. A pilot randomized coronary patency trial of double-bolus recombinant staphylokinase versus front-loaded alteplase in acute myocardial infarction. Am Heart, in press.

22. Vanderschueren S, Stockx L, Wilms G, Verhaeghe R, Lacroix H, Vermylen J, Collen D. Thrombolytic therapy of peripheral arterial occlusion with recombinant staphylokinase. Circulation 92:2050, 1995.

23. Vanderschueren SMF, Stassen JM, Collen D. On the immunogenicity of recombinant staphylokinase in pa-

tients and in animal models. Thromb Haemost 72:297, 1994.

24. Declerck PJ, Vanderschueren S, Billiet J, Moreau H, Collen D. Prevalence and induction of circulating antibodies against recombinant staphylokinase. Thromb Haemost 71:129, 1994.

25. Collen D, Bernaerts R, Declerck P, De Cock F, Demarsin E, Jenné S, Laroche Y, Lijnen HR, Silence K, Verstreken M. Recombinant staphylokinase variants with altered immunoreactivity. I. Construction and characterization. Circulation 94:197, 1996.

26. Collen D, Moreau H, Stockx L, Vanderschueren S. Recombinant staphylokinase variants with altered immunoreactivity. II. Thrombolytic properties and antibody induction. Circulation 94:207, 1996.

27. Vanderschueren S, Stassen JM, Collen D. Comparative antigenicity of wild-type staphylokinase (SakSTAR) and a selected mutant (SakSTAR.M38) in a baboon thrombolysis model. J Cardiovasc Pharmacol 27:809, 1996.

28. Collen D, De Cock F, Demarsin E, Jenné S, Lasters I, Laroche Y, Warmerdam P, Jespers L. Recombinant staphylokinase variants with altered immunoreactivity. III. Species variability of antibody binding patterns. Circulation 95:455, 1997.

29. Collen D, Stockx L, Lacroix H, Suy R, Vanderschueren S. Recombinant staphylokinase variants with altered immunoreactivity. IV. Identification of variants with reduced antibody induction but intact potency. Circulation 95:463, 1997.

19. NOVEL TISSUE PLASMINOGEN ACTIVATORS: RETEPLASE (R-PA)

Christoph Bode, Thomas K. Nordt, Benedikt Kohler, W. Douglas Weaver, and Richard W. Smalling

Introduction

Thrombolytic therapy has become an accepted form of treatment for acute myocardial infarction. The GUSTO I trial showed that mortality reduction correlates with early, complete, and sustained patency of the infarct-related coronary artery [1,2]. Current thrombolytic regimens achieve patency 90 minutes after initiation of treatment in only about 81% of cases, and only about 54% experience complete (TIMI grade 3) reperfusion. These results are obtained 90 minutes after initiation of therapy, and earlier patency rates are even more disappointing. Early reocclusion further limits the preservation of left ventricular function. In addition, even though patients are carefully selected, bleeding, especially intracranial bleeding, is a feared side effect, limiting the applicability of this form of treatment. In order to improve the risk/benefit ratio of thrombolytic therapy for patients, a number of new thrombolytic agents are being developed, primarily with the aim of reducing mortality by establishing more rapid, more complete, and more stable coronary patency.

This review summarizes the molecular characteristics and pharmacological properties of reteplase, obtained in vitro and in experimental animal studies, as well as the clinical results obtained in patency and mortality studies using this new drug. Although most studies of reteplase have expressed doses in megaunits (MU), on the basis of an amidolytic assay, doses in this review are cited in units (U) based on a new clot lysis assay. One MU equals one U in the new system.

Molecular Characteristics of Reteplase

Reteplase, which is alternatively referred to as r-PA (recombinant plasminogen activator) or BM 06.022, is a genetically engineered deletion mutant of human tissue-type plasminogen activator (t-PA). Reteplase is produced by expression of an appropriately constructed plasmid in *Escherichia coli*, where it is localized in inclusion bodies. Like many proteins expressed in prokaryotic cells, the fully functional, nonglycosylated protein becomes available after an in vitro refolding process. SDS-polyacrylamide electrophoresis and amino acid analysis reveal a single-chain, nonglycosylated protein of 39.6 kd, which consists of amino acids 1–3 and 176–527 of human t-PA. Reteplase consists of the kringle-2 and protease domains of human t-PA, whereas the kringle-1, finger, and epidermal growth factor domains have been deleted. The one-chain form can be cleaved by plasmin to a two-chain form [3,4]. The structural changes of reteplase relative to human t-PA result in markedly different properties in vitro and in vivo.

Functional Studies with Reteplase In Vitro

The structure and function of the enzymatic domain of human t-PA (alteplase) are largely retained by reteplase. Reteplase was shown to have only low affinity for fibrin; however, it acts as a fibrin-specific protein in vivo at appropriate dosages [3]. The plasminogenolytic activity of reteplase, in the absence of stimulatory CNBr fibrinogen fragments, is similar to that of alteplase; however, in the presence of stimulator, its activity is about fourfold less when compared on a molar basis [3]. Plasminogen activator inhibitor (PAI)-1 inhibition was similar for reteplase and t-PA, indicating that the responsible structures of the kringle 2 and protease domains were identical in the two molecules [5]. Presumably because of the lack of glycosylation and/or the lack of the finger and growth factor domains, a lower affinity for endothelial cells as compared with t-PA has been reported [3].

Extensive studies on the in vitro lysis of fresh, aged, platelet-poor, and plateletet-rich clots, as well as whole blood clots, have been performed [6]. To achieve 50% clot lysis at 4 hours into the experiment, 6.4 times higher molar concentrations of reteplase (vs. alteplase) had to be used. The data suggest that, in vitro, reteplase achieved a lower thrombolytic potency, especially in lysing aged clots and platelet-rich clots, when compared with alteplase on a molar basis. In further experiments, clots incubated with reteplase or alteplase were transferred to plasminogen activator–free plasma. Clot lysis continued for 3 hours with alteplase; in contrast, no further lysis occurred with reteplase.

Evaluation of Reteplase in Experimental Animals

The intended prolongation in half-life of reteplase relative to t-PA was demonstrated in rats, dogs, and nonhuman primates [7]. In the rabbit model of jugular vein thrombosis, reteplase proved to be 5.3 times more effective than alteplase when each activator was given as a bolus. The plasma clearance was 4.3-fold lower than that of alteplase; thus, the apparent higher potency may well be the result of the lower clearance rate. At equipotent dosages, residual fibrinogen was similar for both activators; thus no relative loss in specificity was observed [8]. In a canine model of coronary thrombosis, reteplase was compared with alteplase, anistreplase, urokinase, and streptokinase. Reperfusion was achieved significantly more rapidly with reteplase than with the other tested plasminogen activators, and, remarkably, bleeding time was least affected [9]. To achieve 50% recanalization in another study utilizing a dog model of coronary thrombosis, the required dose of intravenous reteplase was 11.6-fold lower than that for intravenous alteplase [10]. Further experiments suggest that an antithrombotic adjunct may be useful for preservation of patency after fibrinolysis with reteplase [11,12]. Double-bolus administration of reteplase was shown to be more effective than infusion or single-bolus dose regimens [13]. Reteplase also proved useful in reversing pulmonary hypertension in a dog model of pulmonary embolism. Because of its bolus application, reteplase acted faster than other plasminogen activators in these experiments [14]. Reteplase and alteplase had no effect on platelet count or, when given alone, on ex vivo platelet aggregation. In animals pretreated with aspirin, reteplase significantly reduced platelet aggregation in comparison with alteplase [15], a difference that was not observed in patients [16].

Clinical Studies with Reteplase

Phase I studies evaluating the effects of reteplase on healthy volunteers provided no data mitigating against phase II testing [17,18].

GRECO I AND II STUDIES

The first phase II trial with reteplase (the first German RECOmbinant Plasminogen Activator Study or GRECO I) was designed as an open, sequential dose-finding study in patients with acute myocardial infarction [19]. With the first tested dose of 10 units (U) of reteplase, the predefined minimal 90-minute patency of 70% was not achieved, as indicated by a sequential probability ratio test after treatment of 42 patients. The 90-minute patency rate (TIMI grade 2 or 3) was 67%. An increased dose of 15 U of reteplase, administered as a single bolus, resulted in a patency at 90 minutes (TIMI grade 2 or 3) of 76% in the following 100 patients (74% at 60 minutes). Complete patency (TIMI grade 3) after 90 minutes was achieved in 69% of patients in the 15 U group and in 52% of those treated with 10 U. To increase the efficacy further, the concept of a double-bolus administration was investigated in an open, noncontrolled, dose-finding study in 50 patients (GRECO II). Sixty- and 90-minute patency (TIMI grade 2 or 3) after a 10 U + 5 U (30 minutes apart) double-bolus regimen was 72% and 78%, respectively, and TIMI grade 3 patency was 50% and 58% [20].

RAPID I STUDY

The 15 U bolus regimen, the 10 + 5 U double bolus regimen and a new 10 + 10 U regimen of reteplase were compared with conventional alteplase (100 mg over 3 hours) in an international, randomized study enrolling 606 patients with acute myocardial infarction (Reteplase vs. Alteplase Patency Investigation During acute myocardial infarction, or RAPID I trial) [21]. The 10 + 10 U reteplase regimen was superior to the other reteplase regimens and also achieved better 60 and 90-minute TIMI grade 3 patency than alteplase (reteplase vs. alteplase at 60 minutes, 51.0% vs. 32.7%, $P < 0.01$; and at 90 minutes, 62.7% vs. 49.3%; $P < 0.05$). Similarly, overall patency (TIMI grade 2 and 3) was better under treatment with reteplase 10 + 10 U, although not significantly so (reteplase vs. alteplase at 60 minutes, 77.6% vs. 66.3%; and at 90 minutes, 85.2% vs. 77.8%). Patency was achieved more rapidly with reteplase than with alteplase. TIMI grade 3 patency at 60 minutes for reteplase (51.0%) was similar to that for alteplase at 90 minutes (49.3%). Superior speed and completeness of reperfusion resulted in better preservation of left ventricular function in the

10 + 10 U reteplase group [22]. The risk of bleeding was not significantly different for reteplase and conventional alteplase [23]. There was no significant difference between reteplase and alteplase with respect to platelet aggregation or thrombin activity during and up to 12 hours after treatment of patients with acute myocardial infarction [16].

INJECT STUDY

In an effort to assess the safety and efficacy of reteplase in a larger study population, the International Joint Efficacy Comparison of Thrombolytics (INJECT) study was performed [24]. Reteplase 10 + 10 U was compared with streptokinase in 6010 patients with acute myocardial infarction in a double-blind, randomized trial, with 35-day mortality as the primary endpoint. The primary aim of the INJECT study was to demonstrate that the 10 + 10 U double-bolus regimen of reteplase is at least equivalent to the standard regimen of streptokinase in terms of mortality. Equivalence was defined as a 35-day mortality rate for reteplase not more than 1% higher than for streptokinase. The trial was not powered to demonstrate superiority and had design features (recruitment up to 12 hours, trial confined to Europe) that made it difficult to compare it with other trials (e.g., GUSTO I).

Death up to 35 days after the index infarction occurred in 9.02% of 2994 patients in the reteplase group and 9.53% of 2992 patients in the streptokinase group. The difference of −0.51% (90% confidence interval, −1.74 to 0.73) in favor of reteplase was nonsignificant. Thus, reteplase showed equivalent efficacy to that of streptokinase using the above-mentioned definition. Mortality at 6 months was also equivalent, with 11.02% in the reteplase group and 12.05% in the streptokinase group (difference, −1.03%; 90% confidence interval, −2.65 to 0.59%). Patient follow-up was 99.6% complete. The incidence of cardiac shock (reteplase vs. streptokinase, 4.7% vs. 6.0%), heart failure (23.6% vs. 26.3%), hypotension (15.5% vs. 17.6%), and atrial fibrillation (7.2% vs. 8.8%) was lower in the reteplase group.

The INJECT study also provided data comparing the safety and tolerability of reteplase and streptokinase. The overall incidence of bleeding (reteplase vs. streptokinase, 15.0% vs. 15.3%) and significant bleeding (4.6% vs. 4.7%) were very similar. Also, there was no significant difference in the total incidence of stroke (1.23% vs. 1.00%) or hemorrhagic stroke (0.77% vs. 0.37%). Data from the invasive RAPID I and II studies support these findings in showing no excess side effects for reteplase versus alteplase.

RAPID II STUDY

After the GUSTO I study [1,2] had shown that an accelerated dose regimen for alteplase (100 mg over 90 minutes) was superior to streptokinase, and possibly also to conventional alteplase therapy with respect to efficacy and safety, the RAPID II study was undertaken. The 10 + 10 U reteplase regimen was compared with the GUSTO regimen of alteplase in an open, randomized trial enrolling 324 patients. The study design differed from the RAPID I study in that there was no age limit (RAPID I <75 years) and patients were included until up to 12 hours after the onset of pain (RAPID I <6 hours). Infarct-related coronary artery patency (TIMI grade 2 and 3) and complete patency (TIMI grade 3) at 90 minutes were significantly higher in the reteplase-treated patients (TIMI grade 2 and 3, reteplase vs. alteplase, 83.4% vs. 73.3%, $P = 0.03$; TIMI grade 3, 59.9% vs. 45.2%, $P = 0.01$). At 60 minutes, the incidences of both patency and complete patency were also significantly higher in reteplase-treated patients (TIMI grade 2 and 3, 81.8% vs. 66.1%, $P = 0.01$; TIMI grade 3, 51.2% vs. 37.4%, $P = 0.03$; Figure 19-1). Reteplase-patients required fewer additional acute coronary interventions (13.6% vs. 26.5%, $P < 0.01$) and there was no apparent increase in death at 35 days (reteplase vs. alteplase, 4.1% vs. 8.4%), stroke (1.8% vs. 2.6%), hemorrhagic stroke (1.2% vs. 1.9%), in-hospital reocclusion (9.0% vs. 7.0%), or bleeding rate (12.4% vs. 9.7%) (Figure 19-2) [25]. The GUSTO III study is currently investigating whether the apparent advantages of reteplase over alteplase in achieving early and complete patency translate into a lower mortality.

Implications for Clinical Practice and Future Research

Double-bolus administration (10 + 10 U) of reteplase results in effective, rapid, and complete lysis of coronary thrombi in the majority of patients. With respect to these parameters, the 10 + 10 U regimen was superior to established alteplase regimens in the RAPID studies. The GUSTO III study is currently investigating whether the improved patency data translate into reduced mortality. There is reason to believe that this will indeed be the case based on the results of the GUSTO I trial and its angiographic substudy [1,2]. Patency appears to be an appropriate surrogate endpoint for mortality, but only when investigated in large, multicenter, randomized trials with blinded, centralized assessment of results. That these requirements appear mandatory may be delineated from two examples: Double-bolus

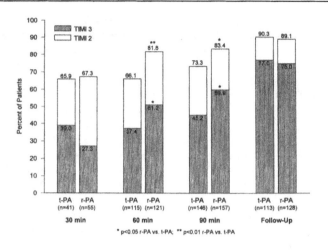

FIGURE 19-1. Coronary patency rates at different time points achieved with alteplase (t-PA) or reteplase (r-PA). (From RAPID II, with permission.)

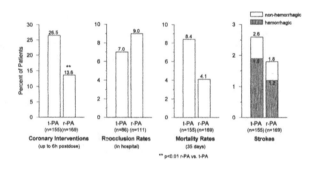

FIGURE 19-2. Important clinical endpoints after therapy with alteplase (t-PA) and reteplase (r-PA). (From RAPID II, with permission.)

administration of alteplase was first investigated in a relatively small, single-center, nonrandomized study [26] suggesting very high patency rates, superior to those achievable with an accelerated alteplase infusion. In a larger study, the alteplase double bolus, in fact, turned out to be slightly less effective than the accelerated alteplase infusion [27].

A similar pattern could be noted when the GUSTO IIB investigators showed patency results for acute percutaneous transluminal coronary angioplasty (PTCA) to be much inferior to those previously reported in smaller trials [28,29]. In fact, the patency rates for reteplase-treated patients recruited within 6 hours in the RAPID II study (TIMI grade 2 and 3, 86.5%; TIMI grade 3, 65%) are closer to those re-

ported for acute PTCA in the GUSTO IIB trial (TIMI grade 2 and 3, 82%; TIMI grade 3, 75%) than to those of other thrombolytic regimens, so that a large trial comparing prehospital thrombolysis with double-bolus reteplase (exploiting this logistic advantage of thrombolysis) with acute PTCA offers an interesting comparison.

New thrombolytic agents, such as antibody-targeted plasminogen activators, have been produced as conjugates [30] and recombinant molecules [31], and may further improve thrombolytic therapy. The potency and specificity of these agents compare favorably with conventional plasminogen activators in different animal models [31,32]. More specific thrombolytic agents, which leave the clotting system largely intact, may well require equally specific anti-coagulants as adjuncts [33].

While many new approaches are under investigation, reteplase has proven, at present, to be a potent and safe thrombolytic agent in patients with acute myocardial infarction, with the convenience of double-bolus injection. If the GUSTO III study substantiates the clinical results obtained thus far, reteplase may well become the standard against which other thrombolytic agents — and also mechanical reperfusion strategies — will have to prove their usefulness. Constant advancement in mechanical strategies (e.g., newer stent generations) and possible combinations of both thrombolytic and "rescue" mechanical strategies deserve further attention.

References

1. The GUSTO Investigators. An international randomized trial comparing four thrombolytic strategies for acute myocardial infarction. N Engl J Med 329:673, 1993.
2. The GUSTO Angiographic Investigators. The effects of tissue plasminogen activator, streptokinase, or both on coronary-artery patency, ventricular function and survival after acute myocardial infarction. N Engl J Med 329:1615, 1993.
3. Kohnert U, Rudolph R, Verheijen JH, Weening-Verhoeff EJ, Stern A, Opitz U, Martin U, Lill H, Prinz H, Lechner M. Biochemical properties of kringle 2 and protease domains are maintained in the refolded t-PA deletion variant BM 06.022. Protein Eng 5:93, 1992.
4 Martin U, Bader R, Böhm E, Kohnert U, von Möllendorf E, Fischer S, Sponer G. BM 06.022: A novel recombinant plasminogen activator. Cardiovasc Drug Rev 11:299, 1993.
5. Madison EL, Goldsmith EJ, Gerard RD, Gething MJ, Sambrook JF. Serpin-resistant mutants of human tissue-type plasminogen activator. Nature 339:721, 1989.
6. Martin U, Sponer G, Strein K. Differential fibrinolytic properties of the recombinant plasminogen activator BM 06.022 in human plasma and blood clot systems in vitro. Blood Coagul Fibrinolysis 4:235, 1993.
7. Martin U, Köhler J, Sponer G, Strein K. Pharmacokinetics of the novel recombinant plasminogen activator BM 06.022 in rats, dogs, and non-human primates. Fibrinolysis 6:39, 1992.
8. Martin U, Fischer S, Kohnert U, Opitz U, Rudolph R, Sponer G, Stern A, Strein K. Thrombolysis with an Escherichia coli-produced recombinant plasminogen activator (BM 06.022) in the rabbit model of jugular vein thrombosis. Thromb Haemost 65:560, 1991.
9. Martin U, Sponer G, Strein K. Evaluation of thrombotic and systemic effects of the novel recombinant plasminogen activator BM 06.022 compared with alteplase, anistreplase, streptokinase and urokinase in a canine model of coronary artery thrombosis. J Am Coll Cardiol 19:433, 1992.
10. Martin U, Fischer S, Kohnert U, Rudolph R, Sponer G, Stern A, Strein K. Coronary thrombolytic properties of a novel recombinant plasminogen activator (BM 06.022) in a canine model. J Cardiovasc Pharmacol 18:111, 1991.
11. Martin U, Sponer G, Strein K. Hirudin and sulotroban improve coronary blood flow after reperfusion induced by the novel recombinant plasminogen activator BM 06.022 in a canine model of coronary artery thrombosis. Int J Hematol 56:143, 1992.
12. Martin U, Fischer S, Sponer G. Influence of heparin and systemic lysis on coronary blood flow after reperfusion induced by novel recombinant plasminogen activator BM 06.022 in a canine model of coronary thrombosis. J Am Coll Cardiol 22:914, 1993.
13. Martin U, Sponer G, König R, Smolarz A, Meyer-Sabellek W, Strein K. Double bolus administration of the novel recombinant plasminogen activator (BM 06.022) improves coronary blood flow after reperfusion in a canine model of coronary thrombosis. Blood Coagul Fibrinolysis 3:139, 1992.
14. Martin U, Sponer G, Strein K. Rapid reversal of canine thromboembolic pulmonary hypertension by bolus injection of the novel recombinant plasminogen activator BM 06.022. J Cardiovasc Pharmacol 7:365, 1993.
15. Martin U, Dalchau H, Sponer G. Effects of the novel recombinant plasminogen activator BM 06.022 on platelets and bleeding time in rabbits. Platelets 3:247, 1992.
16. Bode C, Kohler B, Nordt T, Peter K, Ruef J, von Hodenberg E, Smalling RW and the RAPLD Investigators. Thrombin activity during and after thrombolysis with reteplase or alteplase in patients with acute myocardial infarction (abstr). Circulation 90(Suppl. I):563, 1994.
17. Martin U, von Möllendorf E, Akpan W, Kientsch-Engel R, Kaufmann B, Neugebauer G. Dose-ranging study of the novel recombinant plasminogen activator BM 06.022 in healthy volunteers. Clin Pharmacol Ther 50:429, 1991.
18. Martin U, von Möllendorf E, Akpan W, Kientsch-Engel R, Kaufmann B, Neugebauer G. Pharmacokinetic and hemostatic properties of the recombinant plasminogen activator BM 06.022 in healthy volunteers. Thromb Haemost 66:569, 1991.
19. Neuhaus KL, von Essen R, Vogt A, Tebbe U, Rustige J, Wagner HJ, Appel KF, Stienen U, König R, Meyer-Sabellek W. Dose finding with a novel recombinant plasminogen activator (BM 06.022) in patients with acute myocardial infarction: Results of the German Recombinant Plasminogen Activator Study. J Am Coll Cardiol 24:55, 1994.

20. Tebbe U, von Essen R, Smolarz A, Limbourg P, Rox J, Rustige J, Vogt A, Wagner J, Meyer-Sabellek W, Neuhaus KL. Open, noncontrolled dose-finding study with a novel recombinant plasminogen activator (BM 06.022) given as a double bolus in patients with acute myocardial infarction. Am J Cardiol 72:518, 1993.

21. Smalling RW, Bode C, Kalbfleisch J, Sen S, Limbourg P, Forycki F, Habib G, Feldman R, Hohnloser S, Seals A, and the RAPID Investigators. More rapid, complete, and stable coronary thrombolysis with bolus administration of reteplase compared with alteplase infusion in acute myocardial infarction. Circulation 91:2725, 1995.

22. Smalling RW, Bode C, Kalbfleisch J, Sen S, Limbourg P, Forycki F, Habib G, Feldman R, Hohnloser S and Seals A for the RAPID Investigators. Improvement of global and regional LV-function by the bolus administration of recombinant plasminogen activator (r-PA) in acute myocardial infarction: A comparison with standard dose alteplase (abstr). Circulation 90(Suppl. I):562, 1994.

23. Bode C, Smalling RW, Sen S, Kalbfleisch J, Feldman R, Forycki F, Limbourg P, Mann D, Böhm E, Odenheimer DJ and the RAPID Investigators. Safety profile of reteplase (r-PA) as compared to alteplase (rt-PA): Will there be fewer strokes? (abstr) Eur Heart J 15(Suppl. I):P3096, 1994.

24. The INJECT Study Group. Randomized, double-blind comparison of reteplase double-bolus administration with streptokinase in acute myocardial infarction (INJECT): Trial to investigate equivalence. Lancet 346:329, 1995.

25. Bode C, Smalling RW, Berg G, Burnett C, Lorch G, Kalbfleisch J, Chernoff R, Christie L, Feldman R, Seals A, Weaver WD, and the RAPID Investigators. Randomized comparison of coronary thrombolysis achieved with double bolus reteplase (r-PA) and front-loaded "accelerated" alteplase (rt-PA) in patients with acute myocardial infarction. Circulation 94:891, 1996.

26. Purvis JA, McNeill AJ, Siddequi RA, Roberts MJD, McClements BM, McEneaney D, Campbell NPS, Khan MM, Webb SW, Wilson CM, Adgey AAJ. Efficacy of 100 mg of double-bolus alteplase in achieving complete perfusion in the treatment of acute myocardial infarction. J Am Coll Cardiol 23:6, 1994.

27. Bleich SD, Adgey AAJ, Pickering E, Hillis WS, Ghali M, Blankenship I, Madigan P, Bates E, Rees A, Love T, for the DOUBLE-Trial Investigators. An angiographic assessment of the efficacy and safety of front-loaded and bolus regimens of activase (Alteplase recombinant). The Double Bolus Lytic Efficacy Trial (abstr). Circulation 92(Suppl. I):415, 1995.

28. Verheugt FWA. Primary angioplasty for acute myocardial infarction: Is the balloon half full or half empty? Lancet 347:1276, 1996.

29. Grines CL, Browne KF, Marco J, Rothbaum D, Stone GW, O'Keefe J, Overlie P, Donohue B, Chelliah N, Timmis GC, Vlietstra RE, Strzelecki M, Pughrowicz-Ochocki S, O'Neill WW for the Primary Angioplasty in Myocardial Infarction Study Group. A comparison of immediate angioplasty with thrombolytic therapy for myocardial infarction. N Engl J Med 328:673, 1993.

30. Bode C, Matsueda GR, Hui KY, Haber E. Antibody-directed urokinase: A specific fibrinolytic agent. Science 229:765, 1985.

31. Runge MS, Quertermous T, Zavodny PJ, Love TW, Bode C, Freitag M, Shaw SY, Huang PL, Chou CC, Mullins D. A recombinant chimeric plasminogen activator with high affinity for fibrin has increased thrombolytic potency in vitro and in vivo. Proc Natl Acad Sci USA 88:10337, 1991.

32. Runge MS, Harker LA, Bode C, Ruef J, Kelly AB, Marzec UM, Allen E, Caban R, Shaw SY, Haber E, Hanson SR. Enhanced thrombolytic and antithrombotic potency of a fibrin-targeted plasminogen activator in baboons. Circulation 94:1412, 1996.

33. Bode C, Hudelmayer M, Mehwald P, Bauer S, Freitag M, von Hodenberg E, Newell JB, Kübler W, Haber E, Runge MS. Fibrin targeted recombinant hirudin inhibits thrombus growth more efficiently than recombinant hirudin in vitro. Circulation 90:1956, 1994.

20. CHEMISTRY, PHARMACOKINETICS, AND PHARMACODYNAMICS OF t-PA, TNK AND DSPA ALPHA 1

Steffen P. Christow and Dietrich C. Gulba

Introduction

Tissue-type plasminogen activator (t-PA), the principal physiological human plasminogen activator, has been expressed in large quantities by recombinant technologies and, thus, has been available for therapeutic use for almost a decade. Despite the initial expectations, subsequent experience with this substance has somewhat reduced clinicians' early enthusiasm; as a result, attempts have been made to engineer the molecule and to search for alternate and better plasminogen activators.

Site-directed mutagenesis of tissue-type plasminogen activator has produced a molecule (the TNK variant of t-PA) with resistance to the specific plasminogen activator inhibitor-1 and with a threefold prolongation of its plasma half-life. Further search for molecules with improved thrombolytic properties has led to the identification of a bat plasminogen activator (DSPA) that shares a greater than 70% homology with tissue-type plasminogen activator, has a half-life in the range of hours, and seems to offer almost complete fibrin specificity. Tissue-type plasminogen activator, the TNK variant thereof, and the plasminogen activator of the vampire bat have close structural and functional similarities. For this reason, these three agents are reviewed in a single chapter.

Tissue-Type Plasminogen Activator

CHEMICAL PROPERTIES

Tissue-type plasminogen activator (alteplase) is a 70-kD, fourfold glycosylated serine proteinase consisting, in its native form, of a single polypeptide chain of 527 amino acid residues [1–4] (Table 20-1; Figure 20-1). On cleavage of the plasmin-sensitive Arg^{275}–Ile^{276} peptide bond, the molecule is converted to a two-chain derivative composed of a heavy N-terminal chain and a light C-terminal chain, linked by a single disulfide bond (Ser^{264}–Ser^{395}) [1–3]. The native single-chain form and the two-chain product of limited proteolysis share the same pharmacological properties. The N-terminal region is composed of a signal peptide followed by four domains: a finger domain, which mediates fibrin binding; a growth factor domain; and two kringles, the second of which also contributes to fibrin binding. The catalytic active site is located in the C-terminal portion of the molecule.

BIOCHEMICAL AND PHARMACOLOGICAL PROPERTIES

Tissue-type plasminogen activator is produced by various cell types and is widely distributed physiologically in body fluids and tissues [5–10] (see Table 20-1). It has been detected in large amounts in the lungs and uterus. The bulk of t-PA, however, seems to be synthesized and secreted in plasma by endothelial cells, both constitutively and in response to various stimuli [6,9,11–15].

In blood, there is a highly sensitive balance between coagulation and fibrinolysis, which guarantees blood fluidity. Plasma levels and local secretion of t-PA are major contributors to this balance. In humans, the measured plasma concentration of t-PA averages $5\,\mu g/L$ but, with locally applied stimuli, the concentrations can rise to much higher levels, for example, after thrombus formation [11,12,15,16].

t-PA is reported to activate plasminogen to plasmin with a K_m of $65–100\,\mu M$ and a k_{cat} of $0.06/s$ [11,17,18]. Other authors, have found K_m and k_{cat} values of 2.1 mM and 11.4/s, or of $3.9\,\mu M$ and 0.58/min, respectively, in the presence of fibrinogen, depending on the analytic systems used [19,20]. The catalytic activity (K_m/k_{cat}) of t-PA on circulating plasminogen is very weak but is increased by two orders

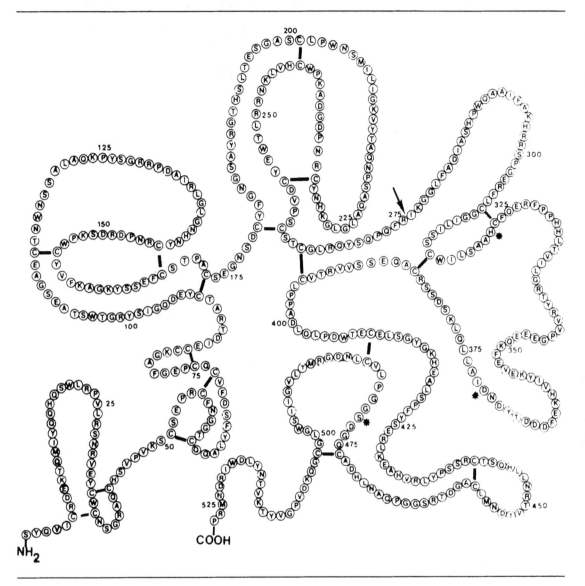

FIGURE 20-1. Secondary structure of tissue-plasminogen activator. Arrow-site of conversion into the two-chain form; black bars = disulfide bonds; asterisks = active site of the protease domain. The four glycosylation side chains are not shown.

of magnitude (K_m 2.4 μM, k_{cat} 0.02/s) [3,17,21] in the presence of fibrin or its fragments, endowing t-PA with a largely specific, plasmin-mediated, lytic activity toward fibrin (Figure 20-2). The plasminogenolytic activity of t-PA on Lys-plasminogen, in the presence of fibrin, is reported to be 10- to 15-fold higher than on Glu-plasminogen (K_m 19 μM, k_{cat} 0.2/s) [11,17,18]. Lys-plasminogen, in turn, binds preferentially to fibrin, contributing to the fibrin specificity of t-PA. This relative fibrin specificity [17,22,23] is mediated by a mechanism in which fibrin provides a surface to which t-PA and Lys-plasminogen adsorb, thus yielding a cyclic ternary complex [11,17,24]. The constant release of fibrin fragments causes increasing plasminogenolysis in a time-dependent manner. This leads to a progressive loss of fibrin specificity during the process of thrombolysis (see Figure 20-2).

TABLE 20-1. Chemical, biochemical, and pharmacological properties of tissue-type plasminogen activator (t-PA), the TNK-variant of tissue-type plasminogen activator (TNK-t-PA), and the plasminogen activators from vampire bat (DSPA) in comparison with streptokinase

Plasminogen activator	Streptokinase	t-PA	TNK-t-PA	DSPA
Generic name	Streptokinase	Alteplase	?	?
Molecular weight (kD)	47	70	70	52
Direct PA	No	Yes	Yes	Yes
Main $t_{1/2}$ (min)	10–25	4–9	15–19	170
k_{cat}/K_m $(s^{-1}\mu M^{-1})$				
+ fibrin	6×10^3	10	2.5×10^{-2}	684
− fibrin	6×10^3	10^{-3}	0.3×10^{-3}	0.06
Stimulation by vascular β-amyloid	No	Yes	Yes (?)	No
Production	Bacteria	Hamster ovarian cells	Hamster ovarian cells	COS-1 cells
Procedure	Isolation	Recombinant	Recombinant	Recombinant

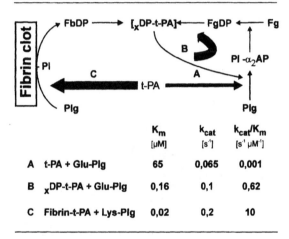

		K_m [µM]	k_{cat} [s⁻¹]	k_{cat}/K_m [s⁻¹ µM⁻¹]
A	t-PA + Glu-Plg	65	0,065	0,001
B	ₓDP-t-PA + Glu-Plg	0,16	0,1	0,62
C	Fibrin-t-PA + Lys-Plg	0,02	0,2	10

FIGURE 20-2. The pharmacokinetic properties of tissue-type plasminogen activator that convey relative fibrin specificity. t-PA = tissue-type plasminogen activator; Plg = plasminogen; Pl = plasmin; FbDP = fibrin degradation products; Fg = fibrinogen; FgDP = fibrinogen degradation products; Pl-α₂AP = plasmin–α₂-antiplasmin complex. (Adapted from Hoylaerts et al. [17], with permission.)

β-Amyloid also enhances the fibrinolytic activity of t-PA. Whether this β-amyloid–dependent stimulation of plasmin generation can be related to the increased hemorrhagic stroke rate observed with t-PA as compared with streptokinase currently remains a matter of speculation [58].

The fibrinolytic system is controlled by plasminogen activator inhibitors (PAI). The main antagonist of t-PA is PAI-1 [11,12]. During the inhibition reaction, PAI-1 binds irreversibly to the amino acid sequence $Lys^{296}–His^{297}–Arg^{298}–Arg^{299}–Ser^{300}–Pro^{301}–Gly^{302}–Arg^{303}$ of the light chain of t-PA, containing the active site of the molecule [25–27]. After binding to PAI-1, the structure of the active site is modified, so that plasminogen activation is completely prevented.

The specific activities of alteplase and duteplase (a nonglycosylated variant of t-PA, in which Met^{245} is substituted for Val^{245} [28]) are reported to be 80,000–90,000 U/mg protein [2,29] and about 300,000 U/mg protein [28], respectively. However, the activity of duteplase may vary considerably (±100,000 U/mg protein), depending on different conditions during the production phase. This has led to the expression of alteplase doses in mg/kg body weight and of duteplase doses in U/kg body weight.

t-PA is rapidly cleared from the circulation by metabolism in the liver [30] and subsequent secretion into the bile. Thus, the half-life of the substance is increased in patients with severe hepatic failure. In healthy subjects and in patients with acute myocardial infarction, t-PA has a half-life of 4–9 minutes [31–34].

PRODUCTION

Recombinant human t-PA is currently expressed and synthesized in large amounts in bacterial cells (duteplase) and mammalian cell cultures (alteplase) [1,2,8,35]. In contrast to mammalian t-PA, the t-PA produced in bacteria is nonglycosylated [36] and, therefore, has a lower molecular weight (about 47 kD). Alteplase, which has been commercially available for thrombolytic therapy since 1987, is produced in hamster ovarian cells.

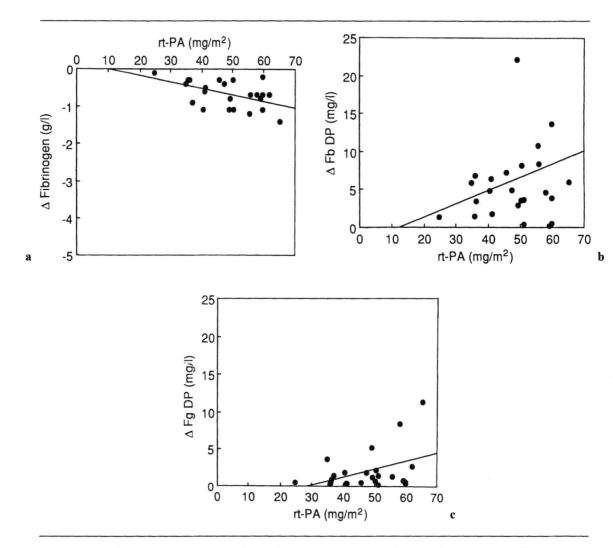

FIGURE 20-3. Effect of increasing doses of recombinant human t-PA (rt-PA) on plasma levels of fibrinogen and of specific fibrin degradation products (Fb DP) or on fibrinogen degradation products (Fg DP) during thrombolysis in acute myocardial infarction.

PRECLINICAL AND CLINICAL PROPERTIES

Tissue-type plasminogen activator has been compared with streptokinase and urokinase [37–41] in various in vitro [3,42,43], ex vivo and animal models (Table 20-2). In contrast to streptokinase and urokinase, the thrombolytic efficacy of t-PA is probably strongly dose-dependent, as suggested by the dose-related decrease in plasma fibrinogen, plasminogen, and α_2-antiplasmin levels, and by the simultaneous increase in the levels of fibrin and of fibrinogen degradation products (Figure 20-3). A threshold dose of 20–30 mg/m² body surface area exists, below which thrombolysis with t-PA seems to be completely fibrin selective. Only at very high doses does the fibrin specificity of t-PA slowly vanish, giving rise to systemic plasminogen activation. Extremely high doses of t-PA are capable of inducing fibrinogen degradation, comparable with that observed with streptokinase [44]. The thrombolytic efficacy of t-PA, on the other hand, is dependent on the constant supply of new plasminogen molecules with circulating blood. A sharp decline of t-PA–related thrombolysis occurs when plasminogen is depleted below a certain threshold (less than 30% of normal; Figure 20-4) [44]. This phenomenon, first recognized by Sobel et al., is called *plasminogen steal* [44].

TABLE 20-2. Preclinical and clinical properties of tissue-type plasminogen activator (t-PA), the TNK-variant of tissue-type plasminogen activator (TNK-t-PA), and the plasminogen activator from vampire bat (DSPA α1) in comparison with streptokinase

Plasminogen activator	Streptokinase	t-PA	TNK-t-PA	DSPA α1
Generic name	Streptokinase	Alteplase	?	?
Bolus administration possible	(Yes)	?	(Yes)? (Double bolus)	Yes
Fibrin specificity	−	+	++	+++
Antigenicity	+++	−	± (?)	+ (?)
Hypotensive effect	++	−	−	−
Recommended dose in AMI	1.5×10^6 U over 1 h	100 mg over 1.5 h	?	?
Clinical experience	++++	+++	(−)	−
Evaluated for	AMI, DVT, PE, APVD, (stroke)	AMI, DVT, PE, (stroke)	AMI	—

Assessment: ++++ strong to − lacking.
AMI = acute myocardial infarction; DVT = deep venous thrombosis; PE = pulmonary embolism; APVD = acute peripheral vascular disease; ( ) = not definitely accepted procedure; ? = questionable or not defined.

Plasminogen Steal

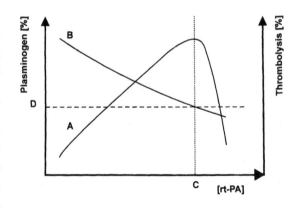

FIGURE 20-4. The plasminogen steal phenomenon. Relation between thrombolysis (A), dose of rt-PA, and plasma plasminogen concentrations (B). Critical value of rt-PA concentration (C) beyond which the thrombolytic activity of rt-PA is exhausted. Threshold of plasminogen concentration (D) required for sufficient plasminogen delivery to warrant maximum thrombolysis.

With today's most effective approved dose regimen for thrombolysis in patients with acute myocardial infarction (the Neuhaus regimen, i.e., an intravenous bolus of 15 mg of alteplase, followed by a continuous infusion of 50 mg over 30 minutes and of 35 mg over the next 60 minutes [45,46]), only little systemic fibrin degradation is observed. This regimen yields t-PA plasma levels of approximately two or three orders of magnitude above physiological concentrations. Clinical trials suggest that changes in this regimen of t-PA may further improve its thrombolytic efficacy [47,48].

Administration of high doses of t-PA leads to partial loss of fibrin specificity [46,49–54]. The effect is more pronounced with prolonged infusion regimens, such as those used in the treatment of deep venous thrombosis and peripheral arterial occlusions, or with accelerated regimens involving high initial bolus doses. Acceleration by fibrin of t-PA's plasminogen activation is similar to that caused by crosslinked β-amyloid (K_m 1.8 μM, k_{cat} 0.06/s). β-Amyloid is detectable in cerebral amyloid angiopathy, a regular finding in the arteries of patients over the age of 70, and in Alzheimer's disease [55–57]. Therefore, one might speculate that a substance-specific mechanism is responsible for the observed higher rate of cerebral hemorrhage with t-PA compared with streptokinase [58].

The results of the Global Utilization of Streptokinase and Tissue Plasminogen Activator for Occluded Coronary Arteries (GUSTO) I trial undoubtedly support the overall superiority of t-PA (alteplase) over streptokinase [59,60]. In over 40,000 patients with evolving myocardial infarction randomized to four thrombolytic treatments, 30-day mortality was 6.3% in over 10,000 patients randomized to accelerated t-PA versus 7.4% in over 10,000 streptokinase recipients. (Patients allocated to a combination of streptokinase and t-PA, or to streptokinase with subcutaneous instead of intravenous heparin, showed intermediate 30-day mortality rates). Coronary arteriography, performed after 90 minutes of treatment onset in approximately 300 patients of each of the four treatment groups, showed complete vessel patency in 54% of t-PA versus 32% of streptokinase recipients, respectively. Nevertheless, the greater thrombolytic efficacy of t-PA is accompanied by a higher risk of hemorrhagic stroke, compared with streptokinase (0.72% vs. 0.54%) [60]. In ISIS-3 (Third International Study of Infarct Survival), mortality rates were similar in the streptokinase and duteplase groups [61], but bleeding complications and the frequency of stroke were higher in patients receiving duteplase (1.39% vs. 1.04%).

TNK Variant of Tissue-Type Plasminogen Activator

The efficacy and safety of currently available thrombolytic agents, including t-PA, cannot be regarded as wholly satisfactory; moreover, in the treatment of patients with acute myocardial infarction, these agents now compete with angioplasty. Thus, the demand for improved thrombolytic drugs continues. Many animal and patient studies indicate that the time required to reperfuse occluded coronary arteries influences infarct size and left ventricular function, which, in turn, alter survival rates after myocardial infarction. This has stimulated the search for agents that can reduce the time to reperfusion. The management of patients with acute myocardial infarction would also benefit from a lytic substance cleared from plasma more slowly than t-PA, which could therefore be administered as a bolus injection.

Gene technology has allowed the molecular structure of t-PA to be changed, endowing it with more desirable pharmacological properties. Using site-directed mutagenesis, the glycosylation site in kringle 1, important for hepatic clearance [62], has been deleted; this prevents binding to hepatic receptors and substantially prolongs the half-life of the substance [20]. Further mutagenesis of the PAI-1 binding site prevents interaction with PAI-1. Although other t-PA mutants, for example, lacking the finger, epidermal growth factor, and/or first kringle domain, have a substantially slower plasma clearance than native t-PA, most of these substances exhibit low specific fibrinolytic activity. Prolongation of t-PA's half-life can also be obtained by substitution or deletion of one or more selected amino acids in the finger or epidermal growth factor domains. Such mutants preserve specific fibrinolytic activity.

From a variety of several mutations of the t-PA molecule, a variant (TNK-variant of t-PA) has been selected for further development because it is more potent, has greater fibrin specificity, is cleared more slowly from plasma, and has an improved resistance to inactivation by PAI-1 compared with native t-PA.

CHEMICAL PROPERTIES

The combination of three mutations (T 103 N, N 117 Q, KHRR 296–299 AAAA) of recombinant human t-PA in a single molecule is referred to as rt-PA-TNK [20] (Figure 20-5; see Table 20-1). The first mutation consists of the replacement of threonine by asparagine at position 103 (T103N: rt-PA-T); this introduces a new glycosylation site in kringle 1 and prevents receptor binding in the liver. In rt-PA-K, the amino acids $Lys^{296}–His^{297}–Arg^{298}–Arg^{299}$ of the PAI-1 binding site are replaced with alanine (K296A, H297A, R298A, R299A: rt-PA-K), leading to both half-life prolongation and resistance to PAI-1 [20,25,63,64]. This tetra-alanine substitution also confers enhanced fibrin specificity and increased potency on platelet-rich arterial thrombi (rich in PAI-1). Additional substitution of asparagine by glutamine at position 117 (N117Q: rt-PA-N) results in deletion of the glycosylation site in kringle 1, with a further reduction of plasma clearance and enhanced resistance to inhibition by PAI-1 [20].

BIOCHEMICAL AND PHARMACOLOGICAL PROPERTIES

In the presence of fibrinogen, the TNK-variant of t-PA exhibits only a 10-fold lower specific fibrinolytic activity relative to rt-PA (K_m 3.9 vs. 4.8 µM, k_{cat} 0.58 vs. 0.08/min) [20]. In contrast, upon stimulation with fibrin, this activity rises 2-fold (K_m 0.3 vs. 1.5 µM, k_{cat} 0.071 vs. 2.27/min) [20], resulting in a 10- to 20-fold enhancement of fibrin specificity [20]. Moreover, inactivation of the TNK-variant by PAI-1 is 10-fold lower than that of native t-PA, which results in a 100-fold greater plasminogen activation activity (k_{cat}/K_m 120 × 10^5 vs. 1.4 × 10^5 $s^{-1}M^{-1}$) [20] (see Table 20-1).

PRECLINICAL AND CLINICAL PROPERTIES

In in-vitro models of clot lysis, the TNK variant of t-PA was shown to have similar specific fibrinolytic activity [65], but a 2.6-fold increased potency towards platelet-rich plasma clots (rich in PAI-1) compared with t-PA (see Table 20-2). In rabbit and rat models, the TNK variant of t-PA is 8–10 times more potent than human recombinant t-PA [66]. In a rabbit arterial thrombosis model, TNK caused more rapid and more durable reperfusion, reducing the

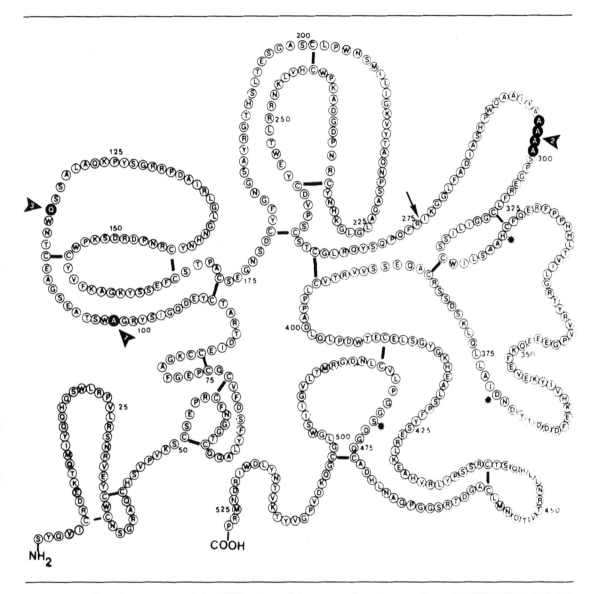

FIGURE 20-5. Secondary structure of the TNK variant of tissue-type plasminogen activator (T103N, KHRR 296–299 AAAA, N117Q-mutant of t-PA). Arrow-site of conversion into the two-chain form; black bars = disulfide bonds; asterisks = active site of the protease domain. The glycosylated side chains are not shown. The three mutated sites are in bold.

time to reperfusion to less than 40% and prolonging reperfusion by 60% of the reference values obtained with recombinant human t-PA [67]. Despite the greater thrombolytic potency, it seemed to cause less surgical bleeds. In a combined arterial and venous thrombosis model in dogs, the time to vessel recanalization was shortened, whereas the duration of reperfusion was substantially prolonged, compared with t-PA [68]. A 20-mg bolus injection did not

reduce the plasma levels of fibrinogen, plasminogen, and α_2-antiplasmin. A single- or double-bolus TNK regimen, with or without heparin, in a rabbit femoral arterial occlusion model, led to recanalization in 28 out of 30 cases, after an average of 16–36 minutes [69].

The plasma clearance of the TNK variant is five to six times slower than that of t-PA [20]. Like recombinant human t-PA, TNK is predominantly cleared by the liver [70]. Clearance kinetics in dogs, however, seem saturable at a concentration of 10 mg/kg. Coadministration of high molecular weight heparin does not affect its pharmacokinetics [71]. The plasma half-life of TNK in patients with acute myocardial infarction was 15–19 minutes, and the clearance was 198 ± 42 mL/min, compared with 550–680 mL/min for alteplase [72].

Presently, initial results are available from pilot studies in patients with acute myocardial infarction. In a phase I dose-finding study (TIMI 10A), patients with acute myocardial infarction were treated with escalating doses of TNK (5–50 mg each, given as a single IV bolus). These studies provided encouraging pharmacokinetic, efficacy, and safety data to warrant further clinical testing of the substance [89]. Two further dose-finding studies (TIMI 10B and ASSENT 1) are currently underway, testing a single 30-mg bolus versus a single 50-mg bolus of the substance (unpublished data). While TIMI 10B is designed as an angiographically controlled patency study, AS-SENT 1 is designed to give reliable safety data. With the 50-mg bolus in TIMI 10B, but not in ASSENT 1, however, an alarming frequency of cerebral bleeds was noticed (unpublished results). Both studies, therefore, will be continued, comparing a single 30-mg bolus to a 40-mg bolus dose.

In general, the TNK variant of rt-PA appears to achieve rapid coronary artery patency, with little systemic effects when moderate doses are used. Confirmation of these preliminary results in large randomized trials is awaited in the near future.

DSPA: The Plasminogen Activator of the Vampire Bat, Desmodus rotundus

Various organisms synthesize substances that can interfere with the hemostatic system of mammals; the best known are streptococci, which produce streptokinase. More developed organisms, especially those feeding on fresh blood, also produce substances that interfere with the hemostatic system of the blood donor. The saliva of the vampire bat *Desmodus rotundus* contains a variety of such proteins [73].

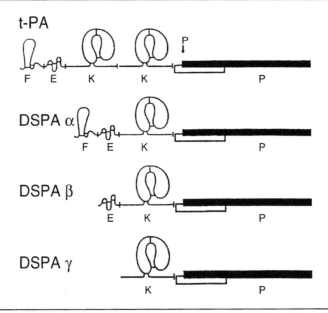

FIGURE 20-6. Schematic structure of the *Desmodus* salivary plasminogen activator (DSPA) family compared with that of tissue-type plasminogen activator. Structural domains: F = finger domain; E = epidermal growth factor domain; K = kringle domain; P = protease domain. Arrow with P = cleavage site for proteases leading to conversion into the two-chain form. (Adapted from Petri et al. [74], with permission.)

CHEMICAL PROPERTIES

Different molecular forms of the *Desmodus* salivary plasminogen activators (DSPA) have been isolated [73] (Figure 20-6 and Table 20-1). Variations in the cDNA encoding the amino acid composition of these different proteins suggest that they are not mere deletion derivatives and that different genes encode for the different variants [73]. Compared with the endogenous human tissue-type and urokinase-type plasminogen activators, DSPA α1 and DSPA α2 contain a signal peptide, a finger, an epidermal growth factor, and a kringle domain, but neither a second kringle nor a plasmin-sensitive processing site. The kringle domain of DSPA α1 resembles kringle 1 rather than kringle 2 of t-PA [74]. DSPA β and DSPA γ, the two smaller forms, lack the finger domain and the finger and epidermal growth factor domains, respectively [73] (see Figure 20-6).

DSPA α1 (or DSPA) and DSPA α2 (bat-PA) are closely related proteins, each consisting of 477 amino acid residues with 89% homology in their amino acid sequence. Their cDNAs differ in only 80 of 2245 base pairs. Both proteins have an apparent molecular weight of 52 kD. DSPA β and DSPA γ are composed of 431 and 394 amino acid residues, and have apparent molecular weights of 42 and 40 kD, respectively. The two high molecular weight forms of DSPA exhibit about 85% homology with human t-PA. The finger, epidermal growth factor, and kringle 1 domains are particularly highly conserved. All four DSPA variants lack the plasmin-sensitive region found in t-PA and u-PA [22]. Thus, they act exclusively as single-chain molecules [73].

BIOCHEMICAL AND PHARMACOLOGICAL PROPERTIES

DSPA at appropriate doses activates plasminogen only in the presence of a fibrin clot (polymeric fibrin as a cofactor) [75]. DSPA α1 and DSPA α2 both actively bind weakly to fibrin, whereas fibrin binding is not detected with the other two variants (DSPA β and DSPA γ) that lack the finger domain. For the fibrin specificity of DSPA, however, fibrin binding is apparently not necessary. Furthermore, DSPA α1 and DSPA α2 are endowed with prolonged dominant plasma half-lifes: 190 minutes in the dog (α1) and 17 minutes in the rabbit (α2), compared with 5–8 minutes and 1 minute, respectively, with t-PA [86,83]. Unlike t-PA, the half-life of DSPA is not dose-dependent, which adds to the favorable pharmacological profile of this agent. Given its long circulating half-life, bolus administration of DSPA α1 is possible.

Of the four DSPA variants, DSPA α1 seems to have the most promising thrombolytic properties

[76] (see Table 20-1). Its fibrin specificity has been confirmed in several kinetic studies. In the absence of any cofactor, it is almost inert against Glu-plasminogen, as reflected by the catalytic rate constants K_m (9.5 μM) and k_{cat} (0.6/s) [22]. Stimulation with fibrinogen alters these constants only marginally (K_m 16.3 μM, k_{cat} 0.86/s), whereas stimulation with fibrin causes dramatic changes (K_m 0.38 μM, k_{cat} 260/s, k_{cat}/K_m 684 $s^{-1}\mu M^{-1}$). This shift represents a 100,000-fold increase in activity [22]. Therefore, with DSPA α1, almost complete fibrin specificity can be expected [22].

In an in vitro model of clot lysis, DSPA α1 shows thrombolytic activities comparable with t-PA [22]. As expected, fibrinolysis with this agent is almost completely fibrin specific and occurs without any fibrinogen degradation [75,77,78]. In contrast to streptokinase and t-PA, which both significantly attenuate ADP- and collagen-induced platelet aggregation, virtually no inhibition of platelet function is detected with DSPA α1. The thrombolytic efficacy of DSPA α1, unlike that of t-PA, is not reduced by the presence of platelet-rich thrombi [76]. Furthermore, in contrast to streptokinase, urokinase, and t-PA, DSPA α1 does not induce paradoxical thrombin generation [76]. Because of its unique properties (prolonged plasma half-life and almost complete fibrin specificity), DSPA α1 has been selected for development as a third-generation thrombolytic agent.

PRODUCTION

DSPA can be isolated in small amounts from the saliva of the vampire bat [79,80]. Recently, cDNAs of all four DSPA variants have been cloned and the related proteins have been expressed in, and isolated from, COS-1 cells (baby hamster kidney cells) [73,81]. DSPA α1 is currently being produced in large quantities in mammalian cells (COS-1 cells).

PRECLINICAL AND CLINICAL PROPERTIES

The thrombolytic properties of all DSPA variants have been studied in various animal models of thrombosis, including rats [82], dogs [83], rabbits [84–86], and primates [76] (see Table 20-2). In these models, DSPA α1 has induced high rates of rapid and persistent reperfusion, compared with t-PA [83]. Reocclusions, regularly seen in the canine copper-coil model of arterial thrombosis after reperfusion with t-PA, were observed in only a few cases [83]. While lysis with t-PA is accompanied by consumption of plasminogen and α_2-antiplasmin, DSPA α1 in equimolar doses has almost no systemic effect. As with t-PA, a marked prolongation of the bleeding time is observed [84,87]. The severity of bleeds, however, is usually mild and, in contrast to t-PA, the duration is shorter.

Clinical studies, however, are required before any firm conclusion can be drawn on the safety of DSPA α1 in a clinical setting. In a pilot study of eight healthy volunteers, the pharmacokinetic properties of DSPA α1 were investigated. Doses of 0.03 to 0.05 mg/kg body weight were administered as a single bolus injection. The dominant half-life was determined to be 2.8 hours [90].

Because DSPA α1 is a protein of nonhuman origin, it may induce antibody production in humans. In rats and primates, antibodies have been detected in a fraction of the animals tested when doses of more than 10 mg were given as a single bolus [88]. Repeated administration of lower doses was also accompanied by antibody production in some, but not all, animals; the generation of antibodies was mostly seen when DSPA α1 was given a second time after at least 9 days [90]. DSPA α1 may booster antibody titers, especially when antibodies are still present in the circulation. Antibodies have been detected up to 49 weeks after the first administration of DSPA. This booster reaction may be accompanied by an inflammatory response, as indicated by simultaneous elevations of fibrinogen levels [90]. Thus, treatment with DSPA α1 may cause allergic reactions and, although not observed in animal models, including primates, it cannot be excluded that repeated administration may cause severe or even life-threatening anaphylactic shock.

Because of the high degree of structural homology between t-PA and DSPA [73], there has been concern that antibodies against DSPA α1 may neutralize the physiologic activity of t-PA through cross-reacting antibodies. Studies in sensitized primates revealed almost complete suppression of the thrombolytic activity of DSPA α1, but did not indicate that any of the thrombolytic activity of natural or exogenous t-PA was quenched by the increased antibody titers [90]. Despite these favorable results from animal studies, this question of crucial importance remains to be settled. Future clinical trials will need to determine whether potential antibodies against DSPA α1 have such neutralizing properties and how long these may persist.

Clinical testing of DSPA α1 is planned in patients with acute myocardial infarction and stroke. The first patient with acute myocardial infarction was given DSPA in September 1996, with complete restoration of coronary blood flow (TIMI grade 3) after 90 minutes (unpublished results).

References

1. Pennica D, Holmes WE, Kohr W, Harkins RN, Vehar GA, Ward CA, Bennett WF, Yelverton E, Seeburg PH, Heyneker HL, Goeddel DV, Collen D. Cloning and expression of human tissue-type plasminogen activator cDNA in E. coli. Nature 301:214, 1983.
2. Rijken DC, Collen D. Purification and characterization of the plasminogen activator secreted by human melanoma cells in culture. J Biol Chem 256:7035, 1981.
3. Rijken DC, Hoylaerts M, Collen D. Fibrinolytic properties of one-chain and two-chain human extrinsic (tissue-type) plasminogen activator. J Biol Chem 257:2920, 1982.
4. Ny T, Elgh F, Lund B. The structure of human tissue-type plasminogen activator gene: Correlation of intron and exon structures to functional and structural domains. Proc Natl Acad Sci USA 81:5355, 1984.
5. Kok P, Astrup T. Isolation and Purification of a tissue plasminogen activator and its comparison with urokinase. Biochemistry 8:79, 1969.
6. Aoki N, von Kaulla KN. The extraction of vascular plasminogen activator from human cadavers and description of some of its properties. Am J Clin Pathol 55:171, 1971.
7. Cole ER, Bachmann FW. Purification and properties of a plasminogen activator from pig heart. J Biol Chem 252:3729, 1977.
8. Collen D, Rijken DC, van Damme J, Billiau A. Purification of human tissue-type plasminogen activator in centigram quantities from human melanoma cell culture fluid and its conditioning for use in vivo. Thromb Haemost 48:294, 1982.
9. Radcliffe R, Heinze T. Isolation of plasminogen activator from human plasma by chromatography on lysine-Sepharose. Arch Biochem Biophys 189:185, 1978.
10. Wallén P, Kok P, Ranby M. The tissue activator of plasminogen. In Magnusson S, Ottesen M, Foltman B, Dano K, Neurath H (eds). Regulatory Enzymes and their Control. Oxford: Pergamon Press, 1978:127.
11. Bachmann F. Fibrinolysis. In Verstraete M, Vermylen J, Lijnen R, Arnout J (eds). Thrombosis and Haemostasis 1987. Leuven: University Press, 1987:227.
12. Collen D. On the regulation and control of fibrinolysis. Thromb Haemost 43:77, 1980.
13. Goldsmith GH, Ziats NP, Robertson AL. Studies on plasminogen activator and other proteases in subcultured human vascular cells. Exp Mol Pathol 35:257, 1981.
14. Levin EG. Latent tissue plasminogen activator produced by human endothelial cells in culture: Evidence for an enzyme-inhibitor complex. Proc Natl Acad Sci USA 1991.
15. Rijken DC, Wijngaards G, Collen D. Tissue-type plasminogen activator from human tissue and cell cultures and its occurrence in plasma. In Collen D, Lijnen HR, Verstraete M (eds). Thrombolysis, Biological and

Therapeutic Properties of New Thrombolytic Agents. Edinburgh: Churchill Livingstone, 1985:15.

16. Bode C, Schönermark S, Schuler G, Zimmermann R, Schwarz F, Kübler W. Efficacy of intravenous pro-urokinase and a combination of pro-urokinae and urokinase in acute myocardial infarction. Am J Cardiol 61:971, 1988.

17. Hoylaerts M, Rijken DC, Lijnen HR, Collen D. Kinetics of the activation of plasminogen by human tissue plasminogen activator. Role of fibrin. J Biol Chem 257:2912, 1982.

18. Norrman B, Wallén P, Ranby M. Fibrinolysis mediated by tissue plasminogen activator. Disclosure of a kinetic transition. Eur J Biochem 149:193, 1985.

19. Kohnert U, Rudolph R, Verheijen JH, Jacoline E, Weening-Verhoeff D, Stern A, Opitz U, Martin U, Lill H, Prinz H, Lechner M, Gress G-B, Buckel P, Fischer S. Biochemical properties of the kringle 2 and protease domains are maintained in the refolded t-PA deletion variant BM 06.022. Protein Eng 5:93, 1992.

20. Paoni NF, Keyt BA, Refino CJ, Chow AM, Nguyen HV, Berleau LT, Badillo J, Pena LC, Brady K, Wurm FM, Ogez J, Bennett WF. A slow clearing, fibrin-specific, PAI resistant variant of t-PA (T103N, KHRR 296–299 AAAA). Thromb Haemost 70:307, 1993.

21. Zamarron C, Lijnen HR, Collen D. Kinetics of the activation of plasminogen by natural and recombinant tissue-type plasminogen activator. J Biol Chem 259:2080, 1983.

22. Bringmann P, Gruber D, Liese A, Toschi L, Krätzschmar J, Schleuning W-D, Donner P. Structural features mediating fibrin selectivity of vampire bat plasminogen activator. J Biol Chem 270:25596, 1995.

23. Williams GT, Neuberger MS. Production of antibody-tagged enzymes by melanoma cells: Application to DNA polymerase I Klenow fragment. Gene 43:319, 1986.

24. Gulba DC, Westhoff-Bleck M, Reil G-H. Thrombolysetherapie des akuten Herzinfarktes — Ergebnisse und neue Entwicklungen. Dtsch Med Wochenschr 115:187, 1990.

25. Bennett WF, Paoni NF, Keyt BA, Botstein D, Jones AJS, Presta L, Wurm FM, Zoller MJ. High resolution analysis of functional determinants on human tissue-type plasminogen activator. J Biol Chem 266:5191, 1991.

26. Eastman D, Wurm FM, van Reis R, Higgins DL. A region of tissue plasminogen activator that affects plasminogen activation differentially with various fibrin(ogen)-related stimulators. Biochemistry 31:419, 1992.

27. Paoni NF, Refino CJ, Brady K, Pena LC, Nguyen HV, Kerr EM, Johnson AC, Wurm FM, van Reis R, Botstein D, Bennett WF. Involvement of residues 296–299 in the enzymatic activity of tissue-type plasminogen activator. Protein Eng 5:259, 1992.

28. Christophodoulides M, Boucher DW. The potency of tissue-type plasminogen activator (TPA) determined with chromogen and clot lysis assay. Biologicals 18:103, 1990.

29. Martin U, Fischer S, Kohnert U, Rudolph R, Sponer G, Stern A, Strein K. Coronary thrombolytic properties of a novel recombinant plasminogen activator (BM 06.022) in a canine model. J Cardiovasc Pharmacol 18:111, 1991.

30. Emeis JJ, van den Hoogen CM, Jense D. Hepatic clearance of tissue-type plasminogen activator in rats. Thromb Haemost 54:661, 1985.

31. Tiefenbrunn AJ, Robison AK, Kurnik PB, Ludbrook PA, Sobel BE. Clinical pharmacology in patients with evolving myocardial infarction of tissue plasminogen activator produced by recombinant DNA technology. Circulation 71:110, 1985.

32. Verstraete M, Bounameaux H, de Cock F, van de Werf F, Collen D. Pharmacokinetics and systemic fibrinogenolytic effects of recombinant human tissue-type plasminogen activator (rt-PA) in humans. J Pharmacol Exp Ther 235;506, 1985.

33. Verstraete M, Su CAPF, Tanswell P, Feuerer W, Collen D. Pharmacokinetics and effects on fibrinolytic and coagulation parameters of two doses of recombinant tissue-type plasminogen activator (rt-PA) in healthy volunteers. Thromb Haemost 56:1, 1986.

34. Tanswell P, Tebbe U, Neuhaus KL, Gläsle-Schwarz L, Wojcik J, Seifried E. Pharmacokinetics and fibrin specificity of alteplase during accelerated infusions in acute myocardial infarction. J Am Coll Cardiol 19:1071, 1992.

35. Brone MJ, Dodd I, Carey JE, Chapman CG, Robinson JH. Increased yield of human tissue-type plasminogen activator obtained by means of recombinant DNA technology. Thromb Haemost 54:422, 1985.

36. Martin U, Bader R, Böhm E, Kohnert U, von Möllendorf E, Fischer S, Sponer G. BM 06.022: A novel recombinant plasminogen activator. Cardiovasc Drug Rev 11:299, 1993.

37. Matsuo O, Bando H, Okada K, Tanaka K, Tsukada M, Iga Y, Arimura H. Thrombolytic effect of single-chain pro-urokinase in a rabbit jugular vein thrombosis model. Thromb Res 42:187, 1986.

38. Matsuo O, Rijken DC, Collen D. Thrombolysis by human tissue plasminogen activator and urokinase in rabbits with experimental pulmonary embolus. Nature 291:590, 1981.

39. Korninger G, Matsuo O, Suy R, Stassen JM, Collen D. Thrombolysis with human extrinsic (tissue-type) plasminogen activator in dogs with femoral thrombosis. J Clin Invest 69:573, 1982.

40. Collen D, Stassen JM, Verstraete M. Thrombolysis with human extrinsic (tissue-type) plasminogen activator in rabbits with experimental jugular vein thrombosis. Effect of molecular form and dose of activator, age of the thrombus, and route of administration. J Clin Invest 71:368, 1982.

41. Bergmann SR, Fox AA, Ter-Pogossian MM, Sobel BE, Collen D. Clot-selective coronary thrombolysis with tissue-type plasminogen activator. Science 220:1181, 1983.

42. Matsuo O, Rijken DC, Collen D. Comparison of the relative fibrinogenolytic, fibrinolytic and thrombolytic properties of tissue plasminogen activator and urokinase in vitro. Thromb Haemost 45:225, 1981.

43. Lijnen HR, Marafino BJ, Collen D. In vitro fibrinolytic activity of recombinant tissue-type plasminogen activator in the plasma of various primate species. Thromb Haemost 52:308, 1984.

44. Sobel BA, Nachowiak DA, Fry ETA, Bergmann SR, Torr SR. Paradoxical attenuation of fibrinolysis attributable to "plasminogen steal" and its implication for coronary thrombolysis. Cor Art Dis 1:111, 1990.

45. Neuhaus K-L, Feuerer W, Jeep-Tebbe S, Niederer W, Vogt A, Tebbe U. Improved thrombolysis with a modified dose regimen of recombinant tissue-type plasminogen activator. J Am Coll Cardiol 14:1566, 1989.

46. Neuhaus K-L, von Essen R, Tebbe U, Vogt A, Roth M, Riess M, Niederer W, Forycki F, Wirtzfeld A, Maeurer W, Limbourg P, Merx W, Haerten K. Improved thrombolysis in acute myocardial infarction with front-loaded administration of alteplase: Results of the rt-PA-APSAC patency study (TAPS). J Am Coll Cardiol 19:885, 1992.

47. Purvis JA, McNeill AJ, Siddiqui RA, Roberts MJ, McClements BM, McEneaney D, Campbell NP, Khan MM, Webb SW, Wilson CM, and the GREAT Study Group. Efficacy of 100 mg of double-bolus alteplase in achieving complete perfusion in the treatment of acute myocardial infarction. J Am Coll Cardiol 23:6, 1994.

48. Gulba DC, Dechend R, Hauck S, Osterziel KJ, Barthels M, Lichtlen PR, Dietz R. An accelerated "frontloaded" rt-PA thrombolysis regimen achieves higher TIMI III patency rates in acute myocardial infarction (abstr). Fibrinolysis 8(Suppl. 1):100, 1994.

49. Topol EJ, Califf RM, George BS, Kereiakes DJ, Rothbaum D, Candela RJ, Abbotsmith CW, Pinkerton CA, Stump DC, Collen D, Lee KL, Pitt B, Kline EM, Boswick JM, O'Neill WW, Stack RS, and the TAMI Study Group. Coronary arterial thrombolysis with combined infusion of recombinant tissue-type plasminogen activator and urokinase in patients with acute myocardial infarction. Circulation 77:1100, 1988.

50. Stump DC, Topol EJ, Chen AB, Hopkins A, Collen D. Monitoring of haemostasis parameters during coronary thrombolysis with recombinant tissue-type plasminogen activator. Thromb Haemost 59:133, 1988.

51. Eisenberg PR, Sobel BE, Jaffe AS. Characterization in vivo of the fibrin specificity of activators of the fibrinolytic system. Circulation 78:592, 1988.

52. Smalling RW, Schumacher R, Morris D, Harder K, Fuentes F, Valentine RP, Batty LL, Merhige M, Pitts DE, Lieberman HA, Nishikawa A, Adyanthaya A, Hopkins A, Grossbard E. Improved infarct-related arterial patency after high dose, weight adjusted, rapid infusion of tissue-type plasminogen activator in myocardial infarction: Results of a multicenter randomized trial of two dosage regimens. J Am Coll Cardiol 15:915, 1990.

53. Topol EJ, George BS, Kereiakes DJ, Candela RJ, Abbottsmith CW, Stump DC, Boswick JM, Stack RS, Califf RM, and the TAMI Study Group. Comparison of two dose regimens of intravenous tissue plasminogen activator for acute myocardial infarction. Am J Cardiol 61:723, 1988.

54. Khan MI, Hackett DR, Andreotti F, Davies GJ, Regan T, Haider AW, McFadden E, Halson P, Maseri A, Kluft C. Effectiveness of multiple bolus administration of t-PA. Am J Cardiol 65:1051, 1990.

55. Li K. The role of beta-amyloid ion the development of Alzheimer's disease. Drugs Aging 7:97, 1995.

56. Kimura T, Takamatsu J, Araki N, Goto M, Kondo A, Miyakawa T, Horiuchi S. Are advanced glycation end-products associated with amyloidosis in Alzheimer's disease? Neuroreport 6:866, 1995.

57. Coria F, Rubio I, Bayon C. Alzheimer's disease, beta amyloidosis, and aging. Rev Neurosci 5:275, 1994.

58. Kingston IB, Castro MJM, Andersonb S. In vitro stimulation of tissue-type plasminogen activator by Alzheimer amyloid β-peptide analogues. Nature Med 1:138, 1995.

59. The GUSTO Angiographic Investigators. The effects of tissue plasminogen activator, streptokinase, or both on coronary-artery patency, ventricular function, and survival after acute myocardial infarction. N Engl J Med 329:1615, 1993.

60. The GUSTO Investigators. An international randomized trial comparing four thrombolytic strategies for acute myocardial infarction. N Engl J Med 329:673, 1993.

61. ISIS-3 (Third International Study of Infarct Survival) Collaborative Group. ISIS-3: A randomised comparison of streptokinase vs. tissue plasminogen activator vs. anistreplase and of aspirin plus heparin vs. aspirin alone among 41,299 cases of suspected acute infarction. Lancet 339:753, 1993.

62. Hotchkiss A, Refino CJ, Leonard CK, O'Connor JV, Crowley C, McCabe J, Tate K, Nakamura G, Powers D, Levinson A, Mohler M, Spellman MW. The influence of carbohydrate structure on the clearance of recombinant tissue-type plasminogen activator. Thromb Haemost 60:255, 1988.

63. Madison EL, Goldsmith EJ, Gerard RD, Gething MJH, Sambrook JF, Basel-Duby RS. Amino acid residues that affect interaction of tissue type plasminogen activator with plasminogen activator inhibitor 1. Proc Natl Acad Sci USA 87:3530, 1990.

64. Madison EL, Goldsmith EJ, Gerard RD, Gething MJH, Sembrook JF. Serpin-resistant mutants of human tissue-type plasminogen activator. Nature 339:721, 1989.

65. Refino CJ, Paoni NF, Keyt BA, Pater CS, Badillo JM,

Wurm FM, Ogez J, Bennett WF. A variant of t-PA (T103N, KHRR 296–299 AAA) that, by bolus, has increased potency and decreased systemic activation of plasminogen. Thromb Haemost 70:313, 1993.

66. Keyt BA, Paoni NF, Refino CI, Berleau L, Nguyen H, Chow A. A faster acting and more potent form of tissue plasminogen activator. Proc Natl Acad Sci USA 91:3670, 1994.

67. Benedict CR, Refino CJ, Keyt BA, Pakala R, Paoni NF, Thomas GR. New variant of tissue human plasminogen activator (t-PA) with enhanced efficacy and lower incidence of bleeding compared with recombinant human t-PA. Circulation 92:3032, 1995.

68. Collen D, Stassen J-M, Yasuda T, Refino C, Paoni N, Key B, Roskams T, Guerrero JL, Lijnen HR, Gold HK, Bennett WF. Comparative thrombolytic properties of tissue-type plasminogen activator and of a plasminogen activator inhibitor-1-resistant glycosylation variant, in a combined arterial and venous thrombosis model in the dog. Thromb Haemost 72:98, 1994.

69. Garabedian HD, Svizzero TA, Guerrero JL, Pena LC, Love TW, Leinbach RC, Gold HK. A new dosing strategy for TNK variant of tissue plasminogen activator eliminates heparin and reduces bleeding without loss of thrombolytic efficacy (abstr). Circulation 92(Suppl I):740, 1995.

70. Eppler S, Modi NB. Pharmacokinetics of TNK and activase t-PA in beagle dogs. Genentech report no. 94-434-0218, 1994.

71. Modi NB. Acute intravenous toxicity study with GN 0218 in dogs — pharmacokinetic analysis. Genentech report no. 94-090-0218, 1994.

72. Cannon CP, Love TW, McCabe CH, Kirshenbaum JM, Henry T, Sequira R, Schweiger M, Breed J, Cutler D, Tracy R, for the TIMI 10 investigators. TNK-tissue plasminogen activator in myocardial infarction (TIMI) 10: Results of the initial patients in the TIMI 10 pilot — a phase 1, pharmacokinetics trial (abstr). Circulation 92(Suppl. I): 415, 1995.

73. Krätzschmar J, Haendler B, Langner G, Boidol W, Bringmann P, Alagon A, Donner P, Schleuning W-D. The plasminogen activator family from salivary gland of the vampire bat Desmodus rotundus: Cloning and expression. Gene 105:229, 1991.

74. Petri T, Baldus B, Boidol W, Bringmann P, Cashion L, Donner P, Haendler B, Kreatzschmar J, Langer G, Siewert G, Witt W, Schleuning W-D. Novel plasminogen activators from the vampire bat Desmodus rotundus. In Spier RE, Griffiths JB, MacDonald C (eds). Animal Cell Technology: Developments, Processes and Products. European Society for Animal Cell Technology, 1991:599.

75. Bergum PW, Gardell SJ. Vampire bat salivary plasminogen activator exhibits a strict and fastidious requirement for polymeric fibrin as its cofactor, unlike human tissue-type plasminogen activator. J Biol Chem 267:17726, 1994.

76. Gulba DC, Praus M, Witt W. DSPA alpha — proper-ties of the plasminogen activator of the vampire bat Desmodus rotundus. Fibrinolysis 9(Suppl. I):91, 1995.

77. Schleuning W-D, Alagon A, Boidol W, Bringmann P, Petri T, Krätzschmar J, Haendler B, Langer G, Baldus B, Witt W, Donner P. Plasminogen activation in fibrinolysis, on tissue remodeling and in Development. Ann N Y Acad Sci 667:395, 1992.

78. Hare TR, Gardell SJ. Vampire bat salivary plasminogen activator promotes robust lysis of plasma clots in a plasma millieu without causing fluid phase plasminogen activation. Thromb Haemost 68:165, 1992.

79. Cartwright T, Hawkey C. Activation of the blood fibrinolytic mechanism in birds by saliva of the vampire bat (Diaemus youngi). Physiological Society 45P, 1968.

80. Hawkey C. Plasminogen activator in saliva of the vampire bat Desmodus rotundus. Nature 211:434, 1966.

81. Gardell SJ, Dupe RJ, Diehl RE, York JD, Hare TR, Register RB, Jacobs JW, Dixon RAF, Friedman PA. Isolation, characterization, and cDNA cloning of a vampire bat salivary plasminogen activator. J Biol Chem 264:17947, 1989.

82. Witt W, Baldus B, Bringmann P, Cashion L, Donner P, Schleuning W-D. Thrombolytic properties of Desmodus rotundus (vampire bat) salivary plasminogen activator in experimental pulmonary embolism in rats. Blood 79:1213, 1992.

83. Witt W, Maass B, Baldus B, Hildebrand M, Donner P, Schleuning W-D. Coronary thrombolysis with Desmodus salivary plasminogen activator in dogs — fast and persistent recanalization by intravenous bolus administration. Circulation 90:421, 1994.

84. Gardell SJ, Ramjit DR, Stabilito II, Fujita T, Lynch JJ, Guca GC, Jain D, Wang S, Tung J, Mark GE, Shebuski RJ. Effective thrombolysis without marked plasminemia after bolus intravenous administration of a vampire bat salivary plasminogen activator in rabbits. Circulation 84:244, 1991.

85. Mellott MJ, Stabilito II, Holahan MA, Cuca GC, Wang S, Li P, Gardell SJ. Vampire bat salivary plasminogen activator promotes rapid and sustained reperfusion without concomitant systemic plasminogen activation in a canine model of arterial thrombosis. Arterioscler Thromb 12:212, 1992.

86. Muschick P, Zeggert D, Donner P, Witt W. Thrombolytic properties of Desmodus (vampire bat) salivary plasminogen activator DSPA-alpha-1, alteplase and streptokinase following intravenous bolus injection in a rabbit model of carotid artery thrombosis. Fibrinolysis 7:284, 1993.

87. Burton G, Graichen G, Witt W. Effect of the novel thrombolytic DSPA alpha 1 on venipuncture bleeding time in the rat: Comparison to anistreplase and t-PA. Thromb Haemost 69:842, 1993.

88. Witt W, Kirchhoff D, Woy P, Zierz R, Bhargava AS. Antibody formation and effects on endogenous fibrinolysis after repeated administration of DSPA alpha 1 in rats. Fibrinolysis 8(Suppl. 1):66, 1994.

89. Cannon CP, McCabe CH, Gibson CM, Ghali M, Sequeira RF, McKendall GR, Breed J, Modi NB, Fox NL, Tracy RP, Love TW, Braunwald E, TIMI 10 A investigators. TNK-tissue plasminogen activator in acute myocardial infarction Results of the Thrombolysis in Myocardial Infarction trial Circulation 95:351, 1997.

90. Gulba DC, Praus M, Dechend R, Dietz R. Update on the toxicology and pharmacology of rDSPA-alpha-1 (bat-PA) in animals and humans. Fibrinolysis 1997, suppl, in press.

SECTION VII: NATIONAL GOALS AND PERSPECTIVES FOR IMPROVING PATIENT CARE: THE NATIONAL HEART ATTACK ALERT PROGRAM

Costas T. Lambrew

There is clear evidence from clinical studies and registries that early treatment of patients with ST-segment elevation acute myocardial infarction results in a significant mortality reduction compared with late treatment. Yet patient-mediated delays, delays in getting the patient promptly to the hospital for reperfusion therapy, and significant delays in the identification and Treatment of these patients significantly compromises outcome. The National Heart Attack Alert Program (NHAAP) is the latest of the National Heart, Lung and Blood Institute's Educational Programs. Its goals are to have more patients with ST-segment elevation acute myocardial infarction treated with reperfusion therapy, if appropriate, and to have reperfusion therapy delivered as early as possible after the onset of symptoms and arrival in the emergency department. This section addresses issues related to all three phases of delay, provides a perspective on treatment of sudden cardiac death in the community, and presents an evaluation of diagnostic interventions used in the identification of acute cardiac ischemia in the emergency department.

21. NATIONAL GOALS AND PERSPECTIVES FOR IMPROVING PATIENT CARE: THE NATIONAL HEART ATTACK ALERT PROGRAM

Costas T. Lambrew

The National Heart Attack Alert Program (NHAAP) is the most recent of the National Education Programs developed and promoted by the National Heart, Lung and Blood Institute (NHLBI). The primary goal of this educational initiative is to reduce morbidity and mortality associated with acute myocardial infarction (AMI), including infarct-related sudden death. The NHAAP is similar in scope to the institute's other well-known programs, including the National High Blood Pressure Education Program and the National Cholesterol Education Program. It was developed on the recommendation of a symposium of experts convened by the NHLBI in October 1990 to discuss barriers to early identification and treatment of individuals with symptoms and signs of AMI, and to present specific recommendations to the NHLBI for addressing and resolving these issues within the context of a National Education Program. Three phases of delay in the treatment of these patients were identified:

- Patient and bystander recognition of symptoms and signs of AMI, and delayed actions in response to these symptoms
- Prehospital actions by health care professionals and emergency medical service (EMS) providers
- Hospital actions by health care professionals at the hospital

In the past 10 years, thrombolytic therapy has become the standard of care for patients with AMI, with significant, substantial reduction of mortality in all clinical trials with each of the currently available thrombolytic agents. Furthermore, these clinical trials have supported the early laboratory observation that the benefit of thrombolytic therapy appears to be related to early opening of the infarct-related artery, resulting in rapid reperfusion of jeopardized myocardium, thereby limiting infarct size, decreasing left ventricular dysfunction, and resulting in improved survival. The time–benefit curve, however, is very steep, and the most dramatic benefit from myocardial salvage accrues to those patients treated within the first hour after the onset of symptoms. The incremental benefit after 2 hours is smaller, may be related to mechanisms other than myocardial salvage, but outweighs risk out to approximately 12 hours after the onset of symptoms.

Therefore, the primary focus of the NHAAP at the present time is to develop educational programs that would reduce delays in patient presentation, early identification and treatment of patients presenting to the EMS systems with chest pain, and earlier identification and treatment of such patients in the hospital emergency department. The ultimate, albeit currently unachievable, goal would be to offer reperfusion therapy to as many AMI patients as possible within 60 minutes after the onset of chest pain. The greatest period of delay, related to recognition of symptoms by patients and their health-seeking behaviors, has not been modified significantly over the last 20 years by multiple community intervention strategies, both in this country and abroad. The RE-ACT Program, a recently funded project of the NHLBI will, over the next 5 years, attempt to develop and test community interventions that would promote recognition of cardiac symptoms by patients and earlier calls for help. Interim recommendations for educational strategies to prevent prehospital delay in patients who are at high risk for acute myocardial infarction that can be offered by physicians and other health professionals will be published in the course of the next year. In this section, Dr. Robert Goldberg addresses factors associated with patient delay and gives an overview of community trials designed to reduce the duration of this delay in seeking care.

Recommendations related to the use of universal medical access (911), an appropriate response by medical dispatchers who receive calls from patients with chest pain, and an appropriate response by prehospital providers is presented by Dr. James Atkins. These recommendations from the NHAAP are in the process of publication. The problem of sudden death in the community, the use of the automatic external defibrillator (AED), and questions related to the effectiveness of prehospital thrombolysis are addressed by Dr. Joseph Oronato.

The first recommendations from the NHAAP addressed delays in the early identification and treatment of such patients in the emergency department, and approaches to reducing those delays through application of the concepts of quality improvement. This report recommended that all patients with typical symptoms for AMI, no contraindications, and findings of ST elevation consistent with injury on the ECG be treated with a thrombolytic drug within 30 minutes of their arrival in the hospital emergency department. Dr. Harry Selker discusses approaches to the screening and identification of patients with unstable ischemic syndromes. Dr. Costas Lambrew discusses barriers to the early identification and treatment of the patient in the emergency department and strategies whereby these barriers can be identified and the process modified to meet the goal of 30 minutes to treatment.

22. DELAYS IN TREATMENT OF ACUTE MYOCARDIAL INFARCTION IN THE EMERGENCY DEPARTMENT: REDUCING DOOR TO DRUG TIME

Costas T. Lambrew

Introduction

Delays related to recognition of symptoms by the patient and prompt initiation of a call for help to the Emergency Medical Services System (EMSS) have yet to be effectively addressed and are subject to ongoing studies. Recommendations relating to reducing delays in EMSS response and transport times to hospital have been addressed in Chapter 24. Reducing inappropriate delays in the emergency department is within the purview of physicians, nurses, and hospital staff and should be achievable through application of the process of continuous quality improvement.

Most physicians and hospital staff involved in the care of patients with acute myocardial infarction generally underestimate the time required to identify and initiate reperfusion therapy in patients with ST-segment elevation acute myocardial infarction (AMI). Yet, when time from the emergency department arrival to initiation of a lytic drug (door-drug time) is actually recorded and tracked, median time delays of 70–90 minutes are common [1–4].

The National Heart Attack Apert Program (NHAAP) Working Group, considering potential sources of delay in the identification of patients with AMI and their treatment with thrombolytic drugs, identified four critical time points in the process, referred to as the 4 Ds, which are defined as follows:

- Door: time of arrival in the emergency department
- Data: time of acquisition of the ECG showing ST elevation
- Decision: time when the order is written to administer a thrombolytic agent
- Drug: time when the infusion of the thrombolytic drug is begun [5]

These time points are recorded for every patient and are easily retrievable. It is recommended that these time points be tracked for every patient with nontraumatic chest pain coming to an emergency department to be evaluated for the possibility of an unstable ischemic syndrome and eligibility for a reperfusion strategy. These time points enclose three intervals in the process of identification and treatment of such patients that include actions and reflect policies that need to be continually examined for the purpose of reducing delays while ensuring a high standard of care. These time points, intervals, and secondary time points that might be collected for the purpose of identifying actual sources of delay, are shown in Figure 22-1. Critical review of emergency department process can occur only through actual recording of these time points and regular review of door to drug time in relationship to emergency department process and policies. Major causes of delay, generic to many emergency departments, include outdated emergency department protocols for the identification and treatment of patients with acute myocardial infarction (AMI), poor coordination between the emergency department and other hospital departments (such as the ECG service and pharmacy), and disputes among medical staff related to policies of consultation on such patients, authority to order the ECG, and who may order the thrombolytic drug.

The NHAAP recommends that all patients with typical symptoms of AMI, no contraindications, and findings of ST elevation consistent with injury on the ECG be treated with a thrombolytic drug within 30 minutes of their arrival in the hospital emergency department [5]. This recommendation of a 30-

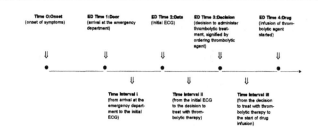

FIGURE 22-1. Process time points and intervals through which the Acute MI patient passes until treatment in the emergency department.

TABLE 22-1. Guidelines for emergency department
registration clerk's and/or triage nurse's identification of AMI patients

REGISTRATION/CLERICAL STAFF
patients over 30 years of age with the following chief complaints require immediate assessment by the triage nurse and *should be referred for further evaluation*:

Chief Complaint
• Chest pain, pressure, tightness, or heaviness. Radiating pain in neck, jaw, shoulders, back, or one or both arms
• Indigestion or "heartburn"/nausea and/or vomiting
• Persistent shortness of breath
• Weakness/dizziness/lightheadedness/loss of consciousness

TRIAGE NURSE
Patients with the following symptoms and signs require immediate assessment by the triage nurse *for initiating the AMI protocol*:

Chief Complaint
• Chest pain. Patients over 30 years of age with chest pain or severe epigastric pain, nontraumatic in origin, having components typical of myocardial ischemia or infarction:
  — Central/substernal compression or crushing chest pain
  — Pressure, tightness, heaviness, cramping, burning, aching sensation
  — Unexplained indigestion/belching
  — Radiating pain in neck, jaw, shoulders, back, or one or both arms
• Associated dyspnea
• Associated nausea/vomiting
• Associated diaphoresis

If these symptoms are present, obtain stat ECG.

Medical History
The triage nurse should do a brief, targeted initial history assessing for current or past history of:

• Coronary artery bypass grafting, angioplasty, coronary artery disease, or AMI
• Nitroglycerin use to relieve pain
• Risk factors, including smoking, hyperlipidemia, hypertension, diabetes mellitus, family history, cocaine use

This brief history **must not delay** entry into the AMI protocol.

Special Considerations
• Questions have been raised as to whether women may present most frequently with atypical chest pain and symptoms.
• Diabetic patients may have atypical presentations due to autonomic dysfunction.
• Elderly patients may have stroke, syncope, or change in mental status.

minute door to drug time is based on an analysis of emergency department process that is framed within the long-term goal of 60 minutes to treatment after onset of symptoms once patient and prehospital delays are addressed. It is consistent with the American Heart Association recommendation that such patients be treated within 30–60 minutes of emergency department arrival [6]. The data supporting this recommendation, a detailed discussion of barriers to early treatment in the emergency department, and recommendations for reducing door to drug time have been previously published [5].

In addition to the general causes of delay noted earlier, each emergency department has its own unique barriers to early treatment. Emergency departments must develop a multidisciplinary team that includes emergency physicians, cardiologists, nurses, ECG technicians, pharmacists, and registration clerks, who would review door to drug time on a regular basis and identify problems for the purpose of developing and implementing effective department policies, protocols, and guidelines that would facilitate early therapeutic intervention. Each emergency department must adopt a protocol to this end based on the input from this multidisciplinary group.

Door

There are many causes for delay as the patient enters the emergency department. Those patients who come in by private conveyance as opposed to ambulance — up to 50% of patients with AMI in some studies — may not be triaged as promptly as those who arrive by ambulance [7]. These patients may be perceived as non-urgent and put in a queue for registration. In some instances, registration clerks are trained to gather demographic information prior to eliciting a chief complaint from patients who are ambulatory, inappropriately delaying triage and identification of patients with an unstable ischemic syndrome. It is recommended that the chief complaint always be elicited on all patients prior to recording of demographic information, which can be gathered at a later, more appropriate time.

Registration representatives should elicit a focused history from any patient presenting to the emergency department. Should the complaint be among those listed in Table 22-1, the patient should be immediately referred to the triage nurse, who should proceed along the suggested guideline for the purpose of determining whether the AMI protocol should be initiated. Identification and treatment of patients with AMI has been facilitated by developing a fast track for

such patients or by assigning such patients a higher triage category, thereby having them assessed professionally in a shorter period of time. Both of these strategies have resulted in a significant decrease in the interval between the emergency department entry and recording of a 12-lead ECG [8]. In those relatively few communities in which emergency department staff has a prehospital 12-lead ECG available for patients being transported to the hospital by ambulance, ST-segment elevation on the ECG or, indeed, ST-segment depression, identified prior to arrival has significantly reduced door to drug time [9,10]. The triage nurse should immediately communicate the presence of a patient with suspected myocardial infarction to the emergency department physician.

At the least, communications from prehospital personnel transporting patients in an ambulance might include a description of symptoms and history, which would alert emergency department receiving staff to the need for early triage and workup of the patient coming to them. However, detailed information from the prehospital care provider should not preclude efficient, rapid, and safe transport of the patient to the hospital.

Data

The finding of ST-segment elevation on the 12-lead ECG in a patient with symptoms consistent with cardiac ischemia is clearly the trigger that leads to consideration of reperfusion therapy. The triage nurse should have authority by protocol to order a 12-lead ECG on patients suspected of having myocardial ischemia, thereby obviating any delay related to restricting the authority to order the ECG to the physician. Delays in ECG availability of up to 20 minutes, once the order is entered, have been reported [3]. It is recommended that an ECG should be available no later than 5 minutes after it is ordered. An ECG machine should be located in the emergency department for use by the person acquiring the ECG and for availability during the night when an ECG technician may not be available. Technicians being paged to acquire the ECG must respond within this time frame on an emergency basis. If this is not possible, then emergency department personnel must be trained to acquire the ECG. Once the ECG is recorded, it should be given to a caregiver, either the nurse or the physician. Emergency department nurses should be trained to recognize ECG changes consistent with AMI. The ECG should not be sequestered at the desk and should be seen by the evaluating physician as soon as it is available.

In addition to having standard orders to obtain an ECG, the emergency nurse should, by protocol, have authority to initiate

- Administration of aspirin for patients with clinically suspected unstable angina or AMI who are not allergic to salicylates
- ECG monitoring for disturbances in rhythm
- Oxygen therapy
- Intravenous access
- Appropriate baseline laboratory studies, such as myocardial enzymes
- Sublingual or topical nitrates as appropriate

Once again, none of these activities should in any way delay a decision about initiation of thrombolytic therapy.

Decision

Many factors may affect the capacity of the treating emergency physician to diagnose AMI, and to decide if thrombolytic therapy is indicated and if other therapy should be initiated. There should be a clear, concise treatment algorithm that specifies inclusion criteria, including ECG criteria, that would qualify a patient for thrombolytic therapy, as well as relative and absolute contraindications to thrombolytics. That algorithm should also specify other interventions in the patient with an unstable ischemic syndrome, including AMI, such as aspirin, heparin, beta blockers, nitrates, and ACE inhibitors, so as to ensure that these agents are promptly administered. However, no intervention should delay prompt initiation of thrombolytic therapy when the diagnosis is established. The algorithm should reflect the results of large trials. Care should be taken not to list contraindications or exclusion criteria that would inappropriately exclude select patient groups from treatment with thrombolytics. Age, surprisingly, continues to be used as an absolute exclusion criterion in some protocols, while others continue to limit the administration of thrombolytic drugs to patients with onset of chest pain within 6 hours [11]. Agreements between physicians in cardiology, internal medicine, and emergency medicine, as well as with emergency department nurses and appropriate technologists, should result in a protocol that will be used by all and will, by virtue of familiarity, facilitate care.

Clear-cut ST-segment elevation meeting the inclusion criteria for thrombolysis in a patient with typical symptoms without contraindications should result in an immediate decision to initiate thrombolytic therapy. ECG findings that are equivocal, confusing, or open to differing interpretations, may significantly prolong decision time. Use of more sophisticated algorithms for computerized interpretation of electrocardiograms, which are highly sensitive and specific for myocardial injury, could assist the emergency physician in making the diagnosis of AMI and in initiating prompt protocol-driven therapy [12,13]. This technology is currently being evaluated in the clinical setting. Atypical clinical presentation, and nonconclusive or nondiagnostic findings on the 12-lead ECG require immediate cardiology consultation. Frequently, this can be effectively accomplished by telephone or facsimile transmission of the 12-lead ECG for evaluation by a cardiologist. Use of telephone and fax consultation has been found to significantly reduce delay over bedside consultation by the cardiologist [11].

The emergency physician should have delegated authority from the medical staff to initiate thrombolytic therapy in patients with clear-cut symptoms of AMI, diagnostic electrocardiograms, and no contraindications, without mandatory bedside consultation from a cardiologist or contact of the primary care physician as a matter of policy. A surprising number of hospitals require the primary care physician to be called and the cardiologist to perform a bedside consultation despite clear-cut findings, and both of these practices, in the patient who fulfills all protocol criteria, in no way contribute to the decision or the quality of care, but significantly compromise early treatment by imposing a substantial delay on the initiation of thrombolytic therapy [3,11,14]. The primary care physician may be notified once the decision is made and the drug is initiated. The cardiologist may appropriately assume care of the patient once the patient reaches the cardiac care unit.

Other routine studies or diagnostic interventions are not necessary in the patient with classic ECG findings of ST-elevation AMI as defined by the protocol. Patients with unclear symptomatic presentations and/or equivocal ECG findings may benefit from cardiac consultation, and selective application of other diagnostic studies, including, possibly, echocardiography, to assess the presence or absence of wall-motion abnormality, or nuclear imaging studies. The sensitivity of continuous ST-segment monitoring and the application of rapidly available assays for enzymes that are released soon after onset of necrosis in making the diagnosis of AMI are also being evaluated, but the role of all of these studies has not been clearly defined, and they should be restricted in their application to the evaluation of selected patients.

Drug

Once the decision is made to treat a patient with thrombolytic therapy, the drug should be made available and administered promptly. Delays in mixing the drug and receiving the drug from the pharmacy, where they occur, may be obviated by maintaining the drug and preparing it for administration in the emergency department itself [14]. The greatest contributor to delay in administration of drug is imposed by policy that requires that the drug be administered only after the patient is transported to the cardiac care unit. Initiation of the drug in the emergency department cuts door to drug time by 25–50 minutes [2,11,14].

Written informed consent continues to be required from patients receiving a thrombolytic drug in a significant number of hospitals [11]. It is recommended that these patients can be adequately informed of their condition and the benefits as well as the risks of thrombolytic therapy in a concise verbal communication [5]. It is probable that patients with severe chest pain are not in a position to fully comprehend a lengthy written informed consent that they are required to read, which, again, inappropriately delays treatment and is probably not valid under the circumstances, even when signed [11].

Standard protocols for the actual administration of the thrombolytic, adjunctive agents, such as beta blockers, nitrates, and ACE inhibitors, as well as conjunctive agents such as aspirin and heparin, should be available so as to facilitate prompt administration. The emergency department record would facilitate review of care of these patients were it to include a check-off that these drugs have been given and provisions for entry of each of the 4D time points.

Evaluation of Treatment for Acute Myocardial Infarction

It is recommended that there be a multidisciplinary group that continually reviews the process and quality of care of patients with AMI. The W. Edwards Deming model of continuous quality improvement (CQI) involves repetitive sequences of evaluation, corrective intervention, and re-evaluation that continuously improve quality. The process requires an explicit knowledge of the process of care. Changes cannot be made in a system that functions poorly unless there is an understanding of how the system works.

Each emergency department and hospital is unique. The analysis of process should result in an efficient, effective process, with measurable changes

as reflected in significant reductions in door to drug time and an increasing percentage of patients who are treated within the recommended standard of 30 minutes from hospital arrival. This evaluation and follow-up of these data need to occur on a regular basis. It is clear that just because a goal is met, it is not necessarily maintained if close follow-up and monitoring of data are not performed on a regular basis.

Other components of the evaluation process are as follows:

- Currency of protocols. Do the protocols reflect current recommendations as results of clinical trials are published?
- Eligible patients treated. What percent of patients eligible for thrombolytic therapy according to the protocol actually receive thrombolytic therapy?
- Are patients being inappropriately excluded on the basis of age, time from onset of symptoms, or perceived contraindications that are not reflected in the protocol?
- Accuracy of ECG interpretation. Are patients being treated with lytics on the basis of overinterpretation of the ECG? Do the ECGs of patients treated with lytics meet the ST-segment elevation criteria as specified on the protocol? What percentage of patients treated have enzyme-confirmed myocardial injury?
- Appropriate use of adjunctive and conjunctive drugs. What percent of patients receive aspirin, heparin (in patients treated with t-PA), beta blockers if no contraindication, nitrates for pain, ACE inhibitors, and/or magnesium? Are calcium channel blockers being inappropriately used?
- Outcomes. Mortality, morbidity, and, perhaps, an assessment of myocardial salvage, as reflected by ejection fraction, should be reviewed on a regular basis. All complications should be reviewed from the perspective of whether presenting characteristics might have predicted the possibility of a complication such as a bleed.

Feedback should continually be given to members of the medical staff in all departments, nursing staff, as well as ECG and pharmacy staff that would reinforce positive behavior or result in modification of the process to further reduce the door to drug time or improve compliance to protocol. Application of this process in a number of institutions has been reported. It is clear that door to drug time can be reduced substantially toward the goal of improving outcomes for patients with AMI while maintaining safety and increasing the use of effective drugs when appropriate. Reduction of door to drug time to 20–25 minutes is possible in most emergency departments [15,16].

References

1. Kereiakes DJ, Weaver WD, Anderson JL, Feldman T, Gibler B, Aufderheide T, Williams DO, Martin LH, Anderson LC, Martin JS, et al. Time delays in the diagnosis and treatment of acute myocardial infarction: A tale of eight cities. Report from the Pre-hospital Study Group and the Cincinnati Heart Project. Am Heart J 120:773, 1990.
2. Sharkey SW, Brunette DD, Ruiz E, Hession WT, Wysham DG, Godenberg IF, Hodges M. An analysis of time delays preceding thrombolysis for acute myocardial infarction. JAMA 262:3171, 1989.
3. Kline EM, Smith DD, Martin JS, Dracup K, Woodlief LH, Granger CB, Califf RM. In-hospital treatment delays in patients treated with thrombolytic therapy: A report of the GUSTO Time to Treatment Substudy (abstr). Circulation 86(Suppl. 1):702, 1992.
4. Moses HW, Bartolozzi JJ, Koester DL, Colliver JA, Taylor GJ, Mikell FL, Dove JT, Katholi RE, Woodruff RC, Miller BD, et al. Reducing delay in the emergency room in administration of thrombolytic therapy for myocardial infarction associated with ST elevation. Am J Cardiol 68:251, 1991.
5. National Heart Attack Alert Coordinating Committee, 60 Minutes to Treatment Working Group. Emergency Department: Rapid Identification and Treatment of Patients with Acute Myocardial Infarction. Ann Emerg Med 23:311, 1994.
6. American Heart Association/Emergency Cardiac Care Committee and Subcommittees. Guidelines for cardiopulmonary resuscitation and emergency cardiac care, III: Adult advanced cardiac life support. JAMA 268:2199, 1992.
7. Weaver WD, Cerqueira M, Hallstrom AP, Litwin PE, Martin JS, Kudenchuk PJ, Eisenberg M (for the Myocardial Infarction Triage and Intervention Project Group). Prehospital-initiated vs. hospital-initiated thrombolytic therapy: The Myocardial Infarction Triage and Intervention Trial. JAMA 270:1211, 1993.
8. Higgins GL, Lambrew CT, Hunt E, et al. Expediting the early hospital care of the adult patient with nontraumatic chest pain: Impact of a modified ED triage protocol. Am J Emerg Med 11:576, 1993.
9. Kereiakes DJ, Gibler WB, Martin LH, Pieper KS, Anderson LC, Cincinnati Heart Project Study Group. Relative importance of emergency medical system transport and the prehospital electrocardiogram on reducing hospital time delay to therapy for acute myocardial infarction: A preliminary report from the Cincinnati Heart Project. Am Heart J 123:835, 1992.
10. Weaver WD, Eisenberg MS, Martin JS, Litwin PE, Shaeffer SM, Ho MT, Kudenchuk P, Hallstrom AP, Cerqueira MD, Copass MK. Myocardial infarction triage and intervention project — phase I: Patient characteristics and feasibility of prehospital initiation of thrombolytic therapy. J Am Coll Cardiol 15:925, 1990.
11. Lambrew CT, Weaver WD, French WJ, Bowlby L, Rubison M for the National Registry of Myocardial Infarction. Impact of hospital protocols on time to treatment with thrombolytic therapy. J Am Coll Card 23(Suppl. A):14A, 1994.
12. Kudenchuk PJ, Ho MT, Weaver WD, Litwin PE, Martin JS, Eisenberg MS, Hallstrom AP, Cobb LA (for the MITI Project Investigators). Accuracy of computer-interpreted electrocardiography in selecting patients for thrombolytic therapy. J Am Coll Cardiol 17:1486, 1991.
13. Selker HP. Coronary care unit triage decision aids: How do we know when they work [editorial]? Am J Med 87:491, 1989.
14. Gonzalez ER, Jones LA, Ornato JP, Bleecker GC, Strauss MJ (Virginia Thrombolytic Study Group). Hospital delays and problems with thrombolytic administration in patients receiving thrombolytic therapy: A multicenter prospective assessment. Ann Emerg Med 21:1215, 1992.
15. Cannon CP, Antman EM, Walls R, Braunwald E. Time as an adjunctive agent to thrombolytic therapy. J Thromb Thrombolys 1:27, 1994.
16. Lambrew CT. Emergency department triage of patients with nontraumatic chest pain. ACC Curr J Rev 4:61, 1995.

23. FACTORS ASSOCIATED WITH PREHOSPITAL DELAY AND OVERVIEW OF COMMUNITY TRIALS TO REDUCE THE DURATION OF PREHOSPITAL DELAY IN PATIENTS WITH SYMPTOMS OF ACUTE CORONARY DISEASE

Robert J. Goldberg and Voula Osganian

Introduction

Death rates from coronary heart disease (CHD) in the United States increased dramatically at the beginning of the 20th century, reaching epidemic proportions by the mid-1960s [1–4]. Since the peak in CHD death rates in 1968, during which approximately 675,000 persons died from CHD and nearly 370,000 from acute myocardial infarction (AMI), age-adjusted mortality rates attributed to CHD have leveled off and have exhibited a consistent downward trend, declining by approximately 2–3% annually. Despite these encouraging declines in CHD mortality rates over the past 25 years, CHD remains the major cause of death and disability in the United States and other industrialized countries; approximately 1.25 million persons experience an AMI in the United States each year, and almost 500,000 CHD deaths occur annually, with nearly half of these deaths attributed to AMI alone [5]. CHD is a major health concern for both men and women.

A paucity of population-based data exist to explain the observed temporal trends in CHD mortality rates. While reasons for the decline in mortality rates attributed to CHD in the United States, as well as in a number of other industrialized countries, are incompletely understood, it is likely that this decline is due to factors affecting the risk of developing and/or dying from CHD, including changes in the prevalence and/or levels of the major coronary risk factors and improvements in the medical management of pa-

tients with established coronary artery disease [5]. In general, national estimates of population changes in the commonly accepted risk factors for CHD have demonstrated consistent improvements over the past two decades. For example, overall population prevalence rates of cigarette smoking have declined in adults since the issuance of the Surgeon General's first report on smoking and health in 1964, marked increases in the population awareness and control of high blood pressure have been observed since the late 1960s, and declines in the average population cholesterol levels have been seen in health surveys of the noninstitutionalized population of the United States since the early 1960s to the late 1970s [5].

Striking advances in the management of AMI have also taken place during the past decade [5,6]. The medical management of AMI has evolved from a strategy of watchful waiting with primarily hemodynamic support to one of active intervention with thrombolytic agents and aggressive mechanical interventions, such as coronary angioplasty, that are designed to restore perfusion to the ischemic myocardium. These measures are utilized to prevent or reduce the risk of complications associated with acute myocardial necrosis. The results of a number of secondary prevention trials employing thrombolytic therapies such as streptokinase or tissue plasminogen activator (t-PA) have demonstrated a significant reduction in mortality following AMI [7–11].

Thrombolytic Therapy for Acute Myocardial Infarction

The advent, introduction, and success of thrombolytic therapy has held out considerable promise for reducing the high morbidity and mortality associated with AMI and has dramatically changed the delivery of care in the early hours of this disease process. A meta-analysis of 14 published randomized clinical trials has shown that the early administration of thrombolytic therapy is associated with an approximate 25% reduction in in-hospital case-fatality rates following AMI [9]. These studies have also shown that the earlier thrombolytic therapy is initiated, the greater the reduction in mortality, or conversely, the efficacy of thrombolytic therapy in altering the course of AMI decreases rapidly with time since the onset of the acute event.

Despite the clear benefits associated with use of thrombolytic therapy in patients with AMI, several studies suggest that less than one quarter of AMI patients receive a thrombolytic agent, primarily due to delays in seeking medical care as well as due to real or perceived contraindications to use of this therapy [10,11]. Although data from the multihospital, population-based Worcester Heart Attack Study showed a marked increase in the use of thrombolytic agents in community residents hospitalized with validated AMI between 1986 and 1990, only 23% of AMI patients received thrombolytic therapy in 1990 [12]; use of these agents was directly related to the duration of patient delay in presentation to the hospital after the appearance of AMI symptoms [13]. Patients arriving at the emergency department in any of 16 university-affiliated and community hospitals in the Worcester metropolitan area within 1 hour of the onset of AMI symptoms were approximately 6.5 times more likely to receive thrombolytic therapy than were those presenting to these emergency departments 6 or more hours after the onset of acute symptoms. Of patients presenting to the hospital within 1 hour of the onset of AMI symptoms, 32% received thrombolytic therapy; this percentage decreased to 22%, 13%, and 8% in those presenting between 2 and 3 hours, 4 and 6 hours, and greater than 8 hours, respectively, after the onset of AMI symptoms [13].

Delay in Seeking Medical Care Following Onset of Acute Coronary Symptoms and Factors Associated with Delay

Given the magnitude of CHD in the United States, the availability of therapies that have been shown to reduce infarct size and to improve short-term survival following AMI, data suggesting that the timing of administration of these agents is related to efficacy, and that delays in seeking definitive medical care may result in increased risk of sudden cardiac death and poorer in-hospital survival, compelling reasons are put forth for community-wide efforts to further understand and reduce the extent of delay in individuals seeking medical care after the onset of symptoms suggestive of AMI. While a number of investigations are attempting to streamline the delivery of thrombolytic therapy in the emergency department and to reduce hospital-associated delays in the administration of this therapy, the vast majority of the delay time associated with administration of thrombolytic therapy is related to patient-associated factors that occur before the patient reaches the hospital setting. Several studies have, therefore, attempted to define the stages of delay in seeking medical care following the onset of symptoms of acute CHD, to assess the magnitude of delay associated with these various stages, and to determine factors associated with delay.

A number of phases may occur when one delays the decision to seek medical treatment following the onset of acute CHD symptoms, and these phases do not necessarily follow in a logical ordered sequence [14]. Using the framework constructed by Alonzo [15] from previous work done by others on stages of illness [16], the following phases of delay may exist: the prodromal phase, the definition phase of self-evaluation, the lay consultation phase, the medical consultation phase, the hospital travel phase, and the hospital procedural phase from arrival at the emergency department to the initiation of treatment. Delay can occur during any of these phases, impacting on the receipt of thrombolytic therapy or mechanical revascularization upon hospital arrival.

The major component of total delay time is patient decision time; transportation time to the hospital represents only a small percentage of the overall extent of delay. Table 23-1 reviews several published studies that have examined the extent of prehospital delay in patients hospitalized with AMI [17]. Although considerable variation in the magnitude of delay exists, there is substantial delay from the time of perceived symptom onset to hospital arrival noted. Median delay times ranging from less than 2 hours to as much as 8 hours, and mean delay times ranging from 1.6 hours to longer than 1 day have been observed in these observational studies carried out between the early 1960s and the mid to late 1980s. A number of these studies have found that approximately one half of patients delay seeking treatment

TABLE 23-1. Characteristics of study samples and delay times in
patients with confirmed acute myocardial infarction (AMI) in selected studies

Author	Study years	n	Mean age (yr.)	% Men	Selection of cases	Previous history of AMI (%)	Ascertainment of delay time data	Delay time (h)	
								Mean	Median
Olin et al. (29)	1962–63	31	53	78	Random sample	10	Interview	5.2	2.0
Moss et al. (30)	1968–69	160	61	72	Emergency dept.	24	Interview	42.4	3.5
Tjoe et al. (31)	1970	48	N.R.	59	Successive admissions to CCU	29	Interview	25.8	8.0
Turi et al. (32)	1978–83	778	57	73	Patients randomized into a clinical trial (5 CCUs)	23	Medical record	3.6	2.0
Cooper et al. (33)	1983–84	111	60	56	Admissions to a medical service emergency dept.	23	Interview	22.5	6.0
Mitic et al. (19)	1984	101	58	64		N.R.	Medical record	1.6	N.R.
Ho et al. (20)	1986–87	135	63	57	Admissions to 9 CCUs	N.R.	Interview	N.R.	2.6
Herlitz et al. (23)	1986–87	762	N.R.	N.R.	Emergency dept.	N.R.	Medical record	N.R.	3.0
Ridker et al. (34)	1982–88	258	>40	100	Patients with initial AMI in Physicians Health Study	0	Medical record	N.R.	1.8
Ridker et al. (34)	1982–88	240	>40	100	Patients with initial AMI in ISIS-2	0	Medical record	N.R.	4.9
Schmidt et al. (35)	1988–89	126	60	75	Admitted and transferred patients	25	Questionnaire	5.9	2.2
Moses et al. (21)	1991	66	57	45	Emergency dept.	N.R.	Medical record	3.6	1.7
Yarzebski et al. (17)	1986–90	1279	N.R.	62	Community-based survey of 16 teaching and community hospitals	32	Medical record	4.2	2.0
Ell et al. (36)	1988–90	448	N.R.	51	African-American patients admitted to a public and a private hospital for suspect AMI	N.R.	Interview	14.9	2.7

N.R. = not reported.

for 4 or more hours after acute symptom onset. In the most recent and largest of these studies of metropolitan Worcester MA, residents [17], the average (4.2 hours) and median (2.0 hours) delays between onset of symptoms suggestive of AMI and hospital presentation did not change significantly over the periods examined (1986–1990). This variability across studies is likely to be a result of several factors, including differences in the definition and components of delay time, acute symptom onset, patient inclusion criteria and diagnosis of AMI, variability in the number of subjects studied, and differences in patient demographic and clinical characteristics. In particular, a number of questions have been raised concerning the ability of patients to accurately recall the time of onset of AMI-related symptoms and to interpret the nature and seriousness of more nonspecific signs and symptoms.

A variety of factors have been examined surrounding the decision to act and respond to the symptoms of AMI [14]. The majority of studies examining sources of delay have shown that lengthy decision making and inappropriate responses, or failure to recognize the onset of acute CHD-related symptoms, are the principal contributors to prehospital delay. While inconsistent findings have been reported concerning the association of age and gender with prehospital delay, several studies have shown that the elderly delay longer than younger individuals. Racial differences in the extent of prehospital delay have not been systematically examined; the few studies that have examined this relationship have shown African Americans to delay longer than whites in seeking care for AMI symptoms. Neither socioeconomic status nor level of education has been shown to be associated with care-seeking behavior [14]. A prior history of

CHD does not appear to be associated with reduced delay and may actually increase delay in seeking care.

Seeking the assistance of a spouse or physician in making the decision to go to the hospital for AMI symptoms has been associated with prolonged delay, as has the use of self-treatment measures for cardiac symptoms. Onset of cardiac symptoms during the daytime hours and on the weekend is typically associated with an increase in delay times. Inability to interpret symptoms suggestive of acute coronary disease, slowly developing symptoms, confusion in the recognition of these symptoms, as well as denial or fear have been suggested as reasons for patient delay in seeking treatment. Availability of medical care, perceived quality of care, and cost-related issues may also impact on the duration of prehospital delay.

Overview of Studies Designed to Reduce Extent of Prehospital Delay

While a number of national and international intervention programs have been designed and carried out to modify the major risk factors for CHD by encouraging individuals at increased risk for CHD and entire communities to modify their lifestyle practices, there have been surprisingly few community-based attempts to alter the health care–seeking behavior of individuals once the signs and symptoms of acute coronary disease have developed [18–25]. The descriptive characteristics of several of these trials and their results are summarized in Table 23-2.

The earliest of these studies, in Nottingham, England, asked adult patients registered with three general medical practices to telephone a special hospital number if they were having chest pain lasting for more than 10 minutes [18]. Patients from three intervention practices reported chest pain earlier than patients in 10 comparison practices selected as convenience samples. This initial investigation was followed by a study in Canada that utilized an 8-week "Signals and Actions" television and radio media campaign. Two concepts were emphasized in this program: that the symptoms of a heart attack can be clearly described and recognized and the importance of seeking immediate professional help [19]. This study observed a significant increase (16% precampaign to 29% postcampaign) in the percentage of patients presenting to the emergency department within 2 hours of symptom onset from before, during, and after the mass media campaign.

This program was followed by a public education campaign in Seattle, Washington, which was carried out in collaboration with the local American Heart Association affiliate [20]. The primary message of the 2-month educational campaign emphasized the symptoms of AMI, the importance of acting quickly in response to AMI symptoms, and for the need to call 911 to activate the EMS system. The print media as well as radio and television public service announcements were used to disseminate the health education messages. The results of this study showed a favorable, albeit nonsignificant, trend in reduction of patient delay from before to after the campaign.

The sole study carried out in a small rural setting used patient education brochures, television and newspaper advertisements, posters, radio spots, and talks to the general public for their education program [21]. These approaches were extensively utilized during the first 2 months of this 2-year campaign, with the message then staggered throughout the remainder of the study. No changes in either patient response or emergency department visits were seen in this campaign. During the first week of a 1-year media campaign in Geneva, Switzerland, hospital visits for chest pain due to cardiac and noncardiac causes increased significantly [22]. Utilization of thrombolytic therapy also increased from baseline levels.

The most extensively reported study was carried out in Göteborg, Sweden, in which a 3-week intensive media campaign was followed by a maintenance phase of nearly 1 year, primarily using print materials [23–25]. A simple rhythmic slogan. Hjarta-Smarta-90000, was developed for this campaign. The primary intent of this campaign was to inform individuals who were having prolonged chest pain to immediately call this emergency number. This public education campaign resulted in a 40-minute average reduction in the median delay time from a baseline level of 3.0 hours. A similar positive finding was observed in Australia, although the intervention effects were not maintained [26]. In this study a public education media campaign was conducted three times for 1 week each in 1975, 1985, and 1989. The results of a 6-month community-wide media campaign in the greater Heidelberg area of Germany have been reported in preliminary abstract form [27]. From pre to post intervention assessment, median delay time decreased from 4.0 to 2.1 hours, while hospital admissions within 4 hours of symptom onset increased substantially.

The collective results of these studies suggest that while informational campaigns may increase knowledge and awareness of AMI in patients at risk for CHD, they do not demonstrate a significant reduc-

TABLE 23-2. Summary of community campaigns designed to reduce the delay between onset of chest pain and hospital treatment for acute myocardial infarction

Author	Year published	Community	No. of hospitals included in surveillance network	Educational interventions	Evaluation	Results
Mitic et al. (19)	1984	Population of 300,000 residing in eastern Canada	1	8-week media campaign of "Signals and Actions" Television, radio spots and public service announcements (PSAs) used	Pre-post comparison of delay times in 4-week period before media campaign (pre) with during the campaign and 3 months after completion of media campaign (post)	Significant increases in delay times of ≤2 hours from pre (16% of all individuals studied), to during the campaign (32%), and at the postdata collection period (29%)
Ho et al. (20)	1989	King County, Washington	9	Two-month public education campaign in association with AHA Campaign message emphasized symptoms of AMI, importance of acting quickly and calling 911 to activate EMS Television, radio spots, and newspapers utilized	Comparison of delay time between premedia period (4–5 months), message period (2 months), and post-message period (4–5 months)	Patient delay times did not change significantly between premessage period (median = 2.6 hours) and postmessage period (median = 2.3 hours)
Moses et al. (21)	1991	Population of 26,000 residing in Jacksonville, Illinois	1	Two-year public education program consisting of brochures, television and newspaper ads, PSAs, and public talks and posters	Pre-post evaluation of educational campaign	No significant change in mean delay time pre and post (mean = 105 minutes) educational campaign among patients with angina, AMI, noncardiac chest pain. Small increase in emergency dept. visits
Blohm et al. (24)	1991	Population of 450,000 residing in Götebörg, Sweden	1	Three-week intensive period of radio and television ads, leaflets to healthy individuals and those with AMI, posters on buses and trains, articles on AMI in local newspaper, and talks to local district clinics, hospital, and pharmacy Maintenance media phase followed acute intervention period	Evaluation of patients seen in emergency dept. 21 months before (pre) and 13 months after (post) the campaign	Decrease in median delay time from 3.0 hours (pre) to 2.3 hours during campaign Increase in percentage of patients receiving thrombolysis No change in hospital or 1 year mortality following AMI

tion in prehospital delay among those with confirmed CHD or an increased or selective use of the EMS system in comparison with the preintervention period. These studies do, however, suggest the feasibility and potential success of short-term public education interventions on prehospital delay times. As a number of investigators have noted [28], more attention must be given to interpersonal education strategies rather than the mass media as the major intervention approach.

Each of these investigations, however, suffers from a number of methodological problems that limit their interpretation and potential generalizability. These problems include sample size considerations of both the number of communities under study and the number of individuals with AMI surveyed, inability to examine potential differential effects of the educational intervention on sociodemographically or clinically defined subgroups, the relatively short duration of the educational campaigns, and failure to target high-risk subgroups and to tailor the intervention approaches. Of greatest methodological concern, none of the studies utilized an experimental design in which there was a comparative assessment with communities that did not receive the interventions. In addition, study endpoints were limited, few studies examined the effect of the public education interventions on the receipt of thrombolytic therapy among those with confirmed AMI, or of the impact of these programs on short-term survival associated with AMI. These studies do, however, provide insights to approaches that might be utilized or needed in developing an effective population-based educational campaign and of the types of measures to be utilized in assessing the impact of these programs.

Based on the review of existing studies, the Consensus Conference on the Rapid Identification and Treatment of AMI recommended several areas for further study in order to promote reductions in prehospital delay time in patients with symptoms of evolving acute coronary disease [14]. These areas included the identification of individuals perceived to be at high risk for prolonged delay (e.g., the elderly, blacks, individuals with a history of cardiovascular disease); provision of specific instructions on how to access and effectively use EMS systems; development of public educational campaigns to increase the knowledge and awareness of the signs and symptoms of AMI; and the development of educational programs for family members and coworkers of those with prior AMI, specifically targeting family members of patients with a history of CHD.

National Heart, Lung and Blood Institute–Sponsored Randomized Trial of Community-Wide Efforts to Influence Patient Care-Seeking Behavior Following The Onset of Acute Coronary Symptoms

In response to these and additional concerns, in June 1993 the National Heart, Lung, and Blood Institute (NHLBI) released a request for applications for a multicenter collaborative research program to study the effects of community-wide education on seeking care following the symptoms of acute coronary disease through use of a randomized controlled study design. The purpose of this experimental study, called the Rapid Early Action for Coronary Treatment (REACT) trial, is to evaluate the effects of a public education campaign on patient delay time in seeking medical care following the onset of symptoms of acute coronary disease, the use of emergency medical services and the emergency department, the use of thrombolytic agents in those with confirmed AMI, and in-hospital case fatality rates following AMI. A number of additional hypotheses are being examined in this randomized controlled community trial. Five field centers in Alabama, Massachusetts, Minnesota, Texas, and Washington are included, and the coordinating center for REACT is the New England Research Institute.

The design of this study is based on the model of community intervention research. Each of the five field centers have recruited two sets of pair-matched communities to this trial, with one half of each community pair randomly assigned to intervention or control status; a total of 10 communities have thereby been chosen to receive the educational intervention approaches, while the other 10 communities will serve as the comparison or reference sites and will not be exposed to the public, patient, and healthcare provider intervention strategies.

The intervention approaches that are being applied from a community-wide perspective are based on a number of conceptual theories, including the theory of reasoned action, community diffusion of information theory, social learning and stages of change theory, the health belief model, attribution theories, and social marketing principles designed to favorably affect overall behavioral change. Health professionals in each of the intervention communities are being educated regarding the rapid diagnosis and treatment of patients with AMI. Individuals considered at high risk for coronary disease, as well as the general public, are being exposed to a variety of educational messages about the symptoms of acute coronary disease, the importance of early treatment, and the appropriate actions that should be taken in the event of a possible heart attack. Community-based surveys of the general population are being carried out, follow-up interviews of patients presenting with suspect and confirmed acute coronary disease completed, and monitoring of trends in community mortality rates from CHD will be performed to examine the effects of the educational programs on selected study outcomes.

The REACT trial is being conducted over a 4-year period. Baseline data for a 4 month period has been collected during the fall of 1995. Following this baseline period, an 18-month phased-in educational campaign has been applied in the 10 intervention committies which will end in the fall of 1997. Following the completion of intervention activities, the remaining time will be devoted to the write up, analysis and evaluation of study results. The results of this collaborative, multisite, community-based trial will provide insights to intervention approaches that can be successfully utilized to reduce the duration of prehospital delay following the onset of symptoms of acute CHD and will result in more favorable outcomes in individuals with acute ischemic coronary syndromes.

References

1. Havlik RJ, Feinleib M (eds). Proceedings of the Conference on the Decline in Coronary Heart Disease Mortality. Washington, DC: Government Printing Office, 1979. DHEW Publication No. (NIH) 79.

2. Higgins MW, Luepker RV (eds). Trends in Coronary Heart Disease Mortality. The Influence of Medical Care. New York: Oxford University Press, 1988.

3. Stern M. The recent decline in ischemic heart disease mortality. Ann Intern Med 91:630, 1979.

4. Goldman L, Cook EF. The decline in ischemic heart disease mortality rates. An analysis of the comparative effects of medical interventions and changes in lifestyle. Ann Intern Med 101:825, 1984.

5. Goldberg RJ. Temporal trends and declining mortality rates from coronary heart disease in the United States. In Ockene IS, Ockene JK (eds). Prevention of Coronary Heart Disease. Boston: Little, Brown, 1992:42.

6. Braunwald E. The aggressive treatment of acute myocardial infarction. Circulation 71:1087, 1985.

7. ACC/AHA Task Force Report. Guidelines of the early management of patients with acute myocardial infarction. Circulation 82:664, 1990.

8. ACC/AHA Task Force Report. Guidelines for the early management of patients with acute myocardial infarction. J Am Coll Cardiol 16:249, 1990.

9. Yusuf S, Wittes J, Friedman L. Overview of results of randomized clinical trials in heart disease. I. Treatments following myocardial infarction. JAMA 260:2088, 1988.

10. Grines CL, DeMaria AN. Optimal utilization of thrombolytic therapy for acute myocardial infarction: Concepts and controversies. J Am Coll Cardiol 16:223, 1990.

11. Anderson HV, Willerson JT. Thrombolysis in acute myocardial infarction. N Engl J Med 329:703, 1993.

12. Pagley PR, Yarzebski J, Goldberg RJ, Chen Z, Chiriboga D, Dalen P, Gurwitz J, Alpert JS, Gore JM. Gender differences in the treatment of patients with acute myocardial infarction: A multi-hospital, community-based perspective. Arch Intern Med 153:625, 1993.

13. Goldberg RJ, Gurwitz J, Yarzebski J, Landon J, Gore JM, Alpert JS, Dalen PM, Dalen JE. Patient delay and receipt of thrombolytic therapy among patients with acute myocardial infarction from a community-wide perspective. Am J Cardiol 70:421, 1992.

14. Dracup K, Moser DK. Treatment-seeking behavior among those with symptoms and signs of acute myocardial infarction. Proceedings of the NHLBI Symposium on Rapid Identification and Treatment of Acute Myocardial Infarction. U.S. Department of Health and Human Services, September, 1991.

15. Alonzo AA. Acute illness behavior: A conceptual exploration and specification. Soc Sci Med 14A:515, 1980.

16. Suchman EA. Stages of illness and medical care. J Health Soc Behav 6:114, 1965.

17. Yarzebski J, Goldberg RJ, Gore JM, Alpert JS. Temporal trends and factors associated with extent of delay to hospital arrival in patients with acute myocardial infarction: The Worcester Heart Attack Study. Am Heart J 128:255, 1994.

18. Rowley JM, Hill JD, Hampton JR, Mitchell JRA. Early reporting of myocardial infarction: Impact of an experiment in patient education. Br Med J 284:1741, 1982.

19. Mitic WR, Perkins J. The effect of a media campaign on heart attack delay and decision times. Can J Public Health 75:414, 1984.

20. Ho MT, Eisenberg MS, Litvin PE, Schaeffer SM, Damonsk. Delay between onset of chest pain and seeking medical care: The effect of public education. Ann Emerg Med 18:727, 1989.

21. Moses HW, Engelking N, Taylor GJ, Prabhakar C, Vallala M, Colliver JA, Silberman H, Schneider JA. Effect of a two-year public education campaign on reducing response time of patients with symptoms of acute myocardial infarction. Am J Cardiol 68:249, 1991.

22. Gaspoz JM, Under PF, Urban P, Chevralet JC, Rutishauser W, Heliot C, Sechaud L, Mischier S, Waldvogel F. Impact of a public campaign on prehospital delay times in suspected acute myocardial infarction (abstr). Circulation, Vol 88, 4, Part 2, 63: I-13, 1993.

23. Herlitz J, Hartford M, Blohm M, Karison BW, Ekstrom L, Risenfors M, Wennerblom B, Luepker RV, Holmberg S. Effects of a media campaign on delay

times and ambulance use in suspected acute myocardial infarction. Am J Cardiol 64:90, 1989.

24. Blohm M, Herlitz J, Hartford M, Karison BW, Risenfors M, Luepker RV, Sjolin M, Holmberg S. Consequences of a media compaign focusing on delay in acute myocardial infarction. Am J Cardiol 69:411, 1992.

25. Herlitz J, Blohm M, Hartford M, Karison BW, Luepker R, Holmberg S, Risenfors M, Wennerblom B. Follow-up of a 1 year media campaign on delay times and ambulance use in suspected acute myocardial infarction. Eur Heart J 13:171, 1992.

26. Bett N, Aroney G, Thompson P. Impact of a national educational campaign to reduce patient delay in possible heart attack. Aust N Z J Med 23:157, 1993.

27. Rustige JM, Burczyk U, Schiele R, et al. Media campaign on delay times in suspected myocardial infarction — the Ludwigshafen Community Project (abstr). Eur Heart J 11(Suppl.):171, 1990.

28. Kennedy GT. Strategies for change: Patient educaton. Proceedings of the NHLBI Symposium on Rapid Identification and Treatment of Acute Myocardial Infarction, U.S. Department of Health and Human Services, Public Health Service, 1991.

29 Olin HS, Hackett TP. The denial of chest pain in 32 patients with acute myocardial infarction. JAMA 190:977, 1994.

30 Moss AJ, Wynar B, Goldstein S. Delay in hospitalization during the acute coronary period. Am J Cardiol 24:659, 1969.

31. Tjoe SL, Luria MH. Delays in reaching the cardiac care unit: an analysis. Chest 61:617, 1972.

32. Turi ZG, Stone PH, Muller JE, Parker C, Rude RE, Raabe DE, Jaffe AS, Hartwell TD, Robertson TL, Braunwald E, and the MILIS Study Group. Implications for acute intervention related to time of hospital arrival in acute myocardial infarction. Am J Cardiol 58:203, 1986.

33. Cooper RS, Simmons B, Castaner A, Prasad R, Franklin C, Ferlinz J. Survival rates and prehospital delay during myocardial infarction among black persons. Am J Cardiol 57:208, 1986.

34. Ridker PM, Manson JE, Goldhaber SZ, Hennekens CH, Buring JE. Comparison of delay times to hospital presentation for physicians and nonphysicians with acute myocardial infarction. Am J Cardiol 70:10, 1992.

35. Schmidt SB, Borsh WA. The pre-hospital phase of acute myocardial infarction in the era of thrombolysis. Am J Cardiol 65:1411, 1990.

36. Ell K, Haywood LJ, Sobel E, De Guzman M, Blumfield D, Ning JP. Acute chest pain in african americans: factors in delay in seeking emergency care. Am J Public Health 84:965, 1994.

24. EMERGENCY MEDICAL SERVICES

James M. Atkins

Introduction

Emergency medical services can aid the rapid reperfusion of patients with an acute myocardial infarction as well as speed the care for other patients with acute cardiac ischemia. The importance of emergency medical services in the care of the patient with acute cardiac ischemia is best understood when one considers the critical nature of time. The various syndromes produced by acute cardiac ischemia present many challenges, and time is a major component of those challenges. Acute cardiac ischemia can present with any of three major syndromes — sudden cardiac death, acute myocardial infarction, and angina pectoris (stable or unstable). In patients with asymptomatic coronary atherosclerosis, the first symptom of acute cardiac ischemia is sudden death in about 25% of patients, acute myocardial infarction in about 45% of patients, and angina pectoris in the remainder of the patients [1–3]. A small percentage also present with heart failure initially. The importance of time, accuracy, and costs must permeate decision making when dealing with a patient with chest discomfort. Time also becomes a critical determinant in the outcome of cardiac arrest victims.

The critical nature of time is obvious when the patient suffers a cardiac arrest. When out-of-the-hospital cardiac arrest is examined, 93% of the long-term survivors had witnessed cardiac arrests and ventricular fibrillation [4–6]. Time to defibrillation and cardiopulmonary resuscitation (CPR) seem to be the most important determinants of survival [7]. The *Textbook of Advanced Cardiac Life Support* contains a composite of several different studies showing that time to defibrillation and time to CPR as well as time to advanced cardiac life support (epinephrine) are very critical [7]. The shorter the duration of each of these key time intervals, the greater is the survival.

As previously stated, time is also a critical factor in dealing with a patient with an acute myocardial infarction. A patient with an acute myocardial infarction can have a cardiac arrest at any time. With the advent of thrombolytic therapy and, more recently, with acute angioplasty of the occluded artery in infarcted patients, time to treatment has also become very important [8–11]. The MITI trial [12] has shown that thrombolytic therapy given within 70 minutes of the onset of pain can reduce mortality from acute myocardial infarction to less than 2%. The MITI trial also showed that very early thrombolytic therapy can reduce the amount of tissue lost to 0–1% of muscle mass in 40% of patients and to 2–10% loss of muscle mass in another 40% of patients. These results were obtained due, in part, to a rapid, highly efficient emergency medical services (EMS) system.

Therefore, it is obvious that time to treatment is very critical when looking at many of these patients. When we closely examine the time to treatment issue, there are three major sets of interactions that determine the amount of delay to treatment. The patient must make a decision to obtain medical care. Because the patient frequently asks a lay person for advice, this has been called the patient/bystander portion of the delay. Once the patient decides to obtain medical care, there is the transportation phase or emergency medical service phase, if that is used. Once the patient has arrived at the hospital, there are further delays; these delays are usually in the emergency department. This chapter deals only with the EMS portion of this delay.

This chapter discusses the role of emergency services and its components, as well as the role of automated external defibrillators and first responder defibrillation. Special technologies that can be used in the prehospital arena to aid in the rapid diagnosis and treatment of patients follow. Prehospital therapy, adjunctive therapy to reperfusion, and the possible use of prehospital thrombolytic therapy are reviewed. The final portion deals with triage and regional planning for reperfusion therapy.

Emergency Medical Service Systems

The development of modern EMS in the United States was sparked in the late 1960s and early 1970s by the occurrence of several different events. The year 1966 was a pivotal year in the development of EMS. The National Research Council of the National Academy of Sciences issued two major policy statements. The first dealt with trauma, the neglected disease [13]. The second contained the recommendation that health professionals learn CPR [14]. The development of CPR followed Dr. Kouwenhoven's description of closed-chest cardiac massage in 1960 [15]. Also in 1966, the first portable battery-powered defibrillator (74 lbs) became available.

Over the next 5 years, many governmental agencies developed standards for training, ambulances, and every aspect of prehospital care. The American Heart Association developed training programs in resuscitation. The American College of Surgeons developed standards for trauma facilities. The American College of Orthopedic Surgeons developed training courses for a new breed of personnel: the Emergency Medical Technician — Ambulance.

These factors pushed the development of emergency medical services from many angles. On the other hand, the old system of having multiple ambulance companies, usually owned by funeral homes, was starting to collapse for many different reasons. People began to expect that an ambulance would come to their aid within 10 minutes, not 30 minutes. There was an increased recognition by the public that there was a better system for treating patients.

Between 1969 and 1973, the pioneers in this field — Pantridge from Belfast, Cobb from Seattle, Nagel from Florida and Baltimore, Grace from New York, as well as many others — showed that patients could be resuscitated in the field and could later return to a useful, functional life. Successful resuscitations were demonstrated at large gatherings of people, such as at football games [16–20]. Pantridge and others in Ireland and Britain published data that indicated physicians and nurses on the ambulances could salvage a number of patients in the field [21–28]. In the United States, Grace also showed that patients could be resuscitated in the field [29,30]. A number of studies, particularly in the United States, demonstrated the effectiveness of telemetry of electrocardiograms, which brought about the establishment of paramedics and nurses providing prehospital care without a physician being present [31–37]. Finally, the success of these systems was demonstrated by Crampton, Nagel, Pantridge, Cobb, and others [18,38–48].

It is important to understand the history of EMS in order to comprehend the wide variation that occurs in these services in different communities. The EMS systems developed locally with no strong state or national standards. The guidelines that were written were more permissive rather than dictating a system. For these reasons there are wide variations in the types of systems and the levels of service provided from one community to the next.

In order for there to be rapid delivery of EMS, there must be rapid access, effective dispatch, and rapid transport to an appropriate facility. Though EMS are usually accessed for cardiac arrest, less than half of patients with an acute myocardial infarction utilize them.

ACCESS

Because time is a critical factor for the cardiac patient, it is essential that access to EMS be uniform and quick. A single, nationwide emergency number for emergency services — fire, police, and medical — is essential, and the number should be the same everywhere, 9-1-1. Today 75–80% of the population is covered by 9-1-1, mostly in urban areas. There are two types of 9-1-1 systems available. One version is the phone number 9-1-1, which connects the caller with an operator or dispatcher. A more sophisticated version is the enhanced 9-1-1 system, which has automatic identification of the caller's telephone number and address. This latter variety has great advantages when dealing with an emergency situation in which people may not be able to communicate calmly the information required to obtain an emergency response. A nationwide enhanced 9-1-1 system should be the goal [49–50]. There is a need for enhanced 9-1-1 because this shortens the time and decreases the likelihood for errors. Relatives and friends may give their home address and not the address where they are located in times of stress. All delays add to the total delay.

DISPATCH

Centralized dispatch is required to provide fast and efficient EMS. With centralized dispatch, a quick and efficient response can be obtained by ensuring that the closest available unit(s) respond. This is particularly important in areas where there are multiple agencies providing similar or the same service. The dispatcher should be trained to determine what services are needed. The need for a centralized dispatch can also be illustrated by the needs of a cardiac arrest victim. A cardiac arrest victim needs quick and efficient CPR as well as defibrillation. Two individuals on an ambulance cannot quickly and efficiently handle a cardiac arrest victim; but with centralized dispatch of an integrated system, a fire engine or other first responder could be sent to provide CPR and early defibrillation with an automated defibrillator, while the paramedic crew can provide the drug and other advanced therapy required in a rapid, efficient manner. For dispatch to be effective, dispatchers need to be trained. There is a need for Emergency Medical Dispatchers (EMDs). These dispatchers can determine the types of equipment and personnel required for the problem and can even provide first aid via the telephone. It has been shown that untrained telephone callers can be told how to do CPR until the system can respond. Thus, trained personnel can greatly improve the quality of dispatch [51–60]. Efficient, centralized dispatch with trained dispatchers should be a national goal.

TYPES OF SERVICE

In the United States there are four major types of EMS that are utilized. These are fire department–based systems, third city service systems, public utility systems, and competitive private systems. There is marked variability in the configuration of these systems. Additionally, many areas have marriages of two different types of service.

The fire department–based system probably affects more citizens than any other system because it is the dominant system in major urban areas. The fire department system uses fire and rescue officers as dual-trained personnel who can work with the fire side of the operation as well as the medical side. These systems vary widely. In some cities the fire department provides both the paramedics for the city as well as all transportation to the hospital. In other cities, the fire department provides the paramedics, but transportation is done by a different entity. In still other cities, the fire department may provide both roles as a basic transport service as well as a paramedic service (two levels service system). Even when the paramedic service and transportation are provided by another entity, the fire department frequently serves as a first responder.

A major advantage of the fire department–based system is the personnel. Employees of the fire service are looking for a permanent career, not a temporary job. Fire services are often very competitive for good personnel. In suburban areas, these individuals provide dual service. In many suburbs of large cities, there is a relatively low volume of fire calls and EMS calls. Firefighter/paramedics can serve two functions simultaneously, taking the appropriate piece of equipment that is needed for the case because the chance of simultaneous events is very rare. This dual function is very cost effective. However, in the inner city both services are extensively used, and the personnel cannot fill a dual function as easily, although they can rotate from one function to the other to reduce stress. Another advantage of the fire service is more extensive training in dangerous environments, such as fire and hazardous materials management, and in extrication and rescue.

The major disadvantage of the fire department–based system is political. The fire department–based systems struggle for funding with other city services and within the fire departments. Fire departments also live in a very public arena and have to contend with differing goals of governmental leaders, news media, and unions. Also, there is competition within the fire department for resources and, at times, hard feelings between fire suppression and EMS. The leadership may favor one side over the other. Promotion may totally favor one side. The civil service system sometimes makes discipline difficult.

Third city services generally provide paramedic or basic service with transportation. This model is frequently used when the city owns the public hospital, such as in New York City or Austin, Texas. Often the third service is operated as a division of the city hospital. The major advantage of this system over the fire department–based system is political. It circumvents intradepartmental politics and gives EMS the same footing as the police and fire department. The major disadvantages are similar to the fire department. Another major cost may be housing and locations for the units. Seldom does a third service system use fire stations for locations. They usually rent facilities in which they base their vehicles. Extra funds are needed for adding alert alarms to these facilities. Turnover of personnel is somewhat greater than in the fire service systems.

In the public utility model a single private provider is given a virtual monopoly by the city in exchange for services. This service provides all ambulance transport, including all contracts with health maintenance organizations (HMOs) or preferred provider organizations (PPOs), non-emergency transfers, and emergency runs. Because the contracts and non-emergency transfers are profitable, the city frequently has to pay less into this system. The advantage of this system is that everyone gets transported for a fee. The tax base does not support the system to the same degree of the other models. A disadvantage is that the cost to the patient is often double the other systems and can run as high as $1200 per call. Service to some areas may not be as good because the system is operated as a cost-efficient business and not as a service. The response time tends to be slightly higher than for the first two systems. Because units are not needed at night, very few units may be available at these times. The highest number of units are available at the highest load times. In case of disaster or an unusual number of calls, the system may either not have enough units available to do the job or may have to call in off-duty personnel for the crisis.

The final model is the competitive private model. In this model competing companies either vie for business or are centrally dispatched on a rotating basis. The only advantage of this system is that it tends to be less expensive. However, response times tend to be long, and the level of service varies and is often minimal.

PUBLIC SERVICE VERSUS BUSINESS

Fire department and third city service systems tend to be run as a public service, whereas public utility systems and competitive private systems tend to be run as businesses. The billing systems tend to be quite different. As a public service, the bulk of the service is usually paid by the taxpayer, with the individual patient or victim paying only a portion of the cost. Cities vary in how much the citizen has to pay for usage. Some cities charge nothing. Other cities charge nonresidents but provide the service free to residents. Still others charge fees. These fees are generally flat fees. Public service systems tend to respond to the victim and to obtain only essential information. Thus, most public service systems only obtain adequate billing information for a limited number of patients. On the other hand, public utility and competitive private systems obtain their funding from the patient, with only a small subsidy coming from the city for indigent losses. The bills are itemized with a response fee, a mileage fee for transport, and fees for any service rendered, similar to a hospital bill and physician's bill combined. These systems tend to provide more billable services for a far greater number of patients than public service systems.

When a system is managed as a public service, there are a number of differences in service that may not be noticed by the casual observer. A public service system tends to offer uniform levels of service. A public service system will position units so that response time is uniform for most of the citizens of the system. A system operated as a business will operate the ambulances so that the load per ambulance is about the same. For a citizen at the periphery of the city in a more sparsely developed area, a public service system would probably have a rapid response time (5–6 minutes), while a business-type system might be considerably longer. Neither the average response times nor the percentage of calls handled within a time period might reveal these differences, but they could greatly affect some citizens.

Another difference between the two major approaches is the problem of unusual load. The business type of system keeps the number of ambulances on the road to handle the usual volume of calls efficiently. If there is an unusually high number of calls, there may be inadequate resources. At the time of a storm or disaster, business types of systems may not be able to respond promptly. Public service systems tend to staff for the disaster, so that they have greater flexibility should the unusual arise. Fire department systems often have extra personnel who can be moved quickly from fire suppression to emergency medical services should the need arise.

Business types of systems can respond more quickly to changes in technology. Because most new technology can be billed, a business type of system would add a new drug or technology to the service quickly. Because public service systems are a part of the governmental bureaucracy, it is difficult to add new technology. If a new service is very advantageous, it takes a minimum of 2 years to add it to the service. It takes 6 months of education to convince the fire service or others of the need for the new technology. Once convinced of the usefulness, it must be added to the city budget. The departmental budget request must be submitted internally at least 6 months prior to the budget year. It must then compete against the priorities within the ambulance division, and then against other priorities within the fire department. It must also compete with police priorities before an assistant city manager, and again against all other city services before the city manager. Then it can be submitted to the city council, where it competes against the various agendas of the elected officials. It is a difficult, uphill battle to obtain new technology. Once it is approved, it then takes months to prepare specifications for bids, bids to be received, and then justification of the vendor selected. Business types of systems can quickly obtain the equipment that they wish.

Public service systems are in a fishbowl. Public service personnel more freely admit mistakes and, because most records are open records, the news media can freely criticize the system. Business types of systems tend to keep mistakes internal; because they are privately owned, the open records rules do not apply. Some business systems have better quality control because they are not under governmental immunity as a public service system is. Most business types of systems are willing to pay for quality control systems; it is difficult to obtain funds for quality control in public service systems. In Europe ambulance service is a public service.

LEVELS OF SERVICE

In the United States there are several different levels of service provided by EMS. The two most common levels of service are the EMT-A, Emergency Medical Technician-Ambulance (or Basic) and the EMT-P, Emergency Medical Technician-Paramedic, commonly called the *paramedic* [63–67].

An EMT-A has between 81 and 176 hours of training in basic first aid skills; the exact number of hours depends on the date of certification and varies from state to state. An EMT-A is trained to provide CPR, oxygen therapy, and other types of first aid. Most ambulance personnel are EMT-As [63–67]. Recently, automated external defibrillation has been added to the national curriculum for the basic level.

The EMT-P, or paramedic, has more extensive training, varying from 400 to 2000 hours. Paramedics can provide advanced therapy, including defibrillation, administration of certain cardiac drugs, infusion of intravenous fluids, and endotracheal intubation. Though EMT-Ps comprise a minority of ambulance personnel on a national basis, this level makes up the majority of personnel in cities. Because most Americans live in cities, the majority of the prehospital patients probably receive their prehospital care from paramedics [63,64,66,67].

There are other levels of prehospital personnel, which vary from state to state. Many states have an EMT-I, which is an intermediate from of EMT. An EMT-I may be able to infuse intravenous fluids or intubate a patient, and may be able to give a few drugs, such as 50% dextrose. The EMT-D, EMT-Defibrillation, is another certification level found in some states. The EMT-D initially used a manual defibrillator with a minimum amount of training. Recently, the development of automated defibrillators has allowed major expansion of this concept. Automated defibrillation can be taught with a 4-hour course and can be used by EMTs with few problems. Automated defibrillators may be less expensive than standard types of defibrillators [68–76].

Emergency medical service crews can be augmented with first responders. These are personnel who will arrive first at a scene and initiate treatment, such as CPR and even automated defibrillation. They may be volunteers, firemen, police, security, or other types of personnel. First responders can provide earlier defibrillation, thus increasing survival [63,64,66,67].

Automated External Defibrillation

The need for early defibrillation is well known [7]. The ability to provide early defibrillation has been enhanced by the development of automated external defibrillators. Patients who have had a cardiac arrest may be candidates for thrombolytic therapy if the resuscitation has not been too traumatic. The faster a patient is defibrillated, the more likely it is that the patient will survive. The earlier a patient is defibrillated, the less likely it is the resuscitation will be traumatic. Hence, faster defibrillation will increase the number of candidates for thrombolytic therapy and for other forms of reperfusion. Although the need for early defibrillation is obvious, the majority of ambulances in the United States are not equipped with defibrillators, either of the standard manual type or of the automated external type. The need for having defibrillators on ambulances is obvious, and this goal needs to be established in local areas [7,68–76].

Automated external defibrillators allow minimally trained individuals to successfully defibrillate patients. These devices can be used where there are only basic level emergency medical technicians to make defibrillation available on every ambulance. Even in systems that have paramedics, automated external defibrillation in the hands of first responders may make early defibrillation possible. First responders may be firemen on fire engines, police, security, or other personnel. Many cities have added automated external defibrillators to their fire engines [7,68–76].

Although programs of early defibrillation can be very successful, logistics still play a major role. The number of cardiac arrests varies widely across a community. There are different population densities that affect the number of arrests. Different areas of a community have different ages of people living in the area. Younger aged populations do not have as many cardiac arrests as an older age population. Hence, some areas of a community may have only one cardiac arrest per year in several square miles, while other areas of the community may have one a week in a single square mile. The American Heart Association has had conferences to make early defibrillation a high priority; it has been suggested that high-rise buildings might have automated external defibrillators with trained individuals in the building to use them [7,68–76].

Prehospital Technologies

There are methods by which the EMS system can facilitate rapid hospital administration of reperfusion therapy. Obviously rapid transport to the hospital is one method. The EMS system can also aid the hospital in determining the need for the type of reperfusion as well as reduce the time to reperfusion once the patient has arrived at the hospital. Technologies that can support early hospital reperfusion include a 12-lead electrocardiogram obtained before the patient has arrived at the hospital, asking directed questions to help in determining the type of reperfusion therapy, and possibly helping with rapid enzyme determination if that is needed.

PREHOSPITAL 12-LEAD ELECTROCARDIOGRAMS FOR CARDIAC PATIENTS

One recent advance in technology is the use of 12-lead electrocardiograms (ECGs) in the prehospital arena. Paramedics can be taught to quickly perform ECGs both accurately and quickly. High-quality 12-lead ECGs with computerized interpretation can be transmitted by cellular phone or radio. This will be useful to the receiving hospital. If the receiving hospital receives a 12-lead ECG that reveals an acute myocardial infarction (AMI) along with an appropriate history, the personnel in the hospital can be ready to give thrombolytic agents, beta-blocking agents, nitroglycerin, or other agents as soon as the patient arrives, rather than being delayed while the hospital obtains those data after arrival. This is of benefit.

Seattle has shown that this is of marked benefit to the patient, greatly reducing the time to thrombolytic therapy and decreasing the morbidity and mortality [12,61,62]. Computerized 12-lead ECGs have the advantage that they can be transmitted without distortion. Because they have been digitized, there is no wave distortion with transmission via a cellular telephone or radio. Standard analog ECGs, on the other hand, are distorted during radio or cellular telephone transmission, making the ST-segment less reliable. Some systems have taught their paramedics to recognize ST-segment elevation on a standard analog ECG and to transmit the information verbally. It remains to be seen whether physicians in the emergency department will rely on this type of information verbally transmitted by a paramedic. For these reasons, a computerized ECG has tremendous advantages. In Seattle and other areas, having an ECG before arrival has greatly reduced the time to treatment in the emergency department. Several areas of the United States using this technology have reported median door-to-needle times of less than 30 minutes [12,61,62].

PREHOSPITAL QUESTIONNAIRE

Prehospital questionnaires can also be of benefit. Several communities have used a standardized questionnaire to determine the indications for thrombolytic therapy and the major contraindications. These questionnaires usually have very structured questions that are asked of the patient, and the results are reported via radio or telephone to the control or receiving hospital. The report is usually divided into indications and contraindications. The report given by the paramedic is usually that the indications are "all present" or "present with the exception of," followed by which indication is not present. Then the report follows with "no contraindications present" or "contraindication of previous GI bleed." Because the majority of patients have no contraindications, this helps the hospital make the decision as to the probability of need for thrombolytic therapy.

The emergency department armed with a 12-lead ECG, the knowledge of indications, and absence of contraindications may then prepare to administer thrombolytic therapy prior to arrival so that only a brief and quick assessment is needed in the emergency department prior to administration. If the patient has contraindications for thrombolytic therapy but does have a positive 12-lead ECG and indications, the emergency department may activate the angioplasty team prior to patient arrival. Seattle has shown that these strategies may be of benefit [12].

Prehospital use of structured questioning in combination with the ECG may also be of benefit. The ACI Predictive Instrument might be a significant improvement. This technique uses a handheld calculator into which a number of variables are placed. The variables include:

- Chest pain or left arm pain/discomfort
- Chest or left arm discomfort as the most important presenting symptom
- History of a previous myocardial infarction
- History of use of nitroglycerine for chest pain
- ECG ST-segment flattening ("straightening") in two or more leads
- ECG ST elevation or depression of ≥ 1 mm in two or more leads
- ECG T-wave elevation ("hyperacute") or ≥ 1 mm inversion in two or more leads

The technique may be very helpful in the prehospital assessment of patients. Studies of this type of system are needed in the prehospital environment [140–146].

PREHOSPITAL ENZYME DETERMINATION

With the development of rapid bedside devices that can analyze creatine kinase (CK), MB-CK, troponin, and myoglobin, this technology may be of benefit in the prehospital setting. The usefulness of this type of device has not been studied. Paramedics could also draw a blood sample enroute, so that it could be quickly analyzed on arrival at the hospital. Most patients who are candidates for reperfusion do not need the determination of enzymes prior to the reperfusion therapy; however, there is a subset for which enzymes are needed to make the decision. Obtaining the specimen or running the assay in the prehospital arena might be of benefit. However, these strategies need to be studied to see if they are of benefit.

Prehospital Therapy

Emergency medical services can provide drug therapy to patients with an acute myocardial infarction. These therapies include routine advanced cardiac life support (ACLS) as well as therapies specifically for the acute myocardial infarction patient.

ADVANCED CARDIAC LIFE SUPPORT
Paramedic systems deliver advanced cardiac life support to patients. These systems not only handle cardiac arrests, but also treat symptomatic bradycardia and tachycardia as well as hypotension and congestive heart failure. ACLS has been a standard of paramedic systems for many years [7].

SPECIFIC THERAPIES
Patients with acute cardiac ischemia can benefit from several prehospital therapies. The administration of oxygen, nitroglycerin, morphine, and aspirin are frequent portions of the prehospital therapy provided by many emergency medical service systems. The most significant question is whether these systems can administer thrombolytic therapy.

There are two major studies that need to be examined. The European Myocardial Infarction Project studied 5469 patients. Of these, 2750 patients were randomized to prehospital therapy. The prehospital therapy group received anistreplase on the ambulance followed by a placebo administration on arrival in the emergency department. In the hospital group, 2719 patients received placebo in the ambulance followed by anistreplase after arrival in the emergency department. This very large study revealed a 13% decrease in 30-day mortality in the group receiving prehospital thrombolytic therapy; however, this difference was nonsignificant ($P = 0.08$). Cardiac death was of borderline significance, with a 16% decrease ($P = 0.049$) for prehospital therapy. These borderline findings in a very large study need to be considered. It is important to realize that the difference in time to thrombolytic therapy was 55 minutes between those patients who received active drug in the ambulance versus those who received active drug in the emergency department [84].

The Myocardial Infarction Triage and Intervention Trial (MITI) was performed in Seattle and revealed no difference between those patients treated in the ambulance versus those receiving thrombolytic therapy after arrival in the hospital. In this trial, computerized ECGs where transmitted to the hospital. The transmission of patient information and ECGs greatly shortened the door-to-needle time of those patients who received active drug in the emergency department. The difference in time to treatment was only 20–25 minutes in this study [12].

Thus, the European trial showed borderline advantages of prehospital thrombolytic therapy, whereas the MITI trial did not show benefit of prehospital thrombolysis. The greatest difference in these trials is that the time to treatment variation between the two arms was much less in MITI when an ECG was transmitted. Another major difference that should be considered is that in the European studies the decision in the field was made by a physician being physically present, not by paramedics talking over the telephone or radio to a physician.

The decision to use prehospital thrombolysis should be determined by logistical considerations. If the difference in time to treatment is long due to long transportation times or other factors, then prehospital thrombolytic therapy may be of benefit. However, if the transportation times are not long, the difference between prehospital therapy and hospital therapy may not be of benefit if the necessary information and ECGs are obtained and transmitted to the hospital.

Another consideration for prehospital thrombolytic therapy is the medicolegal risk. It may be more difficult to defend a paramedic obtaining the information and assisting in the decision versus a physician directly seeing the patient and making the decision. Because there is no case law in this area at the present time, it is hard to determine how the American judicial system will handle this problem. Those patients with long response times unfortunately are often in rural areas. Rural areas are less likely to have paramedics or the necessary equipment to obtain or transmit ECGs to the hospital. Many of these rural systems do not have communication with the hospital or physician.

For these reasons, prehospital thrombolytic therapy with the presently available agents will not be a widely utilized strategy in the United States. In other countries, it may be used more frequently.

If newer agents are developed that are safer and easier to administer, this may change the usefulness of thrombolytic therapy in the prehospital arena.

Regional Planning and Triage

A final consideration that should be examined is the need for regional planning and development of a triage plan. Regional planning has not been used extensively in the prehospital care of cardiac patients, other than determining the destination of patients with cardiac arrests. Not all hospitals are comfortable with giving thrombolytic therapy, although this is decreasing. Some hospitals do not have intensive care capability.

One strategy that has been used in rural areas, where the local hospital lacks intensive care capability, has been to transfer the patient. The local hospital physician administers thrombolytic therapy with the advice and assistance of a distant cardiologist. The patient is then transferred to a facility with intensive care. This allows the early administration of thrombolytic therapy followed by adequate intensive care in areas that are distant from a hospital with intensive care. The same thing could also be done in a distant rural area that does not have a hospital. The local physician could administer the therapy in his or her office and then transfer the patient.

In urban areas, triage decisions need to be planned. The patient may wish to go to a distant hospital, bypassing several closer facilities. The reasons for this include being closer to family or home, going to the facility where their physician has privileges, and going to a facility that is covered by their insurance plan. Emergency medical services often prefer to take the patient to the closest facility. Transporting to the closer facility means that the ambulance can be back in service more quickly, reducing the need and cost for additional ambulances. Paramedics do not like a patient to get into trouble in the back of their ambulance; therefore, they prefer to transport to the closest facility. Closer facilities may be able to shorten the time to thrombolytic therapy. Thus, these issues need to be closely examined on a regional basis to determine how these situations will be handled.

Another potential use of a regional plan is to determine the appropriate facility for hospital destination. Using the information and the ECG, it might be determined that the patient needs reperfusion but has a major contraindication for thrombolytic therapy. This patient might well deserve emergent angioplasty. Thus, transportation to a facility that can provide acute angioplasty might be of benefit. The system could also help with the triage of patients when logistical problems exist. An area might develop a system to triage a patient to a hospital with an available intensive care bed or available angioplasty. If a hospital's intensive care beds are full, the system might be directed to take the patient to another facility. If the patient needs angioplasty and the catheterization laboratory is not available, the system might be directed to take the patient to a facility that does have a catheterization laboratory available. Two hospitals might decide to share calls for angioplasty; in this situation the two hospitals might alternate days when they will accept acute angioplasty patients and/or thrombolytic therapy candidates. Thus, regional planning might be of benefit. Many local areas are familiar with this type of regional planning because they have done regional planning for the care of trauma patients.

Conclusions

Emergency medical services can be an important adjunct to the reperfusion of patients with acute myocardial infarction. They can provide resuscitation for the cardiac arrest victim. They can provide ACLS therapy for patients needing this level of care. They can provide critical information and therapy that will aid in the diagnosis and treatment of patients with acute myocardial infarction. The rapidity of reperfusion can be greatly influenced by careful planning and coordination of the prehospital system with the hospital system. To be most effective, there needs to careful planning and integration of the prehospital and hospital systems. However, for this system to have its greatest impact, patients and their families need to be taught to use the EMS system properly; today less than one half of patients in the United States with an acute myocardial infarction are transported by EMS.

References

1. Guidelines for Cardiopulmonary Resuscitation and Emergency Cardiac Care. Emergency Cardiac Care Committee and Subcommittee, American Heart Association. JAMA 268:2171, 1992.
2. Morbidity and Mortality Chartbook on Cardiovascular, Lung and Blood Disease 1990. Bethesda, MD: National Heart, Lung, and Blood Institute, 1990.
3. Goldman L, Cook EF. The decline in ischemic heart disease mortality rates: An analysis of the comparative effects of medical interventions and changes in lifestyle. Ann Intern Med 101:825, 1984.
4. Callaham M, Madsen CD, Barton CW, Sàunders CE, Pointer J. A randomized clinical trial of high-dose epinephrine and norepinephrine vs. standard-dose epi-

nephrine in prehospital cardiac arrest. JAMA 268:2667, 1992.

5. Brown CG, Martin DR, Pepe PE, Stveven H, Commins RO, Gonzalez E, Jastremshi M, and the Multicenter High-Dose Epinephrine Study Group. A comparison of standard-dose and high-dose epinephrine in cardiac arrest outside the hospital. N Engl J Med 327:1051, 1992.

6. Stiell IG, Hebeit PC, Weitzman BN, Wells GA, Roman S, Stork RM, Higginson LAJ, Ahuja J, Dickinson GL. High-dose epinephrine in adult cardiac arrest. N Engl J Med 327:1045, 1992.

7. Cummins RO. Textbook of Advanced Cardiac Life Support. 1994:4.

8. Tiefenbrunn AJ, Sobel BE. Timing of coronary recanalization: Paradigms, paradoxes, and pertinence. Circulation 85:2311, 1992.

9. National Heart Attack Alert Program Coordinating Committee 60 Minutes to Treatment Working Group. Emergency department: Rapid identification and treatment of patients with acute myocardial infarction. US Department of Health and Human Services, publication #93-3278, 1993.

10. National Heart Attack Alert Program Coordinating Committee 60 Minutes to Treatment Working Group. Emergency department: Rapid identification and treatment of patients with acute myocardial infarction. Ann Emerg Med 23:311, 1994.

11. Granger CB. Califf RM, Topol EJ. Thrombolytic therapy for acute myocardial infarction: A review. Drugs 44:293, 1992.

12. Weaver WD, Cerqueira M, Hallstrom AP, Litwin PE, Martin JS, Kudenchoti PJ, Eisenberg M. For the Myocordial Infarction Triage and Intervention Group. Prehospital-initiated vs. hospital-initiated thrombolytic therapy: The Myocardial Infarction Triage and Intervention Trial JAMA 270:1211, 1993.

13. Accidental Death and Disability: The Neglected Disease of Modern Society. Committee on Trauma and Committee on Shock, Division of Medical Sciences. Washington, DC: National Academy of Sciences, National Research Council, 1966.

14. Cardiopulmonary Resuscitation: Statement by the Ad Hoc Committee on Cardiopulmonary Resuscitation of the Division of Medical Sciences, National Academy of Sciences, National Research Council. JAMA 198:372, 1966.

15. Kouwenhoven WB, Jude JR, Knickerbocker GG. Closed-chest cardiac massage. JAMA 173:1064, 1960.

16. Schlicht J, Mitcheson M, Henry M. Medical aspects of large outdoor festivals. Lancet 1:948, 1972.

17. Kassanoff I, Whaley W, Walter WH III, Burge D, Harrison C, Hurst JW, Wenger NK. Stadium coronary care; a concept in emergency health care delivery. JAMA 221:397, 1972.

18. Carveth SW, Reese HE, Buckman RJ, et al. A life support unit at Nebraska football stadium. Emerg Med Serv 3:26, 1974.

19. Carveth SW. Cardiac resuscitation program at the Nebraska football stadium. Dis Chest 53:8, 1968.

20. Pace NA. An approach to emergency coronary care in industry. J Occup Med 15:793, 1973.

21. Pantridge JF, Adgey AAJ. Pre-hospital coronary care; the mobile coronary care unit. Am J Cardiol 24:666, 1969.

22. Pantridge JF. Mobile coronary care. Chest 58:229, 1970.

23. Dewar HA, McCollum JPK, Floyd M. A year's experience with a mobile coronary resuscitation unit. Br Med J 4:226, 1969.

24. Gearty GF, Hickey N, Bourke GJ, Mulcahy R. Prehospital coronary care service. Br Med J 3:33, 1971.

25. Sandler J, Pistevos A. Mobile coronary care; the coronary ambulance. Br Heart J 34:1283, 1972.

26. Robinson JS, McLean ACJ. Mobile coronary care. Med J Aust 2:439, 1970.

27. Kernohan RJ, McGucken RB. Mobile intensive care in myocardial infarction. Br Med J 3:178, 1968.

28. Staff of the Cardio-Vascular Units at St. Vincent's Hospital and the Prince of Wales Hospital Sydney. Modified coronary ambulances. Med J Aust 1:875, 1972.

29. Grace WJ, Chadbourn JA. The mobile coronary care unit. Dis Chest 55:452, 1969.

30. Grace WJ. The mobile coronary care unit and the intermediate coronary care unit in the total systems approach to coronary care. Chest 58:363, 1970.

31. Anderson GJ, Knoebel SB, Fisch C. Continuous prehospitalization monitoring of cardiac rhythm. Am Heart J 82:642, 1971.

32. Nagel EL, Hirschman JC, Nussenfeld SR, Rankin D, Lundblad E. Telemetry-medical command in coronary and other mobile emergency care systems. JAMA 214:332, 1970.

33. Nagel EL, Hirschman JC, Mayer PW, Dennis F. Telemetry of physiologic data: An aid to fire-rescue personnel in a metropolitan area. South Med J 61:598, 1968.

34. Uhley HN. Electrocardiographic telemetry from ambulances; a practical approach to mobile coronary care units. Am Heart J 80:838, 1970.

35. Lambrew CT, Schuchman WL, Cannon TH. Emergency medical transport systems: Use of ECG telemetry. Chest 63:477, 1973.

36. White NM, Parker WS, Binning RA, Kimber ER, Ead HW, Chamberlain DA. Mobile coronary care provided by ambulance personnel. Br Med J 2:618, 1973.

37. Honick GL, Nagel T, Daniels A. A nurse staffed mobile coronary care unit. Oklae State Med Ass J 63:565, 1970.

38. Adgey AAJ, Nelson PG, Scott ME, Geddes JS, Allen JD, Zaidi SA, Pantridye JF. Management of ventricular fibrillation outside hospital. Lancet 1:1169, 1969.

39. Kernohan RJ, McCucken RB. Mobile intensive care in myocardial infarction. Br Med J 3:178, 1968.

40. Gearty GF, Hickey N, Bourke GJ, Mulchy R. Prehospital coronary care service. Br Med J 3:33, 1971.

41. Rose LB, Press E. Cardiac defibrillation by ambulance attendants. JAMA 219:63, 1972.

42. White NM, Parker WS, Binning RA, Kimber ER, Ead HW, Chamberlain DA. Mobile coronary care provided by ambulance personnel. Br Med J 3:618, 1973.

43. Baum RS, Alvarez H, Cobb LA. Mechanisms of out-of-hospital sudden cardiac death and their prognostic significance. Circulation 48(Suppl. IV):IV40, 1973.

44. Crampton RS, Aldrich RF, Stillerman R, et al. Reduction of community mortality from coronary artery disease by the community-wide emergency cardiac care system. Circulation 48(Suppl. IV):IV94, 1973.

45. Lewis RP, Warren JV. Factors determining mortality in the prehospital phase of acute myocardial infarction. Am J Cardiol 33:152, 1974.

46. Gorsuch TL, Nichols C, Driver E, Beard EJ. Mobile prehospital coronary care in Waynesboro, Virginia. Virginia Med Monthly 101:121, 1974.

47. Liberthson RR, Nagel EL, Hirschman JC, Nussemfeld SR, Blactibourne BD, Davis JH. Pathophysiologic observations in prehospital ventricular fibrillation and sudden cardiac death. Circulation 49:790, 1974.

48. Liberthson RR, Nagel EL, Hirschman JC, Nussenfeld SR. Prehospital ventricular defibrillation; prognosis and follow-up. N Engl J Med 291:317, 1974.

49. National Heart Attack Alert Program Coordinating Committee Access to Care Subcommittee. 9-1-1: Rapid identification and treatment of acute myocardial infarction. US Dept of Health and Human Services, NIH Publication #94-3302, 1994.

50. National Heart Attack Alert Program Coordinating Committee Access to Care Subcommittee. 9-1-1: Rapid identification and treatment of acute myocardial infarction. Am J Emerg Med 13:188, 1995.

51. National Heart Attack Alert Program Coordinating Committee Access to Care Subcommittee. Emergency medical dispatching: Rapid identification and treatment of acute myocardial infarction. US Dept of Health and Human Services, NIH Publication #94-3287, 1994.

52. National Heart Attack Alert Program Coordinating Committee Access to Care Subcommittee. Emergency medical dispatching: Rapid identification and treatment of acute myocardial infarction. Am J Emerg Med 13:67, 1995.

53. Clawson J. Emergency medical dispatching. In Roush WR (ed). Principles of EMS Systems, a Comprehensive Text for Physicians. Dallas: American College of Emergency Physicians, 1989.

54. Clawson JJ. Dispatch priority training — strengthening the weak link. J Emerg Med Serv 6:32, 1981.

55. Eisenberg MS, Carter W, Hallstrom A, Commins RO, Litwin PE, Hearne T. Identification of cardiac arrest by emergency dispatchers. Am J Emerg Med 4:299, 1986.

56. Clawson JJ, Dernocoeur KB. Principles of Emergency Medical Dispatching. Englewood Cliffs, NJ: Brady/Prentice Hall, 1988.

57. Clawson J. Regulations and standards for emergency medical dispatchers: A model for state or region. Emerg Med Serv 13:25, 1984.

58. Clawson J. Telephone treatment protocols: Reach out and help someone. J Emerg Med Serv 11(6):43, 1986.

59. Slovis C, Carnuth TB, Seitz WJ, Thomas CM, Elsez WR. A priority dispatch system for emergency medical services. Ann Emerg Med 14:1055, 1985.

60. National Standard Curriculum for EMS Dispatchers, 2nd ed. Washington DC: United States Department of Transportation, 1983.

61. National Heart Attack Alert Program Coordinating Committee Access to Care Subcommittee. Staffing and equipping emergency medical services systems: Rapid identification and treatment of acute myocardial infarction. US Dept of Health and Human Services, NIH Publication #94-3304, 1994.

62. National Heart Attack Alert Program Coordinating Committee Access to Care Subcommittee. Staffing and equipping emergency medical services systems: Rapid identification and treatment of acute myocardial infarction. Am J Emerg Med 13:58, 1995.

63. Kuehl AE (ed). National Association of EMS Physicians: EMS Medical Director's Handbook. St. Louis, MO: C.V. Mosby, 1989.

64. Roush WR (ed). Principles of EMS Systems: A Comprehensive Text for Physicians. Dallas: American College of Emergency Physicians, 1989.

65. Congress of the United States, Office of Technology Assessment. Rural Emergency Medical Services. Special report. OTA-H-445, November 1989.

66. Department of Transportation Training Guidelines. Emerg Med Serv 15:165, 1986.

67. Department of Transportation, National Highway Traffic Safety Administration. Emergency Medical Technician — Paramedic National Standard Curriculum, 1987.

68. Atkins JM. The use of automated defibrillators in the prehospital arena. In Kuehl AE (ed). EMS Medical Directors Handbook. National Association of EMS Physicians. St. Louis, MO: Morton Publishing, 1989:291.

69. Atkins JM. New option: Automated defibrillation for sudden cardiac death. Contemp Intern Med 2(1):11, 1990.

70. Cummins RO, Eisenberg MS, Bergner L, Hallstrom A, Hearne T, Mnrray JA. Automatic external defibrillation: Evaluations of its role in the home and in emergency medical services. Ann Emerg Med 13:798, 1984.

71. Cummins RO, Eisenberg MS, Moore JE, Hearne TR, Andersen E, Wendt R, Litwin PE, Graves JR, Hallstrom AP, Pierce J. Automatic external defibrillators: Clinical, training, psychological, and public health issues. Ann Emerg Med 14:755, 1985.

72. Cummins RO, Eisenberg MS, Stults KR. Automated external defibrillators: Clinical issues for cardiology. Circulation 73:381, 1986.

73. Cummins RO, Eisenberg MS, Litwin PE, Graves JR, Hearne TR, Hallstrom AP. Automatic external defibrillators used by emergency medical technicians: A controlled clinical trial. JAMA 257:1605, 1987.

74. Jacobs L. Medical, legal and social implications of automatic external defibrillators [editorial]. Ann Emerg Med 15:863, 1986.

75. Weigel A, Atkins JM, Taylor J. Automated Defibrillation. Englewood, CO: Morton Publishing, 1988.

76. Automated external defibrillation. Textbook of Advanced Cardiac Life Support. Dallas: American Heart Association, 1990:287.

77. Pozen MW, D'Agostino RB, Mitchell JB, Rosenfeld DM, Guglierno JT, Schwartz MS, Teebagy N, Valentine JM, Hoad WB. The usefulness of a predictive instrument to reduce inappropriate admissions to the coronary care unit. Ann Intern Med 92:238, 1980.

78. Pozen MW, D'Agostino RB, Selker HP, Sytkowski PA, Hood WB. A predictive instrument to improve coronary-care-unit admission practices in acute ischemic heart disease. N Engl J Med 310:1273, 1984.

79. McNutt RA, Selker HP. How did the acute ischemic heart disease predictive instrument reduce unnecessary coronary care unit admissions? Med Decision Making 8:90, 1988.

80. Selker HP, Griffith JL, D'Agostino RB. A tool for judging coronary care unit admission that is appropriate for both real-time and retrospective use: A time-insensitive predictive instrument (TIPI) for acute cardiac ischemia: A multicenter study. Med Care 29:610, 1991.

81. Selker HP, D'Agostino RB, Laks MM. A predictive instrument for acute ischemic heart disease to improve coronary care unit admission practices: A potential on-line tool in a computerized electrocardiography. J Electocardiogr 21:S11, 1988.

82. Holthof B, Selker HP. A cost-benefit analysis of the use of a predictive instrument for coronary-care-unit admission decisions: A projection of potential national savings based on hospital costs. Health Care Manag Rev 17:45, 1992.

83. Selker HP. Coronary care unit triage decision aids: How do we know when they work? Am J Med 87:491, 1989.

84. Boissel JP. The European Myocardial Infarction Project: An assessment of pre-hospital thrombolytics. Int J Cardiol 49(Suppl.):S29, 1995.

25. PREHOSPITAL APPROACHES TO TREATING SUDDEN CARDIAC DEATH AND ACUTE MYOCARDIAL INFARCTION

Joseph P. Ornato and Mary Ann Peberdy

Introduction

In the last 25 years, most communities in the United States have developed sophisticated emergency medical services (EMS) systems that are designed to minimize death and disability from a variety of medical conditions. Sudden cardiac death (SCD) and acute myocardial infarction (AMI) account for the majority of life-threatening, nontraumatic, community emergencies affecting adults. The purpose of this chapter is to describe the pathophysiology and epidemiology of SCD and AMI, and to review the ways in which the EMS system design and function can maximize survival from these conditions.

Sudden Cardiac Death in the Community

Most initial episodes of unexpected SCD in adults occur in the home or workplace [1–3]. The most common victim is a male who is 50–75 years of age [1,3]. Although only 2–4% of all runs in a typical EMS system are due to cardiac arrest [4], such calls represent a large proportion of the incidents in which field intervention can make a life or death difference in outcome. EMS systems are the most effective means presently known to deal with the problem of sudden cardiac death because they can provide (1) initial rescue and a source of referral for electrophysiological testing and therapeutic intervention in patients who experience their first episode of pulseless ventricular tachycardia (VT) or fibrillation (VF); and (2) salvage of patients who go into cardiac arrest again despite treatment.

The initiating event is a ventricular tachyarrhythmia (VT degenerating rapidly to VF in 62%, torsade de pointes in 13%, and "primary" VF in 8%) in over 80% of patients who develop out-of-hospital, primary cardiac arrest during ambulatory electrocardiographic monitoring [5]. Fewer than 70% of patients are in VT or VF by the time rescue personnel arrive on the scene (typically 5–10 minutes after the onset of collapse in most efficient EMS systems) [6]. Most of the remaining patients (31%) are in a pulseless, bradycardic rhythm or asystole.

The outcome of field resuscitation is strongly influenced by the patient's initial cardiac rhythm. In one series of 352 consecutive out-of-hospital cardiac arrest patients, 67% of the patients with VT and 23% of those who were initially in VF survived to hospital discharge [6]. None of the patients who presented with a an initial bradyarrhythmia survived to hospital discharge, Similar observations have been made by others [7,8]. One plausible hypothesis is that pulseless bradycardia or asystole may be a marker for a prolonged downtime interval or a more severe underlying disease process [9]. Because ventricular tachyarrhythmias represent the most common, potentially treatable mechanism of sudden cardiac arrest in adults, the best prehospital emergency cardiac care programs have been designed to deliver rapid defibrillation to as many patients as possible.

CHAIN OF SURVIVAL CONCEPT
Survival from pulseless VT or VF is inversely related to the time interval between its onset and termination [10]. Each minute that a patient remains in VF, the odds of survival decrease by 7–10% [11]. Survival is highest when cardiopulmonary resuscitation (CPR) is started within the first 4 minutes of arrest and advanced cardiac life support (ACLS), including defibrillation and drug therapy, is started within the first 8 minutes [12]. The American Heart Association's Emergency Cardiac Care Committee and its Advanced Cardiac Life Support Subcommittee began to widely publicize the *chain of survival* concept in 1991. This symbolic phrase represents a sequence of events that should occur in most cardiac arrest cases to

maximize the odds of successful resuscitation [13]. The steps includes early recognition of the problem and activation of the EMS system by a bystander, early CPR, rapid provision of defibrillation for patients who need it, and advanced cardiac life support (e.g., intubation, administration of medications) [13]. Schematically, this sequence can be depicted by a chain of survival (Figure 25-1).

EARLY ACCESS

Because most out-of-hospital cardiac arrests occur suddenly and without immediate premonitory symptoms, the victim is rarely in a position to activate the EMS system prior to his or her collapse. Bystanders who witness the event can significantly improve the victim's chance of surviving by alerting the community EMS system to the presence of the emergency. All too often, the untrained citizen only further delays treatment by attempting to inform relatives, call the neighbors, or contact the patient's personal physician instead of calling the local community emergency telephone number (in most places it is 9-1-1) [14,15].

Before EMS rescuers can aid the victim, the bystander must recognize that there is a problem, locate a telephone, make a correct call, and give accurate and precise information to the dispatcher. Once the alarm has been sounded, rescuers must travel to the scene, physically arrive at the patient's side, and perform an initial, cursory assessment. Public education can significantly improve the behavior of bystanders when a cardiac emergency occurs in the community. Citizens can be trained to quickly summon help and to initiate lifesaving CPR. For example, bystanders in Seattle initiated CPR in only 5% of cardiac arrests in 1970–71, but by 1976, 34% of cardiac arrest victims were receiving bystander CPR as a result of a widespread, pioneering, public education campaign [16]. Since then, the American Heart Association and the American Red Cross have trained millions of citizens to recognize cardiac emergencies, call for help, and perform CPR [17].

Availability of the simple three digit 9-1-1 emergency number in the United States can reduce confusion and decrease delay in activating the EMS system. In Minneapolis, the percentage of emergency callers who could activate the EMS system in less than 1 minute rose from 63% before, to 82% after, institution of a 9-1-1 number [18]. Only two states currently have 9-1-1 available everywhere within their borders. One community in North Carolina lists 85 different emergency numbers in the local telephone book [19,20]. The American Heart Association has recommended that all communities implement an enhanced 9-1-1 system, which displays the caller's

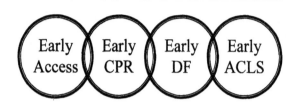

FIGURE 25-1. The chain of survival concept. CPR = cardiopulmonary resuscitation; DF = defibrillation; ACLS = advanced cardiac life support.

location automatically on the dispatcher's terminal when the call is received [13].

EARLY CPR

The next link in the chain is early initiation of CPR, preferably by bystanders. With rare exceptions, EMS system response time characteristics are not good enough to provide CPR within the first few minutes after the patient's collapse [21,22]. One way to ensure initiation of early CPR is to educate and train a "critical mass" of the general population. The effectiveness of such training has varied widely. In Seattle, approximately 50% of the population has been trained to perform CPR [23], while in Minneapolis only 23% of adults surveyed have received such training [24]. In smaller cities and in less affluent areas, the number of trained citizens is often much lower. What percentage of adults needs to be trained in CPR to provide reasonable protection in the community is difficult to determine with certainty. As a rule of thumb, the American Heart Association recommends that at least 20% of the adult population should be trained in basic CPR to reduce mortality from out-of-hospital cardiac arrest [25].

There are a number of problems associated with training the public to perform CPR. For example, it can be argued that we have trained the wrong rescuers. The typical cardiac arrest victim is male, 60–65 years old, and usually arrests at home, often in the presence of a spouse of similar age [26]. Most citizens who have taken CPR training are younger than 30 years of age; typically, fewer than 10% live with family members known to have heart disease [27]. Most citizens who have received CPR training never actually witness or participate in managing a cardiac arrest; conversely, bystanders who witness a cardiac arrest usually do not know how to perform CPR [23,28]. For example, only 10% of CPR-trained citizens in Minneapolis have witnessed an arrest, while only 30% of citizens present at the site of a cardiac arrest were trained in CPR [24]. The majority of "lay" persons who attempt to perform CPR out-of-hospital are actually employed or volunteer their services as health professionals [29]. The best solution to the problem may be to target CPR training to "high-risk" individuals, such as middle-aged persons, senior center residents and staff, and family members (particularly the spouse) of patients who are survivors of myocardial infarction or cardiac arrest, or who have other risk factors for cardiac arrest [27,30,31].

Skill retention is also a problem because CPR is a psychomotor technique that deteriorates rapidly over time unless practiced or used. In Belgium, 46% of bystanders who performed CPR forgot to perform mouth-to-mouth breathing; chest compressions were not done 17% of the time [32]. It is important for lay persons or health care professionals who perform CPR infrequently to receive at least annual reinforcement. However, only about 20% of trainees return for annual training in the United States [24,28]. Fear of communicable disease, particularly infection with the human immunodeficiency virus (HIV), which is disproportionate to the known minimal risk of diseases transmission, may decrease the likelihood that trained rescuers will actually perform mouth-to-mouth ventilation on strangers [33].

Although the value of bystander CPR was once debatable, virtually all recent studies have shown that initiation of bystander CPR within 4 minutes of the patient's collapse results in up to a 12-fold improvement in the odds for survival [13]. The mechanism by which early CPR improves outcome is unclear but may be due to CPR's ability to keep coarse ventricular fibrillation from degenerating to asystole for a few extra minutes until rescuers arrive.

EARLY DEFIBRILLATION LINK
The rationale for the use of early defibrillation stems from four observations: (1) ventricular tachyarrhythmias are the commonest cause of sudden, out-of-hospital cardiac arrest in adults; (2) defibrillation is the most effective treatment for pulseless ventricular tachyarrhythmias; (3) the effectiveness of defibrillation diminishes rapidly over time; and (4) unless treated promptly, VF becomes less coarse and eventually converts to the less treatable rhythm of fine VF or asystole. The best outcomes from sudden, arrhythmic cardiac arrest in adults have been reported from cardiac rehabilitation programs, where defibrillation can be performed within the first minute or two. In such "ideal" settings, as many as 85–90% of patients are resuscitated and return to their prearrest neurological status [34–36]. Sur-

vival from out-of-hospital cardiac arrest treated by EMS personnel has been considerably lower, averaging 15–20% or less, with a maximum survival of 30%, depending on the EMS system configuration [13].

The best survival is attained in EMS systems that can provide early defibrillation to a large percentage of patients. In most cases, this is most cost effectively accomplished by a *tiered-response* system, in which large numbers of rapid *first-response* firefighters or emergency medical technicians (EMT)s are trained and equipped to provide first aid, CPR, and early defibrillation using an automated external defibrillator (AED).

Unfortunately, not all communities in the United States have yet implemented a comprehensive, tiered EMS system. Many systems, particularly in suburban or rural areas, have only EMTs who are neither trained nor equipped to defibrillate. For such areas, adding rapid defibrillation capability offers a cost-effective alternative that can significantly improve survival from out-of-hospital VF or pulseless VT [37,38].

The American Heart Association has recently issued a position statement advocating the widespread implementation of rapid defibrillation programs throughout the nation. The American Heart Association endorses the position that

All emergency personnel should be trained and permitted to operate an appropriately maintained defibrillator if their professional activities require that they respond to persons experiencing cardiac arrest. This includes all first responding emergency personnel, both hospital and nonhospital (e.g., emergency medical technicians (EMTs), non-EMT first responders, fire fighters, volunteer emergency personnel, physicians, nurses, and paramedics).

To further facilitate early defibrillation, it is essential that a defibrillator be immediately available to emergency personnel responding to a cardiac arrest. Therefore, all emergency ambulances and other emergency vehicles that respond to or transport cardiac patients should be equipped with a defibrillator [39].

More novel strategies have also been tried to increase the availability of rapid defibrillation in the community. The most innovative idea is termed *public access defibrillation*, so named because the intent is to have non-healthcare citizens perform early defibrillation.

Early attempts to train family members of high-risk patients or community workers in the use of automated external defibrillators (AEDs) have met with variable success. For example, Eisenberg et al. trained family members of 59 patients who had survived out-of-hospital cardiac arrest in King County, Washington [40]. Only 6 of the 10 cardiac arrests that occurred in these patients were defibrillated successfully, and only one patient survived for few months and sustained new neurological impairment. In contrast, Swenson et al. reported 3 successful resuscitations out of 5 cardiac arrests in 48 patients whose families had been trained to use an AED [41]. More encouraging results have been obtained when community first responders have been trained to use automated defibrillators. For example, 160 security officers were trained to use these devices at Vancouver's World Expo 1986. Five cardiac arrests occurred among the 22.1 million visitors. The AED was correctly applied in all cases by security personnel. In two cases, the initial rhythm was VF and defibrillation was successful. Both patients had a pulse and were regaining consciousness by the time EMS personnel arrived on the scene [42]. Other experimental approaches to rapid defibrillation in the workplace include use on commercial aircraft, British rail stations, oil platforms in the North Sea, electricity plants, passenger cruise ships, and merchant marine vessels [43–45].

EARLY ACLS LINK
Physicians provide prehospital ACLS by staffing specially equipped ambulances in many countries (e.g., western Europe, Scandinavia, Canada). In the United States, "intermediate" level EMTs or paramedics provide most prehospital ACLS intervention (e.g., defibrillation or synchronized cardioversion, endotracheal intubation, intravenous fluid therapy, drug administration). Intermediate EMTs (often called *cardiac technicians*) typically receive several hundred hours of training; paramedics usually receive 1000 or more hours. Adding field ACLS capability appears to favorably impact survival from out-of-hospital cardiac arrest [13,46].

Some EMS systems have upgraded all transporting ambulances to ACLS status to eliminate the possibility that dispatchers might send a basic life support unit on a call that needs a higher level of care. An "all-ACLS" system eliminates the potential "failure point" in the 9-1-1 center because there is no triage of calls to an ACLS or basic cardiac life support (BCLS) response. Existing BCLS ambulances or first-responding vehicles can be upgraded to automated defibrillation capability with minimal expense. Automated defibrillators cost approximately $5000–8000 and require only 2–4 hours of additional training for first responders or emergency medical technicians. This is nominal expense compared with the cost of a typical ambulance ($50,000–100,000) or fire truck ($250,000–500,000). In Richmond, Virginia, upgrading from a half-BCLS/half-ACLS system to an all-ACLS system added less than 1% to the cost of ambulance service (only $2.88 per patient transported) [47].

Acute Myocardial Infarction

Intravenously administered thrombolytic therapy reduces the mortality rate by approximately 25% in patients with acute transmural myocardial infarction (AMI) [48–52]. However, not all patients benefit equally from its use. Administration of a thrombolytic agent within the first hour after the onset of AMI symptoms reduces the mortality rate by 40% or more compared with that seen with later dosing and often results in substantial myocardial salvage [53]. There is less mortality reduction in patients who receive later treatment. Patients with AMI who qualify for thrombolytic therapy should receive it expeditiously.

Prehospital evaluation and transport can account for significant time delay in patients with AMI who need thrombolytic therapy. The time from emergency medical services system activation to arrival of the patient at the hospital ED averaged 46 ± 8 minutes in 3715 patients from eight major centers [54]. In the same study, the door-to-drug time interval (defined as the number of minutes between the time that the patient arrives at the emergency department and the time that the thrombolytic drug is administered) was 84 ± 55 minutes. Thus, the time interval required to evaluate, stabilize, transport, and initiate thrombolytic therapy precludes initiation of treatment within the first hour of symptoms in the majority of patients with AMI.

In many countries, especially throughout Europe and Scandinavia, physicians staff ambulances and make house calls frequently. Prehospital administration of thrombolytic drugs by physicians has been demonstrated to be feasible in limited trials [55–57]. In the United States, thrombolytic therapy is administered to most AMI patients after they arrive at the hospital. Long median door-to-needle times in many hospitals have prompted some to consider the prehospital administration of thrombolytics by paramedics.

The Myocardial Infarction Triage and Intervention (MITI) Trial in Seattle, Washington studied the safety and efficacy of this strategy in a prospective, randomized comparison of tissue plasminogen activator (t-PA) administered by paramedics in the field or by physicians on emergency department arrival. Paramedics used a prehospital checklist and computerized 12-lead interpretation backed up by cellular telephone transmission to hospital-based physicians [58].

Although the study confirmed the value of very early (<70 minutes after onset of AMI symptoms) compared with "early" thrombolysis (70–180 minutes after onset of AMI symptoms), there was no difference in survival or myocardial salvage when paramedics gave t-Pa in the field compared with when physicians and nurses gave it shortly after hospital ED arrival.

In addition to these results, there are significant limitations to the widespread application of prehospital thrombolysis by paramedics in the United States [59]. Regardless of how effective, safe, or practical prehospital thrombolytic therapy proves to be, it only can be used to treat the half of all patients with AMI who choose to call for an ambulance [59]. Efforts to improve the public's use of the emergency care system have thus far been unsuccessful. Public education programs in Seattle, Washington [60] and in Göteborg, Sweden [61] did not significantly increase the number of patients with AMI who were brought to the hospital by ambulance.

Other shortcomings of prehospital thrombolytic therapy include the high cost of equipping all ambulances with electrocardiographic equipment, cellular telephones, expensive thrombolytic agents, refrigeration equipment or the daily rotation of stock to prevent decomposition of the drug under hot environmental conditions, maintenance of paramedic skills, and medicolegal risk [59]. The theoretical appeal of prehospital thrombolytic therapy does not appear to be justified relative to the time, money, and effort required for its use in most U.S. EMS systems at present. Even with generous estimates of the potential impact of prehospital thrombolysis on AMI mortality, in most EMS systems it is more cost effective to equip first-responding fire or EMS vehicles with automated defibrillators. In Richmond, Virginia, it would cost 25 times more dollars per life saved to add prehospital thrombolysis on all paramedic ambulances than to equip all first-responding fire vehicles with automated defibrillators [59].

Based on this kind of analysis, in 1993 the American College of Emergency Physicians issued a Policy Statement on the prehospital use of thrombolytic agents:

The use of thrombolytic agents by nonphysicians in the prehospital setting should currently be considered investigational. The College believes that sound scientific research and further examination of the use of these agents is needed, using carefully designed and properly approved research protocols in EMS systems with strong medical supervision. These studies should seek to determine the feasibility, efficacy, cost-effectiveness, and safety of these agents when administered by prehospital personnel. Until more data is available, the routine use of thrombolytic agents by prehospital emergency medical services should be discouraged [62].

Although expensive, the addition of computer-interpreted, 12-lead ECG capability on paramedic ambulances is accurate in confirming the diagnosis of AMI and does speed the door-to-needle time after the patient is transported to the hospital [63,64]. Technology including 12-lead ECG capability on monitor-defibrillators carried by paramedics is now available, providing the most efficient and cost-effective way of enhancing field diagnosis, with minimal addition of weight to the paramedic's field equipment. Paramedics can achieve a high success rate (almost 99%) in obtaining diagnostic quality prehospital 12-lead ECGs in sophisticated EMS systems, resulting in a diagnostic specificity of 99% for patients with AMI. Acquisition of a prehospital ECG only increases the paramedic on-scene time by an average of 5 minutes. If signs of ischemia or infarction are present, paramedics can administer analgesics for pain relief, oxygen, aspirin, and nitroglycerin.

Conclusions

High-quality prehospital emergency care by trained paramedics and EMTs can make an enormous difference for many patients with cardiac arrest or myocardial infarction. Cardiologists and emergency care practitioners need to work together to provide strong medical leadership and oversight of these highly complex systems. At the present time, most communities should strive to provide a strong chain of survival. Once that is accomplished, prehospital 12-lead electrocardiography is the next logical, cost-effective step. Finally, prehospital thrombolytic therapy appears to have limited value for most nonrural EMS environments in which the transport time to the hospital is relatively rapid.

References

1. Bossaert L, Van Hoeyweghen R, Cerebral Resuscitation Study Group. Bystander cardiopulmonary resuscitation (CPR) in out-of-hospital cardiac arrest. Resuscitation 17(Suppl.):S55, 1989.
2. Cobb LA, Hallstrom AP. Community-based cardiopulmonary resuscitation: What have we learned? Ann N Y Acad Sci 382:330, 1982.
3. Litwin PE, Eisenberg MS, Hallstrom AP, Cummins RO. The location of collapse and its effect on survival from cardiac arrest. Ann Emerg Med 16:787, 1987.
4. Ornato JP, McNeill SE, Craren EJ, Nelson NM. Limitation on effectiveness of rapid defibrillation by emergency medical technicians in a rural setting. Ann Emerg Med 13:1096, 1984.

5. Bayes de Luna A, Coumel P, Leclercq JF. Ambulatory sudden cardiac death: Mechanisms of production of fatal arrhythmia on the basis of data from 157 cases. Am Heart J 117:151, 1989.

6. Myerburg RJ, Conde CA, Sung RJ, Mayooga-Cortes A, Mallon SM, Sheps DS, Appel RA, Castellanos A. Clinical, electrophysiologic and hemodynamic profile of patients resuscitated from prehospital cardiac arrest. Am J Med 68:568, 1980.

7. Hinkle LE, Argyros DC, Hayes JC, Robinson T, Alonso DR. Pathogenesis of an unexpected sudden death: Role of early cycle ventricular contractions. Am J Cardiol 39:873, 1977.

8. Klein RC, Vera Z, Mason DT, DeMaria AN, Awan NA, Amsterdam EA. Ambulatory Holter monitor documentation of ventricular tachyarrhythmias as mechanisms of sudden death in patients with coronary artery disease (abstr). Clin Res 27:7A, 1979.

9. Schaffer WA, Cobb LA. Recurrent ventricular fibrillation and modes of death in survivors of out-of-hospital ventricular fibrillation. N Engl J Med 293:260, 1975.

10. Weaver WD, Cobb LA, Hallstrom AP, Fahrenbruch C, Copass MK, Ray R. Factors influencing survival after out-of-hospital cardiac arrest. J Am Coll Cardiol 7:754, 1986.

11. American Heart Association. Standards and guidelines for cardiopulmonary resuscitation (CPR) and emergency cardiac care (ECC). JAMA 255:2905, 1986.

12. Eisenberg MS, Bergner L, Hallstrom A. Cardiac resuscitation in the community. Importance of rapid provision and implications for program planning. JAMA 241:1905, 1979.

13. Cummins RO, Ornato JP, Thies WH, Pepe PE. Improving survival from sudden cardiac arrest: The "chain of survival" concept. Circulation 83:1832, 1991.

14. Walters G, Gluckman F. Planning a pre-hospital cardiac resuscitation programme: An analysis of community and system factors in London. JR Coll Physic Lond 23:107, 1989.

15. Stults KR. Phone first. J Emerg Med Services 12:78, 1987.

16. Alvarez H, Cobb LA. Experience with CPR training of the general public. In Proceedings of the National Conference on Standards for Cardiopulmonary Resuscitation and Emergency Cardiac Care. Dallas: American Heart Association, 1975:33.

17. American Red Cross. Adult CPR. Boston, MA: American National Red Cross. 1987.

18. Mayron R, Long RS, Ruiz E. The 911 emergency telephone number: Impact on emergency medical systems access in a metropolitan area. Am J Emerg Med 2:491, 1984.

19. Hunt RC, Allison EJ Jr, Yates JG III. The need for improved emergency medical services in Pitt county. N C Med J 47:39, 1986.

20. Hunt RC, McCabe JB, Hamilton GC, Krohmer JR. Influence of emergency medical services systems and prehospital defibrillation on survival of sudden cardiac death victims. Am J Emerg Med 7:68, 1989.

21. Thompson BM, Stueven HA, Mateer JR, Aprahamian CC, Tucker JF, Darin JC. Comparison of clinical CPR studies in Milwaukee and elsewhere in the United States. Ann Emerg Med 14:750, 1985.

22. Kowalski R, Thompson BM, Horwitz L, Stueven H, Aprahamian C, Darin JC. Bystander CPR in prehospital coarse ventricular fibrillation. Ann Emerg Med 13:1016, 1984.

23. Cobb LA, Werner JA, Trobaugh GB. Sudden cardiac death: 1. A decade's experience with out-of-hospital resuscitation. Mod Concepts Cardiovasc Dis 49:31, 1980.

24. Murphy RJ, Luepker Rv, Jacobs DR Jr, Gillum RF, Folsom AR, Blackburn H. Citizen cardiopulmonary resuscitation training and use in a metropolitan area: The Minnesota Heart Survey Am J Public Health 74:513, 1984.

25. Selby ML, Kautz JA, Moore TJ, Gombeski WR Jr, Ramirez AG, Farge EJ, Forthofer RN. Indicators of response to a mass media CPR recruitment campaign. Am J Public Health 72:1039, 1982.

26. Litwin PE, Eisenberg MS, Hallstrom AP, Cummins RO. The location of collapse and its effect on survival from cardiac arrest. Ann Emerg Med 16:787, 1987.

27. Mandel LP, Cobb LA. CPR training in the community. Ann Emerg Med 14:669, 1985.

28. Gombeski WR, Jr, Effron DM, Ramirez AG, Moore TJ. Impact on retention: Comparison of two CPR training programs. Am J Public Health 72:849, 1982.

29. Muelleman RL, Ornato JP. Factors affecting the likelihood that CPR will be used by trained rescuers. Nebraska Med J 70:172, 1985.

30. St. Louis P, Carter WB, Eisenberg MS. Prescribing CPR: A survey of physicians. Am J Public Health 72:1158, 1982.

31. Goldberg RJ. Physicians and CPR training in high-risk family members. Am J Public Health 77:671, 1987.

32. Bossaert L, Van Hoeyweghen R, and the Cerebral Resuscitation Study Group. Evaluation of cardiopulmonary resuscitation (CPR) techniques. Resuscitation 17(Suppl.):S99, 1989.

33. Ornato JP, Hallagan LF, McMahon SB, Peeples EH, Rostafinski AG. Attitudes of BCLS instructors about mouth-to-mouth resuscitation during the AIDS epidemic. Ann Emerg Med 19:151, 1990.

34. Van Camp SP, Peterson RA. Cardiovascular complications of outpatient cardiac rehabilitation programs. JAMA 1160, 1986.

35. Haskell WL. Cardiovascular complications during exercise training in cardiac patients. Circulation 57:920, 1978.

36. Hossack KF, Hartwig R. Cardiac arrest associated with supervised cardiac rehabilitation. J Cardiac Rehab 2:402, 1982.

37. Ornato JP, McNeill SE, Craren EJ, Nelson NM. Limitations on effectiveness of rapid defibrillation by emergency medical technicians in a rural setting. Ann Emerg Med 13:1096, 1984.

38. Eisenberg MS, Copass MK, Hallstrom AP, Blake B, Bergner L, Short FA, Cobb LA. Treatment of out-of-hospital cardiac arrest with rapid defibrillation by emergency medical technicians. N Engl J Med 302:1379, 1980.

39. Kerber RE. Statement on Early Defibrillation from the Emergency Cardiac Care Committee, American Heart Association. Circulation 83:2233, 1991.

40. Eisenberg MS, Moore J, Cummins RO, Andresen E, Litwin PE, Hallstrom AP, Hearne T. Use of the automatic external defibrillator in home of survivors of out-of-hospital ventricular fibrillation. Am J Cardiol 63:443, 1989.

41. Swenson RD, Hill DL, Martin JS, Wirkus M, Weaver WD. Automatic external defibrillators used by family members to treat cardiac arrest (abstr). Circulation 76(Suppl. IV):IV463, 1987.

42. Weaver WD, Sutherland K, Wirkus MJ, Bachman R. Emergency medical care requirements for large public assemblies and a new strategy for managing cardiac arrest in this setting. Ann Emerg Med 18:155, 1989.

43. Chadda KD, Kammerer RJ, Kuphal J, Miller K. Successful defibrillation in the industrial, recreational, and corporate settings by laypersons (abstr). Circulation 76(Suppl. IV):IV12, 1987.

44. Wilson BD, Graton MC, Overton J, Watson W. Unexpected ALS procedures on nonemergency ambulance calls: The value of a single tier system. Prehosp Disaster Med 6:382, 1991.

45. Cummins RO. From concept to standard-of-care? Review of the clinical experience with automated external defibrillators. Ann Emerg Med 18:1269, 1989.

46. Pepe PE, Abramson NS, Brown CG. ACLS—Does it really work? Ann Emerg Med 23:1037, 1994.

47. Ornato JP, Racht EM, Fitch JJ, Berry JF. The need for ALS in urban and suburban EMS systems. Ann Emerg Med 19:151, 1990.

48. Gruppo Italiano per lo Studio della Streptochinasi Nell'Infarto Miocardico (GISSI). Effectiveness of intravenous thrombolytic treatment in acute myocardial infarction. Lancet 1:379, 1986.

49. Gruppo Italiano per lo Studio della Streptochinasi Nell'Infarto Miocardico (GISSI). Effectiveness of intravenous thrombolytic treatment in acute myocardial infarction. Lancet 1:397, 1986.

50. ISIS (Second International Study of Infarct Survival) Collaborative Group. Randomized trial of intravenous streptokinase, oral aspirin, both or neither among 17,187 cases of suspected acute myocardial infarction. ISIS-2. Lancet 2:349, 1988.

51. Wilcox RG, Olsson CG, Skene AM, Vonder Lippe G, Jensen G, Hampton JR (for the ASSET Study Group). Trial of tissue plasminogen activator for mortality reduction in acute myocardial infarction. Lancet 2:525, 1988.

52. AIMS Trial Study Group. Effect of intravenous APSAC on mortality after acute myocardial infarction: Preliminary report of a placebo-controlled clinical trial. Lancet 1:545, 1988.

53. Weaver WD, Cerqueira M, Hallstrom AP, Litwin PE, Martin JS, Kudenchuk PJ, Eisenberg M, for the Myocardial Infarction Triage and Intervention Project Group. Prehospital-initiated vs. hospital-initiated thrombolytic therapy: The myocardial infarction triage and intervention trial.

54. Kereiakes DJ, Weaver WD, Anderson JL, et al. Time delays in the diagnosis and treatment of acute myocardial infarction: A tale of eight cities. Report from the pre-hospital study group and the Cincinnati Heart Project. Am Heart J 120:773, 1990.

55. Castaigne AD, Duval AM, Dubois-Rande JL, et al. Prehospital administration of anisoylated plasminogen streptokinase activator complex in acute myocardial infarction. Drugs 33(Suppl. 3):231, 1987.

56. European Myocardial Infarction Project (E.M.I.P) Subcommittee. Potential time savings with pre-hospital intervention in acute myocardial infarction. Eur Heart J 9:118, 1988.

57. Castaigne AD, Herve C, Duval-Moulin A, et al. Prehospital use of APSAC: Results of a placebo-controlled study. Am J Cardiol 64:30A, 1989.

58. Kennedy JW, Weaver WD. Potential use of thrombolytic therapy before hospitalization. Am J Cardiol 64:8A, 1989.

59. Ornato JP. The earliest thrombolytic treatment of acute myocardial infarction: Ambulance or emergency department? Clin Cardiol 13:VIII27, 1990.

60. Ho MT, Eisenberg MS, Litwin PE, et al. Delay between onset of chest pain and seeking medical care: the effect of public education. Ann Emerg Med 18:727, 1989.

61. Herlitz J, Hartford M, Blohm M, et al. Effect of a media campaign on delay times and ambulance use in suspected acute myocardial infarction. Am J Cardiol 64:90, 1989.

62. American College of Emergency Physicians Board of Directors. American College of Emergency Physicians Policy Statement: Prehospital use of thrombolytic agents. Dallas: American College of Emergency Physicians, October 1993.

63. Aufderheide TP, Hendley GE, Thakur RK, Mateer JR, Stueven HA, Olson DW, Hargarten KM, Laitinen F, Robinson N, Preuss KC, Hoffman RG. The diagnostic impact of prehospital 12-lead electrocardiography. Ann Emerg Med 19:1280, 1990.

64. Kowalenko T, Kereiakes DJ, Gibler WB. Prehospital diagnosis and treatment of acute myocardial infarction: A critical review. Am Heart J 123:181, 1991.

26. IDENTIFICATION OF ACUTE CARDIAC ISCHEMIA IN THE EMERGENCY DEPARTMENT

Harry P. Selker and Robert J. Zalenski

Introduction

Chest pain and other symptoms suggestive of acute cardiac ischemia (ACI, including acute myocardial infarction [AMI] and unstable angina pectoris) account for over 6 million emergency department (ED) visits per year. Of these, the approximately 30% who truly have ACI (just under half of whom will prove to have AMI) [1] must be quickly and accurately separated from the majority of ED patients who do not have ACI and then promptly treated and admitted to the hospital. This is not an easy task, the environment in which this must be done is not often optimal, and there are no perfect tests that completely handle all possible cases. However, as reviewed in this chapter, there are a number of tests and strategies, that, when combined with good clinical judgement, can be of significant assistance.

There are a number of countervailing forces buffeting the ED clinician evaluating patients with symptoms suggestive of ACI. The pressure to make the diagnosis quickly in order to institute the increasing quiver of time-sensitive treatments is one such force. As detailed elsewhere in this volume, for the institution of interventions to prevent and/or reverse fatal arrhythmias, as well as for medical and angioplasty thrombolysis and other acute interventions, passing time represents passing opportunities to benefit, and potentially to save the life of, the patient.

Another force influencing physicians' ED triage is their concern over missing ACI. Although primarily concerned about the patients' welfare, all ED physicians are aware that the failure to properly identify ACI in association with sending a patient home who then has an AMI and/or dies is among the commonest and largest causes of malpractice litigation in this country. Thus, although ED physicians do not intend to hospitalize patients without ACI, they are con-

cerned that being too restrictive in their admission practices would increase the numbers of patients with ACI mistakenly sent home, currently about 7% of those with ACI [2] and about 2–4% of those presenting with AMI [2–5]. Thus there is an understandable "If in doubt, admit!" response to ambiguous ED presentations.

Yet another force increasingly evident in the ED triage process is pressure to reduce costs. It has not gone unnoticed that of the approximately 1.5 million admitted yearly to coronary care units (CCUs), half prove not to have true ACI [2,6], and of those with ACI, their presumably unnecessary hospitalizations may represent direct costs on the order of $3 billion annually [7]. Thus, among the growing pressures on physicians to avoid hospitalization, admission for suspected ACI are one of the largest targets.

These contravailing influences, combined with the difficulty in definitively diagnosing ACI in the ED, make clear the need for reliable diagnostic tools and strategies. Although there is interest in decreasing the false-negative discharge rate yet further, and a clear interest in more rapid diagnosis in order to maximize benefits of thrombolysis and other interventions, there is also an understanding that the typically 10-fold higher false-positive admission rate (ca. 50%) needs to be reduced in the increasingly cost-driven healthcare system. Methods proposed for decreasing false-positive rates (i.e., increase specificity) and/or false-negative rates (i.e., increase sensitivity) of ED triage for patients with symptoms suggestive of ACI have included special attention to certain high-risk clinical indicators [8,9], rapid determination of cardiac enzymes [10,11], two-dimensional echocardiography [12], imaging myocardial perfusion scans using thallium-201 [13] and Tc99m-sestamibi [14–18], and mathematically based decision aids [1,2,19–22]. However, to date few of these have been shown *prospectively* in a controlled trial to improve CCU or hospital admission practice [2,23], or to result in actual cost savings associated with projections of reduced hospitalizations. In the following, after a brief review of the methodologic issues that surround the studies of such diagnostic approaches, the available and developing ED diagnostic technologies and decision aids for this area are reviewed.

Methodologic Issues in the Study of ED Triage of Patients with Suspected Acute Cardiac Ischemia

A number of issues must be kept in mind when considering the literature on methods of identifying ACI that limit applicability to the actual ED setting [6]. First, the predictive value of a particular symptom, sign, or test result in a particular study is very dependent on the prevalence of ACI in its study population [24]. For example, electrocardiogram (ECG) ST-segment abnormalities and echocardiographic regional wall abnormalities may appear very predictive of infarction among *CCU patients*, among whom the prevalence of AMI is relatively high, but they will be much less predictive among *ED patients*, among whom the prevalence of AMI is much lower. Even ED-based studies, especially if not including a variety of ED settings, may not apply to EDs with populations with substantially different prevalences of ACI than in the study, or to EDs with different settings or roles (e.g., urban vs. rural, or teaching vs. community hospital) than the study hospital(s).

Second, the applicability to actual practice of studies of ED triage also depends heavily on study inclusion criteria. For example, if only patients with chest pain are studied, the results may not apply to the 13–25% of patients with ACI who do not present with chest pain [2,25–27]. Indeed, given that patients without clear-cut chest pain are those for whom diagnostic and therapeutic decisions can be most difficult, the studies most useful to the ED clinician are those with broad entry criteria to include, along with those presenting with typical pain, and all patients with potential ACI who present *without chest pain* (e.g., with shortness of breath, epigastric discomfort, dizziness, etc).

Third, the choice of diagnostic endpoint is critical to the study of ED diagnostic performance and triage. Many studies have focused on identifying only AMI rather than all ACI [3,6,28]. Identifying unstable or new-onset angina is also important, because it can lead to hospital monitoring and early therapy that

may prevent progression to AMI, and the institution of longer term secondary prevention strategies. Indeed, as many as 9% of patients admitted with new-onset or unstable angina pectoris have been reported to progress to AMI [29,30]. Thus, the clinically most useful studies will be those seeking to identify for potential hospitalization those ED patients ultimately found to have *either* AMI *or* non-AMI ACI (i.e., new or unstable angina). It is helpful for AMI to be studied and reported as an outcome, but ideally as a *subgroup* in a study of the primary outcome ACI.

Fourth, to be believable, studies of ED triage studies must have convincing completeness of follow-up for all eligible patients. Loss of patients to follow-up can lead to biases in the study sample, especially when the participation rate among eligible patients also is not high. Even more important is the potential impact of incomplete follow-up on the analysis of outcomes. For example, it may be that some of patients for whom follow-up was missed was because of death of a missed ED diagnosis of AMI, and their failure to be included in the analysis would mislead regarding the safety of those sent home. Even with 100% follow-up of subjects, the incidence of AMI still may be underestimated among discharged patients if follow-up evaluations do not include repeated ECGs and cardiac enzyme tests. Unfortunately, to avoid these problems with home follow-up, some studies just do not study those patients sent home. This renders the results less helpful, because the safety of sending a patient home based on the diagnostic technology in question is never actually tested.

Finally, to be able to know if a proposed diagnostic method truly will improve ED triage, actual testing of its *clinical impact* is necessary [31]. Although assessment of a method's diagnostic performance characteristics is important, the effectiveness, safety, generalizability, and economic impact of a diagnostic technology's use can only truly be known by performing a *prospective trial of its impact on patient care* in diverse settings [6,31]. This is particularly important for such high-technology, high-cost tests as echocardiography and radionuclide scanning, with which there is the hope that their considerable investments will be more than repaid by improvements in cost effectiveness in triage. It is even more important to carefully consider any diagnostic technology that might lead to an increase in discharges home of patients with ACI, that might appear promising in a hypothetical study on a test data set but in actual use might lead to adverse outcomes due to mistaken discharges of patients with ACI to home.

Presenting History in the ED Setting

Since the classic initial descriptions of angina pectoris by Heberden [32] and of AMI by Herrick [33], there have been many descriptions of the diagnostic features of ACI, including explicit searches for the key clinical features that might help improve physicians' ED assessment of patients with possible ACI [6]. Clearly chest pain and discomfort itself, and equivalent symptoms, such as left arm and jaw pain, when associated with typical kinetics related to exertion or other conditions, and when accompanied by such signs and symptoms as diaphoresis, dyspnea, dizziness, weakness, etc, raise ACI, and especially AMI, to the top of diagnostic considerations. However, often the symptoms are not definitive. The past history can be especially helpful if there is coronary artery disease prior (CAD) or if similar symptoms have already had their etiology identified. Lee et al. [34] found that certain non-ACI characteristics of the chest pain (stabbing, pleuritic, and positional), and the lack of prior cardiac history, conveyed a very low risk of AMI, but these findings applied to only a small portion of patients.

One commonly acquired aspect of the history that, in fact, has little true bearing on the likelihood of ACI is the classical (i.e., Framingham) CAD risk factors, as was shown by Jayes and colleagues [35]. In their study of ED patients with suspected but without obvious coronary disease, none of the risk factors of diabetes, family history of AMI, smoking, hypertension, or hypercholesterolemia raised the relative risk of ACI in women, and only the presence of diabetes or family history slightly increased the relative risk in men (2.4 and 2.1, respectively). By contrast, the finding of chest pain or pressure increased the relative risk of ACI to 25.0 and 12.1 for women and men, respectively; the findings of ST-segment elevation or flattening increased the relative risk of ACI to 8.7 and 3.9 for men and women, respectively. This empirical study makes clear that the degree of increased risk associated with Framingham risk factors over many years is, when considered on a single day when chest pain or other symptoms motivate a patient to seek emergency evaluation, of only minor importance. Thus the clinician should not put undue weight on them. Generally, the presenting clinical signs and symptoms will raise the question of ACI, which additional tests will either support or not, leading to the diagnostic impression of ACI, which will dominate the ED triage decision.

Electrocardiogram

Bacause clinical features are often not diagnostic, the ED physician relies heavily on the ECG. Unfortunately, although an essential tool for identifying ACI, the ECG itself has significant limitations. Particularly for unstable angina, in which ischemia can come and go, the ECG can be nondiagnostic or even misleading if the patient's ischemia has temporarily abated. Moreover, some patients have an abnormal baseline ECG, which complicates recognizing new changes. Left bundle branch block and paced rhythm, and left ventricular hypertrophy, render the interpretation very difficult. Studies have shown the sensitivity of the resting ECG for AMI to range from 65 to 88% [19,20,34,36,37]. Lee et al. [34] found that among patients presenting to an ED with chest pain, a normal ECG conveyed very low risk of having an AMI; however, only 19% of patients of all patients with chest pain met their criterion for a normal ECG, thus providing limited opportunity to improve diagnostic specificity. The ECG can operate with high sensitivity when any non-normal tracing is interpreted as positive. However, at that cutoff level it is poorly specific. When high specificity is attained by requiring the presence of ST-segment displacement, sensitivity is considerably lower.

Moreover, in general, ECG interpretation is not a precise science, and this inaccuracy in the ED ECG identification of ACI has been shown to impact on care. A prospectve study by Jayes et al. examined the sensitivity and specificity of physicians' ECG readings on 2320 ED patients with possible ACI in 1979–1981 [38]. Using the readings of expert electrocardiographers as the gold standard, the study found that for ST-segment displacement ≥ 1 mm, the ED physicians had high false-negative rates (10–16%) and false-positive rates (25–32%). Overall sensitivity and specificity for and major (≥ 1 mm) and minor (<1 mm) ST-segment findings were 59% and 86%, respectively. Such false-negative and false-positive readings were found to have consequences for clinical care: False-negative and false-positive readings were both statistically significantly associated with suboptimal triage to the CCU or home. The recognition of ECG findings of left ventricular hypertrophy (LVH) is also poor. A multicenter study by Larsen and colleagues demonstrated that "admitting physicians" only recognized ECG findings of LVH 22% of the time. In 70% of patients with ECG-LVH, secondary ST-segment and T-wave findings were interpreted as primary changes of ACI [39].

Recently attempts have been made to improve the ECG by expanding the number of sampled leads to include posterior and right ventricular leads or by increasing the number of recorded ECG tracings. The addition of posterior (V_7–V_9) leads has been shown to modestly increase the sensitivity of the ECG for posterior ST-segment elevation [40,41]. Right ventricular infarction is also detected by the addition of V_{4R} to the ECG. As manifested by ST-segment elevation on V_{4R}, it occurs in about half of cases with inferior AMI [42], and this subgroup has a worse prognosis and warrants aggressive interventions to establish reperfusion [43]. Repeat ECGs have been shown to increase the ED sensitivity for AMI [44] and to identify a larger proportion of thrombolytic candidates [45], but there are no data available at this time on the value of continuous 12-lead monitoring in the ED.

Electrocardiographic Excercise Tolerence Testing

There has been increasing interest in the use of ECG exercise tolerance testing [46,47], (ETT) in the ED (or Chest Pain Center) in selected groups of patients. The rationale for this approach is that in patients for whom AMI has been ruled out with clinical, ECG, and/or serial enzyme testing and who are at low to moderate probability of CAD, a predischarge ETT would identify patients at higher risk of coronary artery disease and an untoward outcome. Kerns et al. [48] studied 32 young ED patients (women 18–49 years, men 18–39 years) presenting during the daytime with atypical chest pain, normal ECGs, and one or no CAD risk factors, and no medications, for whom he calculated a pretest probability of CAD of approximately 20%. All tests were interpreted as normal, and there were no cardiac events in 6 months of follow-up. The difference was that for those in the control group, the average length of stay was 2 days at a cost of $2340, whereas for those receiving ETTs, the cost was $467 for an average stay of 5.5 hours.

Tsakonis et al. [49] also tested ETT in selected ED patients with chest pain in 28 low-risk patients with normal ECGs and found it to be safe and to predict being CAD-free at 6 months. Although all patients were admitted despite negative test results, it was suggested that the negative test could preclude unnecessary hospitalizations. More recent studies have shown that such early ETT testing does raise the sensitivity for the detection of coronary artery disease [50,51], but also raises questions about whether ETT is a good discriminator in the populations to which it is applied. In one large study [46], the test's positive rate was only 1%, half of which were false positives.

The ETT is attractive to the ED physician because, if negative, it suggests that the patient has a low likelihood of CAD, and then by inference, a low likelihood of ACI, and can safely be sent home. This is not faulty logic. The advantage of doing this is the effi-ciency provided to the overall healthcare system by having the follow-up test for CAD performed on the first visit. Difficulties arise in the selection of patients who have a high enough probability to benefit from the test but a sufficiently low enough probability to make the test both safe and helpful. If active ACI is likely, then the ETT is neither necessary nor safe; if the patient has a very low likelihood of disease, then a test with only moderate sensitivity and specificity will be unlikely to further discriminate into diseased and nondiseased subgroups. Also, a significant number of patients will be excluded from this method of testing due to an uninterpretable baseline ECG or poor exercise tolerance. Although there are certainly cases for which the use of an ETT will be helpful, whether the current trend to include them in ED/Chest Pain Center is justified by improvements in triage, medical outcomes, or even cost effectiveness remains to be proven in a controlled trial in the ED setting.

Cardiac Enzymes

Long a key part of the diagnostic criteria for AMI in hospitalized patients, serum tests for creatine kinase (CK), and the more cardiac-specific MB-CK isoenzyme, have been increasingly used in the evaluation of ED patients with symptoms suggestive of ACI, especially in those with nondiagnostic ECGs. However, in addition to the well-appreciated issue of the lack of perfect correspondence of even MB-CK serum levels to myocardial necrosis alone, there are a number of issues specific to the ED that limit its use in actual emergency practice. Indeed, there are the increasing panoply of more accurate, sensitive, and rapid MB-CK assays and other cardiac markers [52]. For example, a newer assay for MB-CK subforms appears to maintain the very desirable specificity of MB-CK, but increases its early sensitivity to within 6 hours of symptom onset [53]. A full review of this rapidly changing field is beyond the scope of this chapter and has been provided elsewhere [52]. However, what follows are the more general conclusions about the utility of a single (MB-)CK or other assay in the ED, regardless of the (increasing) excellence of the assay method.

A classic tenet of the use of CK in the ED setting is the importance of *serial* testing over the first 24 hours after ED presentation [54] as opposed to a *single* MB-CK test, due to the kinetics of AMI-related CK release into the serum. Due to the fact that CK and MB-CK do not begin to rise until 4–6 hours after myocardial injury, and peak at 12–24 hours, an early test will be misleadingly negative. Also, due to the fact that CK tests return to normal within 2–3 days (or earlier in a small AMI) in a patient who may have had an AMI several days prior, with preceding and subsequent anginal symptoms, a single measurement could miss the CK rise. Thus, if MB-CK, or any biochemical marker for AMI, is to be used in the ED setting, serial rather than single measures are necessary. Newer assays of MB-CK have only modified this classic tenet in that they have substantially shortened the time period needed for serial testing [55–57].

A more fundamental problem with the use of even serial MB-CK testing is that, by definition, these results are negative when a patient is having non-infarction ACI, that is, unstable angina pectoris. Given that over half of patients presenting with ACI will have new-onset or unstable angina, and given that the failure to recognize ACI in such patients could lead to subsequent AMI or other life-threatening consequences, an ED triage decision predicated on negative MB-CK testing will often be incorrect.

There have been many studies of the diagnostic performance of MB-CK for AMI in the ED. Viskin et al. [58] found that among ED patients presenting within 4 hours of symptom onset, the ECG identified 66% of patients who proved to have AMI, whereas CK tests identified only 9%. However, among patients with more than at greater than 4 hours from the onset of chest pain, the ECG confirmed AMI in 37%, whereas serum CK levels were elevated in 64%. Lee et al. [59] demonstrated the sensitivity of a single CK or MB-CK sample to be low (34–38%), and further demonstrated the importance of timing and repeated determinations, especially the improved sensitivities and specificities of CK and MB-CK when tested more than 4 hours after symptom onset. Hedges et al. [44] demonstrated serial MB-CK testing to have a sensitivity of 68% for AMI and a specificity of 95% (compared with serial ECGs' sensitivity of 39% and specificity of 88%). Marin and Teichman [60] showed that two MB-CK tests done 2 hours apart have a sensitivity of 94% for AMI and a specificity of 91%. Puleo [53] reported on 1110 patients with chest pain who had MB-CK subforms done every 30–60 minutes for at least 6 hours after the onset of symptoms. The diagnosis of AMI was established using quantitative MB-CK criteria. The sensitivity for AMI at 4 hours was 56%, and the specificity was 93%; by 6 hours they were 96% and 94%, respectively. Finally, Gibler et al. found that serial measurement of MB-CK over the first *24 hours* after ED presentation had 100% sensitivity and 98% specificity for AMI [54].

Unfortunately, these and other studies have failed to follow up on AMI ED patients not admitted, thus the test's true sensitivity may be lower than reported due to the failure to include patients with an AMI inadvertently sent home. Moreover, although giving insight into the diagnostic performance of CK and MB-CK, they do not provide information on how physicians' decision making might actually change if the tests were used in real-time ED practice; this will require an interventional controlled clinical trial with complete follow-up of all ED patients evaluated for possible ACI. In 1979, Eisenberg et al. [10] demonstrated that the use of cardiac enzyme determinations could worsen both false-positive and false-negative ED triage decisions. The data generated over the ensuing decade and a half still leave unanswered important questions about the safety and utility of the use of MB-CK in the ED setting. The advocates of making a decision based only on using a positive result but not a negative result, that is, admitting a patient with a positive MB-CK but not necessarily not admitting a patient with a negative test. Although this has an element of logic, in actual decision making the lack of a positive *is* a negative, and to act differently on the lack of a positive result *is* to act on a negative result. Because of the limitations of biochemical testing, as outlined earlier, such decisions can be dangerous. Indeed, the authors have been asked to review a number of malpractice cases for ED patients sent home who subsequently suffered ACI-related deaths in which a MB-CK was obtained, was negative, and presumably had some influence on the (incorrect) triage decision. Given the above-mentioned theoretical problems and the failure of ED studies of MB-CK use to follow up patients sent home and to actually test the strategy in a controlled study, at this point, except in special cases, it would seem unwise to use MB-CK test results until the decision to hospitalize has already been made.

The recent availability of assays of cardiac troponin T and I, which are specific for AMI and minimal myocardial damage, has not yet led to a proven increase in the identification of patients with ACI in the ED or had an impact on clinical care. [52] They have been shown to be effective in the risk stratification of patients with known cardiac disease enrolled for trials of therapy for coronary ischemia [61–62], a very small proportion of ED patients with symptoms of possible ACI.

Visualizing Abnormalities in Ventricular Function or Perfusion: Echocardiography and Radionuclide Scanning

Because of the difficulties inherent in the ECG and in cardiac markers as aids to ED diagnosis and triage, methods that more clearly demonstrate abnormalities of regional cardiac perfusion or regional ventricular function as signs of ACI have been proposed. These approaches are based on the understanding that myocardial ischemia is part of an evolving series of changes. The earliest phenomenon is an abnormality in myocardial perfusion, followed by increasing degrees of myocardial oxygen/blood flow supply/demand mismatch, resulting in regional ventricular functional abnormality, and then in ECG signs of ischemia, and finally, in chest pain and other symptoms of ACI. Abnormalities in regional perfusion can be visualized by imaging radionuclide myocardial perfusion tracers, and abnormalities in regional ventricular function can be demonstrated by echocardiography.

Ideally, direct non-invasive imaging of regional myocardial perfusion, allowing identification of the initial diminution of regional myocardial blood flow, would be most attractive. Thallium-201, a potassium analogue that is taken up by the myocardium in relation to myocardial blood flow, has been the most commonly used agent to demonstrate myocardial blood flow [63]. In 1976, Wackers et al. [64] showed thallium-201 defects in 100% of selected patients with AMI who were studied within 6 hours of symptom onset, but the sensitivity was markedly diminished with increased time beyond 6 hours. Moreover, in a study of patients with unstable angina, Wackers et al. [65] found (planar) thallium-201 scintigraphy to have 76% sensitivity and 67% specificity for AMI or severe coronary disease. Among patients with abnormal baseline ECGs with transient changes, the sensitivity of a positive thallium-201 scan was 94%, but the specificity was only 46%. There are logistic problems with the use of thallium. In addition to the need for expensive on-site equipment and ready access to technicians and trained and experienced interpreters, the isotope is not readily available for acute imaging, because it typically is produced in central facilities and shipped to hospital laboratories once daily, and its "redistribution" properties require that imaging be *completed* in a short time (i.e., within approximately 15 minutes) after injection. Thus, although thallium-201 scanning has found wide use in non-urgent settings for diagnosing coronary artery disease (CAD), it is not of practical use in the ED setting [52].

Recently, technetium-labeled radioisotopes such as TC-99m-sestamibi have been shown to reflect myocardial blood flow [66]. Sestamibi has several advantages over thallium-201: Its physical characteristics are better suited to gamma camera imaging, it is less subject to tissue attenuation, and it may be generator-produced on site, making it readily available for acute imaging. Also, there is minimal redistribution after its initial coronary flow-related distribution in the myocardium; thus images made up to *several hours after injection* [66], will still reflect myocardial blood flow as it was *at the time of injection*. Indeed, it has been reported that myocardial perfusion defects can be accurately identified even when sestamibi *injection* is delayed up to 2–4 hours after resolution of chest pain [18], further enhancing its practicality for ED use.

There have been several small studies of the use of sestamibi scanning in patients presenting with symptoms suggesting ACI. Among 45 patients hospitalized for suspected unstable angina, Bilodeau et al. [15] demonstrated that Tc-99m sestamibi single photon emission computed tomography (SPECT) imaging performed during an episode of chest pain demonstrated 96% sensitivity and 79% specificity for the detection of CAD, while the predictive value of a negative scan to exclude CAD was 94%. However, this study was performed in patients already hospitalized for suspected unstable angina, and the treating physicians were blinded to the imaging results, and thus prospective testing of clinical impact on triage was not assessed. Varetto et al. [17] tested Tc-99m-sestamibi SPECT imaging in 64 ED patients who presented with symptoms suggesting ACI and with nondiagnostic ECGs. The sensitivity and specificity for the detection of AMI or significant CAD were 100% and 92%, respectively, and the predictive value of a negative scan to exclude CAD or a subsequent cardiac event was 100%. While these data support the potential of sestamibi imaging in the ED population, especially among those with otherwise nondiagnostic presentations, again, admitting physicians were blinded to scan results, and thus the potential impact of sestamibi in reducing unnecessary admissions (53% of patients were admitted to the CCU) could not be tested.

An unresolved issue is the potential cost impact of the ED use of sestamibi scanning. The typical cost (not charge) of a sestamibi scan is $400 *plus* physician interpretation fees, which is far more than the currently used ED tests. However, if used on patients with relatively low likelihoods of ACI but who would otherwise have been hospitalized, its use could reduce overall health care costs by reducing unnecessary hospitalizations. At this point, still lacking a substantial prospective intervention trial using generalizable inclusion criteria, projections about its likely impact in actual care and about its likely impact on costs cannot be made [52].

Soon following diminution of myocardial blood flow, there occur ACI-related left ventricular wall motion abnormalities [67], often prior to the onset of ECG signs. Thus, echocardiographic detection of regional ventricular dysfunction has been studied as an ED test for ACI. In a small study, Peels et al. [68] found echocardiography to be highly sensitive for the detection of AMI and ACI in the ED setting (92% and 88%, respectively), but highly dependent on the presence of symptoms *during the echocardiographic study*, a condition that often is not extant, especially for those very patients about whom there is the most question. Others have also demonstrated a poor sensitivity of echocardiography in the absence of ongoing symptoms [69]. Moreover, specificity was only modest, 53% for AMI and 78% for ACI [68]. Sabia et al. [70] reported a sensitivity of 93% for echocardiographically detected regional wall motion abnormalities to correctly identify AMI, but low specificity (57%) and the lack of detected wall motion abnormalities in the patients ultimately diagnosed as having non–Q-wave AMI [70], a problem also found by others [71]. Finally, and probably most problematic, in these studies, echocardiography had to be limited to patients with normal conduction systems and without prior myocardial infarction, because conduction disturbances and prior areas of infarct can both cause regional wall motion abnormalities in the absence of ACI, thereby limiting its use for just the patients in whom diagnostic uncertainty is greatest. Thus, although if diagnoses involving structural problems of the heart, its valves, its surroundings, or the great vessels are entertained, echocardiography may well be critical and very helpful. At this point there are no studies demonstrating its salutary impact on ED triage, and it cannot be supported for this use as part of routine care [52].

Computer-Based Decision Aids

Based on the disappointing results of using customarily available clinical data and the lack, so far, of clearly useful diagnostic tests, a number of mathematically based decision aids aimed at optimizing ED triage of patients with symptoms suggestive of ACI have been developed [52]. These diagnostic aids seek to improve physicians' use of clinical information by quantifying risk in the face of uncertainty [6,72–73].

The first such diagnostic aid was Säwe's *clinical diagnostic index*, which predicted AMI based on nine clinical variables [74]. Tested prospectively, it was 100% sensitive for AMI, but its very poor specificity (16%) made it not useful for actual practice. Tierney et al. [20] created a multivariable model predicting AMI based on the clinical presentations and ECGs of 655 ED patients with chest pain that was more specific (86% vs. 78%), but less sensitive (81% vs. 87%), than physicians. Hypothetical integration of its predictions with physicians' triage decisions did not significantly improve accuracy [20], and the prospective trial on it has not been reported.

Goldman et al. [19,28] developed computer-derived protocols for triage of ED patients with chest pain based on their clinical presentations and ECGs, putting them into subgroups with different likelihoods of AMI. In a hypothetical test on prospectively collected data from 4770 patients presenting with chest pain to six hospitals, their most recent protocol's 88% sensitivity in predicting AMI was equal to that of physicians, but its specificity was slightly better (74% vs. 71%). However, to date the only reported results of a prospective clinical trial of its actual impact on clinical care has shown that it has no impact on care [75].

Using logistic regression, Pozen et al. [2,23] and Selker et al. [1,22,76] developed "predictive instruments" to provide ED physicians with patients' probabilities of ACI based on clinical and ECG findings. In addition to the use of ACI as the clinical endpoint, instead of just AMI, this work also differs from prior work in that, instead of only including patients, with chest pain, it included all ED patients presenting with symptoms suggestive of ACI, including chest pain or left arm pain, abdominal pain or nausea, shortness of breath, and dizziness or lightheadedness. (These inclusion criteria were based on the Imminent Rotterdam MI [IMIR] Criteria, which have been shown to capture more than 90% of all patients in a community with ACI [73]. In controlled prospective trials of the instrument's use, first at Boston City Hospital [23], and then in the Multicenter Predictive Instrument Trial [2], it reduced false-positive CCU admissions by 30% without an increase in false-negative discharges to home. Data collection for the 10-hospital clinical trial of our newer electrocardiograph-based version, the ACI-TIPI, was just completed, and results of its impact will presumably be available later this year. Despite the publication of the results of the original predictive instrument trial a decade ago [2], the use of this technology has not become widespread. It is hoped that the convenience afforded by the reporting of the ACI-TIPI result on the presenting ECG will lead to widespread use and improved triage practices.

Conclusions and Recommendations

The previous discussion summarizes some of more important diagnostic technologies for ACI/AMI in the ED. The *standard 12-lead ECG* has been shown in many studies to have very good, although not perfect, diagnostic performance in the ED. But, despite its key role in the diagnosis of ACI in the ED, the use of the ECG has provided the needed high sensitivity only at the expense of poor specificity. As an extension of the standard ECG, *nonstandard ECG leads* interrogating the posterior and right ventricle have undergone testing in the ED for detecting ACI. Published data at this point indicate modest increases in sensitivity with posterior leads and valuable prognostic data with the use of right ventricular leads in inferior infarction. A different extension of the standard ECG, the *ECG exercise stress test*, has also been evaluated, to some extent, in the ED. Its diagnostic performance in this setting has been only modest. Given this, and that its actual impact on triage has not been tested, its routine ED use cannot be recommended as of this writing.

Although they have not yet been demonstrated to actually improve the ED triage of symptomatic patients, *blood biochemical tests of myocardial necrosis, particularly creatine kinase*, including a variety of assay types and protocols, have undergone prospective testing of their diagnostic performance for the detection of AMI. Available data suggest that the use of a *single MB-CK* test yields performance insufficient for use in ED triage but that *multiple MB-CK* tests over several or more hours have very good diagnostic performance for AMI. Although the data are less complete, the same pattern appears to be emerging for newer biochemical tests, such as *troponin*, which indicate performance of a single test is not satisfactory, but the use of multiple tests over time has promise. Whether their ability to risk stratify in patients with known ACI will assist in the ED triage of patients is unknown. Finally, none of these tests are useful in detecting unstable angina pectoris, which raises the possibility of missing this form of ACI if triage depends on them. This is one of the reasons that, in the absence of prospective trials of the impact of this technology on ED triage, although very useful for inhospital care, these tests cannot yet be recommended for general ED triage use at this time.

Echocardiography, well studied in other settings, has been investigated in several studies in the ED. These studies have generally shown modest diagnostic performance for initial ED evaluation. Given this, and that its actual impact on ED care has not been evaluated, this technology cannot be recommended for ED use at this time.

Radionuclide imaging, although generally used in non-ED settings, has been studied in terms of diagnostic performance in the ED. *Thallium scanning's* characteristics are not appropriate for ED use.

Sestamibi scanning has been studied in the ED setting, and thus far its overall diagnostic performance has been promising in preliminary and limited ED studies. Whether sestamibi will be found to be helpful when evaluated for special subgroups, and when tested for its actual impact on care, remains to be seen.

The *Goldman AMI protocol* has a diagnostic accuracy for AMI that has been demonstrated to be excellent; however, it is not intended to detect unstable angina as a form of ACI. In prospective clinical trial evaluation, it so far has not been shown to have an impact on care, and thus, at this point and in its current form its general use cannot be recommended.

To date, the only diagnostic technology with published clinical trial–based diagnostic performance and demonstrated salutary clinical impact is the *original ACI predictive instrument*. Its accuracy and demonstrated improvement in ED triage make it possible to recommend it for general use in the ED evaluation and triage of patients with symptoms suggestive of ACI. Its main drawback has been that its use requires a programmed calculator or chart, which has been an obstacle to its widespread use. Having very similar diagnostic performance as the original ACI instrument, it successor, the electrocardiograph-based *ACI-TIPI*, has been anticipated to have an analogous impact with greater ease of use. The results of a multicenter prospective trial are anticipated to provide more definitive information about its use.

Thus the diagnostic approach to ED patients presenting with chest pain or other symptoms suggestive of ACI starts with the history, physical examination, and ECG (except for the small subset of patients for whom the clinical evaluation excludes the diagnosis of ACI). Patients at moderate or high risk of having ACI will need hospitalization. The group of patients at low risk (but not low enough to be discharged without further workup) may well benefit from a short stay (<24 hours) for evaluation. Serial cardiac enzyme determinations can be used to diagnose AMI. However, these markers do not detect or exclude unstable angina pectoris. Thus, even after an AMI is ruled out in the stable patient without evidence of ischemia at rest, further workup with early stress testing, either before or shortly after discharge, will serve to complete the workup for ACI. In the future, more structured strategies incorporating a number of the above-mentioned diagnostic technologies may well further streamline the ED evaluation and triage process.

References

1. Selker HP, Griffith JL, D'Agostino RB. A tool for judging coronary care unit admission that is appropri-

ate for both real-time and retrospective use: A time-insensitive predictive instrument (TIPI) for acute cardiac ischemia: A multicenter study. Med Care 29:610, 1991.

2. Pozen MW, D'Agostino RB, Selker HP, Sytkowski PA, Hood WB. A predictive instrument to improve coronary care unit admission practices in acute ischemic heart disease. N Engl J Med 310:1273, 1984.

3. Schor S, Behar S, Modan B, Barell V, Drory J, Kariv I. Disposition of presumed coronary patients from an emergency room. A follow-up study. JAMA 236:941, 1976.

4. Lee TH, Rouan GW, Weisberg MC, Brand DA, Acampora D, Stasiulewicz C, Walshon J, Terranova G, Gottlieb I, Goldstein-Wayne B. Clinical characteristics and natural history of patients with acute myocardial infarction sent home from the emergency room. Am J Carciol 60:219, 1987.

5. McCarthy BD, Beshansky JR, D'Agostino RB, Selker HP. Missed diagnoses of acute myocardial infarction in the emergency department: Results from a multicenter study. Ann Emerg Med 22:579, 1993.

6. McCarthy BD, Wong JB, Selker HP. Detecting acute cardiac ischemia in the emergency department: A review of the literature. J Gen Intern Med 5:365, 1990.

7. Fineberg HV, Scadden D, Goldman L. Care of patients with a low probability of acute myocardial infarction: Cost-effectiveness of alternatives to coronary-care-unit admission. N Engl J Med 310:1301, 1984.

8. Fuchs R, Scheidt S. Improved criteria for admission to cardiac care units. JAMA 246:2037, 1981.

9. Nattel S, Warnica JW, Ogilvie RI. Indications for admission to a coronary care unit in patients with unstable angina. Can Med Assoc J 122:180, 1980.

10. Eisenberg JM, Horowitz LN, Busch R, Arvan D, Rawnsley H. Diagnosis of acute myocardial infarction in the ER: A prospective assessment of clinical decision making and the usefulness of immediate cardiac enzyme determination. J Commun Health 4:190, 1979.

11. Seager SB. Cardiac enzymes in the evaluation of chest pain. Ann Emerg Med 9:346, 1980.

12. Horowitz RS, Morganroth J. Immediate detection of early high-risk patients with an acute myocardial infarction using two-dimensional echocardiographic evaluation of left ventricular regional wall motion abnormalities. Am Heart J 103:814, 1982.

13. Wackers FJ, Lic KI, Liem KL, Sokole EB, Samson G, van der Schoot J, Durrer D. Potential value of thallium-201 scintigraphy as a means of selecting patients for the coronary care unit. Br Heart J 41:111, 1979.

14. Gibbons RJ, Verani MS, Behrenbeck T, Pellikka PA, O'Connor MK, Mahmarian JJ, Chesebro JH, Wackers FJ. Feasibility of tomographic 99m-Tc-hexakis-2-methoxy-2-methylpropyl-isonitrile imaging for the assessment of myocardial area at risk and the effect of treatment in acute myocardial infarction. Circulation 80:1277, 1989.

15. Bilodeau I, Theroux P, Gregoire J, Gagnon D, Arsenault A. Technetium-99m sestamibi tomography in patients with spontaneous chest pain: Correlations with clinical, electrocardiographic and angiographic findings. J Am Coll Cardiol 18:1684, 1991.

16. Verani MS. Technetium-99m sestamibi imaging in acute ischemic syndromes. Prim Cardiol 18:56, 1992.

17. Varetto T, Cantalupi D, Altieri A, Orlandi C. Emergency room technetium-99m sestamibi imaging to rule out acute myocardial ischemic events in patients with nondiagnostic electrocardiography. J Am Coll Cardiol 22:1804, 1993.

18. Varetto T, De Cicco Cantalupi D, Altieri A, Leone G, Devoti G, Orlandi C. Tc99m sestamibi perfusion imaging allows detection of unstable angina after chest pain remission. Circulation 86:I46, 1992.

19. Goldman L, Cook EF, Brand DA, Lee TH, Rouan GW, Weisberg MC, Acampora D, Stasiulewicz C, Walshon J, Terranova G. A computer protocol to predict myocardial infarction in emergency department patients with chest pain. N Engl J Med 318:797, 1988.

20. Ticrney WM, Roth BJ, Psaty B, McHenry R, Fitzgerald J, Stump DL, Anderson FK, Ryder KW, McDonald CJ, Smith DM. Predictors of myocardial infarction in emergency room patients. Crit Care Med 13:526, 1985.

21. Baxt WG. Use of an artificial neural network for the diagnosis of myocardial infarction. Ann Intern Med 115:843, 1991.

22. Selker HP, Griffith JL, Patil S, Long WJ, D'Agostino RB. A comparison of performance of mathematical predictive methods for medical diagnosis: Identifying acute cardiac ischemia among emergency department patients. J Invest Med 43:468, 1995.

23. Pozen MW, D'Agostino RB, Mitchell JB, Selker HP, Sytkowski PA, Hood WB. The usefulness of a predictive instrument to reduce inappropriate admissions to the coronary care unit. Ann Intern Med 92:238, 1980.

24. Rifkin RD, Hood WB Jr. Bayesian analysis of electrocardiographic exercise stress testing. N Engl J Med 297:681, 1979.

25. Kinlen LJ. Incidence and presentation of myocardial infarction in an English community. Br Heart J 35:616, 1973.

26. Margolis JR, Kannel WB, Feinleib M, Dawber TR, McNamara PM. Clinical features of unrecognized myocardial infarction—silent and symptomatic. Eighteen year follow-up: The Framingham Study. Am J Cardiol 32:1, 1973.

27. Uretsky BF, Farquhar DS, Berezin AF, Hood WB Jr. Symptomatic myocardial infarction without chest pain: Prevalence and clinical course. Am J Cardiol 40:498, 1977.

28. Goldman L, Weinberg M, Weisberg M, Olshen R, Cook EF, Sargent RK, Lamas GA, Dennis C, Wilson C, Deckelbaum L, Fineberg H, Stiratelli R. A computer-derived protocol to aid in the diagnosis of ER patients with acute chest pain. N Engl J Med 307:588, 1982.

29. Russell RO, et al. Unstable angina pectoris: National Cooperative Study Group to compare medical and surgical therapy: IV. Results in patient with left anterior descending coronary artery disease. Am J Cardiol 48:517, 1981.

30. Krause KR, Hutter AM Jr, DeSanctis RW. Acute coronary insufficiency. Course and follow-up. Circulation 45/46(Suppl. I):166, 1972.

31. Selker, HP. Coronary care unit triage decision aids: How do we know when they work? Am J Med 87:491, 1989.

32. Heberden W. Some account of disorder of the breast. Med Trans R Coll Phys Lond, 1772.

33. Herrick JB. Clinical features of sudden obstruction of the coronary arteries. JAMA 199:156, 1912.

34. Lee TH, Cook F, Weisberg M, Sargent RK, Wilson C, Goldman L. Acute chest pain in the emergency room: Identification and examination of low risk patients. Arch Intern Med 145:65, 1985.

35. Jayes RL, Beshansky JR, D'Agostino RB, Selker HP. Do patients' coronary risk factor reports predict acute cardiac disease in the Emergency Department? A multicenter study. J Clin Epidemiol 45:621, 1992.

36. Behar S, Schor S, Kariv I, Barell V, Modan B. Evaluation of electrocardiogram in emergency room as a decision-making tool. Chest 71:486, 1977.

37. Rude RE, Poole WK, Muller JE, Turi Z, Rutherford J, Parker C, Roberts R, Raabe DS Jr, Gold HK, Stone PH. Electrocardiographic and clinical criteria for recognition of acute myocardial infarction based on analysis of 3697 patients. Am J Cardiol 52:936, 1983.

38. Jayes RL, Larsen GC, Beshansky JR, D'Agostino RB, Selker HP. Physician electrocardiogram reading in the emergency department: Accuracy and effect on triage decisions -- findings from a multicenter study. J Gen Intern Med 7:387, 1992.

39. Larsen GC, Griffith JL, Beshansky JR, D'Agostino RB, Selker HP. Electrocardiographic left ventricular hypertrophy in patients with suspected acute cardiac ischemia— Its influence on diagnosis, triage, and short term prognosis: A multicenter study. J Gen Intern Med 9:666, 1994.

40. Zalenski RJ, Cooke D, Rydman R, Sloan EP, Murphy DG. Assessing the diagnostic value of an ECG containing leads V_{4R}, V_8, and V_9: The 15 lead ECG. Ann Emerg Med 22:786, 1993.

41. Zalenski RJ, Rydman R, Sloan E, Hahn K, Cooke D, Fagan J, Fligner DJ, Hessions W, Justis D, Kampe LM, Shah S, Tucker J, Zwicke D. Value of posterior and right ventricular leads in comparison to the standard 12-lead electrocardiogram in evaluation of ST segment elevation in suspected acute myocardial infarction. Am J Cardiol 79, 1997 in press.

42. Zehender M, Kasper W, Kauder E, Geibel A, Schonthaler M, Olschewski M, Just H. Right ventricular infarction as an independent predictor of prognosis after acute inferior myocardial infarction. N Engl J Med 328:981, 1993.

43. Zehender M, Kasper W, Kauder E, Geibel A,

Schonthaler M, Olschewski M, Just H. Eligibility for and benefit of thrombolytic therapy in inferior myocardial infarction: Focus on the prognostic importance of right ventricular infarction. J Am Coll Cardiol 24:362, 1994.

44. Hedges JR, Young GP, Henkel GF, Gibler WB, Green TR, Swanson JR. Serial ECGs are less accurated than serial CK-MB results for emergency department diagnosis of myocardial infartion. Ann Emeg Med 21:1445, 1992.

45. Sharkey SW, Berger CR, Brunette DD, Hentry TD. Impact of the electrocardiogram on the delivery of thrombolytic therapy for acute myocardial infarction. Am J Cardiol 73:550, 1994.

46. Gibler WB, Runyon JP, Levy RC, Sayre MR, Kacich R, Hattemer CR, Hamilton C, Gerlach JW, Walsh RA. A rapid diagnostic treatment center for patients with chest pain in the emergency depratment. Ann Emerg Med 25:1, 1995.

47. Gaspoz JM, Lee TH, Cook EF, Weisberg MC, Goldman L. Outcome of patiens who were admitted to a new short-stay unit to rule-out AMI. Am J Cardiol 68:145, 1991.

48. Kerns JR, Shaub TF, Fontanarosa PB. Emergency cardiac stress testing in the evaluation of emergency department patients with atypical chest pain. Ann Emerg Med 22:794, 1993.

49. Tsakonis JS, Shesser R, Rosenthal R, Bittar GD, Smith M, Wasserman AG. Safety of immediate treadmill testing in selected emergency department patients with chest pain — a preliminary report. Am J Emerg Med 9:557, 1991.

50. Lewis WR, Amsterdam EA. Utility and safety of immediate exercise testing of low-risk patients admitted to the hospital for suspected acute myocardial infarction. Am J Cardiol 74:987, 1994.

51. Zalenski RJ, McCarren M, Roberts R, Rydman RJ, Jovanovic B, Das K, Mendez J, El-Khadra M, Fraker L, McDermott M. An evaluation of an emergency department chest pain diagnostic protocol to exclude acute myocardial infarction and ischemia. Arch Intern Med 157, 1997, in press.

52. Selker H, Zalenski R, Antman E, Aufderheide T, Bernard S, Bonow R, Gibler WB, Hagen M, Johnson P, Lau J, McNutt R, Ornato J, Schwartz JS, Scott J, Tunick P, Weaver WD. Working Group of the National Heart Attack Alert Program, National Heart Lung and Blood Institute, National Institutes of Health. An evaluation of technologies for identifying acute cardiac ischemia in the Emergency Department. Ann Emerg Med 29:13, 1997.

53. Puleo PR, Meyer D, Wathen C, Tawa CB, Wheceler S, Hamburg RJ, Ali N, Obermueller SD, Triana JF, Zimmerman JL. Use of a rapid assay of subforms of creatine kinase MB to diagnose or rule out acute myocardial infarction. N Engl J Med 331:561, 1994.

54. Gibler WB, Lewis LM, Erb RE, Makens PK, Kaplan BC, Vaughn RH, Biagini AV, Blanton JD, Campbell WB. Early detection of acute myocardial infarction in

patients presenting with chest pain and non-diagnostic ECGs: Serial CK-MB sampling in the emergency department. Ann Emerg Med 19:1359, 1990; erratum 20:420, 1991.

55. Gibler WB, Young GP, Hedges JR, Lewis LM, Smith MS, Carleton SC, Aghababian RV, Jorden RO, Allison EJ, Otten EJ, Makens PK, Hamilton C. Acute myocardial infarction in chest pain patients with nondiagnostic ECGs: Serial CK-MB sampling in the emergency department. Ann Emerg Med 2:504, 1992.

56. Lee TH, Juarez G, Cook EF, Weisberg MC, Rouan GW, Brand DA, Goldman L. Ruling out acute myocardial infarction: A prospective multicenter validation of a 12-hour strategy for patients at low risk. N Engl J Med 324:1239, 1991.

57. deWinter RJ, Koster RW, Sturk A, Sanders GT. Value of myoglobin, troponin T, and CK-MB$_{mass}$ in ruling our an acute myocardial infarction in the emergency department. Circulation 92:3401, 1995.

58. Viskin S, Heller K, Gheva D, Hassner A, Shapira I, Meyer M, Sarfatti E, Lucksman D, Shibolet S. The importance of creatine kinase determination in identifying acute myocardial infarction among patients complaining of chest pain in an emergency room. Cardiology 74:100, 1987.

59. Lee TH, Weinberg M, Cook F, Daley K, Brand DA, Goldman L. Evaluation of creatine kinase and creatine kinase-MB for diagnosing myocardial infarction: Clinical impact in the emergency room. Arch Intern Med 147:115, 1987.

60. Marin MM, Teichman SL. Use of rapid serial sampling of creatine kinase MB for very early detection of myocardial infarction of patients with acute chest pain. Am Heart J 123:354, 1992.

61. Antman EM, Tanasijevic MJ, Thompson B, Schactman M, McCabe CH, Cannon CP, Fischer GA, Fung AY, Thompson C, Wycnga D, Braunwald E. N Engl J Med 335:1342, 1996.

62. Ohman EM, Armstrong PW, Christenson RH, Granger CB, Katus HA, Hamm CW, O'Hanesian MA, Wagner GS, Klciman NS, Harrell FE, Califf RM, Topol EJ. Cardiac troponin T levels for risk stratification in acute stratification in acute myocardial ischemia. N Engl J Med 335:1333, 1996.

63. Strauss HW, Harrison K, Langan JK, Lebowitz E, Pitt B. Thallium-201 for myocardial imaging: Relation of thallium-201 to regional myocardial perfusion. Circulation 51:641, 1975.

64. Wackers FJ, Sokole EB, Samson G, Schoot JB, Lie KL, Wellens HJ. Value and limitations of thallium-201 scintigraphy in the acute phase of myocardial infarction. N Engl J Med 295:1, 1976.

65. Wackers FJ, Lie KI, Liem KL, Sokole EB, Samson G,

van der School JB, Durrer D. Thallium-201 scintigraphy in unstable angina pectoris. Circulation 57:738, 1978.

66. Okada RD, Glover D, Gaffney T, Williams S. Myocardial kinetics of technetium-99m-hexakis-2-methoxy-2-methylpropyl-isonitri Ic. Circulation 77:491, 1988.

67. Hauser AM, Gangadharan V, Ramos R, Gordon S, Timmis GC. Sequence of mechanical, electrocardiographic and clinical effects of repeated coronary artery occlusion in human beings: Echocardiographic observations during coronary angioplasty. J Am Coll Cardiol 5:193, 1985.

68. Peels CH, Visser CA, Kupper AJF, Visser FC, Roos JP. Usefulness of two-dimensional echocardiography for immediate detection of myocardial ischemia in the emergency room. Am J Cardiol 65:687, 1990.

69. Sasaki H, Charuzi Y, Beeder C, Sugiki Y, Lew AS. Utility of echocardiography for the early assessment of patients with non-diagnostic chest pain. Am Heart J 112:494, 1986.

70. Sabia P, Abbott RD, Afrooktch A, Keller MW, Touchstone DA, Kaul S. Value of regional wall motion abnormality in the emergency room diagnosis of acute myocardial infarction. Circulation 84:I85, 1991.

71. Loh IK, Charuzi Y, Beeder C, Marshall LA, Ginsburg JH. Early diagnosis of non-transmural myocardial infarction by two-dimensional echocardiography. Am Heart J 104:963, 1982.

72. McNutt RA, Selker HP. How did the acute ischemic heart disease predictive instrument reduce unnecessary coronary care unit admissions? Med Decis Making 8:90, 1988.

73. Wasson JH, Sox HC, Neff RK, Goldman L. Clinical prediction rules: Applications and methodological standards. N Engl J Med 313:793, 1985.

74. Sawe U. Early diagnosis of acute myocardial infarction with special reference to the diagnosis of the intermediate coronary syndrome: A clinical study. Acta Med Scand 520(Suppl.):I76, 1972.

75. Lee TH, Pearson SD, Johnson PA, Garcia TB, Weisberg MC. Guadagnoli E, Cook EF, Goldman L. Failure of information as an intervention to modify clinical management: A time-series trial in patients with acute chest pain. Ann Intern Med 122:434, 1995.

76. Selker HP, D'Agostino RB, Laks MM. A predictive instrument for acute ischemic heart disease to improve coronary care unit admission practices: A potential on-line tool in a computerized electrocardiograph. J Electrocardiol 88:S11, 1988.

77. Van der Does E, Lubsen J, Pool J. Acute coronary events in a general practice: Objectives and design of the Imminent Myocardial Infarction Rotterdam Study. Heart Bull 7:91, 1976.

SECTION VIII: PREHOSPITAL STRATEGIES FOR THE TREATMENT OF ACUTE MYOCARDIAL INFARCTION

W. Douglas Weaver and Richard C. Becker

The time from symptom onset to treatment has been shown to be an important factor in the outcome of individuals treated with thrombolytic therapy. The outcomes of patients treated in the emergency department with thrombolytic therapy were considerably better then was seen in earlier trials in which treatment was initiated first in the angiography laboratory and secondly in the coronary care unit. A logical extension of this effort to reduce the time to treatment includes extending and permitting the diagnosis of acute myocardial infarction outside the hospital, as well as the initiation of treatment. A review of the findings from clinical trials and community experience on the use of prehospital initiation, thrombolytic therapy, and implementation of a diagnostic strategy in the out-of-hospital setting is reviewed in this section.

27. THE SCIENTIFIC BASIS AND RATIONALE FOR EARLY THROMBOLYTIC THERAPY

Arie Roth

Thrombolytic Treatment and Left Ventricular Function

There are vast amounts of data that support the use of thrombolytic treatment in evolving acute myocardial infarction, and the evidence to justify early treatment is substantial. In the landmark GISSI trial [1], the administration of streptokinase within the first 3 hours was associated with a remarkable improvement in mortality (12.0% controls vs. 9.2% streptokinase), whereas in those treated within the first hour, mortality was reduced in as much as 47% (15.4% controls vs. 8.2% streptokinase). A similar relation with time was shown in the Second International Study of Infarct Survival (ISIS-2) [2]: Treatment within the first hour resulted in 13.4% mortality with placebo and 8.1% with streptokinase treatment.

Although placebo-controlled thrombolytic trials have shown improvement in both left ventricular ejection fraction and regional wall motion in most [3–5] but not all [6] series, and because there is a correlation between the individual left ventricular ejection fraction and survival, it is imperative to assess the impact of thrombolytic treatment and the time of its application both on infarct size and residual left ventricular function.

Ischemia and Reperfusion

Although only as late as 1977 did Reimer et al. [7] establish the relationship between the duration of coronary occlusion and the degree of myocardial necrosis in dogs, Tennant and Wiggers [8] carried out the pioneer experiments in 1935 and were followed by Blumgart and coworkers [9], who reported on the effects of occlusion and reperfusion in animals. They demonstrated that the temporary acute closure of epicardial coronary arteries in open-chest dogs resulted

in left ventricular dysfunction and that early restoration of blood flow often resolved left ventricular dysfunction and prevented myocardial infarction. Additional animal data have shown that, although a brief period of coronary occlusion results in temporary impairment of contraction that outlasts the electrocardiographic evidence of ischemia by several hours [10], it was early reperfusion that ultimately limited infarct size [11–13].

The canine subendocardium, like that in humans, is prone to severe ischemia after coronary occlusion, which, together with its greater metabolic requirements, makes it usceptible to infarction. In anesthetized open-chest dogs, cardiac myocytes remain viable for at least 15 minutes following coronary occlusion, and if reperfusion occurs, myocardial infarction may be prevented and there is complete recovery of contractile function. If the arterial occlusion is not resolved, the process of necrosis expands gradually at the cost of jeopardized, but still salvageable, myocardial cells. However, after 15 minutes of coronary occlusion, progressively more cardiac myocytes become irreversibly injured, and thus reperfusion cannot prevent the occurrence of some cell death.

After 40 minutes, although much of the subendocardial zone has been irreversibly injured, the midepicardial and subepicardial regions are still viable. Reperfusion at this stage prevents infarction of these zones, because, in contrast to myocytes of the endocardium, subepicardial cardiac myocytes are capable of recovering after 3–6 hours of ischemia. Thus, while ischemia that is relieved after 1–3 hours is followed by some recovery, a wavefront of cell death progresses from the endocardium to the epicardium following a long duration of ischemia, and a permanent loss of viability and function occurs to the extent determined by the duration of occlusion [7,14] and the speed, which depends primarily on the residual blood flow in the ischemic area. If the residual blood flow is poor, the infarction process may be complete within a few hours, whereas it may continue for several hours in the presence of a good residual flow. Moreover, the presence and recruitment of collateral flow may extend the time window before necrosis occurs.

The driving theory behind thrombolytic therapy in acute myocardial infarction is that early restoration of infarct artery patency can "salvage" ischemic muscle, preserve left ventricular function, and hence decrease mortality. It was shown by Popovic et al. [15] that rapid and early administration of thrombolytic agents limited ventricular enlargement, with higher ejection fractions being seen as early as 1 day after acute myocardial infarction, thereby suggesting that myocardial salvage is directly related to the achievement of early infarct artery patency.

It should be borne in mind that although infarct size, preservation of ventricular function, and survival are related to coronary flow [16,17], epicardial blood flow does not necessarily mean there is microvascular perfusion, and there may be no reflow at a cellular level. Ischemia and reperfusion may result in injury to the microvasculature of the heart, which may compromise the return of normal coronary perfusion [18].

In humans, data regarding ventricular recovery following acute myocardial infarction are conflicting, showing both improvement or lack of it over a short time period despite angiographically documented reperfusion at 90 minutes after initiation of therapy [19,20]. Other reports provide variable results in more extended measurements carried out within 24 hours of thrombolytic administration [21]. Progressive improvement in regional wall motion may occur in some patients after 24 hours [22,23]. In addition, there is evidence that the full recovery of left ventricular function may be delayed for several months [24]. Delayed recovery of ventricular function has also been noted in patients undergoing "rescue" coronary angioplasty [25].

Time Effect on Left Ventricular Function

Because evolution of myocardial damage following coronary artery occlusion is rapid, and in light of the evidence in experimental coronary occlusion showing that infarct size and residual dysfunction are related to the time until reperfusion [7,13,14,26], it became apparent that very early thrombolytic treatment may result in significant myocardial "salvage" or may actually abort infarction. The feasibility of prehospital thrombolysis was first evaluated in several small-scale

pioneer studies. Treatment with streptokinase was initiated in the prehospital phase by Koren [27], Weis [28], and Villemant [29] and their colleagues. Anistreplase (APSAC) was given both by Castaigne [3] and in the Belgian study [30], Roth et al. used tissue plasminogen activator (t-PA) [31] and Schofer et al. used urokinase [32].

These investigations were then followed by larger scale studies (MITI, EMIP, GREAT). The conclusions of all these studies were that there were no additional complications compared with patients being treated under the usual protocol in hospitals or when compared with patients given placebo, if it was given before hospitalization and while allowing initiation of thrombolysis 25 to >60 minutes earlier than would have taken place after admission.

Assessment of Thrombolytic Impact

INFARCT SIZE
The direct effects of thrombolytic therapy in terms of limitation of infarct size can be evaluated by quantitative measurments of cardiac enzyme release [33–36], whereas the use of maximal creative kinase (CK) activity as an index of infarct size may be less appropriate because this measure is known to be further elevated when thrombolysis is effective. In three randomized controlled trials of thrombolytic therapy in 1374 patients enrolled in the European Cooperative Study Group, very early treatment with intravenous t-PA resulted in a substantial (30–70%) reduction in infarct size [37]. More than half of this effect was lost when treatment was delayed more than 60–75 minutes. Similarly, infarct size was reduced more notably in patients with anterior wall infarction treated up to 2 hours compared with 2–4 hours from symptom onset [27,38].

The Netherlands Interuniversity Trial [34] showed that infarct size, as evaluated from myocardial enzyme release, was reduced by 51% in patients treated within 1 hour, by 31% in those treated between 1 and 2 hours, and by 13% in patients treated later than 2 hours. It was equal in the treated and control patients when the symptoms had been present for over 3 hours. Also, infarct size was measured from cumulative release of alpha-hydroxybutyrate-dehydrogenase, and left ventricular function was assessed by contrast angiography [39]; all showed beneficial effects of very early treatment.

The Intravenous Streptokinase in Acute Myocardial Infarction ISAM Study Group [33] found that patients treated within 1.5 hours of the onset of chest pain had a smaller area under the MB-CK curve and a higher global or infarct-related regional ejection fraction compared with patients treated 1.5–4 hours after acute myocardial infarction.

In the MITI trial, myocardial infarct size and global left ventricular function were determined by quantitative thallium single-photon emission computed tomography and radionuclide ventriculography [40]. This relatively small trial did not show any advantage of prehospital thrombolysis compared with in-hospital treatment with respect to infarct size or ejection fraction. However, when all patients were included in an analysis of the effects of very early treatment (<70 minutes), there was substantial evidence of benefit expressed by a reduction of infarct size, augmentation of ejection fraction, and improvement in survival. Of special note was that 40% of patients treated very early had no evidence on the thallium scintigraph of a myocardial infarction.

In contrast to the mortality, wherein the relation between the benefit derived from thrombolytic therapy and the time to onset of myocardial infarction is not linear, there does appear to be a linear relation between time to treatment and infarct size, as measured by thallium uptake, after myocardial infarction. The Western Washington IV Streptokinase Trial, in which the mean time to treatment was more than 270 minutes, reported that infarct size was 19% of the left ventricle. In the MITI trial, those patients who had been treated within 70 minutes had a 50% reduction in infarct size. Thus, there appears to be a good relationship between time to treatment and infarct size according to these and other studies [6,41–45].

GLOBAL LEFT VENTRICULAR EJECTION FRACTION

Several indices of left ventricular function were used to evaluate left ventricular "salvage." In the prethrombolytic era, global left ventricular ejection fraction, which correlates well with functional capacity, was found to be an important predictor of late survival after infarction. As a result, it was advocated as being a surrogate endpoint for mortality in clinical thrombolytic trials [46]. This index, which became the most commonly used, is easily calculated from end-diastolic and end-systolic ventricular contours using single or biplane area lengths, or volumetric or radionuclide methods.

In accordance with their results in experimental models, several studies have suggested that very early administration of a thrombolytic agent causes maximal recovery of left ventricular function, particularly when the thrombolytic agent is given within 2 hours of symptom onset [38,47–49]. Some reports, however, failed to demonstrate a relationship between

time to treatment and recovery of left ventricular function [20,50,51], but few patients in these studies actually received thrombolytic agents within 2 hours of symptom onset. Topol et al. [52] demonstrated a higher immediate ejection fraction for patients who received intravenous rt-PA therapy in a community hospital compared with patients who received delayed therapy. Fine et al. [53] treated the majority of their patients by <2 hours from symptom onset and demonstrated a nearly intact ventricular ejection fraction, as determined by ventriculography performed at 6 days.

Although many large, well-designed randomized trials have proven the beneficial effect of thrombolytic agents on survival and, on average, ejection fraction for patients treated with thrombolytics was five points higher than control patients, the evidence that myocardial "salvage" occurred with early thrombolytic treatment, judged by global ejection fraction, is not impressive [4–6,43,54–58]. Moreover, randomized trials of prehospital thrombolytics that resulted in improved door-to-needle time have shown either improved survival without improved residual left ventricular function [59], improved left ventricular function with no difference in survival [3,27], or no significant difference in survival or left ventricular function [32].

The use of left ventricular ejection fraction as the sole index of myocardial salvage after thrombolytic therapy may be plagued by limitations within series, and its measurement requires meticulous attention to details if it is to be reproducible between centers. For example, estimation of myocardial salvage using single-plane ventriculographic methods may be problematic, particularly in patients with circumflex occlusion [60].

Contrast or isotope ventriculography may not always be obtainable, and imputed values for missing patients, quite likely to be those patients with extreme values or who have died, have been used in some [61], although not all, assessments [62]. Incomplete ventriculographic follow-up is commonplace due to refusal on the part of patients or physicians, medical contraindications, and technical exclusions, which are frequently caused by patient movements. measurements also depend on loading conditions, different medications, arrhythmia, or inadequate ventricular opacification with contrast.

In technically adequate studies, clinically effective thrombolysis may not change global ventricular function despite its improving the regional function of a jeopardized ischemic myocardium because the initially compensatory hyperkinesis of the noninfarct zone, driven by adrenergic stimulation, may, to a certain extent, counterbalance akinesis or dyskinesis of "stunned" but reversibly ischemic tissue wall motion asynergy and result in a near-normal global left ventricular ejection fraction [49,63,64]. With recovery of infarct-related regional wall motion over a period of days to weeks, non–infarct-related hyperkinesis lessens and little or no net change in global ejection fraction may be noted over time.

The relation between outcome and time of administration of treatment is not a true reflection of therapeutic efficacy at different times for several reasons. The outcome will be biased against an indication of greater efficacy with earlier administration because of the greater severity of infarction in patients who present earlier [65]. A trend tooward a larger sum of initial ST-segment deviation [39] was shown in the early treatment groups, and this may reflect an even potentially larger infarction at baseline [66,67].

If left ventricular function is measured early, the myocardium will not have recovered from stunning and, for human or technical reasons, measurements may not be possible in the sickest patients [68]. Moreover, van der Werf [69] has pointed out that because thrombolytic therapy may be particularly beneficial in patients with the largest amount of damaged myocardium, patients with the worst left ventricular function are more likely to survive if a comparison is made among those treated early, and thus who have a preponderance of low ejection fraction.

If left ventricular function is measured later than when recovery from stunning might be expected, a selection bias is introduced because the majority of deaths will already have occurred, eliminating from the study a subgroup with a worse-than-average ejection fraction, with the result that the average ejection fraction of those in whom it is measured becomes misleadingly high. Alternatively, patients with poor function who are treated later may die before the follow-up left ventricular assessment, thus increasing the average ejection fraction value in this group. The final outcome for patients with myocardial infarction who are given thrombolytic therapy at the earliest possible moment will, therefore, comprise the balance of two opposing influences: greater severity of infarction with earlier presentation, but greater efficacy of thrombolytic therapy with earlier administration.

Another parameter in need of consideration is age. Advanced age correlates with increased prehospital time [70], and the elderly also do poorly despite having an infarct size similar to that of younger patients [71]. When many of the early trials of prehospital thrombolytic therapy were performed, eligibility for thrombolytic therapy was not well defined, and an age of more than 70 years generally excluded the individual from prehospital thrombolytic treatment. Administration of thrombolytic drugs to patients older than 70 years has been cautioned against because of a possible higher incidence of major intracranial bleeding [72].

However, many trials have confirmed a possible greater benefit in saving more lives with an acceptable incidence of complications in the aged [1,2,73]. The GUSTO trial actually showed a benefit for those patients older than 75 years of age [74]. Thus, a possible combination of various factors that lead to late arrival in potentially poor survivors, who do get life-saving thrombolytics, may increase the population that otherwise would have died, but have survived, albeit with low ventricular function.

The time window in studies that compare early versus late thrombolysis is a major determinant of ventricular function. In the largest prehospital thrombolytic trial, the EMIP [75], more than one half of patients in the prehospital group received thrombolysis after the first hour of chest pain. Furthermore, in most randomized studies of prehospital thrombolysis, there was considerable overlap in the times of prehospital and in-hospital treatments, and a high proportion of patients in the hospital groups received thrombolytic therapy within 2 hours of symptom onset, that is, at the time of enhanced efficacy. The shortened home-to-hospital delays brought about by conducting these trials prevented demonstrating the benefit of prehospital thrombolysis. In addition, several trials were too small to produce conclusive evidence of benefit.

Thus, although some patients may be treated significantly earlier than others, they may still be in the same time frame in which an appreciable significance may not have been reached. It was only in the GREAT trial, designed and carried out in a rural area, wherein patients were randomly allocated to receive treatment immediately on presentation or after a considerable delay, that the importance of delay could be determined. In this more definitive trial, it was clearly shown that the efficacy of thrombolytic therapy is enhanced when administered within 2 hours of the onset of symptoms.

As noted earlier, the relation between outcome and time of administration of thrombolytic therapy is not a true reflection of its efficacy at different times because the outcome will be biased against manifesting greater efficacy at an earlier time of administration by the greater severity of infarction in patients presenting at that time. This may explain why placebo-controlled trials of thrombolytic therapy have not consistently shown greater benefit with earlier treatment.

In experimental models of coronary reperfusion, brief periods of ischemia may result in marked delays in the recovery of regional left ventricular function [10]. For example, in the canine model 4–7 days may be required for regional wall motion recovery after a 60-minute occlusion and 4 weeks may be required when occlusion lasts for more than 3 hours [13]. This delayed recovery of left ventricular function, termed myocardial *stunning*, has been attributed to alterations in oxidative metabolism, calcium flux, and accumulation of leukocytes within the ischemic myocardium [76–78].

Recovery of function measured at rest is mostly complete within 1 week of occlusion, but improvement in the contractile response to stress may continue for up to 1 month [13]. The same probably applies to humans in whom recovery of global left ventricular function measured at rest is seen within 1 week [79] and is largely accomplished by the time of discharge [80], although recovery may take longer in patients whose left ventricular function is severely depressed [81]. Nevertheless, because the correlation between left ventricular ejection fraction and survival is imperfect [69], some authors have recommended that left ventricular ejection fraction be abandoned as a surrogate mortality endpoint in comparative thrombolytic trials [68].

REGIONAL LEFT VENTRICULAR
EJECTION FRACTION
For the reasons cited earlier, clinical trials using global left ventricular ejection fraction as the sole index of myocardial preservation may underestimate the overall efficacy of the agent under evaluation, while quantitation of infarct-related regional wall motion may provide a more sensitive index of myocardial salvage. However, accurate use of this system requires precise computer-assisted analysis. Nevertheless, in TIMI 1 patients, treatment within 4 hours of the onset of symptoms resulted in greater improvement in regional wall motion abnormalities than treatment given at 4–10 hours [82].

LEFT VENTRICULAR VOLUMES
AND REMODELING
Left ventricular dilatation occurs in up to one third of patients within 6 months of myocardial infarction in the absence of thrombolytic therapy [83]. Dilatation, which is most pronounced in patients with anterior infarction [83,84] and in those with extensive infarct-related regional wall-motion abnormalities,

results from infarct expansion, slippage of myofibrils, and lengthening of the necrotic myocytes. Left ventricular dilation may begin within hours of infarction and progresses during the subsequent weeks to months [83–86].

The magnitude of left ventricular dilatation, shown to have prognostic significance, particularly when the ejection fraction is less than 50% [87], may be ameliorated by early spontaneous or pharmacologically induced coronary reperfusion. Left ventricular volumes measured 1 month after myocardial infarction were unchanged in patients with early reperfusion but increased significantly in those without spontaneous reperfusion [88].

Patients randomized to receive intracoronary streptokinase therapy had significantly lower end-diastolic and end-systolic ventricular volumes 7–10 days after infarction in comparison with those assigned to conservative measures [49,89]. In addition, left ventricular volumes were significantly higher in patients with infarct-artery coronary occlusion than in those with sustained reperfusion [49].

STROKE DISTANCES
Rawles et al. [90], in presenting their data from the GREAT study, used stroke distance, the systolic velocity integral of blood flow, in the aortic arch using a Doppler ultrasound technique, which was shown to be a good and reproducible modality [91] for assessing left ventricular function. This technique, its limitations notwithstanding [92,93], was suggested by the authors because of its benign nature, which allows its performance even on the sickest of patients and may be repeated as often as required. It was shown that mean stroke distance on the last inpatient day was significantly greater in the home-treated group than in the hospital group in the subgroup of patients assigned randomly to treatment within 2 hours, but not in those assigned to treatment after that timeframe.

COMBINED CLINICAL AND
LABORATORY MEASURES
Although clinical indices of left ventricular dysfunction may serve as valuable qualitative endpoints, it is hard to estimate them quantitatively, and an apparently objective attempt to combine clinical, electrocardiographic, and echocardiographic endpoints, as in the GISSI-2 trial [94], resulted in conclusions of limited clinical applicability.

Q-WAVE INFARCTION
Left ventricular function reflects infarct size [95], which, in turn, is reflected in the proportion of pa-

tients with new Q waves. Fewer Q-wave infarctions were observed in those treated early at home [31,90].

Comments

The original salvage paradigm cannot be considered as the single most beneficial mechanism of action of thrombolytic therapy. Surprisingly, survival benefit derived from achieving infarct artery patency several hours after symptom onset, in a time frame beyond which myocardial salvage could be expected, was first demonstrated in the Western Washington Intracoronary Streptokinase Trial [96]. As attractive as it seems, the open-artery hypothesis alone may not explain the survival benefit seen with thrombolytic therapy. A 5-year follow-up in the Netherlands Interuniversity trial [97] did not find arterial patency predictive of outcome; rather, left ventricular function and significant multivessel disease were again the important determinants.

In spite of these uncertainties, a definite impression persists that there is a quantitative, and possibly a qualitative, difference in the patency-left ventricular function survival relationship between patients who receive very early restoration of patency and patients in whom reperfusion is delayed beyond 3 hours or so. In the former, there is a good chance of preserving ventricular function as well as there being a major survival benefit. In the latter, there is still a worthwhile improvement in survival, but permanent ventricular impairment is likely and there is a disparity between survival and functional data. In order to explain this, it is important to remember that both the increase in mortality risk with loss of ventricular function and the loss of myocardium with increasing ischemia time are highly nonlinear functions.

Concluding Remarks

Very early treatment has the potential to maximize the beneficial effects of thrombolytic treatment. The critical issue is time lag rather than place of initiation. The outcome of thrombolytic therapy, wherever applied first, is ultimately the result of the salutary effects of early treatment, on the one hand, and the greater severity of infarction with early presentation, on the other hand. The time effect is not linear and a stepup in efficiency of thrombolytic therapy, when it is given within 2 hours, is especially pronounced within 1 hour of the onset of symptoms.

References

1. GISSI. Long-term effects of intravenous thrombolysis in acute myocardial infarction: Final report of the GISSI study. Lancet 2:871, 1987.
2. ISIS-2 (Second International Study of Infarct Survival) Collaborative Group. Randomised trial of intravenous streptokinase, oral aspirin, both, or neither among 17,187 cases of suspected acute myocardial infarction. Lancet 1:349, 1988.
3. Castaigne AD, Herve C, Duval-Moulin AM, Gaillard M, Dubois-Rande JL, Boesch C, Wolf M, Lellouche D, Jan F, Vernant P, Huguenard P. Prehospital use of APSAC: Results of a placebo-controlled study. Am J Cardiol 64:30A, 1989.
4. National Heart Foundation of Australia Coronary Thrombolysis Group. Coronary thrombolysis and myocardial salvage by tissue plasminogen activator given up to 4 hours after onset of myocardial infarction. Lancet 1:203, 1988. [Published erratum appears in Lancet 27:519, 1988.]
5. White HD, Norris RM, Brown MA, Takayama Morimasa, Maslowski A, Bass NM, Ormiston JA, Whitlock T. Effect of intravenous streptokinase on left ventricular function and early survival after acute myocardial infarction. N Engl J Med 317:850, 1987.
6. Ritchie JL, Davis KB, Williams DL, Caldwell J, Kennedy JW. Global and regional left ventricular function and tomographic radionuclide perfusion: The western Washington intravenous streptokinase in myocardial infarction trial. Circulation 70:867, 1984.
7. Reimer KA, Lowe JE, Rasmussen MM, Jennings RB. The wave front phenomenon of ischemia cell death: Myocardial infarct size vs. duration of coronary occlusion in dogs. Circulation 56:786, 1977.
8. Tennannt R, Wiggers CJ. The effect of coronary occlusion on myocardial contraction. Am J Physiol 112:351, 1935.
9. Blumgart HL, Gilligan R, Schlesinger MJ. Experimental studies on the effect of temporary occlusion of a coronary artery II. The production of myocardial infarction. Am Heart J 22:374, 1941.
10. Heyndrickx GR, Millard RW, McRitchie RJ, Maroko PR, Vatner SF. Regional myocardial functional and electrophysiological alterations after brief coronary artery occlusion in concious dogs. J Clin Invest 56:978, 1975.
11. Jennings RB, Sommers HM, Smyth GA, Flack HA, Linn H. Myocardial necrosis induced by temporary occlusion of a coronary artery in dog. Arch Pathol Lab Med 70:68, 1960.
12. Bergmann SR, Fox KAA, Ludbrook PA. Determinants of salvage of jeopardized myocardium after coronary thrombolysis. Cardiol Clin 5:67, 1987.
13. Lavallee M, Cox D, Patrick TA, Vatner SF. Salvage of myocardial function by coronary artery reperfusion 1, 2 and 3 hours after occlusion in concious dogs. Circ Res 53:235, 1983.
14. Baughman KL, Maroko PR, Vatner SF. Effects of

coronary artery reperfusion on myocardial infarct size and survival in conscious dogs. Circulation 63:317, 1981.

15. Popovic AD, Neskovoic AN, Babic R, Obradovic V, Bozinovic L, Marinkovic J, Lee JC, Tan M, Thomas JD. Independent impact of thrombolytic therapy and vessel patency on left ventricular dilation after myocardial infarction. Serial echocardiographic follow-up. Circulation 90:800, 1994.

16. Lincoff AM, Topol EJ. Trickle down thrombolysis J Am Coll Cardiol 21:1396, 1993.

17. Anderson JL, Karagounis LA, Becker LC, Sorenson SG, Menlove RL, for the TEAM-3 investigators. TIMI perfusion grade 3 but not grade 2 results in improved outcome after thrombolysis for myocardial infarction: Ventriculographic, enzymatic, and electrocardiographic evidence from the TEAM-3 study. Circulation 87:1829, 1993.

18. Hearse DJ, Maxwell L, Saldanha C, Gavin JB. The myocardial vasculature during ischemia and reperfusion: A target for injury and protection. J Mol Cell Cardiol 25:759, 1993.

19. Khaja F, Walton JA, Brymer JF, Lo E, Osterberger L, O'Neill WW, Colfer HT, Weiss R, Lee T, Kurian T, Goldberg D, Pitt B, Goldstein S. Intracoronary fibrinolytic therapy in acute myocardial infarction. Report of a prospective randomized trial. N Engl J Med 308:1305, 1983.

20. Reduto LA, Smalling RW, Freund GC, Gould KL. Intracoronary infusion of streptokinase in patients with acute myocardial infarction: Effects of reperfusion on left ventricular performance. Am J Cardiol 48:403, 1981.

21. Wackers FJ, Berger HJ, Weinberg MA, Zaret BL. Spontaneous changes in left ventricular function over the first 24 hours of acute transmural myocardial infarction: Implications for evaluating early therapeutic interventions. Circulation 66:748, 1982.

22. Sheehan FH, Doerr R, Schmidt WG, Bolson EL, Uebis R, von Essen R, Effert S, Dodge HT. Early recovery of left ventricular function after thrombolytic therapy for acute myocardial infarction: An important determinant of survival. J Am Coll Cardiol 12:289, 1988.

23. Bourdillon PDV, Broderick TM, Williams ES, Davis C, Dillon JC, Armstrong WF, Fineberg N, Ryan T, Feignbaum H. Early recovery of regional left ventricular function after reperfusion in acute myocardial infarction assessed by serial two-dimentional echocardiography. Am J Cardiol 63:641, 1989.

24. Schmidt WG, Sheehan FH, von Essen R, Uebis R, Effert S. Evolution of left ventricular function after intracoronary thrombolysis for acute myocardial infarction. Am J Cardiol 63:497, 1989.

25. Grines CL, O'Neill WW, Anselmo BG, Juni JE, Topol EJ. Comparison of left ventricular function and contractile reserve after successful recannalization by thrombolysis versus rescue percutaneous transluminal coronary angioplasty for acute myocardial infarction. Am J Cardiol 62:352, 1988.

26. Bergmann SR, Lerch RA, Fox KAA, Ludbrook PA, Welch MJ, Ter-Pogossian MM, Sobel BE. Temporal dependence of beneficial effects of coronary thrombolysis characterized by positron tomography. Am J Med 73:573, 1982.

27. Koren G, Weiss AT, Hasin Y, Appelbaum D, Welber S, Rozenman Y, Lotan C, Mosseri M, Sapoznikov D, Luria MH, Gotsman M. Prevention of myocardial damage in acute myocardial ischemia by early treatment with intravenous streptokinase. N Engl J Med 313:1384, 1985.

28. Weiss AT, Fine DG, Appelbaum D, Welber S, Sapoznikov D, Lotan C, Mosseri M, Hasin Y, Gotsman MS. Prehospital coronary thrombolysis: A new strategy in acute myocardial infarction. Chest 92:124, 1987.

29. Villemant D, Barriot P, Riou B, Bodenan P, Brunet F, Noto R, Monsallier JF. Achievement of thrombolysis at home in cases of acute myocardial infarction it [letter]. Lancet 1:228, 1987.

30. Belgian Eminase Prehospital Study (BEPS) Cooperative Group. Prehospital thrombolysis in acute myocardial infarction. The Belgian Eminase Prehospital Study (BEPS) Eur Heart J 12:965, 1991.

31. Roth A, Barbash GI, Hod H, Miller HI, Rath S, Modan M, Har-Zahav Y, Keren G, Bassan S, Kaplinsky E, Laniado S. Should thrombolytic therapy be administered in the mobile intensive care unit in patients with evolving myocardial infarction? A pilot study. J Am Coll Cardiol 15:932, 1990.

32. Schofer J, Buttner J, Geng G, Gutschmidt K, Herden HN, Mathey DG, Moecke HP, Ploster P, Raftopoulo A, Sheehan FH, Voelz P. Prehospital thrombolysis in acute myocardial infarction. Am J Cardiology 66:1429, 1990.

33. The ISAM Study Group. A prospective trial of intravenous streptokinase in acute myocardial infarction (ISAM). N Engl J Med 314:1465, 1986.

34. Simoons ML, Serruys PW, van den Brand M, Res J, Verheugt PW, Krauss XH, Remme WJ, Bar F, de Zwaan C, van der Laarse, Vermeer F, Lubsen J, for the working group on thrombolytic therapy in acute myocardial infarction of the Netherlands interuniversity cardiology instituite. Early thrombolysis in acute myocardial infarction: Limitation of infarct size and improved survival. J Am Coll Cardiol 7:717, 1986.

35. Van de Werf F. Lessons from the European Cooperative Recombinant Tissue-Type Plasminogen Activator (rt-PA) Versus Placebo Trial. J Am Coll Cardiol 12:14A, 1988.

36. McNeill AJ, Cunningham SR, Flannery DJ, Dalzell GW, Wilson CM, Campbell NP, Khan MM, Patterson GC, Webb SW, Adgey AA. A double blind placebo controlled study of early and late administration of recombinant tissue plasminogen activator in acute myocardial infarction. Br Heart J 61:316, 1989.

37. Hermens WT, Willems GM, Nijssen KM, Simoons ML. Effect of thrombolytic treatment delay on myocardial infarct size [letter]. Lancet 340:1297, 1992.

38. Mathey DG, Sheehan FH, Schofer J, Dodge HT. Time

from onset of symptoms to thrombolytic therapy: A major determinant of myocardial salvage in patients with acute transmural infarction J Am Coll Cardiol 6:518, 1985.

39. Linderer T, Schroder R, Arntz R, Heineking ML, Wunderlich W, Kohl K, Forycki F, Henzgen R, Wagner J. Prehospital thrombolysis: Beneficial effect of very early treatment on infarct size and left ventricular function. J Am Coll Cardiol 22:1304, 1993.

40. Weaver WD, Cerqueira M, Hallstrom AP, Litwin PE, Martin JS, Kudenchuk PJ, Eisenberg M. For the Myocardial Infarction Triage and Intervention Project Group. Prehospital-initiated vs hospital-initiated thrombolytic therapy. JAMA 270:1211, 1993.

41. Ritchie JL, Cerqueira M, Maynard C, Davis K, Kennedy JW. Ventricular function and infarct size: The western Washington intravenous streptokinase in myocardial infarction trial. J Am Coll Cardiol 11:689, 1988.

42. Maynard C, Althouse R, Olsufka M, Ritchie JL, Davis KB, Kennedy W. Early versus late hospital arrival for acute myocardial infarction in the Western Washignton Thrombolytic therapy trials. Am J Cardiol 63:1296, 1989.

43. Armstrong PW, Baigrie RS, Daly PA, Haq A, Gent M, Roberts RS, Freeman MR, Burns R, Liu P, Morgan CD. Tissue plasminogen activator: Toronto (TPAT) placebo-controlled randomization trial in acute myocardial infarction. J Am Coll Cardiol 13:1469, 1989.

44. Bassand JP, Cassagnes J, Machecourt J, Lusson JR, Anguenot T, Wolf JE, Maublant J, Bertrand B, Schiele F. Comparative effects of APSAC and rt-PA on infarct size and left ventricular function circulation 84:1107, 1991.

45. Cerqueira MD, Maynard C, Ritchie JL. Radionuclide assessment of infarct size and left ventricular function in clinical trials of thrombolysis. Circulation 84:1100, 1991.

46. Norris RM, White HD. Therapeutic trials in coronary thrombosis should measure left ventricular function as primary end-point of treatment. Lancet 1:104, 1988.

47. Schwarz F, Schler G, Katus H, Hofmann M, Manthey J, Tillmanns H, Mehmel HC, Kubler W. Intracoronary thrombolysis in acute myocardial infarction: Duration of ischemia as a major determinant of late results after recanalization. Am J Cardiol 50:933, 1982.

48. Schroder R, Biamino G, von Leitner ER, Linderer T, Bruggemann T, Heitz J, Vohringer HF, Wegscheider K. Intravenous short-term infusion of streptokinase in acute myocardiial infarction. Circulation 67:536, 1983.

49. Serruys PW, Simoons ML, Suryapranata H, Vermeer F, Wijns W, van den Brand M, Bar F, Zwaan C, Krauss XH, Remme WJ, Res J, Verheught FWA, van Domburg R, Lubsen J, Hugenholtz PG, for the working group on thrombolytic therapy in acute myocardial infarction of the Netherlands interuniversity cardiol-

ogy instituite. Preservation of global and regional left ventricular function after early thrombolysis in acute myocardial infarction. J Am Coll Cardiol 7:729, 1986.

50. Rogers WJ, Hood WP, Mantle JA, Baxley WA, Kirklin JK, Zorn GL, Nath HP. Return of left ventricular function after reperfusion in patients with myocardial infarction: Importance of subtotal stenosis or collaterals. J Am Coll Cardiol 69:338, 1984.

51. Marzoll U, Kleiman NS, Dunn JK, Verani MS, Minor ST, Roberts R, Raizner AE. Factors determining improvement in left ventricular function after reperfusion therapy for acute myocardial infarction: Primacy of baseline ejection fraction. J Am Coll Cardiol 17:613, 1991.

52. Topol EJ, Bates ER, Walton Jr. JA, Baumann G, Wolfe S, Maino J, Bayer L, Gorman L, Kline EM, O'Neill WW, Pitt B. Community hospital administration of intravenous tissue plasminogen activator in acute myocardial infarction: Improved timing, thrombolytic efficacy and ventricular function. J Am Coll Cardiol 10:1173, 1987.

53. Fine DG, Weiss AT, Sapoznikov D, Welber S, Applebaum D, Lotan C, Hasin Y, Ben-David Y, Koren G, Gotsman MS. Importance of early initiation of intravenous streptokinase therapy for acute myocardial infarction. Am J Cardiol 58:411, 1986.

54. Guerci AD, Gerstenblith G, Brinker JA, Chandra NC, Gottlieb SO, Bahr RD, Weiss JL, Shapiro EP, Flaherty JT, Bush DE, Chew PH, Gottlieb SH, Halperin HR, Ouyang P, Walford GD, Beli WR, Fatterpaker AK, Llwellyn M, Topol EJ, Healy B, Siu CO, Becker LC, Weisfeld ML. A randomized trial of intravenous tissue plasminogen activator for acute myocardial infarction with subsequent randomization to elective coronary angioplasty. N Engl J Med 317:1613, 1987.

55. Van de Werf F, Arnold AE. Intravenous tissue plasminogen activator and size of infarct, left ventricular function, and survival in acute myocardial infarction. Br Med J 297:1374, 1988.

56. O'Rourke M, Baron D, Keogh A, Kelly R, Nelson G, Barnes C, Raftos J, Graham K, Hillman K, Newman H, Healy J, Woolridge J, Rivers J, White H, Whitlock R, Norris R. Limitation of myocardial infarction by early infusion of recombinant tissue-type plasminogen activator. Circulation 77:1311, 1988.

57. Kennedy JW, Martin GV, Davis KB, Maynard C, Stadius M, Sheehan FH, Ritchie JL. The Western Washington Intravenous Streptokinase in Acute Myocardial Infarction Randomized Trial [Published erratum appears in Circulation 77:1037, 1988.] Circulation 77:345, 1988.

58. Bassand JP, Machecourt J, Cassagnes J, Anquenot T, Lusson R, Borel E, Peycelon P, Wolf E, Ducellier D. Multicentric trial of intravenous anisoylated plasminogen streptokinase activator complex (APSAC) in acute myocardial infarction: Effects on size and left ventricular function. J Am Coll Cardiol 13:988, 1989.

59. Barbash GI, Roth A, Hod H, Miller H, Modan M, Rath S, Har-Zahav Y, Shachar A, Basan S, Batler A,

Rabinowitz B, Kaplinsky E, Seligsohn U, Laniado S. Improved survival but not left ventricular function with early and pre-hospitsal treatment with tissue plasminogen activator in acute myocardial infarction. Am J Cardiol 66:261, 1990.

60. Sheehan FH. Left ventricular dysfunction in acute myocardial infarction due to isolated left circumflex coronary artery stenosis. Am J Cardiol 64:440, 1989.

61. The TIMI Research Group. Immediate vs. delayed catheterization and angiography following thrombolytic therapy for acute myocardial infarction. TIMI IIA results. JAMA 260:2849, 1988.

62. White HD, Rivers JT, Maslowski AH, Ormiston JA, Takayama M, Hart HH, Sharpe DN, Whitlock RML, Noris RM. Effect of intravenous streptokinase as compared with that of tissue plasminogen activator on left ventricular function after first myocardial infarction. N Engl J Med 320:817, 1989.

63. Sheehan FH, Mathey DG, Schofer J, Krebber HJ, Dodge HT. Effect of interventions in salvaging left ventricular function in acute myocardial infarction: A study of intracoronary streptokinase. Am J Cardiol 52:431, 1983.

64. Stack RS, Phillips HR, Grierson DS, Behar VS, Kong Y, Peter RH, Swain JL, Greenfield JC Jr. Functional improvement of jeopardized myocardium following intracoronary streptokinase infusion in acute myocardial infarction. J Clin Invest 72:84, 1983.

65. Rawles JM, Metcalf MJ, Shirreffs C, Jennings K, Kenmure ACE. Association of patient delay with symptoms, cardiac enzymes, and outcome in acute myocardial infarction. Eur Heart J 11:643, 1990.

66. Willems JL, Wilems RJ, Willems GM. Arnold AE, Van de Werf F, Verstraete M for the European Cooperative Study Group for Recombinant Tissue-Type Plasminogen Activator. Significance of initial ST segment elevation and depression for management of thrombolytic therapy in acute myocardial infarction. Circulation 82:1147, 1990.

67. Schroder R, Linderer T, Briggemann T, Neuhaus KL, Tebbe U, Wegscheider K. Controversial indications. Rational for thrombolysis: Later than 4–6h from symptom onset, and in patients with smaller myocardial infarction. Eur Heart J 11:19, 1990.

68. Califf RM, Harrelson-Woodlief L, Topol EJ. Left ventricular ejection fraction may not be useful as an end point of thrombolytic therapy comparative trials. Circulation 82:1847, 1990.

69. Van de Werf F. Discrepancies between the effects of coronary reperfusion on survival and left ventricular function. Lancet 1:1367, 1989.

70. Schmidt SB, Borsch MA. The prehospital phase of acute myocardial infarction in the era of thrombolysis. Am J Cardiol 65:1411, 1990.

71. Maggioni AP, Maseri A, Fresco C, Franzosi MG, Mauri F, Santoro E, Tognoni G on behalf of GISSI-2. Age related increase in mortality among patients with first myocardial infarction treated with thrombolysis. N Engl J Med 329:1442, 1993.

72. Braunwald E. Optimizing thrombolytic therapy of acute myocardial infarction. Circulation 82:1510, 1990.

73. Fibrinolytic Therapy Trialists Collaborative Group. Indications for fibrinolytic therapy in suspected acute myocardial infarction: Collaborative overview of early mortality and major morbidity results from all randomised trials over 1000 patients. Lancet 343:311, 1994.

74. The GUSTO investigators. An international randomized trial comparing four thrombolytic strategies for acute myocardial infarction. N Engl J Med 329:673, 1993.

75. Prehospital thrombolytic therapy in patients with suspected acute myocardial infarction. The European Myocardial Infarction Project Group. N Engl J Med 329:383, 1993.

76. Sheehan FH. Determinants of improved left ventricular function after thrombolytic therapy in acute myocardial infarction. J Am Coll Cardiol 9:937, 1987.

77. Braunwald E, Kloner RA. The stunned myocardium: Prolonged, postischemic ventricular dysfunction. Circulation 66:1146, 1982.

78. Kloner RA, Przyklenk K, Petel B. Altered myocardial status. The stunned and hibernating myocardium. Am J Med 86:14A, 1989.

79. Sheehan FH, Thery C, Durand P, Bertrand ME, Bolson EL. Early beneficial effect of streptokinase on left ventricular function in acute myocardial infarction. Am J Cardiol 67:555, 1991.

80. Henzlova MJ, Bourge RC, Papaietro SE, Maske LE, Morgan TE, Tauxe L, Rogers WJ. Long-term effect of thrombolytic therapy on left ventricular ejection fraction after acute myocardial infarction. Am J Cardiol 67:1354, 1991.

81. Pfisterer M, Zuber M, Wenzel R, Burkart F. Prolonged myocardial stunning after thrombolysis: Can left ventricular function be assessed definitely at hospital discharge? Eur Heart J 12:214, 1991.

82. Sheehan FH, Braunwald E, Canner P, Dodge HT, Gore J, Van Natta P, Passamani ER, Williams DO, Zaret B. The effect of intravenous thrombolytic therapy on left ventricular function: A report on tissue-type plasminogen activator and streptokinase from the Thrombolysis in Myocardial Infarction (TIMI Phase I) trial. Circulation 755:817, 1987.

83. Jeremy RW, Allman KC, Bautovitch G, Harris PJ. Patterns of left ventricular dilatation during the six months after myocardial infarction. J Am Coll Cardiol 13:304, 1989.

84. Seals AA, Pratt CM, Mahmarian JJ, Tadros S, Kleiman N, Roberts R, Verani MS. Relation of left ventricular dilation during acute myocardial infarction to systolic performance, diastolic dysfunction, infarct size and location. Am J Cardiol 61:224, 1988.

85. McKay RG, Pfeffer MA, Pasternak RC, Markis JE, Comep C, Nakao S, Alderman JD, Ferguson JJ, Safian RD, Grossman W. Left ventricular remodeling after

myocardial infarction: A corollary to infarct expansion. Circulation 74:693, 1986.

86. Warren SE, Royal HD, Markis JE, Grossman W, McKay RG. Time course of left ventricular dilation after myocardial infarction: Influence of infarct-related artery and success of coronary thrombolysis. J Am Coll Cardiol 11:12, 1988.

87. White HD, Norris RM, Brown MA, Brandt PWT, Whitlock RML, Wild CJ. Left ventricular end-systolic volume as the major determinant of survival after recovery from myocardial infarction. Circulation 76:44, 1987.

88. Shen WF, Cui LQ, Gong LS, Lesbre JP. Beneficial effect of residual flow to the infarct region on left ventricular volume changes after acute myocardial infarction. Am Heart J 119:525, 1990.

89. van der Laarse A, Kerkhof PLM, Vermer F, Serruys PW, Hermes WMT, van der Wall EE, Simoons ML, for the working group on thrombolytic therapy in acute myocardial infarction of the Netherlands interuniversity cardiology instituite. Relation between infarct size and left ventricular performance assessed in patients with first acute myocardial infarction randomized to intracoronary thrombolytic therapy or to conventional treatment. Am J Cardiol 61:1, 1988.

90. Rawles JM, on behalf of the GREAT group. Recovery of left ventricular function after acute myocardial infarction: Efficacy of domiciliary thrombolysis in the Grampian Region Early Anistreplase Trial. Cor Art Dis 4:801, 1993.

91. Mowat DHR, Haites NE, Rawles JM. Aortic blood velocity measurement in healthy adults using a simple ultrasound technique. Cardiovasc Res 17:75, 1983.

92. Haites NE, McLennan FM, Mowat DHR, Rawles JM. Assessment of cardiac output by the Doppler ultrasound technique alone. Br Heart J 53:123, 1985.

93. Metcalfe MJ, Rawles JM. Stroke distance in acute myocardial infarction: A simple measurment of left ventricular function. Lancet 1:1371, 1989.

94. Gruppo Italiano per lo Studio della Streptochinasi nell'Infarto Miocardico (GISSI-2). A factorial randomised trial of alteplase versus streptokinase and heparin versus no heparin among 12,490 patients with acute myocardial infarction. Lancet 336:65, 1990.

95. Christian TF, Behrenbeck T, Gersh BJ, Gibbons RJ. One year after acute myocardial infarction to infarct size determined by technetium-99m sestamibi. Am J Cardiol 68:21, 1991.

96. Kennedy JW, Ritchie JL, Davis KB, Stadius ML, Maynard C, Fritz JK. The Western Washington randomized trial of intracoronary streptokinase in acute myocardial infarction. A 12-month follow-up report. N Engl J Med 312:1073, 1985.

97. Simoons ML, Vos J, Tijssen JGP, Vermeer F, Verheught F, Krauss AK. Long-term benefit of early thrombolytic therapy in patients with acute MI. 5-year follow-up of trial conduction by the Interuniversity Cardiology Institute of the Netherlands. J Am Coll Cardiol 14:1609, 1989.

28. PATIENT SELECTION FOR THROMBOLYTIC THERAPY FOR EVOLVING MYOCARDIAL INFARCTION

Alfred E.R. Arnold, Eric Boersma, Maureen van der Vlugt, and Maarten L. Simoons

From Clinical Trial to Individual Patient

"ONE REGIMEN FITS ALL?"

Initially, investigators recommended a "standard" thrombolytic regimen for all patients with evolving myocardial infarction [1,2]. Although thrombolytic therapy will be beneficial in most patients with evolving myocardial infarction, the overall results of clinical trials are not directly applicable to all individual patients [3,4]. Complying with the inclusion criteria of the thrombolysis trials is not enough because patients included in the trials are heterogeneous regarding their profile of both cardiac and bleeding risks. Let us focus on a patient with an evolving myocardial infarction who is at very low risk for death without thrombolytic therapy for example, 1–2% in the first year. He will probably not benefit from thrombolytic therapy because mortality reduction is maximally 0.5–1 per hundred patients treated and is likely to be offset by intracranial bleeding in 0.5–2% patients, 50% of which are lethal [5–9]. Therefore, careful weighing of the benefits and risks in individual patients is necessary, especially in patients with risk factors for intracerebral bleeding with little expected benefit from thrombolytic therapy.

IN WHICH PATIENTS SHOULD THROMBOLYTIC THERAPY BE CONSIDERED?

In early thrombolysis trials, evolving myocardial infarction was defined as prolonged chest pain (more than 30 minutes) with ST-segment elevation suggesting transmural infarction on the admission electrocardiogram [10,11]. No specific electrocardiographic patterns were required in the ISIS trial [5] and in ASSET [6]. In these trials the prognosis of patients with a normal admission ECG was good, with no apparent benefit from thrombolytic therapy. This group may include patients without acute thrombotic occlusion and with nonischemic chest pain. In patients with ST-segment depression, the prognosis is poor, with 19% mortality in the first 5 weeks, but was not improved by thrombolytic therapy [5]. Apparently, the pathophysiology in these patients is different, and most of these patients probably have no occlusive intracoronary thrombus that might be resolved by thrombolytic therapy. On the other hand, patients with complete bundle branch block (left or right) are at increased risk with a 5-week mortality of 23.6% in the collaborative overview of the Fibrinolytic Therapy Trialists Group and do benefit from thrombolytic therapy [3]. Therefore, thrombolytic therapy should be considered in patients with ST-segment elevation or complete bundle branch block.

WHICH THERAPEUTIC OPTIONS SHOULD BE CONSIDERED?

The therapeutic options for reperfusion strategies are listed in Table 28-1, with a semiquantitative summary of efficacy, bleeding risk, and costs. Inceasing efficacy runs parallel to higher costs and more complex logistics (direct PTCA).

Aspirin. Aspirin produces a 21% reduction in mortality independent of the effect of thrombolytic therapy [5]. Unlike thrombolytic therapy, there is no clear relation between treatment delay and treatment effect for aspirin, possibly because it acts primarily by preventing reocclusion [12]. Because aspirin in a dose of 80–160 mg is associated with few side effects and is also effective in patients with unstable angina, all patients with suspected myocardial infarction should receive aspirin, irrespective of the admission electrocardiogram.

TABLE 28-1. Reperfusion strategies for
patients with evolving myocardial
infarction (in order of increasing intensity)

Strategy	Benefit	Bleeding risk	Costs
1. None	−	−	−
2. ASA	+	+/−	−
3. ASA + SK	++	+	+
4. ASA + alteplase	+++	++	+++
5. ASA + direct PTCA	++++	+/−	++++

ASA = acetylsalicylic acid (aspirin); SK = streptokinase; PTCA = percutaneous transluminal coronary angioplasts.

Intravenous Heparin. The value of intravenous heparin in patients with evolving transmural myocardial
infarction who do not receive thrombolytic therapy is
still unknown, but its administration should be recommended in patients with a large area at risk to
prevent left ventricular thrombi. In patients receiving
streptokinase, heparin did not improve the clinical
outcome [13]. In the setting of alteplase administration, however, coronary patency was better in patients
receiving intravenous heparin [14].

Various intravenous regimens of thrombolytic
therapy have been tested using different thrombolytic
agents (streptokinase, alteplase, anistreptase, and
urokinase) [5,6,10,11,15–17]. Two large trials,
GISSI-2 and ISIS-3, compared the first three agents,
and no difference in survival rates was found [18–20].
In contrast, in the GUSTO trial, a further reduction
in mortality was observed by an accelerated alteplase
regimen with aspirin and intravenous heparin [13].
This additional benefit of alteplase was related to
superior early coronary patency. Indeed, other studies
have emphasized the need for adequate heparinization
to maintain coronary patency in patients receiving
alteplase [14,21]. Other regimens of thrombolytic
therapy, with and without new antithrombin or
antiplatelet therapy, are currently under investigation. The clinical benefit, of these approaches have yet
to be determined and are not relevant for clinical
practice.

*Percutaneous Transluminal Coronary Angioplasty
(PTCA).* Routine immediate PTCA is not beneficial
when performed in combination with thrombolytic
therapy [22,23], due to early reocclusion and recurrent ischemia [24]. The role of angioplasty in patients
with failed reperfusion after thrombolytic therapy
(rescue PTCA) has been poorly studied. According to
the RESCUE trial (n = 151), this strategy may be

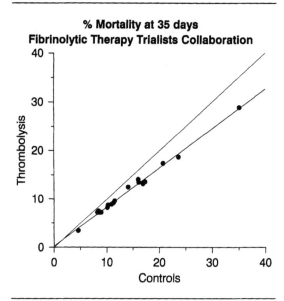

FIGURE 28-1. Regression line representing the relation
between mortality in thrombolysis patients and among controls in various subgroups of 58,600 patients of the Fibrinolytic Therapy Trialists Collaborative Group [3]. The
number of deaths prevented in the first 35 days after myocardial infarction per hundred patients treated is proportional to the mortality in the control group (= cardiac
baseline risk).

beneficial within 8 hours after the start of thrombolytic therapy, with a better late ejection fraction on
exercise, less mortality (5.1% vs. 9.6%), and less severe heart failure (1.3% vs. 7.0) [25]. In the TAMI-5
trial (n = 575), a composite clinical endpoint (death,
stroke, heart failure, reinfarction, reocclusion, or recurrent ischemia) occurred less frequently in patients
with an aggressive strategy with rescue PTCA than
without it (33% vs. 45%) [26]. Direct PTCA with
aspirin and heparin, but without thrombolytic
therapy, was shown to be promising [27,28] and is
the strategy of choice in patients with the largest
expected benefit of reperfusion therapy and/or excessive bleeding risk.

THERAPEUTIC PROFILE OF
REPERFUSION THERAPY
The interplay between cardiac baseline risk and the
benefit of thrombolytic therapy is illustrated in Figure 28-1 for the pooled analysis of the Fibrinolytic
Therapy Trialists Collaborative Group [3]. The
baseline risk for various subsets of patients varies
considerably, and the benefit is directly proportional

TABLE 28-2. Prediction of 1-year mortality after myocardial infarction and number of deaths prevented during the first year of follow-up per hundred patients treated with thrombolytic therapy [32]

No. of risk factors	Prevalence (%)	ST-segment deviation ≥2.0 m Vᵃ	Probability of death (%) in 1st year without thrombolysis	No. of deaths prevented in 1st year per 100 patients treated		
				<3 hours	3–6 hours	6–12 hours
None	25	−	3.1 (1.9–5.2)	1.6	0.8	0.4
		+	4.5 (2.6–7.6)	2.2	1.1	0.6
1	42	−	6.9 (4.7–10.1)	3.5	1.7	0.9
		+	9.8 (6.6–14.4)	4.9	2.4	1.2
2	24	−	15.6 (10.8–21.9)	7.8	3.9	1.9
		+	21.3 (14.9–29.3)	10.6	5.3	2.7
3+	9	−	35.2 (25.4–46.4)	17.6	8.8	4.4
		+	44.3 (33.0–56.3)	22.2	11.1	5.5
Relative mortality reduction (%)				50%	25%	12.5%

Probability of death without thrombolysis predicted from the following risk factors: age greater than 60 years, a history of previous infarction, anterior localization of the current infarct, heart failure on admission, QRS duration ≥120 ms, and total ST-segment deviation in admission ECG. Increased survival with thrombolytic therapy was predicted from these data, assuming 50%, 25%, and 12.5% mortality reduction for treatment within 3, 3–6, and 6–12 hours after the onset of symptoms.
3+ indicates three or more risk factors; −, absent; and +, present.

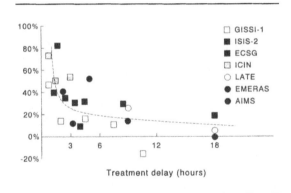

FIGURE 28-2. Mortality reduction by thrombolysis in the major placebo-controlled mortality trials as a function of treatment delay. The dotted curvilinear line represents the assumed relation based on animal experiments.

to that baseline risk in a large spectrum of cardiac baseline risk. In the Fibrinolytic Therapy Trialists Collaborative Group analysis, patients with a blood pressure under 100 mmHg on hospital admission had the highest mortality (35.1% at 5 weeks in the control group), with the same proportional mortality reduction as in the other subgroups. In GISSI-1, pa-

tients with Killip IV had 72.4% mortality without benefit of thrombolytic therapy. It might, therefore, be the case that for the highest levels of cardiac baseline risk, the proportional mortality does not hold. In all age categories up to 75 years, mortality reduction was proportional [3]. For patients above 75 years, the relative and absolute mortality reduction was less [3]. An excess of strokes in 0.8% of patients ≥75 years in the thrombolysis group provided only a partial explanation [3]. Another factor is the higher prevalence of complicating illness [29]. Also, for alteplase relative to streptokinase, such a proportional mortality reduction (more benefit in high-risk subgroups) was found in the GUSTO-1 trial [13].

TIME DELAY FROM ONSET OF SYMPTOMS
TO START OF REPERFUSION TREATMENT
The number of cardiac deaths prevented in the first year per hundred patients treated is strongly related to the time from onset of symptoms to the start of thrombolytic treatment (Figure 28-2) [30]. The benefit of reperfusion therapy 12–24 hours after the onset of symptoms is small and is only relevant in patients with ongoing ischemia [5,31]. There is evidence that the additional benefit of up to 50% mortality reduction might be achieved by very early treatment (the "first golden hour") [10,11,15].

It should be noted that the patient characteristics in the subgroup analyses that were used in Figure 28-2 differ between those with a short treatment delay (patients with large infarcts) and those who were treated later (older patients) [29]. Therefore, for a reliable assessment of the relation between treatment delay and mortality reduction, trials randomizing between early and late treatment are needed. Such trials are available in the setting of prehospital versus in-hospital thrombolysis, but the information contained in these trials is limited due to their small size. In Table 28-2 is given a quick reference to the number of cardiac deaths prevented in the first year per hundred patients treated with reperfusion therapy for several categories of treatment delay.

NEED FOR AN INDIVIDUALIZED APPROACH

As outlined earlier, a multifactorial approach is needed to the candidate for reperfusion therapy. A clinician should decide whether reperfusion therapy should be given. This decision should be based on the expected benefit of thrombolytic treatment, the risk of intracranial bleeding, and economic and logistic considerations. In addition, one should decide which reperfusion regimen (streptokinase, alteplase, or direct PTCA) should be given and whether rescue PTCA should be attempted in the case of thrombolytic therapy failure. To integrate all these variables a stepwise approach called *tailored thrombolytic therapy*, was proposed [32], of the various steps which are described later. Tailored thrombolytic therapy provides the means to score the expected benefit of each patient and to assign, in a consistent manner, the most costly and most benificial strategies to those patients with most expected benefit.

Tailored Thrombolytic Therapy

STEP 1: ASSESS BENEFITS OF THROMBOLYTIC THERAPY FROM PATIENT CHARACTERISTICS, THE ESTIMATED MYOCARDIAL AREA AT RISK, AND TREATMENT DELAY (Figure 28-3)

Demographics. Important determinants of survival after acute myocardial infarction are demographics such as age, sex, and impaired left ventricular function due to previous infarctions [5]. Although these parameters cannot be altered by thrombolytic therapy, the number of patients in whom death is prevented by thrombolytic therapy is greater in subgroups with a higher mortality (see Figure 28-1). Therefore, these demographics are important predictors of the benefit of thrombolytic therapy.

Myocardial Area at Risk for Necrosis. In patients with evolving myocardial infarction, part of the ischemic myocardium can be salvaged by timely reopening of the coronary artery. The amount of myo-

Step 1: Estimate benefit of thrombolytic therapy

Assess the number of cardiac risk factors   no   yes
   previous infarction
   anterior localization
   inferior + RV infarction (ST elevation in V4R)
   QRS >120 msec
   heart failure
                number of cardiac risk factors

Number of cardiac risk factors	ST dev >=2.0mV	Life exp (yrs) without therapy	Benefit, expected life months added by reperfusion therapy		
			<3hrs	3-6hrs	6-12hrs
Age <50 yrs					
0	no	13.6	3	1	0
0	yes	13.4	4	2	<1
1	no	13.1	7	3	1
1	yes	12.7	10	5	2
2	no	10.8	15	7	3
2	yes	10.1	20	10	5
3+	no	7.7	30	15	7
3+	yes	6.7	39	19	9
Age 50-59 yrs					
0	no	11.6	2	<1	0
0	yes	11.5	3	1	0
1	no	11.2	5	2	<1
1	yes	10.9	7	3	1
2	no	9.4	10	5	2
2	yes	8.8	14	7	3
3+	no	6.8	21	11	5
3+	yes	5.9	27	13	6
Age 60-69 yrs					
0	no	8.8	2	<1	0
0	yes	8.6	3	1	0
1	no	7.6	6	3	1
1	yes	7.1	8	4	1
2+	no	5.6	12	6	3
2+	yes	4.9	16	8	3
Age 70-79 yrs					
0	no	5.5	2	<1	0
0	yes	5.1	3	1	0
1+	no	4.2	5	2	<1
1+	yes	3.6	7	3	1

FIGURE 28-3. Schematic representation of the first step of tailored thrombolytic therapy: Estimation of the benefit of thrombolytic therapy. The cardiac baseline risk of a patient is given in terms of "life expectancy without therapy." The benefit of thrombolytic therapy is expressed in months of life expectancy and depends on the age of the patient, the number of cardiac risk factors present at baseline, the amount of ST-segment elevation and depression in the J-point of the baseline electrocardiogram. The life expectancy without therapy and the benefit of thrombolytic therapy are discounted at 5% to account for patients' preference for early life years in comparison with life years in the distant future. (Data are derived from Boersma et al. [30] and Simoons et al. [32].)

cardium saved depends on the territory that is ischemic, which can be measured from the amount of ST-segment elevation or the number of leads with ST-segment elevation [33,34].

Prognosis After Myocardial Infarction With and Without Thrombolysis. A model to predict 1-year mortality after myocardial infarction was derived from a combined analysis of data from 3179 patients in the ICIN, ECSG, and ISAM studies. In a multivariate analysis, advanced age, a history of previous infarction, anterior location of the current infarct, heart failure during admission, intraventricular conduction delay, and the sum of ST-segment deviation on the admission ECG were identified as predictors of 1-year mortality without thrombolysis [32]. This prediction model is summarized in Table 28-2. This is the only recent prediction model for patients not treated with thrombolytic therapy. Other prediction models proved to be very similar when the effect of thrombolytic therapy was taken into account [35, 36].

Proportional Mortality Reduction. In many thrombolysis trials, the benefit of thrombolytic therapy was proportional to the baseline risk of the patients (see Figure 28-1). Patients with a low baseline risk have little benefit, and patients with a high baseline risk have a large benefit. This was also found for other treatment modalities, such as secondary prevention with beta-blocker therapy after myocardial infarction [37], coronary bypass surgery for angina pectoris [38], and carotid surgery for transient ischemic attacks [39].

One-Year Mortality versus Life Expectancy. Initially, 1-year mortality was chosen in this analysis because lifelong follow-up is not yet available for thrombolysis trials. However, 1-year mortality has the disadvantage that the benefit in older patients is overestimated because the large 1-year benefit lasts only for a few years due to the limited life expectancy in that subgroup. Life expectancies have been calculated assuming that the survival curves of myocardial infarction patients with and without thrombolytic therapy run parallel after the first year, exceeding the mortality rates of the normal reference populations with a constant difference [30]. In clinical decision analysis, it is customary to discount future life years at 5% per year to account for the greater value of the near future. The assessment of benefit of thrombolytic therapy based on discounted life expectancy is summarized in Figure 28-3.

STEP 2: ASSESS THE RISKS OF THROMBOLYTIC THERAPY (Figure 28-4)

Contraindications. The risks of thrombolytic therapy are mainly bleeding risks. Contraindications to the use of thrombolytic therapy are listed in Figure 28-4. The quantitative contribution of these factors to the risk of life-threatening bleeding is still unknown but

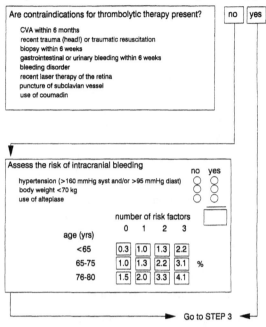

FIGURE 28-4. Flow chart for step 2: Assessment of the risk of thrombolytic therapy. All generally accepted contraindications for thrombolytic therapy are related to bleeding complication, the extent of which is unknown. If one or more contraindications are present, the risk of thrombolytic therapy is assumed to outweigh the benefits (go immediately to step 3). If no contraindication for thrombolytic therapy is present, estimate the intracerebral bleeding risk specifically for age, blood pressure on admission, body weight, and use of alteplase.

is assumed to be too high to allow for the application of thrombolytic therapy.

Overall Incidence of Intracerebral Bleeding. In a pooled analysis of thrombolysis trials, the incidence of intracranial bleeding after thrombolytic therapy was 0.2% for intravenous streptokinase and 0.5% for alteplase [7]. According to a registry of 61 hospitals in The Netherlands, intracranial bleeding occurred in 1% of patients [7]. This difference indicates that the population in the clinical trials was more selected.

Risk Factors for Intracerebral Bleeding. Intracranial bleeding risk depends on the absence or presence of the following risk factors: older age, low body weight, hypertension on admission, and the use of alteplase [8]. The age-specific risk of intracranial bleeding is listed in Figure 28-4 for patients without risk factors and with one or more of these risk factors. Intracranial hemorrhage is lethal in 50% of patients in the first few days after its occurrence [5–9].

STEP 3: SELECTION OF A REPERFUSION STRATEGY (Figure 28-5)

Net Benefits of Thrombolytic Therapy. The benefit of thrombolytic therapy is the net effect of a reduction in cardiac death and an increase in death due to intracranial bleeding, with the latter being small, except when one or more risk factors for bleeding are present [7,8].

Allocation of Limited Health Care Resources. Because the financial resources in health care are restricted, the most costly (and most effective)

strategies should be allocated to patients who are expected to benefit most of the treatment. The proposed stepwise approach was tested in clinical practice in 500 consecutive patients [30]. Patients with very little expected net benefit from thrombolytic therapy were treated with aspirin only (10% of patients). The 20% of patients with the largest expected net benefit and/or at increased bleeding risk were treated with direct angioplasty. The remaining 70% of patients were treated with thrombolytic therapy — half with streptokinase (lower expected benefit) and half with alteplase (higher expected benefit).

The thresholds for expected benefit in Figure 28-5 can be adjusted to local circumstances, depending on the availability of the various treatment strategies. Two scenarios are given. If one chooses for the first option, direct PTCA is performed in 30% of patients. The second option results in direct PTCA in 16%, as was shown in our hospitals in over 700 patients with acute myocardial infarction. However, with option 2 a specific subset of patients with a high bleeding risk is still treated with intravenous streptokinase.

STEP 4: MONITOR EFFECT OF INTERVENTION BY CONTINUOUS ST-SEGMENT RECORDING (Table 28-3)

ST-Segment Monitoring Systems. The effect of thrombolytic therapy can be assessed safely with immediate coronary angiography, even shortly after hospital admission (90 minutes). However, this approach is cumbersome, and a laboratory for coronary angiography is not always available. Continuous multilead ST-segment monitoring is a safe, rather inexpensive way to predict reperfusion, persistent and recurrent ischemia in patients with evolving myocardial infarction [40–42]. Three systems have been validated [43]. The continuously updated 12-lead ECG recording system of Mortara Instrument is based on the conventional 12-lead electrocardiogram. Every 15 seconds the median electrocardiogram of 12 beats is updated and compared with the baseline electrocardiogram. The second system is the dynamic vector–derived 12-lead electrocardiographic recording system (MIDA, Ortivus Medical), in which averaged QRS-T vectors from the Frank orthogonal leads are acquired every minute and transformed into 12-lead electrocardiograms. The third method is based on a three-lead Holter recording system, with a special bipolar lead configuration that mimics the XYZ axes of the Frank lead system.

The temporal relation between ST-segment deviation and coronary occlusion is close in patients with acute myocardial infarction [44]. The classical ECG

Step 3: Selection of a reperfusion strategy

OPTION 1   ASA : SK : rt-PA : direct PTCA = 9 : 36 : 25 : 30 %

Gain in life expectancy (months)	Bleeding risk		
	risk ICH <1.5% and NO other contraindication	risk ICH 1.5-2.5% and NO other contraindication	risk ICH >2.5% or other contraindication
<1	ASA	ASA	ASA
1	streptokinase	ASA	ASA
2-4	streptokinase	streptokinase	■
5-11	■	■	■
>=12	■	■	■

OPTION 2   ASA : SK : rt-PA : direct PTCA = 8 : 38 : 38 : 16 %

Gain in life expectancy (months)	Bleeding risk	
	risk ICH <3% and NO other contraindication	risk ICH >=3% or other contraindication
<1	ASA	ASA
1	streptokinase	ASA
2-4	streptokinase	streptokinase
5-11	■	■
>=12	■	■

FIGURE 28-5. Step 3: Selection of a reperfusion therapy. A reperfusion strategy is proposed for each combination of the expected gain in life expectancy and bleeding risk. The various treatment modalities are allocated in such a way that patients with the most expected benefit receive the most effective (and most expensive) treatment. (See the text for a more detailed explanation.)

TABLE 28-3. Additional reperfusion strategies based on ST-segment monitoring

ST-segment amplitude	Initial treatment strategy	Suggested action	Initial intracranial bleeding risk
Decrease ≥50% within 90 min	Alteplase (or SK[a])	STOP infusion of thrombolytic [53]	—
<50% within 90 min	Alteplase or SK	Rescue PTCA [25,26]	—
Re-elevation of >0.1 mm/lead for at least 20 min	Alteplase or SK	Alteplase (50 mg in 1 h if <24 h after first dose) [54–56]	<1.5%
		PTCA	≥1.5%

ST-segment monitoring should start as soon as possible after hospital admission to give reliable results. Reassessment should be done 60–90 minutes after the start of thrombolytic therapy and only when the initial ST-segment deviation is at least 0.2 mV in at least one ECG lead. Follow steps 1–3 again, considering, the treatment delay +90 minutes.
[a] No clinical data available.
SK = streptokinase; PTCA = percutaneous transluminal coronary angioplasts.

criterion of reperfusion, that is a 50% decrease of the amount of the initial ST-segment deviation, is most reliable if the initial ST-segment elevation is high (0.4 mV per lead) and ST-segment recovery occurs early within 45–90 minutes [43]. In 100% of such patients an open (TIMI 2 or 3) infarct-related coronary artery was found at 90–180 minutes if, after a 50% ST-segment decrease, a short (<20-minute) temporal re-elevation of up to 100% of the initial ST-segment elevation was found. In 85% of patients without such a temporal ST-segment re-elevation, a patent infarct-related coronary artery was found. In patients with little initial ST-segment elevation (<0.2 mV per lead) and ST-segment normalization after 90 minutes, coronary patency was only about 50%. In patients without ST-segment recovery, coronary occlusion was 80%. The reliability of ST-segment monitoring can be further improved by including the occurrence of accelerated idioventricular rhythms and the relief of chest pain, but to what extent is still unknown. An idioventricular rhythm occurred infrequently in a patient with failed thrombolytic therapy (false positives in a pooled analysis of six studies only 3%) [45–50]. However, idioventricular rhythms are found in only 45% of patients with an open infarct-related vessel at 90 minutes [45–50].

Stopping the Infusion of Thrombolytic Therapy on Signs of Reperfusion. One of the main drawbacks of thrombus-resolving therapy is bleeding in the brain in 1% of patients. This risk is dose related for alteplase [51]. Another drawback to the widespread use of alteplase is the unit price of US $2000. A 6-hour prolongation of rt-PA infusion did not decrease the reocclusion rate [52]. Therefore, normalization of

the ST-segment elevation within 90 minutes after the start of treatment has been used to identify patients in whom alteplase infusion could be stopped in order to reduce the bleeding risk and cost [53]. These patients were treated early with alteplase infusion within 3 hours after the start of symptoms. All patients had very small infarcts after treatment, measured from blood heart enzyme levels, although the amount of heart muscle at risk for infarction was extensive. Twenty-two percent of treatment costs were saved in these patients. This first study has to be confirmed in larger patient populations.

Failed Thrombolytic Therapy. Knowledge about coronary vessel patency is relevant for the identification of those patients in whom thrombolytic therapy fails and who could benefit from additional reperfusion strategies, both chemical, such as new thrombin inhibitors, and invasive (rescue PTCA). The stepwise approach that was discussed earlier may help to select patients for such additional interventions that are associated with increasing bleeding risk. This is illustrated in Table 28-3. Although knowledge about the benefit of these approaches is limited, it is likely that most of the benefit is to be expected in those patients with a large cardiac baseline risk and with a small treatment delay.

Reocclusion of the Infarct-Related Coronary Vessel. Although transient ST-segment re-elevation of <20 minutes is prognostic for an open infarct-related coronary artery at 90 minutes after the start of thrombolytic therapy, persistent ST-segment re-elevation is a sign of reocclusion [43]. Possible strategies are depicted in Table 28-3. The clinical experience of repeated thrombolytic therapy is limited (n =

109) but is promising for centers without angioplasty or surgical facilities. Patency rates varied from 54% to 73% and bleeding rates form 13% to 23% [54–56].

FURTHER ADVANTADGES OF THE STEPWISE
APPROACH

Clinical Trials. The stepwise approach might also be helpful for designers of clinical trials to set inclusion criteria in such a manner that the treatment strategy under investigation is tested in those patients who might receive the maximal possible benefit of the treatment. Too often ethical committees agree on protocols to assess therapies only in low-risk patients. Examples are thrombolytic therapy in patients with unstable angina, and thrombin inhibtors and potent platelet inhibitiors, together with thrombolytic therapy, in low-risk infarction patients.

Conclusions

In conclusion, in our experience the stepwise approach appears to be very useful for tackling the sometimes complicated questions of whether a patient should be treated and which reperfusion strategy should be chosen. Clinicians are urged to consider all determinants of the benefits and risks of thrombolytic therapy. With regard to whether the proposed approach is better or worse than clinical judgement alone in treating the right patient, much depends on the clinical judgement of the specific clinician. We know from the literature that some investigators have admitted patients to thrombolysis trials without the benefit of thrombolytic treatment (e.g., those at very low risk with a normal admission electrocardiogram). Others have been too selective, thereby withholding the possible benefit of thrombolytic therapy. A similar interphysician variation is found in clinical practice. An individual physician sometimes becomes more "bleeding risk averse" for a period of time after having a patient suffer intracranial bleeding or more "bleeding risk seeking" when thrombolytic therapy has been successful in a series of patients. This can be avoided by application of the proposed systematic approach.

References

1. Braunwald E. Optimizing thrombolytic therapy of acute mycardial infarction. Circulation 82:1510, 1990.
2. ACC/AHA Task Force Report. Guidelines for the early management of patients with acute myocardial infarction. J Am Coll Cardiol 16:249, 1990.
3. Fibrinolytic Therapy Trialists' (FTT) Collaborative Group. Indications for fibrinolytic therapy in suspected acute myocardial infarction: Collaborative overview of early mortality and major morbidity results from all randomised trials of more than 1000 patients. Lancet 343:311, 1994.
4. Arnold AER, Simoons ML. Thrombolytic therapy for evolving myocardial infarction needs an approach that integrates beefit and risk. Eur Heart J 16:1502, 1995.
5. ISIS-2 Collaborative Group. Randomised trial of intravenous streptokinase, oral aspirin, both or neither among 17,187 cases of suspected acute myocardial infarction. Lancet 2:349, 1988.
6. Wilcox RG, von der Lippe G, Olsson CG, et al. Effects of alteplase in acute myocardial infarction, 6 month results from the ASSET study. Lancet 335:175, 1990.
7. De Jaegere P, Arnold AER, Balk A, Simoons ML. Intracranial hemorrhage in association with thrombolytic therapy. J Am Coll Cardiol 19:289, 1992.
8. Simoons ML, Maggioni AP, Knatterud G, Leimberger JD, de Jaegere P, Domburg R van, Boersma E, Franzosi MG, Califf R, Schroeder R, Braunwald E. Individual risk assessment for intracranial haemorrhage during thrombolytic therapy. Lancet 342:1523, 1993.
9. Maggioni AP, Franzosi MG, Santoro E, et al. The risk of stroke in patients with acute myocardial infarction after thrombolytic and antithrombotic treatment. N Engl J Med 327:1, 1992.
10. Simoons ML, Servuys PW, Brand vd M, et al. Early thrombolysis in acute myocardial infarction: Limitation of infarct size and improved survival. J Am Coll Cardiol 7:717, 1986.
11. Van de Werf F, Arnold AER, for the European Cooperative Study Group. Intravenous tissue plasminogen activator and size of infarct, left ventriclar function, and survival in acute myocardial infarction. Br Med J 297:1374, 1988.
12. Roux S, Christeller S. Effects of aspirin on coronary reocclusion and recurrent ischemia after thrombolysis: A meta-analysis. J Am Coll Cardiol 19:671, 1992.
13. The GUSTO Investigators. An international randomized trial comparing four thrombolytic strategies for acute myocardial infarction. N Engl J Med 329:673, 1993.
14. de Bono DP, Simoons ML, Tijssen JGP, Arnold AER, et al. The effect of intravenous heparin on coronary thombolysis with rt-PA in acute myocardial infarction. Br Heart J 67:122, 1992.
15. Gruppo Italiano per lo Studio della Streptochinasi nell' Infarto miocardico (GISSI). Long-term effects of intravenous thrombolysis in acute myocardial infarction: Final report of the GISSI study. Lancet 1:871, 1987.
16. AIMS Trial Study Group. Long-term effects of intravenous anistreplase in acute myocardial infarction: Final report of the AIMS study. Lancet 335:427, 1990.
17. Arnold AER, Simoons ML, Van de Werf F, et al. Alteplase and immediate angioplasty in acute myocar-

dial infarction, one year follow-up. Circulation 86:111, 1992.

18. GISSI-2. A factorial randomized trial of alteplase vs. streptokinase and heparin vs. no heparin among 12,490 patients with acute myocardial infarction. Lancet 336:65, 1990.

19. The International Study Group. In-hospital mortality and clinical course of 20,891 patients with suspected acute myocardial infarction randomised between alteplase and streptokinase with and without heparin. Lancet 336:71, 1990.

20. ISIS-3. A randomised trial of streptokinase versus tissue plasminogen activator versus anistreplase and of aspirin plus heparin versus aspirin alone among 41,299 cases of suspected acute myocardial infarction. Lancet 339:753, 1992.

21. Bleich SD, Nichols TC, Schumacher RR, Cooke DH, Tate DA, Teichman SL. Effect of heparin on coronary arterial patency after thrombolysis with tissue plasminogen activator in actue myocardial infarction. Am J Cardiol 66:1412, 1990.

22. Simoons ML, Arnold AER, Betriu A, et al. Thrombolysis with tissue plasminogen activator in acute myocardial infarction: No additional benefit from immediate percutaneous coronary angioplasty. Lancet 1:197, 1988.

23. The TIMI Research Group. Comparison of invasive and conservative strategies after treatment with intravenous tissue plasminogen activator in acute myocardial infarction. N Engl J Med 320:618, 1989.

24. Arnold AER, Serruys PW, Rutsch W, et al. Reasons for the lack of benefit of immediate angioplasty during recombinant tissue plasminogen activator therapy for acute myocardial infarction: A regional wall motion analysis. J Am Col Cardiol 17:11, 1991.

25. Ellis SG, Ribeiro da Silva E, Heyndrickx G, et al. Randomized comparison of rescue angioplasty with conservative management of patients with early failure of thrombolysis for acute anterior myocardial infarction. Circulation 90:2280, 1994.

26. Califf RM, Topol EJ, Stack RS, et al. Evaluation of combination thrombolytic therapy and timing of cardiac catheterization in acute myocardial infarction. Results of Thrombolysis and Angioplasty in Myocardial Infarction-Phase 5 randomized trial. Circulation 83:1543, 1991.

27. Grines CL, Browne KF, Marco J, et al. A comparison of immediate angiophasty with thombolytic therapy for acute myocardial infarction. N Engl J Med 328:673, 1993.

28. Zijlstra F, Boer MJ de, Hoorntje JCA, Reiffers S, Reiber JHC, Suryapranata H. A comparison of immediate coronary angioplasty with intravenous streptokinase in acute myocardial infarction. N Engl J Med 328:680, 1993.

29. Weaver WD, Litwin PE, Martin JS, et al. Effect of age on use of thrombolytic therapy and mortality in acute myocardial infarction. J Am Coll Cardiol 18:657, 1991.

30. Boersma H, van der Vlugt MJ, Arnold AER, Deckers JW, Simoons ML. Estimated gain in life expectancy. A simple tool to select optimal reperfusion treatment in individual patients with evolving myocardial infarction. Eur Heart J 17:64, 1996.

31. LATE Study Group. Late Assessment of Thrombolytic Efficacy (LATE) study with alteplase 6–24 hours after onset of acute myocardium infarction. Lancet 342:759, 1993.

32. Simoons ML, Arnold AER. Tailored thrombolytic therapy — a perspective. Circulation 88:2556, 1993.

33. Vermeer F, Simoons ML, Baer FW, et al. Which patients benefit most from early thrombolytic therapy with intracoronary streptokinase. Circulation 74:1379, 1986.

34. Mauri F, Gasparini M, Barbonaglia L, et al. Prognostic significance of the extent of myocardial injury in acute myocardial infarction treated by streptokinase (the GISSI trial). Am J Cardiol 63:1291, 1989.

35. Hillis LD, Forman S, Braunwald E, and the Thrombolysis in Myocardial Infarction (TIMI) Phase II Co-investigators. Risk stratification before thrombolytic therapy in patients with acute myocardial infarction. J Am Coll Cardiol 16:313, 1990.

36. Lee Kl, Woodlief LH, Topol EJ, et al. for the GUSTO-1 investigators. Prediction of 30 day mortality in the era of reperfusion for acute myocardial infarction: Results from an international trial of 41.021 patients. Circulation 91:1659, 1995.

37. Ollson G, Rehnqvist N, Sjogren A, et al. Long-term treatment with metoprolol after myocardial infarction: Effect on 3 year mortality and morbidity. J Am Coll Cardiol 5:1428, 1985.

38. Yusuf S, Zucker D, Peduzzi P, et al. Effect of coronary artery bypass graft surgery on survival: Overview of 10-year results from randomised trials by the coroanry artery bypass graft study trialists collaboration. Lancet 344:563, 1994.

39. Rothwell PM. Can overall results of clinical trials be applied to all patients? Lancet 345:1616, 1995.

40. Dellborg M, Riha M, Swedberg K. Dynamic QRS-complex and ST-segment monitoring in acute myocardial infarction during recombinant tissue-type plasminogen activator therapy. Am J Cardiol 67:343, 1991.

41. Krucoff MW, Green CE, Satler LF, et al. Non-invasive detection of coronary artery patency using continuous ST-segment monitoring. Am J Cardiol 57:916, 1986.

42. Krucoff MW, Croll MA, Pope JE, et al. Continuously updated 12-lead ST-segment recovery analysis for myocardial infarct artery patency assessment and its correlation with multiple simultaneous early angiographic observation. Am J Cardiol 71:145, 1993.

43. Klootwijk P, Langer A, Meij S, Green C, Veldkamp RF, Ross AM, Armstrong PW, Simoons ML. Non-invasive prediction of reperfusion and coronary artery patency by continuous ST-segment monitoring in the GUSTO-1 trial. Eur Heart J 17:689, 1996.

44. Hacket D, Davies G, Chiercha S, Maserie A. Intermittent coronary occlusion in acute myocardial infarction: Value of combined thrombolytic and vasodilator therapy. N Engl J Med 317:1055, 1987.

45. Goldberg S, Greenspan AJ, Urban PL, et al. Reperfusion arrhythmia: A marker of restoration of antegrade flow during intracoronary thrombolysis for acute myocardial infarction. Am Heart J 105:26, 1983.

46. Miller FC, Krucoff MW, Satler LF, et al. Ventricular arrhythmias during reperfusion. Am Heart J 112:928, 1986.

47. Gorgels APM, Vos MA, Letsch IS, et al. Usefulness of the accelerated idioventricular rhythm as a marker for myocardial mecrosis and reperfusion during thrombolytic therapy in acute myocardial infarction. Am J Cardiol 61:231, 1988.

48. Gore JM, Ball SP, Corrao JM, et al. Arrhythmias in the assessmect of coronary artery reperfusion following thrombolytic therapy. Chest 94:727, 1988.

49. Hohnloser Sh, Zabel M, Kasper W, et al. Assessment of coronary artery patency after thrombolytic therapy: Accurate prediction utilizing the combined analysis of three noninvasive markers. J Am Coll Cardiol 18:44, 1991.

50. Gressin V, Louvard Y, Pezzano M, et al. Holter recording of ventricular arrhythmias during intravenous thrombolysis for acute myocardial infarction. Am J Cardiol 69:152, 1992.

51. Braunwald E, Knatterud GL, Passamani ER, Robertson TL. Announcement of protocol change in thrombolysis in myocardial infarction trial. J Am Coll Cardiol 9:467, 1987.

52. Verstraete M, Arnold AER, Brower RW, et al. Acute coronary thrombolysis with rt-PA: Initial patency and influence of maintained infusion on reocclusion rate. Am J Cardiol 60:231, 1987.

53. Arnold AER, van der Vlugt MJ, Boersma H, Barret MJ, Burgersdijk. Tailored thrombolytic therapy for evolving myocardial infarction: Stopping alteplase infusion on signs of reperfusion (abstr). Eur Heart J 16:11, 1995.

54. Simoons ML, Arnout J, van den Brand M, Nyssen K, Verstraete M for the European Cooperative Study Group. Retreatment with alteplase for early signs of reocclusion after thrombolysis. Am J Cardiol 71:524, 1993.

55. Barbash GI, Hod H, Roth A, et al. Repeat infusions of recombinant tissue-type activator in patients with acute myocardial infarction and early recurrent myocardial infarction. J Am Coll Cardiol 16:779, 1990.

56. White HD, Cross DB, Williams BF, Norris RM. Safety and efficacy of repeat thrombolyric treatment after acute myocardial infarction. Br Heart J 64:177, 1990.

SECTION IX: ADJUNCTIVE ANTITHROMBOTIC STRATEGIES

Harvey D. White and Hans J. Rapold

The major goals of treatment for acute myocardial infarction are to reduce infarct size and to preserve left ventricular function by salvage of myocardium with reperfusion of the infarct-related artery. Several thrombolytic agents are available that have been shown to be effective in reducing mortality. However, these agents achieve normal reperfusion in just over half of the patients who receive them, and reocclusion occurs in 5–15%. The challenge is to improve sustained reperfusion rates without significantly increasing the incidence of intracranial hemorrhage. This section discusses experimental and clinical studies with concomitant antiplatelet and antithrombotic agents, which have the potential to greatly improve the outcome after myocardial infarction.

29. ASPIRIN, HEPARIN, AND NEW ANTITHROMBOTIC DRUGS AS ADJUNCTS TO THROMBOLYTIC THERAPY FOR ACUTE MYOCARADIAL INFARCTION

Hans J. Rapold

Introduction

Early intravenous thrombolysis has been firmly established as the therapy of choice for acute myocardial infarction. There is room, however, for an important improvement: Between 15% and 50% of coronary thrombi cannot be lysed with the currently available drugs, 10–25% of successfully recanalized vessels reocclude, and 0.5–1% of the treated patients suffer an intracerebral hemorrhage. Dispute over the thrombolytic agent of choice, including pharmacoeconomic aspects, has continued despite megatrials involving over 100,000 patients [1–5]. While the overall benefit of thrombolytic therapy has been confirmed, questions remain with respect to optimal adjuvant antithrombotic treatment, the validity of surrogate endpoints, and the mechanism through which thrombolysis translates into clinical benefit [6–10].

Although alteplase (recombinant tissue-type plasminogen activator, rt-PA), judged on comparative 90-minute patency, recanalizes infarct-related arteries more efficiently and more rapidly than streptokinase (SK) [11,12], and early treatment correlates with the greatest reduction in mortality [1,2], survival from myocardial infarction did not appear to differ with the thrombolytic drug used in early comparative trials [4,5]. Explanations for this paradox followed several lines. The validity of the 90-minute patency rate in documenting efficient recanalization has been be questioned [8]. Late reperfusion and factors independent of reopening an occluded infarct vessel have been shown to contribute to survival [13]. Most importantly, only sustained recanalization can be expected to provide clinical benefit; reocclusion after initial reperfusion is associated with increased mortality and reduced left ventricular function [14]. Adequate concomitant anticoagulation, both for reperfusion and to protect from reocclusion, was found to be particularly important for fibrin-specific thrombolytic agents [15–17]. Finally, the therapeutic paradigm linking early complete vessel patency to clinical outcome was established beyond a reasonable doubt [18], allowing future investigation to focus on improving early coronary flow quality.

Thrombolytic therapy for acute myocardial infarction can no longer be considered to be monotherapy with a single thrombolytic agent but has rather become a conjunctive pharmacological effort to achieve stable reperfusion of an occluded vessel [19–21]. Primary or rescue angioplasty may be considered in subgroups of patients [22]. The concept is based on experimental and biochemical evidence that reperfusion and reocclusion are the net result of simultaneous competing and interacting processes that result in clot lysis and thrombosis. Whereas the clinical benefit of adding aspirin and heparin to thrombolytic drugs has emerged from several trials, the potential advantages of new antithrombotic compounds, such as low molecular weight heparins, specific antithrombins, novel anticoagulants, and platelet GPIIb/IIIa antagonists, as adjuncts to thrombolysis have yet to be shown in the clinical setting. The present review summarizes the experience with established antithrombotic drugs as well as the potential for new compounds to overcome the remaining limitations of thrombolytic therapy. A careful risk/benefit evaluation will ultimately determine the optimal conjunctive therapeutic approach.

Experimental Evidence for the Enhancement of Thrombolysis with Concomitant Antithrombotic Drugs

The efficacy of thrombolytic or antithrombotic agents depends, to a large extent, on the depth and extent of the arterial lesion and, hence, on the experimental model used. For deep arterial injury, the central role of thrombin for platelet activation as well as for fibrin formation is well established. While arterial thrombi on superficial endothelial damage can be prevented by aspirin [23], and more specific platelet inhibition by serotonin antagonists [24], thromboxane-synthase inhibitors [25], or thromboxane-receptor antagonists [24,26–28] may accelerate thrombolysis and reduce reocclusion rates in certain animal models, thrombin inhibition is needed to prevent thrombosis on deep arterial injury, representing plaque rupture [29–33]. In addition to its dominant role as a platelet activator, thrombin interacts with a number of coagulation factors (IX, VIII, V, XIII, protein C), amplifying both the extrinsic and intrinsic pathways of coagulation;

thrombin initiates fibrin generation [34]; and it presumably orchestrates the vascular response to injury, also influencing the endothelial release of procoagulant factors, as well as cell adhesion, proliferation, and migration [35]. Inhibition of thrombin and its interaction with platelets has thus become a central target in the prevention of acute arterial thrombosis, particularly in the context of fibrinolysis [36].

Heparin [17] and heparin fragments [37] have been shown to potentiate venous lysis induced by alteplase or scu-PA in animal models of femoral or jugular vein thrombosis. Pretreatment [38] or simultaneous infusion of heparin [17,39] or heparin fragments [40] also enhances alteplase-induced reperfusion in arterial thrombosis models (Table 29-1). Specific thrombin inhibitors, such as hirudin [30,39,41], hirulog [42], or PPACK [39], have been shown to be superior to heparin as adjuvants to alteplase in various models. In vivo data indicating an interaction between streptokinase and heparin are scarce. But the observation that the antithrombotic effects of various thrombolytic agents, including alteplase, alteplase mutants, rscu-PA (recombinant single chain urokinase-type plasminogen activator), UK (two-chain urokinase), streptokinase, and STAR (recombinant staphylokinase), parallels their

TABLE 29-1. Alteplase with or without heparin: Results of experimental arterial and venous thrombolysis in dogs

	Group I Heparin (n = 10)	Group II No heparin (n = 10)	Level of significance (P)
Blood flow through stenosis (% of baseline)	41 ± 2	37 ± 2	n.s.
Arterial reperfusion (n)			
Within 30 minutes	7	1	0.018
After 30 minutes	2	3	
None	1	6	
Venous clot lysis (%)	81 ± 4	49 ± 7	0.001
Fibrinogen levels (g/L)			
Baseline	1.4 ± 0.3	1.5 ± 0.2	
At 60 minutes	1.2 ± 0.3	1.2 ± 0.2	n.s.
At 150 minutes	1.3 ± 0.2	1.2 ± 0.3	
APTT(s)			
Baseline	21 ± 1	20 ± 1	
At 30 minutes	177 ± 3	24 ± 1	
At 60 minutes	180 ± 0	29 ± 2	<0.001
At 150 minutes	178 ± 2	24 ± 2	

Data represent mean ± SEM.
n.s., not significant ($P > 0.05$).
From Rapold HJ et al. [17], with permission.

fibrinogenolytic effect and not their thrombolytic potency [43] suggests that non–fibrin-specific thrombolysis depends to a lesser degree on concomitant anticoagulation. The main mechanism by which heparin potentiates thrombolysis is thought to be the prevention of new fibrin formation on the lysing thrombus.

Residual thrombi, indeed, appear to be the basis of reocclusion [36]; they were found to be more thrombogenic than deep arterial injury, especially when combined with the high shear rate of a residual stenosis [44]. During thrombolysis, fibrin-bound thrombin is re-exposed and may again generate fibrin and activate platelets. Fibrin-bound thrombin is protected from inactivation by heparin, but not by specific thrombin inhibitors, which might explain the antithrombotic supremacy of the latter [45].

Neutralization of fibrinogen binding to the activated platelet GPIIb/IIIa receptor represents the most potent mechanism for inhibiting platelet aggregation. Acceleration of arterial thrombolysis and prevention of reocclusion following alteplase have been shown experimentally with a number of these compounds that are either monoclonal antibodies [46–49], snake venoms [50,51], synthetic peptides containing the RGD recognition sequence of fibrinogen [52–55], or peptidomimetic inhibitors [56,57] (Figure 29-1).

Biochemical Evidence for Enhanced Prothrombotic Activity During Therapeutic Thrombolysis

Fibrin generation or thrombin levels can be monitored by sensitive biochemical markers, such as fibrinopeptide A (FPA) [58,59] or thrombin–antithrombin III (TAT) complexes [60], as shown in patients with venous thrombosis and pulmonary embolism [58,61], unstable angina [62,63], or acute myocardial infarction [64,65]. The effect of alteplase with and without intravenous heparin on fibrin generation was quantified in patients with acute myocardial infarction [15,16] (Figure 29-2). Initially raised FPA plasma levels increased further under alteplase without heparin before falling almost to normal as soon as intravenous heparin was added. This sustained fibrin formation under thrombolysis, despite reperfusion, might be due to a release of coagulation factors bound to clots, to re-exposure of thrombotic subendothelium, or to infarct vessel–unrelated ischemia. FPA may also be released from fibrinogen by t-PA directly; it is therefore not a specific marker of thrombin activity. Finally, increased levels of pro-

thrombin fragment 1.2 suggest ongoing thrombin generation [66] under heparin, which might explain the rebound in thrombin activity and associated ischemic events observed in patients with acute coronary syndromes after cessation of heparin [67,68].

The sixth ECSG trial confirmed that the enhanced thrombin activity (but not necessarily its generation) under alteplase and aspirin can be suppressed by adequate anticoagulation, resulting in higher early patency rates of the infarct vessel [69] (Figure 29-3). While FPA plasma levels could not be shown to be sensitive markers of thrombotic events or reocclusion, as initially suggested [15], the intensity of anticoagulation appears to have a pivotal role for a sustained reperfusion by alteplase [69,70]. Although high FPA plasma levels were also measured in SK-treated patients [71], the origin and clinical significance of high FPA concentrations in hypofibrinogenemia remains unclear.

Plasminogen activator inhibitor-1 (PAI-1) is an important regulator of fibrinolytic activity under physiologic conditions [72], which might also influence therapeutic thrombolysis. Plasma levels of active PAI-1 were shown to increase markedly, early after thrombolytic therapy, suggesting an antifibrinolytic rebound phenomenon independent of physiologic diurnal fluctuation [73]. Other prothrombotic effects related to thrombolytic therapy include plasmin-induced stimulation of factor V [74] or X [75] as well as plasmin-induced platelet activation [76–78]. On the other hand, plasmin-dependent platelet inhibition, apparently not involving the GPIIb/IIIa receptor, was shown in vitro by streptokinase, but not by alteplase [79].

Clinical Experience with Current Antithrombotic Drugs as Adjuncts to Thrombolytic Therapy

The independent beneficial effect of oral aspirin (160 mg daily) on mortality following thrombolytic therapy of acute myocardial infarction with streptokinase has been established by the ISIS 2 trial [2]; it is likely to be due to prevention of reocclusion and recurrent ischemia, and probably also applies to alteplase, although the latter evidence is only based on retrospective meta-analysis of smaller trials [80]. Aspirin was not associated with excess cerebral hemorrhage or bleeding requiring transfusion. It has therefore become a gold standard for the treatment of acute myocardial infarction, both with and without thrombolytic therapy.

Clinical trials have also confirmed that fibrin-

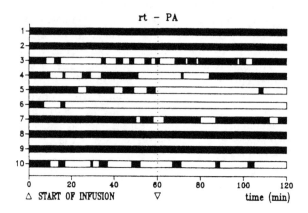

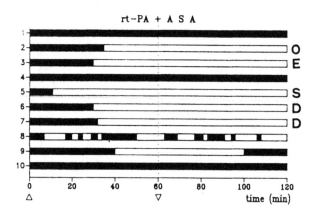

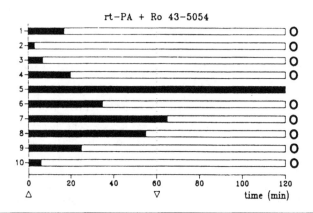

FIGURE 29-1. Alteplase, aspirin and Ro 43-5054, a peptidominetic platelet GPIIb/IIIa inhibitor for experimental thrombolysis in dogs. Schematic representation of the patency status (occluded [■] or permeant [□]) of stenosed and thrombosed coronary arteries in dogs treated with alteplase alone (30 μg/kg/min) over 1 hour (alteplase), alteplase + aspirin (ASA; 10 mg/kg), and alteplase + Ro 43-5054 (3 μg/kg-min). △ and ▽, start and end of alteplase infusion. When the coronary artery did not reocclude during the 120-minute observation period, additional thrombogenic challenges were undertaken. The coronary artery could then reocclude by increasing the degree of the coronary stenosis (S), infusion of epinephrine (E), or subendothelial damage (D), or not reocclude by either stimulus (O). (From Roux et al. [56], with permission.)

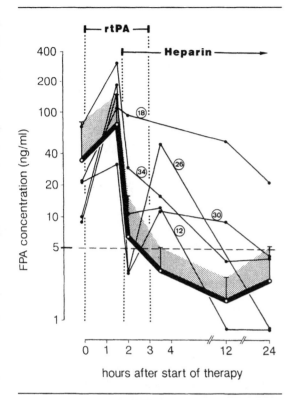

FIGURE 29-2. Fibrinopeptide A (FPA) plasma levels in patients with acute myocardial infarction before, during, and after thrombolytic therapy with alteplase. FPA plasma levels in mean values (ng/mL ± SD). ○■■○, patients without reocclusion (n = 25); •—•, patients with reocclusion (n = 5) at 45 minutes (patient 12), 4 hours (patient 34), 7 hours (patient 26), 8 days (patient 18), and repeatedly over 4 hours (patient 30) after primary success of thrombolytic therapy. (From Rapold et al. [15], with permission.)

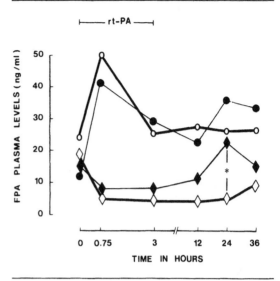

FIGURE 29-3. FPA plasma levels in patients with acute myocardial infarction with respect to treatment allocation (alteplase + IV heparin or alteplase + IV placebo) and subsequent coronary patency at 48–120 hours. Fibrinopeptide A (FPA) plasma levels in median values (ng/mL): —◊—, heparin, patent (n = 129); —◆—, heparin, occluded (n = 30); —○—, placebo, patent (n = 106); —•—, placebo, occluded (n = 41). *P < 0.05. (From Rapold et al. [69], with permission.)

specific thrombolytic agents, such as alteplase, require adequate concomitant anticoagulation, in addition to platelet inhibtion by aspirin, for rapid and sustained reperfusion of occluded infarct vessels. Early trials showed a significant benefit of alteplase over streptokinase for coronary patency at 90 minutes [11,12]. Concomitant heparin seemed of minor importance for early patency with alteplase in a smaller trial [81]. These data, as well as the fear of bleeding complications, led to the design of two comparative megatrials with delayed subcutaneous rather than concomitant intravenous anticoagulation, resulting in identical mortality for alteplase- and streptokinase-treated acute myocardial infarction [4,5]. With emerging experimental and biochemical evidence that fibrin-specific thrombolytic drugs depend on

concomitant anticoagulation for optimal efficacy, three trials focused on the role of intravenous heparin for alteplase-induce thrombolysis. All of the trials documented significantly improved coronary patency with concomitant intravenous heparin, 7–24 hours [82], 48–72 hours [83], as well as 48–120 hours [69,84] following thrombolytic therapy, irrespective of aspirin.

Additionally, the sixth ECSG trial linked coronary patency with in vivo fibrin generation [69] and the intensity of anticoagulation [69,70]. With optimal anticoagulation (defined as activated partial thromboplastin times [APTTs] at least doubled constantly with respect to baseline over 36 hours), 90% 90-minute patency rates (TIMI 2 or 3) were achieved with alteplase (Figure 29-4). The study thus underlined that intravenous heparin warrants individual dose titration for optimal efficacy [69,70]. The final gap linking early vessel patency to outcome in terms of mortality, a therapeutic paradigm that was not apparent from earlier trials [4,5], has been closed by the GUSTO 1 study [18], comparing a front-loaded regimen of alteplase + concomitant intravenous

TABLE 29-2. GUSTOV-1:

	Alteplase + IV H	SK + IV H	SK + SC H	t-PA + SK	P value t-PA vs. SK
No. patients	10,344	10,377	9796	10,328	
90-minute coronary patency (TIMI 2 or 3; %)	80.8	61.0	55.6	73.1	<0.001
24-hour coronary patency (%)	87.1	80.4	77.5	94.7	n.s.
5–7 day coronary patency (%)	86.2	86.0	73.3	78.0	n.s.
24-hour mortality (%)	2.3	2.9	2.8	2.8	0.005
30-day mortality (%)	6.3	7.4	7.2	7.0	0.001
Stroke, total (%)	1.6	1.4	1.2	1.6	n.s.
Stroke, hemorrhagic (%)	0.7	0.5	0.5	0.9	0.03
Net clinical benefit (death or nonfatal stroke) (%)	6.9	7.9	7.7	7.6	0.006

H = heparin; SK = streptokinase; t-PA = tissue plasminogen activator; IV = intravenous; SC = subcutaneous.

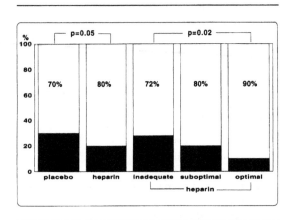

FIGURE 29-4. Alteplase, intensity of concomitant anticoagulation, and coronary patency in acute myocardial infarction. Coronary perfusion status (□ open, TIMI 2–3, ■ occluded, TIMI 0–1) at angiography 48–120 hours after alteplase therapy of acute myocardial infarction in patients randomized to additional heparin (n = 149) or placebo (n = 132). The heparin-treated group is further subdivided into optimally (n = 48), suboptimally (n = 40), and inadequately (n = 61) anticoagulated patients over 36 hours on the basis of sequential aPTT values: Optimal = all aPTT values >200% of baseline; suboptimal = lowest aPTT value 130–200% of baseline; inadequate = lowest aPTT value <130% of baseline. (From Arnout et al. [70], with permission.)

heparin with streptokinase + intravenous heparin, with streptokinase + subcutaneous (delayed) heparin and with (lower dosed) alteplase + streptokinase in 41,021 patients (Table 29-2). A gain in early coronary patency with alteplase and intravenous heparin did translate into improved infarct survival compared with streptokinase with either intravenous or subcutaneous heparin.

Several important concepts were confirmed: (1) early thrombolytic treatment for acute myocardial infarction is associated with an incremental reduction in 30-day mortality. The rates were 4.3% for patients receiving alteplase within 2 hours after the onset of symptoms, 5.5% at 2–4 hours after onset, and 8.9% at 4–6 hours after onset. For streptokinase-treated patients, the mortality rates for the same time intervals were 5.4%, 6.7%, and 9.3% [18]. (2) only complete (TIMI 3) coronary reperfusion at 90 minutes is associated with a significant reduction of mortality at 30 days: the rates, irrespective of treatment, were 4% for TIMI 3, 7.9% for TIMI 2, 9.2% for TIMI 1, and 8.4% for TIMI 0 flow [85]. (3) Fibrin-specific thrombolytic drugs, such as alteplase, warrant a well-controlled concomitant anticoagulation (ideally with aPTTs between 50 and 75 seconds), in addition to aspirin, for optimal efficacy [86]. For thrombolytic drugs inducing hypofibrinogenemia, such as streptokinase, there is no evidence as yet that concomitant intravenous or delayed sc anticoagulation, in addition to aspirin, is beneficial. Delayed subcutaneous heparin, however, is safer and may be recommended.

Future Prospects for Conjunctive Thrombolytic and Antithrombotic Treatment

Current antithrombotic drugs, although widely used and proven to be efficacious, still have important limitations.

UNFRACTIONATED HEPARIN

Unfractionated heparin is a mixture of sulfated polysaccharides with a molecular weight range between 5000 and 30,000 d [86]. A specific pentasaccharide sequence present in approximately one third of the molecules binds with high affinity to antithrombin III (AT III) [87–89], thereby potentiating the ability of this natural anticoagulant to inactivate the circulating factors IXa, Xa, and IIa (thrombin) [90]. Whereas factor Xa may be inactivated by heparin–AT III [88,91] directly, the inactivation of thrombin by heparin–AT III requires the formation of a ternary complex [92–94]. Heparin molecules with <18 saccharides (<5400 d) cannot bind to AT III and thrombin simultaneously and lose their ability to potentiate thrombin inactivation by AT III while retaining their anti–factor Xa activity [94,95].

Due to the large size of the AT III molecule (58,000 d), complex formation with heparin and thrombin is hindered within a thrombus. Thrombin bound to fibrin [45] or extracellular matrix [96] is not inhibited by heparin–AT III; likewise, phospholipid-bound factor Xa is protected from heparin–AT III inactivation [97,89]. Hence, heparin has only a limited anticoagulant effect in the presence of preformed or residual thrombogenic clots. Furthermore, platelet factor-4, released by activated platelet [99] or displaced from the endothelial surface [100], as well as fibrin monomers II and thrombospondin, hinder the heparin–AT III complex formation.

Finally, a major drawback of heparin is a dose-dependent pharmacokinetic profile due to its binding to endothelial cells [101,102] and plasma proteins [103], resulting in considerable dose-response variability, a narrow therapeutic window, and the need for close monitoring.

LOW MOLECULAR WEIGHT HEPARINS

Low molecular weight heparins (LMWHs) are heterogeneous heparin fragments (1000–10,000 d) obtained by chemical or enzymatic depolymerization of unfractionated heparin [104]. With only 25–50% of the fragments containing 18 or more saccharide units required for thrombin inhibition, LMWHs exhibit an anticoagulant profile different from heparin, with in vitro anti–factor Xa/anti–factor IIa ratios between 4:1 and 2:1. The anti–factor Xa activity of LMWHs is not inhibited by platelet factor-4 [105] nor membrane binding of factor Xa [106]; fibrin-bound thrombin, however, remains protected from both unfractionated heparin and LMWHs.

The main advantage of LMWHs is their good bioavailability at low doses, coupled with a more predictable anticoagulant response [107], which is due to less protein and endothelial cell binding [99,102,103,106,108]. The longer half-life allows once-a-day administration without laboratory monitoring for prophylactic clinical indications.

While most randomized trials in general surgery failed to show a significant advantage of LMWHs over heparin in terms of efficacy and safety [109–112] LMWHs may be more efficacious than low-dose heparin [113,114], or as efficacious but safer than higher dosed heparin [115], for the prevention of venous thrombosis in orthopedic surgery. However, because LMWHs have a reduced antithrombin activity and share with unfractionated heparin AT III dependency and a poor anticoagulant effect in the presence of clots, their potential as adjuvants to fibrinolytic therapy would seem limited. In the FRAMI trial, Fragmin post acute MI did reduce the incidence of left ventricular thrombi, but not reinfarction or mortality when compared with aspirin [116].

SPECIFIC OR DIRECT ANTITHROMBINS

Specific or direct antithrombins do not depend on AT III for their activity. Rapid clot penetration and inhibition of fibrin-, platelet-, or matrix-bound thrombin [45,96] explain the antithrombotic supremacy of specific antithrombins over heparin or heparin-related substances. Hirudin, a 7000-d (65-residue) protein derived from leech salivary glands or produced by recombinant DNA technology, binds to thrombin's active site as well as to its anion-binding exosite with unique affinity and specificity [116–118]. It prevents not only fibrin formation but, in contrast to heparin [119], albeit at a higher concentration, also platelet deposition following deep arterial injury [33,120]. Hirugen, a 12-residue fragment of hirudin, binds to the anion-binding exosite of thrombin with lower affinity than hirudin [121,122]. Hirulogs are bifunctional peptides (20 residues) with intermediate thrombin affinity. Their hirudin moiety that associates with thrombins anion-binding exosite is coupled with a synthetic tripeptide that binds to the active site [123]. Among the synthetic low molecular weight thrombin inhibitors interacting directly with the active site serine, PPACK (D-Phe-Pro-Arg-CH$_2$CL) and its derivatives bind irreversibly to thrombin [124] but also inhibit other serine proteases, including t-PA, urokinase, and factor Xa. A number of boroarginine derivatives of high thrombin affinity but lower selectivity are currently in preclinical development [125–127].

Direct antithrombins seem well suited as adjuvants to thrombolytic therapy, given their inhibition of clot-bound thrombin and of thrombin-induced platelet aggregation. As outlined earlier, hirudin [30,39,41], hirulog [44], PPACK [39], as well as argatroban [128,129] were experimentally shown to accelerate the lysis of platelet-rich thrombi better than heparin. However, in the context of acute myocardial infarction and despite encouraging clinical dose-finding trials, specific antithrombins have failed to fulfill their experimental promises. Indeed, three large studies (GUSTO 2a, TIMI 9, HIT 3) comparing hirudin with heparin as adjuncts to alteplase or streptokinase had to be interrupted because of an excess in hemorrhagic strokes [130–132]. At a lower dose, hirudin proved to be as safe, but not significantly more efficacious, than heparin in preventing death and reinfarction at 1 month [133,134].

The preliminary results of GUSTO 2b in patients with acute coronary syndromes, including 4860 patients with ST-segment elevation at entry (75% of which underwent thrombolytic therapy by either alteplase or streptokinase) and over 8000 patients without ST-segment elevation, although consistently favoring hirudin over heparin, were clinically less impressive than anticipated [135]. These studies, as well as the lack of longer term (6-month) benefit following PTCA of either hirudin (HELVETICA) [136] or hirulog (HAS) [137], have, in the context of arterial thrombosis, tempered the high initial hopes raised by specific thrombin inhibitors. It has indeed become apparent that the therapeutic window of thrombin inhibition (including conventional anticoagulation) remains narrow. There is also some concern about a rebound of thrombin activity after discontinuation of drugs that specifically inhibit thrombin but no superordinate factors. In a small clinical trial argatroban was associated with biochemical and clinical evidence of rebound coagulation [138]. Limiting prothrombin activation rather than thrombin activity may avoid this effect.

NOVEL ANTICOAGULANTS

Novel anticoagulants inhibit early biochemical steps in the coagulation pathway and inhibit thrombin generation more efficiently by interrupting its self-amplification process. Tissue factor (TF)–initiated coagulation appears to play a critical role in the pathogenesis of coronary artery restenosis following PTCA [139,140], in acute myocardial infarction [141], in sepsis with or without disseminated intravascular coagulation [142,143], and in deep vein thrombosis [144,145]. The TF–factor VIIa complex, catalyzing the extrinsic activation of factor X as well as the intrinsic activation of factor IX, can be inhibited by TF pathway inhibitors (TFPI, formerly lipoprotein associated coagulation inhibitors [LACI] or

extrinsic pathway inhibitors [EPI], by recombinant hybrid proteins with moieties of TFPI and of factor X, by DEG–factor VIIa, or by monoclonal antibody fragments against TF [141,146,147]. The natural TFPI, a 276 amino acid glycoprotein present in platelets and associated with plasma lipoproteins and the vascular endothelium [146–149], forms an inhibitory quaternary complex with TF, factor VIIa, and factor Xa, thereby preventing the formation of the prothrombokinase complex, that is, the formation of thrombin from prothrombin.

Recombinant TFPI (rTFPI), expressed in E. coli and in mammalian cells [150,151] has been studied in pig and rabbit models of restenosis following PTCA [152,153], in dog models of alteplase-induced thrombolysis [146,154], in a myocardium ischemia/reperfusion model [155], and in sepsis models [156]. In general, and particularly without additional antiplatelet agent, substantial prolongation of coagulation times (PT, APTT) was needed to obtain the experimental antithrombotic effect.

Inhibition of the factor IXa–factor VIIIa complex, catalyzing intrinsic factor X activation, may be achieved by active-site blocked factor IXa [157] and by activated protein C [158], or its recombinant form [159], which, in the presence of its cofactor protein S, also inactivates factor Va and increases fibrinolytic activity by inhibiting plasminogen activators inhibitor-1 (PAI-1).

Specific inhibition of factor Xa is possible by tick or nematode anticoagulant peptide (TAP, NAP) [160] or its recombinant form [161], as well as by fragments of factor Xa [162]. Synthetic compounds targeting these steps of coagulation are in early development.

The potential efficacy of these novel anticoagulants as adjuncts to thrombolytic therapy has been experimentally shown for TF pathway inhibitors [146,154], activated protein C [163], and tick anticoagulant peptide [164]. The first studies with r-TFPI in humans are underway.

ANTIPLATELET AGENTS

Because resistance to thrombolysis, as well as reocclusion, are to some extent platelet-related phenomena [165,166] and plasmin generation may lead to additional platelet activation [76,77], antiplatelet agents remain a logical alternative or adjunct to antithrombins and anticoagulants in the context of thrombolysis.

Aspirin, which irreversibly inhibits the cyclooxigenases of both platelet and endothelial cell is now standard treatment for AMI. The ISIS-2 [2] trial has shown its independent effect on survival after streptokinase-induced thrombolysis, which is likely to be due to a significant protection from rethrombosis. Experimentally [128,167] as well as clinically [82], aspirin does not enhance thrombolysis.

Thromboxane A_2 synthase inhibitors block the platelet activating thromboxane A_2 (TxA_2) production specifically, while preserving the endothelial inhibitory prostanoid production (prostaglandin D2, prostacyclin). But accumulating prostaglandin endoperoxides may occupy TxA_2 receptors and activate platelets [168]. Thromboxane A_2 synthase inhibitors could not be shown to enhance arterial fibrinolysis significantly [25,169].

Thromboxane A_2/prostaglandin endoperoxide receptor antagonists competitively inhibit platelet activation by both TxA_2 and endoperoxides without increasing the production of platelet-inhibiting prostanoids. High local TxA_2 levels, however, may dislocate the drug from the receptor. Thromboxane A_2/prostaglandin endoperoxide receptor antagonists were shown experimentally to have a moderate effect on thrombolysis and reocclusion, especially in combination with a thrombin inhibitor [26,27,170].

Thromboxane A_2 synthase and thromboxane A_2/prostaglandin endoperoxide receptor inhibitors combine both pharmacologic principles, while a theoretical and experimental advantage over either intervention alone [28,171], while heparin remains mandatory to optimize the effect [172]. The first drug to be tested clinically [173], however, could not improve the reperfusion rate, reperfusion time, or reocclusion rate of alteplase [174].

Serotonin receptor antagonists represent an alternative approach to inhibiting platelet activation. Although a rather weak platelet inhibitor [175], especially in the context of deep arterial injury, combination with a thromboxane/prostaglandin endoperoxide receptor antagonist was shown experimentally to enhance thrombolysis and to prevent reocclusion with alteplase [24,176].

In view of the importance of thrombin as a platelet agonist in deep arterial injury, specific thrombin receptor antagonists not interfering with fibrin generation might be potent inhibitors of platelet thrombi at plaque rupture sites.

Prostacyclin is not only a platelet aggregation inhibitor but also a strong vasodilator. Additional protection could be anticipated during acute myocardial infarction by inhibiting oxygen free radicals and neutrophil function. However, acceleration of experimental reperfusion by prostacyclin [177], or its more stable analogue iloprost [178], was not demonstrated unequivocally, and clinical experience with prostacyclin analogues as adjuncts to thrombolysis remained disappointing [179,180].

GPIIb/IIIa INHIBITION

Following adhesion of a platelet monolayer to subendothelial glycoproteins, platelet aggregation is mediated exclusively by the binding of circulating glycoproteins (mainly fibrinogen and von Willebrand factor) to the activated platelet surface receptor GPIIb/IIIa. Neutralizing this agonist-independent last step, therefore, represents the most potent pharmacological intervention to inhibit platelet thrombus formation [181].

Inhibition of GPIIb/IIIa was first achieved by monoclonal antibodies [182]. Subsequently snake venom proteins were identified, which compete, with their arginine (or lysine)-glycine-aspartic acid (RGD or KGD) sequence, with fibrinogen or von Willebrand factor for receptor occupancy. Snake venoms have a high affinity but low selectivity for GPIIb/IIIa, also interfering with other related cellular surface receptors (integrins). A number of smaller synthetic RGD (or KGD) peptides were developed with increased selectivity and intermediate affinity for GPIIb/IIIa. Finally, peptidomimetics, organic molecules based on the RGD structure, without peptide bonds and therefore of potential oral activity, are now available.

As anticipated, GPIIb/IIIa inhibition is particularly effective in conjunction with experimental thrombolysis. The moncolonal antibody fragment $7E_3$-F(ab')$_2$ shortens the time to lysis and effectively abolishes reocclusion [46–48,183–185], even when administered after thrombolysis [48,185] or in stringent models, such as everted artery preparations [186,187]. Additional thrombin inhibition, for example by heparin, nevertheless seems beneficial [57]. In a direct comparison, the combination of $7E_3$-F(ab')$_2$ and heparin, added to alteplase, offered better protection from reocclusion than the combination of argatroban and aspirin [129]. Snake venoms were also shown to be potent adjuncts to alteplase and heparin in various animal models of platelet-rich clot lysis [50,51,188,189]. While some weaker RGD peptides, especially without heparin, were less effective than hirudin + aspirin [30,52], others [53,54], including at least one peptidomimetic [56,190], appeared to be as potent as $7E_3$-F(ab')$_2$. Again, caution is warranted when comparing data from different animal models.

Clinical studies with GPIIb/IIIa inhibitors have first focused on preventing thrombotic events following percutaneous coronary revascularization procedures (PTCA, atherectomy, stenting) and in unstable angina. In patients undergoing percutaneous coronary revascularization at incremental risk of acute thrombotic complications, $7E_3$-F(ab')$_2$ (ReoPro) significantly reduced the incidence of death, MI, or reintervention at 1 month from 12.8% to 9.8% (EPIC [191]) and became the first new antithrombotic agent to be approved for clinical use. This benefit was recently shown to remain significant at 6 months [192] and to extend to elective PTCA, with two comparative studies stopped prematurely because of an impressive (albeit perhaps overestimated) reduction in death and AMI (EPILOG, 3.1% vs. 8.1% [193]; CAPTURE, 5.4% vs. 10.9% [194]; preliminary results) at 1 month.

While the KGD-peptide Integrelin (IMPACT-2 [195]) and the peptidomimetic Tirofiban (RESTORE [196]) showed a significant early benefit in patients undergoing PTCA as well, this effect, similar to what was experienced with hirudin [136], was not sustained (9.5% vs. 11.6% [195] and 10.3% vs. 12.2% [196], respectively, for death, AMI, or reintervention at 1 month, data preliminary), leaving the question of an adequate duration of intravenous or oral follow-up treatment open. Indeed, RGD or KGD-related substances that compete with fibrinogen for receptor occupancy have a much shorter pharmacodynamic half-life than a monoclonal antibody blocking the receptor irreversibly. In patients with unstable angina, the peptidomimetic Lamifiban looked promising in a small randomized trial (death and MI at 1 month 2.5% vs. 8.1% [197]). Lamifiban (PARAGON), as well as Tirofiban (PRISM, PRISH PLUS) and Integrelin (PERSUIT), are currently being evaluated in large-scale trials of unstable angina.

Based on experimental evidence, GPIIb/IIIa antagonists seem particularly effective adjuncts to thrombolytic therapy in AMI [183–190], with the aim of optimizing reperfusion quality (TIMI 3 flow rate), which was shown to correlate with the clinical outcome in GUSTO-1 [18]. $7E_3$-F(ab')$_2$ (ReoPro) has been given to a limited number of patients following treatment with alteplase [198]. Integrelin (IMPACT-AMI [199]), as well as Lamifiban (PARADIGM [200]), given concomitantly with either alteplase or streptokinase, are currently being evaluated in dose-finding trials of AMI.

With new specific and potent antithrombotic drugs in development, concomitant thrombolytic and antithrombotic treatment now faces particularly interesting opportunities and challenges. Ultimately, large clinical trials will have to determine the benefit to risk ratios of well-selected regimens, which might also include lower dose combinations of thrombolytics, antithrombins, and antiplatelet drugs. However, accelerating the process of lysis. although experimentally attractive, will have much less clinical impact than shortening the delay between vessel oc-

clusion and the start of therapy. Infarct mortality rates of 4% in patients obtaining early complete (TIMI 3) reperfusion [18] indicate both the therapeutic advance as well as the limits of validating futher progress with this endpoint in reasonably sized studies. Mortality rates among patients with acute myocardial infarction not reaching the hospital are still considerably higher

Future efforts will, therefore, focus on safe ambulatory thrombolysis as well as secondary, if not primary, prevention of plaque rupture. Protection from reocclusion beyond the time of immediate drug effect, without increased bleeding risk, remains an important goal, called *vessel passivation*. Increasing awareness of health costs will probably focus interest on synthetic compounds, if equivalent to biotechnology products, when new antithrombotic drugs become available clinically for the conjunctive treatment of acute myocardial infarction.

Since submission of this manuscript in early 1996 several important clinical trials using new antithrombotic agents in the setting of PTCA and unstable angina were completed. Although they could not be included and referenced here, these studies have not, as yet, changed the clinical practice in the conjunctive antithrombotic-thrombolytic treatment of AMI.

References

1. Gruppo Italiano per lo Studio della Streptokinasi nell Infarto Miocardico (GISSI). Effectiveness of intravenous thrombolytic treatment in acute myocardial infarction. Lancet 1:397, 1986.

2. ISIS-2 (Second International Study of Infarct Survival) Collaborative Group. Randomized trial of intravenous streptokinase, oral aspirin, both, or neither among 17,187 cases of suspected acute myocardial infarction: ISIS-2. Lancet 2:349, 1988.

3. The International Study Group. Inhospital mortality and clinical course of 20,891 patients with suspected acute myocardial infarction randomised between alteplase and streptokinase with or without heparin. Lancet 1:71, 1990.

4. Gruppo Italiano per lo Studio della Streptokinasi nell Infarto Miocardico (GISSI). A factorial randomized trial of alteplase versus streptokinase and heparin versus no heparin among 12,490 patients with acute myocardial infarction. Lancet 2:336, 1990.

5. International Study of Infarct Survival. Collaborative Group. ISIS-3: A randomized comparison of streptokinase vs. tissue plasminogen activator vs. anistreplase and of aspirin plus heparin vs. aspirin alone among 41,299 cases of suspected myocardial infarction. Lancet 1:339, 1992.

6. Collen D. Coronary thrombolysis: Streptokinase or recombinant tissue-type plasminogen activator? Ann Intern Med 112:529, 1990.
7. White D. GISSI-2 and the heparin controversy. Lancet 2:297, 1990.
8. Sherry S, Marder V. Streptokinase and recombinant tissue-type plasminogen activator (alteplase) are equally effective in treating acute myocardial infarction. Ann Intern Med 114:417, 1991.
9. Sobel BE, Hirsh J. Principles and practice of coronary thrombolysis and conjunctive treatment. Am J Cardiol 68:382, 1991.
10. Collen D. Thrombolysis: Is there a future for thrombolytic therapy in acute myocardial infarction? Curr Opin Cardiol 6:552, 1991.
11. The TIMI Study Group. The thrombolysis in myocardial infarction (TIMI) trial. Phase I findings. N Engl J Med 312:932, 1985.
12. Verstraete M, Bernard R, Bory M, for the European Co-operative Study Group. Randomized trial of intravenous recombinant tissue-type plasminogen activator versus intravenous streptokinase in acute myocardial infarction. Lancet 1:842, 1985.
13. Lamas GA, Flaker GC, Mitchell G, Smith S, Gersh BJ, Wun CC, Moye L, Rouleau JL, Rutherford JD, Pfeffer, MA, Braunwald E for the SAVE Investigators. Effect of infarct artery patency on prognosis after acute myocardial infarction. Circulation 92:1101, 1995.
14. Ohman EM, Califf RM, Topol EJ, Candela R, Abbottsmith C, Ellis S, Sigmon KN, Kereiakes D, George B, Stack R. Consequences of reocclusion after successful reperfusion therapy in acute myocardial infarction. Circulation 82:781, 1990.
15. Rapold HJ, Kuemmerli H, Weiss M, Baur H, Haeberli A. Monitoring of fibrin generation during thrombolytic therapy of acute myocardial infarction with recombinant tissue-type plasminogen activator. Circulation 79:980, 1989.
16. Rapold HJ. Promotion of thrombin activity by thrombolytic therapy without simultaneous anticoagulation. Lancet 1:481, 1990.
17. Rapold HJ, Lu HR, Wu Z, Nijs H, Collen D. Requirement of heparin for arterial and venous thrombolysis with recombinant tissue-type plasminogen activator. Blood 77:1020, 1991.
18. The GUSTO Investigators. An international randomized trial comparing four thrombolytic strategies for acute myocardial infarction. N Engl J Med 329:673, 1993.
19. Gold HK. Conjunctive antithrombotic and thrombolytic therapy for coronary artery occlusion. N Engl J Med 323:1483, 1990.
20. Rapold HJ, Collen D. Conjunctive antithrombotic and thrombolytic therapy for acute myocardial infarction. Fibrinolysis 6:137, 1992.
21. Sobel BE (ed). Conjunctive therapy for thrombolysis. Review in depth. Cor Art Dis 3:987, 1992.
22. International Society and Federation of Cardiology and World Health Organization Task Force on Myocardial Reperfusion. Reperfusion in acute myocardial infarction. Circulation 90:2091, 1994.
23. Folts JD, Criwell EB, Row GG. Platelet aggregation in partially obstructed vessels and its elimination with aspirin. Circulation 54:365, 1976.
24. Golino P, Ashton JH, McNatt J, Glas-Greenwalt P, Yao SK, O'Brien RA, Buja LM, Willerson JT. Simultaneous administration of thromboxane A2 and serotonin S2 receptor antagonists markedly enhances thrombolysis and prevents or delays reocclusion after tissue-type plasminogen activator in a canine model of coronary thrombosis. Circulation 79:911, 1989.
25. Michelson JK, Simpson PJ, Gallas MT, Lucchesi BR. Thromboxane synthase inhibition with CGS13080 improves coronary blood flow after streptokinase-induce thrombolysis. Am Heart J 113:1345, 1987.
26. Shebuski RJ, Smith JM Jr, Storer BL, Granett JR, Bugelski PJ. Influence of selective endoperoxide/thromboxane A2 receptor antagonism with sulotroban on lysis time and reocclusion rate after tissue plasminogen activator-induced coronary thrombolysis in the drug. J Pharmacol Exp Ther 246:790, 1988.
27. Kopia GA, Kopaciewicz LJ, Ohlstein EH, Horohonich S, Storer BL, Shebuski RJ. Combination of the thromboxane receptor antagonist, sulotroban, with streptokinase: Demonstration of thrombolytic synergy. J Pharmacol Exp Ther 250:887, 1989.
28. Golino P, Rosolowsky M, Sheng-Kun Yao, Buja LM, Willerson JT. Blockade of TxB_2 synthase enhances thrombolysis and prevents reocclusion more efficiently than either intervention alone. Circulation 80:(Suppl II):II113, 1989.
29. Jang IK, Gold HK, Ziskind AA, Leinbach RC, Fallon JT, Collen D. Prevention of platelet-rich arterial thrombosis by selective thrombin inhibition. Circulation 81:219, 1990.
30. Haskel EJ, Prager NA, Sobel BE, Abendschein DR. Relative efficacy of antithrombin compared with antiplatelet agents in accelerating coronary thrombolysis and preventing early reocclusion. Circulation 83:1048, 1991.
31. Lam JYT, Chesebro JH, Badimon L, Fuster V. Serotonin and thromboxane A_2 receptor blockade decreases vasoconstriction but not platelet deposition after deep arterial injury (abstr). Circulation 74(Suppl. II):II97, 1986.
32. Chesebro JH, Badimon L, Fuster V. Importance of antithrombin therapy during coronary angioplasty. J Am Coll Cardiol 17:96B, 1991.
33. Heras M, Chesebro JH, Penny WJ, Bailey KR, Badimon L, Fuster V. Effects of thrombin inhibition on the development of acute platelet-thrombus deposition during angioplasty in pigs: Heparin versus recombinant hirudin, a specific thrombin inhibitor. Circulation 79:657, 1989.
34. Bettelheim FR. The clotting of fibrinogen: II. Frac-

tionation of peptide material liberated. Biochim Biophys Acta 19:121, 1956.

35. Bar-Shavit R, Benezra M, Sabbah V, Bode W, Vlodovsky I. Thrombin as a multifunctional protein: Induction of cell adhesion and proliferation. Am J Respir Cell Mol Biol 6:123, 1992.

36. Chesebro JH, Fuster V. Dynamic thrombosis and thrombolysis. Role of antithrombins. Circulation 83:1815, 1991.

37. Stassen JM, Juhan-Vague I, Alessi MC, De Cock F, Collen D. Potentiation by heparin fragments of thrombolysis induced with human tissue-type plasminogen activator. Thromb Haemost 58:947, 1987.

38. Cercek B, Lew AS, Hod H, Yano J, Reddy NK, Ganz W. Enhancement of thrombolysis with tissue-type plasminogen activator by pretreatment with heparin. Circulation 74:583, 1986.

39. Agnelli G, Pasucci C, Cosmi B, Nena G. Effects of therapeutic doses of heparin on thrombolysis with tissue-type plasminogen activator in rabbits. Blood 76:2030, 1990.

40. Stassen JM, Rapold HJ, Valinthout I, Collen D. Comparative effects of Enoxaparin and Heparin on arterial and venous clot lysis with alteplase in dogs. Thromb Haemost 69:454, 1993.

41. Rudd MA, George D, Johnstone MT, Moore RT, Collins L, Robbiani LE, Loscalzo J. Effect of thrombin inhibition on the dynamics of thrombolysis and on platelet function during thrombolytic therapy. Circ Res 70:829, 1992.

42. Klement P, Borm A, Hirsh J, Maraganore J, Wilson G, Weitz J. The effect of thrombin inhibitors on tissue plasminogen activator induced thrombolysis in a rat model. Thromb Heamost 68:64, 1992.

43. Stassen JM, Nystrom A, Hoylaerts M, Collen D. Antithrombotic effects of thrombolytic agents in a platelet-rich femoral vein thrombosis model in the hamster. Circulation 91:1330, 1995.

44. Badimon L, Lassila R, Badimon J, Vallabhajosula S, Chesebro JH, Fuster V. Residual thrombus is more thrombogenic than severely damaged vessel wall (abstr). Circulation 78(Suppl. II):II119, 1988.

45. Weitz JI, Hudoba M, Massel D, Maraganore J, Hirsh J. Clot-bound thrombin is protected from inhibition by heparin-antithrombin III but is susceptible to inactivation by antithrombin III-independent inhibitors. J Clin Invest 86:385, 1990.

46. Gold HK, Coller BS, Yasada T, Saito T, Fallon JT, Guerrero JL, Leinbach RC, Ziskind AA, Collen D. Rapid and sustained coronary artery recanalization with combined bolus injection of recombinant tissue-type plasminogen activator and monoclonal antiplatelet GPIIb/IIIa antibody in a canine preparation. Circulation 77:670, 1988.

47. Yasuda T, Gold HK, Fallon JT, Leinbach RC, Guerrero JL, Scudder LE, Kanke M, Shealy D, Ross MJ, Collen D, Coller BS. Monoclonal antibody against the platelet glycoprotein (GP) IIb/IIIa recep-

tor prevents coronary artery reocclusion after reperfusion with recombinant tissue-type plasminogen activator in dogs. J Clin Invest 81:1284, 1988.

48. Mickelson J, Simpson PJ, Cronin M, Homeister JW, Laywel E, Kitzen J, Lucchesi BR. Antiplatelet antibody 7E3 F(ab')₂ prevents rethrombosis after alteplase induced coronary artery thrombolysis in a canine model. Circulation 81:617, 1990.

49. Spriggs D, Gold HK, Hashimoto Y, Vanhoutte E, Bermylen J, Collen D. Absence of potentiation with murine antiplatelet GPIIb/IIIa antibody of thrombolysis with recombinant tissue-type plasminogen activator (alteplase) in a canine venous thrombosis model. Thromb Hemost 61:93, 1989.

50. Shebuski RJ, Stabilito IJ, Sitko GR, Polokoff MH. Acceleration of recombinant tissue-type plasminogen activator-induced thrombolysis and prevention of reocclusion by the combination of heparin and the Arg-Gly-Asp-containing peptide Bitistatin in a canine model of coronary thrombosis. Circulation 82:169, 1990.

51. Yasuda T, Gold HK, Leinbach RC, Yaoita H, Fallon JT, Guerrero L, Napier M, Bunting S, Collen D. Kistrin, a polypeptide platelet GPIIb/IIIa receptor antagonist enhances and sustains coronary arterial thrombolysis with recombinant tissue-type plasminogen activator in a canine preparation. Circulation 83:1038, 1991.

52. Haskel EJ, Adams SP, Feigen LP, Saffitz JE, Gorczynski RJ, Sobel BE, Abenschein DR. Prevention of reoccluding platelet-rich thrombi in canine femoral arteries with a novel peptide antagonist of platelet glycoprotein IIb/IIIa receptors. Circulation 80:1775, 1989.

53. Nichols A, Vasko J, Koster P, Smith J, Barone F, Nelson A, Stadel J, Powers D, Rhodes G, Miller-Stein C, Boppana V, Bennet D, Berry D, Romoff T, Calvo R, Ali F, Sorenson E, Samanen J. SK&F 106760, a novel GPIIb/IIIa antagonist: Antithrombotic activity and potentiation of streptokinase-mediated thrombolysis. Eur J Pharmacol 183:2019, 1990.

54. Lu Hr, Gold HK, Wu Z, Yasuda T, Pauwels P, Rapold HJ, Napier M, Bunting S, Collen D. G4120, a Arg-Gly-Asp containing pentapeptide, enhances arterial eversion graft recanalization with recombinant tissue-type plasminogen activator in dogs. Thromb Haemost 6:686, 1992.

55. Rapold HJ, Gold HK, Wu Z, Napier M, Bunting S, Collen D. Effects of G4120, a ARG-GLY-ASP containing synthetic platelet glycoprotein IIb/IIIa receptor antagonist, on arterial and venous thrombolysis with recombinant tissue-type plasminogen activator in dogs. Fibrinolysis 7:248, 1993.

56. Roux S, Tschopp T, Kuhn H, Steiner B, Hadvary P. Effects of heparin, aspirin and a synthetic platelet GP IIb/IIIa receptor antagonist (Ro 43-5054) on coronary artery reperfusion and reocclusion after thrombolysis with alteplase in the dog. J Pharm Exp Ther 264:501, 1993.

57. Yasuda T, Gold H, Leinbach R, Fellon J, Guerrero L, Yaoita H, Collen D. Effect of reduced heparin on alteplase thrombolysis during platelet IIb/IIIa receptor blockade (abstr). Circulation 81(Suppl. III):III276, 1990.

58. Nossel HL, Yudelman I, Canfield RE, Butler VP Jr, Spanondis K, Wilner GD, Quereshi GD. Measurement of fibrinopeptide A in human blood. J Clin Invest 54:43, 1974.

59. Hofmann V, Straub PA. A radioimmunoassay for rapid measurement of human fibrinopeptide A. Thromb Res 11:171, 1977.

60. Pelzer H, Schwarz A, Heimburger N. Determination of human thrombin-antithrombin-III-complex in plasma with an enzyme-linked immunosorbent assay. Thromb Hemostas 59:101, 1988.

61. Yudelman I, Nossel HL, Kaplan KL, Hirsch J. Fibrinopeptide A levels in symptomatic thromboembolism. Blood 51:1189, 1978.

62. Gallino A, Häberli A, Baur HR, Straub PW. Fibrin formation and platelet aggregation in patients with severe coronary artery disease: Relationship with the degree of myocardial ischemia. Circulation 72:27, 1985.

63. Théroux P, Latour JG, Légier-Gauthier C, De Lara J. Fibrinopeptide A and platelet factor levels in unstable angina pectoris. Circulation 75:156, 1987.

64. Johnsson H, Orinius E, Paul C. Fibrinopeptide A in patients with acute myocardial infarction. Thromb Res 16:255, 1979.

65. Mombelli G, Imhof V, Häberli A, Straub PW. Effect of heparin on plasma fibrinopeptide A in patients with acute myocardial infarction. Circulation 69:684, 1984.

66. Eisenberg PR, Sobel BE, Jaffe AS. Activation of prothrombin accompanying thrombolysis with alteplase. J Am Coll Cardiol 19:1065, 1992.

67. Theroux P, Waters D, Lam J, Juneau M, McCans J. Reactivation of unstable angina after discontinuation of heparin. N Engl J Med 327:141, 1992.

68. Granger CB, Miller JM, Bivill EG, Gruber A, Tracy RP, Krucoff MW, Green C, Berrios E, Harrington RA, Ohman M, Califf RM. Rebound increase in thrombin generation and activity after cessation of intravenous heparin in patients with acute coronary syndromes. Circulation 91:1929, 1995.

69. Rapold HJ, de Bono D, Arnold AER, de Cock F, Arnout J, Collen D and Verstraete M, for the European Co-operative Study Group. Plasma fibrinopeptide A levels in patients with acute myocardial infarction treated with alteplase: correlation with concomitant heparin, coronary artery patency, and recurrent ischemia. Circulation 85:928, 1992.

70. Arnout J, Simoons M, de Bono D, Rapold HJ, Collen D, Verstraete M. Correlation between level of heparin and patency of the infarct-related coronary artery after treatment of acute myocardial infarction with alteplase (alteplase). J Am Coll Cardiol 20:513, 1992.

71. Eisenberg PR, Sherman LA, Jaffe AS. Paradoxic elevation of fibrinopeptide A after streptokinase: Evidence of continued thrombosis despite intense fibrinolysis. J Am Coll Cardiol 10:527, 1987.

72. Kruithof EKO. Plasminogen activator inhibitor type 1: Biochemical, biological and clinical aspects. Fibrinolysis Suppl 2:59, 1988.

73. Rapold HJ, Grimaudo V, Declerck PJ, Kruithof EKO, Bachmann F. Plasma levels of plasminogen activator inhibitor type 1, betathromboglobulin and fibrinopeptide A before, during and following treatment of acute myocardial infarction with tissue-type plasminogen activator. Blood 6:1490, 1991.

74. Lee CD, Mann KG. Activation and inactivation of human factor V by plasmin. Blood 73:185, 1989.

75. Eisenberg PR, Miletich JP, Sobel BE. Factors responsible for the differential procoagulant effects of diverse plasminogen activators in plasma. Fibrinolysis 5:217, 1991.

76. Niewiarowski S, Senyi AF, Gillies P. Plasmin induced platelet aggregation and platelet release reaction. J Clin Invest 52:1647, 1973.

77. Fitzgerald DJ, Catella F, Roy L, Fitzgerald GA. Marked platelet activation in vivo after intravenous streptokinase in patients with acute myocardial infarction. Circulation 77:142, 1988.

78. Ohlstein EH, Stover B, Fujita T, Shebuski RJ. Tissue-type plasminogen activator and streptokinase induce platelet hyperaggregability in the rabbit. Thromb Res 46:575, 1987.

79. Gouin I, Lecompte T, Morel MC, Lebrazi J, Modderman PW, Kaplan C, Samama MM. In vitro effects of plasmin on human platelet function in plasma. Circulation 85:935, 1992.

80. Roux S, Christeller S, Lüdin E. Effects of aspirin on coronary reocclusion and recurrent ischemia after thrombolysis: A meta-analysis. J Am Coll Cardiol 19:671, 1992.

81. Topol EJ, George BS, Kereiakes DJ, Stump DC, Candela RJ, Abbotsmith CW, Aronson L, Pickel A, Boswick JM, Lee KL, Ellis SG, Califf RM, TAMI Study Group. A randomized controlled trial of intravenous tissue plasminogen activator and early intravenous heparin in acute myocardial infarction. Circulation 79:281, 1989.

82. Hsia J, Hamilton WP, Kleiman N, Roberts R, Chaitman BR, Ross AM. A comparison between heparin and low-dose aspirin as adjunctive therapy with tissue-type plasminogen activator for acute myocardial infarction. N Engl J Med 323:1433, 1990.

83. Bleich SD, Nichols TC, Schumacher RR, Cooke DH, Tate DA, Teichman SL. Effect of heparin on coronary arterial patency after thrombolysis with tissue plasminogen activator in acute myocardial infarction. Am J Cardiol 66:1412, 1990.

84. De Bono DP, Simoons ML, Tijssen J, Arnold AER, Betriu A, Burgersdijk C, Baseos LL, Müller E, Pfisterer M, Van de Werf F, Zijlstra F, Verstraete M, for the ESCG. The effect of early intravenous heparin

on coronary patency, infarct size and bleeding complications after alteplase thrombolysis: Results of a randomized double blind European Co-operative Study Group trial. Br Heart J 67:122, 1992.

85. Simes RJ, Topol EJ, Holmes DR, White HD, Rutsch WR, Vahanian A, Simoons ML, Morris D, Betriu A, Califf RM, Ross AM for the Gusto-1 investigators. Link between the angiographic substudy and mortality outcomes in a large randomized trial of myocardial reperfusion. Circulation 91:1923, 1995.

86. Granger C, Hirsh J, Califf R, Col J, White H, Betriu A, Woodlief L, Lee K, Bovill E, Simes RJ. Activated partial thromboplastin time and outcome after thrombolytic therapy for acute myocardial infarction. Results from the GUSTO-I trial. Circulation 93:870, 1996.

87. Johnson EA, Mulloy B. The molecular-weight range of commercial heparin preparations. Carbohydr Res 51:119, 1979.

88. Rosenberg RD, Lam L. Correlation between structure and function of heparin. Proc Natl Acad Sci USA 76:1218, 1979.

89. Lindahl U, Backstrom G, Hook M, Thunberg L, Fransson L-A, Linker A. Structure of the antithrombin-binding site of heparin. Proc Natl Acad Sci USA 76:3198, 1979.

90. Rosenberg RD. The heparin-antithrombin system: A natural anticoagulant mechanism. In Coleman RW, Hirsh J, Marder VJ, Salzman EW (eds). Hemostasis and Thrombosis: Basic Principles and Clinical Practice, 2nd ed. Philadelphia: JB Lippincott, 1987:1373.

91. Chaoy J, Petitou M, Lormeau JC, Sinay P, Casu B, Gatti G. Structure-activity relationship in heparin: A synthetic pentasaccharide with high affinity for antithrombin III and eliciting high anti-factor Xa activity. Biochem Biophys Res Commun 116:492, 1983.

92. Rosenberg RD, Jordan RE, Favreau LV, Lam LH. High active heparin species with multiple binding sites for antithrombin. Biochem Biophys Res Commun 86:1319, 1979.

93. Bjork I, Lindahl U. Mechanism of the anticoagulant action of heparin. Mol Cell Biochem 48:161, 1982.

94. Danielsson A, Raub E, Lindahl U, Bjork I. Role of ternary complexes in which heparin binds both antithrombin and proteinase, in the acceleration of the reactions between antithrombin and thrombin or factor Xa. J Biol Chem 261:15467, 1986.

95. Jordan RE, Costa GM, Gardner WT, Rosenberg RD. The kinetics of hemostatic enzyme-antithrombin interactions in the presence of low molecular weight heparin. J Biol Chem 255:10081, 1980.

96. Bar-Shavit R, Eldor A, Vlodavsky I. Binding of thrombin to subendothelial extracellular matrix; protection and expression of functional properties. J Clin Invest 84:1096, 1989.

97. Marciniak E. Factor Xa inactivation by antithrombin III. Evidence for biological stabilization of factor Xa by factor V-phospholipid complex. Br J Haematol 23:391, 1973.

98. Walker FJ, Esmon CT. The effects of phospholipid and factor Va on the inhibition of factor Xa by antithrombin III. Biochem Biophys Res Commun 90:641, 1979.

99. Lane DA, Pejler G, Flynn AM, Thompson EA, Lindahl U. Neutralization of heparin-related saccharides by histidine-rich glycoprotein and platelet factor 4. J Biol Chem 261:3980, 1986.

100. Dawes J, Smith RC, Pepper DS. The release, distribution and clearance of human β-thromboglobulin and platelet factor 4. Thromb Res 12:851, 1978.

101. Mahadoo J, Hiebert L, Jaques LB. Vascular sequestration of heparin. Thromb Res 12:79, 1977.

102. Glimelius B, Busch C, Hook M. Binding of heparin on the surface of cultured human endothelial cells. Thromb Res 12:773, 1978.

103. Lindahl U, Hook M. Glycosaminoglycans and their binding to biological macromolecules. Ann Rev Biochem 46:385, 1978.

104. Ofosu FA, Barrowcliffe TW. Mechanisms of action of lower molecular weight heparins and heparinoids. In Hirsch J (ed). Antithrombiotic Therapy, Baillere's Clinical Haematology. London: Baillere Tindal, 1990:505.

105. Lane DA, Denton J, Flynn AM, Thunberg L, Lindahl U. Anticoagulant activites of heparin oligosaccharides and their neutralization by platelet factor 4. Biochem J 218:725, 1984.

106. Beguin S, Lindhout T, Hemker HC. The mode of action of heparin in plasma. Thromb Haemost 60:457, 1989.

107. Handeland GF, Abildgaard U, Holm U, Arnesen K-E. Dose adjusted heparin treatment of deep venous thrombosis: A comparison of unfractionated and low molecular weight heparin. Eur J Clin Pharmacol 39:107, 1990.

108. Baru T, Molho P, Tobelem G, Petitou M, Caen JP. Binding of heparin and lower molecular weight heparin fragments to human vascular endothelial cells in culture. Nouv Rev Fr Haematol 26:243, 1984.

109. Kakkar VV, Murray WJG. Efficacy and safety of low molecular weight heparin (CY216) in preventing post-operative venous thromboembolism. Br J Surg 72:786, 1985.

110. Caen JP. A randomised double-blind study between a low molecular weight heparin Kabi 2165 and standard heparin in the prevention of deep vein thrombosis in general surgery. Thromb Haemost 59:216, 1988.

111. Hartle P, Brucke P, Dienstl E, Vinazzer H. Prophylaxis of thromboembolism in general surgery: Comparison between standard heparin and fragmin. Thromb Res 57:577, 1990.

112. Leizorovicz A, Picolet H, Peyrieux JC, Borssel JP. Prevention of perioperative deep vein thrombosis in general surgery: A multicentre double-blind study

comparing two doses of logiparin and standard heparin. Br J Surg 78:412, 1991.

113. Planes A, Bochelle N, Mazas F, Mansat C, Zucman J, Landais A, et al. Prevention of postoperative venous thrombosis: A randomized trial comparing unfractionated heparin with low molecular weight heparin in patients undergoing total hip replacement. Thromb Haemost 60:407, 1988.

114. Estoppey D, Hochretter J, Breyer HG, Jakubek H, Leyvraz PF, Haas S, et al. ORG 10172 (Lomoparin) versus heparin-DHE in prevention of thromboembolism in total hip replacement: A multicentre trial (abstr). Thromb Haemost 61(Suppl.):356, 1989.

115. Levine MN, Hirsh J, Gent M, Turpie AGG, LeClerc J, Powers PJ, et al. Prevention of deep vein thrombosis after elective hip surgery: A randomized trial comparing low molecular weight heparin with standard unfractionated heparin. Ann Intern Med 114:545, 1991.

116. Kontny F, Abildgaard U, Pedersen T for the FRAMI Study Group. Low molecular weight Heparin (Fragmin) in acute myocardial infaction (abstr). J Am Coll Cardiol 27:(Suppl A):166A, 1996.

117. Markwardt F, Nowak G, Stürzebecher J, Griessbach U, Walsmann P, Vogel G. Pharmacokinetics and anticoagulant effect of hirudin in man. Thromb Haemost 52:160, 1984.

118. Stone SR, Hofsteenge J. Kinetics of the inhibition of thrombin by hirudin. Biochemistry 25:4622, 1986.

119. Inauen W, Baumgartner HR, Bombeli T, Haeberli A, Straub PW. Dose and shear rate-dependent effects of heparin on thrombogenesis induced by rabbit aorta subendothelium exposed to flowing human blood. Arteriosclerosis 10:607, 1990.

120. Heras M, Chesebro JH, Webster MWI, Mruk JS, Grill DE, Penny WJ. Hirudin, heparin and placebo during deep arterial injury in the pig. The in vivo role of thrombin in platelet-mediated thrombosis. Circulation 82:1476, 1990.

121. Maraganore JM, Chao B, Joseph ML, Jablonski J, Ramachandran KL. Anticoagulant activity of synthetic hirudin peptides. J Biol Chem 264:8692, 1989.

122. Jakubowski JA, Maraganore JM. Inhibition of coagulation and thrombin-induced platelet activation by a synthetic dodecapeptide modeled on the carboxterminus of hirudin. Blood 75:399, 1990.

123. Maraganore JM, Buordon P, Jablonski J, Ramachandran KL, Fenton JW II. Design and characterization of hirulogs: A novel class of bivalent peptide inhibitors of thrombin. Biochemistry 29:7095, 1990.

124. Collen D, Matsuo O, Stassen JM, Kettner C, Shaw E. In vivo studies of a synthetic inhibitor of thrombin. J Lab Clin Med 99:76, 1982.

125. Kettner C, Mersinger L, Knabb R. The selective inhibition of thrombin by peptides of boroarginine. J Biol Chem 265:18289, 1990.

126. Knabb RM, Kettner CA, Timmermans PB, Reilly

TM. In vivo characterization of a new synthetic thrombin inhibitor. Thromb Haemost 67:56, 1992.

127. Claeson G, Philipp M, Agner E, Sully M, Metternich R, Kakkar V, Desoyza T, Niu L. Benzyloxy-carbonyl-D-phe-pro-methoxyprophyl-boroglycine: A novel inhibitor of thrombin with high selectivity containing a neutral side chain at the P1 position. Biochem J 290:309, 1993.

128. Jang I, Gold HK, Leinbach RC, Fallon JT, Collen D. In vivo thrombin inhibition enhances and sustains arterial recanalization with recombinant tissue-type plasminogen activator. Circ Res 67:1552, 1990.

129. Yasuda T, Gold HK, Yaoita H, Leinbach RC, Guerrero JL, Jang I. Comparative effects of aspirin, a synthetic thrombin inhibitor and a monoclonal antiplatelet glycoprotein IIb/IIIa antibody on coronary artery reperfusion, reocclusion and bleeding with recombinant tissue-type plasminogen activator in a canine preparation. J Am Coll Cardiol 16:714, 1990.

130. The GUSTO 2A investigators. Randomized trial of intravenous heparin versus recombinant hirudin for acute coronary syndromes. Circulation 90:1632, 1994.

131. Antman EM for the TIMI 9a investigators. Hirudin in acute myocardial infarction — safety report from the thrombolysis and thrombin inhibition in myocardial infarction (TIMI) 9A trial. Circulation 90:1624, 1994.

132. Neuhaus KL, v. Essen R, Tebbe U, Jessel A, Heinrichs H. Safety observations from the pilot phase of the randomized r-Hirudin for Improvement of Thrombolysis (HIT 3) study. Circulation 90:1638, 1994.

133. Topol EJ. Global Use of Strategies To Open occluded arteries (GUSTO). The preliminary results of GUSTO 2b in patients undergoing thrombolysis for acute myocardial infarction. Presentation at the American Heart Association, Anaheim, CA, November 12th, 1995.

134. Elliot EM. Heparin Versus hirudin as adjunctive therapy for thrombolysis in acute myocardial infarction. The preliminary results of TIMI 9b. Presentation at the American Heart Association, Anaheim, CA, November 12th, 1995.

135. Van de Werf F. Global Use of Strategies To Open coronary arteries (GUSTO). The preliminary results of GUSTO 2b in patients with acute coronary syndromes. Presentation at the American College of Cardiology, Orlando, FL, March 26th, 1996.

136. Serruys PW, Herrman JP, Simon R, Rutsch W, Bode C, Laarman GJ, Van Dijk R, Van den Bos AA, Uhmans VA, Fox KA, Close P, Deckers JW for the HELVETICA investigators. A comparison of hirudin with heparin in the prevention of restenosis after coronary angioplasty. N Engl J Med 333:757, 1995.

137. Bittl JA, Strony J, Brinker JA, Ahmed WH, Meckel CR, Chaitman BR, Maraganore J, Deutsch E, Adelman B for the Hirulog Angioplasty Study investigators. Treatment with Bivalirudin (hirulog) as

compared with heparin during coronary angioplasty for unstable or postinfarction angina. N Engl J Med 333:764, 1995.

138. Gold HK, Torres FW, Garabedian HD, Werner W, Jang I, Khan A, Hagstrom J, Yasuda T, Leinbach R, Newell J. Evidence for a rebound coagulation phenomenon after cessation of a 4-hour infusion of a specific thrombin inhibitor in patients with unstable angina pectoris. J Am Coll Cardiol 21:1039, 1993.

139. Marmur JD, Rossikhina M, Guha A, Fyfe B, Friedrich V, Mendlowitz M, Nemerson Y, Taubman MB. Tissue factor is rapidly induced in arterial smooth muscle after balloon injury. J Clin Invest 91:2253, 1993.

140. Wilcox JN, Smith KM, Schwartz SM, Gordon D. Localization of tissue factor in normal vessel wall and in the atherosclerotic plaque. Proc Natl Acad Sci USA 86:2839, 1989.

141. Haskel EJ, Torr SR, Day KC, Palmier M, Wun TC, Sobel BE. Prevention of arterial reocclusion after thrombolysis with lipoprotein associated coagulation inhibitor (LACI). Circulation 84:821, 1991.

142. Creasy AA, Chang AC, Feigen L, Wun TC, Taylor FB, Hinshaw LB. Tissue factor pathway inhibitor reduces mortality from Escherichia coli septic shock. J Clin Invest 91:2850, 1993.

143. Mueller Berghaus G. Pathophysiologic and biochemical events in disseminated intravascular coagulation: Dysregulation of procoagulant and anticoagulant pathways. Semin Thromb Hemost 15:58, 1989.

144. Giercksky KE, Bjorklid E, Prydz H, Renck H. Circulating tissue thromboplastin during hip surgery. Eur Surg Res 11:296, 1979.

145. Carson SD, Haire WD, Broze GJ, Novotny WF Pirrucello SJ, Duggan MJ. Lipoprotein associated coagulation inhibitor, factor VII, antithrombin III and monocyte tissue factor following surgery. Thromb Haemost 66:534, 1991.

146. Girard TJ, Macphail LA, Likert KM, Novotny WF, Miletich JP, Broze GJ. Inhibition of factor VVIa-tissue factor coagulation activity by a hybrid protein. Science 248:1421, 1990.

147. Ruf W, Edgington TS. An anti-tissue factor monoclonal antibody which inhibits TF. VIIa complex is a potent anticoagulant in plasma. Thromb Haemost 66:529, 1991.

148. Broze GJ, Girard TJ, Novotny WF, et al. Regulation of coagulation by a multivalent Kunitz-type inhibitor. Biochemistry 29:7539, 1990.

149. Novotny WF, Palmier M, Wun TC, et al. Purification and properties of heparin-releasable lipoprotein-associated coagulation inhibitor. Blood 78:394, 1991.

150. Diaz-Collier JA, Palmier MO, Kretzmer KK. Refold and characterization of recombinant tissue factor pathway inhibitor expressed in Escherichia coli. Thromb Haemost 71:1, 1994.

151. Gustafson ME, Junger KD, Wun TC, et al. Renaturation and purification of human tissue factor pathway inhibitor expressed in recombinant E. coli. Protein Expr Purif, in press.

152. Speidel CM, Eisenberg PR, Ruf W, Edgington TS, Abendschein DR. Tissue factor mediated prolonged procoagulant activity on the luminal surface of balloon-injured aortas in rabbits. Circulation 92:3323, 1995.

153. Yang L, St. Pierre J, Kam G, Thornton D, Eisenberg P, Abendschein D. Tissue factor pathway inhibitor attenuates prothrombinase complex formation on balloon-injured arteries in pigs (abstr). J Am Coll Cardiol 27(Suppl. A):14A, 1996.

154. Abendschein DR, Meng YY, Torr-Brown S, Sobel BE. Maintenance of coronary patency after fibrinolysis with tissue factor pathway inhibitor. Circulation 92:944, 1995.

155. Koudsi B, Ferguson EW, Yu CD, Miller GA, Merkel KD, Wun TC, Money SR, Kraemer BA. The effects of tissue factor pathway inhibitor on myocardial infarct size (abstr). J Am Coll Cardiol 27(Suppl. A):81A, 1996.

156. Carr C, Bild GS, Chang AC, et al. Recombinant E. coli-derived tissue factor pathway inhibitor reduced coagulopathic and lethal effects in the baboon gram-negative model of septic shock. Circ Shock 44:126, 1995.

157. Benedict CR, Ryan J, Wolitzky B, Ramos R, Gerlach M, Tijburg P, et al. Active site-blocked factor Ixa prevents intravascular thrombus formation in the coronary vasculature without inhibiting extravascular coagulation in a canine thrombosis model. J Clin Invest 88:1760, 1991.

158. Marlar RA, Kleiss AJ, Griffin JH. Mechanism of action of human activated protein C, a thrombin-dependent anticoagulant enzyme. Blood 59:1067, 1982.

159. Gruber A, Hanson SR, Kelly AB, Yan BS, Bang N, Griffin JH. Inhibition of thrombus formation by activated recombinant protein C in a primate model of arterial thrombosis. Circulation 82:578, 1990.

160. Waxman L, Smith DE, Arcuri KE, Vlasuk GP. Tick anticoagulant peptide (TAP) is a novel inhibitor of blood coagulation factor Xa. Science 248:593, 1990.

161. Schaffer LW, Davidson JT, Vlasuk GP, Siegl PKS. Antithrombotic efficacy of recombinant tick anticoagulant peptide. A potent inhibitor of coagulation factor Xa in a primate model of arterial thrombosis. Circulation 84:1741, 1991.

162. Nawroth PP, Kisiel W, Stern DM. Anticoagulant and antithrombotic properties of a gamma-carboxyglutamic acid-rich peptide derived from the light chain of blood coagulation factor X. Thromb Res 44:625, 1986.

163. Gruber A, Harker LA, Hanson SR, Kelly AB, Griffin JH. Antithrombotic effects of combining activated protein C and urokinase in non-human primates. Circulation 84:2454, 1991.

164. Sitko GR, Ramjit DR, Stabilito II, Lehman D, Lynch

JJ, Vlasuk GP. Conjunctive enhancement of enzymatic thrombolysis and prevention of thrombotic reocclusion with the selective factor Xa inhibitor, tick anticoagulant peptide. Circulation 85:805, 1992.

165. Richardson SG, Allen DC, Morton P, Murtagh JG, Scott ME, O'Keefe DB. Pathological changes after intravenous streptokinase treatment in eight patients with acute myocardial infarction. Br Heart J 61:390, 1989.

166. Jang IK, Gold HK, Ziskind AA, Fallon JT, Holt RE, Leinbach RC, et al. Differential sensitivity of erythrocyte-rich and platelet-rich arterial thrombi to lysis with recombinant tissue-type plasminogen activator. A possible explanation for resistance to coronary thrombolysis. Circulation 79:920, 1989.

167. Fitzgerald DJ, Wright F, Fitzgerald GA. Increased thromboxane biosynthesis during coronary thrombolysis. Evidence that platelet activation and thromboxane A_2 modulate the response to tissue-type plasminogen activator in vivo. Circ Res 65:83, 1989.

168. Bertele V, Certletti C, Schieppati A, Di Minno G, De Gaetano G. Inhibition of thromboxane synthase does not necessarily prevent platelet aggregation. Lancet 1:1057, 1981.

169. Shebuski RJ, Storer BL, Fujita T. Effect of thromboxane synthase inhibition on the thrombolytic action of tissue-type plasminogen activator, in a rabbit model of peripheral arterial thrombosis. Thromb Res 52:382, 1988.

170. Grover GJ, Parham CS, Schumacher WA. The combined antiischemic effects of the thromboxane receptor antagonist SQ 30741 and tissue type plasminogen activator. Am Heart J 121:426, 1991.

171. Golino P, Rosolowsky M, Sheng-Kun Yao, Buja LM, Willerson JT. Blockade of TXA_2 receptors and inhibition of TXA_2 synthase enhances thrombolysis and prevents reocclusion more efficiently than either intervention alone (abstr). Circulation 80(Suppl. II) II113, 1989.

172. Van De Water A, Xhonneux R, De Clerck F, Willerson JT. Heparin enhances the synergism between platelet TXA_2 synthase inhibition/receptor blockade (ridogrel) and tissue plasminogen activator in lysing canine coronary thrombi (abstr). J Am Coll Cardiol 17:52, 1991.

173. Rapold HJ, Van de Werf F, De Geest H, Arnout J, Sangtawesin W, Vercammen E, De Clerck F, Weber C, Collen D. Pilot study of combined administration of ridogrel and alteplase in patients with acute myocardial infarction. Cor Art Dis 2:455, 1991.

174. Tranchesi B, Caramelli B, Gebara O, Bellotti G, Pileggi F, Van de Werf F, et al. Efficacy and safety of ridogrel versus aspirin in coronary thrombolysis with alteplase for myocardial infarction (abstr). J Am Coll Cardiol 19:92A, 1992.

175. Golino P, Buja LM, Ashton JH, Kulkarni P, Taylor A, Willerson JT. Effect of thromboxane and serotonin receptor antagonists on intracoronary platelet deposi-tion in dogs with experimentally stenosed coronary arteries. Circulation 78:701, 1988.

176. Golino P, Ashton JH, Glas-Greenwalt P, McNatt J, Buja LM, Willerson JT. Mediation of reocclusion by thromboxane A_2 and serotonin after thrombolysis with tissue-type plasminogen activator in a canine preparation of coronary thrombosis. Circulation 77:678, 1988.

177. Schumacher WA, Lee EC, Lucchesi BR. Augmentation of streptokinase-induced thrombolysis by heparin and prostacyclin. J Cardiovasc Pharmacol 7:739, 1985.

178. Nicolini FA, Mehta JL, Nichols WW, Saldeen TGP, Grant M. Prostacyclin analogue iloprost decreases thrombolytic potential of tissue-type plasminogen activator in canine coronary thrombosis. Circulation 81:1115, 1990.

179. Sharma B, Wyeth RP, Gimenez HJ, Franciosa JA. Intracoronary prostaglandin E1 plus streptokinase in acute myocardial infarction. Am J Cardiol 58:1161, 1986.

180. Topol EJ, Ellis SG, Califf RM, George BS, Stump DC, Bates ER, et al. Combined tissue-type plasminogen activator and prostacyclin therapy for acute myocardial infarction. J Am Coll Cardiol 14:877, 1989.

181. Coller BS. Platelets in cardiovascular thormbosis and thrombolysis. In Fozzard HA, Haber E, Jennings RB, Katz AM, Morgan HE (eds). The Heart and Cardiovascular Systems, 2nd ed. New York: Raven Press, 1991:219.

182. Coller BS, Peerschke EI, Scudder LE, Sullivan CA. A murine monoclonal antibody that completely blocks the binding of fibrinogen to platelets produces a thrombasthenic-like state in normal platelet and binds to glycoproteins IIb and/or IIIa. Clin Invest 72:325, 1983.

183. Fitzgerald DJ, Wright F, FitzGerald GA. Increased thromboxane biosynthesis during coronary thrombolysis. Circ Res 65:83, 1989.

184. Fitzgerald DJ, Hanson M, FitzGerald GA. Systemic lysis protects against the effects of platelet activation during coronary thrombolysis. J Clin Invest 88:1589, 1991.

185. Rote WE, Walsh DG, Bates ER, Mu DX, Nedelman MA, Lucchesi BR. Comparison of 7E3 $F(ab')_2$ antibody with hirudin after alteplase induced thrombolysis in a chronic model of coronary thrombosis. FASEB J 6:A1877, 1992.

186. Yasuda T, Gold HK, Leinbach RC, Saito T, Guerrero JL, Jang I-K. Lysis of plasminogen activator-resistant platelet-rich coronary artery thrombus with combined bolus injection of recombinant tissue-type plasminogen activator and antiplatelet GPIIb/IIIa antibody. J Am Coll Cardiol 7:1728, 1990.

187. Lu HR, Gold HK, Wu Z, De Cock F, Jang IK, Pauwels P. Acceleration and persistence of recombinant tissue plasminogen activator induced arterial eversion graft recanalization with a single bolus injec-

tion of F(ab')₂ fragments of the antiplatelet GPIIb/IIIa antibody 7E3. Cor Art Dis 2:1039, 1991.

188. Holahan MA, Mellott MJ, Garsky VM, Shebuski RJ. Prevention of reocclusion following tissue-type plasminogen activator-induced thrombolysis by the RGD-containing peptide, echistatin, in a canine model of coronary thrombosis. Pharmacology 42:340, 1991.

189. Scarborough RM, Rose JW, Hsu MA, Phillips DR, Fried VA, Campbell AM. Barbourin: A GPIIb/IIIa specific integrin antagonist from the venom of Sistrurus M barbouri. J Biol Chem 266:9359, 1991.

190. Alig L, Edenhofer A, Hadvary P, Hürzeler M, Knopp D, Müller M, Steiner B, Trzeciak A, Weller T. Low molecular weight, non-peptide fibrinogen receptor antagonists. J Med Chem 35:4393, 1992.

191. The EPIC investigators. Use of a monoclonal antibody directed against the platelet glycoprotein IIb/IIIa receptor in high-risk coronary angioplasty. N Engl J Med 330:956, 1994.

192. Topol EJ, Califf RM, Weisman HF, Anderson K, Wang A, Willerson JT. Randomized trial of coronary intervention with antibody against platelet IIb/IIIa integrin for reduction of clinical restenosis: Results at six months. The EPIC investigators. Lancet 343:881, 1994.

193. Lincoff AM. Use of the monoclonal antibody against GP IIb/IIIa 7E3-F(ab')2 (ReoPro) in percutaneous coronary interventions. The preliminary results of the EPILOG trial (1500 patients). Presentation at the American College of Cardiology, Orlando, FL, March 27th, 1996.

194. Simoons M. Use of the monoclonal antibody against GP IIb/IIIa 7E3-F(ab')2 (ReoPro) in high risk patients undergoing PTCA. The preliminary results of the CAPTURE trial (2000 patients). Presentation at

the American College of Cardiology, Orlando, FL, March 27th, 1996.

195. Horrigan MC, Tscheng JE, Califf RM, Kitt M, Lorenz T, Sigmon K, Lincoff AM, Topol EJ. Maximal benefit of Integrelin Platelet IIb/IIIa blockade 6–24 hours after therapy: Results of the IMPACT-2 trial (abstr). J Am Coll Cardiol 27(Suppl. A):55, 1996.

196. King S. Administration of Tirofiban (MK 383) will reduce the incidence of adverse cardiac outcome following PTCA/PTA. The preliminary results of the RESTORE trial. Presentation at the American College of Cardiology, Orlando, FL, March 27th, 1996.

197. Theroux P, Kouz S, Nasmith J, Knudtson M, Kells C, Bokslag M, Rapold HJ. Platelet membrane receptor GP IIb/IIIa antagonism in unstable angina. The Canadian Lamifiban study. Circulation 94:899, 1996.

198. Kleiman NS, Ohman EM, Keriakes DJ, Ellis SG, Weisman HF, Topol EJ. Profound platelet inactivation with 7E3 shortly after thrombolytic therapy for acute myocardial infarction: Preliminary results of the TAMI 8 trial (abstr). Circulation 84(Suppl. II):II522, 1991.

199. Ohman EM, Kleiman NS, Gacioch G, et al. For the IMPACT-AMI group. Simultaneous platelet glycoprotein IIb/IIIa integrin blockade and front-loaded tissue plasminogen activator in acute myocardial infarction: Results from a randomized trial (abstr). J Am Coll Cardiol 27(Suppl. A):167, 1996.

200. Moliterno DJ, Harrington RA, Rapold HJ, Califf RM, Topol EJ. Randomized, placebo-controlled study of lamifiban with thrombolytic therapy for the treatment of acute myocardial infarction: Rationale and design for the Platelet Aggregation Receptor Antagonist Dose Investigation and reperfusion Gain in Myocardial infarction (PARADIGM) study. J Thrombos Thromboly 2:16, 1995.

30. NEW ANTIPLATELET STRATEGIES IN THE ADJUNCTIVE TREATMENT OF ACUTE MYOCARDIAL INFARCTION

Christopher J. Ellis and Harvey D. White

Introduction

Platelets play a pivotal role in the pathogenesis of acute coronary syndromes [1]. Platelet activation at the site of arterial injury leads to a cascade of events generating a platelet-rich thrombus, which may occlude vessels with subsequent ischemia or infarction [2,3]. A range of drugs aimed at modifying the actions of platelets are currently being developed for the adjuvant treatment of acute myocardial infarction and unstable angina, and following percutaneous coronary interventions. This chapter reviews the structure and function of platelets during thrombosis, and outlines the previous and current clinical studies of antiplatelet agents in the adjunctive treatment of acute myocardial infarction.

Coronary Thrombosis

Occlusive thrombus in a coronary artery is the predominant cause of acute myocardial infarction [4,5]. Prompt reperfusion of the occluded artery is crucial for limiting the size of the infarct [6] and preserving left ventricular function [7]. Thrombolytic therapy is the most widely applicable therapy [8–10], although both primary and rescue angioplasty following failed thrombolytic therapy are increasingly being advocated [11–13] as alternative means of opening occluded infarct-related arteries. From detailed autopsy studies of patients who died after acute myocardial infarction, it is now well established that atherosclerotic plaque rupture and the exposure of plaque contents and subendothelial material initiate thrombus formation [2,4,14]. It has also been shown that a layer of adherent platelets covers the plaque site [15] and that the accompanying platelet-rich thrombus is often accompanied by both proximal and distal clot, consisting mainly of fibrin and erythrocytes [15]. The understanding that plate-let adhesion and aggregation play a central role in the initiation of arterial thrombosis makes adjuvant antiplatelet therapy a central therapeutic approach for the treatment of unstable coronary syndromes, including acute myocardial infarction.

Platelet Structure and Function

Anatomically, platelets consist of plasma and internal membranes, a cytoskeleton, mitochondria, glycogen granules, storage granules (α granules and dense bodies), lysosomes, and perioxisomes [16]. Mature platelets do not have a nucleus, and hence very little protein synthesis occurs. Their actions are modulated via a variety of surface receptors. In thrombosis both external chemical and mechanical stimuli are able to induce the three major platelet responses of adhesion, activation with secretion from storage granules, and aggregation. These three steps lead to the formation of a platelet hemostatic plug.

PLATELET ADHESION

Platelet adhesion is the first step in the process of hemostasis. It is triggered by damage to the arterial wall and local exposure of the subendothelial matrix, particularly collagen [17]. Coverage of the exposed site by platelets is dependent on the recognition of arterial wall adhesive proteins (ligands) by specific platelet-membrane glycoproteins, many of which are integrins (heterodimeric molecules composed of a series of α and β subunits) [17–19].

Glycoprotein Ib is the principal receptor involved in the initial contact between platelets and the vessel wall, using the von Willebrand factor as the ligand [20]. Other receptors also contribute to the process of adhesion, including glycoprotein Ia/IIa [21,22], glycoprotein Ic/IIa [23], glycoprotein IIb/IIIa (in addition to its major function in platelet aggregation)

TABLE 30-1. Platelet-membrane glycoprotein receptors involved in the adhesion and aggregation of platelets

Receptor	Ligand	Receptor-mediated action	Amino acid sequency recognized
Integrin			
$\alpha_2\beta_1$ (GP Ia/IIa)	Collagen	Adhesion	DGEA[a]
$\alpha_5\beta_1$ (GP Ic/IIa)	Fibronectin	Adhesion	RGD
$\alpha_6\beta_1$	Laminin	Adhesion	Not confined to a short sequence
αIIbβ_3 (GP IIb/IIIa)	Fibrinogen	Aggregation	KOAGDV or RGD
	Fibronectin		RGD[a]
	von Willebrand factor		RGD
	Vitronectin		
αvβ_3	Vitronectin	Adhesion	RGD
	Fibrinogen		RGD
	Fibrinectin		RGD
	von Willebrand factor		RGD
Nonintegrin			
GP Ib	von Willebrand factor	Adhesion	Not confined to a short sequence
GP IV	Thrombospondin	Adhesion	CSVTCG
	Collagen		?

[a]Other amino acid sequences may also be involved.
GP = glycoprotein.
From Lefkovits et al. N Engl J Med 332:1553–1559, 1995, with permission.

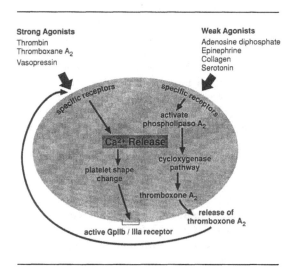

Strong Agonists
Thrombin
Thromboxane A$_2$
Vasopressin

Weak Agonists
Adenosine diphosphate
Epinephrine
Collagen
Serotonin

FIGURE 30-1. Platelet activation (simplified schematic diagram).

[24,25], glycoprotein IV [26,27], and others [17,23]. Their ligands include collagen, fibronectin, von Willebrand factor, vitronectin, and thrombospondin (Table 30-1) [17]. In addition, adhesion under conditions of high shear stress is mediated by glycoproteins Ib and IIb/IIIa using the von Willebrand ligand [28].

PLATELET ACTIVATION

Platelet activation follows adhesion, and can be initiated by several mechanical and chemical stimuli, which can be divided into strong and weak agonists [29,30]. Strong agonists, such as thrombin, thromboxane A$_2$, platelet activating factor, and vasopressin, can cause direct platelet activation, which does not require additional secretion of platelet substances (Figure 30-1). Via specific receptors, these strong agonists activate phospholipase C, leading to the release of stored calcium and the activation of various calcium-dependent enzymes in the platelet [3,31]. These enzymes cause changes in the shape of the platelets, with cytoskeletal reorganization, activation of the IIb/IIIa receptor, secretion of factors from α and dense granules, an increase in procoagulant activity, and arachidonic acid release [32–34]. Because strong agonists induce platelet activation directly, aspirin (a cyclooxygenase inhibitor) is not a particularly effective antagonist, except against the small component derived from secondary thromboxane A$_2$ release.

Weak agonists, such as adenosine diphosphate, epinephrine, collagen, and serotonin, first stimulate platelets to secrete thromboxane A$_2$, which by a feedback loop is then able to directly activate platelets. Hence these agonists bind to specific platelet receptors that activate phospholipase A$_2$ and cause the release of endogenous arachidonic acid from membrane phospholipids. Via the cyclooxygenase pathway, arachidonic acid is ultimately converted to thromboxane A_2, a strong agonist, which then activates other platelets (see Figure 30-1) [32,35]. Platelet activation can also result from shear stress [28].

The release of calcium and other granule products provides feedback amplification of the platelet activation process because the granules contain vasoconstrictor and proaggregatory substances [35]. The α-granule contents include platelet factor-4, β-thromboglobulin, von Willebrand factor, epidermal growth factor, transforming growth factor-β_1, factor V, fibrinogen, immunoglobulin-G, albumin, and possibly platelet-derived growth factor and thrombospondin [30]. The α-granule membrane contains P-selectin and the glycoprotein IIb/IIIa receptor, which represents a storage pool of this platelet surface receptor. With activation and the release of α-granule factors, P-selectin appears on the platelet surface [30]. P-selectin mediates the attachment of platelets to moncytes and neutrophils [36]. With activation, the glycoprotein IIb/IIIa receptor can translocate to the platelet surface. Later return to the storage pool may represent a recycling of this receptor. Dense granules store serotonin, adenosine diphosphate, adenosine triphosphate, and calcium [30].

Specific platelet receptors that mediate the platelet response to agonist activation have been identified. These include receptors to thrombin [37], collagen [38,39], ADP [40,41], epinepherine [42,43], 5HT (serotonin) [44,45], and thromboxane A_2 [46]. The final result of platelet activation is the release of calcium from the sarcoplasmic reticulum into the cytoplasm and a series of reactions resulting in activation of the intracellular contractile apparatus.

Specific receptors to factors that inhibit platelet activation have also been identified, in particular, receptors to the inhibitory prostaglandins PGI_2 (prostacyclin) and PGD_2 [47,48]. Glycoprotein IIb/IIIa receptors that have been activated can return to a resting state when prostacyclin is added to stimulated platelets [49]. In addition, nitric oxide is a platelet inhibitor that has actions independent of a platelet receptor. By diffusing into the platelet and stimulating cyclic GMP (guanosine monophosphate) synthesis, nitric oxide can inhibit platelet adhesion, secretion, and aggregation [50–52].

PLATELET AGGREGATION

Aggregation occurs when platelets that have adhered to the arterial wall and been activated then crosslink to form a mesh. Irrespective of the platelet agonist or pathway responsible for platelet activation, glycoprotein IIb/IIIa receptors mediate the final common step leading to platelet aggregation. These receptors are the most abundant on the platelet surface [53]. Platelet activation initiates conformational changes in the unactivated glycoprotein IIb/IIIa receptors, transforming them into an activated, ligand-competent state. Fibrinogen is the principal adhesive ligand involved in platelet aggregation [54,55], with adhesion to the glycoprotein IIb/IIIa receptors of adjacent platelets. Other crosslinking adhesive proteins, including fibronectin, vitronectin, and von Willebrand's factor, can also bind glycoprotein IIb/IIIa [53,56,57] but play only a minor role [53].

The recognition specificity of the glycoprotein IIb/IIIa receptor is defined by two peptide sequences. The arginine-glycine-asparagine (RGD) sequence is present in fibrinogen, von Willebrand's factor, vitronectin, and fibronectin [34,58]. The KQAGDV recognition sequence is found in fibrinogen [59] and may be the principal sequence for platelet aggregation [60,61]. Following receptor occupancy, a multiprotein cytoskeleton forms, which helps to reinforce and contract the developing clot [62].

SHEAR STRESS

Shear stress is a physical agonist that induces the platelet responses of adhesion, activation with secretion, and aggregation. Shear stress results from forces created at the vessel wall between blood flowing down an artery and the stationary endothelium. With the exposure of the subendothelial matrix by endothelial denudation or plaque rupture, shear stress–induced platelet adhesion may occur at sites of high shear stress, being mediated by the von Willebrand factor ligand and the platelet receptor glycoprotein Ib [63], which also stimulates platelet activation [20,64]. It is likely that the shear stress functionally alters the glycoprotein Ib receptor to induce activation, because the von Willebrand factor itself is unaltered [65].

Platelet aggregation in areas of high shear stress is mediated principally by von Willebrand factor bridging [28,66] between glycoprotein IIb/IIIa receptors on adjacent platelets, with some additional bridging between glycoprotein Ib receptors [65–68]. Shear-induced platelet aggregation occurs more readily in the presence of epinepherine [69] or desmopressin [70].

PROTHROMBOTIC EFFECTS OF PLATELETS

Platelets have direct and indirect prothrombotic effects. They secrete coagulation factor V and calcium, with the result that the prothrombinase complex forms from factor Va, calcium, and factor Xa [71]. When present on the platelet surface, this enzyme complex catalyzes thrombin formation from prothrombin. Thrombin, itself a strong agonist for platelet activation, also catalyzes the formation of fibrin from fibrinogen, with the resulting meshwork necessary for erythrocyte-rich clot.

Indirect prothrombotic effects include the release of potent vasoconstrictors, especially ADP, serotonin, and thromboxane A$_2$, which cause further intravascular stasis and coagulation. Thrombospondin and platelet factor-4, which are also released, may exert antiheparin effects [72], and release of transforming growth factor β leads to plasminogen activator inhibitor-1 (PAI-1) release by hepatocytes and endothelial cells [73,74].

Platelet Activation After Thrombolysis

Using in vitro and animal models of thrombotic occlusion with pharmacologic reperfusion, the addition of various platelet-inhibiting drugs has been shown to increase the rate and incidence of reperfusion, and also to limit reocclusion (Table 30-2) [72]. In vivo pharmacologic lysis of a thrombus with streptokinase or tissue plasminogen activator (t-PA) results in increased platelet activation. During thrombolysis, plasmin-induced platelet activation occurs [75–77]. Streptokinase may also increase platelet activation via an immunological mechanism [78]. Thrombin is generated during thrombolysis and, as the strongest

TABLE 30-2. Platelet-inhibiting agents shown experimentally to decrease time to lysis with plasminogen activators and to decrease the frequency of reocclusion

---

TxA$_2$ inhibition
    TxA$_2$ receptor blockers
    Combined thromboxane synthase and thromboxane
        receptor inhibitors
    Iloprost
    Prostaglandin E$_1$
Serotonin receptor blockade
Combined serotonin and TxA$_2$ receptor blockade
Adhesion receptor blockade
    Aurin tricarboxylic acid
    Monoclonal anti-Ib receptor antibody
Aggregation receptor blockade
    Snake venom–derived RGD peptides
    Synthetic RGD peptides
    Anti-IIb/IIIa monoclonal antibody (7E3)

From Kleiman. Antiplatelet therapy in the setting of acute myocardial infarction. In Califf et al. Acute Coronary Care, 2nd ed. St. Louis, MO: Mosby-Year Book, 1995:341–353.
RGD = arginine-glycine-asparagine; TxA$_2$ = thromboxane A$_2$.

platelet agonist, it probably significantly enhances platelet aggregation [79–81].

Enhanced platelet activity may be a factor in failure to achieve reperfusion after thrombolytic therapy, and in reocclusion. However, thrombolytic drugs may also encourage or inhibit platelet aggregation. t-PA has been reported to disaggregate platelets [82], and plasmin-dependent platelet inhibition has been shown in vitro with t-PA [83].

The constituency of the coronary artery thrombus is important. Jang and colleagues demonstrated in a rabbit arterial model that platelet-rich thrombi are more resistant to thrombolysis than are erythrocyte-rich clots [84]. Furthermore, platelet-rich thrombi are three times more likely to be present in patients who die despite thrombolytic therapy than in those who die without thrombolytic therapy [85,86].

Antiplatelet Treatment in Patients

A variety of platelet inhibitors have been studied in the setting of acute myocardial infarction. Most agents have been tested with pharmacologic thrombolysis, although there have been some studies in the absence of thrombolytic therapy.

Cyclooxygenase Inhibitors

ASPIRIN
Aspirin irreversibly inhibits platelet and endothelial cell enzyme cyclooxygenase [87]. Prostaglandin cyclooxygenase catalyzes the formation of cyclic endoperoxides (which are intermediaries in the formation of thromboxane A$_2$ and prostacyclin) from arachidonic acid. In vitro, aspirin inhibits the reformation of thrombolysed clots formed in platelet-rich plasma but does not accelerate thrombolysis [88]. Aspirin does not reduce shear-induced platelet aggregation [89,90], and in most in vivo models of thrombolysis in a severely stenosed vessel does not prevent reocclusion as effectively as a glycoprotein IIb/IIIa receptor antagonist [91].

The landmark clinical trial demonstrating the efficacy of aspirin in patients with acute myocardial infarction was the Second International Study of Infarct Survival (ISIS-2) [9]. In this study, 17,187 patients with suspected acute myocardial infarction underwent randomization to treatment either with aspirin 162.5 mg chewed immediately, 1.5 million units of intravenous streptokinase over 1 hour, neither, or both. Compared with placebo, there was a significant reduction of mortality with aspirin of 23%, with streptokinase of 25%, and with both of 42%. Unlike the effect seen after streptokinase treatment, the mortality reduction in patients receiving aspirin was independent of time from the onset of symptoms. Treatment with aspirin at any point within the first 24 hours had the same relative effect on 5-week mortality.

No trial has prospectively assessed the benefit of aspirin therapy as adjunctive treatment with t-PA. Two retrospective studies have examined the issue. In the TIMI II study prior ingestion of aspirin did not lead to better arterial patency 18–48 hours after t-PA treatment compared with patients who had not received aspirin prior to the study [92]. The Thrombolysis and Angioplasty in Myocardial Infarction (TAMI) group reported a retrospective review of their data and showed that patients who had previously received aspirin did not have lower rates of reocclusion after successful thrombolysis compared with patients first treated with aspirin at the time of t-PA treatment [93]. However, meta-analysis by Roux and colleagues suggested that for patients treated with either streptokinase or t-PA, reocclusion rates were approximately half those seen in studies in which aspirin was not used [94].

ASPIRIN DOSE

The optimal dose of aspirin required to achieve clinically important inhibition of platelet function is controversial. In healthy volunteers, 20 mg taken once daily over a period of days inhibits cyclooxygenase activity and platelet aggregation [95]. Similar inhibition of platelet aggregation and thromboxane A_2 antagonism after regular daily dosages ranging from 20 to 1000 mg has also been reported [95–98]. Smaller doses than the 160-mg dose used in ISIS-2 may take more than 24 hours to fully inhibit platelet aggregation [99–101]. Virtually complete inhibition of cyclooxygenase occurs with the ISIS-2 dose of aspirin by 1 hour [95,102].

The rationale for avoiding higher daily doses of aspirin is based on the reported frequency of side effects, predominantly gastrointestinal, which are dose dependent [103]. Gastrointestinal symptoms have been reported in 39% of patients on 1200 mg/d [104]. However, low-dose aspirin therapy may be beneficial because it can inhibit platelet cyclooxygenase without suppressing endothelial production of the vasodilator prostacyclin, which is suppressed by higher doses [97,100].

Prostacyclin Analogs

Prostacyclin, a metabolite of arachidonic acid, is a potent vasodilator produced by the vascular endothe-

lium and media. Prostacyclin antagonizes the release of thromboxane A_2 and is potentiated by aspirin [105]. It may also inhibit oxygen free radicals and neutrophil function. In vitro, prostacyclin has a powerful antiaggregatory effect on platelets [106]. However, when given by the intracoronary route to patients with acute myocardial infarction and occluded vessels refractory to streptokinase, prostacyclin (1, 5, and 10 ng/kg/min) did not improve reperfusion rates [107] and, in another small study, did not limit infarct size or the frequency of clinical events [108]. Furthermore, the TAMI 4 investigators found lower patency rates and no improvement in left ventricular ejection fraction when patients treated with t-PA also received an infusion of iloprost (a stable synthetic prostacyclin analog). This double-blind study produced major side effects of fever, nausea, and diarrhea in patients receiving iloprost, and was stopped early [109]. The lower patency rates seen in the TAMI 4 study may be explained by increased catabolism of t-PA, which has been shown at high doses of iloprost in the dog model [110] but has not been shown in humans [111].

Another prostacyclin analogue, taprostene, has recently demonstrated slightly more promise as an adjunctive agent. It was well tolerated in acute myocardial infarction patients treated with single-chain urokinase plasminogen activator (scu-PA). However, it did not enhance the patency achieved with scu-PA, despite being associated with less postinfarction ischemia [112].

PROSTAGLANDIN E_1

Prostaglandin E_1 (PGE_1) is a vasodilator [113]. By stimulating platelet adenylcyclase activity [114], it causes suppression of the calcium-induced release of thromboxane A_2. Hence in vitro it is a mild antagonist of platelet adhesion and aggregation. This effect is potentiated by the phosphodiesterase inhibitors dipyridamole and theophylline [105,115]. High concentrations of PGE_1 have been shown to accelerate thrombolysis with t-PA both in vitro [88] and in vivo [116]. However, a major problem with the therapeutic use of intravenous PGE_1 is that approximately two thirds is metabolized on the first pass through the pulmonary circulation [117,118] and large infused doses are required.

Some benefit was shown in an early trial in which patients receiving intracoronary streptokinase were given 5–20 ng/kg/min of intracoronary PGE_1 [119]. In this small study, there appeared to be more rapid reperfusion and less reocclusion. However, when PGE_1 was given at the same dose with intravenous t-PA, the rate of reperfusion was not improved [120].

THROMBOXANE A₂ SYNTHASE INHIBITORS

These agents block platelet thromboxane A_2 production and preserve endothelial prostaglandin production. However, prostaglandin endoperoxides may activate platelets and also stimulate the thromboxane A_2 receptors [121]. Thromboxane A_2 synthase inhibitors have not been evaluated with respect to patency rates in humans.

THROMBOXANE A₂ PROSTAGLANDIN ENDOPEROXIDE RECEPTOR ANTAGONISTS

These agents block platelet activation by thromboxane A_2 and endoperoxides, but high thromboxane A_2 levels may overcome the effect. They may improve patency rates and also reduce reocclusion, particularly if used in combination with a thrombin inhibitor [122–124].

THROMBOXANE A₂ SYNTHASE AND THROMBOXANE A₂ PROSTAGLANDIN RECEPTOR INHIBITORS

Ridogrel is a thromboxane synthase inhibitor that, like aspirin, inhibits thromboxane A_2 production, with additional antagonism of the thromboxane A_2 receptor. Ridogrel did not improve reperfusion or reocclusion when used with t-PA [125]. Ridogrel was also compared with aspirin in a study of 907 patients treated with streptokinase. There was no additional benefit over aspirin on early reperfusion, assessed noninvasively or by angiographically determined arterial patency at 7–14 days. Interestingly, on post hoc analysis a significant decrease in recurrent ischemia was seen in patients treated with ridogrel (19% vs. 13%, $P < 0.025$) [126].

SEROTONIN RECEPTOR ANTAGONISTS

Ketangenin is a weak platelet inhibitor, which, in combination with a thromboxane A_2 receptor antagonist, has been shown in dogs to increase reperfusion and to decrease reocclusion with t-PA [127].

Glycoprotein IIb/IIIa Receptor Antagonists

A number of glycoprotein IIb/IIIa receptor antagonists are being developed. The effective murine monoclonal antibody m7E3 [128] was cleaved into fragments and m7E3 F(ab⁻)₂ or m7E3 Fab was developed. By removal of the Fc (fragment crystallizable) region, there was avoidance of the potential for complement activation, circulating platelet clearance by the reticuloendothelial system [129], and resulting thrombocytopenia. With m7E3 Fab there was a shorter lysis time [130] and a decrease in reocclusion with t-PA [131]. Gold and colleagues reported that m7E3 Fab enhanced t-PA–induced thrombolysis and

prevented reocclusion in the dog coronary artery thrombosis model [130]. The reperfusion time was shortened from 33 minutes in the heparin group to 6 minutes in the antibody group, and reocclusion did not occur during the follow-up period. Further, after antibody treatment the arterial surface was covered with a monolayer of platelets, and there were no platelet clumps present [132].

The effect of m7E3 Fab on prevention of rethrombosis after t-PA–induced reperfusion was also studied in another dog coronary artery thrombosis model [131]. Rethrombosis occurred in all animals in the saline control group but in only one of nine dogs in the antibody-treated group. The same antibody was further tested with t-PA for lysis of thrombolysis-resistant, platelet-rich coronary thrombus in dogs [133]. The resistance was overcome by the combined use of a reduced dose of t-PA and m7E3 Fab. In this model, m7E3 Fab combined with t-PA induced reperfusion in all five animals, whereas heparin with t-PA reperfused only one of five dogs.

The development of human–antimurine antibodies to m7E3 Fab was detected in 37 of 78 patients in two small dose-finding human studies [134,135]. Abciximab (ReoPro™) was synthetically designed to retain the murine heavy and light chain variable regions, which include the antigen binding site for the GPIIb/IIIa receptor, but human constant region se-

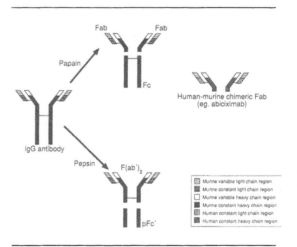

FIGURE 30-2. Diagram of the relationship between the basic murine monoclonal antibody (M7E3) against the glycoprotein IIb/IIIa receptor, murine 7E3 (Fab), and chimeric 7E3 (abciximab or ReoPro™) [143]. Fab = fragment antigen binding; Fc = fragment crystallizable. (From Faulds et al. Drugs 48:583–598, 1994, with permission.)

TABLE 30-3. Glycoprotein IIb/IIIa inhibitors recently evaluated in clinical trials

Agent	Glycoprotein IIb/IIIa inhibitor type
Chimeric 7E3	Monoclonal antibody
MK-852	Cyclic RGD peptide
Integrilin (COR Therapeutics, South San Francisco, CA)	Cyclic KGD peptide
Lamifiban (Hoffman La-Roche, Basel, Switzerland)	Peptide derivative
Tirofiban (Merck & Co, West Point, PA)	Nonpeptide
Xemilofiban	Orally active agent

From Lefkovits et al. N Engl J Med 332:1553–1559, 1995, with permission.

quences were substituted. Abciximab, the chimeric human–murine 7E3 (c7E3) Fab fragment, contains approximately 50% human genetic sequence (Figure 30-2) [136].

However, monoclonal antibodies such as c7E3 Fab have several potential problems besides immunogenicity, such as prolonged duration of action, lack of reversibility, and high production costs [34]. Alternative agents based on the RGD recognition sequence have been developed from naturally occurring RGD peptides from viper, leech, and tick venom, all of which inhibit the glycoprotein IIb/IIIa receptor [137–139]. Nonpeptide oral agents are also being developed (Table 30-3).

Although much experimental work has supported a beneficial role for glycoprotein IIb/IIIa antagonism as an adjunct to thrombolysis, there have been few clinical trials. In the TAMI 8 pilot study [135], the Fab fragment of the murine monoclonal antibody $7E_3$ was administered at escalating bolus doses (0.10, 0.15, 0.20, and 0.25 mg/kg intravenously) at decreasing intervals (15, 6, or 3 hours) after initiation of thrombolysis in 60 patients receiving t-PA, aspirin, and heparin. An additional 10 control patients were studied without receiving $m7E_3$ Fab. The cautious protocol included a decrease in heparin dose for patients treated 3 or 6 hours after t-PA. Administration of $m7E_3$ Fab produced profound dose-dependent inhibition of platelet aggregation to below 20% of normal, with 50% recovery of aggregation 6 hours after the $m7E_3$ Fab bolus. The extent of inhibition was directly proportional to the degree of binding of $m7E_3$ Fab to the GPIIb/IIIa receptor. Importantly, there was no increase in bleeding complications, and there was a trend toward improved coronary patency (92% vs. 56%) among patients receiving $m7E_3$ Fab.

The chimeric form of the GPIIb/IIIa antibody c7E3 has been studied in a small group of patients undergoing primary angioplasty or rescue angioplasty following failed thrombolytic therapy for acute myocardial infarction. From the initial trial of 2099 patients undergoing high-risk angioplasty [140], this subgroup of patients with myocardial infarction demonstrated a dramatic reduction in recurrent ischemic events when treated with the GPIIb/IIIa antagonist antibody. There were no episodes of recurrent infarction or need for revascularization by 6 months in patients treated with a 0.25 mg/kg bolus followed by a 12-hour 0.10 mg/h infusion of c7E3 [141].

A number of GPIIb/IIIa receptor blockers are currently undergoing evaluation in conjunction with thrombolytic drugs. The IMPACT-AMI group compared integrilin with placebo in a double-blind trial of 106 patients receiving accelerated t-PA, aspirin, and heparin. Integrilin was given as a bolus dose of 180 μg/kg followed by a 0.75 μg/kg infusion, which was continued for 24 hours. The rate of severe bleeding was similar in both groups (4% vs. 5%), but there was an incidence of intracranial bleeding of 2% with integrilin. TIMI-3 angiographic flow at 90 minutes was 39% in placebo-treated patients and 66% in integrilin-treated patients ($P < 0.01$) [142].

Conclusions

An understanding of the role of platelets in arterial thrombosis is central to current developments in the treatment of acute myocardial infarction. The most promising antiplatelet agents are the GPIIb/IIIa receptor antagonists, which are likely to provide substantial additional benefits in treatment strategies, with the possibility of improving reperfusion rates and decreasing reocclusion without substantially increasing bleeding.

References

1. Fuster V, Badimon L, Badimon JJ, Chesebro JH. The pathogenesis of coronary artery disease and the acute coronary syndromes. N Engl J Med 326:242, 1992.
2. Davies MJ, Thomas AC. Plaque fissuring: The cause of acute myocardial infarction, sudden ischemic death, and crescendo angina. Br Heart J 53:363, 1985.
3. Kroll MH, Schafer AI. Biochemical mechanisms of platelet activation. Blood 74:1181S, 1989.
4. Davies MJ, Thomas A. Thrombosis and acute coronary lesions in sudden ischemic death. N Engl J Med 310:1137, 1984.
5. DeWood MA, Spores J, Notske R, Mouser LT, Burroughs R, Golden MS, Lang HT. Prevalence of total coronary occlusion during the early hours of transmural myocardial infarction. N Engl J Med 303:897, 1980.
6. Simoons ML, Serruys PW, van den Brand M, Res J, Verheugt FWA, Krauss XH, Remme WJ, Bar F, de Zwaan C, van der Laarse A, Vermeer F, Lubsen J, for the Working Group on Thrombolytic Therapy in Acute Myocardial Infarction of the Netherlands Interuniversity Cardiology Institute. Early thrombolysis in acute myocardial infarction: Limitation of infarct size and improved survival. J Am Coll Cardiol 7:717, 1986.
7. White HD, Norris RM, Brown MA, Takayama M, Maslowski A, Bass NM, Ormiston JA, Whitlock T. Effect of intravenous streptokinase on left ventricular function and early survival after acute myocardial infarction. N Engl J Med 317:850, 1987.
8. Gruppo Italiano per lo Studio della Streptochinasi nell'Infarto Miocardico (GISSI). Effectiveness of intravenous thrombolytic treatment in acute myocardial infarction. Lancet 1:397, 1986.
9. ISIS-2 (Second International Study of Infarct Survival) Collaborative Group. Randomised trial of intravenous streptokinase, oral aspirin, both, or neither among 17, 187 cases of suspected acute myocardial infarction: ISIS-2. Lancet 2:349, 1988.
10. The GUSTO Investigators. An international randomized trial comparing four thrombolytic strategies for acute myocardial infarction. N Engl J Med 329:673, 1993.
11. Stone GW, Grines CL, Browne KF, Marco J, Rothbaum D, O'Keefe J, Hartzler GO, Overlie P, Donohue B, Chelliah N, Timmis GC, Vlietstra R, Strzelecki M, Puchrowicz-Ochocki S, O'Neill WW. Predictors of in-hospital and 6-month outcome after acute myocardial infarction in the reperfusion era: The Primary Angioplasty in Myocardial Infarction (PAMI) trial. J Am Coll Cardiol 25:370, 1995.
12. Michels KB, Yusuf S. Does PTCA in acute myocardial infarction affect mortality and reinfarction rates? A quantitative overview (meta-analysis) of the randomized clinical trials. Circulation 91:476, 1995.
13. Ellis SG, da Silva ER, Heyndrickx G, Talley JD, Cernigliaro C, Steg G, Spaulding C, Nobuyoshi M, Erbel R, Vassanelli C, Topol EJ, for the RESCUE Investigators. Randomized comparison of rescue angioplasty with conservative management of patients with early failure of thrombolysis for acute anterior myocardial infarction. Circulation 90:2280, 1994.
14. Onodera T, Fujiwara H, Tanaka M, Wu J, Matsuda M, Takemura G, Ishida M, Kawamura A, Kawai C. Cineangiographic and pathological features of the infarct related vessel in successful and unsuccessful thrombolysis. Br Heart J 61:385, 1989.
15. Friedman M, Van den Bovenkamp GJ. The pathogenesis of a coronary thrombus. Am J Pathol 48:19, 1966.
16. Lind SE. Platelet morphology. In Loscalzo J, Schafer AI (eds). Thrombosis and Hemorrhage. Boston: Blackwell Scientific, 1994:201.
17. Lefkovits J, Plow EF, Topol EJ. Platelet glycoprotein IIb/IIIa receptors in cardiovascular medicine. N Engl J Med 332:1553, 1995.
18. Hynes RO. Integrins: A family of cell surface receptors. Cell 48:549, 1987.
19. Smyth SS, Joneckis CC, Parise LV. Regulation of vascular integrins Blood 81:2827, 1993. [Published erratum appears in Blood 83:2013, 1994.]
20. Kroll MH, Harris TS, Moake JL, Handin RI, Shafer AI. von Willebrand factor binding to platelet GpIb initiates signals for platelet activation. J Clin Invest 88:1568, 1991.
21. Saelman EU, Nieuwenhuis HK, Hese KM, de Groot PG, Heijnen HFG, Sage EH, Williams S, McKeown L, Gralnick HR, Sixma JJ. Platelet adhesion to collagen types I through VIII under conditions of stasis and flow is mediated by GPIa/IIa ($\alpha_2\beta_1$-integrin). Blood 83:1244, 1994.
22. Kunicki TJ, Nugent DJ, Staats SJ, Orchekowski RP, Waynder EA, Carter WG. The human fibroblast class II extracellular matrix receptor mediates platelet adhesion to collagen and is identical to the platelet glycoprotein Ia-IIa complex. J Biol Chem 263:4516, 1988.
23. Ginsberg MH, Xiaoping D, O'Toole TE, Loftus JC, Plow EF. Platelet integrins. Thromb Haemost 70:87, 1993.
24. Hantgan RR, Hindriks G, Taylor RG, Sixma JJ, de Groot PG. Glycoprotein Ib, von Willebrand factor, and glycoprotein IIb:IIIa are all involved in platelet adhesion to fibrin in flowing whole blood. Blood 76:345, 1990.
25. Lages B, Weiss HJ. Evidence for a role of glycoprotein IIb-IIIa, distinct from its ability to support aggregation, in platelet activation by ionophores in the presence of extracellular divalent cations. Blood 83:2549, 1994.

26. Tandon NN, Kralisz U, Jamieson GA. Identification of glycoprotein IV (CD36) as a primary receptor for platelet-collagen adhesion. J Biol Chem 264:7576, 1989.

27. Asch AS, Barnwell J, Silverstein RL, Nachman RL. Isolation of the thrombospondin membrane receptor. J Clin Invest 79:1054, 1987.

28. Weiss HJ, Hawiger J, Ruggeri ZM, Turitto VT, Thiagarajan P, Hoffman T. Fibrinogen-independent platelet adhesion and thrombus formation on subendothelium mediated by glycoprotein IIb-IIIa complex at high shear rate. J Clin Invest 83:288, 1989.

29. Collen D, Bounameaux H, De Cock F, Lijnen HR, Verstraete M. Analysis of coagulation and fibrinolysis during intravenous infusion of recombinant human tissue-type plasminogen activator (rt-PA) in patients with acute myocardial infarction. Circulation 73:511, 1986.

30. Kamat SG, Kleiman NS. Platelets and platelet inhibitors in acute myocardial infarction. Cardiol Clin 13:435, 1995.

31. Majerus PW, Connolly TM, Deckmyn H, Ross TS, Bross TE, Ishii H, Bansal VS, Wilson DB. The metabolism of phosphoinositide-derived messenger molecules. Science 234:1519, 1986.

32. Kroll MH. Mechanisms of platelet activation. In Loscalzo J, Schafer AI (eds). Thrombosis and Hemorrhage. Boston: Blackwell Scientific, 1994:247.

33. Coller BS. Platelets in cardiovascular thrombosis and thrombolysis. In Fozzard HA, Haber E, Jennings RB, Katz AM, Morgan HE (eds). The Heart and Cardiovascular System: Scientific Foundations, 2nd ed. New York: Raven Press, 1992:I219.

34. Lefkovits J, Topol EJ. Platelet glycoprotein IIb/IIIa receptor inhibitors in ischemic heart disease. Curr Opin Cardiol 10:420, 1995.

35. Stein B, Fuster V, Israel DH, Cohen M, Badimon L, Badimon JJ, Chesebro JH. Platelet inhibitor agents in cardiovascular disease: An update. J Am Coll Cardiol 14:813, 1989.

36. Larsen I, Celi A, Gilbert GE, Furie BC, Erban JK, Bonfant R, Wagner DD, Furie B. PADGEM protein: A receptor that mediates the interaction of activated platelets with neutrophils and monocytes. Cell 59:305, 1989.

37. Hung DT, Vu TKH, Wheaton VI, Ishii K, Coughlin SR. Cloned platelet thrombin receptor is necessary for thrombin-induced platelet activation. J Clin Invest 89:1350, 1992.

38. Fuster V, Badimon L, Cohen M, Ambrose JA, Badimon JJ, Chesebro J. Insights into the pathogenesis of acute ischemic syndromes. Circulation 77:1213, 1988.

39. Niewenhuis HK, Akkerman JWN, Houdijk WPM, Sixma JJ. Human blood platelets showing no response to collagen fail to express surface glycoprotein Ia. Nature 318:470, 1985.

40. Colman RW. Aggregin, a platelet ADP receptor that mediates activation. FASEB J 4:1425, 1990.

41. Greco NJ, Tandon NN, Jackson BW, Tandon NN, Moos M, Jamieson GA. Identification of a nucleotide binding site on glycoprotein IIb. J Biol Chem 266:13627, 1991.

42. Kobilka BK, Matsui H, Kobilka TS, Yang-Feng TL, Francke V, Caron MG, Lefkowitz RJ, Regan JW. Cloning, sequencing, and expression of the gene coding for the human platelet alpha$_2$-adrenergic receptor. Science 238:650, 1987.

43. Regan JW, Nakata H, De Marinis RM, Caron MG, Lefkowitz RJ. Purification and characterization of the human platelet alpha$_2$-adrenergic receptor. J Biol Chem 261:3894, 1986.

44. De Chaffoy de Courcelles D, Leysen JE, De Clerck F, Van Belle H, Janssen PA. Evidence that phospholipid turnover in the signal transducing system is coupled to serotonin S2 receptor sites. J Biol Chem 260:7603, 1985.

45. Saltzman AG, Morse B, Whitman MM, Ivanshchenko Y, Jaye M, Felder S. Cloning of the human serotonin 5-HT2 and 5-HT1C receptor subtypes. Biochem Biophys Res Commun 181:1469, 1991.

46. Hirata M, Hayashi Y, Ushikubi F, Yokota Y, Kageyama R, Nakanishi S, Narumiya S. Cloning and expression of cDNA for a human thromboxane A2 receptor. Nature 349:617, 1991.

47. Schafer AI, Cooper B, O'Hara D, Handin RI. Identification of platelet receptors for prostaglandins I$_2$ and D$_2$. J Biol Chem 254:2914, 1979.

48. Siegel AM, Smith JB, Silver MJ, Nicolaou KC, Ahern D. Selective binding site of [^{3}H]-prostacyclin on platelets. J Clin Invest 63:215, 1979.

49. van Willigen G, Akkerman J-WN. Regulation of glycoprotein IIb/IIIa exposure on platelets stimulated with α-thrombin. Blood 72:82, 1992.

50. Ignarro LJ. Endothelium-derived nitric oxide: Actions and properties. FASEB J 3:31, 1989.

51. Broekman MJ, Eiroa EM, Marcus AJ. Inhibition of human platelet reactivity by endothelium-derived relaxing factor from human umbilical vein endothelial cells in suspension: Blockade of aggregation and secretion by an aspirin-insensitive mechanism. Blood 78:1033, 1991.

52. Radomski MW, Palmer RM, Moncada S. Endogenous nitric oxide inhibits human platelet adhesion to vascular endothelium. Lancet 2:1057, 1987.

53. Phillips DR, Charo IF, Parise LV, Fitzgerald LA. The platelet membrane glycoprotein IIb-IIIa complex. Blood 71:831, 1988.

54. Gogstad GO, Brosstad F, Krutnes M, Hagen I, Solum NO. Fibrinogen-binding properties of the human platelet glycoprotein IIb-IIIa complex: A study using crossed radioimmunoelectropheresis. Blood 60:663, 1982.

55. Plow EF, Ginsberg MH. Glycoprotein IIb/IIIa as a prototypic adhesion receptor. In Coller BS (ed). Progress in Hemostasis and Thrombosis. Philadelphia: WB Saunders, 1989:117.

56. Pytela R, Pierschbacher MD, Ginsberg MH, Plow EF, Ruoslahti E. Platelet membrane glycoprotein IIb/IIIa: Member of a family of Arg-Gly-Asp specific adhesion receptors. Science 231:1559, 1986.

57. Ruggeri ZM, De Marco L, Gatti L, Bader R, Montgomery RR. Platelets have more than one binding site for von Willebrand factor. J Clin Invest 72:1, 1983.

58. Pierschbacher MD, Ruoslahti E. Cell attachment activity of fibronectin can be duplicated by small synthetic fragments of the molecule. Nature 309:30, 1984.

59. Kloczewiak M, Timmons S, Hawiger J. Recognition site for the platelet receptor is present on the 15-residue carboxy-terminal fragment of the gamma chain of human fibrinogen and is not involved in the fibrin polymerization reaction. Thromb Res 29:249, 1983.

60. Weisel JW, Nagaswami C, Vilaire G, Bennett JS. Examination of the platelet membrane glycoprotein IIb-IIIa complex and its interaction with fibrinogen and other ligands by electron microscopy. J Biol Chem 267:16637, 1992.

61. Farrell DH, Thiagarajan P, Chung DW, Davie EW. Role of fibrinogen alpha and gamma chain sites in platelet aggregation. Proc Natl Acad Sci USA 89:10729, 1992.

62. Fox JEB. The platelet cytoskeleton. Thromb Haemost 70:884, 1993.

63. Alevriadou BR, Moake JL, Turner NA, Ruggeri ZM, Folie BJ, Phillips MD, Schreiber AB, Hrinda ME, McIntire LV. Real-time analysis of shear-dependent thrombus formation and its blockade by inhibitors of von Willebrand factor binding to platelets. Blood 81:1263, 1993.

64. Chow TW, Hellums JD, Moake JL, Kroll MH. Shear stress-induced von Willebrand factor binding to platelet glycoprotein Ib initiates calcium influx associated with aggregation. Blood 80:113, 1992.

65. Peterson DM, Stathopoulous NA, Giorgio TD, Hellums JD, Moake JL. Shear-induced platelet aggregation requires von Willebrand factor and platelet membrane glycoproteins Ib and IIb-IIIa. Blood 69:625, 1987.

66. Ikeda Y, Handa M, Kawano K, Kamata T, Murata M, Araki Y, Anbo H, Kawai Y, Watanabe K, Itagaki I, Sakai K, Rugerri ZM. The role of von Willebrand factor and fibrinogen in platelet aggregation under varying shear stress. J Clin Invest 87:1234, 1991.

67. Moake JL, Turner NA, Stathopoulous NA, Nolasco LH, Hellums JD. Involvement of larger von Willebrand factor (vWf) multimers and unusually large vWf forms derived from endothelial cells in shear stress-induced platelet aggregation. J Clin Invest 78:1456, 1986.

68. Roth GJ. Developing relationships: Arterial platelet adhesion, glycoprotein Ib, and leucine-rich glycoproteins. Blood 77:5, 1991.

69. Goto S, Ikeda Y, Murata M, Handa M, Takahashi E, Yoshioka A, Fujimura Y, Fukuyama M, Handa S, Ogawa S. Epinephrine augments von Willebrand factor-dependent shear-induced platelet aggregation. Circulation 86:1859, 1992.

70. Cattaneo M, Lombardi R, Bettega D, Lecchi A, Mannucci PM. Shear-induced platelet aggregation is potentiated by desmopressin and inhibited by ticlopidine. Arterioscler Thromb 13:393, 1993.

71. Monkovic DD, Tracy PB. Functional characterization of human platelet-released factor V and its activation by factor Xa and thrombin. J Biol Chem 265:17132, 1990.

72. Kleiman NS. Antiplatelet therapy in the setting of acute myocardial infarction. In Califf RM, Mark DB, Wagner GS (eds). Acute Coronary Care, 2nd ed. St Louis, MO: Mosby-Year Book, 1995:341.

73. Fujii S, Lucore CL, Hopkins WE, Billadello JJ, Sobel BE. Potential attenuation of fibrinolysis by growth factors released from platelets and their pharmacologic implications. Am J Cardiol 63:1505, 1989.

74. Fujii S, Hopkins WE, Sobel BE. Mechanisms contributing to increased synthesis of plasminogen activator inhibitor type 1 in endothelial cells by constituents of platelets and their implications of thrombolysis. Circulation 83:645, 1991.

75. Fitzgerald DJ, Catella F, Roy L, Fitzgerald GA. Marked platelet activation in vivo after intravenous streptokinase in patients with acute myocardial infarction. Circulation 77:142, 1988.

76. Niewiarowski S, Senyi AF, Gillies P. Plasmin-induced platelet aggregation and platelet release reaction. J Clin Invest 52:1467, 1973.

77. Ohlstein EH, Storer B, Fujita T, Shebuski RJ. Tissue-type plasminogen activator and streptokinase induce platelet hyperaggregability in the rabbit. Thromb Res 46:575, 1987.

78. Terres W, Kruger K, Bleifeld W. Prevalence and mechanism of streptokinase-induced platelet stimulation: Effect of acetylsalicylic acid. Eur Heart J 13:1514, 1992.

79. Eisenberg PR, Sherman LA, Jaffe AS. Paradoxic elevation of fibrin peptide A after streptokinase: Evidence for intense thrombosis despite intense fibrinolysis. J Am Coll Cardiol 10:527, 1987.

80. Winters KJ, Santoro SA, Miletich JP, Eisenberg PR. Relative importance of thrombin compared with plasmin-mediated platelet activation in response to plasminogen activation with streptokinase. Circulation 84:1522, 1991.

81. Aronson DL, Chang P, Kessler CM. Platelet-dependent thrombin generation after in vitro fibrinolytic treatment. Circulation 85:1706, 1992.

82. Loscalzo J, Vaughan D. Tissue plasminogen activator promotes platelet disaggregation in plasma. J Clin Invest 79:1749, 1987.

83. Gouin I, Lecompte T, Morel MC, Lebrazi J, Modderman PW, Kaplan C, Samama MM. In vitro

effects of plasmin on human platelet function in plasma. Circulation 85:935, 1992.

84. Jang IK-K, Gold HK, Ziskind AA, Fallon JT, Holt RE, Leinbach RC, May JW, Collen D. Differential sensitivity of erythrocyte-rich and platelet-rich arterial thrombi to lysis with recombinant tissue-type plasminogen activator: A possible explanation for resistance to coronary thrombolysis. Circulation 79:920, 1989.

85. Gertz SD, Kragel AH, Kalan JM, Braunwald E, Roberts WC, and the TIMI Investigators. Comparison of coronary and myocardial morphologic findings in patients with and without thrombolytic therapy during fatal first acute myocardial infarction. Am J Cardiol 66:904, 1990.

86. Kragel AH, Gertz SD, Roberts WC. Morphologic comparison of frequency and types of acute lesions in the major epicardial coronary arteries in unstable angina pectoris, sudden coronary death, and acute myocardial infarction. J Am Coll Cardiol 18:801, 1991.

87. Roth GJ, Majerus PW. The mechanism of the effect of aspirin on human platelets: I: Acetylation of a particular fraction protein. J Clin Invest 56:624, 1975.

88. Terres W, Beythien C, Kupper W, Bleifeld W. Effects of aspirin and prostaglandin E$_1$ on in vitro thrombolysis with urokinase: Evidence for a possible role of inhibiting platelet activity in thrombolysis. Circulation 79:1309, 1989.

89. Turner NA, Kamat SG, Moake JL, Schafer AI, Kleiman NS, Jordan R, McIntire LV. Comparative real-time effects on platelet adhesion and aggregation under flowing conditions of in vivo aspirin, heparin, and monoclonal antibody fragment against glycoprotein IIb/IIIa. Circulation 91:1354, 1995.

90. O'Brien JR. Shear-induced platelet aggregation. Lancet 335:711, 1990.

91. Bates ER, McGillem MJ, Mickelson JK, Pitt B, Mancini GBJ. A monoclonal antibody against the platelet glycoprotein IIb/IIIa receptor complex prevents platelet aggregation and thrombosis in a canine model of coronary angioplasty. Circulation 84:2463, 1991.

92. Robertson TL, Forman SA, Williams DO, Dodge HT, and TIMI Research Group. Aspirin rt-PA, and reperfusion in AMI: A TIMI observational study (abstr). Circulation 78(Suppl. II): II128, 1988.

93. Ohman EM, Califf RM, Topol EJ, Candela R, Abbottsmith C, Ellis S, Sigmon KN, Kereiakes D, George B, Stack R, and the TAMI Study Group. Consequences of reocclusion after successful reperfusion therapy in acute myocardial infarction. Circulation 82:781, 1990.

94. Roux S, Christeller S, Ludin E. Effects of aspirin on coronary reocclusion and recurrent ischemia after thrombolysis: A meta-analysis. J Am Coll Cardiol 19:671, 1992.

95. Patrignani P, Filabozzi P, Patrono C. Selective cumulative inhibition of platelet thromboxane production

by low-dose aspirin in healthy subjects. J Clin Invest 69:1366, 1982.

96. Kallmann R, Nieuwenhuis HK, Groot PGD, Gijn J, Sixma JJ. Effects of low doses of aspirin, 10 mg and 30 mg daily, on bleeding time, thromboxane production and 6-keto-PGF1α excretion in healthy subjects. Thromb Res 45:355, 1987.

97. Weksler BB, Pett SB, Alonso D, Richter RC, Stelzer P, Subramanian V, Tack-Goldman K, Gay WA. Differential inhibition by aspirin of vascular and platelet prostaglandin synthesis in atherosclerotic patients. N Engl J Med 308:800, 1983.

98. Rasmains G, Vesterqvist O, Green K, Edhag O, Henriksson P. Effects of intermittent treatment with aspirin on thromboxane and prostacyclin formation in patients with acute myocardial infarction. Lancet 2:245, 1988.

99. Patrono C. Aspirin as an antiplatelet drug. N Engl J Med 330:1287, 1994.

100. Clarke RJ, Mayo G, Price P, Fitzgerald G. Suppression of thromboxane A$_2$ but not of systemic prostacyclin by controlled-release aspirin. N Engl J Med 325:1137, 1991.

101. Berglund U, Wallentin L. Persistent inhibition of platelet function during long-term treatment with 75 mg acetylsalicylic acid daily in men with unstable coronary artery disease. Eur Heart J 12:428, 1991.

102. Reilly IAG, Fitzgerald GA. Inhibition of thromboxane formation in vivo and ex vivo: Implications for therapy with platelet inhibitory drugs. Blood 68:180, 1987.

103. Antiplatelet Trialists' Collaboration. Collaborative overview of randomised trials of antiplatelet therapy — I: Prevention of death, myocardial infarction, and stroke by prolonged antiplatelet therapy in various categories of patients. Br Med J 308:81, 1994.

104. Peto R, Warlow C, and the UK-TIA Study Group. United Kingdom transient ischaemic attack (UK-TIA) aspirin trial: Interim results. Br Med J 296:316, 1988.

105. Ball G, Brereton GG, Fulwood M, Ireland DM, Yates P. Effect of prostaglandin E1 alone and in combination with theophylline or aspirin on collagen-induced platelet aggregation and on platelet necleotides including adenosine 3′:5′-cyclic monophosphate. Biochem J 120:709, 1970.

106. Harfenist EJ, Packham MA, Kinlough-Rathbone RL, Mustard JF. Inhibitors of ADP-induced platelet aggregation prevent fibrinogen binding to rabbit platelets and cause rapid deaggregation and dissociation of bound fibrinogen. J Lab Clin Med 97:680, 1981.

107. Hackett D, Davies G, Maseri A. Effect of prostacyclin on coronary occlusion in acute myocardial infarction. Int J Cardiol 26:53, 1990.

108. Armstrong PW, Langevin LM, Watts DG. Randomized trial of prostacyclin infusion in acute myocardial infarction. Am J Cardiol 61:455, 1987.

109. Topol EJ, Ellis SG, Califf RM, George BS, Stump DC, Bates ER, Nabel EG, Walton JA, Candela RJ, Lee KL, Kline EM, Pitt B, and the TAMI 4 Study Group. Combined tissue-type plasminogen activator and prostacyclin therapy for acute myocardial infarction, TAMI (4) Study Group. J Am Coll Cardiol 14:877, 1989.

110. Nicolini FA, Mehta JL, Nichols WW, Saldeen TGP, Grant M. Prostacyclin analogue iloprost decreases thrombolytic potential of tissue-type plaminogen activator in canine coronary thrombosis. Circulation 81:1115, 1990.

111. Kerins DM, Roy L, Kunitada S, Adedoyin A, Fitzgerald GA, Fitzgerald DJ. Pharmacokinetics of tissue-type plasminogen activator during myocardial infarction in men: Effect of a prostacyclin analogue. Circulation 85:526, 1992.

112. Bar FW, Meyer J, Michels R, Uebis R, Lange S, Barth H, Groves R, Vermeer F. The effect of taprostene in patients with acute myocardial infarction treated with thrombolytic therapy: Results of the START study. Saruplase Taprostene Acute Reocclusion Trial. Eur Heart J 14:1118, 1993.

113. Feldman RL, Rose B, Verbust KM. Hemodynamic and angiographic effects of prostaglandin E1 in coronary artery disease. Am J Cardiol 62:698, 1988.

114. Karinguian A, Legrand YJ, Caen JP. Prostaglandins: Specific inhibition of platelet adhesion to collagen and relationship with cAMP level. Prostaglandins 23:437, 1982.

115. Mills DCB, Smith JB. The influence of platelet aggregation on drugs that affect the accumulation of adenosine $3':5'$-cyclic monophosphate in platelets. Biochem J 121:185, 1971.

116. Vaughan DE, Plavin SR, Schafer AI, Loscalzo J. PGE₁ accelerates thrombolysis by tissue plasminogen activator. Blood 73:1213, 1989.

117. Golub M, Zia P, Matsuno M, Horton R. Metabolism of prostaglandins A₁ and E₁ in man. J Clin Invest 56:1404, 1975.

118. Peskar BA, Cawello W, Rogatti W, Rudofsky G. On the metabolism of prostaglandin E₁ in administered intravenously to human volunteers. J Physiol Pharmacol 42:327, 1991.

119. Sharma B, Wyeth RP, Gimenez HJ, Franciosa JA. Intracoronary prostaglandin E₁ plus streptokinase in acute myocardial infarction. Am J Cardiol 58:1161, 1986.

120. Kleiman NS, Tracy RP, Schaaf LJ, Harris S, Hill RD, Puleo P, Roberts R. Prostaglandin E₁ does not accelerate rTPA-induced thrombolysis in acute myocardial infarction. Am Heart J 127:738, 1994.

121. Bertele V, Certletti C, Schieppati A, Di Minno G, De Gaetano G. Inhibition of thromboxane synthase does not necessarily prevent platelet aggregation. Lancet 1:1057, 1981.

122. Shebuski RJ, Storer BL, Fujita T. Effect of thromboxane synthase inhibition on thrombolytic action of tissue-type plasminogen activator in a rabbit model of peripheral arterial thrombosis. Thromb Res 52:381, 1988.

123. Kopia GA, Kopaciewicz LJ, Ohlstein EH, Horohonich S, Storer BL, Shebuski RJ. Combination of the thromboxane receptor antagonist, sulotroban, with streptokinase: Demonstration of thrombolytic synergy. J Pharmacol Exp Ther 250:887, 1989.

124. Grover GJ, Parham CS, Schumacher WA. The combined antiischemic effects of the thromboxane receptor antagonist SQ 30741 and tissue type plasminogen activator. Am Heart J 121:426, 1991.

125. Tranchesi B, Caramelli B, Gebara O, Bellotti G, Pileggi F, Van de Werf F, Verstraete M. Efficacy and safety of ridogrel versus aspirin in coronary thrombolysis with alteplase for myocardial infarction (abstr). J Am Coll Cardiol 19:92A, 1992.

126. The RAPT Investigators. Randomized trial of ridogrel, a combined thromboxane A₂ synthase inhibitor and thromboxane A₂/prostaglandin endoperoxide receptor antagonist, versus aspirin as adjunct to thrombolysis in patients with acute myocardial infarction: The ridogrel versus aspirin patency trial (RAPT). Circulation 89:588, 1994.

127. Golino P, Ashton JH, Glas-Greenwalt P, McNatt J, Buja LM, Willerson JT. Mediation of reocclusion by thromboxane A₂ and serotonin after thrombolysis with tissue-type plasminogen activator in a canine preparation of coronary thrombosis. Circulation 77:678, 1988.

128. Coller BS. A new murine monoclonal antibody reports on activation-dependent change in the conformation and/or microenvironment of the glycoprotein IIb/IIIa complex. J Clin Invest 76:101, 1985.

129. Ellis SG, Bates ER, Schiable T. Prospects for the use of antagonists to the platelet glycoprotein IIb/IIIa receptor to prevent postangioplasty restenosis and thrombosis. J Am Coll Cardiol 17:89B, 1991.

130. Gold HK, Coller BS, Yasuda T, Saito T, Fallon JT, Guerrero JL, Leinbach RC, Ziskind AA, Collen D. Rapid and sustained coronary artery recanalization with combined bolus injection of recombinant tissue-type plasminogen activator and monoclonal antiplatelet GP IIb/IIIa antibody in a canine preparation. Circulation 77:670, 1988.

131. Mickelson JK, Simpson PJ, Cronin M, Homeister JW, Laywell E, Kitzen J, Lucches BR. Antiplatelet antibody [7E3 F(ab)2] prevents rethrombosis after recombinant tissue-type plasminogen activator-induced coronary artery thrombolysis in a canine model. Circulation 81:617, 1990.

132. Yasuda T, Gold HK, Fallon JT, Leinbach RC, Guerrero JL, Scudder LE, Kanbe M, Shealy D, Ross MJ, Collen D, Coller BS. Monoclonal antibody against the platelet glycoprotein (GP) IIb/IIIa receptor prevents coronary artery reocclusion after reperfusion with recombinant tissue-type plasminogen activator in dogs. J Clin Invest 81:1284, 1988.

133. Yasuda T, Gold HK, Leinbach RC, Saito T, Guerrero JL, Jang IK, Holt R, Fallon JT, Collen D. Lysis of

plasminogen activator-resistant platelet-rich coronary artery thrombus with combined bolus injection of recombinant tissue-type plasminogen activator and antiplatelet GP IIb/IIIa antibody. J Am Coll Cardiol 16:1728, 1990.

134. Ellis SG, Tcheng JE, Navetta FI, Muller DW, Weisman HF, Smith C, Anderson KM, Califf RM. Safety and anti-platelet effect of murine monoclonal antibody 7E3 Fab directed against platelet glycoprotein IIb/IIIa in patients undergoing elective coronary angioplasty. Cor Art Dis 4:167, 1993.

135. Kleiman NS, Ohman EM, Califf RM, George BS, Kereiakes D, Aguirre FV, Weisman H, Schaible T, Topol EJ. Profound inhibition of platelet aggregation with monoclonal antibody 7E3 Fab after thrombolytic therapy: Results of the TAMI 8 pilot study. J Am Coll Cardiol 22:381, 1993.

136. Wagner CL, Knight D, McAleer MF, Lance E, Mattis J, Coller B, Weisman HF, Jordan RE. Immunological comparison of murine and chimeric 7E3 Fab fragments in human clinical trials (abstr). J Immunol 150:158, 1993.

137. Gan ZR, Gould RJ, Jacobs JW, Friedman PA, Polokoff MA. Echistatin: A potent platelet aggregation inhibitor from the venom of the viper *Echis carinatus*. J Biol Chem 263:19827, 1988.

138. Dennis MS, Henzel WJ, Pitti RM, Lipari MT, Napier MA, Deisher TA, Bunting S, Lazarus RA. Platelet glycoprotein GPIIb/IIIa protein antagonists from snake venoms: Evidence for a family of platelet-aggregation inhibitors. Proc Natl Acad Sci USA 87:2471, 1989.

139. Musial J, Niewiarowski S, Rucinski B, Stewart G, Cook JJ, Williams JA, Edmunds LH. Inhibition of platelet adhesion to surfaces of extracorporeal circuits by disintegrins: RGD-containing peptides from viper venoms. Circulation 82:261, 1990.

140. The EPIC Investigators. Use of a monoclonal antibody directed against the platelet glycoprotein IIb/IIIa receptor in high-risk coronary angioplasty. N Engl J Med 330:956, 1994.

141. Lefkovits J, Ivanhoe R, Anderson K, Weisman H, Topol EJ. Platelet IIb/IIIa receptor inhibition during PTCA for acute myocardial infarction: Insights from the EPIC trial (abstr). Circulation 90:I546, 1994.

142. Ohman EM, Kleiman NS, Gacioch G, Worley S, Talley JD, Navetta FI, Anderson HV, Spriggs D, Miller M, Cohen M, Kereiakes D, George BS, Sigmon KN, Krucoff M, Califf RM, Topol EJ, for the IMPACT-AMI Group. Simultaneous platelet glycoprotein IIb/IIIa integrin blockade and front-loaded tissue plasminogen activator in acute myocardial infarction: Results from a randomized trial (abstr). J Am Coll Cardiol 27(Suppl. A):167, 1996.

143. Faulds D, Sorkin EM. Abciximab (c7E3 Fab): A review of its pharmacology and therapeutic potential in ischaemic heart disease. Drugs 48:583, 1994.

31. EXPERIMENTAL EVIDENCE FOR ENHANCEMENT OF THROMBOLYSIS BY CONVENTIONAL THROMBOLYTIC DRUGS

Paolo Golino

Introduction

Braunwald et al.'s hypothesis that the extent of myocardial injury reflects the degree of imbalance between myocardial oxygen supply and oxygen requirements gained wide acceptance in the 1970s as a result of observations in both experimental animals and patients [1]. It soon became clear that reduction of myocardial oxygen requirements by itself only modestly attenuated the extent of ischemic injury [2]. Subsequently, major efforts have been made to develop techniques that directly restore nutritive myocardial perfusion. In particular, with the knowledge that thrombotic coronary occlusion occurs in the vast majority of patients in the early phase of acute myocardial infarction [3], a rationale for thrombolytic therapy existed. Administration of drugs capable of lysing the intracoronary thrombus seems particularly attractive because its simplicity makes it applicable to most of the patients with acute myocardial infarction. This review summarizes advances related to thrombolysis and suggests additions to or alterations in thrombolytic therapy that could make it even more effective as a therapeutic intervention in the future.

How Effective Is Thrombolysis?

The ultimate goal of optimal thrombolysis is salvage of jeopardized myocardium by restoration of antegrade perfusion at the tissue level. Although a few investigators have argued that the salutary effects of thrombolytic agents may result from mechanisms other than restoration of infarct artery patency [4], it is almost universally accepted that benefit with this form of therapy is linked to the establishment of an open artery. Failed recanalization after thrombolysis has been associated with higher rates of in-hospital mortality and morbidity, and with minimal recovery of left ventricular function compared with outcome in patients in whom reperfusion is successful [5,6].

Results of numerous studies attest to the efficacy of coronary thrombolysis in achieving recanalization of the infarct-related artery. During the first 24 hours after acute myocardial infarction, angiography reveals a patent infarct-related artery in only 9–29% of patients who have not been treated with thrombolytic agents [7–11]. Thus, conventional angiographic assessment of the efficacy of various thrombolytic agents has focused on the establishment of infarct artery patency, typically at 90 minutes after initiation of therapy. By these criteria, early effective thrombolysis is achieved least frequently after treatment with intravenous streptokinase (43–64%) [9,12–14] or urokinase (53–66%) [15–17] and in nearly equal proportions of patients receiving tissue plasminogen activator (t-PA) in standard dosages (63–79%) [7–18] or anistreplase (55–73%) [19–21]. Superior results have been obtained using accelerated dosing regimens of t-PA, with 90-minute patency rates ranging from 82% to 91% in five studies of a combined more than 500 patients [16,19,22–24].

However, although patency rates appear to be acceptably high at 90 minutes after initiation of therapy, it has been suggested that this parameter may not be an adequate reflection of optimal reperfusion. In particular, it has been reported that patients exhibiting fully restored flow (TIMI grade 3) at 90 minutes after thrombolysis have a 30-day mortality rate less than half (4.0%) that of patients with TIMI grade 2 flow [25]. These observations have persuaded some investigators to designate TIMI grade 2 flow after thrombolysis as reperfusion failure rather than reperfusion success [25]. Considering that with the currently most widely used thrombolytic regimen, accelerated t-PA plus heparin and aspirin, the prevalence of angiographic complete restoration of flow (TIMI grade 3) at 90 minutes is –55%, and that the prevalence of TIMI grade 3 flow after the therapeutic alternative, namely, direct angioplasty, exceeds 90%, it is evident that every effort should be made to identify adjunctive interventions to thrombolysis in order to achieve a similar rate of complete reperfusion.

Potential Pharmacological Interventions for Enhancement of Thrombolysis

The duration of the ischemic period is by far the most important factor that ultimately affects the clinical outcome of thrombolysis. Indeed, as already outlined, using currently employed doses and means of administration of t-PA, about 55% of patients exhibit full recanalization 90 minutes after the initiation of therapy. It seems, therefore, of pivotal importance to identify interventions capable of increasing the reperfusion rate and reducing the interval between the administration of t-PA and the achievement of full reperfusion.

One possibility for overcoming this problem is to enhance the lytic properties of a thrombolytic agent or possibly to use different thrombolytic agents, the combination of which has been shown to be synergistic in lysing intravascular thrombi. It has been suggested that mutant forms of t-PA as well as chimeric molecules containing the fibrin recognition site of t-PA and the protease activity of single-chain urokinase plasminogen activator (scu-PA) may be more potent and fibrin specific than native t-PA [26]. It has been also shown that a mutant form of t-PA with a glycosylation defect and prolonged clearance time causes lysis of experimentally induced coronary thrombi more rapidly than wild-type t-PA and may delay reocclusion, while having similar effects on circulating fibrinogen as wild-type t-PA [27]. Other experimental studies have shown that vampire bat salivary plasminogen activator (bat-PA), a plasminogen activator displaying strict fibrin specificity, is more rapid than t-PA in inducing effective thrombolysis in a rabbit model of femoral artery thrombosis, but is associated with less plasminemia and depletion of circulating fibrinogen [28].

More recently, Markland et al. have studied the thrombolytic effects of fibrolase in a canine model of coronary artery thrombosis [29]. Fibrolase is a direct-acting fibrinolytic enzyme isolated from the southern copperhead snake venom. It does not rely on plasminogen activation or any other bloodborne components for its activity, and is not inhibited by any of the rapidly acting serine proteinase inhibitors present in the blood. In that study, fibrolase effectively lysed experimental coronary artery thrombi within 10 minutes following its administration without causing fibrinogen depletion or excessive hemorrhage [29].

There is also some evidence in studies carried out in vitro or in experimental animals [30] and on a limited number of patients [31–33] that there may be a synergism between the actions of scu-PA and t-PA. Finally, coupling t-PA to antifibrin monoclonal antibodies may also improve fibrin specificity [34]. All of these alterations of thrombolytic agents might be beneficial, but other than the preliminary studies on the combination of t-PA and scu-PA, they have not been tested rigorously as yet. Therefore, their clinical value is presently uncertain and further studies about these new agents are warranted.

Another approach to enhance thrombolysis might be through interfering with the process of thrombus formation. It has been demonstrated that thrombus formation is a dynamic process, with new fibrin and platelets being added to the thrombus for several hours after its formation [35,36]. This growth of the thrombus during the first hours may well proceed during administration of thrombolytic therapy, thus increasing the total amount of the thrombus to be lysed and therefore the time to reperfusion. Starting from the observation of Salimi et al., who showed that arterial thrombi continue to incorporate new fibrin for up to 72 hours after their formation [36], Cercek et al. demonstrated that concomitant treatment with heparin increases the thrombolytic properties of t-PA on experimentally induced coronary thrombi [37]. The authors speculated that heparin may enhance thrombolysis by blocking the formation of new fibrin and by preventing its incorporation into a thrombus during infusion of t-PA. Based on this and other observations [38,39], the majority of clinical trials of intravenous tissue plasminogen activator have been performed with the concomitant use of heparin. In particular, two recent large clinical trials involving more than 41,000 patients have clearly established that both coronary patency rates following t-PA administration and survival benefits are higher with early concomitant systemic heparin treatment [40,41].

In addition to fibrin, another major component of arterial thrombi is platelet aggregates [42]. It has been shown that platelets bind fibrin both through exposure of specific membrane receptors [43] and by nonspecific binding [44]. Furthermore, increased local concentrations of proaggregatory substances, such as thromboxane A_2 (TxA_2), serotonin (5HT), ADP, and platelet activating factor (PAF), secreted by activated platelets already embodied into the thrombus may recruit additional platelets, which, in turn, may contribute to thrombus growth. In a recent study, Gold et al. have shown that intracoronary platelet activation continues after formation of the thrombus and that deposition of additional platelets onto the thrombus may prolong the time to reperfusion during thrombolytic treatment in a canine model of coronary thrombosis [45]. These authors demonstrated that administration of a monoclonal antibody directed against the platelet glycoprotein IIb/IIIa receptor (a specific receptor for fibrinogen and fibrin as well as other adhesive plasma proteins), together with t-PA, caused a more rapid recanalization of the occluded vessel as compared with animals treated with t-PA alone [45].

It is known that platelets aggregate in response to a variety of substances in vivo. In particular, TxA_2 and 5HT are two important mediators of platelet activation in stenosed, endothelially injured canine coronary arteries [46–48]. We have shown that TxA_2 and 5HT cooperatively mediate intracoronary platelet activation during administration of t-PA and that simultaneous administration of TxA_2 and 5HT receptor antagonists markedly reduces the time to reperfusion as compared with that in control animals and animals treated with either antagonist alone [49]. Alterations in prostaglandin synthesis have also been shown to be a useful intervention in potentiating the thrombolytic properties of t-PA. In the same animal preparation, simultaneous blockade of TxA_2 receptors and inhibition of TxA_2 synthase is more effective than either intervention alone in shortening the time to thrombolysis by t-PA because of a redirection of prostaglandin endoperoxides toward the synthesis of antiaggregatory prostaglandins, such as PGI_2, PGE_1, or PGD_1 [50,51].

Because PGH_2 shares the same receptor on platelet membranes with TxA_2 and it has a proaggregatory effect, inhibition of TxA_2 synthase results in a potentiation of the thrombolytic effects of t-PA in the presence of concomitant blockade of TxA_2/PGH_2 receptors. Recently, two experimental studies have suggested that a marked improvement in the thrombolytic properties of t-PA may be obtained when t-PA is administered with either clopidogrel, a potent inhibitor of ADP-induced platelet aggregation [52], or VCL, a recombinant fragment of human von Willebrand factor that binds to platelet glycoprotein Ib [53]. Both of these interventions have been shown to markedly shorten the lysis time of experimental coronary artery thrombi in a canine model with respect to aspirin or heparin alone [52,53]. In particular, VCL, because of its mechanism of action

(see also later), seems particularly attractive for a potential use in the clinical setting.

The importance of concomitant antiplatelet therapy in patients undergoing coronary thrombolysis was emphasized by the results of the ISIS-2 trial [54]. In this study, 17, 187 patients with suspected acute myocardial infarctions were randomized to receive either streptokinase or aspirin, the combination of the two drugs, or neither. Streptokinase alone decreased early cardiovascular mortality by 25%, while the combination of aspirin and streptokinase decreased the death rate by 42% as compared with the placebo group. The benefits of these agents appeared to be independent of one another, and the addition of aspirin to streptokinase reduced the clinical reinfarction rate by approximately 50%.

The phenomenon of reocclusion of the infarct-related artery after successful thrombolysis remains an important problem facing the clinician because it may blunt or even negate the benefits of early reperfusion. Just as the rate of successful recanalization has varied from study to study, the angiographically documented reocclusion rate has ranged from 0% to 45%. It is, however, evident that no thrombolytic agent so far studied offers complete protection against reocclusion. It can be speculated that preservation of higher fibrinogen levels might be a contributing factor to reocclusion because fibrinogen is essential for platelet aggregation to occur [55] and fibrin (ogen) degradation products exert a potent antiplatelet effect [56]. For the 100 mg t-PA dose, the expected rate of reocclusion is 10–33%.

In understanding the pathophysiological mechanisms involved in reocclusion after thrombolysis, it is worth emphasizing that the causes of coronary artery thrombosis are not well established as yet, although it is widely accepted that the trigger for thrombotic occlusions is often related to plaque fissure, rupture, and/or endothelial disruption, with consequent exposure of collagen, tissue factor, and other substances of the subendothelial matrix, such as fibronectin and von Willenbrand factor, all of which may activate both circulating platelets and the coagulation cascade [57,58]. Furthermore, these events typically occur in a coronary artery with moderate to severe atherosclerotic stenosis, in which the shear rate is markedly increased. As a consequence, a rapid growth of platelet-rich thrombi occurs [59–61]. Subsequently, a fibrin mesh is added to the platelet thrombus as a result of thrombin activation through activation of the extrinsic pathway [62,63], as well as the rise of thrombin-like activity on the platelet surface [64]. Keeping this in mind, reocclusion of the infarct-related artery after discontinuation of thrombolytic therapy is not a surprising event if one considers that thrombolytic agents might dissolve the thrombus but usually will not alter or remove the factors primarily involved in causing thrombus formation. Included among these factors are severe residual stenosis and injury to the coronary endothelium, with continuing exposure of circulating blood to the subendothelium and, therefore, potential platelet aggregation and activation of the coagulation cascade.

Several studies have provided evidence for an increase in platelet activation and in thrombin activity after administration of streptokinase or t-PA. In particular, Fitzgerald et al. observed a marked elevation of plasma and urinary metabolites of thromboxane A_2 (as an index of platelet activation) in patients with acute myocardial infarction who were successfully reperfused with streptokinase [65] or with t-PA [66]. This effect was not seen in patients pretreated with aspirin or in those patients in whom reperfusion was not achieved [65,66], thus suggesting that platelet activation was possibly the consequence of their reexposure to the subendothelium of a fissured or ulcerated atherosclerotic plaque rather than an effects of streptokinase or t-PA per se. Furthermore, Eisenberg et al. showed an increase in fibrinopeptide A (which is released by the action of thrombin on fibrinogen) immediately after thrombolytic therapy in patients with acute myocardial infarction [67].

Several experimental studies have emphasized the importance of platelet activation in mediating reocclusion after successful thrombolysis. In dogs with experimentally induced coronary thrombosis successfully reperfused with t-PA, reocclusion occurs early after discontinuation of the thrombolytic agent [45,49–51,68,69], providing that the thrombogenic stimulus is not removed (a condition that mimics the situation occurring in patients with occluding coronary thrombi successfully reperfused with thrombolytic therapy). In all these studies, reocclusion occurred despite the administration of a full dose of heparin (i.e., sufficient to induce a 2.5- to 3-fold increase in activated coagulation time), and it is known that reocclusion may occur also in patients receiving heparin during the post-thrombolytic state. These observations suggest that platelet activation plays an important role in mediating coronary artery reocclusion following thrombolytic therapy.

As previously stated, in spite of high rates of reperfusion achieved with different thrombolytic agents, the incidence of acute reocclusion is unacceptably high, and it occurs even in the presence of full anticoagulant therapy. Active research is underway to indentify better antithrombotic interventions that will reduce the rate of reocclusion of the infarct-related artery. As discussed earlier, platelet activation following thrombolytic therapy in an artery in which altered hemodynamics and exposure of a residual thrombogenic surface coexist is an important contributor to coronary artery reocclusion.

Platelet thrombus formation in vivo is a complex phenomenon, involving initially platelet adherence at sites of vascular injury. The components modulating this response include adhesive proteins in the subendothelial extracellular matrix, such as von Willebrand factor (vWF), and the platelet membrane glycoprotein (Gp) Ib [70]. Binding of vWF to platelet GpIb results in activation of platelets through a series of intracellular biochemical reactions [70]. Activated platelets then release a number of chemical mediators, including TxA_2, 5HT, ADP, and PAF, all of which promote the recruitment of additional platelets from the circulation via hydrolysis of platelet membrane phosphatidylinositol by phospholipase C, which results in a decrease in the intracellular concentration of cAMP and a consequent mobilization of calcium from the platelet-dense tubular system [71,72]. Any or all of these pathways of platelet activation result in the formation of a calcium-dependent heterodimer complex of platelet membrane GPIIb and GPIIIa. This complex expresses a receptor for adhesive proteins responsible for the formation of platelet aggregates, including fibrinogen, vWF, and fibronectin [55]. The dimeric structure and twofold symmetry render fibrinogen uniquely well suited to serve as a molecular bridge from platelet to platelet. The combination of platelet secretion and rheologic changes, resulting in collision of inactivated platelets with those that have undergone shape change, allows interplatelet contact and the formation of platelet aggregates. Thus, there are several potentially different interventions that might interfere with the process of platelet activation.

One possibility is represented by blocking one or more activating receptors present on platelet membranes. For instance, we have shown that post-thrombolysis platelet activation and reocclusion are cooperatively mediated by TxA_2 and 5HT, because simultaneous administration of selective TxA_2 and 5HT receptor antagonists prevents or markedly delays reocclusion following t-PA when administered at the time of reflow in an experimental canine model [69]. This protective effect is also observed when these antagonists are administered *during* thrombolytic therapy [50]. In this case, TxA_2 and 5HT receptor antagonists are also capable of enhancing the thrombolytic properties of t-PA, because lysis time is significantly shorter and the amount of t-PA is substantially less than in those animals receiving t-PA alone [50]. At least one aspect of this previous study deserves further comment. The observation that simultaneous blockade of two different types of receptors (namely, TxA_2 and 5HT) is necessary to enhance thrombolysis and to prevent reocclusion, whereas either intervention alone is relatively ineffective in this experimental model, suggests that the surface exposed after lysis of the thrombus represents a strong thrombogenic stimulus. Indeed, synergistic inhibition of platelet aggregation has been achieved with simultaneous use of TxA_2 and 5HT receptor antagonists in the experimental setting [73] as well as in humans [74].

Interfering with the synthesis of endogenous prostaglandins also seems to be an effective adjunctive therapy to thrombolysis. In principle, inhibition of TxA_2 synthase, the enzyme responsible for the conversion of PGH_2 to TxA_2, should offer more advantages than blockade of TxA_2 receptors because some of the PGH_2 produced during platelet activation can be transformed into PGI_2 by endothelial cells or into PGE_2 and PGD_2 in the plasma by a specific isomerase [75]. These prostaglandins are known to possess antiplatelet effects, which may be of adjunctive usefulness in preventing platelet activation. However, part of the PGH_2 is not transformed into potentially protective prostaglandins, and it may directly stimulate platelet aggregation through activation of TxA_2/PGH_2 receptors.

In this regard, simultaneous inhibition of TxA_2 synthase and blockade of TxA_2 receptors should result in more powerful antiplatelet effects than either intervention alone. To test this hypothesis, we have administered R68070, a drug that has TxA_2 synthase inhibitory and receptor blocking properties [50,51], to dogs with experimentally induced coronary thrombosis in combination with t-PA. The combined interventions resulted in enhancement of thrombolysis and prevention of reocclusion more effectively than blocking TxA_2 receptors [50] or inhibition of TxA_2 synthase separately [51].

However, according to the pathophysiological scheme described earlier, interfering with the binding of platelet GPIb to vWF or of GPIIb/IIIa to fibrinogen should result in more effective antithrombotic interventions than interfering with the various platelet agonists. In fact, GPIb–vWF interaction represents the initial common pathway of platelet activation, at least under conditions of high shear stress, whereas GPIIb/IIIa binding to fibrinogen is the final common pathway of platelet aggregation. Indeed, in a canine model of coronary thrombolysis, Gold et al. showed that administration of a monoclonal GPIIb/IIIa antibody together with t-PA not only shortens the lysis time, but also prevents or delays infarct-related artery reocclusion after discontinuation of t-PA [68]. In addition, recent evidence indicates that inhibiting glycoprotein GPIb–vWF interaction with VCL, a recombinant fragment of human vWF, also results in a marked improvement in thrombolysis and in prevention of reocclusion following discontinuation of t-PA administration [53]. Because of their peculiar mechanisms of action, both of these approaches seem particularly promising to be used in the clinical scenario.

Finally, increasing evidence indicates that thrombin plays a central role in mediating both the continuous growth of the thrombus during thrombolytic therapy and reocclusion of the infarct-related artery [67]. In addition to heparin, new direct thrombin inhibitors have been recently identified, including hirudin and hirulog [76]. These new thrombin inhibitors have the advantage over heparin in that they are antithrombin III independent, inactivate clot-bound thrombin, and prevent thrombin-induced platelet aggregation [76]. Several experimental and clinical studies have shown that these agents might be beneficial when administered in conjunction with thrombolytics [77–81]. However, a potential limitation of these agents is that new formation of thrombin is not affected [76]. This may cause persistence of thrombin activity despite the presence of an inhibitor [76,82]. In addition, these compounds may carry an increased risk of bleeding when administered in conjunction with thrombolytic therapy, which represents the most concerning adverse effect [79–81].

With these possible limitations of thrombin inhibitors, we have tested the efficacy of a monoclonal antibod against rabbit tissue factor (AP-1) when administered in conjunction with t-PA in a rabbit model of carotid artery thrombosis. Tissue factor (TF) is a 47-kd membrane-bound glycoprotein essential for activation of the extrinsic coagulation pathway that is constitutively expressed by cells that are not in contact with blood. Tissue factor complexes with factors VII and VIIa, permitting enzymatic activation of factors X and IX, the substrates for factor VIIa [83], ultimately leading to the generation of thrombin [83]. In this regard, a potential advantage of AP-1 is that it inhibits an early step of the extrinsic coagulation pathway, involving binding of factor VII/VIIa to TF, which ultimately results in inhibition of new thrombin formation, interrupting the positive-feedback loop that autoamplifies thrombin generation. We have shown that AP-1 administration not only significantly shortens lysis time induced by t-PA, but also completely prevented reocclusion after t-PA discontinuation [84].

It should be emphasized that these results were obtained without affecting platelet function and prothrombin time [84]. These data suggest the importance of TF exposure, with the consequent activation of the extrinsic coagulation pathway, in mediating a continuous thrombin generation, leading to growth of the thrombus during thrombolysis, as well as causing reocclusion of the vessel after thrombolytic therapy is discontinued. Further studies are required to elucidate the potential clinical applications of AP-1 as adjunctive therapy with thrombolytic agents.

Conclusions

The initial promising results of thrombolytic therapy in patients with acute myocardial infarction have greatly, and probably permanently, altered the care of such patients. Despite the substantial progress made during the past few years, a number of unresolved issues still exist. Specifically, much more effort needs to be made with regard to shortening the interval between the onset of ischemia and the achievement of full reperfusion, prevention of reocclusion, and prevention of reperfusion injury. The ischemic period may be significantly shortened by using more powerful thrombolytic agents, such as mutants of t-PA, or by using synergistic combinations of thrombolytic agents, such as t-PA and scu-PA. Adjunctive therapy might be provided by a variety of antiplatelet drugs that shorten the time to thrombolysis and delay or prevent reocclusion, including thromboxane A_2 synthase inhibitors and receptor antagonists, serotonin receptor antagonists, thrombin antagonists, ADP receptor antagonists, possibly platelet activating factor antagonists, or monoclonal antibodies to the platelet receptors responsible for platelet attachment or aggregation, that is, monoclonal antibodies or synthetic peptides to platelet GPIb or GPIIb/IIIa. Last but not least, the important question of whether reperfusion injury is clinically important and whether it can be prevented in the clinical setting needs to be addressed as well as the possibility that selected pharmacological interventions, such as beta blockers, phospholipase, lysosomal or protease inhibitors, free radical scavengers, and calcium antagonists, might enhance the infarct-reducing ability of thrombolytic interventions needs to be evaluated.

Acknowledgments

This work was supported in part by grant no. 91.00122.PF41 from the Consiglio Nazionale delle Ricerche, Progetto Finalizzato Prevenzione e Controllo dei Fattori di Malattia, Italy.

References

1. Maroko PR, KjekshusJK, Sobel BE, et al. Factors influencing infarct size following experimental coronary artery occlusions. Circulation 43:67, 1971.
2. Sobel BE, Braunwald E. The management of acute myocardial infarction. In Braunwald E (ed). Heart Disease: A Textbook of Cardiovascular Medicine, 2nd ed. Philadelphia: WB Saunders, 1984:1301.
3. De Wood MA, Spores J, Notske R, et al. Prevalence of total coronary occlusion during the early hours of transmural myocardial infarction. N Engl J Med 303:897, 1980.
4. Chamberlain DA. Unanswered questions in thrombolysis. Am J Cardiol 63:34A, 1989.
5. Califf RM, Topol EJ, George BS, Boswick JM, Lee KL, Stump D, Dillon J, Abbottsmith C, Candela RJ, Kereiakes DJ, ONeill WW, Stack RS. C'haracteristics and outcome of patients in whom reperfusion with intravenous tissue-type plasminogen activator fails: Results of the Thrombolysis and Angioplasty in Myocardial Infarction (TAMI) trial. Circulation 77:1090, 1988.
6. Morgan CD, Roberts RS, Haq A, Baigrie RS, Daly PA, Gent M, Armstrong PW, for the TPAT Study Group. Coronary patency, infarct size and left ventricular function after thrombolytic therapy for acute myocardial infarction: Results from the Tissue Plasminogen Activator Toronto (TPAT) placebo-controlled trial. J Am Coll Cardiol 17:1451, 1991.
7. Topol EJ, Morris DC, Smalling RW, Schumacher RR, Taylor CR, Nishikawa A, Liberman HA, Collen D, Tufte ME, Grossbard EB, O'Neill WW. A multicenter. randomized, placebo-controlled trial of a new form of intravenous recombinant tissue-type plasminogen activator (Activase) in acute myocardial infarction. J Am Coll Cardiol 9:1205, 1987.
8. Anderson JL, Marshall HW, Askins JC, Lutz R, Sorensen SG, Menlove RL, Yanowitz FG, Hagan AD. A randomized trial of intravenous and intracoronary streptokinase in patients with acute myocardial infarction. Circulation 70:606, 1984.
9. Chesebro JH, Knatterud G, Roberts R, Borer S, Cohen LS, Dalen J, Dodge HT, Francis CK, Hillis D, Ludbrook P, Markis JE, Mueller H, Passamani ER, Powers ER, Rao AK, Robertson T, Ross A, Ryan TJ, Sobel BE, Willerson J, Williams DO, Zaret BL, Braunwald E. Thrombolysis in Myocardial Infarction (TIMI) Trial, Phase 1: A comparison between intravenous tissue plasminogen activator and intravenous streptokinase. Circulation 76:142, 1987.
10. Armstrong PW, Baigrie RS, Daly PA, Haq A, Gent M, Roberts RS, Freeman MR, Burns R, Liu P, Morgan CD. Tissue plasminogen activator: Toronto (TPAT) Placebo-Controlled Randomized Trial in Acute Myocardial Infarction. J Am Coll Cardiol 13:1469, 1989.
11. Verstraete M, Brower RW, Collen D, Dunning AJ, Lubsen J, Michel PL, Schofer J, Vanhaecke J, Van de Werf F, Bleifeld W, Charbonnier B, de Bono DP,

Lennane RJ, Mathey DG, Raynaud P, Vahanian A, van de Kley GA, Von Essen R. Double-blind randomized trial of intravenous tissue-type plasminogen activator versus placebo in acute myocardial infarction (ECSG-I). Lancet 1:965, 1985.

12. Stack RS, O'Connor CM, Mark DB, Hinohara T, Phillips HR, Lee MM, Ramirez NM, O'Callaghan WG, Simonton CA, Carlson EB, Morris KG, Behar VS, Kong Y, Peter RH, Califf RM. Coronary perfusion during acute myocardial infarction with a combined therapy of coronary angioplasty and high-dose intra venous streptokinase. Circulation 77:151, 1988.

13. PRIMI Trial Study Group. Randomised double-blind trial of recombinant pro-urokinase against streptokinase in acute myocardial infarction. Lancet 1:863, 1989.

14. Verstraete M, Bory M, Collen D, Erbel R, Lennane RJ, Mathey D, Michels HR, Schartl M, Uebis R, Bernard R, Brower RW, DeBono DP, Huhmann W, Lubsen J, Meyer J, Rutsch W, Schmidt W, VonEssen R. Randomised trial of intravenous recombinant tissue-type plasminogen activator versus intravenous streptokinase in acute myocardial infarction. Lancet 1:842, 1985.

15. Whitlow PL, Bashore TM. Catheterization/Rescue Angioplasty Following Thrombolysis (CRAFT) study: Acute myocardial infarction treated with recombinant tissue plasminogen activator versus urokinase. J Am Coll Cardiol 17:276A, 1991.

16. Neuhaus K, Tebbe U, Gottwik M, Weber M, Feuerer W, Niederer W, Haerer W, Praetorius F, Grosser K, Huhmann W, Howpp H, Alber G, Sheikhzadeh A, Schneider B. Intravenous recombinant tissue plasminogen activator (rt-PA) and urokinase in acute myocardial infarction: Results of the German Activator Urokinase Study (GAUS). J Am Coll Cardiol 12:581, 1988.

17. Califf RM, Topol EJ, Stack RS, Ellis SG, George BS, Kereiakes DJ, Samaha JK, Worley SJ, Anderson IL, Harrelson-Woodlief L, Wall TC, Phillips HR, Abbottsmith CW, Candela RJ, Flanagan WH, Sasahara AA, Mantell SJ, Lee KL. Evaluation of combination thrombolytic therapy and timing of cardiac catheterization in acute myocardial infarction: Results of Thrombolysis and Angioplasty in Myocardial Infarction — phase 5 randomized trial. Circulation 83:1543, 1991.

18. TIMI Research Group. Immediate vs. delayed catheterization and angioplasty following thrombolytic therapy for acute myocardial infarction: TIMI IIA results. JAMA 260:2849, 1988.

19. Neuhaus K-L, von Essen R, Tebbe U, Vogt A, Roth M, Riess M, Niederer W, Forycki F, Wirtzfeld A, Maeurer W, Limbourg P, Merx W, Haerten K. Improved thrombolysis in acute myocardial infarction with front-loaded administration of alteplase: Results of the rt-PA-APSAC Patency Study (TAPS). J Am Coll Cardiol 19:885, 1992.

20. Hogg KJ, Gemmill JD, Burns JMA, Lifson WK, Rae AP, Dunn FG, Hillis WS. Angiographic patency study of anistreplase versus streptokinase in acute myocardial infarction. Lancet 335:254, 1990.

21. Relik-van Wely L, Visser RF, van der Pol J, Bartholomeus I, Couvee JE, Drost H, Vet A, Klomps HC, van Ekelen W, Van der Berg F, Krauss X. Angiographically assessed coronary arterial patency and reocclusion in patients with acute myocardial infarction treated with anistreplase: Results of the Anistreplase Reocclusion Multicenter Study (ARMS). Am J Cardiol 68:296, 1991.

22. Carney RJ, Murphy GA, Brandt TR, Daley PJ, Pickering E, White HJ, McDonough TJ, Vermilya SK, Teichman SL, for the RAAMI Study Investigators. Randomized angiographic trial of recombinant tissue-type plasminogen activator (Alteplase) in myocardial infarction. J Am Coll Cardiol 20:17, 1992.

23. Smalling RW, Schumacher R, Morris D, Harder K, Fuentes F, Valentine RP, Battey LL, Merhige M, Pitts DE, Lieberman HA, Nishikawa A, Adyanthaya A, Hopkins A, Grossbard E. Improved infarct-related arterial patency after high dose, weight-adjusted, rapid infusion of tissue-type plasminogen activator in myocardial infarction: Results of a multicenter randomized trial of two dosage regimens. J Am Coll Cardiol 15:915, 1990.

24. Wall TC, Califf RM, George BS, Ellis SG, Samaha JK, Kereiakes DJ, Worley SJ, Sigmon K, Topol EJ, for the TAMI-7 Study Group. Accelerated plasminogen activator dose regimens for coronary thrombolysis. J Am Coll Cardiol 19:482, 1992.

25. Forrester JS. New standard for success of thrombolytic therapy. Circulation 92:2026, 1996.

26. Collen D. Molecular mechanism of action of newer thrombolytic agents. J Am Coll Cardiol 10:11B, 1987.

27. Eidt JF, McNatt J, Wydro RM, Yao SK, Allison P, Garramone S, Peters L, Livingston DJ, Buja LM, Willerson JT. Coronary thrombolysis with a variant of human tissue-type plasminogen activator in a canine preparation: Slightly enhanced thrombolysis and prolonged time to reocclusion. Cor Art Dis 2:931, 1991.

28. Gardell SJ, Ramjit DR, Stabilito II, Fujita T, Lynch JJ, Cuca GC, Jain D, Wang S, Tung JS, Mark GE, Shebuski RJ. Effective thrombolysis without marked plasminemia after bolus intravenous administration of vampire bat salivary plasminogen activator in rabbits. Circulation 84:244, 1991.

29. Markland FS, Friedrichs GS, Pewitt SR, Lucchesi BR. Thrombolytic effects of recombinant fibrolase or APSAC in a canine model of carotid artery thrombosis. Circulation 90:2448, 1994.

30. Collen D, Stassen JM, Stump DC, Verstraete M. Synergism of thrombolytic agents in vivo. Circulation 74:838, 1986.

31. Collen D, Stump DC, Van de Werf F. Coronary thrombolysis in patients with acute myocardial infarction by intravenous infusion of synergic thrombolytic agents. Am Heart J 112:1083, 1986.

32. Collen D, Van de Werf F. Coronary arterial thrombolysis with low-dose synergistic combinations of recombinant tissue type plasminogen activator (rt-PA) and recombinant single chain urokinase-type plasminogen activator (rscu-PA) for acute myocardial infarction. Am J Cardiol 60:431, 1987.

33. Bode C, Schuler G, Nordt T, et al. Intravenous thrombolytic therapy with a combination of single-chain urokinase-type plasminogen activator and recombinant tissue-type plasminogen activator in acute myocardial infarction. Circulation 81:907, 1990.

34. Bode C, Runge MS, Schonermark S, et al. Conjugation to an antifibrin antibody enhances the fibrinolytic potency of single-chain urokinase (scuPA). Clin Res 36:265A, 1988.

35. Hanson SR, Paxton LD, Harker LA. Iliac artery mural thrombus formation: Effect of antiplatelet therapy on ^{111}In-platelet deposition in baboons. Arteriosclerosis 6:511, 1986.

36. Salimi A, Oliver GC Jr, Lee J, Sherman LA. Continued incorporation of circulating radiolabeled fibrinogen intopreformed coronary artery thrombi. Circulation 56:213, 1977.

37. Cercek B, Lew AS, Hod H, Yano J, Reddy NKN, Ganz W. Enhancement of thrombolysis with tissue-type plasminogen activator by pretreatment with heparin. Circulation 74:583, 1986.

38. Andrade-Gordon P, Strickland S. Interaction of heparin with plasminogen activators and plasminogen: Effects on the activation of plasminogen. Biochemistry 25:4033, 1986.

39. Mickelson JK, Simpson PJ, Lucchesi BR. Effects of heparin and intravenous tissue plasminogen activator or streptokinase in a canine model of coronary artery thrombosis. Clin Res 35:305A, 1987.

40. Hsia J, Hamilton WP, Kleiman N, Roberts R, Chaitman BR, Ross AM for the HART Investigators. A comparison between heparin and low dose aspirin as adjunctive therapy with tissue plasminogen activator for acute myocardial infarction. N Engl J Med 323:1433, 1990.

41. The GUSTO Investigators. An international randomized trial comparing four thrombolytic strategies for acute myocardial infarction. N Engl J Med 329:673, 1993.

42. Chapman I. Morphogenesis of occluding coronary artery thrombosis. Arch Pathol 80:256, 1965.

43. Hantgan RR, Taylor RG, Lewis JC. Platelets interact with fibrin only after activation. Blood 65:1299, 1985.

44. Harfenist EJ, Packham MA, Mustard JF. Comparison of the interactions of fibrinogen and soluble fibrin with washed rabbit platelets stimulated with ADP. Thromb Haemost 53:183, 1985.

45. Gold HK, Coller BS, Yasuda T, et al. Rapid and sustained coronary artery recanalization with combined bolus injection of recombinant tissue-type plasminogen activator and monoclonal antiplatelet GPIIb/IIIa antibody in a canine preparation. Circulation 77:670, 1988.

46. Bush LR, Campbell WB, Buja LM, Tilton GD, Willerson JT. Effects of the selective thromboxane synthetase inhibitor dazoxiben on variations in cyclic blood flow in stenosed canine coronary arteries. Circulation 69:1161, 1984.

47. Ashton JH, Schmitz JM, Campbell WB, et al. Inhibibon of cyclic flow variations in stenosed canine coronary arteries by thromboxane A2/prostaglandin H2 receptor antagonists. Circ Res 59:568, 1986.

48. Ashton JH, Benedict CR, Fitzgerald C, et al. Serotonin as a mediator of cyclic flow variations in stenosed canine coronary arteries. Circulation 73:572, 1986.

49. Golino P, Ashton JH, McNatt J, et al. Simultaneous administration of thromboxane A2 and serotonin S2-receptor antagonists markedly enhances thrombolysis and prevents or delays reocclusion after tissue-type plasminogen activator in a canine model of coronary thrombosis. Circulation 79:911, 1989.

50. Golino P, Yao SK, Rosolowsky M, De Clerck F, Buja LM, Willerson JT. Simultaneous blockade of thromboxane A2 receptors and inhibition of thromboxane A2 synthase is more effective in enhancing thrombolysis and preventing reocclusion after tissue plasminogen activator than blockade of thromboxane A2 receptors alone. Clin Res 37:S18A, 1989.

51. Golino P, Rosolowsky M, Sheng-Kun Y, McNatt J, De Clerck F, Buja I M, Willerson JT. Endogenous prostaglandin endoperoxides and prostacyclin modulate the thrombolytic activity of tissue plasminogen activator. J Clin Invest 86:1095, 1990.

52. Yao SK, Ober JC, Ferguson JJ, Maffrand J-P, Anderson HV, Buja LM, Willerson JT. Clopidogrel is more effective than aspirin as adjuvant treatment to prevent reocclusion after thrombolysis. Am J Physiol 267:H488, 1994.

53. Yao SK, Ober JC, Garfinkel LI, Hagay Y, Ezov N, Ferguson JJ, Anderson HV, Panet A, Gorecki M, Buja LM, Willerson JT. Blockade of platelet membrane glycoprotein Ib receptors delays intracoronary thrombogenesis, enhances thrombolysis, and delays coronary artery reocclusion in dogs. Circulation 89:2822, 1994.

54. ISIS-2 (Second International Study of Infarct Survival) Collaborative Group. Randomised trial of intravenous streptokinase, oral aspirin, both, or neither among 17, 187 cases of suspected acute myocardial infarction: ISIS-2. Lancet 2:349, 1988.

55. Marguerie GA, Plow EF. The fibrinogen-dependent pathway of platelet aggregation. Ann N Y Acad Sci 408:556, 1983.

56. Thorsen Ll, Brosstad F, Gogstad G, Sletten K, Solum NO. Competitions between fibrinogen with its degradation produces for interactions with the platelet-fibrinogen receptor. Thromb Res 44:611, 1986.

57. Davies MJ, Thomas A. Thrombosis and acute coronary-artery lesions in sudden cardiac ischemic death. N Engl J Med 310:1137, 1984.

58. Sherman CT, Litvack F, Grundfest W, et al. Coronary

angioscopy in patients with unstable angina pectoris. N Engl J Med 315:913, 1982.

59. Badimon L, Badimon JJ, Galvez A, Chesebro JH, Fuster V. Influence of arterial damage and wall shear rate on platelet deposition: Ex vivo study in a swine model. Arteriosclerosis 6:312, 1986.

60. Davies MJ, Thomas T. The pathological basis and microanatomy of occlusive thrombus formation in human coronary arteries. Phil Trans R Soc Lond (Series B) 294:225, 1981.

61. Willerson JT, Golino P, Eidt JF, Campbell WB, Buja LM. Specific platelet mediators and unstable coronary artery lesions: Experimental evidence and potential clinical implications. Circulation 80:198, 1989.

62. Fuster V, Badimon L, Cohen M, Ambrose JA, Badimon JJ, Chesebro J. Insights into the pathogenesis of acute ischemic syndromes. Circulation 77:1213, 1988.

63. Vermylen J, Verstraete M, Fuster V. Role of platelet activation and fibrin formation in thrombogenesis. J Am Coll Cardiol 8(Suppl. B): 2B, 1986.

64. Walsh PN. The role of platelets in the contact phase of blood coagulation. Br J Haematol 22:237, 1972.

65. Fitzgerald DJ, Catella F, Roy L, FitzGerald GA. Marked platelet activation in vivo after intravenous streptokinase in patients with acute myocardial infarction. Circulation 77:142, 1988.

66. Kerins DM, Roy L, FitzGerald GA, Fitzgerald DJ. Platelet and vascular function during coronary thrombolysis with tissue type plasminogen activator. Circulation 88:1718, 1989.

67. Eisenberg PR, Sherman LA, Jaffe AS. Paradoxic elevation of fibrinopeptide A after Streptokinase: Evidence for continued thrombosis despite intense fibrinolysis. J Am Coll Cardiol 10:527, 1987.

68. Yasuda T, Gold HK, Fallon JT, et al. Monoclonal antibody against the platelet glycoprotein (GP) IIb/IIIa receptor prevents coronary artery reocclusion after reperfusion with recombinant tissue-type plasminogen activator in dogs. J Clin Invest 81:1284, 1988.

69. Golino P, Ashton JH, Glas-Greenwalt P, McNatt J, Buja LM, Willerson JT. Mediation of reocclusion by thromboxane A_2 and serotonin after thrombolysis with tissue-type plasminogen activator in a canine preparation of coronary thrombosis. Circulation 77:678, 1988.

70. Kroll MH, Harris TS, Moake JL, Handin RI, Schafer AI. von Willebrand factor binding to platelet GpIb initiates signals for platelet activation. J Clin Invest 88:1568, 1991.

71. Ware JA, Smith M, Salzman EW. Synergism of platelet aggregating agents: Role of elevation of cytoplasmic calcium. J Clin Invest 80:267, 1987.

72. Fitzgerald DJ. Platelet inhibition with an antibody to glycoprotein IIb/IIIa. Circulation 80:1918, 1989.

73. Ashton JH, Ogletree ML, Michel IM, Golino P, et al. Cooperative mediation by serotonin S_2 and thromboxane A_2/prostaglandin H_2 receptor activation of cyclic flow variations in dogs with severe coronary artery stenoses. Circulation 76:952, 1987.

74. De Clerck F, Xhonneux L, Van Gorp, et al. S_2-serotonergic receptor inhibition (ketanserin), combined with thromboxane A_2/prostaglandin endoperoxide receptor blockade (BM13.177): Enhanced anti-platelet effect. Thromb Haemost 56:236, 1986.

75. Needleman P, Turk J, Jakschik BA, Morrison AR, Lefkowith JB. Arachidonic acid metabolism. Annu Rev Biochem 55:69, 1986.

76. Lefkovits J, Topol EJ. Direct thrombin inhibitors in cardiovascular medicine. Circulation 90:1522, 1994.

77. Klement P, Hirsh J, Maraganore J, Fenton J, Weitz J. Effects of heparin and hirulog on t-PA induced thrombolysis in a rat model. Thromb Haemost 68:64, 1992.

78. Haskel EJ, Prager NA, Sobel BE, Abenschein DR. Relative efficacy of antithrombin compared with antiplatelet agents in accelerating coronary thrombolysis and preventing early reocclusion. Circulation 83:1048, 1991.

79. Cannon CP, Mc Cabe CH, Henry TD, Schweiger MJ, Gibson RS, Mueller HS, Becker RC, Kleiman NS, Haugland JM, Anderson JL, Sharaf BL, Edwards SJ, Rogers WJ, Williams DO, Braunwald E. A pilot trial of recombinant desolphatohirudin compared with heparin in conjunction with tissue-type plasminogen activator and aspirin for acute myocardial infarction: Results of the Thrombolysis in Myocardial Infarction (TIMI) 5 trial. J Am Coll Cardiol 23:993, 1994.

80. Lee LV, McCabe CH, Antman EM, Koch M, Wilensky R, Stringer K, Hochman J, Mueller HS, Henry TD, Kleiman N, Steingart RM, Wasserman H, for the TIMI 6 Investigators. Initial experience with hirudin and streptokinase in acute myocardial infarction: Results of the TIMI 6 trial. J Am Coll Cardiol (Special issue): 344A, 1994.

81. Topol EJ, Bonan R, Jewitt D, Sigwart U, Kakkar VV, Rothman M, de Bono D, Ferguson J, Willerson JT, Strony J, Ganz P, Cohen MD, Raymond R, Fox I, Maraganore J, Adelman B. Use of a direct antithrombin, hirulog, in place of heparin during coronary angioplasty. Circulation 87:1622, 1993.

82. Eisenberg PR, Sobel BE, Jaffe AS. Activation of prothrombin accompanying thrombolysis with recombinant tissue-type plasminogen activator. J Am Coll Cardiol 19:1065, 1992.

83. Rapaport SI, Rao LVM. Initiation and regulation of tissue factor-dependent blood coagulation. Arterioscler Thromb 12:1111, 1992.

84. Ragni M, Cirillo P, Pascucci I, Scognamiglio A, D'Andrea D, Eramo N, Ezekowitz MD, Pawashe A, Chiariello M, Golino P. A monoclonal antibody against tissue factor shortens tissue-plasminogen activator lysis time and prevents reocclusion in a rabbit model of carotid artery thrombosis. Circulation, in press.

SECTION X: PLASMA MARKERS OF INFARCTION, THROMBOSIS, AND THROMBOLYSIS

Dana R. Abendschein

Rapid treatment with fibrinolytic agents has been an important advance in the acute care of patients with myocardial infarction. However, it has also led to some challenges, including the need to diagnose evolving myocardial infarction unequivocally within the first few hours of its onset and to promptly recognize patients who require additional therapy, either because the infarct-related artery fails to recanalize or because it does not remain patent. Plasma markers of infarction and thrombosis have traditionally served as retrospective indices to confirm the clinical diagnosis and to predict morbidity. Nevertheless, in the context of rapid administration and close monitoring of the outcome of therapy, there has been increased interest in markers that may be used as accurate, prospective indices of myocardial infarction, the results of treatment, and the likelihood of complications.

This section reviews significant recent advances in the use of several potential plasma markers for early, sensitive detection of myocardial infarction, thrombosis, and coronary fibrinolysis. Although many are in the process of individual clinical evaluation, combination panels of these markers may ultimately serve to rapidly and noninvasively identify patients who are candidates for coronary fibrinolysis as well as to predict the outcome of therapy.

32. EARLY DIAGNOSIS OF MYOCARDIAL INFARCTION WITH MB-CK SUBFORMS

Robert Roberts

Introduction

Caring for patients with acute myocardial infarction (AMI) in a dedicated critical care unit was introduced in 1962 and over the next decade became widespread throughout North America and Europe. There was a significant reduction in mortality from between 30% and 35% to about 20% within 5–6 years of introducing the coronary care unit (CCU). As these results became available and more knowledge accrued of the mechanisms involved with sudden death and cardiac failure, it became the accepted norm for patients with AMI to be admitted to the CCU. However, due to the lack of distinguishing features of chest pain and the lack of diagnostic specificity of the electrocardiogram (ECG), it was often necessary to admit the patient to the CCU to subsequently exclude myocardial infarction. Initially the diagnostic enzymatic markers performed in the CCU consisted of serum glutamic oxaloacetic transaminase (SGOT), lactic dehydrogenase (LDH), and creatine kinase (CK), which were performed daily for 3 days for exclusion of infarction [1]. In the latter part of the 1970s, this profile was replaced with mainly LDH isoenzymes and the MB-CK isoenzyme [2]. The daily profile of 3 days was soon replaced by every 6–12 hours for 24–48 hours, and the marker was primarily MB-CK [1,3]. The temporal profile of plasma MB-CK of significant elevation above normal plasma levels within 8–12 hours of the onset of symptoms, with maximal activity around 24 hours, was ideal for triaging patients in the CCU, whether it was for treatment, discharge home, or transfer to a regular hospital bed. The patients in whom AMI was excluded were in the CCU for only a few hours, or at most one night, prior to transfer.

Need for Earlier Diagnosis

Due to recent developments both in diagnosis and therapy, the need to triage patients with chest pain has shifted from the CCU to the emergency room [1,4]. The urgency to triage on admission in the emergency room rather than in the CCU is driven by many factors. The number of patients seen in the emergency room with chest pain, requiring exclusion of AMI, has climbed to over 5 million, while the percentage of patients with AMI is only 10–15% [5]. Patients with AMI comprise less than 20% of all patients admitted to the CCU [5–10]. The CCU cost is particularly expensive for those without infarction or other justifiable reasons [5]. It is estimated that the total cost to the United States alone per year for excluding myocardial infarction is around $12 billion (DRG Handbook, HCIA, 1993). The introduction of acute revascularization for the treatment of AMI, either by thrombolytic therapy and/or primary percutaneous transluminal coronary angioplasty (PTCA), as routine, gave the impetus for people to seek therapy for their chest pain earlier than in previous years. The mean time of patients presenting to the emergency room used to be in the range of 10–12 hours after the onset of symptoms, whereas today more than half of the patients are presenting within 6 hours of the onset of symptoms. It is perhaps very important to recognize that thrombolytic therapy is far more effective if implemented within the initial hours after symptoms appear, with minimal benefit, if any, when given beyond 6 hours from the onset of symptoms [11]. The later observation has significantly accelerated the need for an earlier diagnosis. Thus, the need to triage patients in the emergency room is, in part, to provide for more appropriate therapy and to be more cost effective.

Lack of Sensitivity of Conventional Markers for Acute Myocardial Infarction

The profile of daily enzymes for 3 days in the 1960s was replaced in the 1980s by a profile of every 4–6 hours. However, to meet the needs for triaging in the

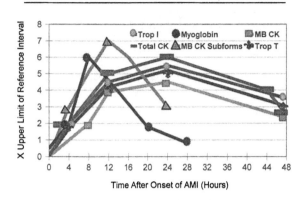

FIGURE 32-1. Plasma temporal profiles of commonly used cardiac diagnostic markers including MB-CK, total CK, troponin I, troponin T, myoglobin, and MB-CK subforms. Early diagnosis of infarction (≤6 hours) is only potentially possible with two of the markers, namely, MB-CK subforms and myoglobin.

emergency room, it would require more frequent sampling and a more rapid diagnosis than afforded by the conventional plasma MB-CK. The dilemma of early detection relates to the lack of specificity of the presenting symptoms and ECG manifestations. The causes of chest pain are numerous, and there is very little in its nature or character to distinguish cardiac pain from pain of noncardiac origin. The ECG exhibits only one specific early manifestation for myocardial infarction, namely, ST-segment elevation, which is present in less than 50% of patients with AMI [12,13]. In the remainder, the ECG changes are nonspecific and cannot distinguish between those originating from cardiac and those from noncardiac causes. In the emergency room it is estimated that only about 15–20% of the patients presenting with chest pain are subsequently shown to have myocardial infarction, and thus an ECG diagnostic of infarction is present in only about 7–10% of patients presenting with chest pain [14,15].

The traditional means of confirming myocardial infarction as routinely performed in the CCU, namely, with biochemical markers such as MB-CK, are not appropriate for early diagnosis in the emergency room because there is an interval of 8–10 hours required between the onset of myocardial infarction and when the marker is released from the injured myocardium in sufficient quantity to exceed the upper plasma limit of normal [16,17]. Elevated plasma MB-CK activity is the gold standard for the diagnosis of myocardial infarction. Plasma MB-CK, as measured by assays based on enzymatic activity, has a

diagnostic sensitivity of about 20–30% within the first 4 hours from the onset of symptoms [18], and 50–70% after 6 hours, reaching 90–100% sensitivity after 10–12 hours from the onset. The sensitivity is increased slightly if MB-CK is detected by immunological methods (preferred and routine today) such that sensitivity is 60–80% at 6 hours, and 99% at 12 hours [19,20]. The specificity is 90–98% at each interval. Troponin T, a newly proposed diagnostic marker, has sensitivities of 50% at 4 hours, 70% at 6 hours, and 90% at 12 hours which, are similar to MB-CK when detected by enzymatic activity assays and less sensitive than MB-CK when detected by immunological assays [20]. Troponin T appears to be somewhat less specific than MB-CK for the diagnosis of AMI, although this may reflect detection of unstable angina by troponin T [20].

It may be predicted from their plasma profiles that neither MB-CK nor troponin T are ideal diagnostic markers for detecting AMI in the first 4–6 hours from the onset of pain (Figure 32-1). Practically all studies involving a significant number of patients performed prior to 1995 compared the sensitivity and specificity of diagnostic markers in relation to the time of presentation rather than the onset of symptoms [20]. In that era, patients presented to the emergency room much later because there was no therapeutic advantage to present within the first 1–2 hours. However, today, as the public has become better educated and early thrombolytic therapy has become widely available, most patients are now presenting to the emergency room within 4–6 hours of the onset of symptoms. Thus, it has only been in the past year or so that diagnostic markers have been compared for sensitivity in relation to onset of symptoms. In two such recent studies, MB-CK and troponin T were compared by hourly sampling in relation to the onset of symptoms, and the investigators concluded that neither MB-CK nor troponin T qualify as markers for early diagnosis [18,20]. The more recent diagnostic marker for AMI is troponin I, which has a similar temporal profile as troponin T, with a similar sensitivity and specificity as MB-CK, and is not a marker for early diagnosis [21,22]. In clinical conditions accompanied by skeletal muscle damage and renal failure, troponin I may be more specific than MB-CK or troponin T [21]. The overall diagnostic problem in the emergency room is very much one of excluding myocardial infarction rather than including myocardial infarction; thus markers that have a sensitivity below 90% within the first 6 hours are less than adequate for excluding myocardial infarction. However, an abnormally elevated plasma level of troponin T, MB-CK, or troponin I at any interval from onset,

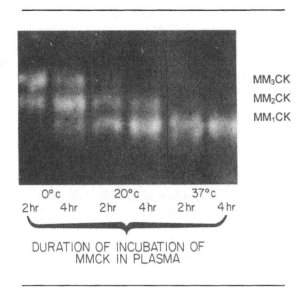

FIGURE 32-2. Effects of in vitro incubation of tissue MM creatine kinase (MMCK) with plasma, as analyzed, by nondenaturing polyacrylamide gel electrophoresis.

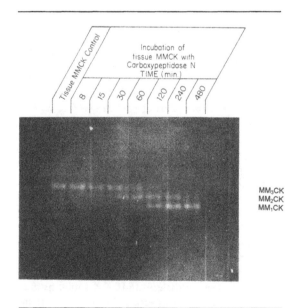

FIGURE 32-3. Effect of incubation of tissue MM creatine kinase (MMCK) with carboxypeptidase-N. The migratory pattern of MM_2 and MM_3 corresponds to that of the in vivo forms of MM_2 and MM_3, with MM_3 corresponding to tissue MM-CK. Analysis was performed by nondenaturing polyacrylamide gel electrophoresis.

whether it is 1 or more hours, is highly specific for infarction. A small percentage of patients may show elevated levels of these markers, even in the first 4–6 hours, because several factors determine their quantitative release into the plasma. The more extensive the area of damage, the earlier the release of the markers and the greater the amount released [20]. Early restoration of coronary flow, whether it is spontaneous, as it seems to be in non–Q-wave infarction [11], or induced pharmacologically, as with thrombolytic therapy, is associated with earlier and greater release of the markers (MB-CK peaks 12–13 hours). Similarly, more extensive collateral coronary flow correlates with early release of markers from the impaired myocardium. However, in those individuals in whom the plasma markers remain in the normal range, one is required to wait until 8–10 hours from the onset to reliably exclude infarction based on MB-CK and 12–16 hours for troponin T and I [20].

MB-CK Subforms: Origin and Mechanism of Production

It is well documented that the cytosolic isoenzymes of MM, MB, and BB CK are derived from two separate genes that encode for the M or B subunits [23–25]. Quantitative analysis of the CK isoenzyme composition of various human tissues, including the myocardium in animals and humans, consistently show only one product for the M gene and one for the B gene, such that tissues have a single form of MM-CK, BB-CK, or the hybrid MB-CK [25]. In the 1970s, the observation was made by Wevers et al. [26] that the plasma obtained from patients undergoing myocardial infarction exhibited what appeared to be multiple forms of MM- and MB-CK. Wevers confirmed that the tissue has only one form of MM-CK and MB-CK, and showed that three forms of MM-CK and two forms of MB-CK were generated in the blood.

Electrophoresis indicated that the newly developed forms in the blood were more negatively charged and migrated faster toward the positive electrode than the parent tissue form (Figure 32-2). According to the International Society for Biochemistry, the molecule with the least mobility is given the high number and thus the tissue MM-CK is designated as MM_3 and the two additional forms observed in the blood are MM_2 and MM_1. In the case of MB-CK, there are only two forms, the one in the tissue, referred to as MB_2CK and the additional form generated in the blood, referred to as MB_1CK. In 1981, using chromatofocusing chromatography, we isolated and purified the three MM subforms [27]. We demonstrated that the subform conversion in the blood is mediated by the plasma

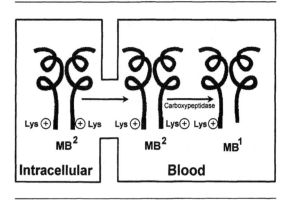

FIGURE 32-4. Molecular mechanism of MB-CK subform converson in the blood. Loss of a single positively charged lysine residue (Lys+) yields a more negatively charged molecule, resulting in faster anodal migration.

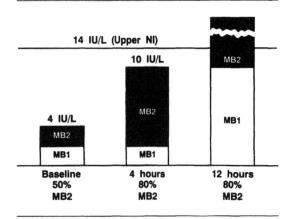

FIGURE 32-5. The upper limit for total MB-CK varies from 10 IU/L to 14 IU/L. In many individuals the baseline is 4 IU/L or less. The ratio of MB_2 to MB_1 at baseline is in equilibrium in a ratio of approximately 1 : 1. Thus, as illustrated here, an increase in the ratio of severalfold, as shown at 4 hours, does not exceed the upper limit of normal for total MB-CK, yet would be highly diagnostic of infarction if one used a 50% or more increase in the MB_2/MB_1 ratio as the diagnostic criterion.

enzyme, carboxypeptidase-N (CP-N). We were able to generate MM-CK subforms in vitro in the absence of serum by incubating purified tissue MM_3CK with CP-N (Figure 32-3).

Using peptide mapping and amino acid sequence analysis, the mechanism of production of other subforms from MM_3CK was shown to be via cleavage

of the positively charged amino acid lysine from the carboxy terminus of the M subunit [27]. This results in a polypeptide chain having a slightly greater net negative charge and therefore a faster rate of migration toward the positive electrode. The conversion reaction progresses rapidly; in vitro, MM_3CK present in excess was converted to MM_1CK within 2 hours at 37°F (see Figure 32-2) [17]. Thus, the sequential appearance of the MM-CK subforms can be explained as follows: Initially, release of MM_3CK from necrotic myocardium makes it the more abundant subform. Subsequent cleavage of the terminal lysine from one of the two M polypeptides of MM_3CK by CP-N yields a heterodimer MM_2CK, which transiently becomes the predominant subform after cessation of CK release. Subsequently, the removal of the remaining terminal lysine from the second M chain by CP-N produces MM_1CK, with the return of the three forms in equilibrium with each other after 16–21 hours [16,17]. A similar mechanism has been postuated for the conversion of MB_2CK to MB_1CK, with only the M-chain lysine undergoing removal (Figure 32-4). However, because both the M and B subunits have lysine as the terminal amino acid, other subforms of MB-CK may exist that cannot be resolved by electrophoresis [28].

Rational for the Use of MB-CK Subforms as a Marker for Early Diagnosis

The failure of conventional markers to detect myocardial infarction early after onset relates to the interval required for the release of the marker into the plasma in sufficient quantity to exceed the upper limits of normal. The upper limit of plasma MB-CK activity detected by enzymatic activity varies from 10 to 14 IU/L and for immunologic activity from 8 to 10 ng/L (Figure 32-5). The background levels of MB-CK vary markedly and in many individuals average only 1–2 IU/L. Thus, the level in some individuals is required to increase severalfold above baseline before providing a plasma level that is considered diagnostic of infarction, which may require 4–12 hours from the onset of symptoms, depending on the extent of myocardial damage and other factors. This is also the same limiting factor for troponin T and troponin I.

The rationale for the use of MB-CK subforms as an early marker relates to assessing the ratio of the tissue form to the plasma form. Under baseline conditions, the ratio of MB_2CK (tissue form) to MB_1CK (plasma form) is about 1 : 1 and the concentration of MB_2 or MB_1 is about 1 or 2 IU/L [16,17]. In contrast to the need for MB-CK to exceed 8–12 units using the conventional total MB-CK assay, even minimal re-

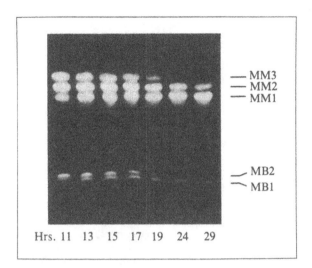

FIGURE 32-6. MM-CK and MB-CK subforms in the blood following acute myocardial infarction (AMI). Progressive conversion from the tissue subforms (of MM-CK and MB-CK) to the faster migrating, modified subforms occurs with increasing time after AMI.

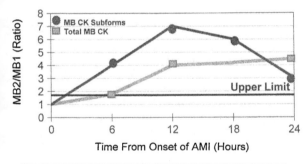

FIGURE 32-7. Plasma MB-CK subform time-activity curve. Illustrated here is the potential for MB-CK subforms to be used to diagnose myocardial infarction despite total MB-CK activity remaining in the normal range. This is a plot of the MB_2/MB_1 ratio (circle) versus the time from the onset of infarction compared with that of the plasma time-activity curve of total MB-CK (square). There is a 50–200% increase in the MB_2/MB_1 ratio between 2 and 6 hours, while there is no significant change in total MB-CK. This illustrates how the ratio of MB_2/MB_1 has increased sensitivity and specificity to diagnose infarction early, as opposed to total MB-CK.

lease of MB_2CK would be expected to change the ratio drastically in favor of MB_2CK, which could provide an early diagnosis. The steady state of baseline values in a normal individual is due to continuous

release of a small amount of MB-CK from skeletal and cardiac muscle that is converted to the modified subforms and cleared from the blood. With the onset of AMI, the rate of myocardial MB_2 release into the blood quickly exceeds the rate of conversion of MB_2 to MB_1, so the ratio of MB_2 to MB_1 increases dramatically [16]. Thus, rapid release of small quantities of MB_2 will be sufficient to increase the ratio before the value for total CK or MB-CK activity is sufficiently increased to exceed the upper limit of normal.

Development of the Rapid MB-CK Subform Assay

Separation of proteins by electrophoresis is normally performed with a voltage of 150–200 V, which provides adequate separation of the MB-CK subforms in about 2 hours. Increased voltage generates heat, which denatures the protein. In an attempt to provide more rapid separation, we worked in conjunction with Helena Laboratories. The temperature of the sample was controlled by jets supplying very cold air, which permitted an increase in voltage, up to 1600 V, without damage to the subforms [16]. The increased voltage provided separation of the MB-CK subforms within about 15 minutes. Following the rapid separation by electrophoresis, it was possible to adjust and develop an automated system in which the sample was applied and the process automated, including automated quantitation of the density of each electrophoretic band with digital display of the results within about 25 minutes (Figure 32-6).

Initially, the MM subform distribution was evaluated for early diagnosis of AMI in animals [29] and in

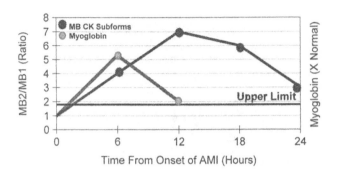

FIGURE 32-8. Plasma temporal profile of MB-CK subforms versus myoglobin. Illustrated here are the plasma temporal profiles of MB-CK subforms and myoglobin, showing that both markers are significantly elevated within the first 6 hours and, thus, potentially provide for the early diagnosis of infarction. The upper limit of normal for the MB_2/MB_1 ratio using the new CardioRep analyzer is 1.7, and the upper limit of normal for myoglobin is 60 µg/L.

several studies involving human subjects [30,31]. Although these results were very promising, with the MM_3/MM_1 ratio rising out of the normal range between 4 and 6 hours after AMI onset, the disadvantage of the MM subforms is the potential lack of specificity. As discussed earlier, assay of total CK activity rather than MB-CK for the diagnosis of AMI may introduce a 20–30% false-positive rate due to release of MM-CK from skeletal muscle [32,33]. Such elevations, occurring due to exercise or myositis, have been shown to be associated with a rise in the percent MM^3 [34–37], thus reducing the diagnostic specificity.

Because of the lack of specificity of MM-CK subform analysis, we evaluated the utility of MB-CK subforms in the early diagnosis of AMI. The rapid electrophoresis system (REP, Helena Laboratories, Beaumont, TX) was validated using purified MB_2 and MB_1 reconstituted in heat-inactivated serum. The assay was shown to be linear for both MB subforms, even at very low levels (r = 0.99 between 1.0 and 10.0 IU/L; n = 70), highly reproducible, and generated the expected MB_2/MB_1 ratio when both subforms were added to plasma (r = 0.95, n = 144). Its sensitivity is 1.0 IU/L, and the total assay time is about 25 minutes. The profile of the MB_2CK to MB_1CK ratio as a diagnostic marker is shown in Figure 32-7. The early portion of the plasma myoglobin temporal profile is very similar to the same portion of the plasma temporal profile of the MB-CK subforms (Figure 32-8).

Evaluation of the MB-CK Subform Assay for Early Diagnosis

Initial application of the rapid electrophoretic assay for MB-CK included a population of 200 patients, of which 100 had myocardial infarction, 50 had ischemia, and 50 were normal [16]. The results showed the assay to be very promising with respect to the sensitivity and specificity for diagnosing myocardial infarction within the first 4–6 hours of the onset of symptoms. A systematic study [18] was then undertaken to properly evaluate the sensitivity and specificity of the MB-CK rapid electrophoretic assay in diagnosing or excluding myocardial infarction in the emergency room in patients with chest pain of cardiac and noncardiac origin. The study was performed over a 14-month period from 1992 to 1993, involved 1110 consecutive patients, and was unique in two ways: first, careful attention was paid to estimate the onset of symptoms in each case, and, secondly, the patients were enrolled consecutively in the emergency room on a 24-hour basis, 7 days per week. Blood samples were obtained every 30–60 minutes until at least 6 hours had elapsed from the onset of chest pain; among patients subsequently admitted to the hospital, blood samples were obtained every 4 hours for up to 48 hours. Blood samples were analyzed for total MB-CK activity using the quantitative glass bead assay [38], which has an upper limit of normal of 14 IU/L, and for MB-CK subforms with the rapid electrophoresis assay. The results of the assay for MB-CK subforms and the conventional assay for total MB-CK were analyzed separately and independently by at least two investigators without any knowledge of clinical findings. The diagnosis of myocardial

TABLE 32-1. Occurrence of myocardial infarction, death, or serious
complications in relationship to time of arrival in the emergency room

Onset to arrival (h)	No. of non-MIs (%)	No. of MIs (%)	No. of deaths (%)	Nonfatal complications (%)
0–6	598 (60.4)	95 (78.5)	13 (72.2)	18 (69.2)
6–12	180 (18.2)	11 (9.1)	3 (16.7)	4 (15.4)
12–24	113 (11.4)	5 (4.1)	0 (0.0)	1 (3.8)
Uncertain	98 (9.9)	10 (8.3)	2 (11.1)	3 (11.5)
Total	989 (89.1)	121 (10.9)	18 (1.6)	26 (2.3)
Male	495 (50.0)	74 (61.3)[a]	10 (55.6)	11 (42.3)
Mean age (SD)	50.8 ± 13.6	56.6 ± 11.4[a]	58.6 ± 13.1	60.0 ± 13.0

[a] $P < 0.0001$ versus no acute myocardial infarction.
MI = myocardial infarction; SD = standard deviation.

TABLE 32-2. Sensitivity and specificity of subform assay[a]

Test results[b]	Myocardial infarction (n = 118)	Death or complications[c] (n = 41)	No MI admitted (n = 539)	No MI discharged from ER[d] (n = 450)
Positive	114 (96.6)	34 (82.9)	33 (6.1)	17 (3.8)
Negative	4 (3.4)	7 (17.1)	506 (93.9)	433 (96.2)

[a] The sensitivity of the assay is indicated by the percentage of patients with myocardial infarction who had positive test results, and the false-negative rate by the percentage who had negative results. The specificity is indicated by the percentage of patients without myocardial infarction ([MI] hospitalized or discharged from the emergency room [ER]) who had negative test results, and the false-positive rate by the percentage who had positive results.
[b] Test results were considered positive if one or more samples had abnormal subform activity, and negative if all samples had normal subform activity and at least one sample was obtained 6 or more hours after the onset of symptoms.
[c] Three patients died before sample collection was complete.
[d] A total of 44 patients were discharged from the ER before 6 hours had elapsed since the onset of symptoms. Plasma subform activity in samples obtained from these patients prior to discharge were evaluated for false-positive results.

infarction was confirmed or excluded on the basis of abnormal or normal total MB-CK activity, respectively, according to previously published criteria [39,40]. The criteria for myocardial infarction were as follows: an MB-CK level $\geq 14\,IU/L$ in two or more sequential blood samples obtained 6–12 hours apart; an MB-CK level of $\geq 14\,IU/L$ in a single sample if the value represented a threefold increase above the previous value; and a single MB-CK level of $\geq 14\,IU/L$ if only one sample was available. In all the patients with myocardial infarction, except the three who died early, serial blood samples were obtained over a period of 24–48 hours. The diagnostic criteria for myocardial infarction, based on the subform levels, were an $MB_2 \geq 1.0\,IU/L$ and a ratio of MB_2 to $MB_1 \geq 1.5$ recurring within 6 hours after the onset of symptoms.

There were a total of 121 patients in whom the diagnosis of myocardial infarction was confirmed. A total of 531 patients (47.8%) were admitted to the coronary care unit; 118 received a subsequent diagno-

sis of myocardial infarction, as confirmed by serial elevation of plasma MB-CK levels; in the other 413, myocardial infarction was excluded. Of the 129 patients (11.6%) admitted to an in-patient unit other than the CCU, three subsequently received the diagnosis of myocardial infarction. A total of 450 patients (40.5%) were discharged home from the emergency room. Thus, 121 patients received a subsequent diagnosis of myocardial infarction, with 65 having Q-wave infarction and 58 non–Q-wave infarction. It is of note that 90% of the 65 patients with Q-wave infarction presented with typical ST-segment elevation, while only 4 of the 56 patients with non–Q-wave infarction presented with ST-segment elevation. The other patients with non–Q-wave infarction presented with either ST-segment depression or T-wave inversion. It is also of some note that patients with myocardial infarction presented significantly earlier after the onset of symptoms than did the patients without myocardial infarction ($P < 0.001$; Table 32-1).

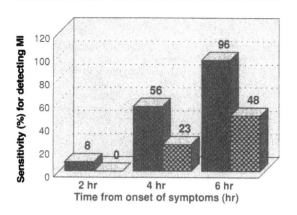

FIGURE 32-9. Comparison of the sensitivity of the assays of total MB-CK (light bars) and its subforms (dark bars) 2, 4, and 6 hours after the onset of symptoms. The diagnosis of myocardial infarction in the study patients was confirmed by the total MB-CK activity during the subsequent 48 hours.

The overall sensitivity and specificity both in patients with infarction and in those without infarction, either admitted or discharged home, are shown in Table 32-2. The sensitivity of the assay for detecting myocardial infarction within the first 6 hours from the onset of symptoms was 96.6%, with a 90–99% confidence interval. This was in marked contrast to the sensitivity of the conventional MB-CK assay, which had a sensitivity of 48%. The mean MB_2CK level at 6 hours in patients with infarction was $5.1 \pm 3.2 \, IU/L$, and the mean ratio of MB_2CK to MB_1CK was 4.4. Only 16 patients with myocardial infarction came to the emergency room more than 6 hours after the onset of symptoms, and each of them had a positive test for MB-CK subforms in the first blood sample obtained. The sensitivity of the MB-CK subforms as compared with that of the conventional assay is shown in Figure 32-9 at various intervals from the onset of symptoms. In patients with myocardial infarction, the average interval from arrival in the emergency room until the plasma MB-CK subform activity was elevated was 1.22 ± 1.17 hours. It is also of note that 50 of the patients with myocardial infarction who came to the emergency room within 6 hours had abnormal MB-CK subform activity in the first blood sample, which was obtained a mean of 3.25 ± 1.70 hours after the onset of symptoms. In the other patients with infarction, MB-CK subform assay was normal in the first sample, which was taken on an average of 2.37 ± 1.07 hours after onset of symptoms and became elevated a mean of 4.22 ± 1.13 hours after the onset of symptoms.

In the 539 patients admitted to the hospital without myocardial infarction, the MB-CK subform assay was abnormal in 33 of these patients, giving a specificity of 93.9%. However, it is of interest that 79% of those patients with possible false-positive results had unstable angina, and of the remaining 21%, two had rabdomyolysis, two had hypothyroidism, and in the remaining three the diagnosis was unknown. Of the 450 patients sent home, 433 were negative for MB-CK subforms (96.2% specificity). Of the 17 patients with abnormal MB-CK subforms, 6 were readmitted and shown to have myocardial infarction and 7 others had no symptoms and appeared to do well. Four patients were lost to follow-up. Thus, the estimated false-positive result of 3.8% is a significant overestimate, but in view of the time lapse, we could not be certain that the two sets of MB-CK values represented the same clinical event. Therefore, no changes were made in the estimate of false-positive results. On utilizing the MB-CK subform assay as a means of triaging patients based on these results, we found that the total number of admissions would have been reduced from 531 to 164, representing a 69.1% reduction. In summary, the sensitivity and specificity of the rapid assay for MB-CK subforms in diagnosing myocardial infarction within 6 hours of the onset of symptoms were 96.6% and 93.9%, respectively, as compared with 48.2% and 48.0%, respectively, for the conventional MB-CK assay.

Limitations of the MB-CK Subform Assay

The MB-CK subform assay, with a sensitivity of 96% and specificity of 94%, accurately identifies patients with myocardial infarction within the first 6 hours after the onset of symptoms. However, in patients with muscular dystrophy [41] or severe skeletal muscle damage [42], MB_2CK is released and thus would give a false-positive diagnosis. The modern assays for MB-CK are based on soluble immunological detection; however, attempts thus far to develop an antibody that distinguishes between the subforms have not been fruitful. In the large prospective study, 79% of 33 patients sent home with abnormal MB-CK subforms had unstable angina. It is possible that several of the patients with unstable angina who were admitted to the hospital had small areas of myocardial necrosis below the threshold detection of the conventional assay [43]. However, the possibility that very small quantities of MB_2CK were released because of cardiac ischemia cannot be excluded [44,45].

Nevertheless, in a recent experimental study, we have shown that release of CK from the heart reflects necrosis [46]. In a series of conscious dogs, the left anterior descending coronary artery was occluded for 10, 15, 20, or 25 minutes followed by reperfusion for at least 48 hours. The dogs were anesthesized and the hearts removed and analyzed for myocardial ischemia (glycogen depletion and swelling) and necrosis (organelle disruption and sarcolemma disruption) with light and electron microscopy. There were seven animals for each duration of coronary occlusion. None of the animals undergoing 10 minutes of occlusion had elevated plasma CK, and histological analysis showed severe depletion of glycogen and cell swelling but no evidence of necrosis. Five of the seven animals undergoing 15 minutes of coronary occlusion exhibited no elevation in plasma CK and no evidence of myocardial necrosis. In contrast, two animals showed a minimal elevation in plasma CK, and the myocardium showed two areas of micronecrosis of about 1 mm in diameter. All animals with 20 minutes or more of coronary occlusion had elevated plasma CK and morphological evidence of myocardial necrosis. These results strongly indicate that release of CK from the heart does not occur with reversible ischemia but is consistently released with myocardial necrosis.

Advantages of MB-CK Subform for Early Diagnosis

The assay is very simple to perform, requiring minimal expertise, because it utilizes electrophoresis, which has been available in clinical laboratories for decades. This technique, with which practically all technicians are acquainted, even in community hospitals, makes the assay available to the medical community regardless of the size of the institution. The assay is rapid, requiring about 25 minutes, and is completely automated. The test is extremely cost effective when performed every hour for the first 6 hours after onset because the majority of the patients with infarction will only need one sample to ascertain the diagnosis, and in the remainder without infarction only two to three samples will be required. It is estimated that using this assay to triage patients with chest pain in the emergency room would save the nation several billion dollars per year. In the patients presenting within 6 hours of onset, in whom infarction is not present, the mean number of samples required to exclude the diagnosis is 2.5. This is, in part, because many patients with chest pain without myocardial infarction present to the emergency room after the first 4 hours, whereas patients with myocar-

dial infarction are more likely to present within the first 4 hours.

MB-CK Subforms Versus Other Markers for Early Diagnosis of AMI

The diagnosis of myocardial infarction within the first 6 hours of onset of symptoms at the 90% confidence level is only feasible at the present time with the MB-CK subform assay. The only other marker that is appropriate for early diagnosis of myocardial infarction is myoglobin [20,47]. Myoglobin is analyzed by a rapid immunological assay, which requires only 20 minutes to perform. In several studies, myoglobin has lacked both sensitivity and specificity for early diagnosis of myocardial infarction. However, myoglobin, when performed within the window of 2–6 hours from onset, if consistently negative, has a high negative predictive value for excluding myocardial infarction [20]. It must be taken into account that the window for myoglobin is very short, becoming elevated within the first 1–2 hours from onset and rapidly declining because of renal clearance after about 6–7 hours from onset. Thus, myoglobin must not be relied upon after 6–7 hours from onset. Also in very small infarcts, if one does not have serial samples from 4–6 hours, the sensitivity may be less than adequate. The specificity is a problem in patients with skeletal muscle injury because the antibody cannot differentiate between myoglobin from the heart and myoglobin from skeletal muscle [35,37]. Nevertheless, myoglobin is the next best assay to perform in excluding myocardial infarction early after admission to the emergency room if the MB-CK subforms are not available. The other markers previously discussed, such as troponin T, troponin I, and total MB-CK, are not released early enough after the onset of pain to provide the necessary sensitivity for exclusion of myocardial infarction within the first 6 hours, even if performed serially [20].

Suggested Protocol for Utilization of MB-CK Subforms

In assessing the patient in the emergency room, it is recommended that a sample be obtained on admission and another at 1 hour. If either of these samples is positive for myocardial infarction, then revert to samping every 4–6 hours for 24 hours. If after 1 hour the sample is negative, it is necessary to do hourly samples until 6 hours from the onset of chest pain. One can only reliably exclude myocardial infarction with MB-CK subforms if the values remain normal up to 6 hours from onset. The necessity for determining samples beyond the 6 hours in those patients with infarctions admitted to the hospital is arguable, although many would prefer to determine the peak MB-CK activity as a rough estimate of the extent of myocardial infarction.

Although knowing these data may not affect the patients' treatment, it is a good prognostic index. In many instances, once the diagnosis of myocardial infarction has been confirmed, additional assays may be omitted to be cost effective. In patients admitted to the hospital 12 or more hours after the onset of symptoms, if the MB-CK subform assay is to be used, then every 4 hours until at least two values are positive is recommended for making the diagnosis of myocardial infarction [1]. In this time interval after infarction, other assays could be equally effective, such as total MB-CK, troponin T, or troponin I. While we recommend every 4–6 hours for 24 hours, once two samples are abnormal and the diagnosis is confirmed, further sampling may be unnecessary. Samples for MB-CK subforms should be collected in EDTA and the plasma separated from the cellular components, preferably within 3 hours if the sample is at room temperature, and if kept on ice, within 8 hours [16]. For storage, samples are preferably frozen at −20°C, and under these conditions they have been found to be stable for at least 3 years [18]. The EDTA removes the calcium, which is a necessary cofactor for CP-N. About six samples can be assayed on the CardioRep (Helena Laboratories) every 20–30 minutes. The criteria used for MB-CK subforms in the evaluation study [18] required MB_1CK to MB_1CK of ≥1 IU/L and a ratio of MB_2CK to MB_1CK of ≥1.5. However, the new updated CardioRep has greater sensitivity, and thus the diagnostic criteria have been adjusted to the following: MB_2CK of ≥2.6 IU/L and a ratio of MB_1CK of ≥1.7. In our own laboratory over the past 4 years, we have routinely used the MB-CK subforms as the only marker and have had experiences in over 20,000 samples. The negative predictive value of a normal MB-CK subform rate at 6 hours from the onset of symptoms is essentially 100%. Total MB-CK can be obtained from the MB-CK subform assay for late diagnosis.

Future Prospects

While the role of MB-CK subforms as a marker for the early diagnosis of myocardial infarction is being established, there is considerable reluctance to adopt the method on a routine basis in many hospitals. The major objection to the MB-CK subforms is the inconvenience of performing electrophoresis despite automation of the assay. Nevertheless, several investigators have confirmed the high sensitivity and specificity of the technique [48–50]. The technique is now employed in countries throughout the world, and in the United States over 200 medical centers are utilizing this technique. Cannon and Walls [51], in a recent editorial, outlined the problems as well as the need for an early diagnosis and indicated that at present the MB-CK subforms appear to be the only marker that offers adequate sensitivity and specificity. In large prospective, multicenter, randomized study, all of the markers (myoglobin, troponin I, troponin T, and total MB-CK) were sampled hourly for the first 6 hours, and then every 6 hours for 24 hours, in 1002 patients seen consecutivly in the emergency room with chest pain. Results showed that the MB-CK subform reliably diagnosed 92% of the patients with myocardial infarction within the first 60 minutes of arrival in the emergency room, and myoglobin reliably diagnosed 81%. In contrast, total MB-CK, troponin T, and troponin I had a sensitivity of 60% at 6 hours from onset, but 95% sensitivity at 16 hours from onset. These studies confirm that the MB-CK subform assay is a reliable marker for diagnosis of infarction within the first 6 hours of onset and troponin T, troponin I, and total MB-CK are reliable markers for late diagnosis after 12–16 hours from onset [52].

References

1. Roberts R. Enzymatic diagnosis of acute myocardial infarction. Chest 93:3S, 1988.
2. Roberts R. Diagnostic assessment of myocardial infarction based on lactate dehydrogenase and creatine kinase isoenzymes. Heart Lung 10:486, 1981.
3. Roe CR, Limbird LE, Wagner GS, Nerenberg ST. Combined isoenzyme analysis in the diagnosis of myocardial injury: Application of electrophoretic methods for the detection and the quantitation of the creatine phosphokinase MB isoenzyme. J Lab Clin Med 80:577, 1972.
4. Roberts R. Reperfusion and the plasma isoforms of creatine kinase isoenzymes: A clinical perspective. J Am Coll Cardiol 9:464, 1987.
5. Selker HP. Coronary care unit triage decision aids: How do we know when they work? Am J Med 87:491, 1989.
6. Lee TH, Weisberg MC, Brand DA, Rouan GW, Goldman L. Candidates for thrombolysis among emergency room patients with acute chest pain. Ann Intern Med 110:957, 1989.
7. Weingarten SR, Ermann B, Riedinger MS, Shah PK, Ellrodt G. Selecting the best triage rule for patients hospitalized with chest pain. Am J Med 87:494, 1989.
8. Young MJ, McMahon LF, Stross JK. Prediction rules

for patients with suspected myocardial infarction. Arch Intern Med 147:1219, 1987.

9. Stark ME, Vacek JL. The initial electrocardiogram during admission for myocardial infarction. Arch Intern Med 47:843, 1987.

10. Fesmire FM, Percy RF, Wears RL, MacMath TL. Risk stratification according to the initial electrocardiogram in patients with suspected acute myocardial infarction. Arch Intern Med 149:1294, 1989.

11. Roberts R. Thrombolysis and its sequelae: Calcium antagonists as potential adjunctive therapy. Circulation 80:IV93, 1989.

12. Brush JE, Brand DA, Acampora D, Chalmer B, Wackers FJ. Use of the initial electrocardiogram to predict in-hospital complications of acute myocardial infarction. N Engl J Med 312:1137, 1985.

13. Yusuf S, Pearson M, Sterry H. The entry ECG in the early diagnosis and prognostic stratification of patients with suspected acute myocardial infarction. Eur Heart J 5:690, 1984.

14. Lee TH, Rouan GW, Weisberg MC, Brand DA, Cook EF, Acampora D, Goldman L. Sensitivity of routine clinical criteria for diagnosing myocardial infarction within 24 hours of hospitalization. Ann Intern Med 106:181, 1987.

15. Lee TH, Juarez G, Cook EF, Weisberg MC, Rouan GW, Brand DA, Goldman L. Ruling out acute myocardial infarction. N Engl J Med 324:1239, 1991.

16. Puleo PR, Guadagno PA, Roberts R, Perryman MB. Sensitive, rapid assay of subforms of creatine kinase MB in plasma. Clin Chem 35:1452, 1989.

17. Puleo PR, Guadagno PA, Roberts R, Scheel MV, Marian AJ, Churchill D, Perryman MB. Early diagnosis of acute myocardial infarction based on assay for subforms of creatine kinase-MB. Circulation 82:759, 1990.

18. Puleo PR, Meyer D, Wathen C, Tawa CB, Wheeler SH, Hamburg RJ, Ali MN, Obermueller SD, Triana JT, Zimmerman JL, Perryman MB, Roberts R. Use of rapid assay of subforms of creatine kinase MB to diagnose or rule out acute myocardial infarction. N Engl J Med 331:561, 1994.

19. Delahunty TJ, Forback CC. Automated creatine kinase-MB estimation by immunoinhibition: A clinical evaluation. Clin Chem 26:568, 1980.

20. de Winter RJ, Koster RW, Sturk A, Sanders GT. Value of myoglobin, troponin T, and CK-MB mass in ruling out an acute myocardial infarction in the emergency room. Circulation 92:3401, 1995.

21. Adams JE, Bodor GS, Davila-Roman VG, Delmez JA, Apple FS, Ladenson JH, Jaffe AS. Cardiac troponin I: A marker with high specificity for cardiac injury. Circulation 88:101, 1993.

22. Adams JE, Sicard GA, Allen BT, Bridwell KH, Lenke LG, Davila-Roman VG, Bodar GS, Ladenson JH, Jaffe AS. Diagnosis of perioperative myocardial infarction with measurement of cardiac troponin I. N Engl J Med 330:670, 1994.

23. Perryman MB, Strauss AW, Olson J, Roberts R. In vitro translation of canine mitochondrial creatine kinase from messenger RNA. Biochem Biophys Res Commun 110:967, 1983.

24. Perryman MB, Kerner SA, Bohlmeyer TJ, Roberts R. Isolation and sequence analysis of a full-length cDNA for human M creatine kinase. Biochem Biophys Res Commun 140:981, 1986.

25. Villarreal-Levy G, Ma TS, Kerner SA, Roberts R, Perryman MB. Human creatine kinase: Isolation and sequence analysis of cDNA clones for the B subunit, development of subunit specific probes and determination of gene copy number. Biochem Biophys Res Commun 144:1116, 1987.

26. Wevers RA, Delsing M, Klein-Gebbink JA, Soons JB. Post-synthetic changes in creatine kinase isoenzymes. Clin Chim Acta 86:323, 1978.

27. George S, Ishikawa Y, Perryman MB, Roberts R. Purification and characterization of naturally occurring and in vitro induced multiple forms of MM creatine kinase. J Biol Chem 259:2667, 1984.

28. Billadello JJ, Fontanet HL, Strauss AW, Abendschein DR. Characterization of MB creatine kinase isoform conversion in vitro and in vivo in dogs. J Clin Invest 83:1637, 1989.

29. Hashimoto H, Abendschein DR, Strauss AW, Sobel BE. Early detection of myocardial infarction in conscious dogs by analysis of plasma MM creatine kinase isoforms. Circulation 71:363, 1985.

30. Jaffe AS, Serota H, Grace A, Sobel BE. Diagnostic changes in plasma creatine kinase isoforms early after the onset of acute myocardial infarction. Circulation 74:105, 1986.

31. Wu AH, Gornet TG, Wu VH, Brockie RE, Nishikawa A. Early diagnosis of acute myocardial infarction by rapid analysis of creatine kinase isoenzyme-3 (CK-MM) subtypes. Clin Chem 33:358, 1987.

32. Grande P, Christiansen C, Pedersen A, Christensen MS. Optimal diagnosis in acute myocardial infarction. A cost effectiveness study. Circulation 61:723, 1980.

33. Klein MS, Shell WE, Sobel BE. Serum creatine phosphokinase (CPK) isoenzymes after intramuscular injections, surgery, and myocardial infarction. Experimental and clinical studies. Cardiovasc Res 7:412, 1973.

34. Apple FS, Rogers MA, Ivy JL. Early detection of skeletal muscle injury by assay of creatine kinase MM isoforms in serum after acute exercise. Clin Chem 34:1102, 1988.

35. Apple FS, Rogers MA, Ivy JL. Creatine kinase isoenzyme MM variants in skeletal muscle and plasma from marathon runners. Clin Chem 32:41, 1986.

36. Clarkson PM, Apple FS, Byrnes WC, McCormick KM, Triffletti P. Creatine kinase isoforms following isometric exercise. Muscle Nerve 10:41, 1987.

37. Annesley TM, Strongwater SL, Schnitzer TJ. MM subisoenzymes of creatine kinase as an index of disease activity in polymyositis. Clin Chem 31:402, 1985.

38. Henry PD, Roberts R, Sobel BE. Rapid separation of plasma creatine kinase isoenzymes by batch absorption with glass beads. Clin Chem 21:844, 1975.

39. Turi ZG, Rutherford JD, Roberts R, Muller JE, Jaffe AS, Rude RE, Parker C, Raabe DS, Stone PH, Hartwell TD, Lewis SE, Parkey RW, Gold HK, Robertson TL, Sobel BE, Willerson JT, Braunwald E, and the MILIS Study Group. Electrocardiographic, enzymatic and scintigraphic criteria of acute myocardial infarction as determined from study of 726 patients (a MILIS Study). Am J Cardiol 55:1463, 1985.

40. MILIS Study Group. National Heart, Lung, and Blood Institute Multicenter Investigation of the Limitation of Infarct Size (MILIS): Design and Methods of the Clinical Trial. An Investigation of Beta-Blockade and Hyaluronidase for Treatment of Acute Myocardial Infarction. Dallas, TX: American Heart Association Monograph 100, 1984.

41. Yasmineh WG, Ibrahim GA, Abbasnezhad MA, Awad EA. Isoenzyme distribution of creatine kinase and lactate dehydrogenase in serum and skeletal muscle in Duchenne muscular dystrophy, collagen disease, and other muscular disorders. Clin Chem 24:1985, 1978.

42. Apple FS, Rogers MA, Sherman WM, Costill DL, Hagerman FC, Ivy JL. Profile of creatine kinase isoenzymes in skeletal muscles of marathon runners. Clin Chem 30:413, 1984.

43. Ohman EM, Sigmon KN, Califf RM. Is diagnostic certainty essential for the use of thrombolytic therapy during myocardial infarction in the 1990s? Circulation 82:1073, 1990.

44. Michael LH, Hunt JR, Weilbaecher D, Perryman MB, Roberts R, Lewis RM, Entman ML. Creatine kinase and phosphorylase in cardiac lymph: Coronary occlusion and reperfusion. Am J Physiol 17:H350, 1985.

45. Heyndrickx GR, Amano J, Kenna T, Fallon JT, Patrick TA, Manders WT, Rogers GG, Rosendorff C, Vatner SF. Creatine kinase release not associated with myocardial necrosis after short periods of coronary artery occlusion in conscious baboons. J Am Coll Cardiol 6:1299, 1985.

46. Ishikawa Y, Saffitz JE, Mealman JE, Grace AM, Roberts R. Reversible myocardial ischemic injury is not associated with increased creatine kinase activites in plasma. Clin Chem 43:467, 1997.

47. Grenadier E, Keidar S, Kahana L, Alpan G, Marmor A, Palant A. The roles of serum myoglobin, total CPK, and CK-MB isoenzyme in the acute phase of myocardial infarction. Am Heart J 105:408, 1983.

48. Bhayana V, Henderson AR. Evaluation of cardio-REP for creatine kinase isoforms analaysis (abstr). Clin Chem 41:S184, 1995.

49. Plebani M, Secchiero S, Altinier S, Lachin M, Sciacovelli L. Evaluation of a new automated system for CK-MB isoforms determination (abstr). Clin Chem 41:S174, 1995.

50. Snow JS, Cohen MB, Morrison J, Ward M, Sama AE, Ryan JG, Tria L, Sun T. CK-MB isoforms as a marker of myocadial infarction (abstr). J Investig Med 43:313, 1995.

51. Cannon CP, Walls RM. Editorial: Waiting for godot: Use of chemical markers in the emergency department evaluation of chest pain. J Emerg Med 13:533, 1995.

52. Roberts R, From R, Beaudreaux A, Zimmerman J, Meyer D, Wun C, Davis B, Smallings R, Habib G. Multi-center blinded trial utilizing multiple diagnostic markers to exclude myocardial infarction in patients presenting consecutively to the ER with chest pain (abstr). Circulation 94:1, 1996.

33. TROPONINS AS EARLY MARKERS OF ACUTE MYOCARDIAL INFARCTION

Sanjay Dixit and Allan S. Jaffe

Introduction

Acute myocardial infarction is a major cause of cardiovascular morbidity and death [1]. The diagnosis of acute myocardial infarction, as formally established by the World Health Organization requires at least two of the following criteria: a history of characteristic chest pain, evolutionary changes on the electrocardiogram, and elevation of serial cardiac enzymes [2]. Unfortunately, these findings are not always present in every patient with infarction. As many as one in three acute myocardial infarctions is not recognized clinically by either the patient or physician because symptoms are often atypical or absent [3,4]. Similarly, electrocardiographic findings in patients with possible acute myocardial infarction are often nonspecific. The electrocardiogram (ECG) has been reported to be misleading in 8% of patients with acute myocardial infarction and can be indeterminate in an additional 12% [5]. Furthermore, only a small percentage (10–20%) of the patients with chest discomfort or other symptoms compatible with cardiac ischemia subsequently have documentation of acute myocardial infarction. During the last quarter century, blood assays of a variety of protein markers of myocardial injury have played a pivotal role in the diagnosis of acute myocardial infarction [6]. These tests have helped to redefine acute myocardial infarction, often revealing degrees of myocardial necrosis that previously could not be detected. Indeed, because marker proteins are so much more sensitive and specific than the clinical presentation or the ECG, some have suggested that elevations alone in the proper clinical setting should be considered diagnostic of acute myocardial infarction [7].

Recently there has been increased emphasis on developing strategies to detect the presence of myocardial injury as early as possible in patients who present with chest discomfort [8]. This effort has been predicated on several presumptions:

1. Early diagnosis will facilitate aggressive intervention with either angioplasty or thrombolysis and thus aid in salvaging myocardium at risk for necrosis;
2. Early diagnosis will permit better triage of patients into critical care units versus less intensively monitored areas; and
3. Early diagnosis will aid in identification of patients not having acute myocardial infarction, ensuring that patients can be sent home from the hospital safely, and thus avoiding liability if such patients subsequently have poor outcomes.

The success of this strategy depends not only on its rapidity and effectiveness, but also on how well it compares with existing measures in terms of the three goals listed earlier. There are substantial questions about whether any marker can accomplish these goals, as well as controversy concerning the appropriateness of the goals themselves. [9].

Molecular Biology of the Troponins

Myofibrillar proteins have been explored extensively as markers of myocardial injury with the hope that they would provide not only comparable sensitivity as established markers, but also be more specific for myocardial injury. On the basis of the current literature, troponin T and troponin I offer the most exciting potential as highly specific markers for the diagnosis of myocardial injury.

Troponins are a complex of regulatory proteins uniquely present in the striated muscle that mediate the interaction of calcium with actin and myosin [10,11]. Contractile activity in vertebrate striated muscle is regulated by the changes in the concentration of free calcium in the sarcoplasm, mediated by changes induced by the interaction of the troponin complex with tropomyosin [11]. The troponin com-

413

plex is composed of three components, troponin I, which inhibits actinmyosin ATPase; troponin C, which binds calcium; and troponin T, which binds to tropomyosin and helps to locate the complex at a repeat of 385 Å along the thin filament [10–12].

These three isoenzymes exist in a number of isoforms, each a product of unique genes. Different isoforms of troponin I and T are expressed in slow-twitch, fast-twitch, and cardiac muscle [14–17]. Troponin C has only a skeletal muscle and a slow-twitch/cardiac isoform [18]. Each form has a unique structure (troponin I has a molecular weight of 23,500 d, whereas troponin T weighs 33,000 d [6]) and different regulatory effects on calcium binding, as well as varying responses, to beta agonists and changes in the pH. During the development of the cardiac and skeletal muscles, some of the isoforms of the troponin components manifest a high degree of tissue specificity. While the exact reason for this is not known, it is believed that a highly complex control mechanism is at work in the gene expression for the different muscle proteins, triggered endogenously or influenced by exogenous factors [19].

Embryonic to adult cardiac troponin T (cTnT) switching has been clearly demonstrated in the mammalian heart, and a similar switch in the cardiac troponin I (cInI) protein has been demonstrated in the rat cardiac muscle [15,17–19]. This switching does not occur in skeletal muscle, because, as far as can be determined, cTnI is not expressed in skeletal muscle at any time during ontogeny [17,19]. Fetal rat, chick, and human heart express both the skeletal and cardiac forms of TnI initially. After the ninth postnatal month, only the cardiac isoform of TnI is expressed. This isoform differs from the others, not only in basic structure but also by virtue of an additional 31 amino acid sequence at the N-terminal end, which is believed to be a post-translational modification [17,20]. In comparison, the specificity of cTnT for myocardium has not been fully delineated. Skeletal muscle troponin T (sTnT) and cTnT are both expressed in fetal heart and skeletal muscle. The skeletal muscle form is suppressed during ontogeny in the heart and is re-expressed in response to stress [21]. In contrast to cTnI, the cardiac isoform of TnT also is expressed in fetal skeletal muscle and is re-expressed in adult rat skeletal muscle after injury or denervation [22].

The notion that proteins initially expressed during ontogeny but suppressed prior to maturation can be re-expressed in response to injury is conceptually important. It is, for example, the reason why the concentration of creatine kinase B chain protein increases after an acute or chronic insult or after extreme exer-

cise [23]. The fact that cTnT is expressed during development suggests that it may be expressed in response to injury.

This was documented recently in humans by immunohistochemical analysis of diseased skeletal muscle by Bodor and colleagues [24]. Even in some putatively normal skeletal muscle, the cardiac form of cTnT is observed, but it is more frequently observed in patients with skeletal muscle myopathies or the myopathy associated with renal failure [25]. Because the cardiac form of cTnI is never expressed in skeletal muscle, it is not observed in either normal or damaged skeletal muscle [26]. Thus, from these basic developmental principles, cTnI should have an advantage over cTnT in terms of cardiac specificity. These differences may be less apparent clinically now, but they may be in the future if the assays for cTnI and cTnT become substantially more sensitive.

Normal Levels

If release of troponin is specific for cardiac injury, there should be no troponin circulating in plasma. Indeed, with the present iteration of assays, values of troponins in normal subjects are undetectable [27–29]. Using a highly sensitive assay, Missov and colleagues have reported a group of "normal controls" with very low levels of cTnI, suggesting either some ongoing turnover of the protein or a small degree of ongoing cardiac injury, whether reversible or irreversible, that leads to release of an epitope that is detectable in plasma [30,31]. However, with the assays presently available, normal subjects should not have detectable levels. Nevertheless, for most measurements, the lowest level of sensitivity is associated with a higher degree of analytic fluctuation, and therefore there are some analytic "false positives" at this level of detection. There will, of course, also be analytic false positives from any assay that depends on a variety of chemicals for stabilization [32].

Levels above the normal range of the present assays represent either release of the protein or abnormal clearance, and therefore should be considered indicative of some pathologic process. However, elevated values do not imply that the pathologic process needs to be ischemic heart disease, only that there is myocardial release or reduced clearance. Thus, myocarditis, occult or overt [33,34], contusion [35], damage related to any other potential injurious substance, for example, catecholamines, could all lead to elevations of troponin. Given the fact that most of the troponin is bound to the myofibrillar apparatus (97% for cTnI [36] and 94% for cTnT [37]), it is likely that release represents irreversible injury. However, early

TABLE 33-1. Duration of elevations (time to normalization for cTnI)

Patient group	n	Range	Day cTnI normalized		
			Median	10%	90%
Intervened					
Q-wave	62	3, >16	9.5	6	10, >16
Non–Q-wave	22	3, >10	6	4	>9
Non-intervened					
Q-wave	23	3, ≥13	8	4	12
Non–Q-wave	56	4, >13	7	4	11

Reproduced with permission from Jaffe et al. [51].

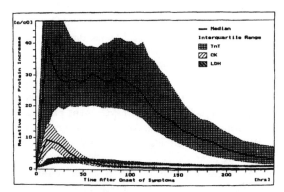

FIGURE 33-1. Biphasic release of cardiac troponin T after acute myocardial infarction. Initial release is predominantly from the "cytosolic pool." Subsequent release is indicative of degradation of structurally bound protein. A similar pattern has been described with cardiac troponin I as well. (Reproduced from Katus et al. [46], with permission.)

release from a "cytosolic pool" is subject to some controversy, which has existed with regard to creative kinase (CK) [38] with regard to whether cytosolic proteins can be released by injury that does not result in cell death.

Release and Kinetics

The release and kinetics of any protein marker depends on

1. The intracellular localization of the protein, because cytosolic proteins are released more rapidly than are structural proteins [39];

2. The molecular weight, because larger molecules diffuse at a slower rate compared to smaller ones [2];
3. Local blood and lymph flow [40]; and
4. The rate of elimination from the blood [36].

Small markers generally are cleared more rapidly than those of greater size [2]. Thus, when myocardial proteins are released, those of small size that are localized on the plasma membrane or in the cytosol are released more rapidly. Structural proteins take longer to be released.

Most of the cardiac troponin is tightly complexed to the contractile apparatus. Circulating levels are normally low, but they rise relatively rapidly after acute myocardial infarction, in a time course comparable with other markers with a cytosolic pool (e.g., CK and MB-CK). These pools have been estimated to be 3% for cTnI [36] and 6% for cTnT [37]. However, the troponins remain elevated for a prolonged period (i.e., a median of 8 days and, in some cases, far beyond 10 days [41–43]), irrespective of the locus of infarction (Q-wave or non–Q-wave) or treatment (Table 33-1) [36]. The duration of elevation may be somewhat longer for cTnT than for cTnI [37]. The likely explanation for the biphasic nature of the troponins (Figure 33-1) is that release occurs early from the cytosolic pool, and subsequently more slowly from the structural pool. This concept is supported by the fact that the half-life of cTnI is short, whether as an isolated peptide [36] or as part of a larger complex (Figure 33-2) (Ladenson, Landt, and Abendschein, unpublished data).

Preliminary data with cTnI suggest that it increases at about the same time after acute infarction as MB-CK (4–6 hours, range 3–19 hours), peaks at about 11 hours (range 6–29 hours), and remains elevated beyond 144 hours, whereas MB-CK normal-

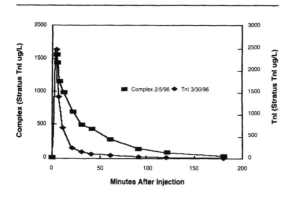

FIGURE 33-2. Half-life of purified cTnI and TnI complexed with cTnT when injected into dogs. The alpha-distributive half-life for the purified form was 4.6 ± 0.9 (SD) minutes, with a beta-distributive half-life of 67.2 ± 29.2 minutes. For the complex, the corresponding values are 4.8 ± 9 minutes and 47.6 ± 6.6 minutes. (Reproduced from Jaffe et al. [51], with permission. With the addition of unpublished data.)

izes by 69 hours (range 32–116 hours) [36,41]. cTnT demonstrates similar kinetics, although it appears to rise a little earlier than MB-CK [29]. In patients with Q-wave infarctions, Katus et al. [29] have reported the diagnostic window for cTnT as 11–140 hours after the onset of pain, with the first peak occurring at 24 hours, a rise as early as 3.5 hours, and sustained elevations for up to 12 days. In patients with non–Q-wave infarctions, the diagnostic sensitivity occurred at 10–131 hours after the onset of pain [29]. Other studies have shown comparable results, with some showing even earlier rises in cTnT during the first hour after symptoms [28,42,43].

Assays

Assays for the detection of the troponins in plasma or serum, in general, depend on antibodies. With the exception of one assay that relies on polyclonal sera [49], all other assays reported for cTnI have relied on monoclonal antibodies that provide highly efficient analytic specificity and good sensitivity [41,45]. A new version of a more sensitive assay that maintains specificity has recently been reported in association with two clinical abstracts [30,31].

Assays for cTnT also have relied on monoclonal antibodies. However, the initial laboratory assay utilized a monoclonal antibody in the "tag position" that

had some degree of cross-reactivity with skeletal muscle troponin T [46]. This led to concern, especially in patients with concomitant skeletal muscle injury and renal failure, that analytic false-positive elevations might be reported [47,48]. This is likely to be true because even minor degrees of cross-reactivity may be important when the upper bound of the reference range is equivalent to detectability, as is the case with cTnT. A new assay utilizing a more specific monoclonal antibody in the tag position reduces many of these analytic false positives [49]. It is still likely, however, that there may be some biologic increases in cTnT due to its presence in normal and abnormal skeletal muscle [24,25].

Use of Troponin as an Early Marker

Studies have confirmed the specificity and the sensitivity of the troponins as reliable markers of myocardial injury [27,29,36,42,50,51]. They have been shown to improve the specificity of diagnosis in patients with concomitant skeletal muscle injury [35,52]. Furthermore, minor elevations in a variety of patients have been shown to have potent prognostic implications, for example, patients who are critically ill [8] and those with unstable angina [53–58]. However, there are conflicting results about the time required to rise to abnormal levels. Some researchers have observed the elevations of troponins (specifically cTnT) very early (by 1 hour) after the onset of acute myocardial infarction [43,59]. Most, however, agree with the report of Katus et al. [29], who observed rises in cTnT within 3 hours after the onset of symptoms in only a small number of patients. For cTnI, elevations appear to occur slightly later than elevations of MB-CK [45]. Thus, the troponins do not compete effectively as early markers with CK isoforms, myoglobin, or fatty acid binding protein, which are often elevated shortly after the onset of infarction [8].

One comparative study used cTnT and myoglobin obtained at the time of admission [59]. cTnT was reported to be more sensitive than myoglobin (51% vs. 36%, respectively) but less specific as a marker of acute myocardial infarction during the first 4 hours after the onset of symptoms. However, cTnT should have greater specificity for myocardial damage than myoglobin. One possibile reason for this finding is that some of the early cTnT elevations reflected small myocardial infarctions that had occurred in the days prior to admission because elevations of the troponins persist for many days after acute events. If recurrent injury was subsequently diagnosed at the time of presentation in response to the new symptoms, cTnT

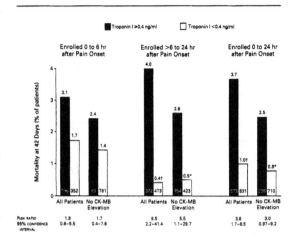

FIGURE 33-3. Mortality rates at 42 days according to the time of onset of pain to study enrollment and baseline cTnI levels, in patient groups separated by time from the onset of symptoms to presentation and those with and without increases in MB-CK. (Reproduced from Antman et al. [57], with permission.)

would appear to be a sensitive early marker. If, on the other hand, infarction was not diagnosed, cTnT would appear to lack specificity. Furthermore, in two studies with cTnI in patients with unstable angina, the data suggest that increases in cTnI in response to myocardial injury have prognostic significance, even when MB-CK remains within the normal range [54,57]. Thus, early elevations of the troponins may be indicative of more sensitive detection, in addition to detecting events that occurred in the days prior to presentation. This may be another reason why a few studies have shown high early sensitivity [43] but most have not [60,61].

Although the troponins may not be as early a marker as myoglobin, CK isoforms, or fatty acid binding protein, elevations, especially in critically ill patients [62] and those with unstable angina, have substantial prognostic value [53–58]. Thus, early assessment of a troponin (I or T) should assist triage of patients into low- and high-risk groups [53–58,62]. Furthermore, recent data in patients with acute infarction suggest that increases in troponin at the time of presentation nearly doubles the risk of subsequent mortality and the complications of acute infarction, such as congestive heart failure, shock, and arrhythmias [62]. These relationships were observed both in patients with non–Q-wave infarction as well as in those with Q-wave myocardial infarction and were only partially explained by differences from the

time of onset of symptoms to presentation [63]. Furthermore, Collinson and associates recently have confirmed that the prognostic significance of elevations of troponins at the time of hospital admission persist as long as 3 years after the acute event, suggesting that elevations of troponin may be indicative of some relatively important finding, perhaps within the coronary vasculature [64].

The initial findings in patients with unstable angina are attributable to Hamm and associates [56]. They reported that patients with unstable angina, especially those with ST-segment changes, had an increased incidence of complications and mortality if they presented with elevated values of cTnT. Thirty-three of the 109 patients (36%) had elevated levels of cTnI on admission. Thirty percent of these 33 patients subsequently had myocardial infarctions and five died. Nearly identical values were reported by Collinson et al. in a series of 400 patients [55]. Ravildke et al. further confirmed these studies but suggested that it was the group of patients who had subsequently had elevated MB-CK values as well (indicative of non–Q-wave infarction) that were at greater risk [53]. For that reason, studies by Galvani et al. [54] and Antman et al. [57] with cTnI in similar patients corrected for this problem by eliminating patients with elevations of MB-CK early after admission. They found a slightly lower incidence of elevations with this strategy, but there was persistence of the adverse prognostic factor associated with elevations (Figure 33-3). In studies with large populations, risk has risen in association with higher troponin values (Figure 33-4) [57,58].

Some elevations of troponins may represent those that persist from previous events. Thus, it would not be surprising if patients with unstable angina superimposed on previous non–Q-wave myocardial infarction were at higher risk than others. However, several lines of data support the contention originally made by Hamm and colleagues [56] that many of the elevations of troponins in plasma represent more sensitive detection of small amounts of myocardial necrosis. For example, in the study by Galvani and colleagues [54], elevations of cTnI were present on admission in only one third of patients who subsequently had elevations. The remainder developed elevations, while values of MB-CK utilizing a sophisticated mass assay performed in a centralized core laboratory remained within the normal range. These data suggest that elevations of troponin are more sensitive than MB-CK for the detection of myocardial injury [54]. Similarly, Antman and colleagues [57] corrected their data to exclude patients with elevations of MB-CK. Their study documented a 1.8-

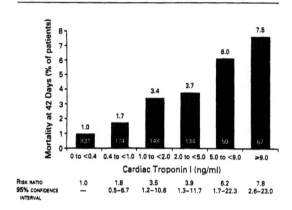

| RISK RATIO | 1.0 | 1.8 | 3.5 | 3.9 | 6.2 | 7.8 |
| 95% CONFIDENCE INTERVAL | — | 0.5–6.7 | 1.2–10.6 | 1.3–11.7 | 1.7–22.3 | 2.6–23.0 |

FIGURE 33-4. Incremental increases in mortality at 42 days associated with increasing levels of cTnI measured at the time of enrollment. (Reproduced from Autman et al. [57], with permission.)

fold increase in mortality in patients who presented early after the onset of symptoms (0–6 hours) and a 9.5-fold increase in patients presenting between 6 and 24 hours after onset. For these patients, risk ratios of 1.7 and 5.5 persisted, even in the subset of patients without MB-CK elevations during their initial period of hospitalization. Overall, the risk ratio of 3.8 was diminished only slightly to 3.0 when patients who developed elevations in MB-CK were excluded. These data suggest, but do not prove, that increases in the troponins may be more sensitive than those of MB-CK for the detection of myocardial injury.

Another important subgroup in whom elevations of troponin may be of significance are patients who are critically ill. In a recent study, Guest and colleagues [62] reported that of 209 consecutive patients admitted to the respiratory and critical care units with a variety of diagnoses, including gastrointestinal bleeding, sepsis, diabetic ketoacidosis, etc., increases in cTnI occurred in 15% of patients and marked a subsequent mortality rate of 40%. Individuals with normal cTnI values had a mortality rate of 15%. In this study, troponin values were not made available to the physicians managing the patients. Thus, it is possible that minor increases in cTnI, which indicate the presence of cardiac involvement with the underlying disease process and/or concomitant ischemic heart disease, render their prognostic significance by indicating the presence of cardiovascular dysfunction. Treating cardiac involvement in these patients may lead to a reduction in mortality.

Conclusions

In conclusion, the troponins should not, from first principles, facilitate an earlier diagnosis of acute myocardial infarction. However, the finding of elevated cardioc troponins in plasma, whether because of their persistence after acute events or because of their increased sensitivity compared with other markers in patients with definite acute MI, suspected acute MI, unstable angina, or those who are critically ill, may add important prognostic information that could optiminze therapy. Such prognostic information due to the persistence of elevations or increased sensitivity should be distinguished from the idea that increases in the cardiac troponins occur earlier than elevations of markers such as myoglobin, CK isoforms, or fatty acid binding protein because with the present generation of assays this does not appear to be the case. However, more sensitive assays that improve detection should be available in the near term. It may well be that once they are available, improved early sensitivity will be achieved allowing a cost-effective strategy of combining the potent prognostic information garnered by cardiac troponins with early sensitivity for the detection of myocardial injury. Such increased sensitivity may be a mixed blessing because very sensitive detection of tiny amounts of myocardial injury may lead to confusion over the etiology and significance of minor amounts of cardiac damage. Such possibilities exist whenever major strides are made in diagnostic or therapeutic efficacy.

References

1. McGovern PG, Pankow JS, Shahar E, Doliszny KM, Folsom A, Blackburn H, Luepker, R. Recent trends in acute coronary heart disease — mortality, morbidity, medical care, and risk factors. The Minnesota Heart Survey Investigators. NEJM 334:884, 1996.
2. Ellis AK. Serum protein measurements and the diagnosis of acute myocardial infarction. Circulation 83:1107, 1991.
3. Kannel WB. Prevalence and clinical aspects of unrecognized myocardial infarction and sudden unexpected death. Circulation 75:114, 1987.
4. Grimm RH Jr, Tillinghast S, Daniels K, Neaton JD, Mascioli S, Crow R, Pritzker M, Prineas RJ. Unrecognized myocardial infarction: Experience in the Multiple Risk Factor Interventional Trial (MRFIT). Circulation 75:116, 1987.
5. Turi ZG, Rutherford JD, Roberts R, Muller JE, Jaffe AS, Jude RE, Parker C, Raabe DS, Stone PH, Hartwell TD, Lewis SE, Parker PW, Gold HK, Robertson TL, Sobel BE, Willerson JT, Braunwald E. Electrocardiographic, enzymatic, and scintigraphic criteria of acute myocardial infarction as determined from study of 726

patients (a MILIS Study). Am J Cardiol 55:1463, 1985.

6. Adams JE, Abendschein DR, Jaffe AS. Biochemical markers of myocardial injury: Is MB creatine kinase the choice for the 1990s? Circulation 88:750, 1993.

7. Roberts R. The two out of three criteria for the diagnosis of infarction. Is it passe? Chest 86:511, 1984.

8. Guest TM, Jaffe AS. Rapid diagnosis of acute myocardial infarction. Cardiol Clin 13:283, 1995.

9. Jaffe AS. More rapid biochemical diagnosis of myocardial infarction: Necessary? Prudent? Clin Chem 39:1567, 1993.

10. Eisenberg E, Kielley WW. Troponin-tropomyosin complex. J Biol Chem 249:4742, 1974.

11. Potter JD, Gergely J. Troponin, tropomyosin, and actin interactions in the Ca^{2+} regulation of muscle contraction. Biochemistry 13:2697, 1974.

12. Ebashi S, Ohnishi S, Maruyama K, Fujii T. Molecular mechanism of regulation of muscle contraction by Ca-troponin system. In: Biro EN, ed. Proteins of Contractile Systems. Amsterdam: North-Holland, 31:71, 1975.

13. Weber A, Murray JM. Molecular control mechanisms in muscle contraction. Physiol Rev 53:612, 1973.

14. MacGeoch C, Barton PJ, Vallins WJ, Bhavsar P, Spurr NK. The human cardiac troponin I locus: Assignment to chromosome 19p 13.2-19q13.2. Hum Genet 88:101, 1991.

15. Wade R, Eddy R, Shows TB, Kedes L. cDNA sequence, tissue specific expression and chromosomal mapping of the human slow twitch skeletal muscle isoform of troponin I. Genomics 7:346, 1990.

16. Wilkinson M, Grand RJA. Comparison of amino acid sequence of troponin I from different striated muscles. Nature 271:31, 1978.

17. Saggin L, Gorza L, Ausoni S, Schiaffino S. Troponin I switching in the developing heart. J Biol Chem 264:16299, 1989.

18. Schreier T, Kedes L, Gahlmann R. Cloning, structural analysis, and expression of the human slow twitch skeletal muscle/cardiac troponin C gene. J Biol Chem 265:21247, 1990.

19. Toyota N, Shimada Y. Differentiation of troponin in cardiac and skeletal muscles in chicken embryos as studied by immunofluorescence microscopy. J Cell Biol 91:497, 1981.

20. Bhavsar PK, Dhoot GK, Cumming DV, Butler-Browne GS, Yacoub MH, Barton PJ. Developmental expression of troponin I isoforms in fetal human heart. FEBS Ltrs 292:5, 1991.

21. Anderson PA, Malouf NN, Oakeley AE, Pagani ED, Allen PD. Troponin T isoform expression in humans. A comparison among normal and failing adult heart, fetal heart, and adult and fetal skeletal muscle. Circulation 69:1226, 1991.

22. Saggin L, Gorza L, Ausoni S, Schiaffino S. Cardiac troponin T in developing regenerating and denervated rat skeletal muscle. Development 110:547, 1990.

23. Sadeh M, Stern LZ, Czyzewski K, Finley PR, Russell DH. Alterations in creatine kinase, ornithine decar-boxylase, and transglutaminase during muscle regeneration. Life Sci 34:483, 1984.

24. Bodor GS, Porterfield D, Voss E, Kelly J, Smith S, Porterfield D, Apple FS. Cardiac troponin-T composition in normal and regenerating human skeletal muscle. Clin Chem 41:S148, 1995.

25. McLaurin M, Apple FS, Voss EM, Herzog CA, Sharkey S. Serum cardiac troponin, I cardiac troponin T and CK MB in dialysis patients without ischemic heart disease: Evidence of cardiac troponin T expression in skeletal muscle. Clin Chem, 43:976, 1997.

26. Bodor GS, Porterfield D, Voss EM, Smith S, Apple FS. Cardiac troponin-I is not expressed in fetal and healthy or diseased adult human skeletal muscle tissue. Clin Chem 41:1710, 1995.

27. Adams JE, Bodor GS, Davila Roman BG, Delmez JA, Apple FS, Ladenson JH, Jaffe AS. Cardiac troponin I: A marker with high specificity for cardiac injury. Circulation 88:101, 1993.

28. Mair J, Artner-Dworzak E, Lechleitner P, Smidt J, Wagner I, Dienstl F, Puschendorf B. Cardiac troponin T in diagnosis of acute myocardial infarction. Clin Chem 37:845, 1991.

29. Katus HA, Remppis A, Neumann FJ, Scheffold T, Diederich KW, Vinar G, Noe A, Matern G, Kuebler W. Diagnostic efficiency of troponin T measurements in acute myocardial infarction. Circulation 83:902, 1991.

30. Missov E, Calzolari C, Pau B. High circulating levels of cardiac troponin I in human congestive heart failure (abstr). J Am Coll Cardiol 27:994, 1996.

31. Missov E, Pau B, Calzolari C. Increased circulating levels of cardiac troponin I in anthracycline-treated patients (abstr). Circulation 94:4283, 1996.

32. Butch AW, Goodnow TT, Brown WS, McClellan A, McClellan A, Kessler G, Scott MG. Stratus automated creatine kinase-MB assay evaluated: Identification and elemination of falsely increased results associated with a high-molecular-mass form of alkaline phosphatase. Chin Chem 35:2048, 1989.

33. Smith SC, Ladenson JH, Mason JW, Jaffe AS. Elevations of cardiac troponin I associated with myocarditis: Experimental and clinical correlates. Circulation 95:163, 1997.

34. Franz WM, Remppis A, Kandolf R, Kubler W, Katus HA. Serum troponin T: Diagnostic marker of acute myocarditis. Clin Chem 42:340, 1996.

35. Adams JE, Davila-Roman VG, Bessey PQ, Blake DP, Ladenson JH, Jaffe AS 1. Improved detection of cardiac contusion with cardiac troponin I. Am Heart J 131:308, 1996.

36. Adams J, Scheckman KB, Landt J, Ladenson JH, Jaffe AS. Comparable detection of acute myocardial infarction by creatine kinase MB isoenzyme and cardiac troponin I. Clin Chem 4017:1291, 1994.

37. Katus HA, Remppis A, Scheffold T, Drederich KW, Kuebler W. Intracellular compartmentation of cardiac troponin T and its release kinetics in patients with reperfused and nonreperfused myocardial infarction. Am J Cardiol 67:1360, 1991.

38. Samarel AM, Ferguson AG, Vander Heide RS, Davison R, Ganote CE. Release of unassembled rat cardiac myosin light chain 1 following the calcium paradox. Circ Res 58:166, 1986.

39. Heyndrickx GR, Amano J, Kenna T, Fallon JT, Fallon JT, Patrick TA, Manders WT, Rogers GG, Rosendorff C, Vatner SF. Creatine kinase release not associated with myocardial necrosis after short periods of coronary artery occlusion in conscious baboons. JACC 6:1299, 1985.

40. Roberts R, Henry PD, Sobel BE. An improved basis for enzymatic estimation of infarct size. Circulation 52:743, 1975.

41. Bodor GS, Porter S, Landt Y, Ladenson JH. Development of monoclonal antibodies for an assay of cardiac troponin-I and preliminary results in suspected cases of myocardial infarction. Clin Chem 38:2203, 1992.

42. Gerhardt W, Katus HA, Ravkilde J, Hamm C, Jorgensen PJ, Peheim E, Ljungdahl L, Lofdahl P. S-troponin-T in suspected ischemic myocardial injury compared with mass and catalytic concentrations of S. creatine kinase isoenzyme MB. Clin Chem 3718:1405, 1991.

43. Mair J, Morandell D, Genser N, Lechleitner P, Dienstl F, Puschendorf B. Equivalent early sensitivities of myoglobin, creatine kinase MB mass, creatine kinase isoform ratios, and cardiac troponins I and T for acute myocardial infarction. Clin Chem 41:1266, 1995.

44. Cummins B, Auckland ML, Cummins P. Cardiac specific troponin I radioimmunoassay in the diagnosis of acute myocardial infarction. Am Heart J 113:1333, 1987.

45. Larue C, Calzolari C, Bertinchant J, Leclerq F, Grolleau R, Pau B. Cardiac specific immunoenzymometric assay of troponin in the early phase of acute myocardial infarction. Clin Chem 39:972, 1993.

46. Katus HA, Looser S, Hallermayer K, Remppis A, Scheffold T, Borgya A, Essig U, Geuss U. Development and in vitro characterization of a new immunoassay of cardiac troponin T. Clin Chem 38:386, 1992.

47. Hafner G, Thome-Kromer B, Schaube J, Kupferwasser I, Ehrenthal W, Cummins P, Prellwitz W, Michel G. Cardiac troponins in serum in chronic renal failure. Clin Chem 40:1790, 1994.

48. Li D, Keffer J, Corry K, Vazquez M, Jialal I. Nonspecific elevation of troponin T levels in patients with chronic renal failure. Clin Chem 41:S199, 1995.

49. Wu AHB, Feng Y-J, Roper L, Herbert K, Schweizer R. Cardiac troponins T and I before and after renal transplantation. Clin Chem 43:411, 1997.

50. Ravkilde J, Horder M, Gerhardt W, Lungdahl L, Pettersson T, Tryding N, Moller BH, Hamfelt A, Graven T, Asberg A, Helin M, Penttila I, Thygessen K. Diagnostic performance and prognostic value of serum troponin T in suspected acute myocardial infarction. Scand J Clin Lab Invest 53:677, 1993.

51. Jaffe AS, Landt V, Pavvin CA, Abendschein DR, Geltman EM, Ladenson JH. Comparative sensitivity of cardiac troponin I and lactate dehydrogenase isoenzymes for diagnosing acute myocardial infarction. Clin Chem 42:1770, 1996.

52. Adams JE, Sicard G, Allan BT, Bridwell KH, Lenke LG, Davila-Roman VG, Bodor GS, Ladenson JH, Jaffe AS. Diagnosis of perioperative myocardial infarction with measurement of cardiac troponin I. N Engl J Med 330:670, 1994.

53. Ravkilde J, Nissen H, Horder M, Thygesen K. Independent prognostic value of serum creatine kinase isoenzyme MB mass, cardiac troponin T and myosin light chain levels in suspected acute myocardial infarction. J Am Coll Cardiol 25:574, 1995.

54. Galvani M, Ottani F, Ferrini D, Ladenson JH, Destro A, Baccos D, Rusticali F, Jaffe AS. Prognostic influence of elevated values of cardiac troponin I in patients with unstable angina. Circulation, 95:2053, 1997.

55. Collinson PO, Stubbs PJ. The prognostic value of serum troponin T in unstable angina. N Engl J Med 327:1760, 1992.

56. Hamm CW, Ravkilde J, Gerhardt W, Jorgenson P, Peheim E, Ljungdahl L, Goldmann B, Katus HA. The prognostic value of serum troponin T in unstable angina. N Engl J Med 327:146, 1992.

57. Antman EM, Tanasijevic MJ, Thompson B, Schactman M, McCabe CH, Cannon CP, Fischer GA, Fung AY, Thompson C, Wybenga D, Braunwald E. Cardiac-specific troponin I levels to predict the risk of mortality in patients with acute coronary syndromes. N Engl J Med 335:1342, 1996.

58. Lindahl B, Venge P, Wallentin L. Relation between troponin T and the risk of subsequent cardiac events in unstable coronary artery disease. The FRISC Study Group. Circulation 93:1618, 1996.

59. Bakker AJ, Koelemay MJ, Gorgels JP, van Vliers B, Smits R, Tijssen JG, Haagen FD. Troponin T and myoglobin at admission: Value of early diagnosis of acute myocardial infarction. Eur Heart J 15:45, 1994.

60. deWinter RJ, Koster RW, Sturk A, Sanders GT. Value of myoglobin, troponin T, and CK-MB mass in ruling out an acute myocardial infarction in the emergency room. Circulation 92:3401, 1995.

61. Brogan GX, Hollander JE, McCluskey CG, Thode HC Jr., Snow J, Sama A, Bock JL. Evaluation of a new assay for cardiac troponin I vs. creatine kinase-MB for the diagnosis of acute myocardial infarction. Acad Emeg Med 4:6, 1997.

62. Guest TM, Ramanathan AV, Schechtman KB, ladenson JH, Jaffe AS. Myocardial injury in critically ill medical patients: A surprisingly frequent complication. JAMA 273:1945, 1995.

63. Ohman EM, Armstrong PW, Christenson RH, Granger CB, Granger CB, Katus HA, Hamm CW, O'Hanesian MA, Wagner GS, Kleiman NS, Harrell FE Jr., Califf RM, Topol EJ. Cardiac troponin T levels for risk stratification in acute myocardial ischemia. GUSTO IIA Investigators. N Engl J Med 335:1333, 1996.

64. Stubbs P, Collinson P, Moseley D, Greenwood T, Noble M. Prognostic significance of admission troponin T concentrations in patients with myocardial infarction. Circulation 94:1291, 1996.

34. MARKERS OF THROMBOSIS AND FIBRINOLYSIS

L. Veronica Lee, Dana R. Abendschein, and Paul R. Eisenberg

Introduction

Thrombosis plays a central role in the pathogenesis of acute coronary syndromes. Currently available therapies, which possess primarily antithrombotic and fibrinolytic properties, have improved the clinical outcome of patients with unstable angina and myocardial infarction. However, because of residual thrombosis, a significant proportion of patients with acute coronary syndromes develop complications such as reocclusion, reinfarction, recurrent ischemia, and stenosis, with clinical manisfestations ranging from stable angina to death. We currently lack critical information regarding the balance between thrombosis and fibrinolysis that would help guide the development of short-term, long-term, and preventive treatments. Plasma markers of thrombosis and fibrinolysis are likely to be crucial to the development and use of current and future therapeutic approaches. The following is an overview of some currently available and novel assays for thrombotic and fibrinolytic activity, and recent clinical data on their potential role in the assessment of acute coronary syndromes and in guiding therapy.

Markers of Activation and Inhibition of Coagulation

TISSUE FACTOR: THE INITIATOR OF THROMBOSIS

Tissue factor is a membrane-associated glycoprotein (263 amino acids, 37 kd) [1] that mediates activation of the coagulation cascade in response to endothelial injury (e.g., atherosclerotic plaque rupture) by binding factor VIIa and promoting activation of factor X (Figure 34-1). In normal arteries tissue factor is expressed by cells in the adventitia, and to a lesser extent the media [2,3], and its expression is increased in atherosclerotic plaques [3,4] and in response to arterial injury [5,6]. Increases in tissue factor have been identified by immunohistochemical methods in atherectomy specimens from patients with unstable coronary syndromes [4], suggesting that tissue factor expression may be a marker of a thrombotic mechanism in these patients [4]. However, there are no data available to suggest that plasma concentrations of tissue factor antigen or measurement of its activity (induced or constitutive) are markers of vascular wall expression of tissue factor.

Tissue factor antigen has been measured in plasma with assays based on specific monoclonal antibodies [7–11] that do not distinguish between procoagulant and potentially inactive forms [12]. A whole-blood assay for measurement of tissue factor antigen concentrations has recently been developed, but it has not been extensively evaluated in a clinical setting [13]. Assays that measure the expression of tissue factor activity induced in cultured circulating monocytes have been used to characterize plasma tissue factor–dependent procoagulant activity. Increases in time-dependent expression have been found in patients with myocardial infarction and in those with unstable and stable angina [13–15]. In these studies, circulating monocytes were collected, cultured, and stimulated in vitro by direct contact with the patient's lymphocytes [14], or by the addition of endotoxin [15]. Increased tissue factor–dependent procoagulant activity has been shown to persist for as long as 4 weeks in patients admitted to the hospital for unstable angina, suggesting a prolonged hypercoagulable state [14]. Monocyte expression of tissue factor in whole blood has also been characterized by flow-activated cell sorting (FACS) with the use of specific fluoroscein-labeled monoclonal antibodies [13]. Whether tissue factor antigen in plasma is membrane bound, possibly on circulating monocytes, or free in solution has not been well defined, and the functional significance of plasma levels is also unclear, because

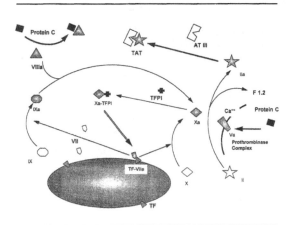

FIGURE 34-1. Activation of the coagulation cascade. Membrane-associated tissue factor (TF) acts as a cofactor to activated factor VII. The TF–factor VIIa complex then promotes the activation of factors IX and X. Factor VIIIa, which can be inhibited by activated protein C, forms a complex with factor IXa to also activate factor X. Tissue factor pathway inhibitor (TFPI) forms a complex with factor Xa that inhibits the membrane-bound TF–factor VIIa complex. Prothrombin is activated by the membrane-associated prothrombinase complex of factors Xa and Va in the presence of calcium. Activated protein C also inhibits the prothrombinase complex. Prothrombin fragment F1.2 is released when thrombin (factor IIa) is activated by factor Xa/factor Va. Factor IIa is inhibited by antithrombin III, forming the thrombin–antithrombin complex (TAT).

tissue factor activity must be closely regulated to prevent intravascular coagulation. Currently available information suggests that plasma tissue factor is either inactive or that its activity is regulated by a mechanism that is as yet undefined.

Increased concentrations of this antigen in urine correlate with the severity of disease in inflammatory bowel disease, as well as breast, colon, and bladder cancer. In patients with cancer, increased plasma tissue factor activity is associated with an elevated risk of thrombosis [16,17]. Endotoxin-mediated increases in tissue factor expression on macrophages and endothelial cells are thought to be a mechanism for disseminated intravascular coagulation [18–20], but plasma levels of tissue factor activity measured by enzyme-linked immunosorbent assay (ELISA) do not directly correlate with the presence of such coagulation [8,12]. Nonetheless, changes in plasma levels of tissue factor may reflect the clinical severity of patients with disseminated intravascular coagulation.

FACTOR VII

Factor VII (56 kd) is activated by factor IXa, factor Xa, or thrombin, and autoactivates when bound to tissue factor [21–24]. The half-life of factor VII is 5 hours and that of activated factor VII (VIIa) is approximately 2 hours [25]. Normally, factor VIIa exists as less than 1% of the total factor VII concentration of 0.5 µg/mL in plasma, unless there is a hypercoagulable state or rapid turnover of clotting factors [26,27]. The tissue factor–factor VIIa complex activates factors IX and X (see Figure 34-1).

The majority of plasma assays for factor VII measure only the activated form and factor VIIa activity against synthetic substrates [25], or factor VIIa coagulant activity [28], but antigen-based assays (e.g., ELISA, RIA) have also been described [29–32]. Assays that detect antigen or coagulant activity may not accurately measure concentrations of factor VII because they may detect it in several forms with variable procoagulant activity (factors VII and VIIa, and in either membrane-bound or tissue factor pathway inhibitor–associated complexes) and because factor VIIa may continue to be generated after plasma sampling [33].

A more promising specific assay for factor VIIa has been developed by the use of site-directed mutations of tissue factor. This technique permits direct detection of factor VIIa coagulant activity in plasma without the need for phospholipid membranes for binding of the tissue factor–factor VIIa complex [34,35]. In the absence of phospholipid membranes, autoactivation of factor VII does not occur, and only factor VIIa activated in vivo is measured [27,36,37]. Using this method factor VIIa concentrations have been measured in normal volunteers and have been found to be in the range of 0.5–8.4 ng/mL (mean 3.6 ng/mL), representing 0.8% of the total circulating factor VII [27]. Levels of factor VIIa are elevated in association with pregnancy and decrease in patients with deep vein thrombosis who are receiving anticoagulants [27]. Elevated factor VIIa concentrations are also present in non–insulin-dependent diabetics and in elderly patients with cardiovascular disease; however, there is no relationship to cholesterol or triglyceride concentrations in the latter group, as previously described with assays based on factor VIIa coagulant activity [38–40].

Elevations of factor VIIa coagulant activity have been reported in patients with complicated myocardial infarction and in those with uncomplicated myocardial infarction, and in patients with unstable angina and peripheral vascular disease; these elevations have been shown to be a risk factor for both fatal and nonfatal cardiac events in prospective population studies [41–47]. In the Northwick Park study, factor VIIa coagulant activity was a risk factor for ischemic heart disease and correlated with early cardiac-related death. Other studies have not found a significant relationship between factor VII concentrations and cardiac events, but this may reflect differences in the assays used [48]. Thus, whether the increase in the concentration of factor VIIa activity or that in factor VII results in increased cardiovascular risk is unclear [28,43].

Although there are data that suggest that increases in factor VII concentrations are correlated with the risk of cardiac events (principally myocardial infarction and death), differences among assays preclude any recommendations for the measurement of either factor VII coagulant activity or antigen. Factor VIIa activity measured with the soluble tissue factor assay appears accurate, but the clinical utility of this assay remains to be defined.

TISSUE FACTOR PATHWAY INHIBITOR

Tissue factor pathway inhibitor (TFPI), a Kunitz-type serine protease inhibitor (both 34 and 41 kd forms have been found), initially binds and inhibits factor Xa, and the factor Xa–TFPI complex inhibits factor VIIa–tissue factor complex (see Figure 34-1) [49,50]. Fifty to 70% of total TFPI in the circulation is bound to endothelial cells, 10% is in platelets and can be released by platelet activation, and the rest circulates bound to low-density lipoproteins [51]. The normal plasma concentration of TFPI is approximately 89 ng/mL. Endothelial release is thought to be responsible for the observed tripling of TFPI concentration in blood when samples are obtained by a template bleeding-time incision [52].

Concentrations of TFPI in plasma are increased in association with sepsis, cancer, exercise, pregnancy, adult respiratory distress syndrome, hypercholesterolemia, and disseminated intravascular coagulation [53–58]. Levels have also been shown to increase in patients with coronary heart disease in association with elevated concentrations of the factor VII–phospholipid complex [59]. After myocardial infarction, increases in the concentration of TFPI have been shown to correlate with increased levels of low-density lipoprotein (LDL), and it has been suggested that binding of TFPI to LDL in hyperlipidemic patients may impair the antithrombotic effects of the former [60,61].

Subcutaneous or intravenous unfractionated heparin results in a twofold to fourfold increase in plasma TFPI concentrations [56,62–64], presumably caused by its displacement from endothelium [61,65], with levels returning to baseline within 24

hours of cessation of dosing [66]. However, TFPI levels have been reported to remain elevated for up to 7 days after exposure to low molecular weight heparin in patients with deep venous thrombosis [67]. From studies in patients with deep venous thrombosis and in normal volunteers, there is some evidence that the absence of an increase in TFPI with heparin is a marker, and possibly the mechanism, of heparin resistance [67,68].

Markers of Thrombin Generation

PROTHROMBIN FRAGMENT 1.2

Prothrombin is cleaved by the factor Xa–factor Va complex to form α-thrombin and prothrombin fragment 1.2 (F1.2; 32 amino acids) [69]. Factor Xa–mediated activation of prothrombin requires the formation of the factor Xa–factor Va complex in the presence of calcium on a membrane surface, probably provided by platelets (prothrombinase complex) [70,71]. Plasma concentrations of F1.2 appear to be a sensitive marker of prothrombin activation and may be a more sensitive marker of the prethrombotic state than measures of thrombin activity, such as fibrinopeptide A (FPA) [72].

F1.2 concentrations have been measured by several immunoassays, but interpretation of the results has been hampered by the dissimilarity of the assays with regard to anticoagulants and antibodies used [73,74]. In general, however, F1.2 concentrations are elevated in the presence of disseminated intravascular coagulation, deep vein thrombosis [75], and promyelocytic leukemia [76]. Concentrations also increase with age, body mass index, and in patients with cardiac risk factors (e.g., smokers, sedentary lifestyle, parental history of heart disease, and hypercholesterolemia) [40].

Concentrations of F1.2 are increased in patients with coronary atherosclerosis, but the degree of elevation does not correlate with the severity of disease [77]. A recent study documented elevations in F1.2 for 6 months after a first episode of unstable angina or acute myocardial infarction, although no association between levels and the risk of cardiac events could be found [78]. Concentrations of FPA normalized in this group of patients over the same time period. The finding of persistently elevated F1.2 levels after acute ischemic events may be a marker of a persistent procoagulant state.

The measurement of F1.2 levels has been proposed for monitoring the adequacy of anticoagulation. Although concentrations of F1.2 decrease in patients with angina and deep venous thrombosis treated with heparin or warfarin, they do not consistently correlate

Markers of Fibrin Formation and Degradation

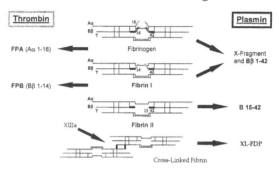

FIGURE 34-2. Markers of fibrin formation and degradation. Proteolytic actions of thrombin are displayed on the left side of the figure and of plasmin on the right. Sequential cleavage of FPA and FPB by thrombin results in the formation of fibrin I and then fibrin II. Factor XIIIa crosslinks the fibrin II monomers to form crosslinked fibrin polymers. Plasmin degrades fibrinogen, forming fragment X and Bβ1-42. Plasmin proteolysis of fibrin II results in the production of fragment β15-42. Plasmin degradation of crosslinked fibrin results in the formation of crosslinked fibrin degradation products (XL-FDP).

with other measures of anticoagulation (e.g., PT, aPTT) or with the intensity of therapy [77,79,80]. In one study of patients undergoing coronary bypass surgery, concentrations of F1.2 were found to peak within 3 hours and to return to baseline within 20 hours after discontinuation of cardiopulmonary bypass, despite treatment with heparin [81]. The increases in F1.2 after surgery correlate with increases in soluble fibrin and thrombin–antithrombin III complex levels over the same interval and with the occurrence of myocardial ischemia, suggesting that inadequate thrombin inhibition may be a mechanism for ischemia in these patients. The use of protamine at the end of surgery to reverse the effects of heparin may also contribute to a procoagulant state [82]. Thus, increases in F1.2 may identify patients at risk for a postoperative myocardial infarction. These findings also suggest a need for improved postoperative anticoagulation, but the value of routine measurement of F1.2 levels as a marker of adequate inhibition of thrombin has not yet been confirmed.

Results of studies using long-term oral anticoagulation with warfarin have suggested that measurement of F1.2 may have a role in monitoring the adequacy of anticoagulation, but concentrations of F1.2 do not correlate with the prothrombin time or

the occurrence of venous and arterial thrombotic events [83,84]. Measurement of F1.2 has recently been suggested for monitoring oral anticoagulation after coronary stent placement [85], and may also have a role in assessing the efficacy of novel anticoagulants, such as inhibitors of factor Xa or the tissue factor pathway. For example, several recent studies have found that F1.2 concentrations are not decreased in patients treated with hirudin, suggesting that persistent thrombin elaboration is occurring despite inhibition of thrombin activity [86–88].

Concentrations of F1.2 increase in association with thrombolytic therapy, due to activation of prothrombin, and are not normalized by administration of heparin [89,90]. These data are consistent with increased procoagulant activity during thrombolytic therapy, attributable in part to plasmin-induced activation of the coagulation system and to exposure of clot-associated factor Xa–factor Va complex [91]. However, increases in F1.2 concentrations in patients treated with coronary thrombolysis do not appear to be associated with an increased risk of adverse events [92].

FIBRINOPEPTIDES

Fibrinopeptide A (FPA) and fibrinopeptide B (FPB) are released by the proteolytic action of thrombin on fibrinogen. FPA is a 16 amino acid peptide from the amino terminus of the fibrinogen α-chain. The concentration of FPA in plasma has been estimated to increase by 4 ng/mL for every 1 mg of fibrinogen converted to fibrin by thrombin [93]. FPA is rapidly cleared by the kidneys, with a half-life of 3–5 minutes [93]. FPA is released more rapidly from fibrinogen than is FPB, resulting in the intermediate fibrin I molecule (des AA-fibrin; Figure 34-2) [94–96]. FPB is released from the amino terminus of the β-chain of fibrinogen or fibrin I, and is a 14-amino acid peptide. The sequential cleavage of FPA and FPB results in the formation of the fibrin II monomer (des AABB-fibrin). Fibrin I forms double-stranded protofibrils that can be crosslinked by factor XIIIa in the presence of calcium [97]. However, crosslinked fibrin usually consists of a complex gel-like matrix of protofibrils formed from fibrin II [98]. Fibrin clots form when the ratio of fibrin to fibrinogen exceeds 1:5 [99].

The concentration of FPA in healthy volunteers is between 0.1 and 1.3 nM, with a mean of 0.6 nM [100]. Three molecular forms of FPA circulate in plasma: FPA-P, in which the serine at position 3 is phosphorylated; unphosphorylated FPA; and FPA-Y, in which the amino-terminal alanine is cleaved [101,102]. The percentage of the phosphorylated form appears to be increased in acute illness and may represent as much as 60% of the total concentration of FPA [103]. The mean urinary excretion of FPA is 1.67 ± 0.1 (SE) μg/24 h or 0.2–0.5% of total FPA released from fibrinogen in 1 day [104]. FPA may be dephosphorylated, and the carboxy terminus may be cleaved by the kidneys before excretion [105]. Concentrations of FPA in urine collected over 24 hours correlate with plasma levels [104,106].

Assays for FPA and FPB. Several plasma assays for FPA have been developed since the initial description of a radioimmunoassay (RIA) by Nossel et al. [93,107,108]. Most assays recognize the amino terminus of the Aα-chain of fibrinogen, and therefore fibrinogen and fibrinogen degradation products must be removed from plasma samples before the assay is performed. This can be accomplished by bentonite adsorption [109,110], C$_{18}$-reversed phase chromatography (SEP-pak), or 50–75% ethanol precipitation. Recovery of FPA from plasma after sample preparation ranges from 70% to more than 90% with these methods [93,111–115]. Antiserum (R2) specific for the carboxy terminus of FPA has also been described by Nossel [107,108], and Kudryk [116] later developed a monoclonal antibody with similar specificity. Because these assays recognize only FPA, removal of fibrinogen from the sample is not necessary.

Measurement of FPA requires meticulous acquisition, collection, and processing of blood samples to avoid thrombin elaboration and ex vivo increases in FPA concentration [117,118]. Thrombin must be rapidly inhibited at the time of sampling or concentrations of FPA will be artificially elevated; therefore, samples must be collected in a mixture that includes both an anticoagulant and a plasmin inhibitor, such as aprotinin, to prevent fibrinogen degradation. In initial studies, high concentrations of heparin were shown to be sufficient to inhibit thrombin during sample acquisition for measurement of FPA under a variety of thrombotic conditions [117,119]. However, in samples from patients treated with tissue plasminogen activator (t-PA), inhibition of t-PA activity against fibrinogen required the addition of d-phe-pro-arg-chloromethylketone (PPACK). PPACK was initially designed as a thrombin inhibitor, but at high concentrations it also inhibits plasmin and t-PA [117].

An assay for FPB was developed initially by Eckhardt et al. [120], but this peptide has been difficult to measure in plasma because of reduced immunoreactivity after cleavage of C-terminal arginine by carboxypeptidase. A radioimmunoassay [96] and an tiserum to des-Arg FPB [76] have also been described, but there is little information on the concentrations of FPB in humans.

Clinical Utility of Measurements of FPA. Concentrations of FPA are increased in patients in thrombotic states, such as those with ischemic stroke [121,122], pulmonary embolism [123], venous thromboembolism [100,124], malignancies [125,126], burns, disseminated intravascular coagulation, systemic lupus erythematosus [111], ischemic chest pain [127], mural thrombosis [128], and sudden cardiac death [112,123,129]. Increases in FPA levels are sensitive markers of thrombosis, but may not reflect a pathologic condition if other inducers of thrombin elaboration are present, such as indwelling catheters or extravascular thrombin activity [130,131].

Concentrations of FPA in plasma have been shown to be more elevated in patients with unstable than in those with stable coronary artery disease, and elevations have been related to increases in the incidence of ischemic events [132]. FPA levels are also elevated in the urine of patients with unstable angina, and the differences in FPA concentrations in those with unstable and those with stable angina are even more marked in urine [133]. Plasma FPA increases soon after the onset of ischemic symptoms and then decreases rapidly in the majority of patients. Elevations may persist in patients with active thrombosis and are a marker for increased risk of complications, such as recurrent infarction [134,135]. The presence of clinical markers of high-risk unstable angina (e.g., symptoms refractory to medical management, ST depression on the ECG, or plaques complicated by thrombosis) is associated with more marked increases in plasma and urine concentrations of FPA [135,136], and concentrations are higher in patients with myocardial infarction and unstable angina than in patients with stable angina, even when the blood samples are drawn from those without clinically active ischemia [78,106,137].

Concentrations of FPA in plasma are decreased by heparin, and the rapid decrease (<15 minutes) in FPA after an intravenous bolus of heparin has been used as a criterion for distinguishing intravascular (fast response) from extravascular thrombin generation (slow response) [100,125]. The effects of heparin are not complete or long lasting. However, in a study by Mombelli et al., patients with myocardial infarction treated with a 5000 IU intravenous bolus of heparin had rapid decreases in plasma FPA, even during a constant intravenous infusion of 20,000 IU daily FPA did not return to normal levels [138]; and once heparin was stopped, the FPA concentration increased significantly.

Persistent increases in FPA despite heparin therapy have been found to be markers of heparin resistance and of an increased risk of thrombosis in several studies. In patients undergoing coronary interventions in whom the activated clotting time (ACT) was maintained above 300 seconds with heparin boluses, concentrations of FPA in samples obtained from the coronary sinus remained above the threshold for suppression of thrombin activity in 45% of patients [139]. There was also a significant relationship between elevations in FPA and the presence of intracoronary thrombus, abrupt closure, postprocedural myocardial infarction, and unsuccessful procedures. In patients with myocardial infarction, concentrations of FPA in samples obtained from a peripheral vein decreased rapidly after administration of intravenous heparin, but more gradually after administration of subcutaneous heparin. As in the study described earlier, neither mode of administration of heparin decreased concentrations of FPA to normal levels, suggesting that patients are more resistant to the effects of heparin after myocardial infarction [140].

Concentrations of FPA are increased in patients treated with fibrinolytic agents, in part because of de novo elaboration of thrombin [89,141,142]. Such increases are attenuated, but not abolished, by concomitant intravenous heparin [143,144]. Increases in FPA levels during treatment with fibrinolytic agents have been associated with inadequate thrombolysis or persistent procoagulant activity, which can result in reocclusion or failure of reperfusion [145–147]. Specifically, high or persistent elevations of FPA concentrations within 30 and 90 minutes of streptokinase (SK) and t-PA therapy, respectively, have been associated with inadequate thrombolysis [141,146]. Elevations of FPA decrease within 30 minutes of the initiation of heparin therapy in patients without clinical evidence of reocclusion who are treated with t-PA [146]. Proteolytic activity of fibrinolytic enzymes at concentrations reached during pharmacologic thrombolysis may result in the formation of FPA (t-PA, plasmin), FPB (t-PA, urokinase), and in the release of fragments with the potential for cross-reactivity in FPA assays, such as fragment Aα1-21 (plasmin, elastase) [148].

THROMBIN–ANTITHROMBIN COMPLEX

Antithrombin III inactivates thrombin by irreversibly binding to its catalytic site. The concentration of antithrombin III in plasma is approximately 2.5 μM, but this does not include that which is bound to

heparin-like molecules on the endothelium [149]. The measurement of concentrations of thrombin–antithrombin III complex (TAT) provides a means of monitoring the elaboration of thrombin and its direct inhibition by antithrombin III [150]. TAT is thought to have a half-life in plasma of approximately 5 minutes [151]. Measurement of TAT may be clinically useful as a marker for thrombin activity, because of this rapid turnover and because blood samples do not appear to be contaminated by elaboration of the complex ex vivo [152,153].

Two assay methods are available to measure TAT levels [154,155]: RIA (normal concentrations, 2.32 ± 0.36 nM [SD]) [150] and ELISA (normal concentrations, 1.45 ± 0.4 ng/ml) [155]. Concentrations of TAT have been shown to be elevated in disseminated intravascular coagulation, deep venous thrombosis [76,156], and pulmonary embolism [157], and tend to be higher in women than in men under basal conditions [158].

Concentrations of TAT are elevated in patients with atherosclerotic heart disease, but the levels do not appear to correlate with the extent of disease [77]. In contrast, there does appear to be a relationship between TAT levels and the severity of peripheral vascular disease [159]. Concentrations of TAT are also increased in patients in whom reperfusion does not occur with coronary thrombolytic therapy [90,151], although it has not been proven that these increases are a sensitive or specific marker of reperfusion in these patients [92]. Heparin therapy does not suppress TAT formation completely, consistent with the hypothesis that thrombin elaboration during treatment with thrombolytics is resistant to heparin antithrombin III–mediated inhibition [89,92,151]. Concentrations of TAT are elevated 3 hours after thrombolysis of a lower limb arterial occlusion and after anticoagulation during coronary pulmonary bypass, and correlate with F1.2 and soluble fibrin levels [81,160]. Interestingly, TAT is decreased after 9 months of oral anticoagulation in patients with coronary artery disease, but is increased in patients treated with aspirin therapy alone [77,161], suggesting an additive role for combining antithrombotic and antiplatelet therapy in coronary artery disease.

SOLUBLE FIBRIN

There has been considerable interest in measuring soluble fibrin species in plasma as a marker of the prethrombotic state, because of its longer half-life (several hours) and decreased susceptibility to sampling artifact. However, the molecular structure of soluble fibrin species in plasma has not been well characterized, and available assays differ considerably in the methods used for detecting soluble fibrin, as will be described later. There is general agreement that soluble fibrin species result when FPA is cleaved and fibrin I associates with fibrinogen in plasma [162], and it has been shown that soluble fibrin is associated with fibrin(ogen) degradation products [162–168]. Levels of soluble fibrin species have been reported to be increased in plasma from patients with myocardial infarction or unstable angina [169–171], but the assays used in these studies were not specific for fibrin moieties so that fibrinogen degradation products may have been measured as well.

Assays for soluble fibrin have been described that measure the extent to which plasma stimulates t-PA–mediated plasminogen activation, reasoning that this stimulation is attributable to the fact that soluble fibrin acts as a cofactor for t-PA. However, this method is not specific, because fibrinogen degradation products also act as cofactors for t-PA [148]. Soluble fibrin can also be characterized by electrophoresis and immunoblotting, but this method, while more specific, is not clinically applicable. One electrophoretic approach that may be feasible for clinical assays involves extraction of fibrin-related antigens from serum with antihuman fibrinogen IgG bound to disk probes. The extracted antigens can be eluted and separated by GPR-phoresis. The proportion of each is then determined by densitometry, with the presence of fibrin monomers and small fibrin polymers confirmed by the ethanol gelation test [170,172–174].

Assays for soluble fibrin based on an ELISA incorporating monoclonal capture antibodies that are specific for neoepitopes on soluble fibrin have recently been developed. One such assay uses an antibody directed against a neoepitope on the γ-chain of fibrin formed after FPA is cleaved [175] and a tag monoclonal antibody specific for the D-region of fibrin in fibrinogen (4D2) [176] conjugated to horseradish peroxidase. In initial studies, the normal range for levels of soluble fibrin in plasma from healthy volunteers was 0.69–1.73 μg/mL, with an upper limit of normal of 1.45–4.5 μg/mL [177,178]. Changes in concentrations of soluble fibrin measured with this assay were as sensitive as measurements of FPA for detection of fibrin elaboration in vitro. In patients with myocardial infarction, soluble fibrin concentrations were increased, and they did not appear to change after treatment with SK or t-PA [178].

PROTEIN C ACTIVATION PEPTIDE

Thrombin, when bound to thrombomodulin on the vascular endothelium in the presence of calcium, activates protein C (62 kd) by cleaving protein C activation peptide, a 12-amino acid polypeptide, from the amino terminus [179]. Activated protein C proteolytically inactivates factors Va and VIIIa [180–182]. Proteolysis of these cofactors results in inactivation of the factor IXa–factor VIIIa and factor Xa–factor Va complexes (see Figure 34-1).

An RIA for protein C activation peptide was developed by Bauer et al., who reported a mean concentration in healthy volunteers of 6.47 pM, with an upper limit of normal of 180 pM [183]. The half-life of protein C activation peptide in primates was found to be approximately 5 minutes. Concentrations of protein C activation peptide were elevated in patients with disseminated intravascular coagulation and deep venous thrombosis, and decreased in response to warfarin therapy [183]. In elderly men, elevated concentrations of protein C activation peptide may be a marker of a prethrombotic state, but there appears to be no correlation with F1.2 or FPA levels [184].

Markers of Plasmin Generation

Characterization of fibrinolytic activity in vivo has been accomplished primarily by measuring the concentration of activators and inhibitors of plasminogen activation and plasmin. Plasminogen (90 kd) is activated by both fibrin-dependent t-PA and urokinase-type plasminogen activator (u-PA), both of which transform it into the double-chain enzyme, plasmin [185]. Physiologic intravascular fibrinolytic activity is attributable to t-PA, which has no catalytic activity toward fibrinogen. However, in the presence of fibrin, both t-PA and plasminogen bind to fibrin, forming a trimolecular complex that induces plasmin formation and fibrinolysis. Urokinase is secreted by cells as a single-chain polypeptide that is relatively inactive in plasma, but the enzyme appears to be the principal regulator of extravascular fibrinolytic activity when bound to specific cell receptors. Plasminogen activation is inhibited by plasminogen activator inhibitor (PAI-1) by the formation of stable complexes with either t-PA or u-PA in a 1:1 stoichiometric relationship [186–189]. Plasmin is inhibited by α_2-antiplasmin, a glycoprotein that forms a 1:1 stoichiometric complex with plasmin [190–192]. Under normal conditions, depletion of fibrinolytic inhibitors has been found to result in an increased production of plasmin and increased fibrin degradation [193].

t-PA AND PAI-1

Plasmin promotes the conversion of t-PA, a 527-amino acid polypeptide, to a two-chain molecule [194]. The one-chain form of t-PA binds fibrin more strongly than its two-chain form, which binds plasminogen and the inhibitors of t-PA more avidly [195–199]. When either t-PA or plasmin is bound to fibrin, it is relatively resistant to inactivation by PAI-1 and α_2-antiplasmin. Complexes of t-PA with PAI-1 or α_2-antiplasmin have recently been shown to be cleared from the liver by low-density lipoprotein receptor–related protein (LRP) [200–202]. The hepatic clearance of t-PA may only be initiated after complex formation with PAI-1 [203–206]. Release of t-PA is thought to be primarily from the vascular endothelium [207–209], and its concentration in plasma exhibits circadian variation and varies with age, the presence of altered hepatic clearance, or increased catecholamines [210–213].

PAI-1 (50 kd) is a serine protease inhibitor [186,201] that has the potential to inhibit plasmin, thrombin, and factors Xa, XIa, and XIIa, in addition to its primary substrates, t-PA and u-PA [214,215]. PAI-1 is synthesized by endothelial cells, and is stored in platelets [215–217], vascular smooth muscle cells, adipocytes [218], and hepatocytes [214,219]; it exists in two functionally different molecular conformations: active and latent [220–223]. The latent form can be converted to the active conformation by treatment with guanidine chloride, sodium dodecyl sulfate, or urea (denaturing conditions) ex vivo, but whether conversion occurs in vivo is not known [222,224,225]. In the α-granules of platelets, PAI-1 concentrations are high (100–200 ng/mL), but it is unclear whether this is attributable to the active or the latent form [226]. The plasma concentration of PAI-1 is 10–20 ng/mL [186,227].

Free PAI-1 has a half-life of 4 hours in plasma [224], but PAI-1 binds to the glycoprotein vitronectin with 1:1 stoichiometry, both in plasma and at extravascular sites, increasing the half-life of the complex (75 kd) to more than 24 hours, and PAI-1 remains in the active conformation when bound to the complex [228–231]. It is present at a concentration of 0.25–0.45 mg/mL in blood [231]. It is an obligatory cofactor for PAI-1 inhibition of thrombin [232,233] and potentiates PAI-1 inhibition of t-PA sixfold. Other cofactors for PAI-1 inhibition of t-PA are fibrin(ogen) and unfractionated heparin [234], but not low molecular weight heparin [235]. Heparin attenuates PAI-1 binding to vitronectin, which may make PAI-1 less stable, resulting in enhanced fibrinolytic activity [236].

Assays for PAI-1 and t-PA. Recent assays to characterize PAI-1 activity in plasma have measured the residual t-PA activity after addition of a known quan-

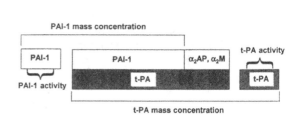

FIGURE 34-3. Assays of the fibrinolytic system. Current assays measure either mass concentration or activity. Mass concentration assays measure total PAI-1 or t-PA concentrations, whereas assay of the activity of t-PA does not measure the inactive fraction of t-PA bound to PAI-1 or other inhibitors. α_2-M = α_2-macroglobulin; α_2-AP = α_2-antiplasmin. (From Jansson JH, Boman K, Nilsson TK. Enalapril-related changes in the fibrinolytic system in survivors of myocardial infarction. Eur J Clin Pharmacol 44:485–488, 1993, with permission.)

tity of t-PA to the sample, or the activity of PAI-1 directly after addition of single-chain t-PA (Figure 34-3) [201,237–242]. Measured concentrations of PAI-1 and t-PA may be falsely high or low when measured by these methods, because of formation of t-PA–PAI-1 complexes, inhibition of t-PA by other inhibitors, concurrent thrombolysis, or platelet activation with release of active PAI-1, plasminogen, or α_2-antiplasmin during sample acquisition [239,243].

Mass concentrations of t-PA and PAI-1 have been assayed by RIA and ELISA methods (see Figure 34-3) [211,239,244–247]. These assays are more sensitive than activity-based assays and are able to detect t-PA and PAI-1, whether they are free or bound in a complex, but they may not be sufficiently sensitive for measuring minimal increases in the concentration of t-PA antigen above baseline levels [211,238,248].

Accurate measurement of PAI-1 requires rapid separation of plasma and analysis of fresh samples, because it is unstable and sensitive to repeated freezing/thawing, which may cause the release of additional PAI-1 from platelets [249]. Similar rapid handling is required before measurement of t-PA in plasma because of its instability and increased activity in the presence of fibrin. Assay of t-PA activity requires the addition of anticoagulants to prevent fibrin formation, and acidification to prevent inhibition by PAI-1, C-1 esterase inhibitor, or α_2-antiplasmin [185,201]. Samples should be obtained at the same time of day to standardize measurements when used for comparison within or between individuals, because there is a significant diurnal variation in PAI-1 and t-PA concentrations: the concentration of PAI-1 is increased and that of t-PA is decreased in the morning [250]. Some data suggest that the resulting potential for a decrease in fibrinolytic activity correlates with an increased risk of coronary thrombosis in the morning [213,249–253].

Clinical Utility of Measurements of PAI-1 and t-PA Several factors increase the synthesis of PAI-1, including endotoxemia [237,254], administration of insulin [255,256], elevations of very low density lipoproteins (VLDL) [257], and increased concentrations of low density lipoproteins (LDL) [258,259]. PAI-1 is also increased in thrombotic disorders such as myocardial infarction, deep venous thrombosis, and pulmonary embolism [237,241,260–263], but PAI-1 is not a specific marker of thromboembolic disease because it is also an acute-phase reactant and concentrations are increased after the first trimester of pregnancy, and in patients with hepatitis, pancreatitis, and malignancies [239,264–266].

PAI-1 concentrations are higher in patients with cardiovascular risk factors, such as diabetes, hypertriglyceridemia, obesity, and hypertension, and in postmenopausal women. Several investigators have found that PAI-1 is increased and correlates with high insulin levels in diabetic patients with insulin resistance syndrome, which is characterized by elevations of serum triglycerides, body mass index (BMI), and the waist-to-hip ratio (WHR) [238,267,268]. A genetic link between PAI-1 concentration and the presence of coronary artery disease in diabetic patients is suggested by the predominance of the PAI-1 genotype 4G/4G in non–insulin-dependent diabetes mellitus patients with coronary artery disease. This genotype is associated with increased PAI-1 levels [269]. Reduction of insulin levels by exercise, weight loss, or metformin therapy has been shown to decrease both insulin resistance and PAI-1 concentrations [270,271], although corresponding increases in insulin levels do not lead to an analogous increase in PAI-1 concentrations [249]. Treatment of hypertriglyceridemia with diet, weight loss, or gemfibrizol therapy decreases fibrinolytic capacity, as measured by changes in the concentration of D-dimer in response to infusion of 1-deamino-8-d-arginine vasopressin and increases in PAI-1 concentrations [272–274].

Obesity is associated with increased PAI-1 concentrations, which also correlate with BMI and WHR [275]. Concentrations of both fibrinogen and PAI-1 correlate with glucose and insulin levels [276], and

inversely correlate with BMI and t-PA activity [277]. Both WHR and PAI-1 concentrations have been found to be independent risk factors for left ventricular dysfunction [278], confirming the importance of obesity and PAI-1 as measures of the risk of heart disease.

There is evidence that estrogen increases fibrinolytic potential, possibly providing a mechanism for its cardioprotective effects [279]. Women have lower PAI-1 levels than men of the same age. In rats, the sex-related difference in PAI-1 concentration disappears after orchiectomy [280]. Women receiving oral or transdermal hormone replacement have lower PAI-1 concentrations than those not receiving treatment, irrespective of their endogenous hormone levels [281].

In patients with established hypertension, PAI-1 and t-PA antigen concentrations have been reported to be increased and t-PA activity decreased, but this relationship could be the result of preexisting atherosclerosis or the coexistence of other factors such as obesity or diabetes [277,282–284]. PAI-1 concentrations increase in a dose-dependent manner after intravenous administration of angiotensin II in both normotensive and hypertensive patients, perhaps representing a mechanism for the increased risk of thrombotic events observed in hypertensive patients with elevated renin concentrations [285,286]. In the SAVE study, PAI-1 concentrations and renin activity were compared after myocardial infarction (mean 12 days) [287]. Treatment of patients after myocardial infarction with angiotensin-converting enzyme inhibitors reduces t-PA and PAI-1 concentrations, and increases the t-PA antigen concentration [243,288,289].

The use of increased plasma levels of PAI-1 as a marker of atherosclerosis has been proposed based on the increased expression of PAI-1 in atherosclerotic tissue. Increased expression of PAI-1 mRNA has been documented in intimal smooth muscle cells, macrophages, and the fibrous cap of atherosclerotic plaques, as well as in the surrounding neovessel formation [290–292]. In patients with well-documented atherosclerosis, plasma PAI-1 and t-PA concentrations are elevated. However, the sensitivity of PAI-1 for atherosclerosis may be limited by the decreases in concentration that occur with advancing age [293]. In a case-control study, patients with atherosclerotic disease and a thrombotic event within 1 year of follow-up had significantly elevated levels of PAI-1, t-PA, and crosslinked fibrin(ogen) degradation products compared with those in patients in whom a thrombotic event did not occur [294].

However, in two other case-control studies, no association between the presence of coronary artery disease and t-PA and PAI-1 concentrations was found [295,296]. Elevations of PAI-1 and t-PA were demonstrated in patients with coronary artery disease documented by coronary angiography, but no relationship between the severity of coronary artery disease and altered fibrinolytic activity was apparent [297]. In another study, patients with exercise-induced ischemia and angiographically documented coronary disease were found to have increases in PAI-1 concentration and reductions in t-PA activation that corresponded to those associated with more severe ischemia or multivessel disease [298].

PAI-1 concentrations are higher in patients with angina without a prior myocardial infarction compared with control patients, but are even higher in patients with angina and a prior myocardial infarction, and are highest in patients with acute myocardial infarction [299,300]. Nonetheless, in several studies of patients with angina, the correlation between PAI-1 concentrations and the severity of coronary artery disease was unclear [301–304]. Whether the increases in PAI-1 observed reflect ongoing thrombosis or a risk of thrombosis has not been established, but in one study of patients with myocardial infarction without significant coronary artery disease, PAI-1 concentrations were elevated and were associated with an increased risk of spontaneous thrombosis. These patients also demonstrated decreased t-PA activity, suggesting inhibited fibrinolytic activity [305]. After myocardial infarction, concentrations of PAI-1 and t-PA remain elevated, but t-PA activity is reduced for up to 3 years [306–309]. These results suggest long-term inhibition of fibrinolytic activity in patients with coronary artery disease who have had a myocardial infarction.

It is possible that the measurement of t-PA and PAI-1 could be useful in identifying patients at high risk for future myocardial infarction [308,310,311]. In prospective studies of patients with myocardial infarction and/or severe angina for a minimum of 4 years who later developed a reinfarction, PAI-1 and t-PA antigen concentrations were elevated and t-PA activity was reduced compared with that in controls, and there was a correlation between increased t-PA antigen and mortality [312–315].

Patients exhibiting restenosis after angioplasty have higher t-PA concentrations 6 hours after the procedure, and increased free PAI-1 and t-PA concentrations at 1 week and 3 months, compared with levels in those without restenosis [302,316–318]. In patients with myocardial infarction, PAI-1 or t-PA antigen concentrations do not increase after angioplasty of arteries that have failed to recanalize with intravenous t-PA, whereas successful reperfusion after emergency catheterization and intracoronary urokinase is associated with an increase in PAI-1 concentration [319,320]. In patients with myocardial infarction treated with t-PA, PAI-1 concentrations increase more rapidly and are higher at 4 hours than those in patients treated with primary angioplasty [321]. Before initiation of therapy in patients with myocardial infarction, spontaneous intermittent myocardial reperfusion, as measured by Holter ST-segment recording, is associated with reduced levels of t-PA and C-reactive protein compared with levels in patients with myocardial infarction without evidence of intermittent reperfusion [322].

It has also been shown that patients with intermittent reperfusion exhibit increased thrombin activity (increased concentration of F1.2) and high soluble fibrin levels, even when coronary artery patency at 90 minutes after thrombolytic therapy is similar to that in patients without intermittent reperfusion [322]. It has been hypothesized that resistance to thrombolysis and reocclusion may be the result of release of PAI-1 from activated platelets and exposure of thrombus-associated procoagulants during thrombolysis [323]. Resistance to clot lysis may also be the result of α_2-antiplasmin and factor XIII–mediated fibrin crosslinking [226,324–328].

PLASMIN–α_2-ANTIPLASMIN COMPLEXES

Several assays have been developed to measure α_2-antiplasmin concentrations in plasma [329]. A latex agglutination assay developed by Collen et al. [330] has been shown to be a measure of fibrinolytic activity in patients with disseminated intravascular coagulation and after thrombolytic therapy. However, this assay is not specific for the complex; it detects free α_2-antiplasmin as well as plasmin–antiplasmin complex (PAP) [331]. With a more specific RIA, measured concentrations of free α_2-antiplasmin are shown to decrease more markedly in patients treated with SK than in those receiving t-PA, consistent with differences between these activators with regard to the extent of activation of free plasminogen [332,333]. An ELISA specific for free α_2-antiplasmin, and another specific for the complex, have also been developed, but have not been used extensively in clinical trials [329,334]. A recent study with another ELISA specific for the PAP complex has shown significantly higher levels of PAP in the presence of sepsis, malignancy, pregnancy, diabetes, myocardial infarction, and thrombolytic therapy, but it is still unclear whether the measurement of concentrations of free α_2-antiplasmin or plasmin–α_2-antiplasmin complexes is useful for defining risk in patients with acute coronary syndromes [335].

CROSSLINKED FIBRIN(OGEN) DEGRADATION PRODUCTS

Fibrin(ogen) degradation products are a heterogeneous group of polypeptides that result from the degradation by plasmin of fibrinogen, fibrin I monomer, fibrin II monomer, or crosslinked fibrin polymers (see Figure 34-2) [336,337]. Fibrinogen is composed of three polymerized chains and is a homodimer. Plasmin-induced proteolysis of fibrinogen produces the well-characterized fragments containing the amino terminus (E fragment) and carboxy terminus (D fragment; see Figure 34-2) [337,338]. Crosslinking of the γ- and α-chains of fibrin render it more resistant to further catabolism [339]. Proteolysis of crosslinked fibrin results in the release of numerous crosslinked fragments, the best characterized of which is D-dimer, which contains D regions crosslinked at the γ-chains. The plasma concentration of crosslinked fibrin degradation products (XL-FDP; half-life of 3–6 hours) [175] reflects plasmin turnover of crosslinked fibrin, which is also a sensitive marker of ongoing thrombosis; concentrations measured by most immunoassays are attributable to D-dimer and larger fragments containing D-dimer regions.

Assays for XL-FDP. Early assays for serum fibrin(ogen) degradation products were based on measurement of fibrinogen immunoreactivity with the use of polyclonal antiserum and did not distinguish between fibrin and fibrinogen degradation products. Immunoassays have been developed that are specific for fibrin degradation product neoantigens, such as fragment D and E, but these also do not distinguish between fibrin and fibrinogen degradation (see Figure 34-2).

Measurement of D-dimer may be the most specific marker of fibrinolytic activity [340]. However, early D-dimer assays varied in the absolute specificity of antibodies for XL-FDP, because non–cross-linked products of fibrinogenolysis were also measured [341–343]. Development of monoclonal antibodies specific for D-dimer has permitted accurate quantification of XL-FDP in a variety of assay formats. Immunoassays recognizing the D-D region and γ-crosslinks can distinguish crosslinked fibrin from the non–crosslinked fragments [176,344–347], and also can detect fragments DDE, DDX, and DDY (see Figure 34-2) [176]. Nonetheless, ELISAs in which one of the antibodies is not specific for fibrin degradation products can overestimate concentrations of XL-FDP, because in plasma the crosslinked fibrin species

may be associated with both crosslinked and non–crosslinked fibrin(ogen) [348–350].

Recently, more fibrin-specific crosslinked fibrin degradation product ELISAs have been described in which both the capture and tag antibodies are fibrin specific [351]. These assays do not appear to overestimate concentrations of XL-FDP in the presence of marked fibrinogenolysis [348,352]. One such assay uses a capture monoclonal antibody specific for the crosslinked D region of fibrin (3B6; Agen Biomedical Limited, Brisbane Australia) [176,347], and a fibrin-specific tag antibody (1D2; D-dimer Gold, Agen Biomedical Limited, Brisbane, Australia) conjugated to horseradish peroxidase [353]. Concentrations of XL-FDP in normal patients vary from 40 to 50 ng/mL depending on the ELISA used, reflecting differences in the specificity of monoclonal antibodies against D-dimer [351,354–356].

Rapid latex bead D-dimer tests have also been developed. Initial studies did not show them to be sufficiently sensitive for clinical use [357], but subsequent trials have shown them to be useful in the detection of deep vein thrombosis [358–361]. A rapid whole-blood assay for XL-FDP (SimpliRED D-dimer) has been recently reported to be sufficiently sensitive to exclude deep venous thrombosis, pulmonary embolism, and endotoxemia [359,362–366].

Clinical Utility of Measurements of XL-FDP. Concentrations of XL-FDP are increased in patients with thromboembolic disease, such as pulmonary embolism [157,367–370], arterial embolism, and peripheral vascular disease [159,358,371–373], and in those with disseminated intravascular coagulation, neoplasia [356], and brain trauma [374]. However, increases in XL-FDP are not specific for thrombosis; they occur in hospitalized patients without clinically evident thrombosis, likely reflecting increased fibrin turnover.

Concentrations of XL-FDP are significantly elevated in some patients with unstable angina and myocardial infarction, compared with levels in healthy volunteers and patients with stable angina [356,375–377]. Marked increases in the concentrations of XL-FDP are indicative of thrombotic complications in patients with myocardial infarction (such as severe congestive heart failure, ventricular tachycardia, mural thrombus, or death), particularly those who present more than 8 hours after the onset of symptoms, probably reflecting physiologic fibrinolysis in response to ongoing thrombosis, or a more pronounced fibrinolytic response to coronary thrombosis and infarction [348]. Thus, elevated XL-FDP may be a marker for increased risk of developing myocardial infarction-related complications and may be predictive of outcome in patients with coronary artery disease. Although not an independent risk factor for myocardial infarction, these levels are a marker of increased physiologic fibrinolysis before the development of infarction [378], and they remain elevated for 1 month after myocardial infarction [379]. In addition, elevated XL-FDP is indicative of an increased likelihood of infarction in patients with peripheral arterial disease [380], is a risk factor for rethrombosis after angioplasty [381,382], and may be an indicator of poor prognosis in patients with myocardial infarction who are treated medically (e.g., warfarin) [161].

Levels of XL-FDP increase in patients receiving fibrinolytic therapy for venous or arterial disease [356,375–377]. However, because of the lack of specificity of most ELISAs used in earlier studies [352,376], quantitative interpretation of the results of the assays for characterization of the extent of crosslinked fibrin degradation is not possible. Measurement of XL-FDP appears useful for excluding venous thrombosis in some clinical settings, and as a marker of complications in patients with coronary artery disease. The most recently available rapid bedside assays for XL-FDP offer the potential for extensive clinical use of this marker of thrombosis and fibrinolysis.

β FIBRINOPEPTIDES: Bβ1-42, β15-42

Fibrinopeptides are measures of plasmin activity on fibrin and fibrin(ogen) degradation products (see Figure 34-2) [336]. Bβ1-42 is cleaved from fibrinogen or fibrin I by plasmin. The median concentration is 1.2 pmol/mL in healthy volunteers [383]. Plasmin proteolysis of fibrin II, which lacks FPB, results in the formation of β15-24 [116,384–386], the half-life of which is 10–20 minutes. β15-42 is not detected in plasma unless there is fibrinolysis [387,388].

Several assays based on polyclonal antisera have been developed to measure Bβ1-42; however, most detected β15-42 as well [116,336]. Specific ELISAs have been developed to Bβ1-42 and β15-42 using monoclonal antibodies [116]. In renal failure patients, concentrations of all Bβ fragments were shown to be elevated because of decreased clearance [389]. Increases in β15-42 have also been reported in patients with venous thrombosis, disseminated intravascular coagulation, liver disease, pancreatitis, pregnancy-related fibrinolytic disorders, malignancies, after exercise, and with the use of either antithrombotics or thrombolytic therapy [376,390]. However, β15-24 concentrations do not appear to be significantly elevated in patients with uncomplicated myocardial infarction. Bβ1-42 is a specific and sensitive marker of fibrinolysis and has been used to characterize the fibrin specificity of fibrinolytic agents, particularly with t-PA and other fibrin-specific activators [391].

Future Role for Markers of Thrombosis and Fibrinolysis

The value of markers of procoagulant and fibrinolytic activity in vivo in the routine clinical evaluation of patients with ischemic heart disease remains to be defined. Although assays of plasma concentrations of fibrinopeptide A, prothrombin fragment 1.2, and thrombin–antithrombin III complexes have been shown to be useful in well-defined populations in clinical studies, the value of these assays in unselected populations, even when performed with optimal techniques, has not been well characterized. Nonetheless, the potential value of such markers in assessing the response to novel anticoagulant therapies is considerable. Further development of assays of soluble fibrin or measurement of fibrinopeptide A in urine are potential novel approaches for characterizing thrombin activity that should be considered in the future. In addition, recently developed rapid assays for measurement of XL-FDP appear to be very sensitive for the detection of these markers of venous thrombosis and of increased risk for thrombotic complications in patients with acute ischemia. If these results are confirmed, it is likely that rapid assays of XL-FDP will be more widely used clinically for detection of thombosis in vivo.

There is considerable evidence that fibrinolysis may be impaired in patients with atherosclerosis and ischemic heart disease, and several studies have shown that increases in plasma concentrations of PAI-1 are markers of increased risk in patients with ischemic heart disease. The clinical application of these observations will depend on whether future studies define the role of measurements of PAI-1 in guiding therapeutic interventions. Other methods, such as measurement of XL-FDP, may also have prognostic value in such patients and may be more clinically applicable.

In summary, the potential value of markers of thrombosis and fibrinolysis in identifying patients at high risk of thrombotic events and in evaluating the response to therapeutic interventions is widely appreciated. The biochemical and physiologic validity of these markers appears well established, and there are now considerable data regarding the validity of specific assays. However, additional clinical studies focusing on the value of these assays in guiding therapeutic interventions are necessary before widespread clinical application can be advocated.

Acknowledgments

This work was supported in part by a SCOR in Coronary and Vascular Disease, grant no. HL-17646, National Heart, Lung, and Blood Institute, National Institutes of Health, Bethesda, MD.

References

1. Bach RR. Initiation of coagulation by tissue factor. CRC Crit Rev Biochem 23:339, 1988.
2. Drake TA, Morrissey JH, Edgington TS. Selective cellular expression of tissue factor in human tissues. Am J Pathol 134:1087, 1989.
3. Wilcox JN, Smith KM, Schwartz SM, Gordon D. Localization of tissue factor in the normal vessel wall and in the atherosclerotic plaque. Proc Natl Acad Sci USA 86:2839, 1989.
4. Annex BH, Denning SM, Channon KM, Sketch MH Jr, Stack RS, Morrissey JH, Peters KG. Differential expression of tissue factor protein in directional atherectomy specimens from patients with stable and unstable coronary syndromes. Circulation 91:619, 1995.
5. Marmur JD, Rossikhina M, Guha A, Fyfe B, Friedrich V, Medlowitz M, Nemerson Y, Taubman MB. Tissue factor is rapidly induced in arterial smooth muscle after balloon injury. J Clin Invest 91:2253, 1993.
6. Taubman MB. Tissue factor regulation in vascular smooth muscle: A summary of studies performed using in vivo and in vitro models. Am J Cardiol 72:55C, 1993.
7. Albrecht S, Luther T, Grossman H, Flossel C, Kotzsch M, Muller M. An ELISA for tissue factor using monoclonal antibodies. Blood Coagul Fibrinolysis 3:263, 1992.
8. Takahashi H, Satoh N, Wada K, Takakuwa E, Seki Y, Shibata A. Tissue factor in plasma of patients with disseminated intravascular coagulation. Am J Hematol 46:333, 1994.
9. Koyama T, Nishida K, Ohdama S, Sawada M, Murakami N, Hirosawa S, Kuriyama R, Matsuzawa K, Hasegawa R, Aoki N. Determination of plasma tissue factor antigen and its clinical significance. Br J Haematol 87:343, 1994.
10. Fukada S, Iijima K, Nakamura K. Measuring tissue factor (factor III) activity in plasma. Clin Chem 35:1897, 1989.
11. Iijima K, Fukuda C, Nakamura K. Measurements of tissue factor-like activity in plasma of patients with DIC. Thromb Res 61:29, 1991.
12. Francis JL, Carvalho M, Francis DA. The clinical value of tissue factor assays. Blood Coagul Fibrinolysis 6:S37, 1995.
13. Leatham EW, Bath PMW, Tooze JA, Camm AJ. Increased monocyte tissue factor expression in coronary disease. Br Heart J 73:10, 1995.
14. Serneri GGN, Abbate R, Gori AM, Attanasio M, Martini F, Giusti B, Dabizzi P, Poggesi L, Modesti PA, Trotta F, Rostagno C, Boddi M, Gensini GF. Transient intermittent lymphocyte activation is responsible for the instability of angina. Circulation 86:790, 1992.
15. Jude B, Agraou B, McFadden EP, Susen S, Bauters C, Lepelley P, Vanhaesbroucke C, Devos P, Cosson A, Asseman P. Evidence for time-dependent activation of monocytes in the systemic circulation in unstable angina but not in acute myocardial infarction or in stable angina. Circulation 90:1662, 1994.
16. Edwards RL, Silver J, Rickles FR. Human tumor procoagulants: Registry of the Subcommittee on Haemostasis and Malignancy of the Scientific and Standardization Committee, International Society on Thrombosis and Haemostasis. Thromb Haemost 69:205, 1993.
17. Andoh K, Kubota T, Takada M, Tanaka H, Kobayashi N, Maekawa T. Tissue factor activity in leukemia cells. Special reference to disseminated intravascular coagulation. Cancer 59:748, 1987.
18. Nawroth PP, Handley DA, Esmon CT, Stern DM. Interleukin 1 induces endothelial cell procoagulant while suppressing cell surface anticoagulant activity. Proc Natl Acad Sci USA 83:3460, 1986.
19. Archipoff G, Beretz A, Freyssinet J, Klein-Soyer C, Brisson C, Cazenave JP. Heterogeneous regulation of constitutive thrombomodulin or inducible tissue factor activities on the surface of human saphenous vein endothelial cells in culture following stimulation by interleukin-1, tumor necrosis factor, thrombin or phorbol ester. Biochem J 273:679, 1991.
20. Wada H, Wakita Y, Shiku H. Tissue factor expression in endothelial cells in health and disease. Blood Coagul Fibrinolysis 6:S26, 1995.
21. Nakagaki T, Foster DC, Berkner KL, Kisiel W. Initiation of the extrinsic pathway of blood coagulation: Evidence for the factor dependent autoactivation of human coagulation factor VII. Biochemistry 30:10819, 1991.
22. Seligsohn U, Casper CK, Osterud B, Rapaport SI. Activated factor VII: Presence in factor IX concentrates and persistence in the circulation after infusion. Blood 53:828, 1979.
23. Nemerson Y, Repke D. Tissue factor accelerates the activation of coagulation factor VII: The role of a bifunctional coagulation cofactor. Thromb Res 40:351, 1985.
24. Nemerson Y, Esnouf MP. Activation of a proteolytic system by a membrane lipoprotein: Mechanism of action of tissue factor. Proc Natl Acad Sci USA 70:310, 1973.
25. Seligsohn U, Osterud B, Rapaport SI. Coupled amidolytic assay for factor VII: Its use with a clotting assay to determine the activity state of factor VII. Blood 52:978, 1978.

26. Morrissey J. Tissue factor interactions with factor VII: Measurement and clinical significance of factor VIIa in plasma. Blood Coagul Fibrinolysis 6:S14, 1995.

27. Morrissey JH, Macik BG, Neuenschwander PF, Comp PC. Quantitation of activation factor VII levels in plasma using a tissue factor mutant selectively deficient in promoting factor VII activation. Blood 81:734, 1993.

28. Hultin MB. Fibrinogen and factor VII as risk factors in vascular disease. Prog Hemost Thromb 10:215, 1991.

29. Broze GJ, Hickman S, Miletich JP. Monoclonal anti-human factor VII antibodies. Detection in plasma of a second protein antigenically and genetically related to factor VII. J Clin Invest 76:937, 1985.

30. Takase T, Tuddenham E, Chand S, Goodall AH. Monoclonal antibodies to human factor VII: A one step immunoradiometric assay for VII:Ag. J Clin Pathol 41:337, 1988.

31. Bom VJJ, van Tilburg NH, Krommenhoek-van Es C, Bertina RM. Immunoradiometric assays for human coagulation factor VII using polyclonal antibodies against the Ca(II)-dependent and Ca(II)-independent conformation. Thromb Haemost 56:343, 1986.

32. Kitchen S, Malia RG, Preston FE. A comparison of methods for the measurement of activated factor VII. Thromb Haemost 68:301, 1992.

33. Mann KG. Factor VII assays, plasma triglyceride levels, and cardiovascular disease risk. Arteriosclerosis 9:783, 1989.

34. Waxman E, Ross JB, Laue TM, Guha A, Thiruvikraman SV, Lin TC, Konigsberg WH, Nemerson Y. Tissue factor and its extracellular soluble domain: The relationship between intermolecular association with factor VIIa and enzymatic activity of the complex. Biochemistry 31:3998, 1992.

35. Waxman E, Laws WR, Laue TM, Yale N, Ross JBA. Human factor VIIa and its complex with soluble tissue factor: Evaluation of asymmetry and conformational dynamics by ultracentrifugation and fluorescence anisotropy decay methods. Biochemistry 32:3005, 1993.

36. Paborsky LR, Caras IW, Fisher KL, Gorman CM. Lipid association, but not the transmembrane domain, is required for tissue factor activity. Substitution of the transmembrane domain with a phosphatidylinositol anchor. J Biol Chem 32:3005, 1991.

37. Neuenschwander PF, Morrissey JH. Deletion of the membrane-anchoring region of tissue factor abolishes autoactivation of factor VII, but not cofactor function: Analysis of a mutant with a selective deficiency in activity. J Biol Chem 267:14477, 1992.

38. Kario K, Sakata T, Matsuo T, Miyata T. Factor VII in non-insulin-dependent diabetic patients with microalbuminuria. Lancet 342:1552, 1993.

39. Kario K, Miyata T, Sakata T, Matsuo T, Kato H. Fluorogenic assay of activated factor VII: Plasma factor VIIa levels in relation to arterial vascular diseases in Japanese. Arterioscler Thromb 14:265, 1994.

40. Rugman FP, Jenkins JA, Daguid JK, Maggs PB, Hay CRM. Prothrombin fragment F1+2: Correlations with cardiovascular risk factors. Blood Coagul Fibrinolysis 5:335, 1994.

41. Meade TW, Brozovic M, Chakrabarti RA, Haines AP, Imeson JD, Mellows S, Miller GJ, North WRS, Stirling Y, Thompson SG. Haemostatic function and ischaemic heart disease: Principal results of the Northwick Park Heart Study. Lancet 2:533, 1986.

42. Balleisen L, Schulte H, Assmann G, Epping PH, Loo JVD. Coagulation factors and the progress of coronary heart disease. Lancet 2:461, 1987.

43. Hoffman C, Shah A, Sodums M, Hultin MB. Factor VII activity state in coronary artery disease. J Lab Clin Med 111:475, 1988.

44. Carvalho de Sousa J, Azevedo J, Soria C, Barros F, Ribeiro C, Parreira F, Caens JP. Factor VII hyperactivity in acute myocardial thrombosis: A relation to the coagulation activation. Thromb Res 51:165, 1988.

45. Cortellaro M, Boschetti C, Cofrancesco E, Zanussi C, Catalano M, Gaetano GD, Gabrielli L, Lombardi B, Specchia G, Tavazzi L, Tremoli E, Volpe AD, Polli E, for The PLAT Study Group. The PLAT study: Hemostatic function in relation to atherothrombotic ischemic events in vascular disease patients — principal results. Arterioscler Thromb 12:1063, 1992.

46. Heinrich J, Balleisen L, Schulte H, Assmann G, Loo JVD. Fibrinogen and factor VII in the prediction of coronary risk: Results from the PROCAM study in healthy men. Arterioscler Thromb 14:54, 1994.

47. Ruddock V, Meade TW. Factor-VII activity and ischaemic heart disease: Fatal and non-fatal events. Q J Med 87:403, 1994.

48. Miller G, Stirling Y, Esnouf MP, Heinrich J, Loo JVD, Kienast J, Wu KK, Morrissey JH, Meade TW, Martin JC, Imeson JD, Cooper JA, Finch A. Factor VII-deficient substrate plasmas depleted of protein C raise the sensitivity of the factor VII bioassay to activated factor VII: An international study. Thromb Haemost 71:38, 1994.

49. Broze GJ, Girard TJ, Novotony WF. Regulation of coagulation by a multivalent Kunitz-type inhibitor. Biochemistry 29:7539, 1990.

50. Rappaport SI. The extrinsic pathway inhibitor: A regulator of tissue factor-dependent blood coagulation. Thromb Haemost 66:6, 1991.

51. Novotny WF, Girard TJ, Miletich JP, Broze GJ. Platelets secrete a coagulation inhibitor functionally and antigenically similar to the lipoprotein associated coagulation inhibitor. Blood 72:2020, 1988.

52. Erhardtsen E, Ezban M, Madsen MT, Diness V, Glazer S, Hedner U, Nordfang O. Blocking of tissue factor pathway inhibitor (TFPI) shortens the bleeding time in rabbits with antibody induced haemophilia A. Blood Coagul Fibrinolysis 6:388, 1995.

53. Lindahl AK, Odegaard OR, Sandset PM, Harbitz TB.

Coagulation inhibition and activation in pancreatic cancer: Changes during progress of disease. Cancer 70:2067, 1992.

54. Sandset PM, Lund H, Norseth J, Abilgaard U, Ose L. Treatment with hydroxymethylglutaryl-coenzyme A reductase inhibitors in hypercholesterolemia induces changes in the components of the extrinsic coagulation system. Arterioscler Thromb 11:138, 1991.

55. Hansen JB, Olsen JO, Osterud B. Physical exercise enhances plasma levels of extrinsic pathway inhibitor. Thromb Haemost 64:124, 1990.

56. Novotny WF, Brown SG, Miletich JP, Rader DJ, Broze GJ. Plasma antigen levels of the lipoprotein-associated coagulation inhibitor in patient samples. Blood 78:387, 1991.

57. Warr TA, Rao LV, Rapaport SI. Human plasma extrinsic pathway inhibitor activity: II. Plasma levels in disseminated intravascular coagulation and hepatocellular disease. Blood 74:994, 1989.

58. Sabharwal AK, Ameri A, Bajaj M, Hyers TM, Tricomi SM, Taylor FB, Bajaj SP. Tissue factor pathway inhibitor levels in plasma and lavage fluids in acute lung injury. Am Rev Respir Dis 145:453a, 1992.

59. Sandset PM, Sirnes PA, Abilgaard U. Factor VII and extrinsic pathway inhibitor in acute coronary disease. Br J Haematol 72:391, 1989.

60. Moore E, Hamsten A, Karpe F, Bavenholm P, Blomback M, Silveria A. Relationship of tissue factor pathway inhibitor activity to plasma lipoproteins and myocardial infarction at a young age. Thromb Haemost 71:707, 1994.

61. Hansen JB, Huseby KR, Huseby NE, Sandset PM, Hanssen TA, Nordoy A. Effect of cholesterol lowering on intravascular pools of TFPI and its anticoagulant potential in type II hyperlipoproteinemia. Arterioscler Thromb Vasc Biol 15:879, 1995.

62. Sandset PM, Abilgaard U, Larsen ML. Heparin induces release of extrinsic coagulation pathway inhibitor (EPI). Thromb Res 50:803, 1988.

63. Valentin S, Ostergaard P, Kristensen H, Nordfang O. Simultaneous presence of tissue factor pathway inhibitor (TFPI) and low molecular weight heparin has a synergistic effect in different coagulation assays. Blood Coagul Fibrinolysis 2:692, 1991.

64. Hoppensteadt DA, Jeske W, Fareed J, Bermes EWJ. The role of tissue factor pathway inhibitor in the mediation of the antithrombotic actions of heparin and low-molecular-weight heparin. Blood Coagul Fibrinolysis 6:S57, 1995.

65. Broze GJ. Tissue factor pathway inhibitor and the revised theory of coagulation. Ann Rev Med 46:103, 1995.

66. Anderson S, Cohen AT, Melissari E, Scully MS, Kakkar VV. Loss of heparin-releasable tissue factor pathway inhibitor in patients undergoing PTCA. Thromb Haemost 73:324, 1995.

67. Kijowski R, Hoppensteadt D, Walenga J, Borris L, Lassen NR, Fareed J. Role of tissue factor pathway inhibitor in post surgical deep venous thrombosis (DVT) prophylaxis in patients treated with low molecular weight heparin. Thromb Res 74:53, 1994.

68. Jeske W, Hoppensteadt D, Klauser R, Kammereit A, Eckenberger P, Haas S, Wyld P, Fareed J. Effect of repeated aprosulate and enoxaparin administration on tissue factor pathway inhibitor antigen levels. Blood Coagul Fibrinolysis 6:119, 1995.

69. Teitel JM, Bauer KA, Lau HK, Rosenberg RD. Studies of the prothrombin activation pathway utilizing radioimmunoassays for the F2/F1+2 fragment and thrombin-antithrombin complex. Blood 59:1086, 1983.

70. Miletich JP, Jackson CM, Majerus PW. Properties of the factor Xa binding site on platelets. J Biol Chem 253:6908, 1978.

71. Mann KG, Nesheim ME, Church WR, Haley P, Krishnaswamy S. Surface-dependent reactions of the vitamin K-dependent enzyme complexes. Blood 76:1, 1990.

72. Bauer KA, Rosenberg RD. Activation markers of coagulation. Bailliere's Clin Haematol 7:523, 1994.

73. Lau HK, Rosenberg JS, Beeler DL, Rosenberg RD. The isolation and characterization of a specific antibody population directed against the prothrombin activation fragments F2 and F1+2. J Biol Chem 254:8751, 1979.

74. Tripoldi A, Chantarngkul V, Bottasso B, Mannucci PM. Poor comparability of prothrombin fragment 1 + 2 values measured by two commercial ELISA methods: Influence of different anticoagulants and standards. Thromb Haemost 71:605, 1994.

75. Boneu B, Bes G, Pelzer H, Sie P, Boccalon H. D-dimer, thrombin antithrombin III complexes, and prothrombin fragments 1 + 2: Diagnostic value in clinically suspected deep vein thrombosis. Thromb Haemost 65:28, 1991.

76. Boisclair MD, Ireland H, Lane DA. Assessment of hypercoagulable states by measurement of activation fragments and peptides. Blood Rev 4:25, 1990.

77. Kienast J, Thompson SG, Raskino C, Pelzer H, Fechtrup C, Ostermann H, Loo JVD. Prothrombin activation fragment 1 + 2 and thrombin antithrombin III complexes in patients with angina pectoris: Relation to the presence and severity of coronary atherosclerosis. Thromb Haemost 70:550, 1993.

78. Merlini PA, Bauer KA, Oltrona L, Ardissino D, Cattaneo M, Belli C, Mannucci PM, Rosenberg RD. Persistent activation of coagulation mechanism in unstable angina and myocardial infarction. Circulation 90:61, 1994.

79. Bruhn HD, Liebsch J, Wagner C. Documentation of hypocoagulability by measurement of prothrombin fragment F1+2 when introducing oral anticoagulant therapy. Thromb Res 68:317, 1992.

80. Estivals M, Pelzer H, Sie P, Pichon J, Boccalon H, Boneu B. Prothrombin fragment 1 + 2, thrombin-antithrombin III complexes and D-dimers in acute

deep vein thrombosis: Effects of heparin treatment. Br J Haematol 78:421, 1991.

81. Slaughter TF. Characterization of prothrombin activation during cardiac surgery by hemostatic molecular markers. Anesthesiology 80:520, 1994.

82. Smith RC, Leung JM, Mangano DT, The SPI Research Group. Postoperative myocardial ischemia in patients undergoing coronary artery bypass graft surgery. Anesthesiology 74:464, 1991.

83. Bauer KA, Rosenberg RD. The pathophysiology of the prethrombotic state in humans: Insights gained from studies using markers of hemostatic system activation. Blood 70:343, 1987.

84. Li Z, Wu J, Mammen EF. Prothrombin fragment F1+2 and oral anticoagulant therapy. Thromb Res 75:601, 1994.

85. Hafner G, Swars H, Erbel R, Ehrenthal W, Rupprecht HJ, Lotz J, Meyer J, Prellwitz W. Monitoring prothrombin fragment 1 + 2 during initiation of oral anticoagulant therapy after intercoronary stenting. Ann Hematol 65:83, 1992.

86. van den Bos AA, Deckers JW, Heyndrickx GR, Laarman GJ, Suryapranata H, Zijlstra F, Close P, Rijnierse JJMM, Buller HR, Serruys PW. Safety and efficacy of recombinant hirudin (CGP 39 393) versus heparin in patients with stable angina undergoing coronary angioplasty. Circulation 88:2058, 1993.

87. Kaiser B, Fareed J, Walenga JM, Hopensteadt D, Markwardt F. In vitro studies in thrombin generation in citrated, r-hirudinized and heparinized whole blood. Semin Thromb Res 64:589, 1991.

88. Gallitz S, Muntean W. Thrombin-hirudin complex formation, thrombin-antithrombin III complex formation, and thrombin generation after intrinsic activation of plasma. Thromb Haemost 72:387, 1994.

89. Eisenberg PR, Sobel BE, Jaffe AS. Activation of prothrombin accompanying thrombolysis with recombinant tissue-type plasminogen activator. J Am Coll Cardiol 19:1065, 1992.

90. Merlini PA, Bauer KA, Oltrona L, Ardissino D, Spinola A, Cattaneo M, Broccolino M, Mannuci PM, Rosenberg RD. Thrombin generation and activity during thrombolysis and concomitant heparin therapy in patients with acute myocardial infarction. J Am Coll Cardiol 25:203, 1995.

91. Ewald GA, Eisenberg PR. Plasmin-mediated activation of the contact system in response to pharmacologic thrombolysis. Circulation 91:28, 1995.

92. Scharfstein JS, Abendschein DR, Eisenberg PR, George D, Cannon CP, Becker RC, Sobel BE, Cupples LA, Braunwald E, Loscalzo J, for the TIMI-5 Investigators. Fibrino(geno)lytic and procoagulant markers during thrombolytic therapy with rt-PA and adjunctive antithrombotic therapy predict clinical outcomes. Am J Cardiol 78:503, 1996.

93. Nossel HL, Yudelman RE, Canfield VP, Butler VP, Spanondis K, Wilner GD, Qureshi GD. Measure-ment of fibrinopeptide A in human blood. J Clin Invest 54:43, 1974.

94. Blomback B, Hessel B, Hogg D, Therkidsen L. A two-step fibrinogen-fibrin transition in blood coagulation. Nature 275:501, 1978.

95. Blomback B, Vestermark A. Isolation of fibrinopeptides by chromatography. Arkiv Kemi 12:173, 1958.

96. Bilizekian SB, Nossel HL, Butler VP, Canfield R. Radioimmunoassay of human fibrinopeptide B and kinetics of fibrinopeptide cleavage by different enzymes. J Clin Invest 6:438, 1975.

97. Laudano AP, Doolittle RF. Influence of calcium ion on the binding of fibrin amino terminal peptides to fibrinogen. Science 212:457, 1981.

98. Hermans J, McDonagh J. Fibrin: Structure and interactions. Semin Thromb Hemost 8:11, 1982.

99. Shainoff J, Page T. Significance of cryoprofibrin in fibrinogen-fibrin conversion. J Exp Med 116:687, 1962.

100. Yudelman IM, Nossel HL, Kaplan KL, Hirsh J. Plasma fibrinopeptide A levels in symptomatic venous thromboembolism. Blood 51:1189, 1978.

101. Blomback B, Blomback M, Edman P, Hessel B. Human fibrinopeptides: Isolation, characterization and structure. Biochim Biophys Acta 115:371, 1966.

102. Koehn JA, Canfield RE. Purification of human fibrinopeptides by high performance liquid chromatography. Anal Biochem 116:349, 1981.

103. Seydewitz HH, Witt I. Increased phosphorylation of human fibrinopeptide A under acute phase conditions. Thromb Res 40:29, 1985.

104. Alkjaersig N, Fletcher AP. Catabolism and excretion of fibrinopeptide A. Blood 60:148, 1982.

105. Leeksma OC, Meijer-Huizinga F, Stoepman-van Dalen EA, van Aken WG, van Mourik JA. Fibrinopeptide A in urine from patients with venous thromboembolism, disseminated intravascular coagulation and rheumatoid arthritis — evidence for dephosphorylation and carboxyterminal degradation of the peptide by the kidney. Thromb Haemost 54:792, 1985.

106. Wilensky RL, Zeller JA, Wish M, Tulchinsky M. Urinary fibrinopeptide A levels in ischemic heart disease. J Am Coll Cardiol 14:597, 1989.

107. Nossel H, Younger L, Wilner G, Procupez T, Canfield R, Butler VPJ. Radioimmunoassay of human fibrinopeptide A. Proc Natl Acad Sci USA 68:2350, 1971.

108. Wilner GD, Nossel HL, Canfield RE, Butler VPJ. Immunochemical studies of human fibrinopeptide A using synthetic peptide homologues. Biochemistry 15:1209, 1976.

109. Soulier J. A new adsorption agent for coagulation factors. J Clin Pathol 12:303, 1959.

110. Soulier JP, Prou-Wartelle O. Action de divers "adsorbants" sur les facteurs de coagulation. Nouv Rev Fr Hematol 15:195, 1975.

111. Cronlund M, Hardin J, Burton J, Lee L, Haber E,

Bloch K. Fibrinopeptide A in plasma of normal subjects and patients with disseminated intravascular coagulation and systemic lupus erythematosis. J Clin Invest 58:142, 1976.

112. Kockum C. Radioimmunoassay of fibrinopeptide A: clinical applications. Thromb Haemost 8:225, 1976.

113. Gerrits W, Flier O, Meer JVD. Fibrinopeptide A immunoreactivity in human plasma. Thromb Res 5:197, 1974.

114. Budzynski A, Marder V. Determination of human fibrinopeptide A by radioimmunoassay in purified systems and in the blood. Thromb Diath Haemorrh 34:709, 1975.

115. Nossel HL, Butler VP, Wilner GD, Canfield RE, Harfenist EJ. Specificity of antisera to human fibrinopeptide A used in clinical fibrinopeptide A assays. Thromb Haemost 35:101, 1976.

116. Kudryk B, Robinson D, Netre C, Hessel B, Blomback M, Blomback B. Measurement in human blood of fibrinogen/fibrin fragments containing the Bβ15–42 sequence. Thromb Res 25:277, 1982.

117. Nossel HL, Butler VP, Canfield AG, Yudelman I, Kalliope-Spanondis MT, Soland T. Potential use of fibrinopeptide A measurement in the diagnosis and management of thrombosis. Thromb Diathes Haemorrh 33:426, 1975.

118. Eisenberg PR. Novel antithrombotic strategies for the treatment of coronary artery thrombosis: A critical appraisal. J Thromb Thrombolysis 1:237, 1995.

119. Hotchkiss KA, Chesterman CN, Hogg PJ. Inhibition of heparin activity in plasma by soluble fibrin: Evidence for ternary thrombin-fibrin-heparin complex formation. Blood 84:498, 1994.

120. Eckhardt J, LaGama KS, Nossel HL. Measurement of des arginine fibrinopeptide B (des-arg-FPB) in plasma by radioimmunoassay. Thromb Haemost 42:97, 1979.

121. De Boer AC, Turpie AGG, Butt RW, Duke RJ, Bloch RF, Genton E. Plasma betathromboglobulin and serum fragment E in acute partial stroke. Br J Haematol 50:327, 1982.

122. Lane DA, Wolff S, Ireland H, Gawel M, Foadi M. Activation of coagulation and fibrinolytic systems following stroke. Br J Haematol 53:655, 1983.

123. Hofmann V, Straub PW. A radioimmunoassay technique for the rapid measurement of human fibrinopeptide A. Thromb Res 11:171, 1977.

124. Peuscher FW, van Aken WG, Flier OTN, Stoepman-van Dalen EA, Cremer-Goote TM, van Mourik JA. Effect of anticoagulant treatment measured by fibrinopeptide A (fpA) in patients with venous thromboembolism. Thromb Res 18:33, 1980.

125. Rickles FR, Edwards RL, Barb C, Cronlund M. Abnormalities of blood coagulation in patients with cancer. Fibrinopeptide A and tumor growth. Cancer 51:301, 1983.

126. Ireland H, Lane DA, Wolff S, Foadi M. In vivo platelet release in myeloproliferative disorders. Thromb Haemost 48:41, 1982.

127. Douglas JT, Lowe GDO, Forbes CD, Prentice CRM. Plasma fibrinopeptide A and β-thromboglobulin in patients with chest pain. Thromb Haemost 50:541, 1983.

128. Eisenberg PR, Sherman LA, Dickens J, Perez J, Jaffe AS. Detection of mural thrombus by assay of fibrinopeptide A (FPA) in plasma. Circulation 72:249, 1985.

129. Meade TW, Howarth DJ, Stirling Y, Welch TP, Crompton MR. Fibrinopeptide A and sudden coronary death. Lancet 2:607, 1984.

130. Nichols AB, Owen J, Kaplan KL, Sciacca AR, Cannon PJ, Nossel HL. Fibrinopeptide A, platelet factor 4, and betathromboglobulin levels in coronary heart disease. Blood 60:650, 1982.

131. Wilner GD, Chatpar P, Arnanda T, Horowitz J. Effects of extravascular clotting on fibrinopeptide A levels in blood. J Lab Clin Med 91:205, 1978.

132. Serneri GGN, Gensini GF, Carnovali M, Prisco D, Rogasi PG, Casolo GC, Fazi A, Abbate R. Association between time of increased fibrinopeptide A levels in plasma and episodes of spontaneous angina: A controlled prospective study. Am Heart J 113:672, 1987.

133. Ardissino D, Gamba MG, Merlini PA, Rolla A, Barberis P, Demicheli G, Testa S, Bruno N, Specchia G. Fibrinopeptide A excretion in urine: A marker of the cumulative thrombin activity in stable versus unstable angina patients. Am J Cardiol 68:58B, 1991.

134. Eisenberg PR, Sherman LA, Schectman K, Perez J, Sobel BE, Jaffe AS. Fibrinopeptide A: A marker of acute coronary thrombosis. Circulation 71:912, 1985.

135. Eisenberg PR, Kenzora JL, Sobel BE, Ludbrook PA, Jaffe AS. Relation between ST segment shifts during ischemia and thrombin activity in patients with unstable angina. J Am Coll Cardiol 18:898, 1991.

136. Wilensky RL, Bourdillon PDV, Vix VA, Zeller JA. Intracoronary artery thrombus formation in unstable angina: A clinical, biochemical, and angiographic correlation. J Am Coll Cardiol 21:692, 1993.

137. van Hultsteijn H, Kolff J, Briet E, van der Laarse A, Bertina R. Fibrinopeptide A and beta thromboglobulin in patients with angina pectoris and acute myocardial infarction. Am Heart J 107:39, 1984.

138. Mombelli G, Im Hof V, Haeberli A, Straub PW. Effect of heparin on plasma fibrinopeptide A in patients with acute myocardial infarction. Circulation 69:684, 1984.

139. Oltrona L, Eisenberg PR, Lasala JM, Sewall DJ, Shelton ME, Winters KJ. Association of heparin-resistant thrombin activity with acute ischemic complications of coronary interventions. Circulation 94:2064, 1996.

140. Gallino A, Haeberli A, Hess T, Mombelli G, Straub PW. Fibrin formation and platelet aggregation in patients with acute myocardial infarction: Effects of

intravenous and subcutaneous low-dose heparin. Am Heart J 112:285, 1986.

141. Eisenberg PR, Sherman LA, Rich M, Schwartz D, Schectman K, Geltman EM, Sobel BE, Jaffe AS. Importance of continued activation of thrombin reflected by fibrinopeptide A to the efficacy of thrombolysis. J Am Coll Cardiol 7:1255, 1986.

142. Owen J, Friedman KD, Grossman BA, Wilkins C, Berke AD, Powers ER. Thrombolytic therapy with tissue plasminogen activator or streptokinase induces transient thrombin activity. Blood 72:616, 1988.

143. Eisenberg PR, Sherman LA, Jaffe AS. Paradoxic elevation of fibrinopeptide A: Evidence for continued thrombosis despite intensive fibrinolysis. J Am Coll Cardiol 10:527, 1987.

144. Galvani M, Abendschein DR, Ferrini D, Ottani F, Rusticali F, Eisenberg PR. Failure of fixed dose intravenous heparin to suppress increases in thrombin activity after coronary thrombolysis with streptokinase. J Am Coll Cardiol 24:1445, 1994.

145. Rapold HJ, Kuemmerli H, Weiss M, Baur H, Haeberli A. Monitoring of fibrin generation during thrombolytic therapy of acute myocardial infarction with recombinant tissue-type plasminogen activator. Circulation 79:980, 1989.

146. Rapold HJ. Promotion of thrombin activity by thrombolytic therapy without simultaneous anticoagulation. Lancet 1:481, 1990.

147. Reganon E, Vila V, Aznar J, Lacueva V, Martinez V, Ruano M. Studies on the functionality of newly synthesized fibrinogen after treatment of acute myocardial infarction with streptokinase, increase in the rate of fibrinopeptide release. Thromb Haemost 70:978, 1993.

148. Weitz JI, Cruickshank MK, Thong B, Leslie B, Levine MN, Ginsberg J, Eckhardt T. Human tissue-type plasminogen activator releases fibrinopeptides A and B from fibrinogen. J Clin Invest 82:1700, 1988.

149. Carlson TH, Simon TL, Atencio AC. In vivo behavior of human radioiodinated antithrombin III: Distribution among three physiologic pools. Blood 66:13, 1985.

150. Teitel JM, Rosenberg RD. Protection of factor Xa from neutralization by heparin-antithrombin complex. J Clin Invest 71:1383, 1983.

151. Gulba DC, Barthels M, Westhoff-Bleck M, Jost S, Wolff R, Daniel WG, Hecker H, Lichtlen PR. Increased thrombin levels during thrombolytic therapy in acute myocardial infarction. Relevance for the success of therapy. Circulation 83:937, 1991.

152. Blanke H, Praetorius G, Leschke M, Seitz R, Egbring R, Strauer BE. Die bedeutung des thrombin-antithrombin III-komplexes in der diagnostik der lungenembolie und der tiefen venenthrombose-vergleich mit fibrinopeptide A, plattchenfaktor 4 und β-thrombulin. Klin Wochenschr 65:757, 1987.

153. Seitz R, Blanke H, Pratorius G, Strauer BE, Egbring R. Increased thrombin activity during thrombolysis. Thromb Haemost 59:541, 1988.

154. Lau HK, Rosenberg RD. The isolation and characterization of a specific antibody directed against the thrombin-antithrombin complex. J Biol Chem 255:5885, 1980.

155. Pelzer H, Schwarz A, Heimburger N. Determination of human thrombin-antithrombin III complex in plasma with an enzyme-linked immunosorbent assay. Thromb Haemost 59:101, 1988.

156. Bounameaux H, Schneider PA, Reber G, Moerloose PD, Krahenbuhl B. Measurement of plasma D-dimer for diagnosis of deep venous thrombosis. Am J Clin Pathol 91:82, 1989.

157. Demers C, Ginsberg JS, Johnston M, Brill-Edwards P, Panju A. D-dimer and thrombin-antithrombin III complexes in patients with clinically suspected pulmonary embolism. Thromb Haemost 67:408, 1992.

158. Giansante C, Fiotti N, Cattin L, Col PGD, Calabrese S. Fibrinogen, D-dimer and thrombin-antithrombin complexes in a random population sample: Relationships with other cardiovascular risk factors. Thromb Haemost 71:581, 1994.

159. Lassila R, Peltonen S, Lepantolo M, Saarinen O, Kauhanen P, Manninen V. Severity of peripheral arteriosclerosis is associated with fibrinogen and degradation products of cross-linked fibrin. Arterioscler Thromb 13:1738, 1993.

160. Garcia-Avello A, Garcia-Frade LJ, Gandarias C, Ocana J, Cancelas JA, Lasso M. High F1.2 fragment of prothrombin. Thrombin-antithrombin III complex (TAT) and soluble fibrin plasma levels demonstrate hypercoagulability induced during loco-regional thrombolytic therapy with rt-PA. Thromb Res 73:109, 1994.

161. Eritsland J, Selfjeflot I, Arnesen H, Smith P, Westvik AB. Effects of long-term treatment with warfarin on fibrinogen, FPA, TAT, and D-dimer in patients with coronary artery disease. Thromb Res 66:55, 1992.

162. Wilf J, Minton AP. Soluble fibrin-fibrinogen complexes as intermediates in fibrin gel formation. Biochemistry 25:3124, 1986.

163. Mehs DA, Siebenlist KR, Bergstrom G, Mosesson MW. Sequences of release of fibrinopeptide A from fibrinogen molecules by thrombin or Atraxin. J Lab Clin Med 125:384, 1995.

164. Smith GF. The mechanisms of fibrin-polymer formation in solution. Biochem J 185:1, 1980.

165. Alkjaersig N, Fletcher AP. Formation of soluble fibrin oligomers in purified systems and in plasma. Biochem J 213:75, 1983.

166. Dietler G, Kanzig W, Haeberli A, Straub PW. Experimental tests of a geometrical abstraction of fibrin polymerization. Biopolymers 25:905, 1986.

167. Hunziker EB, Straub PW, Haeberli A. A new concept of fibrin formation based upon linear growth of interlacing and branching polymers and molecular alignment into interlocked single-stranded segments. J Biol Chem 265:7455, 1990.

168. Janmey PA, Erdile L, Bale MD, Ferry JD. Kinetics of

fibrin oligomer formation observed by electron microscopy. Biochemistry 22:4336, 1983.

169. Fletcher AP, Alkjaersig NK, Ghani FM, Tulevski V, Owens O. Blood coagulation system pathophysiology in acute myocardial infarction: The influence of anticoagulant treatment on laboratory findings. J Lab Clin Med 93:1054, 1979.

170. Kruskal JB, Commeford PJ, Franks JJ, Kirsch RE. Fibrin and fibrinogen-related antigens in patients with stable and unstable coronary artery disease. N Engl J Med 317:1361, 1987.

171. Magari Y, Mizunga S, Ito M, Shibata T, Ito H. Molecular marker for detecting hypercoagulable state. Jpn J Clin Pathol 42:22, 1994.

172. Lane DA. Fibrinogen derivatives in plasma. Br J Haematol 47:329, 1981.

173. Eisenberg PR, Jaffe AS, Stump DC, Collen D, Bovill EG. Validity of enzyme-linked immunosorbent assays of cross-linked fibrin degradation products as a measure of clot lysis. Circulation 82:1159, 1990.

174. Shainoff R, Urbanie DA, DiBello PM, Valenzuela V. GPR-phoresis, a novel approach to determining fibrin monomer and other macromolecular derivatives of fibrinogen and fibrin in blood. Blood Coagul Fibrinolysis 4:87, 1993.

175. Nieuwenhuizen W, Nobel EH, Laterveer R. A rapid immunoassay (EIA) for the quantitative determination of soluble fibrin in plasma. Thromb Haemost 68:273, 1992.

176. Rylatt DB, Blake AS, Cottis DA, Massingham DA, Fletcher WA, Masci PP, Whitaker AN, Elms M, Bunce I, Webber AJ, Wyatt D, Bundesen PG. An immunoassay for human D-dimer using monoclonal antibodies. Thromb Res 31:767, 1983.

177. Dinh D, Bolitho J, Bundensen P, Hillyard C, Marsh N, Moore B, Bottenus R, Rylatt D. Detection of soluble fibrin by enzyme immunoassay. Fibrinolysis 8(Suppl. 1):125, 1994.

178. Lee LV, Ewald G, McKenzie C, Eisenberg PR. The relationship of soluble fibrin and cross-linked fibrin degradation products to the clinical course of myocardial infarction. Arterioscler Thromb Vasc Biol 17:628, 1996.

179. Kisiel W. Human protein C: Isolation, characterisation, and mechanism of activation by alpha-thrombin. J Clin Invest 64:761, 1979.

180. Kisiel W, Canfield WM, Ericsson LH, Davie EW. Anticoagulant properties of bovine plasma protein C following activation by thrombin. Biochemistry 16:5824, 1977.

181. Vehar GA, Davie EW. Preparation and properties of bovine factor VIII (antihemophilic factor). Biochemistry 19:401, 1980.

182. Comp PC, Esmon CT. Activated protein C inhibits platelet prothrombin-converting activity. Blood 54:1272, 1979.

183. Bauer KA, Kass BL, Beeler DL, Rosenberg RD. Detection of protein C activation in humans. J Clin Invest 74:2033, 1984.

184. Bauer KA, Weiss LM, Sparrow D, Vokonas PS, Rosenberg RD. Aging-associated changes in indices of thrombin generation and protein C activation in humans: Normative aging study. J Clin Invest 80:1527, 1987.

185. Collen D. On the regulation and control of fibrinolysis. Thromb Haemost 43:77, 1980.

186. Kruithof EKO, Tran-Thang C, Ransijn A, Bachmann F. Demonstration of a fast-acting inhibitor of plasminogen activators in human plasma. Blood 64:907, 1984.

187. Thorsen S, Philips M, Selmer J, Lecander I, Astedt B. Kinetics of inhibition of tissue-type and urokinase-type plasminogen activator by plasmingogen-activator inhibitor type 1 and type 2. Eur J Biochem 175:33, 1988.

188. Lindahl TL, Ohlsson PI, Wiman B. The mechanism of the reaction between human plasminogen-activator inhibitor 1 and tissue plasminogen activator. Biochem J 265:109, 1990.

189. Chmielewska J, Ranby M, Wiman B. Kinetics of the inhibition of plasminogen activator by the plasminogen-activator inhibitor. Evidence for "second-site" interactions. Biochem J 251:327, 1988.

190. Moroi M, Aoki N. Isolation and characterization of α_2-plasmin inhibitor from human plasma. A novel proteinase inhibitor which inhibits activator-induced clot lysis. J Biol Chem 251:5956, 1976.

191. Collen D. Identification and some properties of a new fast-reacting plasmin inhibitor in human plasma. Eur J Biochem 69:209, 1976.

192. Mullertz S, Clemmensen I. The primary inhibitor of plasmin in human plasma. Biochem J 159:545, 1976.

193. Suenson E, Thorsen S. The course and prerequisites of Lys-plasminogen formation during fibrinolysis. Biochemistry 27:2435, 1988.

194. Pennica D, Holmes WE, Kohr WJ, Harkins RN, Vehar GA, Ward CA, Bennett WF, Yelverton E, Seeburg PH, Heyneker HL, Goeddel DV. Cloning and expression of human tissue-type plasminogen activator cDNA in E. coli. Nature 301:214, 1983.

195. Ranby M, Bergsdorf N, Nilsson T. Enzymatic properties of the one- and two-chain form of tissue plasminogen activator. Thromb Res 27:175, 1982.

196. Rijken DC, Hoylaerts M, Collen D. Fibrinolytic properties of one-chain and two-chain human extrinsic (tissue-type) plasminogen activator. J Biol Chem 257:2920, 1982.

197. Tate KM, Higgens DL, Holmes WE, Winkler ME, Heyneker HL, Vehar GA. Functional role of proteolytic cleavage at arginine-275 of human tissue plasminogen activator as assessed by site-directed mutagenesis. Biochemistry 26:338, 1987.

198. Higgins DL, Vehar GA. Interaction of one-chain and two-chain tissue plasminogen activator with intact and plasmin-degraded fibrin. Biochemistry 26:7786, 1987.

199. Higgins DL, Lamb MC. Incorporation of a fluorescent probe into the active sites of one- and two-chain

tissue-type plasminogen activator. Arch Biochem Biophys 249:418, 1986.

200. Wiman B, Collen D. Molecular mechanism of physiological fibrinolysis. Nature 272:549, 1978.

201. Chmielewska J, Ranby M, Wiman B. Evidence for a rapid inhibitor to tissue plasminogen activator in plasma. Thromb Res 31:427, 1983.

202. Bu G, Williams S, Strickland DK, Schwartz AL. Low density lipoprotein receptor-related protein/α_2-macroglobulin receptor is an hepatic receptor for tissue-type plasminogen activator. Proc Natl Acad Sci USA 89:7427, 1992.

203. Nilsson T, Wallen P, Mellbring G. In vivo metabolism of human tissue-type plasminogen activator. Scand J Haematol 33:49, 1984.

204. Nilsson S, Einarsson M, Ekvarn S, Haggroth L, Mattsson C. Turnover of tissue plasminogen activator in normal and hepatectomized rabbits. Thromb Res 39:511, 1985.

205. Fuchs HE, Berger H, Pizzo SV. Catabolism of human tissue plasminogen activator in mice. Blood 65:539, 1985.

206. Morton PA, Owensby DA, Underhill DM, Schwartz AL. Cellular itinerary of t-PA in human hepatocytes (abstr). Thromb Haemost 65:644, 1991.

207. Labarrere CA, Pitts D, Halbrook H, Faulk WP. Tissue plasminogen activator in cardiac allografts. Transplantation 55:1056, 1993.

208. Labarrere CA, Pitts D, Halbrook H, Faulk WP. Tissue plasminogen activator, plasminogen activator inhibitor-1, and fibrin as indexes of clinical course in cardiac allograft recipients: An immunocytochemical study. Circulation 89:1599, 1994.

209. Faulk WP, Labarrere CA, Pitts D, Halbrook H. Vascular lesions in biopsy specimens devoid of cellular infiltrates: Qualitative and quantitative immunocytochemical studies of human cardiac allografts. J Heart Lung Transplant 12:219, 1993.

210. Cash JD, Woodfield DG, Allan AGE. Adrenergic mechanisms in the systemic plasminogen activator response to adrenaline in man. Br J Haematol 18:487, 1970.

211. Ranby M, Bergsdorf N, Nilsson T, Mellbring G, Winblad B, Bucht G. Age dependence of tissue plasminogen activator concentrations in plasma, as studied by an improved enzyme-linked immunosorbent assay. Clin Chem 32:2160, 1986.

212. De Boer A, Kluft C, Kroon JM, Kasper FJ, Schoemaker HC, Pruis J, Breimer DD, Soons PA, Emeis JJ, Cohen AF. Liver blood flow as a major determinant of the clearance of recombinant human tissue-type plasminogen activator. Thromb Haemost 67:83, 1992.

213. Andreotti F, Davies GJ, Hackett DR, Khan MI, De Bart ACW, Aber VR, Maseri A, Kluft C. Major circadian fluctuations in fibrinolytic factors and possible relevance to time of onset of myocardial infarction, sudden cardiac death and stroke. Am J Cardiol 62:635, 1988.

214. Sprengers ED, Kluft C. Plasminogen activator inhibitors. Blood 69:381, 1987.

215. Loskutoff DJ. Regulation of PAI-1 gene expression. Fibrinolysis 5:197, 1991.

216. Emeis JJ, van Hinsbergh VWM, Verheijen JH, Wijngaards G. Inhibition of tissue-type plasminogen activator by conditioned medium from cultures of human and porcine vascular endothelial cells. Biochem Biophys Res Commun 110:392, 1983.

217. Levin EG. Latent tissue plasminogen activator produced by human endothelial cells in culture: Evidence for an enzyme-inhibitor complex. Proc Natl Acad Sci USA 80:6804, 1983.

218. Lundgren CH, Brown SL, Nordt TK, Sobel BE, Fuji S. Elaboration of type-1 plasminogen activator inhibitor from adipocytes. A potential pathogenic link between obesity and cardiovascular disease. Circulation 93:106, 1996.

219. Laug WE. Vascular smooth muscle cells inhibit the plasminogen activators secreted by endothelial cells. Thromb Haemost 20:165, 1985.

220. Sprengers ED, Verheijen JH, Van Hinsbergh VWM, Emeis JJ. Evidence for the presence of two different fibrinolytic inhibitors in human endothelial cell conditioned medium. Biochim Biophys Acta 801:163, 1984.

221. Erickson LA, Hekman CM, Loskutoff DJ. The primary plasminogen-activator inhibitors in endothelial cells, platelets, serum, and plasma are immunologically related. Proc Natl Acad Sci USA 82:8710, 1985.

222. Hekman CM, Loskutoff DJ. Endothelial cells produce a latent inhibitor of plasminogen activators that can be activated by denaturants. J Biol Chem 260:11581, 1985.

223. Sprengers ED, Akkerman JWN, Sansen BG. Blood platelet plasminogen activator inhibitor: Two different pools of endothelial cell type plasminogen activator inhibitor in human blood. Thromb Haemost 55:325, 1986.

224. Lindahl TL, Sigurdardottir O, Wiman B. Stability of plasminogen activator inhibitor 1 (PAI-1). Thromb Haemost 62:748, 1989.

225. Sprengers ED, Van Hinsbergh VWM, Jansen BG. The active and the inactive plasminogen activator inhibitor from human endothelial cell conditioned medium are immunologically and functionally related to each other. Biochim Biophys Acta 883:233, 1986.

226. Fay WP, Eitzman DT, Shapiro AD, Madison EL, Ginsburg D. Platelets inhibit fibrinolysis in vitro by both plasminogen activator inhibitor-1-dependent and -independent mechanisms. Blood 83:351, 1994.

227. Erickson LA, Ginsberg MH, Loskutoff DJ. Detection and partial characterization of an inhibitor of plasminogen activator in human platelets. J Clin Invest 74:1465, 1984.

228. Mimuro J, Schleef RR, Loskutoff DJ. Extracellular matrix of cultured bovine aortic endothelial cells con-

tains functionally active type 1 plasminogen activator inhibitor. Blood 70:721, 1987.

229. Salonen EM, Vaheri A, Pollanen J, Stephens R, Andreasen P, Mayer M, Dano K, Gailit J, Rouslahti E. Interaction of plasminogen activator inhibitor (PAI-1) with vitronectin. J Biol Chem 264:6339, 1989.

230. Sigurdardottir O, Wiman B. Complex formation between plasminogen activator inhibitor 1 and vitronectin in purified systems and in plasma. Biochim Biophys Acta 1035:56, 1990.

231. Preissner KT. Structure and biological role of vitronectin. Annu Rev Cell Biol 7:275, 1991.

232. Ehrlich HJ, Gebbink RK, Keijer J, Linders M, Preissner TK, Pannekoek H. Alteration of serpin specificity by a protein cofactor. Vitronectin endows plasminogen activator inhibitor 1 with thrombin inhibitory properties. J Biol Chem 265:13029, 1990.

233. Naski MC, Lawrence DA, Mosher DF, Podor T, Ginsburg D. Kinetics of inactivation of α-thrombin by plasminogen activator inhibitor-1. Comparison of the effects of native and urea-treated forms of vitronectin. J Biol Chem 268:12367, 1993.

234. Edelberg JM, Reilly CF, Pizzo SV. The inhibition of tissue type plasminogen activator by plasminogen activator inhibitor-1. The effects of fibrinogen, heparin, vitronectin, and lipoprotein (a). J Biol Chem 266:7488, 1991.

235. Rosenberg RD. The heparin-antithrombin system: A natural anticoagulation mechanism. In Coleman RW, Hirsh J, Marder VJ, Salzman EW (eds). Haemostasis and Thrombosis. Philadelphia: JB Lippincott, 1987:1372.

236. Edelberg JM, Sane DC, Pizzo SV. Vascular regulation of plasminogen activator inhibitor-1 activity. Semin Thromb Hemost 20:319, 1994.

237. Colucci M, Paramo JA, Collen D. Generation in plasma of a fast-acting inhibitor of plasminogen activator in response to endotoxin stimulation. J Clin Invest 75:818, 1985.

238. Wiman B, Hamsten A. Impaired fibrinolysis and risk of thromboembolism. Prog Cardiovasc Dis 34:179, 1991.

239. Kruithof EKO, Gudinchet A, Bachmann F. Plasminogen activator inhibitor 1 and plasminogen activator inhibitor 2 in various disease states. Thromb Haemost 59:7, 1988.

240. Takada Y, Takada A. Measurements of the concentration of free plasminogen activator inhibitor (PAI-1) and its complex with tissue plasminogen activator in human plasma. Thromb Res – Suppl 8:15, 1988.

241. Nilsson IM, Ljungner H, Tengborn L. Two different mechanisms in patients with venous thrombosis and defective fibrinolysis: Low concentration of plasminogen activator or increased concentration of plasminogen activator inhibitor. Br Med J 290:1453, 1985.

242. Eriksson E, Ranby M, Gyzander E, Risberg B. Determination of plasminogen activator inhibitor in plasma using t-PA and chromogenic single-point

poly-D-lysine stimulated assay. Thromb Res 50:91, 1988.

243. Jansson JH, Boman K, Nilsson TK. Enalapril related changes in the fibrinolytic system in survivors of myocardial infarction. Eur J Clin Pharmacol 44:485, 1993.

244. Rijken DC, Juhan-Vague I, Collen D. Complexes between tissue-type plasminogen activator and proteinase inhibitors in human plasma, identified with an immunoradiometric assay. J Lab Clin Med 101:285, 1983.

245. Bergsdorf N, Nilsson T, Wallen P. An enzyme linked immunoabsorbent assay for determination of tissue plasminogen activator applied to patients with thromboembolic disease. Thromb Haemost 50:740, 1983.

246. Urden G, Blomback M. Determination of tissue plasminogen activator in plasma samples by means of a radioimmunoassay. Scan J Clin Lab Invest 44:495, 1984.

247. Takada A, Shizume K, Ozawa T, Takahashi S, Takada Y. Characterization of various antibodies against tissue plasminogen activator using highly sensitive enzyme immunoassay. Thromb Res 42:63, 1986.

248. Ranby M, Nguyen G, Scarabin PY, Samama M. Immunoreactivity of tissue plasminogen activator and of its inhibitor complexes: Biochemical and multicenter validation of a two site immunosorbent assay. Thromb Haemost 61:409, 1989.

249. Wiman B. Plasminogen activator inhibitor 1 (PAI-1) in plasma: Its role in thrombotic disease. Thromb Haemost 74:71, 1995.

250. Kluft C, Verheijen JH. Leiden Fibrinolysis Working Party: Blood collection and handling procedures for assessment of tissue-type plasminogen activator (t-PA) and plasminogen activator inhibitor-1 (PAI-1). Fibrinolysis 4:155, 1990.

251. Angleton P, Chandler WL, Schmer G. Diurnal variation of tissue-type plasminogen activator and its rapid inhibitor (PAI-1). Circulation 79:101, 1989.

252. Grimaudo V, Hauert J, Bachemann F, Kruithof EKO. Diurnal variation of the fibrinolytic system. Thromb Haemost 59:495, 1988.

253. Huber K, Rosc D, Resch I, Schuster E, Glogar DH, Kaindl F, Binder BR. Circadian fluctuation of plasminogen activator inhibitor and tissue plasminogen activator levels in plasma of patients with unstable coronary artery disease and acute myocardial infarction. Thromb Haemost 60:372, 1988.

254. Emeis JJ, Kooistra T. Interleukin-1 and lipopolysaccharide induce an inhibitor of tissue-type plasminogen activator in vivo and in cultured endothelial cells. J Exp Med 163:1260, 1986.

255. Alessi M, Juhan-Vague I, Kooistra T, Declerck P, Collen D. Insulin stimulates the synthesis of plasminogen activator inhibitor 1 by the human hepatocellular cell line Hep G2. Thromb Haemost 60:491, 1988.

256. Schneider DJ, Sobel BE. Augmentation of synthesis

of plasminogen activator inhibitor type 1 by insulin and insulin-like growth factor type-1: Implications for vascular disease by hyperinsulinemic states. Proc Natl Acad Sci USA 88:9959, 1991.

257. Stiko-Rahm A, Wiman B, Hamsten A, Nilsson J. Secretion of plasminogen activator inhibitor-1 from cultured human umbilical vein endothelial cells is induced by very low density lipoprotein. Arteriosclerosis 10:1067, 1990.

258. Latron Y, Chautan M, Anfosso F, Alessi MC, Nalbone G, Lafont H, Juhan-Vague I. Stimulating effect of oxidized low density lipoproteins on plasminogen activator inhibitor-1 synthesis by endothelial cells. Arterioscler Thromb 11:1821, 1991.

259. Tremoli E, Camera M, Maderna P, Sironi L, Prati L, Colli S, Piovella F, Bernini F, Corsini A, Mussoni L. Increased synthesis of plasminogen activator inhibitor-1 by cultured human endothelial cells exposed to native and modified LDLs. An LDL receptor-independent phenomenon. Arterioscler Thromb 13:338, 1993.

260. Juhan-Vague I, Moerman B, De Cock F, Aillaud MF, Collen D. Plasma levels of a specific inhibitor of tissue-type plasminogen activator (and urokinase) in normal and pathological conditions. Thromb Res 33:523, 1984.

261. Juhan-Vague I, Valadier J, Alessi MC, Aillaud MF, Ansaldi J, Philip-Joet C, Holvoet P, Serradimigni A, Collen D. Deficient t-PA release and elevated PA inhibitor levels in patients with spontaneous or recurrent deep venous thrombosis. Thromb Haemost 57:67, 1987.

262. Mellbring G, Dahlgren D, Wiman B, Sunnegardh O. Relationship between preoperative status of the fibrinolytic system and occurrence of deep vein thrombosis after major abdominal surgery. Thromb Res 39:157, 1985.

263. Wiman B, Chmielewska J. A novel fast inhibitor to tissue plasminogen activator in plasma, which may be of great pathophysiological significance. Scand J Clin Lab Invest 45:43, 1985.

264. Juhan-Vague I, Aillard MF, DeCock F. The rapid inhibitor of tissue-type plasminogen activator is an acute phase reactant protein. In Darden JF, Donati MB, Coccheri S (eds). Progress in Fibrinolysis, Vol. VII. Edinburgh: Churchill Livingstone, 146, 1985.

265. Kluft C, Verheijen JH, Jie AFH, Rijken DC, Preston FE, Sue-Ling HM, Jespersen J, Aasen AO. The postoperative fibrinolytic shutdown: A rapidly reverting acute phase pattern for the fast-acting inhibitor of tissue-type plasminogen activator after trauma. Scan J Clin Lab Invest 45:605, 1985.

266. Kruithof EKO, Tran-Thang C, Gudinchet A, Hauert J, Nicoloso G, Genton C, Welti H, Bachmann F. Fibrinolysis in pregnancy: A study of plasminogen activator inhibitors. Blood 69:460, 1987.

267. Juhan-Vague I, Thompson SG, Jespersen J. Involvement of the hemostatic system in the insulin resistance syndrome: A study of 1500 patients with angina pectoris. Arterioscler Thromb 13:1865, 1993.

268. Asplund-Carlson A, Hamsten A, Wiman B, Carlson LA. Relationship between plasma plasminogen activator inhibitor-1 activity and VLDL, triglyceride concentration, insulin levels and insulin sensitivity: Studies in randomly selected normo- and hypertriglyceridemic men. Diabetologia 36:817, 1993.

269. Mansfield MW, Stockland MH, Grant PJ. Plasminogen activator inhibitor-1 (PAI-1) promotes polymorphism and coronary artery disease in non-insulin-dependent diabetes. Thromb Haemost 74:1032, 1995.

270. Juhan-Vague I, Alessi MC, Vague P. Increased plasma plasminogen activator inhibitor-1 levels. A possible link between insulin resistance and atherothrombosis. Diabetologia 34:457, 1991.

271. Folsom AR, Qamheih HT, Wing RR, Jeffery RW, Stinson VL, Kuller LH, Wu KK. Impact of weight loss on plasminogen activator inhibitor (PAI-1), factor VII and other hemostatic factors in moderately overweight adults. Arterioscler Thromb 13:162, 1993.

272. Sundell IB, Dahlgren S, Ranby M, Lundin E, Stenling R, Nilsson TK. Reduction of elevated plasminogen activator inhibitor levels during modest weight loss. Fibrinolysis 3:51, 1989.

273. Andersen P, Smith P, Seljeflot I, Brataker S, Arnesen H. Effects of gemfibrozil on lipids and haemostasis after myocardial infarction. Thromb Haemost 63:174, 1990.

274. Mehrabian M, Peter JB, Barnard RJ, Lusis AJ. Dietary regulation of fibrinolytic factors. Atherosclerosis 84:25, 1990.

275. Vague P, Juhan-Vague I, Aillaud MF, Badier C, Viard R, Alessi MC, Collen D. Correlation between blood fibrinolytic activity, plasminogen activator inhibitor level, plasmin insulin level, and relative body weight in normal and obese subjects. Metabolism 35:250, 1986.

276. Landin K, Stigendal L, Eriksson E, Krotkiewski M, Risberg B, Tengborn L, Smith U. Abdominal obesity is associated with an impaired fibrinolytic activity and elevated plasminogen activator inhibitor-1. Metabolism 39:1044, 1990.

277. Wall U, Jern C, Bergbrant A, Jern S. Enhanced levels of tissue-type plasminogen activator in borderline hypertension. Hypertension 26:796, 1995.

278. Licata G, Scaglione R, Avellone G, Ganguzza A, Corrao S, Arnone S, Chiara TD. Hemostatic function in young subjects with central obesity: Relationship with left ventricular function. Metabolism 44:1417, 1995.

279. Gebara OCE, Mittleman MA, Sutherland P, Lipinska I, Matheney T, Xu P, Weltry FK, Wilson PWF, Levy D, Muller JE, Tofler GH. Association between increased estrogen status and increased fibrinolytic

potential in the Framingham offspring study. Circulation 91:1952, 1995.

280. Smokovitis A, Kokolis N, Taitzoglou I. Sex-related differences in plasminogen activator activity and plasminogen activator inhibition of human and animal kidneys: Effect of orchiectomy or ovariectomy. Haemostasis 21:305, 1991.

281. Meilahn E, Cauley JA, Tracy RP, Macy EO, Gutai JH, Kuller LH. Association of sex hormones and adiposity with plasma levels of fibrinogen and PAI-1 in postmenopausal women. Am J Epidemiol 143:159, 1996.

282. Jansson JH, Johansson B, Boman K, Nilsson TK. Hypofibrinolysis in patients with hypertension and elevated cholesterol. J Intern Med 229:309, 1991.

283. Gleerup G, Winther K. Decreased fibrinolytic activity and increased platelet function in hypertension: Possible influence of calcium antagonism. Am J Hypertens 4:168S, 1991.

284. van Wersch JWJ, Rompleberg-Lahaye J, Lustermans FAT. Plasma concentration of coagulation and fibrinolysis factors and platelet function in hypertension. Eur J Clin Chem Clin Biochem 29:375, 1991.

285. Ridker PM, Gaboury CL, Conlin PR, Seely EW, Williams GH, Vaughan DE. Stimulation of plasminogen activator inhibitor in vivo by infusion of angiotensin II: Evidence of a potential interaction between the renin-angiotensin system and fibrinolytic function. Circulation 87:1969, 1993.

286. Alderman MH, Madhavan S, Ooi WL, Cohen H, Sealey JE, Laragh JH. Association of the renin-sodium profile with the risk of myocardial infarction in patients with hypertension. N Engl J Med 324:1098, 1991.

287. Rouleau JL, de Champlain J, Klein M, Bichet D, Moye L, Packer M, Dagenais G, Sussex B, Arnold JM, Sestier F, Parker JO, McEwan P, Bernstein V, Cuddy E, Lamas G, Gottlieb S, McCans J, Nadeau C, Delage F, Hamm P. Activation of neurohumoral systems in postinfarction left ventricular dysfunction. J Am Coll Cardiol 22:390, 1993.

288. Wright RA, Flapan AD, Albert KGMM, Ludlam CA, Fox KAA. Effects of captopril therapy on endogenous fibrinolysis in men with recent, uncomplicated myocardial infarction. J Am Coll Cardiol 24:67, 1994.

289. Vaughn DE, Rouleau JL, Pfeffer MA. Role of the fibrinolytic system in preventing myocardial infarction. Eur Heart J 16:31, 1995.

290. Schneiderman J, Sawdey MS, Keeton MR, Bordin GM, Bernstein EF, Dilley RB, Loskutoff DJ. Increased type 1 plasminogen activator inhibitor gene expression in atherosclerotic human arteries. Proc Nat Acad Sci USA 89:6998, 1992.

291. Lupu F, Bergonzelli GE, Heim DA, Cousin E, Genton CY, Bachmann F, Kruithof EKO. Localization and production of plasminogen activator inhibitor-1 in human healthy and atherosclerotic arteries. Arterioscl Thromb 13:1090, 1993.

292. Chomiki N, Henry M, Alessi MC, Anfosso F, Juhan-Vague I. Plasminogen activator inhibitor-1 expression in human liver and healthy or atherosclerotic vessel walls. Thromb Haemost 72:44, 1994.

293. Mehta J, Mehta P, Lawson D, Saldeen T. Plasma tissue plasminogen activator inhibitor levels in coronary artery disease: Correlation with age and serum triglyceride concentration. J Am Coll Cardiol 9:263, 1987.

294. Cortellaro M, Confrancesco E, Boschetti C, Mussoni L, Donati MB, Cardillo M, Catalano M, Gabrielli L, Lombardi B, Specchia G, Tavazzi L, Tremoli E, Pozzoli E, Turri M. Increased fibrin turnover and high PAI-1 activity as predictors of ischemic events in atherosclerotic patients: A case-control study. Arterioscler Thromb 13:1412, 1993.

295. Oseroff A, Krishnamurti C, Hassett A, Tang D, Alving B. Plasminogen activator and plasminogen activator inhibitor activities in men with coronary artery disease. J Lab Clin Med 113:88, 1989.

296. Vandekerckhove Y, Baele G, de Puydt H, Weyne A, Clement D. Plasma tissue plasminogen activator levels in patients with coronary heart disease. Thromb Res 50:449, 1988.

297. Paramo JA, Colucci M, Collen D, van de Werf F. Plasminogen activator inhibitor in the blood of patients with coronary artery disease. Br Med J 291:573, 1985.

298. Sakata K, Kurata C, Taguchi T, Suzuki S, Kobayashi A, Yamazaki N, Rydzewski A, Takada Y, Takada A. Clinical significance of plasminogen activator inhibitor activity in patients with exercise-induced ischemia. Am Heart J 120:381, 1990.

299. Almer LO, Ohlin H. Elevated levels of the rapid inhibitor of plasminogen activator (t-PAI) in acute myocardial infarction. Thromb Res 47:335, 1987.

300. Aznar J, Estelles A, Tormo G, Sapena P, Tormo V, Blanch S, Espana F. Plasminogen activator inhibitor activity and other fibrinolytic variables in patients with coronary artery disease. Br Heart J 59:535, 1988.

301. ECAT, Angina Pectoris Study Group. ECAT angina pectoris study: Baseline associations of haemostatic factors with extent of coronary arteriosclerosis and other risk factors in 3000 patients with angina pectoris undergoing coronary angiography. Eur Heart J 14:8, 1993.

302. Huber K, Resch I, Stefenelli T, Lang I, Probst P, Kaindl F, Binder BR. Plasminogen activator inhibitor-1 levels in patients with chronic angina pectoris with or without angiographic evidence of coronary sclerosis. Thromb Haemost 63:336, 1990.

303. Olofsson BO, Dahlen G, Nilsson TK. Evidence for increased levels of plasminogen activator inhibitor and tissue plasminogen activator in plasma of patients with angiographically verified coronary artery disease. Eur Heart J 10:77, 1989.

304. Zalewski A, Shi Y, Nardone D, Bravette B, Weinstock P, Fischman D, Wilson P, Goldberg S, Levin DC, Bjornsson TD. Evidence for reduced fibrinolytic activity in unstable angina at rest: Clinical, biochemical and angiographic correlates. Circulation 83:1685, 1991.

305. Verheugt FW, ten Cate JW, Sturk A, Imandt L, Verhorst PM, van Eenige MJ, Verwey W, Roos JP. Tissue plasminogen activator activity and inhibition in acute myocardial infarction and angiographically normal coronary arteries. Am J Cardiol 59:1075, 1987.

306. Johnson O, Mellbring G, Nilsson T. Defective fibrinolysis in survivors of myocardial infarction. Int J Cardiol 6:380, 1984.

307. Hamsten A, Wiman B, de Faire U, Blomback M. Increased plasma levels of a rapid inhibitor of tissue plasminogen activator in young survivors of myocardial infarction. N Engl J Med 313:1557, 1985.

308. Hamsten A, Walldius G, Szamosi A, Blomback M, de Faire U, Dahlen G, Landou C, Wiman B. Plasminogen activator inhibitor in plasma: Risk factor for recurrent myocardial infarction. Lancet 2:3, 1987.

309. Nilsson TK, Johnson O. The extrinsic fibrinolytic system in survivors of myocardial infarction. Thromb Res 48:621, 1987.

310. Meade TW, Ruddock V, Stirling Y, Charkrabarti R, Miller GJ. Fibrinolytic activity, clotting factors and long-term incidence of ischaemic heart disease in the Northwick Park Heart Study. Lancet 342:1076, 1993.

311. Ridker PM, Vaughan DE, Stampfer MJ, Manson JE, Hennekens CH. Endogenous tissue-type plasminogen activator and risk of myocardial infarction. Lancet 341:1165, 1993.

312. Gram J, Jespersen J, Kluft C, Rijken DC. On the usefulness of fibrinolysis variables in the characterization of a risk group for myocardial reinfarction. Acta Med Scand 221:149, 1987.

313. Munkvad S, Gram J, Jespersen J. A depression of active tissue plasminogen activator in plasma characterizes patients with unstable angina pectoris who develop myocardial infarction. Eur Heart J 11:525, 1990.

314. Jansson JH, Nilsson TK, Olofsson BO. Tissue plasminogen activator and other risk factors as predictors of cardiovascular events in patients with severe angina pectoris. Eur Heart J 12:157, 1991.

315. Jansson JH, Olofsson NO, Nilsson TK. Predictive value of tissue plasminogen activator mass concentration on long-term mortality in patients with coronary artery disease. A 7-year follow-up. Circulation 88:2030, 1993.

316. Sakata K, Miura F, Sugino H, Shinobe M, Shirotani M, Yoshida H, Mori N, Hoshino T, Takada A. Impaired fibrinolysis early after percutaneous transluminal coronary angioplasty is associated with restenosis. Am Heart J 131:1, 1996.

317. Kirschstein W, Simianer S, Dempfle CE, Keller H, Stegaru B, Rentrop P, Heene DL. Impaired fibrinolytic capacity and tissue plasminogen activator release in patients with restenosis after percutaneous transluminal coronary angioplasty. Thromb Haemost 62:772, 1989.

318. Saito M, Nakabayashi T, Iuchi K, Ishikawa T, Kaseno K, Yoshida T, Asakura H, Matsuda T. Effects of direct percutaneous transluminal coronary angioplasty treatment of acute myocardial infarction on plasma levels of haemostatic and fibrinolytic factors. Blood Coagul Fibrinolysis 4:801, 1993.

319. Hara M, Ito K, Nawata T, Tsunematsu Y, Shimoyama N, Maeda T, Sato Y, Saikawa T, Sakata T. Plasminogen activator inhibitor-1, tissue plasminogen activator and serum lipoprotein (a) after reperfusion therapy in acute myocardial infarction: Comparison between sequential and direct percutaneous transluminal coronary angioplasty. Cardiology 86:407, 1995.

320. Sakamoto T, Yasue H, Ogawa H, Misumi I, Masuda T. Association of patency of the infarct-related coronary artery with plasma levels of plasminogen activator inhibitor activity in acute myocardial infarction. Am J Cardiol 70:271, 1992.

321. Hirashima O, Ogawa H, Oshima S, Sakamoto T, Honda Y, Sakata S, Masuda T, Miyao Y, Yasue H. Serial changes of plasma plasminogen activator inhibitor activity in acute myocardial infarction: Difference between thrombolytic therapy and direct coronary angioplasty. Am Heart J 130:933, 1995.

322. Haider AW, Andreotti F, Hackett DR, Tousoulis D, Kluft C, Maseri A, Davies GJ. Early spontaneous intermittent myocardial reperfusion during acute myocardial infarction is associated with augmented thrombogenic activity and less myocardial damage. J Am Coll Cardiol 26:662, 1995.

323. van Meijer M, Pannekoek H. Structure of plasminogen activator inhibitor 1 (PAI-1) and its function in fibrinolysis: An update. Fibrinolysis 9:263, 1995.

324. Fay WP, Shapiro AD, Shih JL, Schleef RR, Ginsburg D. Brief report: Complete deficiency of plasminogen-activator inhibitor type 1 due to a frame-shift mutation. N Engl J Med 327:1729, 1992.

325. Torr-Brown SR, Sobel BE. Attenuation of thrombolysis by plasminogen activator inhibitor type-1 from platelets. Thromb Res 72:413, 1993.

326. Robbie LA, Both NA, Croll AM, Bennett B. The roles of α_2-antiplasmin and plasminogen activator inhibitor 1 (PAI-1) in the inhibition of clot lysis. Thromb Haemost 70:301, 1993.

327. Reed GL, Matsueda GR, Haber E. Platelet factor XIII increases the fibrinolytic resistance of platelet-rich clots by accelerating the crosslinking of α_2-antiplasmin to fibrin. Thromb Haemost 68:315, 1992.

328. Sabovic M, Lijnen H, Keber D, Collen D. Effect of

retraction on the lysis of human clots with fibrin specific and non-fibrin specific plasminogen activators. Thromb Haemost 62:1083, 1989.

329. Wiman B, Haegerstrand-Bjorkman M. Plasmin/α_2-antiplasmin complex in plasma — a global fibrinolytic assay (abstr). Thromb Haemost 69:1091, 1993.

330. Collen D, de Cock F, Cambiaso CL, Masson P. A latex agglutination test for rapid quantitative estimation of the plasmin-antiplasmin complex in human plasma. Eur J Clin Invest 7:21, 1977.

331. Plow EF, de Cock F, Collen D. Immunochemical characterization of the plasmin-antiplasmin system. Basis for the specific detection of the plasmin-antiplasmin complex by latex agglutination assays. J Lab Clin Med 93:199, 1979.

332. Collen D, Wiman B. Turnover of antiplasmin, the fast-acting plasmin inhibitor of plasma. Blood 53:313, 1979.

333. Holvoet P, Lijnen H, Collen D. Monoclonal antibody preventing binding of tissue-type plasminogen activator to fibrin: Useful to monitor fibrinogen breakdown during t-PA infusion. Blood 67:1482, 1986.

334. Mimuro J, Koike Y, Sumi Y, Aoki N. Monoclonal antibodies to discrete regions in α_2-plasmin inhibitor. Blood 69:446, 1987.

335. Montes R, Paramo JA, Angles-Cano E, Rocha E. Development and clinical application of a new ELISA assay to determine plasmin-alpha 2-antiplasmin complexes in plasma. Br J Haematol 92:979, 1996.

336. Nossel HL, Wasser J, Kaplan KL, LaGamma KS, Yudelman I, Canfield RE. Sequence of fibrinogen proteolysis and platelet release after intra-uterine infusion of hypertonic saline. J Clin Invest 64:1371, 1979.

337. Marder VJ, Francis CW, Doolittle RF. Fibrinogen Structure and Physiology. In Haemostasis and Thrombosis. Philadelphia: JB Lippincott, 1982.

338. Jaffe AS, Eisenberg PR, Wilner GD. In vivo assessment of thrombosis and fibrinolysis during acute myocardial infarction. Prog Hematol 15:71, 1987.

339. McDonagh RP, McDonagh J, Duckert F. The influence of fibrin crosslinking on the kinetics of urokinase-induced clot lysis. Br J Haematol 21:323, 1971.

340. Gaffney PJ, Creighton LJ, Callus M, Thorpe R. Monoclonal antibodies to crosslinked fibrin degradation products (XL-FDP). II. Evaluation in a variety of clinical conditions. Br J Haematol 68:91, 1988.

341. Kroneman H, Nieuwenhuizen W, Knute A. Monoclonal antibody-based plasma assays for fibrin(ogen) and derivatives and their clinical relevance. Blood Coagul Fibrinolysis 1:91, 1990.

342. Gaffney PJ, Perry MJ. Unreliability of current serum fibrin degradation product assays. Thromb Haemost 53:301, 1985.

343. Merskey C, Kleiner GJ, Johnson AJ. Quantitative estimation of split products of fibrinogen in human

serum, relation to diagnosis and treatment. Blood 28:1, 1966.

344. Budzynski AZ, Marder VJ, Parker ME, Shames P, Brizuela BS, Olexa SA. Antigenic markers on fragment DD, a unique plasmic derivative of human crosslinked fibrin. Blood 54:794, 1979.

345. Lee-Owen V, Gordon YB, Chard T. The detection of neoantigenic sites on the D-dimer peptide isolated from plasmin digested cross linked fibrin. Thromb Res 14:77, 1979.

346. Siefried E, Tanswel P, Rijken DC, Kluft C, Hoegee E, Nieuwenhuizen W. Fibrin degradation products are not specific markers for thrombolysis in myocardial infarction. Lancet 2:333, 1987.

347. Whitaker AN, Elms MJ, Masci PP, Bundesen PG, Rylatt DB, Weber AJ, Bunce IH. Measurement of crosslinked fibrin derivatives in plasma: An immunoassay using monoclonal antibodies. J Clin Pathol 37:882, 1984.

348. Eisenberg PR, Sherman LA, Perez J, Jaffe AS. Relationship between elevated plasma levels of cross-linked fibrin degradation products (XL-FDP) and the clinical presentation of patients with myocardial infarction. Thromb Res 46:109, 1987.

349. Koppert PW, Kuipers W, Hoegee-de Nobel B, Brommer EJP, Koopman J, Nieuwenhuizen W. A quantitative enzyme immunoassay for primary fibrinogenolysis products in plasma. Thromb Haemost 57:25, 1987.

350. Koopman J, Haverkate F, Koppert P, Niewenhuizen W, Brommere JP, van der Werf VGC. New enzyme immunoassay of fibrin-fibrinogen degradation products in plasma using a monoclonal antibody. J Lab Clin Med 109:75, 1987.

351. Declerck PJ, Mombaerts P, Holvoet P, de Mol M, Collen D. Fibrinolytic response and fibrin fragment D-dimer levels in patients with deep vein thrombosis. Thromb Haemost 58:1024, 1987.

352. Lawler CW, Bovill EG, Stump DC, Collen DJ, Mann KG, Tracy RP. Fibrin fragment D-dimer and fibrinogen Bβ peptides in plasma as markers of clot lysis during thrombolytic therapy in acute myocardial infarction. Blood 76:1341, 1990.

353. Hart R, Bate I, Dinh D, Elms M, Bundesen P, Hillyard C, Rylatt DB. The detection of D-dimer in plasma by enzyme immunoassay: Improved discrimination is obtained with a more specific signal antibody. Blood Coagul Fibrinolysis 5:227, 1994.

354. Ballegeer V, Mombaerts P, Declerck PJ, Spitz B, Van Asche FA, Collen D. Fibrinolytic response to venous occlusion and fibrin fragment D-dimer levels in normal and complicated pregnancy. Thromb Haemost 58:1030, 1987.

355. Soria C, Soria J, Mirshashi MC, Mirshashi M, Dunnica S, Bousheix C, Beaufils R, Sluma R, Caen JP. Dynamic coronary fibrinolysis evaluation in patients with myocardial infarction and unstable angina by specific plasma fibrin degradation product determination. Thromb Res 45:383, 1987.

356. Hunt FA, Rylatt DB, Hart RA, Bundesen PG. Serum crosslinked fibrin (XDP) and fibrinogen/fibrin degradation products (FDP) in disorders associated with activation of the coagulation or fibrinolytic systems. Br J Haematol 60:715, 1985.

357. Chapman CS, Akhtar N, Campbell S, Miles K, O'Connor J, Mitchell VE. The use of D-dimer assay by enzyme immunoassay and latex agglutination techniques in the diagnosis of deep vein thrombosis. Clin Lab Haemat 12:37, 1990.

358. Carter CJ, Doyle DL, Dawson N, Fowler S, Devine DV. Investigations into the clinical utility of latex D-dimer in the diagnosis of deep venous thrombosis. Thromb Haemost 69:8, 1993.

359. Koopman MMW, Brandjes DPM, Beek EJR, Turkstra F, Buller HR. Sensitivity and specificity of a bed-side whole blood latex D-dimer assay (SimpliRED®) in outpatients with deep vein thrombosis. Thromb Haemost 73:1100, 1995.

360. Elias A, Aillaud MF, Roul C, Monteil O, Villain PH, Serradimigni A, Juhan-Vague I. Assessment of D-dimer measurement by ELISA or latex methods in deep vein thrombosis diagnosed by ultrasonic duplex scanning. Fibrinolysis 4:237, 1990.

361. Chang-Liem GS, Lustermans FA, van Wersch JWJ. Comparison of the appropriateness of the latex and ELISA plasma D-dimer determination for the diagnosis of deep venous thrombosis. Haemostasis 21:106, 1991.

362. John MA, Elms MJ, O'Reilly EJ, Rylatt DB, Bundesen PG, Hillyard CJ. The SimpliRED D-dimer test: A novel assay for the detection of crosslinked fibrin degradation products in whole blood. Thromb Res 58:273, 1990.

363. Deitcher SR, Eisenberg PR. Elevated concentrations of cross-linked fibrin degradation products in plasma. Chest 103:1107, 1993.

364. Brenner B, Pery M, Lanir N, Jabareen A, Markel A, Kaftori JK, Gaitini D, Rylatt D. Application of a bedside whole blood D-dimer assay in the diagnosis of deep vein thrombosis. Blood Coagul Fibrinolysis 6:219, 1995.

365. Wells PS, Brill-Edwards P, Stevens P, Panju A, Patel A, Douketis J, Massicotte P, Hirsh J, Weitz JI, Kearon C, Ginsberg JS. A novel and rapid whole-blood assay for D-dimer in patients with clinically suspected deep vein thrombosis. Circulation 91:2184, 1995.

366. Ginsberg JS, Wells PS, Brill-Edwards P, Donovan D, Panju A, Beek EJR, Patel A. Application of a novel and rapid whole blood assay for D-dimer in patients with clinically suspected pulmonary embolism. Thromb Haemost 73:35, 1995.

367. Bounameaux H, Cirafici P, Moerloose PD, Slosman D, Reber G, Unger PF. Measurement of D-dimer in plasma as a diagnostic aid in suspected pulmonary embolism. Lancet 337:196, 1991.

368. Goldhaber SZ, Vaughan DE, Tumeh SS, Loscalzo J. Utility of cross-linked fibrin degradation products in the diagnosis of pulmonary embolism. Am Heart J 116:505, 1989.

369. Rowbotham BJ, Egerton-Vernon J, Whitaker AN, Elms MJ, Bunce IH. Plasma cross linked fibrin degradation products in pulmonary embolism. Thorax 45:684, 1990.

370. Lichey J, Reschofski I, Dissmann T, Priesnitz M, Hoffmann M, Lode H. Fibrin degradation product D-dimer in the diagnosis of pulmonary embolism. Klin Wochenschr 69:522, 1991.

371. Rowbotham BJ, Carroll P, Whitaker AN, Bunce IH, Cobcroft RG, Elms MJ, Masci PP, Bundesen PG, Rylatt DB, Webber AJ. Measurement of crosslinked fibrin derivatives — use in the diagnosis of venous thrombosis. Thromb Haemost 57:59, 1987.

372. Ott P, Astrup L, Hartving JR, Nyeland B, Pedersen B. Assessment of D-dimer in plasma: Diagnostic value in suspected deep venous thrombosis of the leg. Acta Med Scand 224:263, 1988.

373. Lee AJ, Fowkes FGR, Lowe GDO, Rumley A. Fibrin D-dimer, haemostatic factors and peripheral arterial disease. Thromb Haemost 3:828, 1995.

374. Bredbacka S, Edner G. Soluble fibrin and D-dimer as detectors of hypercoagulability in patients with isolated brain trauma. J Neurosurg Anesthesiol 6:75, 1994.

375. Eisenberg PR, Sobel BE, Jaffe AS. Characterization in vivo of the fibrin specificity of activators of the fibrinolytic system. Circulation 78:592, 1988.

376. Eisenberg PR, Sherman LA, Tiefenbrunn AJ, Ludbrook PA, Sobel BE, Jaffe AS. Sustained fibrinolysis after administration of t-PA despite its short half-life in the circulation. Thromb Haemost 57:35, 1987.

377. Vaughan DE, Goldhaber SZ, Kim J, Loscalzo J. Recombinant tissue plasminogen activator in patients with pulmonary embolism: Correlation of fibrinolytic specificity and efficacy. Circulation 75:1200, 1987.

378. Ridker PM, Hennekens CH, Cerskers A, Stampfer MJ. Plasma concentration of cross-linked fibrin degradation products (D-dimer) and the risk of future myocardial infarction among apparently healthy men. Circulation 90:2236, 1994.

379. Abe S, Maruyama I, Arima S, Yamaguchi H, Okino H, Hamasaki S, Yamashita T, Nomoto K, Tahara M, Atsuchi Y, Nakao S, Tanaka H. Increased heparin-releasable platelet factor 4 and D-dimer in patients 1 month after the onset of acute myocardial infarction: Persistent activation of platelets and the coagulation/fibrinolytic system. Int J Cardiol 47:S7, 1994.

380. Fowkes FGR, Lowe GDO, Housley E, Rattray A, Rumley A, Elton RA, MacGregor IR, Dawes J. Cross-linked fibrin degradation products, progression of peripheral artery disease, and risk of coronary heart disease. Lancet 342:84, 1993.

381. Ring ME, Vecchione JJ, Fiore LD, Ruocco NA, Jacobs AK, Deykin D, Ryan TJ, Faxon DP. Detection of

intracoronary fibrin degradation after coronary balloon angioplasty. Am J Cardiol 67:1330, 1991.

382. Jorgensen B, Nielsen JD, Norgard J, Helligso P, Baekgaard N, Egeblad M. Cross-linked fibrin degradation products (XL-FDP) as markers of early rethrombosis in percutaneous transluminal angioplasty. Eur J Vasc Surg 7:720, 1993.

383. Weitz JI, Koehn JA, Canfield RE, Landman SL, Friedman R. Development of a radioimmunoassay for the fibrinogen-derived peptide Bβ1-42. Blood 67:1014, 1986.

384. Koehn JA, Hurlet-Jensen A, Nossel HL, Canfield RE. Sequence of plasma proteolysis at the NH$_2$-terminus of the Bβ chain of human fibrinogen. Anal Biochem 133:502, 1983.

385. Hurlet-Jensen A, Koehn JA, Nossel HL. The release of Bβ1-42 from fibrinogen and fibrin by plasmin. Thromb Res 29:609, 1983.

386. Kudryk B, Rohoza A, Ahadi M, Chin J, Wiebe ME. Specificity of a monoclonal antibody for the NH2-terminal region of fibrin. Mol Immunol 21:89, 1984.

387. Eisenberg PR, Miletich JP. Induction of marked thrombin activity by pharmacologic concentrations of plasminogen activators in nonanticoagulated whole blood. Thromb Res 55:635, 1989.

388. Nieuwenhuizen W, Emers JJ, Vermond A. Catabolism of purified rat fibrin(ogen) plasma degradation products in rats. Thromb Haemost 48:59, 1982.

389. Lane DA, Ireland H, Knight I, Wolf S, Kyle P, Curtis JR. The significance of fibrinogen derivatives in plasma in human renal failure. Br J Haematol 56:251, 1984.

390. Walenga JM, Fareed J, Mariani G, Messmore HL, Bick RL, Emanuele RM. Diagnostic efficacy of a simple radioimmunoassay test for fibrinogen/fibrin fragments containing the Bβ15-42 sequence. Semin Thromb Haemost 10:252, 1984.

391. Eisenberg PR, Sherman LA, Jaffe AS. Differentiation of fibrinolysis from fibrinogenolysis with Bβ1-42 and Bβ15-42. Circulation 74:II – 245, 1986.

35. MARKERS OF CORONARY RECANALIZATION AFTER THROMBOLYSIS

Dana R. Abendschein

Introduction

Rapid assessment of coronary patency in patients receiving intravenous fibrinolytic agents for the treatment of acute myocardial infarction is needed to identify those in whom adequate and sustained patency has not been achieved who could benefit from secondary mechanical interventions (e.g., coronary angioplasty and surgical revascularization). Because delayed initiation of secondary interventions will impede salvage of ischemic myocardium, markers chosen to assess the success of fibrinolytic therapy should have (1) sensitivity to coronary recanalization within minutes of its occurrence, facilitating prospective diagnosis; (2) rapidity for virtual on-line acquisition of results; and (3) specificity for persistent and complete recanalization, because those patients exhibiting transitory or incomplete recanalization may benefit from additional interventions as much as those with persistent arterial occlusion. Among these qualities, high specificity for arteries potentially in need of additional intervention is the most important, even if a modest number of patients with patent vessels are falsely identified as having an occluded artery.

LIMITATIONS OF CLINICAL MARKERS AND ANGIOGRAPHY

Clinical markers of coronary recanalization, including resolution of chest pain, changes in the ST segment of the electrocardiogram (ECG) obtained intermittently, and the appearance of reperfusion arrhythmias, although simple and practical to perform, lack sufficient accuracy. Complete resolution of ST-segment changes is associated with a 96% coronary patency rate and complete or partial resolution of chest pain with an 84% patency rate, but these occur in only 6% and 29% of patients, respectively [1]. Arrhythmias such as accelerated idioventricular rhythms and ventricular tachycardias, though common after re-perfusion, are not invariably present and are common also during the evolution of infarction per se [2]. Even when clinical data are used in concert, their predictive value is 100% only when all three are present or absent, a situation that occurs in only 9% of patients with and 34% of patients without reperfusion [3].

Coronary angiography has been regarded as the gold standard for patency, but it is not practical for use in every patient, considering that it would expose the majority in whom intravenous fibrinolytic agents are successful to the risk and expense of an unnecessary procedure. Angiography is also limited by visualizing blood flow in the infarct-related artery for brief intervals that do not reveal cyclic or unstable patency occurring frequently in patients undergoing treatment with fibrinolytic agents [4]. Accordingly, there has been considerable interest in alternative markers of patency, including changes in circulating levels of the MB isoenzyme of creatine kinase (CK) [5–12], subforms of individual CK isoenzymes [13–24], myoglobin [17,19,24–29], cardiac troponins [24,30–34], and changes in the ST segment monitored by continuous computer-assisted analysis [35–40].

PRINCIPLES FOR USE OF BIOCHEMICAL MARKERS

Biochemical markers are particularly attractive for rapid detection of coronary recanalization because restoration of blood flow induces a so-called washout phenomenon, leading to immediate, abrupt increases in the rates of appearance of intracellular proteins in the circulation. Angiographic-based studies have documented that the time of onset of marked increases in the concentration of tissue proteins in blood corresponds closely with the time of onset of vessel reopening [10]. The washout phenomenon has been attributed to restored myocardial blood flow or to transient profound increases in blood flow induced by reactive hyperemia, which facilitates the transfer of protein from necrotic myocytes and interstitial fluid to the circulation [41,42]. It may be also due, in part, to accelerated myocyte necrosis associated with reoxygenation, which hastens sarcolemmal damage and the release of proteins from previously ischemic cells [43].

Whatever the cause of washout, the changes in plasma profiles of proteins induced are unique for reperfusion of myocardium following coronary recanalization and are presumably modulated by the amount and persistence of blood flow, providing an approach to assess the success of therapy. Thus, it is not essential that the proteins employed as markers be specific for myocardium, as in the circumstance of their use for the detection of acute myocardial infarction. Rather, they must have characteristics of low circulating levels before treatment, high intracellular concentrations, and rapid egress from myocardium, facilitating detection of the washout profile in plasma samples obtained serially. This chapter reviews several potential marker proteins, their relative sensitivity and specificity for detection of coronary recanalization, and, more importantly, the absence of recanalization. Although rapid assays for some markers are not yet available for routine clinical use, results of recent studies have elucidated the principles for their application as new technology emerges.

Creatine Kinase Isoenzymes

It is well known that coronary recanalization induces rapid release of cytosolic CK isoenzymes into plasma, resulting in a shortened time to peak activity in the majority of patients (Figure 35-1) [5–8,13]. The time to peak, defined as the interval between the onset of persistent chest pain and the occurrence of peak total CK activity in plasma, ranges from 10 to 14 hours in patients with recanalization 3–4 hours after the onset of symptoms, compared with 18–27 hours in the absence of recanalization [5–7]. Comparable changes are observed for the more cardiac-specific MB isoenzyme (comprising 10–20% of the CK in myocardium, with the MM isoenzyme comprising the remaining 80–90%), considered separately, because both MB-CK and MM-CK are released from myocardium at similar rates [44]. Despite its early appearance, however, the time to achieve peak activities of CK isoenzymes are not useful for monitoring the success of fibrinolytic therapy because of the delay (as much as 16–18 hours) involved in defining whether a peak has occurred. This is true, in general, for other marker proteins as well. In addition, the time of

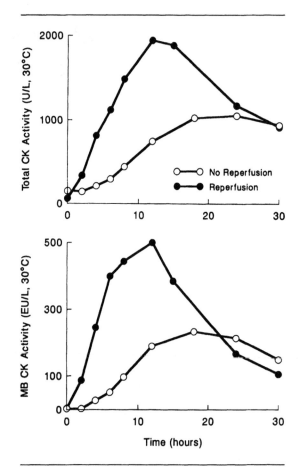

FIGURE 35-1. Time-activity profiles for total CK (top) and MB-CK (bottom) in a patient exhibiting coronary recanalization and a patient who did not exhibit coronary recanalization after intravenous administration of tissue-type plasminogen activator (beginning at time 0).

occurrence of peak CK varies considerably among patients because of differences in the extent of infarction and collateral blood flow [45]. This results in significant overlap of the intervals to peak CK in groups of patients with and without coronary recanalization, precluding reliable diagnosis in individual patients.

An alternative strategy based on analysis of CK isoenzymes involves detection of their accelerated rate of appearance in plasma. Shell et al. [5] initially reported that plasma levels of MB-CK activity were significantly higher and the rate of appearance of CK activity was threefold faster after 2 hours in patients exhibiting recanalization compared with those with persistent coronary occlusion. More recently, increases in plasma MB-CK of 2.2- to 2.5-fold [9], or

TABLE 35-1. Characteristics of biochemical markers of coronary recanalization

Marker	Criteria for recanalization	Sensitivity[a] n (%)	Specificity[b] n (%)	Advantages/ limitations	Refs.
MB-CK activity	$\geq$2.5-fold increase over 90 minutes for left coronary reperfusion	12/13 (92)	3/3 (100)	Easily measured; good apparent specificity after 90 minutes; relatively late compared with other markers; reliability may be affected by variations in infarct size and collateral flow	9
	$\geq$2.2-fold increase over 90 minutes for right coronary reperfusion	10/13 (77)	3/3 (100)		9
	$\geq$10 U/L/h over 90 minutes	(85)	(71)		46
	Appearance rate constant >0.185 over 4 hours	25/29 (86)	33/33 (100)[c]		11
MM-CK subforms	MM$_3$% $\geq$0.18%/min over 60 minutes	11/12 (92)	5/5 (100)	Good sensitivity within 60 minutes; assays are labor intensive and not yet widely applicable	17
	MM$_3$% $\geq$0.18%/min over 90 minutes	124/136 (91)	27/40 (68)		63
	MM$_3$/MM$_1$ >0.35 at 60 minutes	(60)	(100)		19
	MM$_3$/MM$_1$ >2.0 at 90 minutes	(68)	(87)		24
MB-CK subforms	MB$_2$/MB$_1$ $\geq$3.8 over 1–2 hours	18/20 (90)	17/19 (90)	Good sensitivity within 90 minutes; assays are not yet widely applicable	18
	MB$_2$/MB$_1$ $\geq$3.8 over 90 minutes	110/136 (81)	27/40 (68)		63
Myoglobin	>2.6 ng/mL/min over 60 minutes	11/12 (92)	3/5 (60)	Good sensitivity within 60 minutes; reliability may be affected by rapid release and clearance, which limit the diagnostic window	17
	4.6-fold increase over 2 hours	29/34 (85)	6/6 (100)		26
	>5.5 ng/mL/min over 60 minutes	(54)	(83)		19
	$\geq$2.5 ng/mL/min over 90 minutes	(94)	(88)		46
	Ratio of value after to value before fibrinolytic treatment >2.4	(91)	(100)	Distinguishes patency within 15 minutes of recanalization	27
Troponin T	$\geq$0.2 ng/mL/h over 90 minutes	(80)	(65)	Early sensitivity somewhat lower than other markers	46
	$\geq$0.5 ng/mL/h	(92)	(100)		32
Troponin I	$\geq$6 μg/mL over 90 minutes	(82)	(100)		34

[a] Sensitivity is defined as the number of patients identified by the marker as having had adequate reperfusion divided by the total number of patients exhibiting coronary recanalization documented independently (e.g., TIMI grade 2 or 3 flow).
[b] Specificity is the number of patients identified by the marker as having had inadequate reperfusion divided by the total number documented as having persistent occlusion (e.g., TIMI grade 0 or 1 flow).
[c] Adjusted for an estimated 25% rate of spontaneous reperfusion.

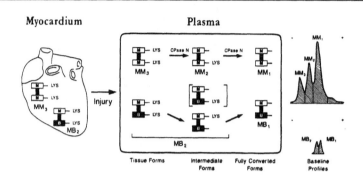

>10 U/L/h [10,46] during the initial 90 minutes of treatment with fibrinolytic agents, or an appearance rate constant >0.185 defined with the use of a multicompartmental model during the first 4 hours after treatment [11] have been shown to separate patients with and without recanalization reasonably well (Table 35-1). Nevertheless, the amount of CK released early after reperfusion is modest, in part because of its large size (molecular weight 80,000 d), and varies with the duration of preceding ischemia, the extent of infarction, and collateral blood flow. Thus, very early (i.e., within 1 hour) identification of patients failing to exhibit recanalization has not been a consistent finding [15,17,20].

ASSAYS

Blood samples should be obtained before administration of the fibrinolytic agent and serially at 30- to 60-minute intervals for 4 hours thereafter. CK activity and/or mass can be assayed in either plasma or serum. Assays based on measurement of CK mass with monoclonal antibodies exhibit high analytical sensitivity and specificity, and have become the method of choice [47–49]. Methods employing automated equipment yield results within 10–20 minutes, facilitating prospective diagnosis [49].

Subforms of CK Isoenzymes

Another approach for the assessment of coronary patency based on CK has emerged because it was learned that CK isoenzymes released from myocardium do not remain homogeneous in the circulation [50,51]. Both MM-CK and MB-CK undergo sequential and irreversible removal of a positively charged lysine residue from the carboxyl terminus of each M and B subunit comprising the dimer during exposure

FIGURE 35-2. Schematic of conversion of subforms of MM-CK and MB-CK. Myocardial subforms are converted in plasma to two other subforms by carboxypeptidase-N (CPase N) catalyzed hydrolysis of the carboxy-terminal lysine from each subunit. A fourth subform of MB-CK with lysine removed from the M but not the B subunit may not be induced in significant quantities because hydrolysis of the B subunit is favored in vivo [58]. Electrophoresis profiles of plasma (**right**) show three bands for MM-CK, but only two bands for MB-CK because of comigration of the tissue and intermediate species.

to circulating carboxypeptidase-N (Figure 35-2) [52–57]. This results in the appearance in the plasma after infarction of the tissue subforms with both carboxy-terminal lysines intact and exhibiting the highest isoelectric points, followed by time-dependent conversion and the appearance of other subforms (Figure 35-3), which retain enzymatic activity but have one or both carboxy-terminal lysine residues removed, and thereby progressively less positive charge and lower isoelectric points (Table 35-2). The subforms are numbered by their relative migration toward the anode during electrophoresis, with those migrating furthest having lower numbers [50]. Thus, for MM-CK, electrophoresis separates three subforms, with the subform comprising >95% of the MM-CK in myocardium [57], MM_3, migrating closest to the cathode; followed by the intermediate subform, with one carboxy-terminal lysine removed, MM_2; and the subform with both carboxy-terminal lysines removed, MM_1, migrating closest to the anode. For MB-CK, considerable confusion has arisen because electrophoresis resolves only two bands, designated MB_2 and MB_1 [50]. However, studies combining chromatographic and immunologic methods have shown that three subforms analogous to MM-CK circulate in vivo [58]; the tissue subform, a subform with the carboxy-

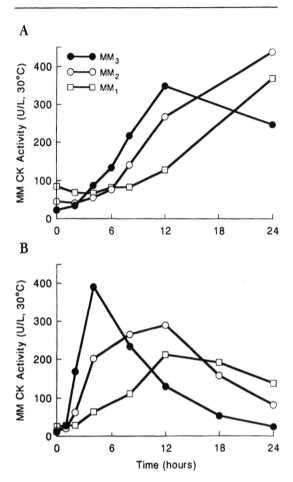

FIGURE 35-3. Time-activity profiles for MM-CK subforms in a patient who did not exhibit coronary recanalization (A) and in a patient who did exhibit coronary recanalization (B) after intravenous administration of tissue-type plasminogen activator (beginning at time 0). Peaks of MM_2 and MM_1 in patients without recanalization (not shown) are typically reached at 24 and 34 hours, respectively [14].

TABLE 35-2. Characteristics of CK subforms

Subform	Isoelectric point[a]	Percentage of total MM-CK or MB-CK isoenzyme activity in normal plasma
MM_3[b]	6.90	15 ± 7[c]
MM_2	6.67	30 ± 10[c]
MM_1	6.45	55 ± 14[c]
(MB_3)[d]	(5.4)	NA
MB_2	5.2	49[e]
MB_1	5.1	51[e]

[a] Determined by isoelectric focusing.
[b] Comprises >95% of MM-CK in the supernatant of extracts of human myocardium [57].
[c] Mean and SD of data from 26 healthy subjects with subforms quantitated by chromatofocusing [66].
[d] Putative tissue subform in extracts of human myocardium [67]. MB_3 and MB_2 together likely comprise the MB_2 band identified by electrophoresis (Figure 35-2).
[e] Average percentages from 56 normal subjects with subforms separated by electrophoresis [91]. The MB_2 fraction is likely to be comprised of both the tissue subform (MB_3) and an intermediate subform lacking one carboxy-terminal lysine (Figure 35-2).

Subform analysis facilitates early detection of coronary recanalization because conversion and plasma clearance of the tissue-specific species occurs rapidly and continuously. Thus, the modest amounts of the tissue subforms released into plasma within the first few hours after the onset of acute myocardial infarction are partially eliminated, keeping the proportions of the tissue subforms in plasma near physiologic concentrations (see Table 35-2). This enhances the sensitivity for the washout of tissue subforms associated with coronary recanalization.

CHARACTERISTICS OF PLASMA PROFILES OF SUBFORMS OF MM-CK ASSOCIATED WITH CORONARY RECANALIZATION

Patients in whom coronary recanalization is induced early (during the 0–6 hour time window) after the onset of symptoms exhibit more rapid appearance and earlier peaking of MM-CK subform activities compared with those in whom recanalization is not achieved (see Figure 35-3). The first manifestation of enzyme washout is the rapid rise in MM_3, which reaches a peak within 9 hours, at least 3 hours before the peak of total CK and MB-CK activities [14,23]. Accelerated rates of increase of MM_3 (expressed as a percentage of total MM-CK activity to eliminate much of the variability seen in CK activity profiles induced by differences in the extent of infarction at the time of reperfusion) have been shown to reliably distinguish animals with release of coronary occlusion

terminal lysine on the M subunit but not the B subunit, and a subform with both carboxy-terminal lysines removed (see Figure 35-2). Thus, cleavage of lysine from the B subunit appears to be favored in vivo. Comigration during electrophoresis of the tissue subform and the subform with lysine removed from the B subunit may account for separation of only two bands, which could blunt the accuracy of analyses based on changes in subform profiles. The physiologic role of subform modifications is unclear because removal of carboxy-terminal lysines from MM-CK delays its clearance from the circulation [59].

from those with persistent occlusion as early as 30 minutes after reperfusion [17,60,61], and to separate patients with and without recanalization within 1 hour after the onset of administration of fibrinolytic agents [15,17,20]. This is remarkable because the average time to recanalization in patients is approximately 45 minutes [62].

The accelerated appearance of $MM_3\%$ after release of coronary occlusions in experimental animals is minimally affected by superimposed flow-limiting, high-grade stenosis (94% reduction of lumen area), typical of that seen in patients [61]. This suggests that any degree of reperfusion may be sufficient to induce striking, early changes in the MM-CK subform profiles, which could make delineation of patients exhibiting only transitory recanalization and early reocclusion more problematic.

Criteria based on accelerated rates of increase of MM_3 appear valid when administration of fibrinolytic agents occurs within 4–6 hours after the onset of symptoms and for acquisition of blood samples up to 2 hours after the onset of reperfusion [21,60], before acceleration of release of MM-CK occurring with nonreperfused infarction overtakes that induced by reperfusion. Preliminary results from the TIMI study group [63] with patency of the infarct-related artery documented angiographically 90 minutes after the onset of fibrinolytic therapy have indicated that a rate of increase of $MM_3\%$ ≥0.18%/min over the first 90 minutes distinguishes the majority of patients with occluded from those with patent arteries (see Table 35-1).

Some investigators have reported criteria for reperfusion based on changes in the ratio of MM_3 to MM_1 [13,14,19,20,23,24], but this index does not appear to improve the reliability compared with MM_3 alone, and it requires measurement of two subform species instead of one. However, inclusion of a criterion that requires $MM_3\%$ to exceed some absolute value indicative of marked and persistent reperfusion (such as $MM_3\%$ ≥54%, equivalent to the mean plus one standard deviation of the peak among patients not exhibiting reperfusion), together with a rate of increase ≥0.18%/min, appears to increase specificity to nearly 90% for Thrombolysis in Myocardial Infarction Trial (TIMI) blood flow grades 0 and 1, indicative of persistent coronary occlusion (Abendschein, unpublished observation). Similarly, Laperche et al. [24], reporting on the performance of criteria applied prospectively in patients treated with fibrinolytic agents, found that the relative increase in absolute value of the ratio of MM_3 to MM_1 over the first 90 minutes exhibited greater specificity for failed reperfusion compared with the slope of the increase.

CHARACTERISTICS OF PLASMA PROFILES OF SUBFORMS OF MB-CK ASSOCIATED WITH CORONARY RECANALIZATION

Changes in profiles of subforms of MB-CK have also been examined for their potential to detect recanalization [16,18], although their utility is presently limited compared with subforms of MM-CK because of the more modest quantity of MB-CK in myocardium and the lack of assays to separate all of the subforms induced in vivo [58]. Based on changes in the two sub-bands separated by electrophoresis, the ratio of MB_2 (the band containing the tissue subform) to MB_1 was shown to increase significantly in the first hour after fibrinolytic therapy, with a peak ratio ≥3.8 permitting reasonable separation of patients identified subsequently as having undergone coronary recanalization (see Table 35-1) [18].

Conjoint analysis of the tissue subforms of both MM-CK and MB-CK may provide even more robust detection of recanalization than is possible with either alone. Very high sensitivity and specificity for detection of recanalization within 30 minutes of its onset was reported with the use of an immunoinhibition assay that quantifies M subunits with intact carboxy-terminal lysines derived from the tissue subforms for both MM-CK and MB-CK, as well as the subform intermediate for MM-CK [22]. Preliminary results also suggest that the rate of increase of $MM_3\%$, considered together with either the ratio of MB_2 to MB_1 [63] or the rate of increase of $MB_2\%$ [64], enhances the sensitivity for the detection of recanalization.

ASSAYS

Blood samples should be obtained before and at 30- to 60-minute intervals for 3 hours after the onset of administration of the fibrinolytic agent. Subforms may be assayed in either plasma or serum, but plasma obtained from blood added directly to ice-cooled tubes containing ethylenediaminetetraacetic acid (EDTA; final concentration 7–10 mmol/L) is preferred to immediately inhibit the carboxypeptidase that induces conversion of the subforms [65].

Because subforms differ with respect to charge, methods including electrophoresis [14,16,18], isoelectric focusing [13,20,23], and chromatofocusing [17,21,65,66] have been used for their separation. Chromatofocusing is the most quantitative method for MM-CK subforms [57,65,66], but it is labor intensive. Electrophoresis, particularly with systems employing high voltage, permits completion of assays within 30 minutes and requires minimal technician time, but it tends to underestimate MM_3 and to overestimate MM_1 compared with chromatofocusing (Abendschein, unpublished observation), and, as described earlier, it does not separate all of the subforms of MB-CK. Isoelectric focusing has been reported to separate MB-CK into three sub-bands [67], but whether the third band represents a true subform or an additional species induced by changes in the redox state, as occurs for subforms of MM-CK separated by isoelectric focusing [68,69], remains to be determined.

More facile assays for rapid quantification of CK subforms currently in development are based on immunologic methods. One commercial assay employs an antibody for M subunits lacking carboxy-terminal lysines to detect the circulating subform species [70]. However, immunodetection of the tissue-specific subforms with intact carboxy-terminal lysines would likely permit even earlier, more reliable detection of new enzyme release associated with coronary recanalization. One such assay in development employs an antibody that recognizes only M subunits with the carboxy-terminal lysines intact [22,71].

Myoglobin

Considerable interest has been shown for myoglobin as a marker of coronary recanalization because of its rapid appearance in plasma, attributable to the small size of the molecule (molecular weight 17,800 d). Like CK, myoglobin is a cytosolic protein found in both skeletal and cardiac muscle, but, as discussed earlier, the lack of specificity for myocardium does not hinder its use to detect the washout response after recanalization. In experimental animals, plasma myoglobin levels peak approximately 30 minutes after the release of coronary occlusions [17,25], which coincides with the time of onset of the peak of MM_3 proportion, but precedes the peak of MB-CK activity by as much as 5 hours [25].

In patients with reperfusion following administration of fibrinolytic agents and/or percutaneous transluminal coronary angioplasty, the peak of myoglobin in plasma occurs within 2 hours after the onset of therapy and the rate of increase is 10-fold higher (13.5 ng/mL/min) than in those with persistent coronary occlusions (peak at 6 hours and rate of 1.2 ng/mL/min) [26]. Criteria for reperfusion based on rates of change of myoglobin concentration >2.5–5.5 ng/mL/min over 60–90 minutes, or a 4.6-fold increase over 2 hours, have been demonstrated to provide reasonably high sensitivities and specificities for recanalization that are comparable with those observed with MM-CK subforms (see Table 35-1) [17,26,46]. Although some have reported that a peak of myoglobin occurring later than 9 hours predicts persistent occlusion with 100% accuracy [72], others have shown considerable overlap of times to peak among patients with and without successful thrombolytic reperfusion precluding reliable diagnosis [19,73]. This limitation, in addition to the delay imposed by delineation of the time at which the peak concentration occurs, suggests that criteria based on rates of increase of plasma concentrations may be most useful.

Because of its smaller size, myoglobin appears in the circulation in significant quantities earlier than CK, which increases its rapidity in diagnosis of recanalization [17,25,27,28]. However, faster release of myoglobin may make the assay less sensitive to transitory or partial reperfusion. Myoglobin also clears from the circulation faster than CK (the clearance half-life in dogs is 38 minutes for myoglobin [25] and 106 minutes for MM-CK [74]), shortening the interval available for detection of the accelerated rates associated with recanalization. Thus, better separation of patients exhibiting recanalization from those with persistent occlusion was observed by analysis of the rate of increase of myoglobin over the first compared with the second hour after the onset of fibrinolytic therapy [17]. Other investigators have suggested that assay of myoglobin every 15 minutes after the onset of treatment may be most useful to yield a high predictive accuracy (≥95%) for reperfusion [27,28].

Because patients with brisk reperfusion blood flow (TIMI grade 3) sometimes develop small infarcts, and therefore may not exhibit a rapid rise in serum myoglobin, leading to a false-negative conclusion, a recent report has suggested the use of a cutoff value for serum myoglobin in addition to the rate of increase [29]. In a modest retrospective study, these investigators observed that an appearance ratio of <2.4 (obtained by dividing the myoglobin concentration at 2 hours by the baseline value), combined with a serum myoglobin value of >200 µg/L at 2 hours, correctly identified patients likely to have had large infarcts and no reperfusion, while patients with ratios <2.4 and serum myoglobin <200 µg/L could have been followed for identification of a peak value within 5 hours indicative of reperfusion of a small infarct. Considering the differences in kinetics between myoglobin and other biochemical markers, conjoint analysis of myoglobin and MB-CK or CK subforms may prove more useful than analysis of individual markers alone, as suggested by preliminary studies [17].

ASSAYS

Blood samples should be obtained before and at 30- to 60-minute intervals for 3 hours after the onset of fibrinolytic therapy. Several assays are commercially available, including a radioimmunoassay, a latex agglutination assay, and an immunonephelometric assay. A quantitative radioimmunoassay was described initially [75], but it takes approximately 2 hours to perform and is therefore unsuitable for prospective analysis. Both the latex agglutination and the immunonephelometric assays are semiquantitative but more rapid, yielding results within 30 minutes [76–78]. Recently, a two-site particle concentration immunofluorescence immunoassay was described that is both rapid (reaction completed in 15 minutes) and sensitive, with a linear analytic range between 20 and 675 µg/L and exhibits good correlation with radioimmunoassay [79].

Troponins

Subunits of the troponin complex (troponin T, the tropomyosin binding subunit, molecular weight 39,000 d; troponin I, the actinomyosin-adenosine triphosphate inhibiting subunit, molecular weight 26,500 d; and troponin C, the calcium binding subunit, molecular weight 18,000 d) have been studied as markers of acute myocardial infarction because they exhibit tissue-specific isoforms [80]. Troponins are primarily bound to the contractile apparatus, accounting for a very low circulating level under physiologic conditions and a protracted release following tissue necrosis.

Nevertheless, patients with coronary recanalization within 6 hours after the onset of symptoms exhibit a more marked early release and peak of troponin T after 12–14 hours compared with a peak after 1–5 days in the absence of reperfusion [30,31,46]. This has been interpreted as reflecting the presence of a mobile pool of troponin, possibly in the cytosol, that is released more rapidly than the bound fraction [30]. Using the rate of increase of plasma troponin T for early diagnosis of coronary recanalization, several studies [32,46] have shown that rates >0.2–0.5 ng/mL/h permit relatively good detection of coronary patency compared with MB-CK and myoglobin (see Table 35-1). More recently, preliminary results [34] with a rate for troponin I of ≥6 µg/mL over the first 90 minutes after the onset of fibrinolytic therapy showed better sensitivity for recanalization compared with either MB-CK or myoglobin (see Table 35-1).

ASSAYS
Optimal sampling intervals have not been defined, but blood samples acquired at intervals similar to those for CK subforms (i.e., 30- to 60-minute intervals over 3 hours) are likely to be useful to identify recanalization. Available assays employ polyclonal or monoclonal antibodies to specific troponin isoforms

and enzyme immunoassays that are suitable for semi-automated analysis to be completed within 30 minutes to 2 hours [30,81,82].

Clinical Implications and Recommendations

Approximately 25% of patients who receive fibrinolytic agents for treatment of acute myocardial infarction do not exhibit sustained coronary recanalization. Thus, rapid, easily performed assays are mandatory to identify during the first 1–2 hours of fibrinolytic therapy, when the majority of vessels reopen, patients with inadequate reperfusion who require alternate interventional procedures. Serial coronary angiography is neither logistically feasible nor required in all patients. Because the kinetics of myocardial protein appearance in the circulation depend on coronary blood flow, monitoring serial changes in selected marker proteins is useful to assess the restoration of blood flow after treatment. Specificity of the marker proteins for myocardium is not as important because their occurrence in abundance in myocardium and in low concentrations in the circulation enhance the analytical sensitivity for protein washout associated with recanalization.

Among potential marker proteins studied thus far, subforms of CK and myoglobin appear to permit the earliest reliable separation of patients with and without coronary recanalization (see Table 35-1) [83–88]. The small quantity of CK released during the first 1–2 hours after the onset of fibrinolytic therapy limits the accuracy of delineation of coronary recanalization from its absence by changes in plasma total CK or MB-CK activity alone, particularly when circulating levels are elevated before therapy begins. However, analysis of subforms permits quantification of the tissue-specific species that increases the sensitivity for even small amounts of released CK. The amount of troponin released early after reperfusion may be even less than for CK, but the low circulating levels of troponins seen initially, and their relatively low molecular weights compared with CK, may facilitate the detection of the washout associated with restored patency. Additional studies are needed to define and test potential criteria for recanalization based on troponin subunits.

For prompt recognition of recanalization by CK subforms or myoglobin, analysis of the rates of increase and the magnitude of change in the tissue protein concentration in blood is preferred over the time to peak concentration because the delay in defining whether a peak has occurred is longer than the time available to rescue unsuccessfully reperfused myocardium. Thus, rates of increase of the tissue subform of MM-CK, $MM_3\%$, $\leq 0.18\%/min$, defined by analysis of two blood samples collected before and 90 minutes after the onset of use of a fibrinolytic agent, have yielded specificities for persistently occluded arteries in the range of 70–100% (see Table 35-1) and nearly 90% when evaluated together with a 90-minute value of $MM_3\%$ of $\leq 54\%$. Comparably high specificity has been observed with the use of rates of increase of myoglobin of $\leq 2.4\,ng/mL/min$ measured over the first 2 hours after the onset of use of a fibrinolytic agent (see Table 35-1). Specificity may be increased further by combining the rate with an absolute value that facilitates the delineation of large, non-reperfused infarcts [29].

Despite the promising results obtained from initial retrospective studies, all of the biochemical markers tested thus far are limited in that they do not adequately distinguish patients with TIMI grade 3 blood flow from those with TIMI grade 2 flow, because any restoration of flow appears to lead to a rapid rise and fall of the marker in plasma. Distinguishing the adequacy of reperfusion blood flow may be important, however, because patients with TIMI grade 2 reperfusion appear to exhibit poor clinical outcomes [89]. Another limitation of currently available markers is that reocclusion occurring after short periods of reperfusion may not be detectable.

Preliminary results suggest that conjoint analysis of multiple markers may be even more sensitive and specific for the adequacy of coronary recanalization than individual markers. Combinations of proteins with different kinetics of release and clearance from plasma, such as myoglobin and subforms of CK or troponin, may be particularly effective [17,63,64]. Another combined approach that is under investigation involves analyses of one or more biochemical markers, together with continuous, computer-assisted monitoring of changes in the QRS complex and ST segments [90], which have been shown to permit rapid, qualitative identification of vessel patency [35–40]. Combinations of biochemical markers and selected clinical variables may be useful as well [12].

Because these approaches are ultimately utilized for virtual on-line detection of arteries requiring additional intervention, results will need to be available within 30–60 minutes of the time of aquisition of blood samples to enable prospective clinical decision making. This is currently a limitation of application of biochemical markers because assays are specific for single analytes, labor intensive, and require processing of plasma or serum samples, which adds to the delay. Subforms of CK are analyzed by semi-automated electrophoresis within 30 minutes of

sample collection, and myoglobin and troponin by immunoassays within 10–20 minutes. However, availability of additional immunologic-based assays, coupled with low-cost automated equipment capable of analysis of multiple markers in whole blood samples, should facilitate STAT laboratory or bedside testing.

References

1. Califf RM, O'Neil W, Stack RS, Aronson L, Mark DB, Mantell S, George BS, Candela RJ, Kereiakes DJ, Abbottsmith C, Topol EJ, and the TAMI Study Group. Failure of simple clinical measurements to predict perfusion status after intravenous thrombolysis. Ann Intern Med 108:658, 1988.

2. Miller FC, Krucoff MW, Satler LF, Green CE, Fletcher RD, Del Negro AA, Pearle DL, Kent KM, Rackley CE. Ventricular arrhythmias during reperfusion. Am Heart J 112:928, 1986.

3. Kircher BJ, Topol EJ, O'Neill WW, Pitt B. Prediction of infarct coronary artery recanalization after intravenous thrombolytic therapy. Am J Cardiol 59:513, 1987.

4. Hackett D, Davies G, Chierchia S, Maseri A. Intermittent coronary occlusion in acute myocardial infarction. Value of combined thrombolytic and vasodilator therapy. N Engl J Med 317:1055, 1987.

5. Shell W, Mickle DK, Swan HJC. Effects of nonsurgical myocardial reperfusion on plasma creatine kinase kinetics in man. Am Heart J 106:665, 1983.

6. Wei JY, Markis JE, Malagold M, Grossman W. Time course of serum cardiac enzymes after intracoronary thrombolytic therapy. Arch Intern Med 145:1596, 1985.

7. Panteghini M, Cuccia C, Calarco M, Gei P, Bozzetti E, Visioli O. Serum enzymes in acute myocardial infarction after intracoronary thrombolysis. Clin Biochem 19:294, 1986.

8. Gore JM, Roberts R, Ball SP, Montero A, Goldberg RJ, Dalen JE. Peak creatine kinase as a measure of effectiveness of thrombolytic therapy in acute myocardial infarction. Am J Cardiol 59:1234, 1987.

9. Garabedian HD, Gold HK, Yasuda T, Johns JA, Finkelstein DM, Gaivin RJ, Cobbaert C, Leinbach RC, Collen D. Detection of coronary artery reperfusion with creatine kinase-MB determinations during thrombolytic therapy: Correlation with acute angiography. J Am Coll Cardiol 11:729, 1988.

10. Lewis BS, Ganz W, Laramee P, Cercek B, Hod H, Shah PK, Lew AS. Usefulness of a rapid initial increase in plasma creatine kinase activity as a marker of reperfusion during thrombolytic therapy for acute myocardial infarction. Am J Cardiol 62:20, 1988.

11. Grande P, Granborg J, Clemmensen P, Sevilla DC, Wagner NB, Wagner GS. Indices of reperfusion in patients with acute myocardial infarction using characteristics of the CK-MB time-activity curve. Am Heart J 122:400, 1991.

12. Ohman EM, Christenson RH, Califf RM, George BS, Samaha JK, Kereiakes DJ, Worley SJ, Wall TC, Berrios E, Sigmon KN, Lee K, Topol EJ, for the TAMI 7 Study Group: Noninvasive detection of reperfusion after thrombolysis based on serum creatine kinase MB changes and clinical variables. Am Heart J 126:819, 1993.

13. Apple FS, Sharkey SW, Werdick M, Elsperger KJ, Tilbury RT. Analyses of creatine kinase isoenzymes and isoforms in serum to detect reperfusion after acute myocardial infarction. Clin Chem 33:507, 1987.

14. Panteghini M, Pagani F. Isoforms of creatine kinase isoenzymes in serum in acute myocardial infarction after intracoronary thromboysis. Clin Chem 33:2039, 1987.

15. Seacord LM, Abendschein DR, Nohara R, Hartzler G, Sobel BE, Jaffe AS. Detection of reperfusion within 1 hour after coronary recanalisation by analysis of isoforms of the MM creatine kinase isoenzyme in plasma. Fibrinolysis 2:151, 1988.

16. Christenson RH, Ohman EM, Clemmensen P, Grande P, Toffaletti J Silverman LM, Vollmer RT, Wagner GS. Characteristics of creatine kinase-MB and MB isoforms in serum after reperfusion in acute myocardial infarction. Clin Chem 35:2179, 1989.

17. Abendschein DR, Ellis AK, Eisenberg PR, Klocke FJ, Sobel BE, Jaffe AS. Prompt detection of coronary recanalization by analysis of rates of change of concentrations of macromolecular markers in plasma. Cor Art Dis 2:201, 1991.

18. Puleo PR, Perryman MB. Noninvasive detection of reperfusion in acute myocardial infarction based on plasma activity of creatine kinase MB subforms. J Am Coll Cardiol 17:1047, 1991.

19. Laperche T, Steg PG, Benessiano J, Dehoux M, Juliard J-M, Himbert D, Gourgon R. Patterns of myoglobin and MM creatine kinase isoforms release early after intravenous thrombolysis or direct percutaneous transluminal coronary angioplasty for acute myocardial infarction, and implications for the early noninvasive diagnosis of reperfusion. Am J Cardiol 70:1129, 1992.

20. Schofer J, Ress-Grigolo G, Voigt KD, Mathey DG, for the PRIMI study group. Early detection of coronary artery patency after thrombolysis by determination of the MM creatine kinase isoforms in patients with acute myocardial infarction. Am Heart J 123:846, 1992.

21. Norris RM, Twigden DG, Williams BF, Johnson RN, White HD. Use of creatine kinase isoforms for diagnosis of infarct artery patency after thrombolytic therapy with streptokinase. Cor Art Dis 4:201, 1993.

22. Abe S, Nomoto K, Arima S, Miyata M, Yamashita T, Maruyama I, Toda H, Okino H, Atsuchi Y, Tahara M, Nakao S, Tanaka H, Suzuki T. Detection of reperfusion 30 and 60 minutes after coronary recanalization by a rapid new assay of creatine kinase isoforms in acute myocardial infarction. Am Heart J 125:649, 1993.

23. Morelli RL, Emilson B, Rapaport E. MM-CK subtypes diagnose reperfusion early after myocardial infarction. Am J Med Sci 293:139, 1987.

24. Laperche T, Steg PG, Dehoux M, Benessiano J, Grollier G, Aliot E, Mossard J-M, Aubry P, Coisne D, Hanssen M, Iliou M-C, for the PERM Study Group. A study of biochemical markers of reperfusion early after thrombolysis for acute myocardial infarction. Circulation 92:2079, 1995.

25. Ellis AK, Little T, Masud ARZ, Klocke FJ. Patterns of myoglobin release after reperfusion of injured myocardium. Circulation 72:639, 1985.

26. Ellis AK, Little T, Masud ARZ, Liberman HA, Morris DC, Klocke FJ. Early noninvasive detection of successful reperfusion in patients with acute myocardial infarction. Circulation 78:1352, 1988.

27. Ishii J, Nomura M, Ando T, Hasegawa H, Kimura M, Kurokawa H, Iwase M, Kondo T, Watanabe Y, Hishida H, Sotohata I, Mizuno Y. Early detection of successful coronary reperfusion based on serum myoglobin concentration: Comparison with serum creatine kinase isoenzyme MB activity. Am Heart J 128:641, 1994.

28. Miyata M, Abe S, Arima S, Nomoto K, Kawataki M, Ueno M, Yamashita T, Hamasaki S, Toda H, Tahara M, Atsuchi Y, Nakao S, Tanaka H. Rapid diagnosis of coronary reperfusion by measurement of myoglobin level every 15 min in acute myocardial infarction. J Am Coll Cardiol 23:1009, 1994.

29. Jurlander B, Clemmensen P, Ohman EM, Christenson R, Wagner GS, Grande P. Serum myoglobin for the early non-invasive detection of coronary reperfusion in patients with acute myocardial infarction. Eur Heart J 17:399, 1996.

30. Katus HA, Remppis A, Scheffold T, Diederich KW, Kuebler W. Intracellular compartmentation of cardiac troponin T and its release kinetics in patients with reperfused and nonreperfused myocardial infarction. Am J Cardiol 67:1360, 1991.

31. Remppis A, Scheffold T, Karrer O, Zehelein J, Hamm C, Grünig E, Bode C, Kübler W, Katus HA. Assessment of reperfusion of the infarct zone after acute myocardial infarction by serial cardiac troponin T measurements in serum. Br Heart J 71:242, 1994.

32. Abe S, Arima S, Yamashita T, Miyata M, Okino H, Toda H, Nomoto K, Ueno M, Tahara M, Kiyonaga K, Nakao S, Tanaka H. Early assessment of reperfusion therapy using cardiac troponin T. J Am Coll Cardiol 23:1382, 1994.

33. Apple FS, Voss E, Lund L, Preese L, Berger CR, Henry TD. Cardiac troponin, CK-MB and myoglobin for the early detection of acute myocardial infarction and monitoring of reperfusion following thrombolytic therapy. Clin Chim Acta 237:59, 1995.

34. Apple FS, Henry TD, Berger CR, Landt YA. Early monitoring of serum cardiac troponin I for assessment of coronary reperfusion following thrombolytic therapy. Am J Clin Pathol 105:6, 1996.

35. Krucoff MW, Green CE, Satler LF, Miller FC, Pallas

RS, Kent KM, Del Negro AA, Pearle DL, Fletcher RD, Rackley CE. Noninvasive detection of coronary artery patency using continuous ST-segment monitoring. Am J Cardiol 57:916, 1986.

36. Dellborg M, Topol EJ, Swedberg K. Dynamic QRS complex and ST segment vectorcardiographic monitoring can identify vessel patency in patients with acute myocardial infarction treated with reperfusion therapy. Am Heart J 122:943, 1991.

37. Krucoff MW, Croll MA, Pope JE, Granger CB, O'Connor CM, Sigmon KN, Wagner BL, Ryan JA, Lee KL, Kereiakes DJ, Samaha JK, Worley SJ, Ellis SG, Wall TC, Topol EJ, Califf RM, for the TAMI 7 study group. Continuous 12-lead ST-segment recovery analysis in the TAMI 7 study. Performance of a noninvasive method for real-time detection of failed myocardial reperfusion. Circulation 88:437, 1993.

38. Krucoff MW, Croll Pope JE, Pieper KS, Kanani PM, Granger CB, Veldkamp RF, Wagner BL, Sawchak ST, Califf RM. Continuously updated 12-lead ST-segment recovery analysis for myocardial infarct artery patency assessment and its correlation with multiple simultaneous early angiographic observations. Am J Cardiol 71:145, 1993.

39. Fernandez AR, Sequeira RF, Chakko S, Correa LF, DeMarchena EJ, Chahine RA, Franceour DA, Myerburg RJ. ST segment tracking for rapid determination of patency of the infarct-related artery in acute myocardial infarction. J Am Coll Cardiol 26:675, 1995.

40. Dellborg M, Steg PG, Simoons M, Dietz R, Sen S, van den Brand M, Lotze U, Hauck S, van den Wieken R, Himbert D, Svensson A-M, Swedberg K. Vectorcardiographic monitoring to assess early vessel patency after reperfusion therapy for acute myocardial infarction. Eur Heart J 16:21, 1995.

41. Blumenthal MR, Wang H-H, Liu LMP. Experimental coronary arterial occlusion and release. Effects on enzymes, electrocardiograms, myocardial contractility and reactive hyperemia. Am J Cardiol 36:225, 1975.

42. Michael LH, Hunt JR, Weilbaecher D, Perryman MB, Roberts R, Lewis RM, Entman ML. Creatine kinase and phosphorylase in cardiac lymph: Coronary occlusion and reperfusion. Am J Physiol 248:H350, 1985.

43. van der Laarse A, van der Wall EE, van den Pol RC, Vermeer F, Verheugt FWA, Krauss XH, Bar FWHM, Hermens WT, Willems GM, Simoons ML. Rapid enzyme release from acutely infarcted myocardium after early thrombolytic therapy: Washout or reperfusion damage? Am Heart J 115:711, 1988.

44. Christenson RH, Ohman EM, Vollmer RT, Clemmensen P, Grande P, Wagner GS. Serum release of the creatine kinase tissue-specific isoforms MM3 and MB2 is simultaneous during myocardial reperfusion. Clin Chim Acta 200:23, 1991.

45. Hirai T, Fujita M, Sasayama S, Ohno A, Yamanishi K, Nakajima H, Asanoi H. Importance of coronary collateral circulation for kinetics of serum creatine kinase in

acute myocardial infarction. Am J Cardiol 60:446, 1987.

46. Zabel M, Hohnloser SH, Koster W, Prinz M, Kasper W, Just H. Analysis of creatine kinase, CK-MB, myoglobin, and troponin T time-activity curves for early assessment of coronary artery reperfusion after intravenous thrombolysis. Circulation 87:1542, 1993.

47. Delanghe JR, De Mol AM, De Buyzere ML, De Scheerder IK, Wieme RJ. Mass concentration and activity concentration of creatine kinase isoenzyme MB compared in serum after acute myocardial infarction. Clin Chem 36:149, 1990.

48. Mair J, Artner-Dworzak E, Dienstl A, Lechleitner P, Morass B, Smidt J, Wagner I, Wettach C, Puschendorf B. Early detection of acute myocardial infarction by measurement of mass concentration of creatine kinase-MB. Am J Cardiol 68:1545, 1991.

49. Landt Y, Vaidya HC, Porter SE, Whalen K, McClellan A, Amyx C, Parvin CA, Kessler G, Nahm MH, Dietzler DN, Ladenson JH. Semi-automated direct colorimetric measurement of creatine kinase isoenzyme MB activity after extraction from serum by use of a CK-MB-specific monoclonal antibody. Clin Chem 34:575, 1988.

50. Wevers RA, Olthuis HP, Van Niel JCC, van Wilgenburg MGM, Soons JBJ. A study on the dimeric structure of creatine kinase (EC 2.7.3.2). Clin Chim Acta 75:377, 1977.

51. Morelli RL, Carlson CJ, Emilson B, Abendschein DR, Rapaport E. Serum creatine Kinase MM isoenzyme sub-bands after acute myocardial infarction in man. Circulation 67:1283, 1983.

52. George S, Ishikawa Y, Perryman MB, Roberts R. Purification and characterization of naturally occurring and in vitro induced multiple forms of MM creatine kinase. J Biol Chem 259:2667, 1984.

53. Billadello JJ, Roman DG, Grace AM, Sobel BE, Strauss AW. The nature of post-translational formation of MM creatine kinase isoforms. J Biol Chem 260:14988, 1985.

54. Billadello JJ, Fontanet HL, Strauss AW, Abendschein DR. Characterization of MB creatine kinase isoform conversion in vitro and in vivo in dogs. J Clin Invest 83:1637, 1989.

55. Abendschein DR, Serota H, Plummer Jr TH, Amiraian K, Strauss AW, Sobel BE, Jaffe AS. Conversion of MM creatine kinase isoforms in human plasma by carboxypeptidase N. J Lab Clin Med 110:798, 1987.

56. Michelutti L, Falter H, Certossi S, Marcotte B, Mazzuchin A. Isolation and purification of creatine kinase conversion factor from human serum and its identification as carboxypeptidase N. Clin Biochem 20:21, 1987.

57. Hashimoto H, Grace AM, Billadello JJ, Gross RW, Strauss AW, Sobel BE. Nondenaturing quantification of subforms of canine MM creatine kinase isoenzymes (isoforms) and their interconversion. J Lab Clin Med 103:470, 1984.

58. Prager NA, Suzuki T, Jaffe AS, Sobel BE, Abendschein DR. Nature and time course of generation of isoforms of creatine kinase, MB fraction in vivo. J Am Coll Cardiol 20:414, 1992.

59. Abendschein DR, Fontanet HL, Markham J, Sobel BE. Physiologic modelling of MM creatine kinase isoforms. Math Comput Modelling 11:621, 1988.

60. Devries SR, Sobel BE, Abendschein DR. Early detection of myocardial reperfusion by assay of plasma MM-creatine kinase isoforms in dogs. Circulation 74:567, 1986.

61. Nohara R, Myears DW, Sobel BE, Abendschein DR. Optimal criteria for rapid detection of myocardial reperfusion by creatine kinase MM isoforms in the presence of residual high grade coronary stenosis. J Am Coll Cardiol 14:1067, 1989.

62. Collen D. Coronary thrombolysis: Streptokinase or recombinant tissue-type plasminogen activator? Ann Intern Med 112:529, 1990.

63. Abendschein DR, Puleo PR, Cannon CP, and the TIMI IV and V investigators. Noninvasive detection of early coronary artery patency based on plasma MM and MB creatine kinase (CK) isoforms. Circulation 86:I267, 1992.

64. Jaffe AS, Eisenberg PR, Abendschein DR. Conjoint use of MM and MB creatine kinase isoforms in detection of coronary recanalization. Am Heart J 127:1461, 1994.

65. Abendschein DR, Fontanet HL, Nohara R. Optimized preservation of isoforms of creatine kinase MM isoenzyme in plasma specimens and their rapid quantification by semi-automated chromatofocusing. Clin Chem 36:723, 1990.

66. Nohara R, Sobel BE, Jaffe AS, Abendschein DR. Quantitative analysis for isoforms of creatine kinase MM in plasma by chromatofocusing, with on-line monitoring of enzyme activity. Clin Chem 34:235, 1988.

67. Kanemitsu F, Okigaki T. Creatine kinase MB isoforms for early diagnosis and monitoring of acute myocardial infarction. Clin Chim Acta 206:191, 1992.

68. Williams J, Williams KM, Marshall T. Heterogeneity of serum creatine kinase isoenzyme MM in myocardial infarction: Clinical significance and post-synthetic conversion of "abnormal" sub-bands. Clin Chem 35:206, 1989.

69. Williams J, Williams KM, Marshall T. Heterogeneity of creatine kinase isoenzyme MM in serum in myocardial infarction: Interconversion of the "normal" and "abnormal" sub-bands by glutathione. Clin Chem 36:775, 1990.

70. Shah VD, Yen S-E, Diorio AF, Hammer PA. Two commercial test kits for CK-MM isoforms evaluated for early recognition of acute myocardial infarction. Clin Chem 35:493, 1989.

71. Suzuki T, Shiraishi T, Tomita K, Totani M, Murachi T. Monoclonal antibody inhibiting creatine kinase MM$_3$ but not isoform MM$_1$. Clin Chem 36:153, 1990.

72. Katus HA, Diederich KW, Scheffold T, Uellner M, Schwarz F, Kubler W. Non-invasive assessment of infarct reperfusion: The predictive power of the time to peak value of myoglobin, CK MB, and CK in serum. Eur Heart J 9:619, 1988.

73. McCullough DA, Harrison PG, Forshall JM, Irving JB, Hillman RJ. Serum myoglobin and creatine kinase enzymes in acute myocardial infarction treated with anistreplase. J Clin Pathol 45:405, 1992.

74. Rapaport E. The fractional disappearance rate of the separate isoenzymes of creatine phosphokinase in the dog. Cardiovasc Res 9:473, 1975.

75. Stone MJ, Willerson JT, Gomez-Sanchez CE, Waterman MR. Radioimmunoassay of myoglobin in human serum: Results in patients with acute myocardial infarction. J Clin Invest 56:1334, 1975.

76. Nørregaard-Hansen K, Hangaard J, Nørgaard-Pedersen B. A rapid latex agglutination test for detection of elevated levels of myoglobin in serum and its value in the early diagnosis of acute myocardial infarction. Scand J Clin Lab Invest 44:99, 1984.

77. Vrenna L, Castaldo AM, Castaldo P, Giardiello D, Di Giacomo C, Esposito LP, Romano F. Comparison between nephelometric and RIA methods for serum myoglobin, and efficiency of myoglobin assay for early diagnosis of myocardial infarction. Clin Chem 38:789, 1992.

78. Uji Y, Okabe H, Sugiuchi H, Sekine S. Measurement of serum myoglobin by a turbidimetric latex agglutination method. J Clin Lab Anal 6:7, 1992.

79. Silva DP Jr, Landt Y, Porter SE, Ladenson JH. Development and application of monoclonal antibodies to human cardiac myoglobin in a rapid fluorescence immunoassay. Clin Chem 37:1356, 1991.

80. Katus HA, Scheffold T, Remppis A, Zehlein J. Proteins of the troponin complex. Lab Med 23:311, 1992.

81. Bodor GS, Porter S, Landt Y, Ladenson JH. Development of monoclonal antibodies for an assay of cardiac troponin-I and preliminary results in suspected cases of myocardial infarction. Clin Chem 38:2203, 1992.

82. Larue C, Calzolari C, Bertinchant J-P, Leclercq F, Grolleau R, Pau B. Cardiac-specific immunoenzymometric assay of troponin I in the early phase of acute myocardial infarction. Clin Chem 39:972, 1993.

83. Adams JE, Abendschein DR, Jaffe AS. Biochemical markers of myocardial injury. Is MB creatine kinase the choice for the 1990s? Circulation 88:750, 1993.

84. Apple FS. Acute myocardial infarction and coronary reperfusion. Serum cardiac markers for the 1990s. Clin Chem 97:217, 1992.

85. Abendschein DR. Detection of recanalization with the use of creatine kinase-MM subforms. Cor Art Dis 3:461, 1992.

86. Grande P, Clemmensen P, Ohman EM, Wagner GS. Biochemical markers of early reperfusion. J Electrocardiol 25:6, 1992.

87. Abendschein DR. Early assessment of the success of thrombolytic therapy by noninvasive markers. Cor Art Dis 4:669, 1993.

88. Klootwijk P, Cobbaert C, Fioretti P, Kint PP, Simoons ML. Noninvasive assessment of reperfusion and reocclusion after thrombolysis in acute myocardial infarction. Am J Cardiol 72:75G, 1993.

89. Anderson JL, Karagounis LA. Becker LC, Sorensen SG, Menlove RL, for the TEAM-3 Investigators. TIMI perfusion grade 3 but not grade 2 results in improved outcome after thrombolysis for myocardial infarction. Ventriculographic, enzymatic, and electrocardiographic evidence from the TEAM-3 study. Circulation 87:1829, 1993.

90. Hohnloser SH, Zabel M, Kasper W, Meinertz T, Just H. Assessment of coronary artery patency after thrombolytic therapy: Accurate prediction utilizing the combined analysis of three noninvasive markers. J Am Coll Cardiol 18:44, 1991.

91. Puleo PR, Guadagno PA, Roberts R, Scheel MV, Marian AJ, Churchill D, Perryman MB. Early diagnosis of acute myocardial infarction based on assay for subforms of creatine kinase-MB. Circulation 82:759, 1990.

SECTION XI: ANTICOAGULATION MONITORING

James J. Ferguson

The safe and effective use of anticoagulant therapy requires that the therapy be adjusted to maintain the delicate balance between the prevention of pathologic thrombosis and the risk of bleeding. As our therapeutic armamentarium expands, so too must our ability to monitor and appropriately titrate the level of anticoagulation. This section describes the commonly used laboratory tests for assessing and adjusting the intensity of anticoagulant therapy, and discusses three major clinical scenarios in which coagulation monitoring is important: interventional procedures in the catheterization laboratory, acute coronary syndromes, and in the setting of chronic anticoagulant therapy for a number of different applications.

36. ANTICOAGULANT MONITORING

James M. Wilson

Introduction

Inhibition of normal hemostatic mechanisms is the cornerstone of medical therapy for many cardiovascular diseases. Inhibition of thrombus growth and development is the goal of antithrombotic therapy, yet it results in an increased risk of spontaneous hemorrhage, which may result in substantial morbidity and even death. Therefore, if antithrombotic therapy is to be of value, a delicate equilibrium must be maintained between prevention of pathologic thrombosis and an excess risk of life-threatening hemorrhage.

The therapeutic administration of antithrombotic drugs must be guided by some assessment of the risk of bleeding or continued thrombosis. While many clinical indicators are useful, the most reliable means of judging the effectiveness of therapy is by laboratory evaluation of drug effect [1]. Platelet function tests, such as the bleeding time, are useful in the diagnosis of specific platelet disorders but are of limited clinical value in judging the efficacy of antiplatelet therapy, which may be directed at a variety of mechanistic targets. However, measurement of blood coagulation is of extraordinary value in guiding drug therapy with conventional anticoagulant agents such as heparin and coumadin. Multiple types of assessment are possible, including individual enzyme inhibition [2–5], quantitation of thrombosis byproducts [6,7], and overall measures of clotting efficiency [8–11].

For years, global measures of coagulation enzyme efficiency, such as the prothrombin time and partial thromboplastin time, have been used as a rough guide to antithrombotic drug dosing. Ease of performance, simple reporting, and abundant clinical experience all contribute to the popularity of coagulation times for the guidance of routine antithrombotic therapy. Beneath the apparent simplicity of the routine coagulation times lies the incredibly complex interplay of enzymes, coenzymes, and inhibitors that combine to produce coagulation. Thorough understanding of these mechanisms and their effect on coagulation testing is a must for proper test interpretation and intelligent management of antithrombotic therapy.

This chapter focuses on the commonly used laboratory tests to assess and adjust the intensity of anticoagulant therapy. A number of different "coagulation times" are presented. For each, the background, theory, methodology, and interpretation are discussed.

Coagulation

In-vivo thrombosis involves platelet activation, aggregation, and the coordinated generation of fibrin, producing a platelet–fibrin polymer meshwork. Blood or plasma coagulation tests are a laboratory reproduction of events resulting in fibrin polymer formation, with or without platelet assistance. As a general rule, the relative speed with which blood or plasma coagulates in the laboratory is a measure of the function of the enzyme pathways, resulting in fibrin generation and thrombosis. However, the two processes are not necesscarily synonymous. Coagulation tests are initiated artificially, within the static confines of a test tube, often without the presence of erythrocytes or platelets. In vivo thrombosis is far more complex and may not be adequately represented, or in some instances may be misrepresented by in vitro coagulation. For example, the presence of a lupus anticoagulant, while prolonging in vitro coagulation, confers an increased risk of thrombosis [12].

Two principles govern laboratory measures of coagulation: the need for activation of an enzyme pathway and the need for a functional cofactor to assist enzyme function [14–17]. The characteristics of an individual test are determined by the activator and whether or not there is an excess of the necessary cofactors, such as phospholipid membrane. In many biological systems, unhindered enzyme cascades achieve their goal within a fraction of a second. Yet, when studied in the laboratory, the coagulation enzyme cascade requires several seconds from activation to the generation of an endpoint. Part of this extra or "lag" time reflects intrinsic regulatory processes in the

TABLE 36-1. Effect of cofactors on enzyme function

Enzyme Complex	Substrate	K_m[a] (μmol/L)	K_{cat}[b] (min^{-1})	K_{cat}/K_m (mol/L-min^1)
VIIa	X	4.87	0.024	4.93×10^3
VIIa/TF/PCPS/Ca^{2+}	X	0.45	69.0	1.53×10^8
IXa	X	299	0.002	6.69
IXa/VIII/PCPS/Ca^{2+}	X	0.063	500.0	7.94×10^9
Xa	II	131	0.6	4.58×10^3
Xa/Va/PCPS/Ca^{2+}	II	1.0	1800.0	1.80×10^9

[a] See Text.
[b] PCPS Phosphatidylcholine-phosphatidylserine vesicles. Adapted with permission [21].

progression of coagulation (see Figure 36-2) [14–16]. In vivo regulation of thrombosis is incredibly complex, with delicate coordination of a vast number of reactions involving the platelet, endothelial cell, procoagulant, anticoagulant, and thrombolytic enzymes. With the activator supplied in a simplified test tube reproduction, which obviates many of the regulatory and counter-regulatory mechanisms, the primary limitation to thrombus initiation and growth is cofactor availability.

For example, to reproduce the intrinsic pathway to thrombin generation in the laboratory, factor XII is activated on a negatively charged surface such as glass or kaolin. The pathway then proceeds with the activation of factor XI and the subsequent generation of an abundance of factor IXa. Factor Ixa works slowly in the absence of factor VIIIa, limiting the velocity and quantity of factor Xa production [15,17–19]. Factor Xa is similarly encumbered, so that after its production by factor IXa, it very slowly produces small amounts of thrombin (Table 36-1) [15,17–20].

Peak function of Factors Ixa and Xa occurs when they are part of an enzyme complex, *Ten-ase* (factor IXa–factor VIIIa–phospholipid membrane–Ca^{2+}) or *prothrombinase* (factor Xa–factor Va–phospholipid membrane–Ca^{2+}) [21–23]. These complexes are made up of an active enzyme (factors IXa and Xa) and the assisting cofactor (factors VIII and Va), interacting with ionized calcium and a catalytic phospholipid surface. In numerical terms, factor Xa alone requires over 100 micromolar concentrations of prothrombin to function at 1/2 V_{max} (a concentration known as the k_m), with a catalytic constant (K_{cat}) of 0.6 min^{-1}. When bound to cofactor Va, the reaction proceeds much faster, with the k_{cat} increasing to 2000 min^{-1}, while the k_m falls to 0.01 nM, making prothrombinase incredibly efficient. All of these reactions proceed upon the surface of a specific type of phospholipid membrane (see Table 36-1) [21].

Factors V and VIII do not circulate in an active form and are not within the stepwise progression leading to thrombin generation; active thrombin must independently activate these necessary cofactors. An activated phospholipid membrane is also not always freely available. It must have specific characteristics and usually be supplied with activated platelets, inflammatory cells. or stimulated endothelial cells [25–33]. Therefore, after maximal contact activation has produced an abundance of factor IXa, the intrinsic pathway is poised, awaiting the generation of factors Va and VIIIa, and perhaps platelet activation, to reach its full potential. When thrombin begins to emerge, it may activate factors VIII and V, thereby releasing the regulatory bottleneck and amplifying its own generation [14,15,18–20,25]. The result is a burst of thrombin activity, quickly reaching concentrations that will produce detectable amounts of fibrin, and timing is stopped.

Performing coagulation or clotting times requires the exposure of blood or plasma to an activator and, in some instances, the addition of calcium and a platelet membrane substitute. The endpoint of the test is the time at which sufficient fibrin has been generated to be detectable. Fibrin polymerization may be detected by a variety of methods, including the appearance of a visible fibrin clot, an increase in the optical density of the specimen, or a change in mechanical resistance (using a magnetic field manipulation or electrical conduction; Figure 36-1) [13].

Prothrombin Time

Near the turn of the century, the understanding of blood coagulation was summarized by:

Prothrombin $\xrightarrow{\text{thrombokinase}}$ thrombin

Fibrinogen $\xrightarrow{\text{thrombin}}$ fibrin

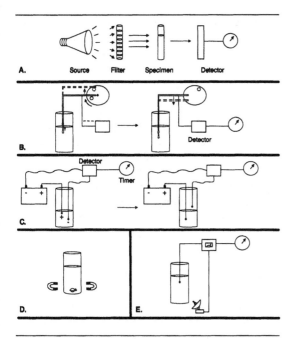

FIGURE 36-1. Fibrin polymer detection methods. **A:** Light transmission of a plasma sample increases as fibrinogen leaves the solution in fibrin polymers. A threshold value or percentage of light transmission may be set to stop the timer. **B:** As fibrin polymers form, specimen viscosity rises. When a plunger is lifted and then allowed to fall, the rate of fall is a measure of specimen viscosity. **C:** Two electrodes may be placed in a specimen and a current established. One of the electrodes may be withdrawn from the specimen at preset intervals. When viscosity rises, contact between the moving electrode and the specimen will not be broken and the timer will stop. **D:** If a ferromagnetic substance is placed in the specimen, motion may be established by an oscillating magnetic field. When motion is restricted to a preset value, timing will stop. **E:** A probe may be placed in the specimen and vibrated at a preset frequency. A sensor, positioned outside the specimen, regulates the output of the probe to maintain a constant value. Fibrin polymerization and increased viscosity decrease sound transmission, increasing the output required of the probe.

The factors necessary to produce coagulation of blood were felt to circulate in an inactive state, awaiting conversion to their active form. The triggering substance for the conversion of prothrombin to active thrombin was termed *thrombokinase* or *thromboplastin*. It was recognized that tissue injury or inflammation promoted blood coagulation; therefore, tissue juice was considered to be a source of thromboplastin. Us-

ing this framework, A.J. Quick devised a method of reproducing in the laboratory what he thought to be physiologic blood coagulation. He reasoned that the efficiency of coagulation would primarily be a function of the prothrombin concentration. The test required a single step, the addition of calcium and tissue-derived thromboplastin to a plasma sample, and observing clot formation; thus it became known as *Quick's one-stage prothrombin time* [34,35]. Our mechanistic understanding of the prothrombin time is a bit more sophisticated than in Quick's time, but with the exception of automation, the methodology is quite similar.

THEORY

When tissue factor and a suitable phospholipid membrane are added to recalcified, platelet-poor plasma, the extrinsic pathway is activated, producing thrombin and a fibrin clot [17,21,31]. In the presence of excess tissue factor, the efficiency of fibrin formation depends on the presence and activity of factors VII, X, and V, and of thrombin and fibrinogen. Drugs or pathologic states resulting in markedly decreased activity of a component of the extrinsic or common pathway may prolong the prothrombin time [35,36].

METHOD

Venous blood is collected in a tube, which, when filled to a predetermined level, will contain nine parts of blood and one part of sodium citrate. Citrate removes ionized calcium, rendering blood incoagulable. The tube is usually a glass vacuum tube, whose inner surface is coated to prevent activation of factor XII. Platelet-poor plasma is prepared by centrifuging the specimen at approximately 2000 g, or more, for 15–30 minutes. Plasma is separated and frozen for storage or tested.

In a separate tube, a suspension of calcium chloride and thromboplastin is incubated at 37°C. One part test plasma is added to two parts calcium chloride/thromboplastin suspension and a timer is started. The calcium chloride solution contains a sufficient quantity of calcium to overcome the chelating potential of citrate, thereby restoring a necessary cofactor for blood coagulation. Fibrin polymerization marks the endpoint of the test. Most automated systems detect the appearance of fibrin polymerization by a change in the optical density of the specimen (see Figure 36-1). Each batch of unknown plasma is compared with a laboratory prepared or commercially available control plasma. The ratio of clotting time of test plasma to control plasma gives an estimate of the efficiency of clotting factor function in the extrinsic pathway.

INTERPRETATION

As previously mentioned, deficiencies or inhibitors of factors VII, V, and X, and of thrombin and fibrinogen, may prolong the prothrombin time in proportion to the severity of the defect [35–37]. In the prothrombin time, an excess of tissue factor (the normally unavailable cofactor) is supplied, allowing factor VII–tissue factor to convert factor X to Xa [17,38,39]. The amount of tissue factor supplied during the test makes the activity of factor VIIa, rather than the amount of tissue factor, the primary determinant of extrinsic pathway activation [40]. The intensity of extrinsic pathway activation affords the prothrombin time complete independence from the intrinsic pathway enzymes [38]. Factor VII has the shortest half-life of all of the vitamin K–dependent procoagulant enzymes, making it the most sensitive to changes in production [41]. In times of limited enzyme production, factor VII activities will fall fastest. Therefore, the prothrombin time, which hinges on factor VII function, can be used to screen for and to estimate the severity of factor production abnormalities, such as liver failure, vitamin K deficiency, or warfarin effect.

One caveat regarding the sensitivity of the prothrombin time to factor VII activity is that in the early stages of initiating oral anticoagulation (the first 4–5 days), a prolonged prothrombin time, representing primarily factor VII depletion, does not accurately reflect the antithrombotic effect. Only after factors with a longer half-life, such as thrombin, have equilibrated (a period of 7–10 days) is the prothrombin time proportional to the antithrombotic effect [40].

Heparin and the specific antithrombins will also prolong prothrombin times [42,43]. However, the plasma activity of heparin required to do so is close to 1 U/mL. Because most commonly used heparin regimens attempt to achieve heparin concentrations, or activities, near 0.4 U/mL (Figure 36-2), this is not of major clinical utility.

Specimen collection and testing methodology may produce abnormal results in the prothrombin time or its ratio to control plasma [44,45]. Collection of blood in improperly prepared tubes, allowing contact between the specimen and glass, which activates the intrinsic pathway, may abbreviate the prothrombin time. An improper relationship between the amount of citrate anticoagulant and collected blood resulting from underfilling (or overfilling) of commercially prepared collection tubes may prolong (or shorten) the prothrombin time. In addition, a similar effect may be seen with blood from patients with polycythemia, in which there is an abnormal ratio of citrate to plasma. Incorrect prothrombin time ratios may result from an incorrect determination of the control plasma prothrombin time, due to aging, improper handling, or an aberrant control plasma [46].

INR. The original source of thromboplastin, which is actually a combination of tissue factor and phospholipid, was a saline extract of pulverized human brain. Commercially available testing kits use nonhuman, mammalian brain as the source of thromboplastin. These individual thromboplastin preparations differ in their capability to initiate and support coagulation factor activity (according to their species of origin and the method of preparation) [47] due to many factors, including the amount and activity of tissue factor supplied and the physical characteristics of the accompanying phospholipid membrane. As a result, there may be substantial interlaboratory variation in the prothrombin time of identical specimens [48–50]. A particularly powerful tissue factor–phospholipid preparation may overcome mild deficiencies in factor activity, producing a normal prothrombin time, whereas a weaker preparation may be

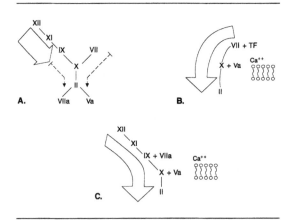

FIGURE 36-2. A: The enzyme cascades producing active thrombin share the principle of tonic inhibition through cofactor deprivation. Provision of VIIIa and Va is the result of thrombin activity. Exposure of tissue factor requires a loss of vascular integrity, activation of certain inflammatory cells, or aberrant production and release (e.g., a tumor). B: In the extrinsic pathway, tissue factor acts as a cofactor for factor VII. Activated factor V, phospholipid, and calcium are also required. C: The intrinsic pathway meets a bottleneck at factor IX, which is dependent on activated factor VIII. Similar to the extrinsic pathway, active factor V, phospholipid, and calcium are required.

produce a prolonged prothrombin time and differences in the ratio of test to control prothrombin times.

At the time that the prothrombin time became popular for guiding warfarin therapy, many laboratories used homemade thromboplastins, derived from human brain. Based on available data, the American Heart Association declared that the therapeutic effect of warfarin was greatest, with the least risk of hemorrhage, when the prothrombin time had prolonged to 2.0–2.5 times the control value. This ratio became the recommended target for oral anticoagulant therapy. Over the ensuing decade, many laboratories began acquiring their testing materials from commercial sources. Most of these thromboplastins were prepared from rabbit brain, which is less sensitive to the effects of factor depletion than a thromboplastin derived from human brain [46]. As a result, warfarin dosing escalated as clinicians continued to follow the AHA recommendations for oral anticoagulant therapy [46,51]. Although long suspected, the effect of these different thromboplastins was clearly established in a multinational study of the treatment of venous thrombosis, which reported an increased risk of bleeding when drug dosing was guided by prothrombin time ratios in North America [52].

A method of controlling of variations in thromboplastin sensitivity to the effect of warfarin was established in 1983 [10,47]. The standardization method employs a mathematical correction of the prothrombin time ratio obtained by an individual laboratory so that the reported result is the same as it would have been if the specimen had been tested using a reference thromboplastin reagent held by the World Health Organization. To calculate this ratio, known as the International Normalized Ratio (INR), the thromboplastin to be used is compared with a reference thromboplastin. When prothrombin times using the different reagents are plotted on a logarithmic scale, there is a linear relationship between the different values. The slope of this relationship is a function of an individual thromboplastin's sensitivity to the effects of factor depletion and is known as the International Sensitivity Index (ISI). Reference thromboplastins have an ISI value of 1.0. Thromboplastin preparations similar to this, which are sensitive to the effect of factor depletion, have a value near 1.0. Less sensitive preparations have a value near 2.0. Using the ISI, an INR can be calculated according to the following formula: INR = (prothrombin time ratio)^{ISI} [10,46].

Errors in the reported INR may arise from an incorrect prothrombin time, prothrombin time ratio, or an ISI (due to the original calibration, change with thromboplastin aging, or choice of reference plasma). Additionally, differences in automated methods may produce some variation in prothrombin times independent of the thromboplastin reagent. This, of course, will produce some variation in the calculated INR [46].

Native Prothrombin Antigen. The realization that coagulation times are an imprecise measure of antithrombotic drug effect and the variation of prothrombin times associated with different reagents prompted a search for an alternative method to guide warfarin therapy that prevents normal carboxylation of factors VII, IX and X, and of prothrombin, rendering them nonfunctional [54]. One such new measurement technique uses immunoassay techniques to quantitate the amount of fully carboxylated biologically active prothrombin by measuring the concentration of functional prothrombin antigen present in plasma [53]. The native prothrombin antigen assay has been compared with the prothrombin time and prothrombin time ratio in its ability to estimate the intensity of drug effect at the time of drug failure, or hemorrhagic complication, with good results [55]. More recently, it was compared with the prothrombin time ratio in managing warfarin therapy and was associated with and 85% reduction in the incidence of complications or drug failure [56]. The consistent test method avoids interlaboratory variation and the need for mathematical manipulation, which may magnify errors in testing. Large-scale testing and comparison with the prothrombin time–INR system has not been performed. Therefore, the role of the native prothrombin antigen assay in the routine management of oral anticoagulant therapy has not been established, but it would appear to be a promising technique for the future.

Whole-Blood Clotting Time

In 1913 Lee and White described the whole blood clotting time, the original method of evaluating the intrinsic capability of blood to clot [57]. This remained the favored method of assessing heparin's anticoagulant effect for a number of years [58]. Among the many derivative tests, the activated partial thromboplastin time and activated clotting time are still widely used in clinical practice.

THEORY

When blood is placed in a glass tube, the intrinsic pathway to thrombin generation is activated. Initial thrombin generation is limited by the availability of cofactors that augment clotting enzyme function, specifically factors VIIIa and Va, calcium, and a phospholipid membrane [14,19–21]. The initial appearance of active thrombin, albeit at low concentrations due to the sluggish nature of unassisted enzyme function, results in the generation of necessary cofactors through its action on factor VIII, factor V, and platelet activation [14,19–25,59]. A burst of thrombin generation and fibrin polymerization follows. This test does not utilize exogenously administered activators (other than the glass tube) or limiting cofactors.

METHOD

The whole blood clotting time is primarily of historical interest because the test methodology and results vary greatly. As usually performed, a blood sample is drawn from a peripheral vein using a 20-gauge or larger needle. Approximately 2–5 mL is withdrawn and discarded. Into a second syringe, the second sample of 5+ mL is withdrawn and the timer started. One-milliliter aliquots are placed in each of three glass tubes, which are incubated at 37°C. The tubes are examined at least every 30 seconds, and timing is stopped at the first appearance of clot in any tube (some methods require that a solid clot be formed). The solid clot may be observed further for evidence of retraction or dissolution [60].

INTERPRETATION

Normal whole-blood clotting times are in the range of 4–20 minutes, depending on the methodology employed and the endpoint chosen. Even with a consistent protocol, there is wide variation in normal values, which are, in part, a function of platelet number and function and the extent of contact activation by the glass tube. This variation limits the utility of the whole blood clotting time for detecting of mild clotting factor aberrations or low-level antithrombin therapy. Historically, when used to guide the administration of heparin, a frequent target range for whole-blood clotting times was about twice the baseline value. Additional assessment of clot retraction and fibrinolysis is also possible. Normal clot retraction is a decrease in the extent of contact along the sides of the tube of more than 50% by 1 hour, and is a function of hematocrit, platelet number, and platelet function. Dissolution of a well-formed clot can also be interpreted as evidence of fibrinolytic activity.

Plasma Recalcification Time

The plasma recalcification time provides similar information as the whole-blood clotting time, without the necessity for making immediate measurements as the time of phlebotomy. A specimen of platelet-rich plasma (prepared from citrate-anticoagulated blood) is placed in a glass tube and contact activation is allowed [61]. Calcium is then added to the preparation to overcome the citrate inhibition of coagulation, and the time to fibrin clot formation is recorded. This test suffers excess variation due to inconsistency of platelet numbers in platelet-rich plasma preparations as well as by variation rising from inconsistencies in the degree of intensity of contact activation.

Activated Partial Thromboplastin Time

In the 1950s, a group of investigators developed a variation of the prothrombin time that used lipophilic extraction of brain for thromboplastin preparation [62]; they used platelet-poor plasma and an excess amount of a membrane substitute. They found that, in contrast to the prothrombin time, their test method gave abnormal results with plasma from hemophiliacs [63]. Concluding that their thromboplastin must be incomplete, they called this test the *partial thromboplastin time* (PTT). Since then other variations have been introduced, but the PTT, in principle, remains the primary clinical means of examining the intrinsic pathway to thrombin activation. The PTT addresses the problems of the plasma recalcification time by separating coagulation from platelet function. It avoids the extrinsic pathway by excluding tissue factor from its reagents. A commonly used modification of the PTT, the *aPTT* (*activated partial thromboplastin time*), avoids variation in the intensity of activation by initiating activation, during a pretest incubation period, with a constant quantity of kaolin or other substances (Table 36-2).

THEORY

When citrated platelet-poor plasma is exposed to strong contact activation, recalcified, and platelet membrane substitute supplied, the time required for a fibrin clot to form is dependent on the presence and function of enzymes and cofactors within the intrinsic pathway to thrombin formation. The partial thromboplastin used to perform the test is simply a phospholipid membrane on which coagulation enzyme reactions may proceed. This serves as a surrogate for activated platelets and is prepared so as not to be contaminated with tissue factor, which would activate the extrinsic pathway. The addition of calcium is required for interaction between several of the activated factors and the phospholipid membrane.

METHOD

Platelet-poor plasma is obtained as described for the prothrombin time. Two parts test plasma are mixed

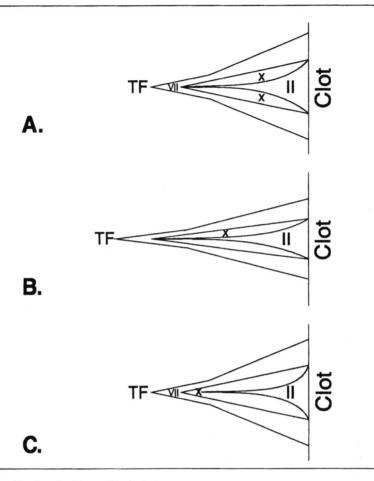

FIGURE 36-3. Prothrombin time. In this graphic depiction of prothrombin time, the diverging lines and the area encompassed by them represent the increasing enzyme activity resulting from the initial activation process. The endpoint is clot formation. A: There is minimal lag time to thrombin production. When active factor VII and tissue factor activate X, thrombin production begins. An avalanche ensues, eventually generating thrombin in concentrations that will form a clot. B: Cofactor depletion, secondary to warfarin, dampens the avalanche, prolonging the time to clot formation. C: In the presence of high concentrations of thrombin scavengers, such as heparin–AT III or hirudin, thrombin is consumed as it is formed, damping and minimally delaying the avalanche effect.

with two parts activator/phospholipid emulsion and incubated for 3 minutes at 37°C. Two parts CaCl₂ solution are then added to the mixture and timing is begun. The endpoint is the detection of fibrin polymerization. Detection methods used for the aPTT are the same as used for the prothrombin time. In both the prothrombin time and the aPTT,

control plasma is tested in conjunction with test plasma.

INTERPRETATION
The aPTT reported by most laboratories is in the range of 20–40 seconds. It is prolonged when any of the factors from contact activation to fibrin polymerization are deficient or are inhibited to less than 30% of normal activity [64–67] (Table 36-3), including high molecular weight kininogen; prekallikrein; factors XII, XI, IX, VIII, X, and V; thrombin; and fibrinogen [62,68–74]. Abbreviated times may be seen when there has been inappropriate contact activation [75], increased availability of factor VIII or VIIIa, and perhaps disseminated intravascular coagulation [76–81] (Table 36-4).

Heparin. When heparin is complexed with antithrombin III (AT III), the ability of heparin–AT

TABLE 36-2. Substances with
the capability for contact activation

Kaolin	Celite
Ellagic acid	Glass
Colloidal silica	Bentonite
Asbestos	Collagen
Spider web	Saturated fatty acid

TABLE 36-3. Causes of a prolonged aPTT

Hereditary factor deficiency	Acquired factor inhibitor
Heparin-antithrombin III	Thrombin inhibitors
Activated protein C[a]	Tick anticoagulant peptide
Liver disease	Vitamin K deficiency
Disseminated intravascular coagulation (DIC)	Warfarin/coumarins
Polycythemia	Dysproteinemia
Gaucher's disease	

[a] In vitro.

TABLE 36-4. Causes of an abbreviated aPTT

Pregnancy (last trimester)
Surgery (postoperative state)
Oral contraceptives
Increased factor VIII
Increased factor V
Myocardial infarction
Disseminated intravascular coagulation (DIC)

III to inhibit thrombin may be increased 1000-fold over that of AT III alone [82]. As a result, the initial steps following contact activation proceed slowly through the regulatory points. The small amount of thrombin produced decays at an accelerated rate, and the activation of factor VIII is impaired. Consequently, more time is required to produce thrombin in sufficient concentrations to effectively overcome the rate-limiting steps in the intrinsic pathway (Figure 36-4). This lag time is the measurable prolongation of clotting times produced by the thrombin inhibitors (such as heparin; Figure 36-5) [14–16,18]. Because the aPTT has a strong contact activation step, it is intermediately sensitive to the presence of thrombin inhibitors. The aPTT is prolonged at a level of thrombin inhibition that correlates with heparin activity of 0.1–0.6U/mL, a range of heparin therapy that has been shown to be effective for the treatment of venous thrombosis and some forms of arterial thrombosis [83–90]. The aPTT has become a widely utilized test for guiding heparin therapy, with a usual target range of 1.5–2.5 times the control value [82–91].

More intense antithrombin therapy is utilized in specific situations, such as percutaneous angioplasty and cardiopulmonary bypass [92–96]. However, when heparin is administered to achieve concentrations greater than the above-quoted ranges, the aPTT is nonlinear in its response to heparin and may be almost infinitely prolonged; the aPTT in these circumstances is no longer a useful test [9,95,97,98]. Because heparin–AT III activity rises above the normal aPTT target ranges, its unchecked activity in a platelet-free environment, and perhaps, serial inhibition of multiple enzymes, may so severely cripple the early phase of enzyme activity that the stimulus dies before thrombin is produced in sufficient quantities to effectively activate factors V and VIII. This phenomenon is not as important in vivo, where platelet participation in the evolving thrombus antagonizes heparin–AT III inhibitory effects (Figure 36-6) [99–101]. Similarly, whole-blood preparations containing platelets will be less susceptible to this problem than platelet-poor plasma.

In the guidance of heparin therapy, particularly for laboratory standardization, the aPTT can be compared with tests of individual enzyme inhibition, such as anti-Xa units or anti-IIa units [5,102]. In these tests, which are often used as an assay of heparin concentrations, plasma samples, to which AT III may or may not have been added (depending on the method employed) are incubated with active factor Xa or thrombin for a prespecified length of time [4]. A chromogenic substrate is used to estimate enzyme activity during that period of time, and comparison with calibration curves provides the measure of enzyme inhibition.

Heparin's action is dependent on endogenous AT III. Therefore, knowledge of the heparin concentration alone would appear to be of little value if the patient's AT III concentration is not known. This is particularly important because AT III concentrations may change during an active thrombotic state or with ongoing heparin therapy [103,104]. Hence, measurement of heparin activity concentrations in which AT III is not added in testing seem more appropriate and more clinically useful in situations in which the aPTT is abnormal at baseline (e.g., lupus anticoagulant or factor deficiencies not associated with an increased risk of hemorrhage). Despite theoretical differences, between testing methods, heparin concentration, heparin activity, and aPTT measurements appear

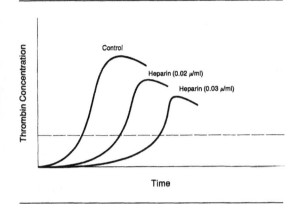

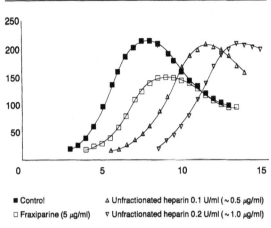

FIGURE 36-4. Thrombin generation in platelet-free plasma. The presence of heparin delays the onset of peak thrombin production and decreases the peak concentration of thrombin that is generated. (Modified from Hemker and Beguin [16], with permission.)

FIGURE 36-6. Influence of heparins on thrombin generation in platelet-rich plasma. In contrast to the platelet-free preparation, heparin cannot limit the peak thrombin concentration generated when platelets are present. Low molecular weight heparins, unaffected by platelet factor-4, continue to limit thrombin production in the presence of platelets. O, control; △, unfractionated heparin 0.1 U/mL (~0.5 μg/mL); ▲, unfractionated heparin 0.2 U/mL (~1.0 μg/mL); •, Fraxiparine (5 μg/mL).

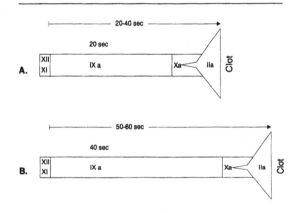

FIGURE 36-5. Lag time of the aPTT. A: In normal plasma, pretest activation produces abundant factor IXa. In the absence of factor VIIIa, production of significant quantities of factor Xa is slow. This is represented by the section labeled IXa. Factor Xa, similarly, is slow to produce active thrombin. When thrombin is produced, it may provide factors VIIIa and Va, resulting in a burst of activity, and clot formation ensues. B: In the presence of heparin or a specific antithrombin, the initial thrombin that is produced is rapidly consumed, impairing factor VIIIa production. Thus, a longer time is required to overcome the bottleneck at factor IXa. At the same time that factor VIIIa appears, improving the function of IXa, factor Va begins to assist factor Xa. As a result, the change in lag time resulting from antithrombin therapy is due to the production rate of factor VIIIa.

to perform equally well in predicting the antithrombotic effect of heparin therapy [4].

Unfortunately the aPTT is also subject to the same pitfalls as the prothrombin time. Different physicochemical effects of the various activators produce variation in activation intensity and clotting times that depend on the type of contact activator and its concentration [105–108]. These variations are magnified when aPTT is measured in the presence of anticoagulants [106,109,110]. The membrane surface supplied by activated platelets or, in the case of the aPTT, by an artificial source, plays an integral role in coagulation enzyme function [21]. Variations in the characteristics of this membrane may also result in test-to-test variability in the sensitivity to factor deficiencies and heparin effect [107,108,111]. Attempts to categorize differences in test results according to reagents and to devise a system of normalization analogous to the INR have not been successful to date [111]. Consequently aPTT values are not interchangeable from site to site, and general recommendations for a particular range of prolongation or ratio of test to control are not precise, and adherence to such guidelines may not provide the desired intensity of anticoagulation. In multicenter studies of antithrombotic therapy, if the aPTT is used to guide therapy, each center should either utilize identical testing apparati/reagents or establish the relationship of their aPTT to heparin activity and "standardize" on the basis of heparin activity.

Specific Thrombin Inhibitors. Specific thrombin inhibitors, in contrast to heparin, are active against fibrin-bound thrombin, which is otherwise resistant to the actions of heparin [101]. Unlike heparin, which is bound to AT III, specific inhibitors not only limit thrombin production and enzyme activity, but may, in addition, inhibit thrombin-induced platelet activation [112,113]. Because direct thrombin inhibitors have different mechanisms of action than heparin, and different dose–effect relationships, the relationship between aPTT prolongation and antithrombotic effect for thrombin inhibitors will not be the same for direct thrombin inhibitors as for heparin. A given aPTT range for a specific thrombin inhibitor may correspond to an equal or greater antithrombotic effect than for heparin, especially in situations in which thrombosis is platelet dependent (i.e., arterial thrombosis) [114,115]. Conversely, in situations in which a thrombotic tendency is due to excessive coagulation enzyme activity (i.e., venous thrombosis), it is conceivable that very mild inhibition, especially of multiple enzymes, beneath the range that may be detectable by the aPTT, may restore normal regulatory influences. Direct comparisons of drug efficacy cannot necessarily be made based on equal prolongation of a clotting time, such as the aPTT [115]. Risk/benefit ratios, with respect to measures of antithrombotic effect, must be determined separately for anticoagulants of different classes. Therefore, antithrombotic recommendations, using the aPTT, must specify not only reagents but also the type of antithrombotic therapy that is utilized.

Activated Coagulation Time

The ACT (*activated coagulation/clotting time*) entails the addition of a contact activator to whole blood and measurement of the time required for a clot to form [117]. The phospholipid surface necessary for coagulation is provided by the patient's own activated platelets. The ACT may be somewhat less sensitive to low levels of heparin anticoagulation than the aPTT. However, it maintains a good correlation with the heparin effect at higher heparin doses [9,97,98] and is popular for guiding heparin therapy in clinical situations such as cardiopulmonary bypass and percutaneous angioplasty [92–96].

THEORY

The ACT is essentially a modified whole-blood clotting time in which an attempt has been made to standardize contact activation by using a constant amount of kaolin or celite. The ACT is similar to the aPTT in its dependence on the contact activation pathway for thrombin generation, but the ACT does not supply an excess of phospholipid membrane. In the aPTT, a phospholipid surface area is supplied in excess so that this will not interfere with the measurement of coagulation enzyme function. The ACT requires that this surface area be developed through platelet activation during the testing process. This introduces an additional variable to the function of coagulation enzymes. In the ACT following contact activation, the first thrombin to appear must activate platelets, in addition to factors V and VIII, and any alterations in endogenous platelet function may also alter activated clotting times. Rather than being a pure test of coagulation enzyme function, the ACT is also a somewhat imprecise measure of the cooperation between the intrinsic pathway and platelet function.

METHOD

Venous blood is withdrawn in a similar manner to that described in the whole-blood clotting time. Although it is common practice to withdraw blood through vascular access devices, some measure of imprecision certainly results. Indwelling catheters, even while patent, form thrombus on their surface. To limit thrombin growth and to prevent catheter closure, these catheters are often flushed with heparin-containing solutions or may be impregnated with heparin. These two factors, heparin and thrombus, which may provide activated platelets, thrombin, and fibrin degradation products, may influence the ACT. Blood samples are placed in commercially prepared containers in which a contact activator and fibrin polymer detection device is present and a timer is started simultaneously. The time from activation to fibrin polymer detection is recorded.

INTERPRETATION

There are currently two systems that perform an automated ACT, Hemochron (International Technidyne, Edison, NJ), and HemoTec (Medtronic HemoTec, Englewood, CO). System activators and fibrin detection mechanisms differ, giving them different sensitivities to factor depletion and inhibitor therapy. The Hemochron system uses a celite activator and detects fibrin polymerization using an oscillating magnetic field (see Figure 36-1). The HemoTec uses a kaolin activator and measures the rate of plunger fall to detect fibrin polymerization (see Figure 36-1). Similar to the prothrombin time and aPTT, any recommendations for anticoagulant intensity, measured by the ACT, must be qualified by the specific type of device used [118]. Although there is a reasonable correlation between the results, the values of one system cannot be extrapolated to the other two systems [119].

In general, the normal ACT is in the range of 90–130 seconds. It may be prolonged in situations in which there is a deficiency or inhibition of any of the factors from contact activation to fibrin polymer formation, including platelet activation [116,120]. Due to the range of variation in normal values of the ACT, small effects will likely go unnoticed in an individual patient. Powerful antiplatelet drugs, such as the glycoprotein IIb/IIIa inhibitors, may prolong the ACT [128]. The ACT may be shortened during ongoing thrombosis, such as surgical procedures or unstable coronary syndromes [121,122], largely as a function of the availability of activated platelets. In vitro addition of platelet activators, such as ADP, epinephrine, and collagen, to the blood of normal volunteers will decrease the ACT by 5–10 seconds compared with the addition of saline diluent (Wilson JM, Ferguson JJ unpublished observations).

The theoretical advantages of the ACT as a test of the entire coagulation cascade may also be viewed as disadvantages. Contamination of the blood sample with activated platelets (as with indwelling catheters) may shorten the ACT. Heparinized blood samples may be particularly sensitive to platelet factor-4 released from contaminating activiated platelets [100]. In vitro addition of platelet-activating agents to heparinized blood has been shown to almost completely normalize ACT values when heparin concentrations are in the range of 0.2 U/mL. When heparin is added to platelet-rich plasma activated by tissue factor, concentrations of 0.5 U/mL are required to affect thrombin concentrations, and even then, do so only slightly [99]. The mere act of phlebotomy has been shown to negate some part of heparin's effect on blood specimens [123]. Although theoretically an excellent global measure of coagulation and the coordination of platelet activation and coagulation, the limitations of the ACT must be kept in mind.

Because the aPTT and ACT measure similar phenomenon (except for the contribution of activated platelets), there is a fair correlation between the tests when assessing heparin therapy [95]. Not surprisingly, the relationship differs when a specific antithrombin is used, in contrast to heparin (Figure 36-7). Specific thrombin inhibitors, in addition to impairing the feedback amplification of coagulation

enzyme function, also prevent thrombin-induced platelet activation [112,113]. The resultant denial of factors VIIIa and Va and a phospholipid surface prolongs the ACT. Unlike heparin, specific antithrombins are not affected as thrombin production begins to overcome regulatory restriction. In drug concentration ranges at which the two tests are responsive, antithrombins produce a proportionately greater rise in the ACT than the aPTT [115]. Thus, at drug concentrations producing an equivalent rise in the aPTT, the ACT increase with specific thrombin inhibitors is significantly longer than that with heparin.

The efficacy of the aPTT and ACT in predicting the antithrombotic effect of heparin and two thrombin inhibitors were compared in a guinea pig carotid thrombosis model [115]. At comparable levels of aPTT prolongation, heparin had virtually no antithrombotic effect, whereas the thrombin inhibi-

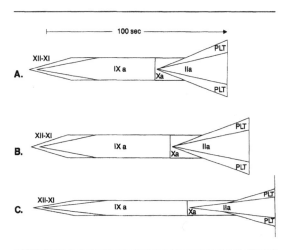

FIGURE 36-7. ACT. **A:** Accumulating contact activation produces factor IXa, which requires factor VIIIa for optimal function. Similar to the aPTT, this produces a bottleneck and a lag time until thrombin generation begins. Thrombin's appearance results in cofactor production and platelet activation, supplying rate-limiting factors for explosive thrombin generation and clot formation. **B:** In the presence of heparin, the early phase of the test is essentially platelet free (in absence of pre-activation) and appears similar to the aPTT. The appearance of thrombin and platelet activation produce an unfavorable environment for heparin. As a result, the eventual amount of thrombin formed and the duration of this final phase of the ACT are unchanged. **C:** The specific antithrombins may prolong the lag phase by limiting the activation of factors VII and V, as well as by inhibiting platelet activation.

tors decreased thrombus formation by 80%. When the ACT was prolonged to similar ranges, the antithrombotic effects were equal. This suggests, at least that the ACT may be more useful that the aPTT in studies that seek to compare the clinical efficacy of direct thrombin inhibitors with heparin.

Limitations aside, the association between platelet activation or inhibition and changes in the ACT suggest that this is the best available test for assessing the intensity of antithrombotic drugs when combinations of anticoagulants and antiplatelet agents are used in a clinical syndrome that may involve endogenous platelet activation or when a single drug may have multiple effects.

Whole-Blood aPTT

The whole-blood aPTT can be thought of as a test that is somewhere between the ACT and the aPTT. It is a global measure of coagulation enzyme function that does not require platelet activation but that can be influenced by the endogenous level of platelet activation.

THEORY
When contact activation is carried out in whole blood (instead of plasma), the intrinsic pathway still functions as previously described. If phospholipid surface and calcium are supplied in excess (as for an aPTT), thrombin production requires only the activation of factors VIII and V. In whole blood, newly generated thrombin goes no to activate platelets, which may additionally participate in enzyme function and fibrin formation. More importantly, the release reaction producing platelet factor-4 from endogenous activated platelets is not impeded.

METHOD
Venous blood is obtained and placed in a prepared test tube containing lyophilized citrate, activator, phospholipid, and buffers. Calcium chloride solution is added and testing is begun [124].

INTERPRETATION
The normal range of the whole-blood aPTT differs according to the test kit manufacturer. The Coaguchek plus system (Boehringer Mannheim Diagnostics, Indianapolis, IN) applies a mathematical conversion to report ranges similar to that of the plasma aPTT (20–40 seconds). The Hemochron system (International Technidyne, Edison, NJ) reports a raw coagulation time (55–85 seconds). In the unfettered

intrinsic pathway, when phospholipid is supplied in excess, the effect of bystander platelet activation is probably minimal and the test result represents coagulation enzyme function. However, in a heparinized whole-blood specimen, the anticoagulant effects of heparin will be reduced by bystander platelet activation and the release of platelet factor-4. As a result, the whole-blood aPTT will respond to heparin in a similar fashion as the ACT, although it may perhaps be a bit more sensitive to heparin's anticoagulant effect [125]. In fact, when the two tests are compared during heparin therapy, there is an extraordinarily good correlation. The rate of rise in coagulation time is almost identical. The primary difference between the two tests is that the whole-blood aPTT is about 45 seconds shorter than the ACT. This may, in fact, represent the lag time of initial platelet activation that is part of an ACT but not a whole-blood aPTT.

Specific antithrombins have the added effect of inhibiting thrombin-mediated platelet activation. The whole-blood aPTT does not require this step. Furthermore, the anticoagulant response to the specific antithrombins is not influenced by the platelet release reaction or platelet factor-4. For the specific antithrombins, the whole-blood aPTT should be considered to be essentially comparable with a standard aPTT.

The whole-blood aPTT, like the ACT, is a test that may be performed at the bedside, decreasing the turnaround time from sample acquisition to a therapeutic decision [125–127]. Its use substantially reduces the time required to achieve adequate heparin anticoagulation when compared with the standard aPTT [127]. The theoretical aspects of this test, including independence from variations initial platelet activation, responsiveness to both high and low concentrations of heparin, and rapid turnaround time, make it an ideal test with which to judge the intensity of the heparin effect. However, its independence from platelet activation makes it very analagous to, and subject to the same drawbacks as, the standard aPTT in evaluating specific thrombin inhibitors or combination antiplatelet/anticoagulant therapy.

Dry Reagent Technology

One of the new techniques for clotting time performance is the use of dry reagent preparations. Rather than using separate solutions that must be added to a test tube, the coagulation activator and cofactors are dried and placed on a card. A very small amount of citrated blood is placed in a reaction chamber; the particular reagent preparation used determines the type of clotting time that is performed. If all of the clotting times use the same type of detection mechanism, a single analyzer may be used for a variety of different tests. There may be variations in the correlations between this type of testing and conventional methods due to differences in the type of activator, thromboplastin (if added), degree of mixing, and detection mechanism. Furthermore, at present there is only limited experience with this technology, although utilization of this type of testing will, in all likelihood, increase as enthusiasm for point-of-care testing grows.

Conclusions

A variety of laboratory methods are available to help guide antithrombotic therapy. Each test has individual strengths and weaknesses (Table 36-5). Therefore, the most appropriate test to use depends on the clinical situation at hand. For example, there is substantial evidence and clinical experience supporting the use of the standard aPTT in guiding heparin therapy for the prevention of pulmonary thromboembolism in patients with acute deep venous thrombosis. In contrast, the aPTT has been supplanted by the ACT for assessing heparinization for angioplasty

TABLE 36-5. Laboratory measures of coagulation

Test	Strength	Weakness	Use	Comment
PT	Sensitive to defects in extrinsic pathway; extensive experience	Interlaboratory variation	Coumadin therapy	Primary weakness is partially corrected by the INR
NPA	Uniform test method; may be superior to the PT in measuring antithrombotic effect	Inadequate clinical experience Awaits widespread testing and acceptance	Coumadin therapy	Narrow utility may limit popularity
WBCT	Bedside test sensitive to intrinsic pathway defects	Non-uniformity requires skill in performance	Heparin therapy	Rarely used
PR	Sensitive to intrinsic pathway defects	Variability	None	
PTT	Very sensitive to defects in intrinsic pathway	Variation in contact activation Unreliable estimate of intense intrinsic pathway inhibition	Heparin therapy	Has been supplanted by the aPTT
aPTT	Sensitive to defects in intrinsic pathway; extensive clinical experience	Measures coagulation enzyme function only; unreliable estimates of intense intrinsic pathway inhibition; interlaboratory variation	Heparin therapy; specific thrombin inhibition therapy	No available correction of interlaboratory variation Prolongation by heparin and thrombin inhibitors may not mean comparable antithrombotic effect
WBPTT	Sensitive to defects in intrinsic pathway; may respond to platelet influence on heparin; bedside test.	Lack of experience	Heparin therapy; thrombin inhibitor therapy	Ease of performance at the bedside may substantially reduce the time required to achieve therapeutic values
ACT	Sensitive to defects in intrinsic pathway; may be responsive to platelets, coagulation enzyme interdependence	Insensitive to low-intensity inhibitor therapy variable	Heparin therapy; thrombin inhibitor therapy	Current role is during high-intensity therapy, such as cardiopulmonary bypass and PTCA; may be the best method to judge comparisons between heparin and thrombin inhibitors

PT prothrombin time, NPA native prothrombin antigen, WBCT whole blood clotting time, PR plasma recalcification time, PTT partial thromboplastin time, aPTT activated PTT, WBPTT whole blood PTT, ACT activated coagulation time.

or bypass surgery, in which rapid determination of the effect of high-dose heparin therapy is required.

The PT and aPTT are designed as measures of coagulation enzyme function. These two tests, although using standardized methods, may be performed with different reagents producing interlaboratory variation in the test results for an identical specimen. To some degree, this variation in the PT is addressed by the INR. Unfortunately, no such correction is available for the aPTT. Additional newer testing methods are becoming available that may be useful in assessing antithrombotic therapy without these concerns.

The current state of anticoagulant monitoring dictates that the application of experience from clinical trials account for variations in testing methods. This may be done by using the INR as a preferred reporting method rather than prothrombin times or ratios (in studies utilizing PTs to guide therapy) and by paying special attention to the type of aPTT or ACT and has been used. Finally, as new antithrombotic drugs and strategies evolve, a relationship between the risk, benefit, and antithrombotic effects measured by individual tests needs to be established independently, rather than relying on traditional values established for older drugs, because the old "therapeutic" ranges may not be applicable to newer compounds.

References

1. Landefield CS, Cook EF, Flatley M, Weisberg M, Goldman L. Identification and preliminary validation of predictors of major bleeding in hospitalized patients starting anticoagulant therapy. Am J Med 82:703, 1987.

2. Hoppensteadt DA, Waling JM, Fareed J. Validity of serine protease inhibition tests in the evaluation and monitoring or the effect of heparin and its fractions. Semin Thromb Hemostas 11:112, 1985.

3. Holm HA, Abildgaard U, Kalvenes S, Anderssen N, Anker E, Arnesen KE, Blikom D, Drivenes A. The antithrombotic effect of heparin in deep venous thrombosis: Relation to four heparin assays. Acta Med Scand 216:287, 1984.

4. Holm HA, Abildgaard U, Larsen ML, Kalvenes S. Monitoring of heparin therapy: Should heparin assays also reflect the patients antithrombin concentration? Thromb Res 46:669, 1987.

5. van den Besselaar AMHP, Meruwisse-Braun J, Bertina RM. Monitoring heparin therapy: Relationships between the activated partial thromboplastin time and heparin assays based on ex-vivo heparin samples. Thromb Haemost 63:16, 1990.

6. Manucci PM, Botasso B, Tripodi A, Bianchi BA. Prothrombin fragment 1 + 2 and intensity of treatment with oral anticoagulants. Thromb Haemost 66:741, 1991.

7. Hoek JA, Nurmohamed MT, tenCate JW, Buller HR, Knipscheer HC, Hamelynck KJ, Marti RK, Stur KA. Thrombin-antithrombin III complexes in the prediction of deep vein thrombosis following total hip replacement. Thromb Haemost 62:1050, 1989.

8. Basu D, Gallus A, Hirsh J, Cade J. A prospective study of the value of monitoring heparin treatment with the activated partial thromboplastin time. N Engl J Med 287:324, 1972.

9. Congdon JE, Kardinal C, Wallin JD. Monitoring heparin therapy on hemodialysis. JAMA 226:1529, 1973.

10. Thompson JM. The implementation of international normalized ratios for standardization of the prothrombin time in oral anticoagulant control. In Thompson JM (ed). Blood Coagulation and Hemostatis. New York: Churchill Livingstone, 1991:261.

11. Bounameaux H, Market GA, Lämmle B, Eichlisberger R, Duckert F. Monitoring of heparin treatment. Comparison of thrombin time, activated partial thromboplastin time, and plasma heparin concentration, and analysis of the behavior of antithrombin III. Am J Clin Pathol 74:68, 1980.

12. Alving BM. Lupus anticoagulants, anticardiolipin antibodies, and the antiphospholipid syndrome. In Loscalzo J, Schaeffer AI (eds). Thrombosis and Hemorrhage. Boston: Blackwell Scientific, 1994:749.

13. Alson JD, Pennell BJ. Automated coagulation systems. In Haven MC, Tetrault GA, Schenken JR (eds). Laboratory Instrumentation Systems, 4th ed. New York: Van Nostrand Reinhold, 1995:391.

14. Hemker HC, Kessels H. Feedback mechanisms in coagulation. Haemostasis 21:189, 1991.

15. Béguin S, Lindhout T, Hemker HC. The mode of action of heparin in plasma. Thromb Haemost 60:457, 1988.

16. Hemker HC, Beguin S. Mode of action of heparin and related drugs. Semin Thromb Hemost 17(Suppl. 1):29, 1991.

17. Rapaport SI, Rao LVM. Initiation and regulation of tissue factor-dependent blood coagulation. Arterioscler Thromb 12:1111, 1992.

18. Ofosu FA, Sie P, Modi GJ, Fernandez F, Buchanan MR, Blajckman MA, Boneu B, Hirsh J. The inhibition of thrombin-dependent positive feedback reactions is critical to the expression of the anticoagulant effect of heparin. Biochem J 243:579, 1987.

19. Jesty J. Interaction of feedback control and product inhibition in the activation of factor X by factors IXa and VIII. Haemostasis 21:208, 1991.

20. Willems GM, Lindhout T, Hermens WT, Hemker HC. Simulation model for thrombin generation in plasma. Haemostasis 21:197, 1991.

21. Mann KG, Krishnaswamy S, Lawson JH. Surface-dependent hemostasis. Semin Hematol 29:213, 1992.

22. Nesheim ME, Taswell JB, Mann KG. The contribu-

tion of bovine factor V and factor Va to the activity of prothrombinase. J Biol Chem 254:10952, 1979.

23. Kane WH, Davie EW. Blood coagulation factors V and VIII, structural and functional similarities and this relationship to hemorrhagic and thrombotic disorders. Blood 71:539, 1988.

24. Rapaport SI, Schiffman S, Patch MJ, Ames SB. The importance of activation of antihemophilic globulin and proaccelerin by traces of thrombin in the generation of intrinsic prothrombinase activity. Blood 21:221, 1963.

25. Pieters J, Lindhout T, Hemker HC. In-situ generated thrombin is the only enzyme that effectively activates factor VIII and factor V in thromboplastin-activated plasma. Blood 74:1021, 1989.

26. Nawroth PP, Handley DA, Esmon CT, Stern DM. Interleukin 1 induces endothelial cell procoagulant activity while suppressing cell-surface anticoagulant activity. Proc Natl Acad Sci USA 83:3460, 1986.

27. Tracy PB, Nesheim ME, Mann KG. Coordinate binding of factor Va and factor Xa to the unstimulated platelet. J Biol Chem 256:743, 1981.

28. Bevers EM, Comfurius P, van Rijn JLML, Hemker HC, Zwaal RFA. Generation of prothrombin converting activity and the exposure of phosphatidyl serine at the outer surface of platelets. Eur J Biochem 122:429, 1982.

29. McGee MP, Li LC. Functional difference between intrinsic and extrinsic coagulation pathways. Kinetics of factor X activation on human monocytes and alveolar macrophages. J Biol Chem 266:8079, 1991.

30. Tracy PB, Rohrback MS, Mann KG. Functional prothrombinase complex assembly on isolated monocytes and lymphocytes. J Biol Chem 258:7264, 1983.

31. Tracy PB, Eide LL, Mann KG. Human prothrombinase complex assembly and function on isolated peripheral blood cell populations. J Biol Chem 260:2119, 1985.

32. Robinson RA, Worfolk L, Tracy PB. Endotoxin enhances the expression of monocyte prothrombinase activity. Blood 79:406, 1992.

33. Altieri D. Coagulation assembly on leukocytes in transmembrane signaling and cell adhesion. Blood 81:569, 1993.

34. Miale JB. Laboratory Medicine: Hematology, 4th ed. St. Louis, MO: Mosby, 1972:1054.

35. Quick AJ, Stanley-Brown M, Bancroft FW. A study of the coagulation defect in hemophilia and jaundice. Am J Med Sci 190:501, 1935.

36. Biggs R, MacFarlane RG. Reaction of hemophilic plasma to thromboplastin. J Clin Pathol 4:445, 1951.

37. Roberts HR, Eberst ME. Other coagulation deficiencies. In Loscalzo J, Schaeffer AI (eds). Thrombosis and Hemorrhage. Boston: Blackwell Scientific, 1994:701.

38. Nemerson Y. The tissue factor pathway of blood coagulation. Semin Hematol 29:170, 1992.

39. Nemerson Y. Tissue factor and hemostasis. Blood 71:1, 1988.

40. Morrissey JH, Macik BG, Neuenschwander PF, Comp PC. Quantitation of activated factor VII levels in plasma using a tissue factor mutant selectively deficient in promoting factor VII activation. Blood 81:734, 1993.

41. Seligsohn U, Kasper CK, Osterud B, Rapaport SI. Activated factor VII: Presence of factor IX concentrates and persistence in the circulation after infusion. Blood 53:828, 1979.

42. Zoldhelyi P, Webster MWI, Fuster V, Grill DE, Gaspar D, Edwards SJ, Cabot CF, Chesebro JH. Recombinant hirudin in patients with chronic, stable coronary artery disease. Safety, half-life, and effect on coagulation parameters. Circulation 88:2015, 1993.

43. Sharma GVRK, Lapsley O, Vita JA, Sharma S, Coccio E, Adelman B, Loscalzo J. Usefulness and tolerability of hirulog, a direct thrombin-inhibitor, in unstable angina pectoris. Am J Cardiol 72:1357, 1993.

44. Palmer RN, Kessler CM, Gralink HR. Warfarin anticoagulation: Difficulties in interpretation of the prothrombin time. Thromb Res 25:125, 1982.

45. Peterson P, Gottfried EL. The effects of inaccurate blood sample volume on prothrombin time and activated partial thromboplastin time (aPTT). Thromb Haemost 47:101, 1982.

46. Poller L, Thompson JM. Problems of international normalized ratio implementation in prothrombin time standardization. In Poller L (ed). Current Advances in Blood Coagulation, No. 6. Churchill Livingstone, 1993:155.

47. Kirkwood TBL. Combination of reference thromboplastins and standardization of the prothrombin time ratio. Thromb Haemost 49:238, 1983.

48. Bussey HI, Force RW, Bianco TM, Leonard AD. Reliance on prothrombin time ratios causes significant errors in anticoagulant therapy. Arch Intern Med 152:278, 1992.

49. Hirsh J, Levine M. Confusion over the therapeutic range for monitoring oral anticoagulant therapy in North America. Thromb Haemost 59:129, 1988.

50. Eckman MH, Levine HJ, Pauker SG. Effect of laboratory variation in the prothrombin-time ratio on the results of oral anticoagulant therapy. N Engl J Med 329:696, 1993.

51. Poller L, Taberner DA. Dosage and control of oral anticoagulants: An international survey. Br J Haematol 51:479, 1982.

52. Hull R, Hirsh J, Jay R, Carter C, Gent M, Turpie AG, McLoughlin D, Dodd P, Thomas M, Raskob G, Ockleford P. Different intensities of oral anticoagulant therapy in the treatment of proximal vein thrombosis. N Engl J Med 307:1676, 1982.

53. Furie B, Liebman HA, Blanchard RA, Coleman M, Kruger SF, Furie BC. Comparison of the native prothrombin antigen and the prothrombin time for monitoring oral anticoagulant therapy. Blood 64:445, 1984.

54. Whitlon DS, Sadowski JA, Suttie JW. Mechanism of

coumarin action: Significance of a vitamin K epoxide reductase inhibition. Biochemistry 17:1371, 1978.

55. Kornberg A, Francis CW, Pellegrini VD, Gabriel KR, Marder VJ. Comparison of native prothrombin antigen with the prothrombin time for monitoring oral anticoagulant prophylaxis. Circulation 88:454, 1993.

56. Furie B, Dinguid CF, Jacobs M, Dinguid DL, Furie BC. Randomized prospective trial comparing native prothrombin antigen with the prothrombin time for monitoring oral anticoagulant therapy. Blood 75:344, 1990.

57. Lee RI, White PD. A clinical study of the coagulation time of blood. Am J Med Sci 145:495, 1913.

58. Pitney WR. Control of heparin therapy. Br Med J 4:139, 1970.

59. Peerschke EIB. Platelet membranes and receptors. In Loscalzo J, Schafer AI (eds). Thrombosis and Hemorrhage Blackwell Scientific, Boston 1994:247.

60. Bauer JD, Ackerman PG, Toro G (eds). Bray's Clinical Laboratory Methods, 7th ed. St. Louis, MO: CV Mosby, 1968:210.

61. Owen C Jr, Mann F, Hurn M, Stickney J. Evaluation of disorders of blood coagulation in the clinical laboratory. Am J Clin Pathol 25:1417, 1955.

62. Langdell RD, Wagner RH, Brinkhous KM. Effect of antihemophilic factor on one stage clotting tests. J Lab Clin Med 41:637, 1953.

63. Nye SW, Graham JB, Brinkhous KM. The partial thromboplastin time as a screening test for the detection of latent bleeders. Am J Med Sci 243:279, 1962.

64. Quick A, Geppert M. Screening for bleeding states – the partial thromboplastin test. Am J Clin Pathol 40:465, 1963.

65. Goulian M, Beck WS. The partial thromboplastin time test. Modification of the procedure and study of the sensitivity and optimal conditions. Am J Clin Pathol 44:97, 1965.

66. Sawitsky A, Boklan BF. Gaucher's disease and coagulation factors. Ann Intern Med 77:150, 1972.

67. Mant MJ, Hirsh J, Pineo GF, Luke KH. Prolonged prothrombin time and partial thromboplastin time in disseminated intravascular coagulation not due to deficiency of factors V and VIII. Br J Haematol 24:725, 1973.

68. Brinkhous KM, Langdell RD, Penick GD, Graham JB, Wagner RH. Newer approaches to the study of hemophilia and hemophilioid states. JAMA 154:481, 1954.

69. Hougie C, Barrow EM, Graham JB. Stuart clotting defect. Segregation of an hereditary hemorrhagic state from the heterogenous group heretofore called "STABLE factor" (SPCA, proconvertin, factor VII) deficiency. J Clin Invest 36:485, 1957.

70. Hathaway WS, Belhasen LP, Hathaway HS. Evidence for a new plasma thromboplastin factor. Case report, coagulation studies and physicochemical properties. Blood 26:521, 1965.

71. Saito H, Ratnoff OD, Waldman R, Abraham JP. Fitzgerald trait — deficiency of a hitherto unrecognized agent, Fitzgerald factor, participating in surface-mediated reactions of clotting, fibrinolysis, generation of kinins, and the property of diluted plasma enhancing vascular permeability (PF-DIL). J Clin Invest 55:1082, 1975.

72. Colman RN, Bagdasarian A, Talamo RC, Scott CF, Seavey M, Guimaraes JA, Pierce JV, Kaplan AP. Williams trait — human kininogen deficiency with diminished levels of plasminogen proactivator and prekallikrein associated with abnormalities of Hageman factor dependent pathways. J Clin Invest 56:1650, 1975.

73. Wuepper KD, Miller DR, Lacombe MJ. Flaujeac trait – deficiency of human plasma kininogen. J Clin Invest 56:1663, 1975.

74. Revak SD, Cochrane CG. Hageman factor: Its structure and modes of activation. Thromb Haemost 35:570, 1976.

75. Hattersly PG, Hayse D. The effect of increased contact activation time on the activated partial thromboplastin time. Am J Clin Pathol 66:479, 1976.

76. Ygge J. Changes in blood coagulation and fibrinolysis during the post operative period. Am J Surg 119:225, 1970.

77. Davidson E, Tomlin S. The levels of plasma coagulation factors in the post operative period. Thromb Diath Hemorrh 10:81, 1963.

78. Pechet L, Alexander B. Increased clotting factors in pregnancy. N Engl J Med 265:1093, 1961.

79. Bonnar J, McNicol GP, Douglas AS. Coagulation and fibrinolytic mechanisms during and after normal childbirth. Br Med J 2:200, 1970.

80. Korsan-Bengsten K, Wilhelmsen L, Elmfeldt D, Tibblen G. Blood coagulation and fibrinolysis in man after myocardial infarction compared with a representative population sample. Atherosclerosis 16:83, 1972.

81. Edson JR, Kiwit W, White JG. Kaolin partial thromboplastin time: High levels of procoagulants producing short clotting times or masking deficiencies of other procoagulants or low concentrations of anticoagulants. J Lab Clin Med 70:463, 1967.

82. Hirsh J. Heparin. N Engl J Med 324:1565, 1991.

83. Basu D, Gallus A, Hirsh J, Cade J. A prospective study of the value of monitoring heparin treatment with the activated partial thromboplastin time. N Engl J Med 287:324, 1972.

84. Spector I, Corn M. Control of heparin therapy with activated partial thromboplastin times. JAMA 201:157, 1967.

85. Hull RD, Raskob GE, Hirsh J, Jay RM, Leclere JR, Geerts W, Rosenbloom D, Sackett DL, Anderson C, Harrison L, Gent M. Continuous intravenous heparin compared with intermittent subcutaneous heparin in the initial treatment of proximal-vein thrombosis. N Engl J Med 315:1109, 1986.

86. Hull RD, Raskob GE, Rosenbloom D, Panju AA, Brill-Edwards P, Ginsbery JS, Hirsh J, Martin GJ, Green D. Heparin for 5 days as compared with 10 days in the initial treatment of proximal venous thrombosis. N Engl J Med 322:1260, 1990.

87. Theroux P, Quimet H, McCans J, Latour JG, Joly P, Levy G, Pelletier E, Juneau M, Stasia KJ, de Guise P. Aspirin, heparin or both to treat acute unstable angina. N Engl J Med 319:1105, 1988.

88. Hsai J, Hamilton WP, Kleiman N, Roberts R, Chaitman BR, Ross AM. A comparison between heparin and low dose aspirin as adjunctive therapy with tissue plasminogen activator for acute myocardial infarction. Am J Cardiol 66:1412, 1990.

89. de Bono DP, Simoons ML, Tijssen J, Arnold AER, Betriu A, Burgersdijk C, Bescos LL, Mueller E, Pfisterer M, Van de Werf F, Zijlstra F, Verstraete M. Effect of early intravenous heparin on coronary patency, infarct size, and bleeding complications after alteplase thrombolysis: Results of a randomized double-blind European Cooperative Study Group trial. Br Heart J 67:122, 1992.

90. Cuccia C, Volterrani M, Volpini M, Musmeci G, Scalvini S, Campana M, Leonzi O, Niccoli L, Pagani M. Relationship between anticoagulation level, ischemic events, and angiographic characteristics of infarct-related artery following streptokinase in patients with acute myocardial infarction (abstr). J Am Coll Cardiol 19:92, 1992.

91. Hirsh J, Fuster V. Guide to anticoagulant therapy. Part 1: Heparin. Circulation 89:1449, 1994.

92. Mattox KC, Guinn GA, Rubio PA, Beall AC Jr. Use of the activated coagulation time in intraoperative heparin reversal for cardiopulmonary operations. Ann Thorac Surg 19:634, 1975.

93. Bull BS, Huse WM, Brauer FS, Korpman RA. Heparin therapy during extracorporeal circulation: II. J Thorac Cardiovasc Surg 69:685, 1975.

94. Young JA, Kisker CT, Doty DB. Adequate anticoagulation during cardiopulmonary bypass determined by activated clotting time and the appearance of fibrin monomer. Ann Thorac Surg 26:231, 1978.

95. Dougherty KG, Gaos CM, Bush HS, Leachman R, Ferguson JJ. Activated clotting times and activated partial thromboplastin times in patients undergoing coronary angioplasty who receive bolus doses of heparin. Cathet Cardiovasc Diagn 26:260, 1992.

96. Ogilby JD, Kopelman HA, Klein LW, Agrawal JB. Adequate heparinization during PTCA: Assessment using activated clotting times. Cathet Cardiovasc Diagn 18:206, 1989.

97. Colman RN, Oxley L, Gianrusa P. Statistical comparison of the automated activated partial thromboplastin time and the clotting time in the regulation of heparin therapy. Am J Clin Pathol 53:904, 1970.

98. Schriever HG, Epstein SE, Mintz MD. Statistical correlation and heparin sensitivity of activated partial thromboplastin time, whole blood clotting time and an automated coagulation time. Am J Clin Pathol 60:323, 1973.

99. Béguin S, Lindhout T, Hemker HC. The effect of trace amounts of tissue factor on thrombin generation in platelet rich plasma, its inhibition by heparin. Thromb Haemost 61:25, 1989.

100. Eitzman DT, Chi L, Saggin L, Schwartz RS, Lucchesi BR, Fay WP. Heparin neutralization by platelet rich thrombi. Role of platelet factor 4. Circulation 89:1523, 1994.

101. Weitz JI, Hudoba M, Massel D, Maraganore J, Hirsh J. Clot-bound thrombin is protected from inhibition by heparin-antithrombin III but is susceptible to inactivation by antithrombin III-dependent inhibitors. J Clin Invest 86:385, 1990.

102. Fey MF, Lang M, Furlan M, Beck EA. Monitoring of heparin therapy with the activated partial thromboplastin time and chromogenic substrate assays. Thromb Haemost 58:853, 1987.

103. de Boer A, van Riel L, den Ottolander GJ. Measurements of antithrombin III, X_2-macroglobulin and X_1 antitrypsin in patients with deep venous thrombosis and pulmonary embolism. Thromb Res 15:17, 1979.

104. Marciniak E, Gockemen J. Heparin-induced decrease in circulating antithrombin III. Lancet 2:581, 1978.

105. Smith LG, Kitchens CS. A comparison between two commercially available activators for determining the partial thromboplastin time. Arch Pathol Lab Med 109:243, 1985.

106. Lenahan JG, Phillips GE. Some variables which influence the activated partial thromboplastin time assay. Clin Chem 12:269, 1966.

107. Bjoinsson TD, Nash PV. Variability in heparin sensitivity of APTT reagents. Am J Clin Pathol 86:199, 1986.

108. Barrowcliffe TW, Gray E. Studies of phospholipid reagents used in coagulation. II. Factors influencing sensitivity to heparin. Thromb Haemost 46:634, 1981.

109. Gawoski JM, Arkin CF, Bovill T, Brandt J, Rock WA, Triplett DA. The effects of heparin on the activated partial thromboplastin time of the College of American Pathologists survey specimens. Arch Pathol Lab Med 111:785, 1987.

110. Brandt JT, Tuplett DA. Laboratory monitoring of heparin: Effect of reagents and instruments on the activated partial thromboplastin time. Am J Clin Pathol 765:530, 1981.

111. Reed SV, Haddon ME, Denson KWE. An attempt to standardize the aPTT for heparin monitoring using the P.T. ISI/INR system of calibration. Results of a 13 center study. Thromb Res 74:515, 1994.

112. Green D, Ts'ao CH, Reynolds N, Kahn D, Kohl H, Cohen I. In vitro studies of a new synthetic thrombin inhibitor. Thromb Res 37:145, 1985.

113. Jakubowski JA, Maraganore JM. Inhibition of coagulation and thrombin-induced platelet activation of a synthetic dodecapeptide modeled on the carboxy-terminus of hirudin. Blood 75:399, 1990.

114. Jang IK, Gold HK, Ziskind AA, Leinbach RC, Fallon JT, Collen D. Prevention of platelet rich arterial thrombosis by selective thrombin inhibition. Circulation 81:219, 1990.

115. Carteaux JP, Gast A, Tschopp TB, Roux S. Activated clotting time as an appropriate test to compare heparin and direct thrombin inhibitors such as hirudin or Ro46-6240 in experimental arterial thrombosis. Circulation 91:1568, 1995.

116. Hattersly PG. Activated coagulation time of whole blood. JAMA 196:437, 1966.

117. Hemker HC, Béguin S. The mode of action of heparins in vitro and in vivo. In Lane et al. (eds). Heparin and Related Polysaccharides. New York: Plenum Press, 1992:221.

118. Ferguson JJ. All ACT's are not the same. THI J19:1, 1992.

119. Avendaño A, Ferguson JJ. Comparison of Hemochron and HemoTec activated coagulation time target values during percutaneous transluminal angioplasty. J Am Coll Cardiol 23:907, 1994.

120. Hattersly P. Program report: The activated coagulation time of whole blood (ACT). Am J Clin Pathol 66:899, 1976.

121. Gravlee GP, Whitaker CL, Mark LJ, Rogers AT, Royster RL, Harrison GA. Baseline activated clotting time should be measured after surgical incision. Anesth Analg 71:549, 1990.

122. Wilson JM, Dougherty KG, Ellis KO, Ferguson JJ. Activated clotting times in acute coronary syndromes and percutaneous coronary angioplasty, Cathet Cardiovasc Diagn 34:1, 1995.

123. van Putten J, Ruit VDM, Beunis M, Hemker HC. Heparin neutralization during collection and processing of blood inhibited by pyridoxal 5'-phosphate. Haemostasis 14:253, 1984.

124. Blakely JA. A rapid bedside method for the control of heparin therapy. Can Med Assoc J 99:1072, 1968.

125. Vacek JL, Hibiya K, Rosamond TL, Kramer PH, Beauchamp GD. Validation of a bedside method of activated partial thromboplastin time measurement with clinical range guidelines. Am J Cardiol 68:557, 1991.

126. Despotis GJ, Santoro SA, Spitznagel E, Kater KM, Barnes P, Cox JL, Lappas DG. On site prothrombin time, activated partial thromboplastin time, and platelet count. A comparison between whole blood and laboratory assays with coagulation factor analysis in patients presenting for cardiac surgery. Anesthesiology 80:338, 1994.

127. Becker RC, Cyr J, Corrao JM, Ball SP. Bedside coagulation monitoring in heparin-treated patients with active thromboembolic disease: A coronary care unit experience. Am Heart J 128:719, 1994.

128. Moliterno DJ, Califf RM, Aguirre FV, Anderson K, Sigmon KN, Weisman HF, Topol EJ. The effect of platelet glycoprotein IIb/IIIa in tcgrin blockade on activated clotting time during percutaneous transluminal coronary angioplasty or directional atherectomy (the EPIC trial). Evaluation of c7E3 Fab in the Prevention of Ischemic Complications trial. Am J Cardiol 75:559, 1995.

37. ANTICOAGULATION MONITORING FOR PERCUTANEOUS TRANSLUMINAL CORONARY ANGIOPLASTY

James J. Ferguson and James M. Wilson

Introduction

Percutaneous transluminal coronary angioplasty (PTCA) relieves coronary obstruction through mechanical disruption of atherosclerotic lesions. It results in focal, traumatic injury, and loss of endothelial integrity, and is an intense stimulus for the formation of thrombus. Thrombus formation at the site of injury may result in reocclusion of the treated vessel and is thought to be a major factor contributing to the process of restenosis. Evidence from the cardiopulmonary bypass literature provides a strong argument that the intensity of anticoagulation influences the frequency with which thrombotic complications may develop. A growing body of evidence suggests that this is true for catheter-based intervention as well. As a result, patients are routinely anticoagulated with intravenous heparin during and immediately after angioplasty, and the degree or intensity of anticoagulation is frequently monitored during PTCA. This chapter presents current views on monitoring the efficacy and adequacy of anticoagulation for catheter-based interventional procedures.

Thrombus and Percutaneous Transluminal Coronary Angioplasty

The presence of thrombus is a major risk factor for adverse outcome following interventional procedures [1-11]. Retrospective studies of several thousand single-vessel angioplasty procedures have shown that angiographic evidence of thrombus prior to intervention may double or triple the likelihood of procedural failure [9–11]. Despite increasing experience and improvements in technology, this risk remained unchanged as late as 1991 [9]. A recent retrospective review of 2699 single-vessel angioplasty procedures

by Reeder et al. [9] identified thrombus as an independent predictor of procedural failure (odds ratio 1.68; $P < 0.0001$). In this study, the degree of risk associated with thrombus-containing lesions appears to have remained relatively constant between 1984 and 1991. A similar study by Tan et al. [10] showed the presence of thrombus, although infrequent (<4%), was a strongly negative independent predictor (odds ratio 0.28, $P = 0.002$) of procedural success. Hillegass et al. [11] showed that patients with unstable angina and angiographic thrombus were more likely to have lower procedural success, higher abrupt closure risk, and worse in-hospital clinical outcome.

An even more powerful predictor of procedural failure is the development of thrombus during a procedure. In a prospective series of 591 consecutive angioplasty procedures at 9 clinical centers, abrupt vessel closure occurred in 65 patients (11%), including both established closure (TIMI grade 0 or 1 flow, 7.1%) and impending closure (>50% stenosis, TIMI grade 0–2 flow, plus use of additional interventions, 3.9%) [12]. Angiographic evidence of thrombus (filling defects) developed in 12.3% of lesions; the presence of newly developed thrombus was associated with significantly lower procedural success (61% vs. 86%) and significantly higher rates of abrupt vessel closure (27.8% vs. 7.2%) and major complications (24.4% vs. 6.4%) (Figure 37-1). Newly developed thrombus was also identified as an independent predictor of procedural failure, abrupt vessel closure, and major complications.

The introduction of new technologies, such as intravascular ultrasound and angioscopy, has emphasized the limitations of contrast angiography in detecting mural thrombus. White et al. [13] used coronary angioscopy to evaluate lesions prior to intervention. Intracoronary thrombi were identified in

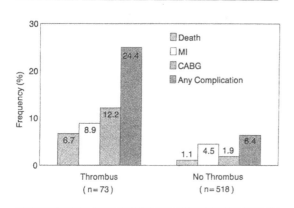

FIGURE 37-1. Newly developed thrombus as a risk factor for procedural complications. The incidences of death, myocardial infarction (MI), emergent coronary artery bypass graft (CABG), and combined adverse events are shown for patients who developed angiographically visible thrombus versus those who did not. (Adapted from Ferguson et al. [12], with permission.)

61% of target lesions with angioscopy, in comparison with only 20% of lesions by angiography. Major in-hospital complications (death, myocardial infarction [MI], emergency coronary artery bypass graft [CABG]) developed in 14% of patients with angioscopically visible thrombi and only 2% of patients without angioscopically visible thrombi. Recurrent ischemia developed in 26% of patients with thrombi, versus 10% without thrombi. There was a definite association (relative risk 3.11, 95% CI 1.28–7.60) between the presence of angioscopic thrombus and adverse outcome. No such relationship was evident for angiographic thrombus. In patients with unstable coronary syndromes, the likelihood of thrombus detectable by angioscopy is even greater (100% in patients with postinfarction angina) and the association with procedural failure even stronger (RR 8.8, 95% CI 1.2–66.9) [14,15]

Thrombus is also a significant risk factor for restenosis following interventional procedures. Violaris et al. [16] retrospectively reviewed data from 2950 patients (3583 lesions) participating in 4 different restenosis studies, and identified 160 lesions with angiographically identifiable thrombus either before or after the procedure. The categorical restenosis rate was significantly higher (43.1%) in lesions with thrombus than in lesions without thrombus (34.4%). This higher rate of restenosis was found to be due primarily to a higher incidence of target lesion occlusion at follow-up (13.8% vs. 5.7%).

Pretreatment with thrombolytic therapy in patients with unstable angina appears to be ineffective in reducing procedural complications and may even increase the incidence of complications in patients with visible thrombus or complex lesions [17]. Heparin infusions prior to PTCA in patients with unstable angina appear to result in a significant decrease in the incidence of thrombotic complications during or after angioplasty [18–20], although prior heparin infusions may make patients relatively heparin resistant.

Intraprocedural Anticoagulation Monitoring

In the early years of angioplasty, the common practice for PTCA was to administer 10,000 U of heparin at the start of the procedure and an additional 5000 U if the procedure lasted for more than an hour [21]. However, this empiric dosing regimen has fallen out of favor, at least in the United States, and has been replaced by close intraprocedural monitoring of heparin therapy [22].

Hattersley [23] first described the activated coagulation time (ACT) in 1966. His method involved drawing whole blood into tubes containing diatomaceous earth, which served as an activator for the coagulation reaction. The tubes were tilted back and forth by hand, and the "coagulation time" was the time that it took for the first visual evidence of thrombus to appear. Further details of the ACT test itself and the current automated techniques employed are discussed in Chapter 36.

With the evolution of extracorporeal bypass support in cardiovascular surgery, dozens of empiric protocols for dosage and reversal of heparin were developed but, in general, failed to provide safe anticoagulation for a significant number of patients. Soon after the introduction of the ACT to control heparin infusion during prolonged extracorporeal bypass, Bull and coworkers [25,26] reviewed the problems with fixed-dose heparin protocols and recommended the use of the ACT to guide the administration and reversal of heparin during cardiopulmonary bypass.

Less blood loss was seen in ACT-monitored patients than in those monitored by the standard empiric protocols [27]. Furthermore, a small percentage of patients in whom anticoagulation was not safely accomplished with the use of standard protocols was recognized [28]. The common problem of heparin resistance was essentially solved by the intraoperative use of ACT, but as late as 1985 articles still appeared in which empiric protocols were compared with ACT-guided anticoagulation in cardiopulmonary by-

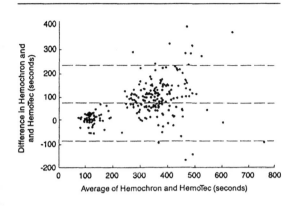

FIGURE 37-2. The difference between Hemochron and HemoTec ACT measurements plotted as a function of the mean value of the two measurements. The degree of variability increases in the higher range of measurements, after the administration of heparin, indicating that measurements on one system cannot be extrapolated to the other. (Adepted from Avendano et al. [38], with permission.)

pass. During the next few years, the focus shifted from the question of whether monitoring was necessary to which method would be the best for monitoring anticoagulation.

In 1986, Scott and associates [29] examined the use of ACT during interventional procedures (i.e., balloon occlusion of the carotid arteries) in which it was used to ensure adequate heparin administration and reversal of its effect prior to sheath removal. Several investigators [30–33] reported the use of anticoagulation monitoring with ACTs for PTCA procedures and documented that standard bolus doses of 10,000 U of heparin do not reliably achieve "adequate" levels of anticoagulation in much the same way that empiric heparin administration for cardiopulmonary bypass was shown to provide inadequate anticoagulation. They recommended that ACT monitoring become standard practice for PTCA procedures. Others [34,35] have documented thrombus development during intravascular procedures associated with low ACTs. Satler and associates [36] emphasized that adequate anticoagulation (defined as ACT greater than 300 seconds) was a primary factor influencing the angioplasty success rate.

As discussed in Chapter 36, a major confounding factor in many of the studies of ACT usage during PTCA is that the data from two different automated systems have been combined. Clear and well-documented differences exist between HemoTec and Hemochron ACTs, and any extrapolations to "target"

ACTs, must remain system specific (Figure 37-2) [37,38]. After a 10,000-U bolus of heparin, 89% of patients achieve an ACT level of 300 seconds measured with a Hemochron system [31]. A much smaller percentage of patients (13.6%) will achieve a "target" ACT of 300 seconds measured on a HemoTec system [33].

To date, a number of published studies have directly examined the relationship between the degree of procedural and postprocedural anticoagulation and the outcome of PTCA (Table 37-1) [39–43], while others have examined this question more indirectly. A retrospective analysis using the aPTT to monitor anticoagulation in 336 patients receiving empiric heparin therapy following PTCA (10,000 U heparin bolus; 2000 U/h infusion) identified two disparate groups [41]. Four percent of patients with aPTTs >3× control suffered abrupt closure or an ischemic event (more than half after withdrawal of heparin) compared with 20% patients with an aPTT <3× control. In contrast, a prospective study [42] of 189 patients undergoing PTCA with fixed doses of heparin and HemoTec ACTs measurements revealed no difference in predilation ACT values, and the authors questioned whether high ACT levels were necessary. However, the low event rate (six episodes of abrupt closure) severely limited their ability to detect any difference in their small study population.

A third study [39] retrospectively examined factors affecting outcomes in patients who developed coronary artery thrombus after a PTCA procedure. Multivariate analysis revealed an association between a postheparin ACT (type not specified) of less than 300 seconds and the occurrence of clinical endpoints of death, CABG, MI, and emergency stent placement to avoid abrupt closure. A total of 92% of uncomplicated cases had a postheparin ACT of >300 second, while only 47% of the complicated cases achieved this level of anticoagulation.

A fourth retrospective analysis [40] compared 103 patients with adverse clinical events (death, emergent CABG, urgent CABG) with 400 comparable event-free patients. Although baseline ACT values (HemoTec) did not differ between patients with and without complications, post-heparin and final ACT values were significantly lower in patients with complications (Figure 37-3). More than three quarters of the patients who remained free of complications had final ACTs of >300 seconds, compared with less than 1% of patients suffering complications who had final ACTs of >300 seconds.

Narins et al. [43] examined more explicitly whether the degree of heparin anticoagulation during

TABLE 37-1.

Design	n	Test	Outcome	Ref.
Retrospective observational	336	aPTT	An aPTT <3× control after PTCA was associated with a fivefold increase in abrupt closure	41
Prospective observational	189	ACT	No correlation between ACT and outcome	42
Retrospective observational	62	ACT	An ACT, after heparin, reached 300 second in only 8% of patients with adverse events compared with 52% without adverse events	39
Case-control	503	ACT	Less than 1% of case patients achieved an ACT >300 seconds compared with 92% of controls	40
Case-control	184	ACT	Inverse relationship between ACT and the likelihood of adverse outcome	43
Prospective observational	59	FPA	Elevated FPA levels were associated with adverse events regardless of ACT results	56

ACT = activated clotting time; aPTT = activated partial thromboplastin time; FPA = fibrinopoptide A; PTCA = percutaneous transluminal coronary angioplasty.

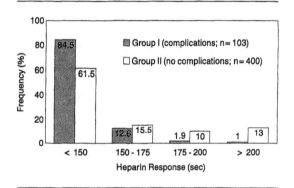

FIGURE 37-3. The relationship between ACT heparin response (in seconds) and the development of major procedural complications. Patients who subsequently develop complications are much more likely to have a lower ACT response to a 10,000 U bolus of heparin. (Adapted from Ferguson et al. [40], with permission.)

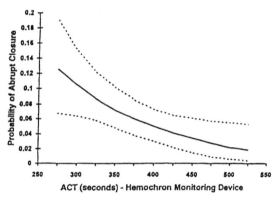

FIGURE 37-4. The probability of abrupt closure (dotted lines indicate upper and lower 95% confidence limits) as a function of the initial postheparin ACT (Hemochron). (From Narins et al. [43], with permission.)

coronary angioplasty (as measured by the activated clotting time) is related to the risk of abrupt vessel closure. Sixty-two cases of in- and out-of-lab abrupt closure in patients undergoing non-emergency coronary angioplasty who had intraprocedure activated clotting times measured were compared with a matched control population of 124 patients who did not experience abrupt closure. Relative to the control population, patients who experienced abrupt closure had significantly lower initial (median 350 vs. 380 seconds) and minimum (345 vs. 370 seconds) activated clotting times. Higher activated clotting times were not associated with an increased likelihood of major bleeding complications. Within this population, a strong inverse linear relationship existed between the activated clotting time and the probability

TABLE 37-2. Outcome of heparin control arms treatment in recent clinical trials

Trial	Date performed	Outcome time points	Heparin dose	Major bleeding	Early death	Early MI	Early revasc. (CABG)	Late death	Late MI	Late revasc.
EPIC [78,79]	1991–1992	30 days 6 months	10,000–12,000 U bolus ACT 300–350	7%	1.7%	8.6%	8.1% (3.6)	3.4%	10.5%	31.8%
HELVETICA [73]	1992–1993	96 hours 30 weeks	10,000 U bolus No ACT titration	6.2%	0.5%	4.2%	7.1% (2.4)	1.0%	5.2%	34%
Hirulog Angioplasty Study [53]	1993–1994	In-hospital 6 months	175 U/kg 15 U/kg/h × 4 hours ACT >350 seconds	9.8%	0.2%	3.9%	9.7%[a] (1.7)	1.1%	6.1%	23.9%
IMPACT II [50]	1993–1994	30 days 6 months	100 U/kg ACT 300–350 seconds	4.8%	1.1%	8.1%	6.1% (2.8)	N/A	N/A	N/A
EPILOG [51,81]	1995	30 days 6 months	100 U/kg ACT 300–350 seconds	3.1%	0.8%	8.7%	5.2% (1.7)	1.7%	9.9%	19.4%
CAPTURE [51,82]	1994–1995	30 days 6 months	10,000 U bolus ACT >300 seconds	1.9%	1.3%	8.2%	10.9%[c] (1.7)	2.2%	9.3%	24.9%
RESTORE [83]	1995	30 days 6 months	100 U/kg ACT >300 seconds	4.2%[b]	0.7%	5.7%	N/A	N/A	N/A	N/A

[a] Incidence of abrupt closure reported.
[b] Including transfusions >2 U.
[c] Includer urgent stenting.
N/A = not available; Revasc. = revascularization; ACT = activated clothing time; MI = myocardial infarction; CABG = coronary artery bypass graft surgery.

of abrupt closure (Figure 37-4). A minimum target activated clotting time could not be identified; rather, the higher the intensity of anticoagulation, the lower the risk of abrupt closure.

The ACT is not the only technique that can be used to assess coagulation status in the catheterization laboratory. Blumenthal et al. Studied the relationship of whole-blood aPTT, ACT, and laboratory aPTT in 166 patients undergoing coronary intervention [44]. Using receiver-operating characteristic (ROC) curves based on laboratory aPTTs as a "standard," they felt that whole-blood aPTTs were superior to ACTs and were a useful potential alternative to ACTs, although additional prospective data are necessary to establish appropriate "target" ranges for whole-blood aPTTs and to further assess the utility of this technique.

There may be a relationship between procedural ACTs and the subsequent development of restenosis [45,46]. This remains purely speculative at present but is a hypothesis that can very easily be tested in future large-scale interventional studies with a 6-month angiographic endpoint.

There are also some reports supporting the use of low-dose heparin for PTCA, without ACT titration. The safety of 5000 IU of heparin was evaluated prospectively in 1375 consecutive elective low-risk PTCA procedures [47]. Success (defined as less than 50% residual stenosis) was obtained in 89.9% of patients. Mortality was 0.3%, and CABG within 24 hours was 1.7%. Prolonged treatment with heparin

was considered necessary in 123 patients (9%). Of the patients selected for prolonged heparinization, 63% had an uncomplicated course; 2.7% had an MI. Re-PTCA for abrupt closure was performed in two patients shortly after sheath removal, and in two patients during prolonged heparin treatment; in five patients re-PTCA within 24 hours was performed for an unsatisfactory re-angiography after heparinization.

A recent study by Boccara et al. [48] randomized 400 patients undergoing PTCA to either a 15,000 bolus or a 100 U/kg bolus of heparin prior to the procedure. There was no difference between the two groups in the incidence of death, MI, unplanned revascularization, or bailout stenting.

A number of trials [49–53] have used weight-based heparin dosing in catheterization laboratories, especially in circumstances in which additional anticoagulants (with concomitant additional bleeding risk) are given. Low body weight has emerged as a significant risk factor for bleeding complications, and weight-based heparin (usually around 100 U/kg) may reduce the risk of overshooting heparin therapy, particularly in lightweight patients. The time to sheath removal and transfer to a stepdown unit were significantly shorter in the weight-adjusted heparin group. However, one study [54] has in fact questioned whether BSA-based or weight-based heparin truly does provide more reliable levels of anticoagulation. Table 37.2 summarizes the outcomes of the heparin control arms of recent major interventional trials utilizing new anticoagulant agents.

The ACT and all similar tests must be viewed as surrogate measures of antithrombotic treatment efficacy. Elevated FPA levels reflecting thrombin activity may be seen in a number of patients (36%), despite "therapeutic" ACTs and high heparin levels. Weight-adjusted heparin did appear to be more effective in this study in achieving adequate (ACT >300s) anticoagulation. Elevated FPA levels (suggesting heparin-resistant thrombus formation) are associated with subsequent adverse clinical events, regardless of whether a "therapeutic" ACT is achieved [56]. Unfortunately there are at present no readily available bedside assays to provide the sophisticated analyses of coagulation activation necessary to identify patients at risk for future adverse events.

Postprocedure Anticoagulation

The proper duration of heparin therapy following PTCA remains controversial [41,57,58–63]. However, inadequate anticoagulation following PTCA was associated with a significant increase in adverse events in at least one study [41]. In complicated cases an overnight heparin infusion is usually recommended, and in cases of unstable coronary syndromes and acute MI it can be continued for up to 5 days, to provide the time necessary for re-endothelization of the injured artery. Postprocedure heparin, if utilized, is probably best titrated to aPTT, and the recent availability of whole-blood bedside testing, which can provide immediate results, may improve the therapeutic efficacy of heparin in this situation.

Pitney et al. [64] have suggested that the "ACT differential" (the difference between the ACT and the heparinase ACT from the same sample — a marker of heparin effect in comparison with heparin-free baseline) may be an alternative technique for monitoring anticoagulation following PTCA. They showed a significant reduction in major and minor bleeding complications when the ACT differential was substituted for the aPTT in adjusting postprocedure heparin.

There are, at present, only preliminary data available on the use of low-molecular weight heparin (which would not require monitoring or titration) following interventional procedures. Low molecular weight heparin may be a reasonable alternative, and it would be an advantage in not requiring anticoagulation monitoring, but much more experience with it will be necessary before its routine use can be advocated.

Current Practice

A recently published survey of interventional cardiologists was designed to assess the current practice patterns (March of 1994) in the United States for anticoagulation during PTCA [65]. A total of 76.8% of respondents routinely started with a 10,000 U bolus of heparin, while only 3.2% of respondents used a weight-adjusted heparin bolus. Fifty-nine percent of respondents routinely used intraprocedure heparin infusions, usually 1000 U/h. Anticoagulation monitoring was used by 92.6% of respondents during PTCA, almost always with activated clotting times (ACTs). Postprocedure heparin infusions (usually titrated to an aPTT >2× control) were used by 70.3% of respondents. Lower volume operators were more likely to use postprocedure heparin infusions.

A survey of 70 sites participating in the IMPACT II study revealed that only 48% of physicians agreed upon a heparin dosing protocol at any given site. Weight-adjusted heparin was used in 10% of cases. Ninety-three percent of sites surveyed used ACTs to adjust heparin dosing. Most physicians surveyed (77%) considered 301–350 (machine unspecified) as a desirable ACT target range.

Thus, heparin therapy for PTCA continues to be largely empiric, although the vast majority of cardiologists surveyed use ACT-guided heparin therapy for the procedure. Weight-based heparin dosing is still relatively uncommon. The usual target levels of anticoagulation for PTCA are 300–350 seconds for Hemochron ACTs and >300 seconds for HemonTec ACTs.

Coagulation Monitoring with Newer Agents

There are a number of antithrombotic agents currently in clinical trials for PTCA. Two specific groups of new drugs have shown particular promise: antithrombins and platelet fibrinogen receptor (GPIIb/IIIa) antagonists.

THROMBIN INHIBITORS

Hirudin, a molecule originally derived from leech saliva, is a direct-acting thrombin inhibitor [67] that prevents thrombin-catalyzed activation of factors V, VIII, and XIII, and thrombin-induced platelet activation. In a randomized study comparing heparin with hirudin in the prevention of thrombotic complications related to PTCA, hirudin significantly reduced the incidence of post-procedural ischemic events [68]. Hirudin has also been shown to decrease the incidence of restenosis in a rabbit angioplasty model [69]. It is currently under investigation as an adjunct to thrombolytic therapy for acute MI [70–72] and as an alternative to heparin for the treatment of unstable angina.

The HELVETICA study [73] showed a significant benefit of hirudin over heparin at 96 hours postprocedure in patients with unstable angina. This initial benefit was not sustained, and at 6-month follow-up there were no differences in event rates between groups. In this study, fixed-dose boluses of heparin (10,000 U) were given in the control group, without titration to ACTs.

Hirulog is a 20 amino-acid synthetic peptide that, like hirudin, binds to thrombin at both the fibrinogen-binding exosite and the active site, and acts to inhibit both free and clot-bound thrombin. Topol et al. [52] recently reported a multicenter dose-ranging study of hirulog; a total of 291 patients undergoing elective PTCA were enrolled in one of five ascending dose groups. The abrupt closure rate in the three lowest dose groups was 11.3%, compared with 3.9% in the two highest dose groups. There was a reproducible dose — response curve of both ACTs and aPTT to hirulog, and there were no thrombotic closures in patients with ACTs >300 seconds. Hirulog was associated with a rapid-onset dose-dependent anticoagulant effect, and in higher doses appeared to provide safe and adequate anticoagulation for PTCA.

In the Hirulog Angioplasty Study [53] 4098 patients undergoing angioplasty for unstable or postinfarction angina were randomized to procedural anticoagulation with either heparin (175 U/kg bolus and an 18–24 hour infusion of 15 U/kg; with procedural ACTs (Hemochron) titrated to >350 seconds) or hirulog (1 mg/kg bolus, a 4-hour infusion of 2.5 mg/kg/h and a 14–20 hour infusion of 0.2 mg/kg/h; no titration of procedural anticoagulation ACT levels). The primary endpoint was the in-hospital incidence of death MI, abrupt vessel closure, or rapid clinical deterioration of cardiac origin. In the total study group (n = 4098), hirulog did not significantly reduce the incidence of the primary endpoint (11.4% vs. 12.2% for heparin) but did result in a lower incidence of bleeding (3.8% vs. 9.8%, P < 0.001). Patients in the hirulog group had slightly lower ACTs after the initial study drug bolus; 37% of the heparin group received additional boluses. In the subgroup of 704 patients with postinfarction angina, hirulog therapy resulted in a lower incidence of the primary endpoint; there was, however, no difference in the primary endpoint or 6-month outcome of the 3194-patient unstable angina subgroup or the total study population.

A recent preliminary report by Ahmed et al. [74] retrospectively examined the relationship between degree of anticoagulation in the Hirulog Angioplasty Study and outcome. They found that with heparin there were decreasing event rates at higher ACT values, but no such relationship existed for hirulog. They speculated that high doses of heparin may overcome local resistance to heparin, but that direct-acting thrombin inhibitors (which are not subject to local resistance) may be effective at a lower intensity of systemic anticoagulation.

Argatroban is an arginine derivative that also directly blocks the action of thrombin. In contrast to hirudin and hirulog, which irreversibly inhibit thrombin binding to both the active site and the fibrinogen binding exosite, argatroban is a competitive inhibitor that binds only to the active site of thrombin. It is a much smaller molecule than hirudin or hirulog, and is currently entering clinical trials as an alternative to heparin for PTCA and unstable angina. Preliminary data have suggested that ACTs and aPTTs do not show parallel changes in patients treated with argatroban and heparin [75]. This suggests that there may be fundamental problems in assessing anticoagulation with these new agents, and that comparisons with heparin at similar levels of ACT or aPTT are not necessarily meaningful. Carteaux et al. [76] have recently suggested that the antithrombotic effect of the direct thrombin inhibitor is more properly assessed by the ACT than the aPTT. However, another recent study [77] has suggested that, in comparison with heparin, argatroban has differential effects on HemoTec and Hemochron ACT's. No comparison data are available at present on other direct thrombin inhibitors.

FIBRINOGEN RECEPTOR ANTAGONISTS

A number of recent studies — EPIC [78,79], PROLOG [80], EPILOG [51,81], CAPTURE [51, 82], IMPACT-II [50], and RESTORE [83] — have suggested that GPIIb/IIIa–blocking drugs may be particularly effective in decreasing the thrombotic complications associated with PTCA. Only limited data on the implications of these agents for intraprocedural coagulation monitoring are available.

In EPIC the platelet GPIIb/IIIa-blocking antibody c7E3 Fab reduced the incidence of ischemic complications by 35%, but was associated with a doubling of the risk for major bleeding complications and red blood cell transfusions [78,79]. Interestingly, c7E3 Fab treatment appeared to independently prolong procedural ACTs by about 30–40 seconds. A small pilot study, PROLOG, was undertaken to investigate whether reduction and weight adjustment of heparin dose, early sheath removal, or both strategies could improve the safety while maintaining the clinical efficacy of c7E3 Fab therapy for PTCA [49]. One hundred and three patients undergoing coronary intervention received c7E3 Fab (0.25 mg/kg bolus, 10 µg/min infusion for 12 hours) and aspirin, and were randomized by a 2 × 2 factorial design to one of two weight-adjusted heparin doses in a blinded fashion and to one of two strategies for heparin discontinuation and vascular sheath removal.

In the "standard-dose heparin" group (n = 52), an initial bolus of 100 U/kg was administered followed by additional bolus doses as necessary to maintain procedural activated clotting time (ACT) ≥300 seconds; in the "low-dose heparin" group (n = 51), an initial bolus of 70 U/kg was administered without adjustment for ACT. In the "late sheath removal" arm (n = 50), heparin infusion was continued for the 12-hour duration of c7E3 Fab infusion, followed by sheath removal 6 hours later; in the "early sheath removal" group (n = 53), heparin was stopped after the interventional procedure and sheaths were removed 6 hours later during the c7E3 Fab infusion. Patients were followed for 7 days or through hospital discharge for the occurrence of the composite efficacy endpoint of death, MI, or urgent revascularization and for the incidence of bleeding complications.

Median Hemochron ACT values immediately prior to coronary interventions were 336 seconds and 257 seconds in the standard-dose and low-dose heparin arms, respectively. There were no differences between patients randomized to standard-dose and low-dose heparin or early and late sheath removal with regard to the occurrence of primary efficacy endpoint events. The maximum decreases in hemoglobin and rates of bleeding, large hematoma formation at the vascular access site, and red blood cell transfusion were all reduced by low-dose heparin and early sheath removal, and were lowest when both strategies were combined.

The large-scale EPILOG trial has investigated this issue further in a much larger population of patients undergoing coronary interventions. EPILOG was halted prematurely because of a positive treatment effect [51,81], and the combination of low-dose heparin (70 U/kg, titrated only to ACTs >200 seconds) and c7E3 Fab was superior to standard doses of heparin alone, and at least as effective (with fewer bleeding complications) as standard-dose heparin plus c7E3 Fab. This may have profound future implications as to how heparin should be dosed with concomitant c7E3 Fab therapy. The data from PROLOG and EPILOG, as well as current clinical experience, strongly suggest that much lower ACT targets (only >200 seconds) are necessary when c7E3 Fab is used.

The CAPTURE trial [51,82], conducted in Europe at the same time, was also halted prematurely because of positive interim results. CAPTURE was originally designed as a placebo-controlled study of c7E3 Fab in 1400 patients with refractory unstable angina scheduled for PTCA. Unlike in EPIC, PROLOG, and EPILOG (in which patients were treated with c7E3 Fab immediately prior to a coronary intervention, and treatment continued for 12 hours following the procedure), in CAPTURE patients were pretreated with c7E3 Fab for 18–24 hours prior to the interventional procedure, and continued for 1 hour following the procedure. An interim analysis of the first 1050 patients showed that the incidence of death, MI, and urgent intervention was significantly reduced by 7E3 Fab (10.8%) versus placebo (16.4%) to a level that exceeded prespecified stopping criteria.

The IMPACT-II study compared two different doses of the cyclic RGD heptapeptide IIb/IIIa blocker Integrilin to placebo in both low- and high-risk PTCA [50]. At 24 hours both doses of Integrelin were effective in reducing procedural complications. At 30 days the benefit appeared somewhat attenuated; even more so at 6 months, when it was no longer statistically significant. At 6-month angiographic follow-up, there was no difference in quantitative coronary angiography–measured treatment-site minimum lethal doses between groups.

Similar to c7E3 Fab, Integrelin also appeared to prolong procedural ACTs, although much less so in heavier patients. Aguirre et al. [84] have noted a paradoxical *increase* in adverse events with increasing ACTs (death, MI, revascularization at 30 days) in placebo-treated patients in IMPACT II, while no such increase was noted in Integrelin-treated patients. This suggests that there may be a point of diminishing returns, at which the documented increase in bleeding events associated with higher levels of anticoagulation may result in worse clinical outcomes.

Another interesting study by Mascelli et al. [85] reports the development of a "bedside" platelet aggregation test to assess the degree of platelet inhibition in patients receiving IIb/IIIa-targeted therapy. While it is unlikely that such devices will be utilized routinely for monitoring antiplatelet therapy during interventional procedures, this technique will no doubt prove useful in identifying appropriate dose ranges for these potent agents as they come into more routine clinical usage.

Conclusions

Interventional procedures such as PTCA injure the endothelium and create an intensely thrombogenic milieu. As a result, anticoagulation antithrombotic therapy is routinely administered to patients undergoing such procedures. The degree of anticoagulation necessary to safely perform PTCA remains controversial. The standard of care in the United Sates currently entails intraprocedural coagulation monitoring, usually with an ACT, and titration of heparin to levels deemed "adequate" for that particular laboratory. A number of new agents show particular promise as adjuncts (IIb/IIIa blockers) or alternatives (hirudin, hirulog, and argatroban) to heparin for PTCA. As we become more conscious of the processes contributing to intraprocedural thrombus formation and the limitations of current therapy with heparin and aspirin, we are moving forward to a new era of aggressive, targeted anticoagulant therapy. Ongoing clinical trials will help to define the optimal anticoagulant strategy of the future.

There are emerging concerns that excessive heparin anticoagulation (and very high ACTs) may be associated not just with more bleeding, but also with more procedural complications. Thus, more recent interventional trials with new, potent anticoagulant agents have attempted not to overshoot the degree of anticoagulation. To some extent procedural complications (and the requirement for more procedural heparin in the setting of complications) may play a confounding role, but it is clear that a number of major questions remain, and that a definitive prospective study to define optimal procedural anticoagulation, particularly with newer anticoagulant agents, needs to be performed.

Acknowledgment

The authors would like to acknowledge the invaluable assistance of Angie Esquivel in the preparation of the manuscript.

References

1. Mabin TA, Holmes DR Jr, Smith HC, et al. Intracoronary thrombus: Role in coronary occlusion complicating percutaneous transluminal coronary angioplasty. J Am Coll Cardiol 3:198, 1985.
2. Ischinger T, Gruentzig AR, Meier B, Galan K. Coronary dissection and total coronary occlusion associated with percutaneous transluminal coronary angioplasty: Significance of initial angiographic morphology of coronary stenoses. Circulation 74:1371, 1986.
3. Laskey MAL, Deutsch E, Hirshfeld JW, Kussmaul WG, Barnathan E, Laskey WK. Influence of heparin therapy on percutaneous transluminal coronary angioplasty outcome in patients with coronary arterial thrombus. Am J Cardiol 65:179, 1990.
4. Sugrue DD, Holmes DR Jr, Smith HC, et al. Coronary artery thrombus as a risk factor for acute vessel occlusion during percutaneous transluminal coronary angioplasty: Improving results. Br Heart J 56:62, 1986.
5. Deligonul U, Gabliani GI, Caralis DG, Kern MJ, Vandormael MG. Percutaneous transluminal coronary angioplasty in patients with intracoronary thrombus. Am J Cardiol 62:474, 1988.
6. Lincoff A, Popma J, Ellis S, Hacker J, Topol E. Abrupt vessel closure complicating coronary angioplasty: Clinical, angiographic and therapeutic profile. J Am Coll Cardiol 19:926, 1992.
7. de Feyter PJ, van den Brand M, Jaarman G, van Domburg R, Serruys PW, Suryapranata H. Acute coronary artery occlusion during and after percutaneous transluminal coronary angioplasty: Frequency, prediction, clinical course, management, and follow-up. Circulation 83:927, 1991.
8. Ellis SG, Roubin GS, King SB III, Douglas JSJ, Weintraub WS, Thomas RG, et al. Angiographic and clinical predictors of acute closure after native vessel angioplasty. Circulation 77:372, 1988.
9. Reeder GS, Bryant SC, Suman VJ, Holmes DR Jr. Intracoronary thrombus: Still a risk factor for PTCA Failure? Cathet Cardiovasc Diagn 34:191, 1995.
10. Tan K, Sulke N, Taub N, Sowton E. Clinical and lesion morphologic determinants of coronary angioplasty success and complications: current experience. J Am Coll Cardiol 25:855, 1995.
11. Hillegass WB, Ohman EM, O'Hanesian MA, Harrington RA, Faxon DP, Fortin DF, Ellis SG, Stack RS, Holmes DR, Califf RM. The effect of preprocedural intracoronary thrombus on patient outcome after percutaneous coronary intervention. J Am Coll Cardiol 25:94A, 1995.
12. Ferguson JJ, Barasch E, Wilson JM, Strony J, Wolfe MW, Schweiger MJ, Leya F, Bonan R, Isner JM, Roubin GS, Cannon AD, Cleman M, Cabin HS, Adelman B, Bittl JA, and the Heparin Registry Investigators. The relation of clinical outcome to dissection and thrombus formation during coronary angioplasty. J Invas Cardiol 7:2, 1995.
13. White CJ, Ramee SR, Collins TJ, Escobar AE, Karsan A, Shaw D, Jain SP, Bass TA, Heuser RR, Teirstein PS, Bonan R, Walter PD, Smalling RW. Coronary thrombi increase PTCA risk. Angioscopy as a clinical tool. Circulation 93:253, 1996.
14. Waxman S, Sassower MA, Mittleman MA, Zarich S, Miyamoto A, Manzo KS, Muller JE, Abela GS, Nesto RW. Angioscopic predictors of early adverse outcome after coronary angioplasty in patients with unstable angina and non-Q wave myocardial infarction. Circulation 93:2106, 1996.
15. Tabata H, Mizuno K, Arakawa K, Satomura K, Shibuya T, Kurita A, Nakamura H. Angioscopic identification of coronary thrombus in patients with postinfarction angina. J Am Coll Cardiol 25:1282, 1995.

16. Violaris AG, Melkert R, Hermann JR, Serruys PW. Role of angiographically identifiable thrombus on long term luminal renarrowing after coronary angioplasty. Circulation 93:889, 1996.

17. Ambrose JA, Almeida OD, Sharma SK, Torre SR, Marmur JD, Israel DM, Ratner DE, Weiss MB, Hjeimdahl-Monsen CE, Myler RK, Moses J, Unterecker WJ, Grunwald AM, Garrett JS, Cowley MJ, Anwar A, Sobolski J. Adjunctive thrombolytic therapy during angioplasty for ischemic rest angina. Results of the thrombolysis and angioplasty in unstable angina (TAUSA) trial. Circulation 90:69, 1994.

18. Lukas MA, Deutsch E, Hirshfeld JW Jr, Kussmaul WG, Barnathan E, Laskey WK. Influence of heparin therapy on percutaneous transluminal angioplasty outcome in patients with coronary arterial thrombus. Am J Cardiol 65:179, 1990.

19. Douglas JS, Lutz JF, Clements SD, Robinson PH, Roubin GS, Lembo NJ, King SB. Therapy of large intracoronary thrombi in candidates for percutaneous transluminal angioplasty (abstract). J Am Coll Cardiol 11(Suppl. A);238A, 1988.

20. Pow TK, Varricchione TR, Jacobs ASK, Ruocco NA, Ryan TJ, Christelis EM, Faxon DP. Does pretreatment with heparin prevent abrupt closure following PTCA? J Am Coll Cardiol 11:238A, 1988.

21. Hollman J, Gruentzig AR, Douglas JS Jr, King SB III, Ischinger T, Meier B. Acute occlusion after percutaneous transluminal angioplasty-a new approach. Circulation 68:725, 1983.

22. Popma JJ, Coller BS, Ohman EM, Bittl JA, Weitz J, Kuntz RE, Leon MB. Antithrombotic therapy in patients undergoing coronary angioplasty. Chest 108:4865, 1995.

23. Hattersley PG. Activated coagulation time of whole blood. JAMA 196:436, 1966.

24. Hill JD, Dontigny L, de Leval M, Mielke CH Jr. A simple method of heparin management during prolonged extracorporeal circulation. Ann Thorac Surg 17:129, 1974.

25. Bull BS, Korpman RA, Huse WM, Briggs BD. Heparin therapy during extracorporeal circulation: I. Problems inherent in existing heparin protocols. J Thorac Cardiovasc Surg 69:674, 1975.

26. Bull BS, Huse WM, Brauer FS, Korpman RA. Heparin therapy during extracorporeal circulation: II. The use of a dose-response curve to individualize heparin and protamine dosage. J Thorac Cardiovasc Surg 69:685, 1975.

27. Babka R, Colby C, El-Etr A, Pifarre R. Monitoring of intraoperative heparinization and blood loss following cardiopulmonary bypass surgery. J Thorac Cardiovasc Surg 73:780, 1977.

28. Roth JA, Cukingnan RA, Scott CR. Use of activated coagulation time to monitor heparin during cardiac surgery. Ann Thorac Surg 28:69, 1979.

29. Scott JA, Berenstein A, Blumenthal D. Use of the activated coagulation time as a measure of anticoagulation during interventional procedures. Radiology 158:849, 1986.

30. Kopelman HA, Klein LW, Agarwal JB. Adequate heparinization during PTCA: Assessment using activated clotting time. J Am Coll Cardiol 11:237A, 1988.

31. Ogilby JD, Kopelman HA, Klein LW, Agarwal JB. Adequate heparinization during PTCA: Assessment using activated clotting times. Cathet Cardiovasc Diagn 18:206, 1989.

32. Rath B, Bennett DH. Monitoring the effect of heparin by measurement of activated clotting time during and after percutaneous transluminal angioplasty. Br Heart J 63:18, 1990.

33. Dougherty KG, Gaos CM, Bush HS, Leachman DR, Ferguson JJ. Activated clotting times and activated partial thromboplastin times in patients undergoing coronary angioplasty who receive bolus doses of heparin. Cathet Cardiovasc Diagn 26:260, 1992.

34. Grayburn PA, Willard JE, Brickner ME, Eichhorn EJ. In vivo thrombus formation on a guidewire during intravascular ultrasound imaging: Evidence for inadequate heparinization. Cathet Cardiovasc Diagn 23:141, 1991.

35. Mooney MR, Mooney JF, Goldenberg IF, Almquist AK, Tassel RAV. Percutaneous Transluminal coronary angioplasty in the setting of large intracoronary thrombi. Am J Cardiol 65:427, 1990.

36. Satler LF, Leon MB, Kent KM, Pichard AD. Strategies for acute occlusion after coronary angioplasty. J Am Coll Cardiol 19:936, 1992.

37. Ferguson JJ. All ACTs are not created equal. Tex Heart Inst J 19:1, 1992.

38. Avendano A, Ferguson JJ. Comparison of Hemochron and HemoTec activated coagulation time target values during percutaneous transluminal angioplasty. J Am Coll Cardiol 23:907, 1994.

39. Vaitkus PT, Hermann HC, Laskey WK. Management and immediate outcome of patients with intracoronary thrombus during percutaneous transluminal coronary angioplasty. Am Heart J 124:1, 1992.

40. Ferguson JJ, Dougherty KG, Gaos CM, Bush HS, Marsh KC, Leachman DR. The relationship between procedural activated clotting times and in-hospital post-PTCA outcome. J Am Coll Cardiol 23:1061, 1994.

41. McGarry TF Jr, Gottlieb RS, Morganroth J, Zelenkofske SL, Kasparian H, Duca PR, Lester RM, Kreulen TH. The relationship of anticoagulation level and complications after successful percutaneous transluminal angioplasty. Am Heart J 123:1445, 1992.

42. Frierson JH, Dimas AP, Simpfendorfer CC, Pearce G, Miller M, Franco I. Is aggressive heparinization necessary for elective PTCA? Cathet Cardiovasc Diagn 28:279, 1993.

43. Narins CR, Hillegass WB Jr, Nelson CL, Tcheng JE, Harrington RA, Phillips HR, Stack RS, Califf RM. Relation between activated clotting time during angioplasty and abrupt closure. Circulation 93:667, 1996.

44. Blumenthal RS, Carter AJ, Resar JR, Coombs V,

Gloth ST, Dalal J, Brinker JA. Comparison of bedside and hospital laboratory coagulation studies during and after coronary intervention. Cathet Cardiovasc Diagn 35:9, 1995.

45. Perin EC, Turner SA, Ferguson JJ. Relationship between the response to heparin and restenosis following PTCA. Circulation 82(Suppl. III):497, 1990.

46. Lins M, Zurborn KH, Dau O, Muurling S, Herrmann G, Simon R. Does coagulation activation cause restenosis in patients undergoing directional coronary atherectomy? (abstr) J Am Coll Cardiol 27(Suppl. A):391, 1996.

47. Koch KT, Piek JJ, Mulder K, Peters RJG, David GK. Safety of low-dose heparin in elective percutaneous transluminal coronary angioplasty. Eur Heart J 16(Suppl.):85, 1995.

48. Boccara A, Benamer H, Juliard JM, Aubry P, Goy P, Himbert D, Karnillon GJ, Steg PG. A radomized trial of a fixed high dose versus a weight-adjusted low dose of intravenous heparin during coronary angioplasty. Circulation, in press.

49. Lincoff AM, Tcheng JE, Bass TA, Popma JJ, Teirstein PS, Kleiman NS, Weisman HF, Musco MH, Cabot CF, Berdan LG, Califf RM, Topol EJ, PROLOG Investigators. A multicenter, randomized, double-blind pilot trial of standard versus low dose weight-adjusted heparin in patients treated with the platelet GP IIb/IIIa receptor antibody c7E3 during percutaneous coronary revascularization. J Am Coll Cardiol 25:80A, 1995.

50. The IMPACT II Investigators: Randomized placebo-controlled trial of effect of eptifibatide on complications of percutaneous coronary intervention: IMPACT II Lancet 349:1422, 1997.

51. Ferguson JJ. EPILOG and CAPTURE trials halted because of positive interim results. Circulation 93:637, 1996.

52. Topol EJ, Bonan R, Jewitt D, Sigwart U, Kakkar VV, Rothman M, de Bonon D, Ferguson J, Willerson JT, Strony J, Ganz P, Cohen MD, Raymond R, Fox I, Maraganore J, Adelman B. Use of a direct antithrombin, hirulog, in place of heparin during coronary angioplasty. Circulation 87:1622, 1993.

53. Bittl JA, Strony J, Brinker JA, Ahmed WH, Meckel CR, Chaitman BR, Maraganore J, Deutsch E, Adelman B, for the Hirulog Angioplasty Study Investigators. Treatment with bivalirudin (hirulog) as compared with heparin during coronary angioplasty for unstable or postinfarction angina. N Engl J Med 333:764, 1995.

54. Wilson JM, Khoshnevis R, Le D, Ferguson JJ, Yaryura RA, Reddy KJ, Waly HM. Are weight-based heparin boluses more predictable? J Invas Cardiol 8:66, 1996.

55. Snitzer R, Miremath YJ, Lee J, Lasala JM, Eisenberg PR, Winters KJ. Suppression of intracoronary thrombin activity by weight-adjusted heparin administration during coronary interventions. Circulation 92(Suppl. I):I609, 1995.

56. Winters KJ, Oltrona L, Hiremath YJ, Lasala JM, Eisenberg PR. Heparin-resistant thrombin activity is associated with acute ischemic events during high-risk

coronary interventions. Circulation 92(Suppl. I):I608, 1995.

57. Hirshfeld JW, Goldberg S, MacDonald R, Vetrovec G, Bass T, Taussig A, Margolis J, Jugo R, Pepine C. Lesion and procedure-related variables predictive of restenosis after PTCA — A report from the M-HEART study. Circulation 76:IV215, 1987.

58. Saenz CB, Baxley WA, Bulle TM, Cherre JM, Dean LS. Early and late effect of heparin infusion following elective angioplasty. Circulation 78:II98, 1988.

59. Ellis SG, Roubin GS, Wilentz J, Douglas JS, King SB. Effect of 18- to 24-hour heparin administration for prevention of restenosis after uncomplicated coronary angioplasty. Am Heart J 117:777, 1989.

60. Walford CD, Midei MM, Aversano TR, Gottlieb SO, Chew PH, Siu CO, Brin KP, Brinker JA. Heparin after PTCA: Increased early complications and no clinical benefit. Circulation 84:II592, 1991.

61. Tanjura L, Pinto I, Centemero M, Chaves A, Mattos L, Feres F, Maldonado G, Cano H, Sousa A, Sousa JE. Use of heparin in coronary angioplasty: Randomized trial for prevention of abrupt closure. Eur Heart J 14:179, 1993.

62. Friedman HZ, Cragg DR, Glazier SM, Gangadharan V, Marsalese DL, Schreiber TL, O'Neill WW. Randomized prospective evaluation of prolonged versus abbreviated intravenous heparin therapy after coronary. J Am Coll Cardiol 24:1214, 1994.

63. Pizzuli L, Zirbes M, Fehske W, Pfeiffer D. Omission of intravenous heparin and nitroglycerin following uncomplicated coronary angioplasty: A prospective. Circulation 92:I74, 1995.

64. Pitney MR, Kelly SA, Allan RM, Giles RW, McCredie M, Walsh WF. Activated clotting time differential is a superior method of monitoring anticoagulation following coronary angioplasty. Cathet Cardiovasc Diagn 37:145, 1996.

65. Ferguson JJ, Dohmen P, Wilson JM, Vaughn WK, Khoshnevis R, Kmonicek P, McKinney AA, Plachetka JR. Results of a national survey on anticoagulation for PTCA. J Invas Cardiol 7:136, 1995.

66. Rund MM, Smith DD, DeLuca SA, Rouse CL, Sigmon KN, Juran NB, O'Brien M, Tcheng JE for the IMPACT II Study Coordinators/Investigators. Heparin during coronary angioplasty: Are there any rules? Circulation 90:I487, 1994.

67. Kaiser B. Anticoagulant and antithrombotic actions of recombinant hirudin. Semin Thromb Hemost 17:130, 1991.

68. van den Bos AA, Deckers JW, Heyndrickx GR, et al. PTCA with hirudin is associated with less acute cardiac complications than with heparin (abstr). Circulation 86(Suppl. I):I372, 1992.

69. Sarembock IJ, Gertz SD, Gimple LW, Owen RM, Powers ER, Roberts WC. Effectiveness of recombinant desulphatohirudin in reducing restenosis after balloon angioplasty of atherosclerotic femoral arteries in rabbits. Circulation 84:232, 1991.

70. The GUSTO IIa Investigators. Randomized trial of intravenous heparin versus recombinant hirudin for

acute coronary syndromes. Circulation 90:1631, 1994.

71. Antman EM, for the TIMI 9A Investigators. Hirudin in acute myocardial infarction. Safety report from the thrombolysis and thrombin inhibition in myocardial infarction (TIMI) 9A trial. Circulation 90:1624, 1994.

72. Neuhaus K-L, v. Essen R, Tebbe U, Jessel A, Heinrichs H, Mäurer W, Döring W, Harmjanz D, Kötter V, Kalhammer E, Simon H, Horacek T. Safety observations from the pilot phase of the radomized r-hirudin for improvement of thrombolysis (HIT-III) study. A study of the Arbeitsgemeinschaft Leitender Kardiologischer Krankenhausärzte (ALKK). Circulation 90:1638, 1994.

73. Serruys PW, Herrman J-PR, Simon R, Rutsch W, Bode C, Laarman G-J, van Dijk R, van den Bos AA, Umans VAWM, Fox KAA, Close P, Deckers JW, for the Helvetica Investigators. A comparison of hirudin with heparin in the prevention of restenosis after coronary angioplasty. N Engl J Med 333:757, 1995.

74. Ahmed WH, Meckel CR, Grines CL, Strony J, Borzak S, Kraft PL, Timmis GC, Ferguson JJ, Adelman B, Bittl JA, on behalf of the Hirulog Angioplasty Study Investigators. Relation between ischemic complications and activated clotting times during coronary angioplasty: Different profiles for heparin and hirulog. Circulation 92(Suppl. I):I608, 1995.

75. Hursting MJ, Joffrion JL, Brooks RL, Swan SK. A comparison of the pharmacodynamics of heparin and argatroban (a direct thrombin inhibitor) in healthy volunteers (abstr). American Society of Hematology, 1996.

76. Carteaux JP, Gast A, Tschopp TB, Roux S. Activated clotting time as an appropriate test to compare heparin and direct thrombin inhibitors such as hirudin or Ro 46-6240 in experimental arterial thrombosis. Circulation 91:1568, 1995.

77. Hursting MJ, Joffrion JL, Brooks RL, Swan SK, Ferguson JJ. Differential effects of Argatroban (a direct thrombin inhibitor) and heparin on the HemoTec and Hemochron activated clotting times (abstr). American Society of Hematology, 1996.

78. The EPIC Investigators. Use of a monoclonal antibody directed against the platelet glycoprotein IIb/IIIa re-

ceptor in high-risk coronary angioplasty. N Engl J Med 330:956, 1994.

79. Topol EJ, Califf RM, Weisman HF, Ellis SG, Tcheng JE, Worley Seth, Ivanhoe R, George BS, Fintel D, Weston M, Sigmon K, Anderson KM, Lee KL, Willerson JT, on behalf of The EPIC Investigators. Randomised trial of coronary intervention with antibody against platelet IIb/IIIa integrin for reduction of clinical restenosis: Results at six months. Lancet 343:881, 1994.

80. Lincoff AM, Tcheng JE, Califf RM, Bass T, Popma JJ, Teirstein PS, Kleiman NS, Hattel LS, Anderson HV, Ferguson JJ, Cabot CF, Anderson KM, Berdan LG, Musco MH, Weisman HF, Topol EJ, for the PROLOG Investigators. A multicenter, randomized, double-blind pilot trial of standard versus low dose weight-adjusted heparin in patients treated with the platelet GP IIb/IIIa receptor antibody fragment c7E3 Fab (Abciximab) during perecutaneous coronary revascularization. Am J Cardiol 79:286, 1997.

81. The EPILOG Investigators: Platelet glycoprotein IIb/IIIa receptor blockade and low-dose heparin during percutaneous coronary intervention. N Engl J Med 336:1689, 1997.

82. The CAPTURE Investigators: Randomized placebo-controlled trial of abciximab before and during coronary intervention in refractory unstable angina: The CAPTURE Study Lancet 349:1429, 1997.

83. Ferguson JJ. Meeting Highlights: American College of Cardiology 45th Annual Scientific Session, Orlando, Florida, March 24 to 27, 1996. Circulation 94:1, 1996.

84. Aguirre FV, Ferguson JJ, Blankenship JC, Pieper KS, Taylor M, Harrington RA, Rund M, Caracciolo EA, Donohue TJ, Califf RM, Lincoff AM, Tcheng JE, Topol EJ, for the IMPACT-II Investigators. Association of pre-intervention activated clotting times (ACT) and clinical outcomes following percutaneous coronary revascularization: Results from the IMPACT-II trial. J Am Coll Cardiol 27(Suppl. A):83A, 1996.

85. Mascelli MA, Lance E, Mack S, Weisman H, Schaible T, Jordan R. Rapid assessment of platelet inhibition using a modified whole blood aggregometer (Aggrestat™) in PTCA patients receiving ReoPro™. J Am Coll Cardiol 27(Suppl. A):361A, 1996.

38. MONITORING CHRONIC ORAL ANTICOAGULANT THERAPY

Reza Khoshnevis and James J. Ferguson

Introduction

The efficacy of oral anticoagulant therapy is well established for preventing and treating venous and arterial thromboembolism in a wide variety of clinical settings. In recent years, standardized laboratory monitoring and recognition of the frequency and hazards of overly intense anticoagulation have resulted in major improvements in the safety and efficacy of oral anticoagulant therapy. In this chapter we briefly review issues relating to monitoring chronic anticoagulant therapy and discuss guidelines for achieving and maintaining an optimal level of anticoagulation in clinical settings in which oral anticoagulant therapy is used, such as deep venous thrombosis, pulmonary embolism, atrial fibrillation, prosthetic heart valves, and following myocardial infarction.

Oral Anticoagulants

Warfarin and other coumarin anticoagulants inhibit vitamin K-2,3-epoxide reductase within hepatic microsomes and thus prevent recycling of vitamin K, a necessary cofactor for the synthesis of γ-carboxyglutamic acid residues needed for post-translational modification and activation of vitamin K–dependent proteins synthesized in hepatocytes (coagulation factors II, VII, IX, and X, proteins C and S) [1]. Warfarin is extremely soluble in aqueous media, is completely absorbed from the gastrointestinal tract, and reaches maximal blood concentrations in healthy volunteers in 90 minutes [2]. Warfarin is metabolized by hepatic microsomal enzymes and is almost totally bound to plasma proteins, which may be partially responsible for its long plasma half-life. The biologic half-life of warfarin ranges from 35 to 45 hours and is independent of the dosage used. It can cross the placental barrier, but there is no firm evidence that the drug appears in breast milk in significant amounts [1,3]. Warfarin is widely used in a variety of clinical circumstances and is the 14th largest selling medication in the United States.

With a dose of warfarin sufficiently large to completely block hepatic synthesis of vitamin K–dependent proteins, each of the involved clotting factors disappear from the blood as a function of its individual half-life. Thus after a latent period the prothrombin time becomes prolonged, mainly from the effect of lowering of the concentration of factor VII, the vitamin K–dependent factor with the shortest half-life (5 hours). The plasma concentration of the other vitamin K–dependent coagulation factors will decrease more slowly because their half-life is longer (20–60 hours for factors IX and X, and 80–100 hours for prothrombin). After 3–5 days of warfarin treatment, all of the affected coagulation factors achieve similar low levels. For effective treatment of thrombosis, the levels of factors II, VII, IX, and X should remain at approximately 25% of normal [4]. With discontinuance of the drug, the clotting factors return to normal, again as a function of their individual intrinsic synthesis rates.

A general clinical approach to warfarin dosing and monitoring is summarized in Table 38-1. If a rapid anticoagulant effect is required, an initial dose of 10 mg/day is administered, often in combination with heparin; heparin is discontinued when the INR has been in the therapeutic range for at least 2 days. In situations in which immediate anticoagulation is not necessary (e.g., in chronic stable atrial fibrillation), treatment can be initiated with an anticipated maintenance dosage of 4–5 mg/day, achieving a steady-state anticoagulant effect in 5–7 days. Prothrombin time (PT) monitoring using International Normalized Ratios (INR) is usually performed daily until a therapeutic effect has been achieved and maintained for at least 2 consecutive days, then two to three times weekly for 1–2 weeks, then less frequently, depending on the stability of the INR. If the INR remains

TABLE 38-1. A practical
approach for anticoagulation with warfarin

Rapid anticoagulation
    Day 1: 10 mg
    Day 2: 10 mg
    Assess INR
    Day 3: 2.5–7.5 mg
    Assess INR until stable and therapeutic

Anticoagulation (rapid effect not required or if there is
bleeding risk)
    Day 1: 5 mg
    Day 2: 5 mg
    Assess INR
    Day 3: 5 mg
    Assess INR until stable and therapeutic

Follow-up INR assessment
    Three times in first week
    Twice in second week
    Weekly for 4 weeks
    Every 2 weeks for 2 months
    Then monthly or longer

stable, the frequency of testing can be reduced to
every 4–6 weeks. If dose adjustments are required,
then the cycle of more frequent monitoring is repeated until a stable dosage is achieved. Some patients
on long-term warfarin therapy may be difficult to
manage because of unexpected fluctuations in the
INR. These fluctuations may be due to a number of
factors (Table 38-2), including changes in diet, inaccurate PT results, poor patient compliance, undis-
closed drug use, surreptitious self-medication, or
intermittent alcohol consumption.

MONITORING ORAL
ANTICOAGULANT THERAPY
A number of different tests have been employed for
laboratory monitoring of oral anticoagulant therapy,
but the test by far the most widely used is the one-
stage prothrombin time (PT) introduced by Quick in
1935 [5]. As discussed in Chapter 37, the interpretation of PT results has been complicated because the
routine commercial thromboplastin reagents vary
markedly in their responsiveness, depending on the

TABLE 38-2. Factors that potentiate or inhibit the anticoagulant effect of warfarin

Enhanced effect	Decreased effect
Drugs	Drugs
Chloramphenicol	Vitamin K
Cimetidine	Oral contraceptives
Anabolic steroids	Rifampin
D-Thyroxine	Griseofulvin
Clofibrate	Glutethimide
Metranidazole	Cholestyramine
Phenylbutazone	Barbiturates
Sulfinpyrazone	
Quinidine	
Disulfiram	
Sulfonamides	
Chloral hydrate	
Alcohol (abuse only)	
Allopurinol	
Amiodarone	
Antibiotics	
Methyldopa	
Omeprazole	
Tamoxifen	
aspirin (in high doses)	
Other	Other
Low Vitamin K intake or absorption	Increased vitamin K intake
Liver disease	Alcohol
Hypermetabolic states (fever, thyrotoxicosis)	

tissue of origin and the method of preparation [6–10]. Consequently, PT results using reagents from different sources are not interchangeable between laboratories. This problem has been largely solved by calibrating PT ratios to a standard, the INR, which is calculated as follows:

$$INR = (\text{observed PT ratio})^C$$

where the PT ratio is (patient PT)/(normal pooled plasma PT) and C is the power value representing the International Sensitivity Index (ISI) for each thromboplastin.

The ISI is a measure of the responsiveness of a given thromboplastin to reduction of vitamin K–dependent coagulation factors; the lower the ISI, the more responsive is the reagent and the closer the derived INR will be to the observed PT ratio. The INR is that PT ratio that would be obtained if the World Health Organization's reference thromboplastin itself (ISI = 1.0) had been used to perform the PT test [7,11]. The value of ISI for thromboplastin reagents used in clinical settings is provided by the manufacturer. A specially designed normogram gives INR values from the PT ratio value for thromboplastins over a range of ISI values [12].

Clinical Settings

TREATMENT OF DEEP VEIN THROMBOSIS AND PULMONARY EMBOLISM

Over the past 20 years, the results of numerous well-designed randomized trials in patients with deep-vein thrombosis (DVT) have helped guide the treatment of this common disorder. In patients with proximal DVT, the goals of therapy are the prevention of pulmonary embolism and prevention of the postphlebitic syndrome by restoration of venous patency and valvular function. Anticoagulation is the first-line of treatment for patients with distal DVT as well as for those with proximal-vein involvement. Therapy should start with an agent that has an immediate anticoagulant effect (e.g., heparin) [13], at an adequate dosage (PTT 1.5–2.5 times the control) [14]. Failure to reach the prescribed intensity of anticoagulation in the first 24 hours of treatment increases the risk of recurrent venous thromboembolism by 15 times [14]. Five days of heparin therapy followed by an oral vitamin K antagonist is usually effective treatment and is generally regarded as conventional therapy [15]. However, asymptomatic extension of DVT to proximal veins or asymptomatic pulmonary emboli can be expected in 8% of the patients so treated [13], and symptomatic

pulmonary emboli may occur in 0.5% [15]. Extending the course of heparin (e.g., 10 days) before warfarin therapy is begun is not beneficial [16,17].

Treatment of DVT with oral anticoagulants alone (without heparin) is not a satisfactory alternative and is followed by symptomatic extension of recurrence of venous thrombosis in 20% of patients [13]. In a study by Hull et al. [18], after initial heparin therapy, patients were randomized to receive subcutaneous low-dose heparin or moderate-intensity warfarin (INR 2.4–4.6). Despite the higher incidence of bleeding in the warfarin group (21%), the recurrence of DVT at 12 weeks was remarkably lower (0% VS. 25.7% in heparin group). In a later study [19] comparing a moderate-dose regimen (INR 2.0–3.0) with a more intense regimen (INR 3.0–4.5), a similar protection from rethrombosis was achieved in both groups, with a significant reduction in the incidence of bleeding in the moderate-dose regimen (4.3% vs. 22.4%). Although substantially less intense anticoagulation may be adequate [20], currently an INR value between 2.0 and 3.0 is a generally accepted target range for this clinical setting [15,21–23].

The optimal duration of anticoagulation therapy is more controversial. There is evidence from prospective studies [25–27] that the risk of recurrence is lower among patients with reversible risk factors (e.g., those with thrombosis secondary to surgery or trauma) than in those with irreversible risk factors (such as cancer) or with idiopathic DVT (thrombosis in the absence of a recognized risk factor). In a recent study by Schulman and associates [28], 897 patients with a first episode of DVT or pulmonary embolism were treated with at least 5 days of unfractionated heparin or low molecular weight heparin and then randomly assigned to receive either 6 weeks or 6 months of warfarin therapy, with a target INR of 2.0–2.85. The incidence of recurrence during 2 years of follow-up was 18.1% among the 443 patients who received 6 weeks of oral anticoagulant therapy, as compared with 9.5% among the 454 patients who received 6 months of therapy ($P < 0.001$). There was no significant difference in the frequency of bleeding or the recurrence of pulmonary embolism between the two groups. An earlier study performed by the Research Committee of British Thoracic Society [25] had also shown that 4 weeks of anticoagulation may be adequate for patients with postoperative venous thrombosis, but a longer course of treatment is necessary for patients without reversible risk factors.

On the basis of these data and other observations [27,28], it is difficult to recommend indefinite anticoagulant therapy for patients with a first episode of venous thrombosis. One reasonable approach is to use anticoagulation therapy for 6 weeks in patients with reversible risk factors and to continue anticoagulation for up to 6 months in patients with no identifiable etiology and presumptive idiopathic venous thrombosis. Anticoagulant treatment for an indefinite period should be considered in patients who have venous thrombosis associated with active cancer, and who may be bedridden and receiving chemotherapy, factors that may contribute to a hypercoagulable state [29]. Long-term anticoagulation therapy should also be considered for patients with recurrent episodes of idiopathic DVT and those with inherited thrombophilia who have had one or more unprovoked episodes of major venous thromboembolism [30].

PREVENTION OF VENOUS THROMBOEMBOLISM

Of the patients who will eventually die of pulmonary emboli, two thirds survive for less than 30 minutes after the event, not long enough for most forms of treatment to be effective [31]. Preventing DVT is clearly clinically preferable to treating the condition after it has happened [32], as well as being cost effective [32–35] if patients at risk can be appropriately identified. The goal of prophylactic therapy in patients with risk factors for DVT is to prevent both its occurrence and its two major consequences: pulmonary emboli and the postphlebitic syndrome.

Multiple clinical studies [36–44] have shown that certain clinical factors clearly predispose patients at risk for venous thromboembolism and identify patients with the most to gain from prophylactic measures [45]. These factors include advanced age; prolonged immobility or paralysis; prior venous thromboembolism; cancer; major surgery (particularly operations involving the abdomen, pelvis, and lower extremities); obesity; varicose veins; congestive heart failure; myocardial infarction; stroke; fractures of the pelvis, hip, or leg; hypercoagulable states; and possibly high-dose estrogen use.

Although the American College of Chest Physicians has recommended that in the majority of cases low-dose unfractionated heparin, low molecular weight heparin (LMWH), dextran, or intermittent pneumatic compression are the agents of choice for DVT prophylaxis, there are potential beneficial effects of oral anticoagulation in certain clinical conditions, including:

1. Selected very high-risk general surgery patients (target perioperative INR of 2.0–3.0) [46,47].

2. As an alternative for LMWH or unfractionated heparin in patients undergoing total hip replacement surgery (target INR of 2.0–3.0, therapy started preoperatively or immediately after operation) [48–67].

3. As an alternative to LMWH in patients undergoing hip fracture surgery (target INR of 2.0–3.0) [68–72].

4. To prevent axillary-subclavian venous thrombosis in patients with long-term indwelling central vein catheters (1 mg daily dose) [73].

5. In selected very high-risk patients will multiple trauma, in whom warfarin may be considered as an alternative to LMWH or intermittent pneumatic compression (target INR not yet well defined)

6. As an alternative for LDUH in patients with myocardial infarction, (duration and intensity of anticoagulation not yet well established)

There is considerable controversy regarding the optimal duration of postoperative prophylaxis. Virtually all reported trials in the setting of elective hip or knee replacement provided prophylaxis for at least 7–10 days postoperatively. Despite data suggesting a significant risk of DVT for at least 2 months following total hip replacement [74–76], it is currently recommended that the duration of postoperative prophylaxis in these settings should be at least 7–10 days regardless of hospital stay (often 5 days or less). There are several ongoing trials addressing the issue of posthospital prophylaxis.

Meta-analysis of the Antiplatelet Trialists' Collaboration [77] has shown a beneficial effect of aspirin in reducing the incidence of DVT by 37% and in reducing the incidence of pulmonary embolism by 71% in general surgical patients; however, multiple other well-designed trials have found aspirin ineffective in preventing DVT in general surgical patients [78] and following total hip [79–84] or knee [79] replacement. Therefore, current recommendations do not advocate aspirin alone for prophylaxis in these settings because other measures have been shown to be more effective [85]. There is no convincing evidence to justify the broad use of routine DVT prophylaxis in all burn patients [86,87]. However, it seems reasonable to recommend prophylaxis in burn patients with additional risk factors for venous thrombosis [88].

ATRIAL FIBRILLATION

Over the past 6 years, five randomized multicenter trials have investigated the safety and efficacy of oral therapy (both anticoagulant and antiplatelet agents) for primary stroke prevention in patients with atrial

TABLE 38-3. Primary prevention trials in atrial fibrillation, baseline characteristics

Clinical trial	Total no. of patients	Mean follow-up (years)	Target INR	Primary outcome measures
AFASAK	1007	1.2	2.8–4.2	S, SE, TIA, ICB
SPAF	1330	1.3	2.0–4.5	S, SE
BAATAF	420	2.2	1.5–2.7	S
CAFA	383	1.3	2.0–3.0	S, SE, ICB, FB
SPINAF	525	1.8	1.4–2.8	S
SPAF II	1100	2.7	2.0–4.5	S, SE

S = stroke; SE = non-CNS systemic embolus; TIA = transient ischemic attack; ICB = intracranial bleed; FB = fatal bleed; AFASAK = trial Fibrillation, Aspirin, Anticoagulation Study [89]; BAATAF = Boston Area Anticoagulation Trial in Atrial Fibrillation study [91]; CAFA = Canadian Atrial Fibrillation Anticoagulation study [92]; SPAF = Stroke Prevention in Atrial Fibrillation study [90]; SPINAF = Veterans Affairs Stroke Prevention In Nonrheumatic Atrial Fibrillation [93].

TABLE 38-4. Event rates for placebo and warfarin in five atrial fibrillation primary prevention trials

	AFASAK (no. = 671)		BAATF (no. = 420)		CAFA (no. = 378)		SPAF (no. = 421)		SPINAF (no. = 525)	
	P no. = 336	W no. = 335	P no. = 208	W no. = 212	P no. = 191	W no. = 187	P no. = 211	W no. = 210	P no. = 265	W no. = 260
Total patient-year observation to death or end of study	417	423	435	487	251	239	259	271	440	465
Stroke	4.8	1.9	3.0	0.4	3.7	2.1	7.0	2.3	4.3	0.9
Non-neurologic systemic embolism	0.2	0	0	0	0.8	0.4	0.8	0	0.4	0.8
Intracerebral hemorrhage	0	0.2	0	0	0	0.4	0	0.4	0	0.2
Subdural hemorrhage	0	0	0	0.2	0	0	0.8	0.4	0	0
Subarachnoid hemorrhage	0	0	0	0	0	0	0	0	0	0
Transient ischemic attack	0.7	0.2	0.9	0.8	0.8	0.8	2.4	1.5	2.6	1.5
Death	6.5	4.7	6.0	2.3	3.2	4.2	3.1	2.2	5.0	3.3
Myocardial infarction	NA	NA	0.7	0.8	NA	NA	0.8	0.4	0.9	1.5
Major bleeds	0	0.3	1.9	1.0	0.8	1.7	0.8	0.4	0.9	1.5

AFASAK = Atrial Fibrillation, Aspirin, Anticoagulation Study [89]; BAATAF = Boston Area Anticoagulation Trial in Atrial Fibrillation study [91]; CAFA = Canadian Atrial Fibrillation Anticoagulation study [92]; SPAF = Stroke Prevention in Atrial Fibrillation study [90]; SPINAF = Veterans Affairs Stroke Prevention In Nonrheumatic Atrial Fibrillation [93]; P = Placebo; W = Warfarin; NA = not recorded.
Adapted from Ezekowiz [198], with permission.

fibrillation [89–93]. The basic characteristics of these trials are summarized in Tables 38-3 and 38-4.

As shown in Figures 38-1 and 38-2, these trials were all remarkably consistent in documenting very low rates of hemorrhagic complications and an approximately 70% reduction in the risk of stroke with low-intensity warfarin therapy. Based on intention to treat analysis, this risk reduction was even higher (greater than 80%) in patients who remained on treatment with warfarin [94], and, in fact, the majority of the strokes that were documented in the "warfarin groups" of the original five trials occurred in patients who were not taking anticoagulant therapy at the time of event. The target ranges for intensity of

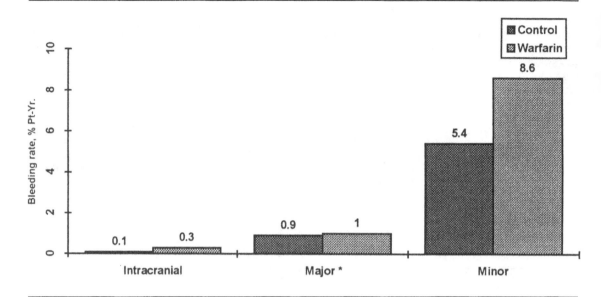

FIGURE 38-1. Summary of bleeding rates in the five atrial fibrillation primary prevention trials. *Bleeding requiring hospitalization of transfusion. (Adapted from Albers et al. [94,95], with permission.)

anticoagulation in these trials are shown in Table 38-3.

Only two of the five trials (AFASAK and SPAF) randomized patients to aspirin versus warfarin for stroke prevention. Warfarin was at least 50% more effective than aspirin therapy for the prevention of ischemic stroke in patients with atrial fibrillation [95] (Figure 38-3). These data are further supported by the results of the current European Atrial Fibrillation Trial (EAFT) [96], which compared anticoagulant therapy, aspirin, and placebo in patients with atrial fibrillation who had sustained a mild stroke or transient ischemic attack within the last 3 months. There was a 68% reduction in stroke with anticoagulant therapy versus a 16% stroke reduction in the aspirin group (a trend that was not significant). Preliminary data from the recent SPAF III study [97], also confirm the superiority of standard-dose warfarin therapy (INR 2–3) over aspirin alone in reducing the risk of stroke in high-risk patients. Low-dose warfarin (INR 1.2–1.5) in combination with aspirin (325 mg/day) also appeared to be less effective in reducing the risk of stroke than standard-dose warfarin therapy.

In a collaborative analysis done by the investigators from the five original atrial fibrillation/stroke prevention studies [98], four independent clinical features were identified on multivariate analysis that identified individuals at increased risk for stroke. These factors included a history of previous stroke of transient ischemic attack (TIA) (relative risk [RR], 2.50), diabetes (RR, 1.7), history of hypertension (RR, 1.60), and increased age (RR, 1.4 for each decade).

Patients with any of these risk factors had an annual stroke risk of at least 4% if untreated. Associated cardiac disorders were also shown to influence stroke risk. Patient whose only risk factor for stroke was congestive heart failure or coronary artery disease (angina or myocardial infarction) had stroke rates approximately three times those in patients without any risk factors.

Probably the most feared complication of anticoagulant therapy is intracranial hemorrhage. This complication is more likely in the very elderly, with excessive anticoagulation [99–101] and with poorly controlled hypertension [100,102,103]. Because approximately half of patients with atrial fibrillation in the United States are over 75 years of age [104], the safety issues associated with anticoagulant therapy become extremely relevant. Unfortunately, to date hard data on the long-term safety of anticoagulant therapy, particularly in very elderly patients with atrial fibrillation, are limited. The prospective randomized trials to date only include data out to 2–3 years, and there were a limited number of patients (only about 25%) over 75 years of age enrolled in these studies [98].

Based on the results of the collaborative analysis of these trials and those of the American College of

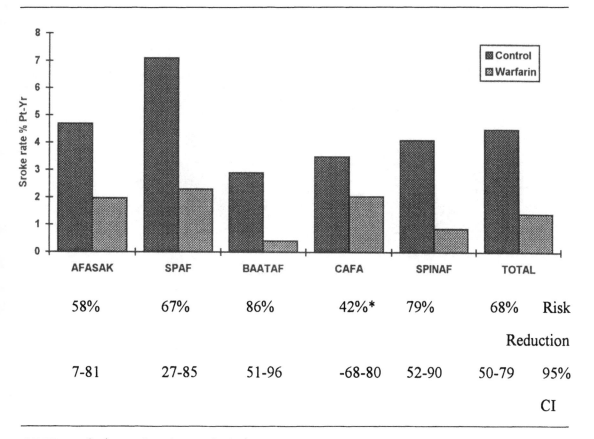

FIGURE 38-2. Stroke rates in patients randomized to warfarin and in control subjects in atrial fibrillation primary prevention trials. Stroke represents all strokes. Transient ischemic attacks, systemic emboli, and intracranial hemorrhages are not included. (Adapted from Albers et al. [94,95], with permission.)

Chest Physicians [105] and the British Society for Hematology [22], it is recommended that long-term oral anticoagulant therapy (INR 2.0–3.0) be strongly considered for all patients older than 65 with atrial fibrillation, and for patients younger than 65 with any of the following risk factors: previous TIA or stroke, hypertension, heart failure, diabetes, clinical coronary artery disease, mitral stenosis, prosthetic heart valves, or thyrotoxicosis, if they are good candidates for anticoagulation. Unreliable individuals or those with other contraindications to anticoagulation should be considered for aspirin treatment (325 mg/d). Despite the higher risk of anticoagulation in very elderly (over 75 years of age), they still appear to benefit from anticoagulation because their risk for stroke is par-

ticularly high; however, this should be done with caution and careful monitoring.

Alternative antithrombotic regimens, such as lower intensity anticoagulation (e.g., an INR of 1.5), or combination therapy with very low-dose warfarin and aspirin in this subgroup, are currently under investigation [95]. Preliminary results from the high-risk arm of SPAF III [97] (which was terminated prematurely) suggest that in high-risk patients with atrial fibrillation, standard-dose warfarin is effective in reducing the risk of stroike below that previously seen with aspirin alone. Low-dose warfarin in combination with aspirin was not an effective therapy in high-risk patients.

Individuals less than 60 years of age without any clinical risk factors (lone atrial fibrillation) do not require antithrombotic therapy for stroke prevention because of their low risk for events (less than 0.5% per year). The stroke rate is also low (about 2% per year) in patients with lone atrial fibrillation between ages 60 and 75 years. These patients appear to be adequately protected from stroke with aspirin therapy. Although secondary analysis of the SPAF data identi-

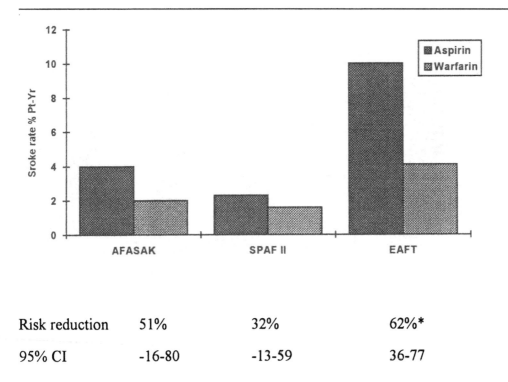

| Risk reduction | 51% | 32% | 62%* |
| 95% CI | -16-80 | -13-59 | 36-77 |

Stroke rates (all strokes regardless of suspected cause) in patients randomized to oral anticoagualtion versus aspirin.

* P < 0.001

Adapted from atrial fibrillation investigators [98]

FIGURE 38-3. Stroke rate in patients randomized to oral anticoagulation versus aspirin.

fied other low-risk subgroups who also appeared to be adequately protected by aspirin [106–108], these findings need to be confirmed in a prospective study prior to making such general clinical recommendations. Although the high-risk arm of SPAF III was terminated prematurely, the low-risk arm is continuing enrollment.

PROSTHETIC HEART VALVES
Despite improvement in valve design, thrombosis and arterial thromboembolism remain major causes of late morbidity and mortality after the replacement of heart valves with mechanical and bioprosthetic pros-

theses [109]. Factors that influence the risk of arterial thromboembolism include the type, site, and number of valves placed [109–114], the presence or absence of atrial fibrillation, treatment with warfarin or other anticoagulants [109], the adequacy of warfarin therapy, and the addition of antiplatelet drugs such as dipyridamole and aspirin [109]. The risk of thrombosis in the mitral position seems to be twice as great as with aortic and tilting-disc valves; bileaflet valves have a lower incidence of major embolism than caged-ball valves [115]. The presence of more than one

TABLE 38-5. Thromboembolic events as a function of INR in patients with St. Jude prosthetic valves

INR	Thrombolic event (% y)		
	Aortic position	Mitral position	>1 prosthetic valve
No anticoagulation [117]	12.3	22.2	91.0
1.8–2.8 [116]	3.9	6.5	7.2
2.5–3.5 [116]	2.8	4.7	4.8
2.8–4.3 [118]	3.0	2.2	0.0
3.0–4.5 [116]	1.9	2.9	4.7
4.0–6.0 [116]	1.4	2.4	4.4

From Horstkotte et al. [116], Bandet et al. [117], and Voget et al. [118].

TABLE 38-6. Effect of antithrombotic therapy on the incidence of valve thrombosis and major and total embolism

Anticoagulation	Incidence rates per 100 patient-years (95% confidence intervals)		
	Valve thrombosis	Major embolism	Total embolism
None	1.8 (0.9–3.0)	4.0 (2.9–5.2)	8.6 (7.0–10.4)
Antiplatelet	1.6 (1.0–2.5)	2.2 (1.4–3.1)	8.2 (6.6–10.0)
Dipyridamole	4.1 (1.9–7.2)	5.4 (2.8–8.8)	11.2 (7.3–15.9)
Aspirin	1.0 (0.4–0.7)	1.4 (0.8–2.3)	7.5 (5.9–9.4)
Warfarin	0.2 (0.2–0.2)	1.0 (1.0–1.1)	1.8 (1.7–1.9)
Warfarin and antiplatelet	0.1 (0.0–0.3)	1.7 (1.1–2.3)	3.2 (2.4–4.1)

Total embolism includes all reported events (valve thrombosis, major and minor embolism). The data represent a meta-analysis of 46 studies, including 13,088 patients.
Reprinted, with permission, from Cannegieter et al. [115].

prosthetic valve is also associated with an increased incidence of thromboembolic events.

For obvious ethical reasons, there are no placebo-controlled clinical trials of oral anticoagulants in patients with prosthetic heart valves. However, observational data [116–119] and meta-analyses [115] strongly support the need for lifelong warfarin treatment with mechanical valves, particularly in the mitral site and probably in the aortic site. The main remaining area of uncertainty is in determining the optimal intensity, specifically the level at which thromboembolic complications are effectively prevented without excessive bleeding [107,120,121]. Table 38-5 presents the incidence of thromboembolic events in relation to the INR from a number of studies [116–119] for St. Jude prosthetic heart valves.

The effect of antithrombotic therapy on the incidence of thromboembolic events in patients with mechanical valve prosthesis [115] are shown in Table 38-6. Without anticoagulation, the risk of major embolism was about 4 per 100 patient-years and was reduced by 75% with anticoagulant therapy to 1.4 per 100 patient-years incidence of major bleeding events. While the beneficial effects of anticoagulants were confirmed in multiple other studies [122,123], the optimal therapeutic range in patients with a mechanical prosthetic valves is still the subject of much debate. In a recent meta-analysis of 12 studies in patients with tilting-disc valves and bileaflet valves [124], when the minimal INR was no lower than 2.5–3.0, there was a low thromboembolic rate with an acceptable hemorrhagic event rate (Figure 38-4). With a lower INR minimum of 1.6–1.9, the rate of thromboembolism increased considerably, while the hemorrhagic events rate decreased slightly. At the other end of the therapeutic range, the thromboembolic rate with a maximal INR of 2.5–3.6 was not different from the thromboembolic rate with a maximal INR of 3.9–4.8. The hemorrhagic rate with a maximal INR or 2.5–3.6 was the same as the hemorrhagic rate with a maximal INR of 3.9–4.8. Increasing the maximal value of the INR to 8.2 had no

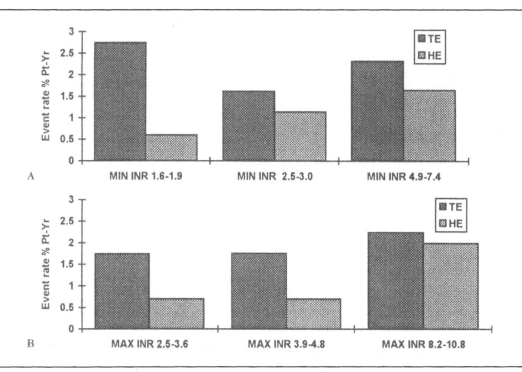

FIGURE 38-4. Thromboembolic and hemorrhagic rates according to minimal (**A**) and maximal (**B**) INR values used in 12 studies analyzed.

further therapeutic benefit, but the hemorrhagic rate increased.

The minimum effective intensity of anticoagulant therapy in the setting of mechanical prosthetic valves has been evaluated in two studies. The first [125] compared a very high-intensity regimen (INR, 7.4–10.8) with a lower intensity regiment (INR, 1.9–3.6) and showed that there was no difference on effectiveness between the two regiments, but the higher intensity regimen produced significantly more bleeding. In the second study [199], the safety and efficacy of a moderate-intensity regimen (INR, 2.0–3.0) was compared with a high-intensity regiment (INR, 3.0–4.5) in patients with mechanical prosthetic valves who were receiving aspirin and dipyridamole. There was no difference in efficacy between the two regimens, but, as in the previous study, the high-intensity regimen was associated with a statistically significant increase in bleeding.

In comparison with anticoagulant agents, the antithrombotic effect of antiplatelet agents in the setting of mechanical prosthetic valves has been less consistent. In Cannegieter's meta-analysis [115], aspirin had a beneficial effect in reducing the risk of major embolism by about 40% compared with no treatment [126–128]. Another meta-analysis showed that aspirin in combination with oral anticoagulants

significantly reduced systemic thromboemboli and mortality [129]. This was offset, however, by increased major bleeding. Yet another meta-analysis showed no benefit of aspirin in combination with oral anticoagulants, and an increased risk of bleeding [115]. Turpie et al. [126] showed that the rate of major bleeding may be reduced by minimizing the dose of aspirin used in combination with warfarin. Regarding dipyridamole in addition to oral anticoagulants, some investigations showed an additive benefit [127,130], one investigation showed no benefit [131], and one investigation showed only a trend [132]. INR data from these studies have not been published.

In conclusion, current data strongly suggest that all patients with mechanical prosthetic heart valves should be orally anticoagulated. A target INR of 2.5–3.5 has been recommended by the American College of Chest Physicians for patients with bileaflet or tilting-disk valves. A higher INR may be considered for patients with caged-ball or caged-disk valves. The addition of aspirin to oral anticoagulants offers additional protection, but with an increased risk of bleed-

TABLE 38-7. Thromboemboli with bioprosthetic valves in patients with sinus rhythm

Medication	No. of patients	Valve position	TE/100 pt-y	Source (ref)
None (after 6 weeks warfarin)	546	AO	1.9	136
None	117	AO	0.2	137
None (after 8 weeks warfarin)	34	AO (Hancock)	2.9	137
None (after 8 weeks warfarin)	45	AO (Carpentier-Edwards	2.0	138
None (after 8 weeks warfarin)		Mitral	1.9	139

TE = thrombolic events; pt. = patient; y = years; AO = .
Adapted from Stein et al. [134], with permission.

ing. Patients with mechanical prosthetic heart valves who suffer systemic embolism despite adequate therapy with oral anticoagulants are good candidates for the addition of low doses of aspirin (80 mg/d). Given conflicting data in favor of and against a role for dipyridamole in reducing the risk of thromboembolism [127,130–132], and in view of the known benefits of low-dose aspirin therapy in combination with oral anticoagulants [126], dipyridamole (400 mg/d) is probably limited to an adjunctive role, with other oral anticoagulants as an alternative to aspirin in patients with systemic embolism despite adequate oral anticoagulation.

For bioprosthetic valves, the frequency of thromboemboli among patients who do not receive antithrombotic therapy except for the first 6–8 weeks, is very low (Table 38-7). In the aortic position, this risk has been further decreased by using aspirin [133,139]. Gonzalez-Lavin and associates [140] have also shown that in the absence of risk factors (such as postoperative atrial fibrillation, an enlarged left atrium, preoperative thromboembolism, and clots in the left atrium), no thrombooembolism occurred during 6 years of follow-up in patients with bioprosthetic valves in the mitral position who received warfarin for only up to 12 weeks. The superiority of warfarin over antiplatelet agents has also been shown in other clinical trials [141].

Because thromboembolism rates as high as 67–80% have been reported in the first 3 months after bioprosthetic valve insertion (particularly in the mitral position) in patients who do not receive antithrombotics [142,144], it has been recommended that all patients with bioprosthetic valves in the mitral position be treated for the first 3 months after valve insertion with less intense warfarin therapy (INR, 2.0–3.0) [145]. Turpie has shown that during the first 3 postoperative months, less intense anticoagulant therapy (INR, 2.0–2.3) was as effective as high-intensity anticoagulation (INR, 2.5–4.5) and was associated with fewer hemorrhagic complications [145]. Anticoagulant therapy in patients with bioprosthetic valves in the aortic position who are in sinus rhythm is optional during the first 3 months. In the presence of atrial fibrillation, with evidence of left atrial thrombus at surgery or with a history of systemic embolization, long-term warfarin therapy with INRs between 2.0 and 3.0 is recommended [146].

Although the appropriate duration of therapy still remains uncertain, the current consensus is to treat patients with a history of systemic embolization for a period of at least 3–12 months. Patients with bioprosthetic valves who have a permanent pacemaker are also at high risk for thromboemboli, but there is no evidence that oral anticoagulants are protective [147]. Anticoagulant therapy (INR, <2.0–3.0) is optional in such patients. Although aspirin (325 mg/d) has been shown to offer protection against thromboembolism among patients in normal sinus rhythm with bioprosthetic valves [139], at present long-term aspirin therapy for prosthetic valve patients is also considered optional [146].

In patients with prosthetic valve endocarditis who are not receiving anticoagulant therapy, CNS thromboembolic events occur in about 50% [4]. There nonrandomized clinical trials [110,148,149] in patients with prosthetic valve endocarditis who were receiving anticoagulant therapy suggest that the thromboembolic rate can be decreased sixfold to ninefold with adequate anticoagulation. It should be noted, however, that the risk of intracranial hemorrhage is substantial and may approach 14% [110,149]. Although the benefits and the risks of anticoagulant in patients with native or bioprosthetic valve endocarditis are not well defined, anticoagulant therapy should not be given in patients with uncomplicated infective endocarditis involving a native valve or a bioprosthetic valve in patients with normal sinus rhythm. This recommendation is based on the increased incidence of hemorrhage in these patients and the lack of demonstrated efficacy of anticoagulation in this setting.

When noncardiac surgery is required in patients with prosthetic valves who are receiving anticoagulants, the risk is minimal when the drug regimen is stopped 4–5 days preoperatively and for a similar period postoperatively. It may be desirable, however, to protect the patient with dipyridamole (300–400 mg/d) and intravenous heparin (to maintain the activated partial thromboplastin time at two times control), continued up to 4–5 hours before the operation. Subcutaneous heparin (15,000 units per day given in two to three divided doses) can also be considered during and early after surgery. Perioperative low molecular weight heparin or dextran are other options in high-risk patients [150].

ACUTE MYOCARDIAL INFARCTION

Approximately one third of patients with acute myocardial infarction develop left ventricular mural thrombi [151]; these tend to occur in the first week, particularly in the first 2 days follwing infarction. Systemic embolism, which occurs in about 10% of cases in which left ventricular thrombi are echocardiographically apparent, is the most important complication [151]. The aims of antithrombotic therapy after myocardial infarction are, therefore, to reduce or prevent cardiac chamber thrombus formation and subsequent thromboembolic complications, as well as to reduce early infarct extension and recurrence of myocardial infarction and death. The initial data regarding the role of anticoagulation in acute myocardial infarction are from three randomized trials performed in 1960s and 1970s. Two of those, the Medical Research Council Study and the Veterans Administration Cooperative Study [152,153], showed a significant reduction in stroke but no effect on mortality with anticoagulants. The third, the Bronx Municipal Study [154], showed a significant reduction in mortality and a nonsignificant trend towards fewer strokes with anticoagulants. There was also a reduction in the incidence of pulmonary embolism in all three studies (presumptive INR 1.5–2.5)

The early evidence that oral anticoagulants are effective in the long-term management of acute myocardial infarction comes from analysis of pooled data from seven randomized trials published between 1964 and 1980, which showed that oral anticoagulant therapy during a 1- to 6-year treatment period reduced the combined endpoints of mortality and nonfatal reinfarction by approximately 20% [155–157]. In Chalmers and coworkers' comprehensive review of 32 trials of anticoagulant agents after myocardial infarction, anticoagulant treatment significantly reduced mortality [158]. Loeliger, in a review of 19 previous trials of oral anticoagulants in the prevention of death and myocardial infarction [159], found that in trials with a level of anticoagulation within an INR range of 2.5–5 [160–167], the average risk of death was lowered by 40% and the average risk of nonfatal reinfarction was reduced by approximately two thirds by the use of anticoagulant agents. In contrast, studies with inadequate or poor documentation of the level of anticoagulation [168–177] found no difference in mortality but identified a trend favoring anticoagulant therapy in the prevention of reinfarction.

Even though the method of pooling data from different trials has been criticized for not taking into account differences in protocols and the quality of the trials [178], analysis with more rigorous methods suggests that anticoagulants reduce mortality by about 22% (95% confidence interval, 8–35%) [179]. The beneficial effects of anticoagulant therapy in the postinfarction period have been re-emphasized by the results of three more recent studies [167,180,181]. In the recent double-blind, placebo-controlled Norwegian Warfarin Reinfarction Study (WARIS), 1214 patients recovering from acute myocardial infarction were randomized to warfarin or placebo group, and were followed for an average of 37 months (target INR 2.8–4.8). At the conclusion of the study there was a highly significant reduction in mortality (24% in the intention-to-treat group and 35% in patients who continued on treatment), rate of nonfatal reinfarctions (50%), and number of tatal cerebrovascular accidents (55%) [180]. The increased risk of intracranial hemorrhage during oral anticoagulant therapy in this study as well as other studies [167] was outweighed by the significant reduction in overall cerebrovascular events.

The study by the Sixty-Plus Reinfarction Study Group was limited to patients older than 60 years who had been treated with oral anticoagulants for at least 6 months [167]. This study also demonstrated a significant reduction in reinfarction and stroke in patients randomized to anticoagulant therapy; however, these findings were limited by its lack of generalizability to the overall population. The Anticoagulants in the Secondary Prevention of Events on Coronary Thrombosis (ASPECT) Trial [181] also reported a greater than 50% reduction in reinfarction and a 40% reduction in stroke with anticoagulants. The INRs used in these trials ranged from 2.7 to 4.5 in the Sixty-Plus Reinfarction study group to 2.8 to 4.8 in the other two studies. There is also indirect evidence, based on studies of patients with peripheral arterial disease [182], that higher intensity anticoagulation (INR of 2.6–4.5) results in a significant (50%) reduction in mortality in patients with coronary artery disease.

The safety and efficacy of aspirin alone (160 mg/d) versus aspirin (80 mg/d) plus a fixed low dose of warfarin (1 or 3 mg/d) started 3 weeks after acute myocardial infarction was also tested in the recent CARS trial. The primary endpoint was the combined incidence of cardiovascular death, nonfatal myocardial infarction, and stroke. There was no significant difference in mortality between groups, and the incidence of ischemic stroke was elevated with warfarin (possibly because of the lower dose of aspirin used in combination with Coumadin) [97].

Considering all these data, the American College of Chest Physicians has recommended that in the setting of acute myocardial infarction, patients with increased risk of systemic or pulmonary embolism (i.e., those with large anterior Q-wave infarcts, severe left ventricular [LV] dysfunction, congestive heart failure, history of systemic or pulmonary embolism, two-dimensional echocardiographic evidence of mural thrombosis, or atrial fibrillation) receive heparin on admission (target APPT to 1.5–2 times control) followed by warfarin (target INR ranges, 2.5–3.5) for up to 3 months. The optimal duration of anticoagulation in the presence of persistent LV dysfunction or mural LV thrombus has not been determined.

OTHER INDICATIONS

Despite the lack of well-designed, placebo-controlled clinical trials, there are certain clinical conditions, such as native valvular heart disease and patients who have suffered at least one episode of systemic embolism, in which the use of oral anticoagulants is reasonable and well accepted.

Valvular Heart Disease. Long-term anticoagulant therapy is indicated in patients with rheumatic valvular heart disease with associated atrial fibrillation. In the absence of atrial fibrillation, based on less rigorous studies, accepted indications for oral anticoagulation in these patients (target INR, 2.0–3.0) include (1) rheumatic mitral valve disease and left atrial size in excess of 5.5 cm [183], (2) patients with mitral valve prolapse who have documented systemic embolism or recurrent TIAs despite aspirin therapy [184–188], and (3) patients with mitral annular calcification complicated by systemic embolism (not documented to be calcific embolism) or with associated atrial fibrillation [183]. The optimal therapeutic range for patients who have sufered one or more systemic em-

bolism is unclear, and until further information is available an INR of 2.0–3.0 has been recommended [183].

Dilated Cardiomyopathy. The incidence of embolic events in patients with idiopathic dilated cardiomyopathy has been reported to be as much as 10 times higher than the incidence in patients with chronic left ventricular aneurysm who are not anticoagulated (3.5/100 patient-years). In Fuster and colleagues' retrospective study [189], the incidence of embolic events was dramatically less in patients on anticoagulation (0% vs. 3.5%). Lacking any prospective trial on antithrombotic therapy in these patients, current evidence supports chronic warfarin administration, particularly in those with overt heart failure or atrial fibrillation [189], independent of any echocardiographic evidence of left ventricular thrombi [190,191]. The intensity of anticoagulation has not been well defined and is usually based on clinical characteristics of these patients.

Chronic Left Ventricular Aneurysm. In contrast to the prevalence of thromboembolism in acute myocardial infarction, the incidence of embolism in chronic left ventricular aneurysm (occurring 3 months or more after myocardial infarction) is significantly lower (0.35% per year) [192]. Thrombi formed within the first few days of infarction are more mobile and friable, and project more into the stream of flowing blood than the organized, laminated ones formed within a chronic aneurysmal sac [193]. Despite the higher prevalence of thrombi in left ventricular aneurysms, these thrombi rarely embolize and anticoagulation treatment has a negligible effect on the development of thrombi or subsequent embolization [194–196]. Therefore, the current recommendation is that routine anticoagulation therapy for patients with chronic left ventricular aneurysms is not indicated. Whether these drugs should be given to patients with echocardiographic evidence of mobile and protruding thrombi, however, remains to be established [4].

Pregnancy. Ideally, in female patients on anticoagulant therapy who wish to bear children, pregnancy should be carefully planned and the regimen of anticoagulant therapy should be modified to avoid the teratogenic effects of the warfarin. Fetal wastage is reported to be approximately 60% in women who receive warfarin therapy at the time of conception and during the first trimester. An incidence of 28.6% of congenital anomalies, predominantly nasal hypoplasia, stippling of bones, mental retardation, optic atrophy, and microcephaly, has been reported with warfarin exposure between the 6th and 12th weeks of gestation [197]. Furthermore, because Coumarin derivatives cross the placental barrier, hemorrhagic complications can also occur in the fetus, especially at the time of delivery. Because heparin does not cross the placental barrier, it can be used as a substitute for warfarin during pregnancy. The most common approach to this clinical situation is to use subcutaneous heparin every 12 hours in doses adjusted to keep the aPTT between 1.5 and 2 times control up until the week before delivery, when the patient should be hospitalized and switched to a heparin infusion, continued until the induction of labor. Another, less common, approach is to use a heparin until the 13th week of pregnancy, then change to warfarin until the middle of third trimester, and then restart heparin therapy until delivery. All antiplatelet agents should be avoided during pregnancy because of the risk of premature closure of the ductus arteriosus and other possible side effects on the fetus.

Conclusions

The efficacy of oral anticoagulant therapy in the treatment and prophylaxis of a wide variety of clinical settings has been established either by double-blind clinical trials (prevention and treatment of venous thromboembolism, atrial fibrillation, prosthetic heart valves, and after acute myocardial infarction) or observational studies (dilated cardiomyopathy, native valvular heart valve disease). The recent widespread use of the INR and recent new clinical trials have helped to further clarify the optimal range of oral anticoagulation for many indications. As a general rule, an INR of 2.0–3.0 is effective in the prevention of venous thrombosis, in the treatment of venous thrombosis after an initial course of heparin, in patients with prosthetic tissue valves, and in patients with chronic atrial fibrillation. A more intense anticoagulation with INR of 2.5–3.5 is recommended for mechanical prosthetic heart valves and survivors of acute myocardial infarction. Using even higher INR ranges appears to increase the hemorrhagic complications without significant reduction of thromboembolic events. Concomitant use of antiplatelet agents (low-dose aspirin, 80–100 mg/d) is usually reserved for situations in which systemic embolic events recur despite adequate therapy with oral anticoagulants. The preliminary results of current studies such as SPAF III argue against the use of lower intensity anticoagulation (INR 1.5–2) in combination with antiplatelet agents in high-risk patients for bleeding complications.

Acknowledgment

The authors would like to acknowledge the invaluable assistance of Angie Esquivel in the preparation of the manuscript.

References

1. Hirsh J, Dakn JE, Deykin D, Poller L. Oral anticoagulants: Mechanism of action, clinical effectiveness and optimal therapeutic range. Chest 102(Suppl.):312S, 1992.
2. Breckenridge AM. Oral anticoagulant drugs: Pharmacokinetic aspects. Semin Hematol 15:19, 1978.
3. Wessler S, Gitel SN. Pharmacology of heparin and warfarin. J Am Coll Cardiol 8:10B, 1986.
4. Fuster V, Ip J, Jang IK, Fay W, Chesebro J. Antithrombotic therapy in cardiac disease. In Parmley W, Chattarjee K (eds). Cardiology. Philadelphia: Lippincott, 1995.
5. Quick AJ. The prothrombin time in haemophilia and obstructive jaundice. J Biol Chem 109:73, 1935.
6. Zucker S, Cathey MH, Sox PJ, Halleck EC. Standardization of laboratory tests for controlling anticoagulant therapy. Am J Clin Pathol 53:348, 1970.
7. Poller L. Progress in standardization in anticoagulant control. Hematol Rev 1:225, 1987.
8. Baily EL, Harper TA, Pinkerton PH. Therapeutic range of one-stage prothrombin time in control of anticoagulant therapy. Can Med Assoc J 105:1041, 1971.
9. Latallo ZS, Thomson JM, Poller L. An evaluation of chromogenic substrates in the control of oral anticoagulant therapy. Br J Hematol 47:307, 1981.
10. Poler L, Taberner DA. Dosage and control of oral anticoagulants: An international survey. Br J Hematol 51:479, 1982.
11. Kirkwood TBL. Calibration of reference thromboplastins and standardization of the prothrombin time ratio. Thromb Haemost 49:238, 1983.
12. Poller L. A simple nomogram for the derivation of International Normalised Ratios for the standardization of prothrombin time. Thromb Haemost 60:18, 1988.
13. Brandjes DPM, Heijboer H, Buller HR, de Rijk M, Jagt H, ten Cate JW. Acenocoumarol and heparin compared with acenocoumarol alone in the initial treatment of proximal-vein thrombosis. N Engl J Med 327:1485, 1992.
14. Hull RD, Raskob GE, Hirsh J, et al. Continuous intravenous heparin compared with intermittent subcutaneous heparin in the initial treatment of proximal-vein thrombosis. N Engl J Med 315:1109, 1986.
15. Hyers TM, Hull RD, Weg JG. Antithrombotic therapy for venous thromboembolic disease. Chest

102(Suppl.):408S, 1992. (Erratum, Chest 103:1636, 1993.)

16. Hull RD, Raskob GE, Rosenbloom D, et al. Heparin for 5 days as compared with 10 days in the initial treatment of proximal venous thrombosis. N Engl J Med 322:1260, 1990.

17. Gallus A, Jackman J, Tillett J, Mills W, Wycherley A. Safety and efficacy of Warfarin started early after submassive venous thrombosis or pulmonary embolism. Lancet 2:1293, 1986.

18. Hull R, Delmore T, Carter C, et al. Warfarin sodium versus low dose heparin in the long term treatment of venous thrombosis. N Engl J Med 301:855, 1979.

19. Hull R, Hirsh J, Carter C, et al. Different intensities of oral anticoagulant therapy in the treatment of proximal vein thrombosis. N Engl J Med 307:1676, 1982.

20. Berdeaux DH, Klein KL, Millhollen JD, et al. Lower dose of anticoagulation is as effective as standard dose of oral anticoagulation (abstr). Blood 80(Suppl.):310, 1992.

21. Hirsh J, Poller L, Deykin D, Levine M, Dalen JE. Optimal therapeutic range for oral anticoagulants. Chest 95(Suppl.):5S, 1989. (Erratum, Chest 96:962, 1989.)

22. British Society for Hematology. Guidelines on oral anticoagulation, 2nd ed. J Clin Pathol 43:177, 1990.

23. Loeliger EA, Poller L, Samama M, et al. Questions and answers on prothrombin time standarisation in oral anticoagulant control. Throm Haemost 54:515, 1985.

24. Hyers T, Hull R, Weg J. Antithrombotic therapy for venous thromboembolic disease. Chest 108(Suppl.):335S, 1995.

25. Research Committee of the British Thoracic Society. Optimum duration of anticoagulation for deep-vein thrombosis and pulmonary embolism. Lancet 340:873, 1992.

26. Prandoni P, Lensing AWA, Büller HR, et al. Deep vein thrombosis and the incidence of subsequent symptomatic cancer. N Engl J Med 327:1128, 1992.

27. Levine MN, Hirsh J, Gent M, et al. Optimal duration of oral anticoagulant therapy: A randomized trial comparing four weeks with three months of Warfarin in patients with proximal deep vein thrombosis. Thromb Haemos 74:606, 1995.

28. Schulman S, Rhedin A-S, Lindmarker P, et al. A comparison of six weeks with six months of anticoagulant therapy after a first episode of venous thromboembolism. N Engl J Med 332:1661, 1995.

29. Levine MN, Gent M, Hirsh J, et al. The thrombogenic effect of anticancer drug therapy in women with stage II breast cancer. N Engl J Med 318:404, 1988.

30. Hirsh J. The optimal duration of anticoagulant therapy for venous thrombosis. N Engl J Med 332:1710, 1995.

31. Donaldson GA, Williams C, Scannell JG, Shaw RS. A reappraisal of the application of the Trendelenburg operation to massive fatal embolism: Report of a successful pulmonary-artery thrombectomy using a cardiopulmonary bypass. N Engl J Med 268:171, 1963.

32. Salzman EW, Davies GC. Prophylaxis of venous thromboembolism: Analysis of cost effectiveness. Ann Surg 19:1207, 1980.

33. Hull RD, Hirsh J, Sackett DL, Stoddart GL. Cost-effectiveness of primary and secondary prevention of fatal pulmonary embolism in high-risk surgical patients. Can Med Assoc J 127:990, 1982.

34. Bergqvist D, Matzch T, Jendteg S, Lindgern B, Persson U. The cost-effectiveness of prevention of post-operative thromboembolism. Acta Chir Scand 556(Suppl.):36, 1990.

35. Paiement GD, Wessinger SJ, Harris WH. Cost-effectiveness of prophylaxis in total hip replacement. Am J Surg 161:519, 1991.

36. Clagett GP. Hematologic factors in arterial thrombotic disease. In Yao JST, Pearce WH (eds). The Ischemic Extremity, Advances in Treatment. East Norwalk, CT: Appleton & Lange, 1995:25.

37. Nachman RL, Silverstein R. Hypercoagulable states. Ann Intern Med 119:819, 1993.

38. Svensson PJ, Dahlbach B. Resistance to activated protein C as a basis for venous thrombosis. N Engl J Med 330:517, 1994.

39. Ridker PM, Hennenkens CH, Lindapaintner K, et al. Mutation in the gene coding for coagulation factor V and the risk of myocardial infarction, stroke, and venous thrombosis in apparently healthy men. N Engl J Med 332:912, 1995.

40. Salzmann EW, Hirsh J. The epidemiology, pathogenesis, and natural history of venous thrombosis. In Colman RW, Hirsh J, Marder VJ, et al. (eds). Hemostasis and Thrombosis, Basic Principles and Clinical Practice, 3rd ed. Philadelphia: JB Lippincott, 1994:1276.

41. NIH Consensus Conference. Prevention of venous thrombosis and pulmonary embolism. JAMA 256:744, 1986.

42. Carter C, Gent M, Leclerc JR. The epidemiology of venous thrombosis. In Coleman RW, Hirsh J, Marder VJ, et al. (eds). Hemostasis and Thrombosis. Philadelphia: JB Lippincott 76:1185, 1987.

43. Coon WW. Epidemiology of venous thromboembolism. Ann Surg 186:149, 1977.

44. Goldhaber SZ, Savage DD, Garrison RJ, et al. Risk factors for pulmonary embolism: The Framingham Study. Am J Med 74:1023, 1983.

45. Kakkar VV, Stringer MD. Prophylaxis of venous thromboembolism. World J Surg 14:670, 1990.

46. Taberner DA, Poller L, Burslem RW, et al. Oral anticoagulants controlled by the British comparative thromboplastin versus low-dose heparin in prophylaxis of deep vein thrombosis. Br Med J 1:1272, 1978.

47. Poller L, McKernan A, Thompson JM, et al. Fixed minidose warfarin: A new approach to prophylaxis against venous thrombosis after major surgery. Br Med J 295:1309, 1987.

48. Francis CW, Pellegrini VD, Marder VJ, et al. Comparison of warfarin and external pneumatic compression in prevention of venous thrombosis after total hip replacement. JAMA 267:2911, 1992.

49. Hull R, Delmore TJ, Hirsh J, et al. Effectiveness of intermittent pulsatile elastic stocking for the prevention of calf and thigh vein thrombosis in patients undergoing elective knee surgery. Thromb Res 16:37, 1979.

50. McKenna R, Galante J, Bachmann F, et al. Prevention of venous thromboembolism after total knee replacement by high-dose aspirin or intermittent calf or thigh compression. Br Med J 280:514, 1980.

51. Haas SB, Insall JN, Scuderi GR, et al. Pneumatic sequential compression boots compared to aspirin prophylaxis of deep-vein thrombosis after total knee arthroplasty. J Bone Joint Surg 72A:27, 1990.

52. Lynch JA, Baker PL, Polly RE, et al. Mechanical measures in the prophylaxis of post-operative thromboembolism in total knee arthroplasty. Clin Orthop 260:24, 1990.

53. Lunceford EM, Patel SJ, Niestat HB, et al. Prevention of thrombophlebitis in total hip arthroplasty by early ambulation. Clin Orthop 33:273, 1978.

54. Prins MH, Hirsh J. A comparison of general anesthesia and regional anesthesia as a risk factor for deep vein thrombosis following hip surgery: A critical review. Thromb Haemost 64:497, 1990.

55. Fullen WD, Miller EH, Steele WF, et al. Prophylactic vena caval interruption in hip fractures. J Trauma 13:403, 1973.

56. Golueke PJ, Garrett WV, Thompson JE, et al. Interruption of the vena cava by means of the Greenfield filter: Expanding the indications. Surgery 103:111, 1988.

57. Vaughn BK, Knezevich S, Lombardi AV, et al. Use of the Greenfield filter to prevent fatal pulmonary embolism associated with total hip and knee arthroplasty. J Bone Joint Surg 71:1542, 1989.

58. Leyvraz PF, Richard J, Bachman F. Adjusted versus fixed-dose subcutaneous heparin in the prevention of deep vein thrombosis after total hip replacement. N Engl J Med 309:954, 1983.

59. Leyvraz PF, Bachmann F, Hoek J, et al. Prevention of deep vein thrombosis after hip replacement: Randomized comparison between unfractionated heparin and low molecular weight heparin. Br Med J 303:543, 1991.

60. Dechavanne M, Ville D, Berruyer M, et al. Randomized trial of a low-molecular-weight heparin (Kabi 2165) versus adjusted-dose subcutaneous standard heparin in the prophylaxis of deep-vein thrombosis after elective hip surgery. Haemostasis 1:5, 1989.

61. Amstutz HC, Friscia DA, Dorey F, et al. Warfarin prophylaxis to prevent mortality from pulmonary embolism after total hip replacement. J Bone Joint Surg 71A:321, 1989.

62. Paiment GD, Wessinger SJ, Hughes R, et al. Routine use of adjusted low-dose warfarin to prevent venous thromboembolism after total hip replacement. J Bone Joint Surg 75A:893, 1993.

63. Hull RC, Raskob GE, Pieno GF, et al. A comparison of subcutaneous low-molecular-weight heparin with warfarin sodium for prophylaxis against deep-vein thrombosis after hip or knee implantation. N Engl J Med 329:1370, 1993.

64. Leclerc JR, Geerts WH, Dwsjardins L, et al. Prevention of venous thromboembolism after knee arthroplasty: A randomized, double blinded trial, comparing a low molecular weight heparin fragment (enoxaparin) to warfarin. Blood 84(Suppl. 1):246A, 1994.

65. Spiro TE, Fitzgerald RH, Trowbridge AA, et al. Enoxaparin a low molecular weight heparin and warfarin for the prevention of venous thromboembolic disease after elective knee replacement surgery. Blood 84(Suppl. 1):246A, 1994.

66. Heit J, Berkowitz S, Bona R, et al. Efficacy and safety of ardeparin (a LMWH) compared to warfarin for prevention of venous thromboembolism following total knee replacement: A double-blind, dose-ranging study (abstr). Thromb Haemost 73:978, 1995.

67. Francis CW, Marder VJ, Evarts CM, et al. Two-step warfarin: Prevention of postoperative venous thrombosis without excessive bleeding. JAMA 249:374, 1983.

68. Borgstrom S, Greitz T, Vand Der Linden W, et al. Anticoagulant prophylaxis of venous thrombosis in patients with fractured neck of femor. Acta Chir Scand 129:500, 1965.

69. Hamilton HW, Crawford JS, Gardiner JH, et al. Venous thrombosis in patients with fracture of the upper end of the femur. J Bone Joint Surg 52:268, 1970.

70. Snook GA, Chrosman OD, Wilson TC. Thromboembolism after surgical treatment of hip fractures. Clin Orthop 155:21, 1981.

71. Bronge A, Dalhlgren S, Lindquist B. Prophylaxis against thrombosis in femoral neck fractures: A comparison between dextran 70 and dicumarol. Acta Chir Scand 137:29, 1971.

72. Berquist E, Bergqvist D, Bronge A, et al. An evaluation of early thrombosis prophylaxis following fracture of the femoral neck. Acta Chir Scand 138:689, 1972.

73. Bern M, Lokich JJ, Wallach SR, et al. Very low doses of warfarin can prevent thrombosis in central venous catheters: A randomized prospective trial. Ann Intern Med 112:423, 1990.

74. Sikarski JM, Hampson WG, Staddon GE. The natural history and etiology of deep vein thrombosis after

total hip replacement. J Bone Joint Surg 63B:171, 1981.

75. Trowbridge A, Boese CK, Woodruff B, et al. Incidence of posthospitalization proximal deep venous thrombosis after total hip arthroplasty. Clin Orthop 299:203, 1994.

76. Lotke PA, Steinberg ME, Ecker ML. Significance of deep vein thrombosis in the lower extremity after total joint arthroplasty. Clin Orthop 299:25, 1994.

77. Antiplatelet Trialists' Collaboration. Collaborative overview of randomized trials of antiplatelet therapy: III. Reduction in venous thrombosis and pulmonary embolism by antiplatelet prophylaxis among surgical and medical patients. Br Med J 308:235, 1994.

78. Kline A, Hughes LE, Campbell H, et al. Dextran 70 in prophylaxis of thromboembolic disease after surgery: A clinically oriented randomized trial. Br Med J 2:109, 1975.

79. Graor RA, Stewart JH, Lotke PA, et al. RD heparin vs. aspirin to prevent deep venous thrombosis after hip or knee replacement surgery (abstr). 58th Annual Scientific Assembly, American College of Chest Physicians, 1992:118S.

80. Harris WH, Salzman EW, Athanasoulis CA, et al. Aspirin prophylaxis of venous thromboembolism after total hip replacement. N Engl J Med 297:1246, 1977.

81. Soreff J, Johnson H, Diener L, et al. Acetylsalicylic acid in a trial to diminish thromboembolic complications after elective hip surgery. Acta Orthop Scand 46:246, 1975.

82. Harris WH, Salzman EW, Athamasoulis C, et al. Comparison of warfarin, low-molecular weight dextran, aspirin, and subcutaneous heparin in prevention of venous thromboembolism following total hip replacement. J Bone Joint Sury 56:1522, 1974.

83. Harris WH, Athanasoulis CA, Waltman AC, et al. Prophylaxis of deep-vein thrombosis after total hip replacement. J Bone Joint Surg 67:57, 1985.

84. Harris WH, Athanasoulis CA, Waltman AC, et al. High and low dose aspirin prophylaxis against venous thromboembolic disease in total hip replacement. J Bone Joint Surg 64:63, 1982.

85. Clagett GP, Anderson FA Jr, Levine MN, et al. Prevention of venous thromboembolism. Chest 102:391S, 1992.

86. Purdue GF, Hunt JL. Pulmonary embolism in burned patients. J Trauma 28:218, 1988.

87. Sevitt S, Gallagher N. Venous thrombosis and pulmonary embolism: A clinico-pathologic study in injured and burned patients. Br J Surg 45:475, 1961.

88. Clagett GP, Heit J, Levine N, Wheeler HB. Prevention of venous thromboembolism. Chest 108:312S, 1995.

89. Peterson P, Godtfredsen J, Boysen G, Anderson ED, Anderson B. Placebo-controlled, randomized trial of warfarin and aspirin for prevention of thromboembolic complications in chronic atrial fibrillation. The Copenhagen AFASAK study. Lancet 1:175, 1989.

90. The Stroke Prevention in Atrial Fibrillation Investigators: The Stroke Prevention in Atrial Fibrillation study: Final results, Circulation 84:527, 1991.

91. The Boston Area Anticoagulation Trial for Atrial Fibrillation investigators. The effect of low-dose warfarin on the risk of stroke in patients with nonrheumatic atrial fibrillation. N Engl J Med 323:1505, 1990.

92. Connoly S, Laupacis A, Gent M. Canadian atrial fibrillation anticoagulation (CAFA) study. J Am Coll Cardiol 18:349, 1991.

93. Ezekowitz M, Bridgers S, James K, et al. VA cooperative study of warfarin in the prevention of stroke associated with nonrheumatic atrial fibrillation. N Engl J Med 327:1406, 1992.

94. Albers GW, Sherman DG, Gress DR, Paulseth JE, Petersen P. Stroke prevention in nonvalvular atrial fibrillation: A review of prospective randomized trials. Ann Neurol 30:511, 1991.

95. Albers GW. Atrial fibrillation and stroke: Three new studies, three remaining questions. Arch Intern Med 154:1443, 1994.

96. EAFT (European Atrial Fibrillation Trial) Study Group. Secondary prevention in nonrheumatic atrial fibrillation after transient ischemic attack or minor stroke. Lancet 342:1255, 1993.

97. Ferguson JJ. Meeting highlights. American College of Cardiology 45th Annual Scientific Session, Orlando, Florida, March 24–27, 1996. Circulation 94:1, 1996.

98. Atrial Fibrillation investigators. Risk factors for stroke and efficacy of antithrombotic therapy in atrial fibrillation: Analysis of pooled data from five randomized controlled trials. Arch Intern Med 154:1449, 1994.

99. Kase CS, Robinson RK, Stein RW, et al. Anticoagulant-related intracerebral hemorrhage. Neurology 35:943, 1985.

100. Wintzer AR, deJonge H, Loeliger EA, Bots GTAM. The risk of intracerebral hemorrhage during oral anticoagulant treatment: A population study. Ann Neurol 16:533, 1984.

101. Albers GW. Intensity of anticoagulant treatment and risk of intracerebral hematoma. Stroke 21:1758, 1990.

102. Levine M, Hirsh J, Landefled S, Raskob G. Hemorrhagic complication of anticoagulant treatment. Chest 102(Suppl.):352S, 1992.

103. Kelton J, Hirsh J. Bleeding associated with antithrombotic therapy. Semin Hematol 17:259, 1980.

104. Philips S, Whisnant J, O'Fallon, Frye R. Prevention of cardiovascular disease and diabetes in residents of Rochester, Minnesota. Mayo Clin Proc 65:344, 1990.

105. Laupacis A, Albers G, Dalen J, et al. Antithrombotic therapy in atrial fibrillation. Chest 108(Suppl.): 352S, 1995.

106. Stroke Prevention in Atrial Fibrillation investigators. Warfarin versus aspirin for prevention of thromboembolism in atrial fibrillation: Stroke prevention in atrial fibrillation II study. Lancet 343:687, 1994.

107. The Stroke Prevention in Atrial Fibrillation investigators. Predictors of thromboembolism in atrial fibrillation II: Echocardiographic features of patients at risk. Ann Intern Med 116:6, 1992.

108. The Stroke Prevention on Atrial Fibrillation investigators. Predictors of thromboembolism in atrial fibrillation, I: Clinical features of patients at risk. Ann Intern Med 116:1, 1992.

109. Stein PD, Collins JJ Jr, Kanatrowitz A. Antithrombotic therapy in mechanical and biological prosthetic heart valves and saphenous vein bypass grafts. Chest 89(Suppl.):46S, 1986.

110. Dale J. Arterial thromboembolic complications in patients with Starr-Edwards aortic ball valve prostheses. Am Heart J 91:653, 1976.

111. Horstkotte D, Körfer R. The influence of prosthetic valve replacement on the natural history of severe acquired heart lesions: A comparison of complications and clinical and hemodynamic findings after implantation of Björk-Shiley, St. Jude Medical, and other heart valve prostheses. In De Bakey ME (ed). Advances in Cardiac Valves: Clinical Perspectives. New York: Yorke Medical Books, 1983:47.

112. Chesebro JH, Ezekowitz M, Badimon L, Fuster V. Intercardiac thrombi and systemic thromboembolism: Detection, incidence, and treatment. Annu Rev Med 36:579, 1985.

113. Christo MC, Souza JM, Stortini MJ, et al. Late complication of cardiac valve replacement with Lillegei-Kaster pivoting disc prosthesis. Artif Organs 4:199, 1980.

114. Yeh TJ, Anabtawi IN, Cornett VE, Ellison RG. Influence of rhythm and anticoagulation upon the incidence of embolization associated with Starr-Edwards prostheses. Circulation 35(Suppl. I):I77, 1967.

115. Cannegieter SC, Rosendaal FR, Briët E. Thromboembolic and bleeding complications in patients with mechanical heart valve prostheses. Circulation 89:635, 1994.

116. Horstkotte D, Schulte HD, Bricks W, et al. Lower intensity anticoagulation therapy results in lower complication rates with the St. Jude Medical Prosthesis. J Thorac Cardiovasc Surg 107:1136, 1994.

117. Baudet EM, Oca CC, Roques XF, et al. A five and half year experience with the St. Jude Medical cardiac valve prosthesis: Early and late results of 737 valve replacements in 671 patients. J Thorac Cardiovasc Surg 90:137, 1985.

118. Vogt S, Hoffmann A, Roth J, et al. Heart valve replacement with the Bjork-Shiley and St. Jude Medical Prostheses: A randomized comparison in 178 patients. Eur Heart J 11:583, 1990.

119. Kopf GS, Hammond GL, Geha AS, et al. Long-term performance of the St. Jude Medical valve: Low incidence of thromboembolism and hemorrhagic complications with modest doses of warfarin. Circulation 76(Suppl. III):III132, 1987.

120. Akbarian M, Austen G, Yurchal PM, Scannell JG. Thromboembolic complications of prosthetic cardiac valves. Circulation 37:826, 1968.

121. Duvoisin GE, Brandenberg RO, McGoon DC. Factors affecting thromboembolism associated with prosthetic heart valves. Circulation 35(Suppl. I):I70, 1967.

122. Douglas PS, Hirshfeld JW, Edie RN, Harken AH, Stephenson LW, Edmunds LH. Clinical comparison of St. Jude and porcine aortic valve prostheses. Circulation 72(Suppl. II):II135, 1985.

123. Wilson DB, Dunn MI, Hassanein K. Low-intensity anticoagulation in mechanical cardiac prosthetic valves. Chest 100:1553, 1991.

124. Stein PD, Gransidon D, Hua TA, et al. Therapeutic levels of oral anticoagulation with warfarin in patients with mechanical prosthetic heart valves: Review of literature and recommendations based on international normalized ratio. Postgrad Med J 70(Suppl. 1):S72, 1994.

125. Saor JN, Sieck JO, Mamo LAR, et al. Trial of different intensities of anticoagulation in patients with prosthetic heart valves. N Engl J Med 322:428, 1990.

126. Turpie AGG, Gent M, Laupacis A, et al. Comparison of aspirin with placebo in patients treated with warfarin after heart-valve replacement. N Engl J Med 329:524, 1993.

127. Rajah SM, Sreeharan N, Joseph A, et al. Prospective trial of dipyridamole and warfarin in heart valve patients (abstr). Acta Thera (Brussels) 6:54, 1980.

128. Yamak B, Karagoz HY, Zorlutuna Y, et al. Low-dose anticoagulant management of patients with a St. Jude medical mechanical valve prostheses. Thorac Cardiovasc Surg 41:38, 1993.

129. Fiore L, Brophy M, Deykin D, et al. The efficacy and safety of the addition of aspirin in patients treated with oral anticoagulants after heart valve replacement: A meta-analysis (abstr). Blood 82(Suppl. I):409, 1993.

130. Sullivan JM, Harken DE, Gorlin R. Effect of dipyridamole on the incidence of arterial emboli after cardiac valve replacement. Circulation 39 (Suppl.):I149, 1969.

131. Groupe de recherche P.A.C.T.E. Prevention des accidents thrombo-emboliques systemiques chez les porteurs de protheses valvulaires artificielles. Coeur 9:915, 1978.

132. Chesebro JH, Fuster V, Elveback LR, et al. Trial of combined warfarin plus dipyridamole or aspirin therapy in prosthetic heart valve replacement: Danger of aspirin compared with dipyridamole. Am J Cardiol 51:1537, 1983.

133. Nunez L, Aguado GM, Celemin D, et al. Aspirin or coumadin as the drug of choice for valve replacement with porcine bioprosthesis. Ann Thorac Surg 33:354, 1982.

134. Stein P, Alpert J, Copeland J, et al. Antithrombotic

therapy in patients with mechanical and biologic prosthetic heart valves. Chest 102(Suppl.):445S, 1992.

135. Cohn LH, Allred EN, DiSesa VJ, et al. Early and late risk of aortic valve replacement: A 12-year concomitant comparison of the porcine bioprosthetic and tilting disc prosthetic aortic valves. J Thorac Cardiovasc Surg 88:695, 1984.

136. Bolooki H, Kaiser GA, Mallon SM, et al. Comparison of long-term results of Carpentier-Edwards and Hancock bioprosthetic valves. Ann Thorac Surg 42:494, 1986.

137. Bloomfield P, Kitchin AH, Wheatley DJ, et al. A prospective evaluation of the Bjork-Shiley, Hancock, and Carpentier-Edwards heart valve prostheses. Circulation 73:1213, 1986.

138. Cohn LH, Allred EN, Cohn LA, et al. Early and late risk of mitral valve replacement. J Thorac Cardiovasc Surg 90:872, 1985.

139. Nunez L, Aguado GM, Larrea JL, et al. Prevention of thromboembolism using aspirin after mitral valve replacement with porcine bioprosthesis. Ann Thorac Surg 37:84, 1984.

140. Gonzalez-Lavin L, Chi S, Blair TC, et al. Thromboembolism and bleeding after mitral valve replacement with porcine valves: Influence of thromboembolic risk factors. J Surg Res 36:508, 1984.

141. Mok CK, Boey J, Wang R, et al. Warfarin versus dipyridamole-aspirin and pentoxifylline-aspirin for the prevention of prosthetic heart valve thromboembolism: A prospective clinical trial. Circulation 72:1059, 1985.

142. Hetzer R, Topalidis T, Borst HG. Thromboembolism and anticoagulation after isolated mitral valve replacement with porcine heterografts. In Cohn LH, Gallucci V (eds). Proceedings, Second International Symposium on Cardiac Bioprostheses. New York: Yorke Medical Books, 1982:170.

143. Oyer PE, Stinson EB, Griepp RB, et al. Valve replacement with the Starr-Edwards and Hancock prostheses: Comparative analysis of later morbidity and mortality. Ann Surg 186:301, 1977.

144. Ionescu MI, Smith DR, Hasan SS, et al. Clinical durability of the pericardial xenograft valve: Ten years experience with mitral replacement. Ann Thorac Surg 34:255, 1982.

145. Turpie AGG, Gunstensen J, Hirsh J, et al. Randomized comparison of two intensities of oral anticoagulant therapy after tissue heart valve replacement. Lancet 1:1242, 1988.

146. Stein P, Alpert J, Copeland J, et al. Antithrombotic therapy in patients with mechanical and biological prosthetic heart valves. Chest 102(Suppl.):445S, 1992.

147. Louagie YA, Jamart J, Eucher P, et al. Mitral valve Carpentier-Edwards bioprosthetic replacement, thromboembolism, and anticoagulants. Ann Thorac Surg 56:931, 1993.

148. Altman R, Boullon F, Rouvier J, Raca R, et al. Aspirin and prophylaxis on thromboembolic complications in patients with substitute heart valves. J Thorac Cardiovasc Surg 72:127, 1976.

149. Karchmer AW, Dismukes WE, Buckley MJ, et al. Late prosthetic valve endocarditis — clinical features influencing therapy. Am J Med 64:199, 1978.

150. Braunwald E. Heart Disease: A Textbook of Cardiovascular Medicine. Philadelphia, ••, 1992:1065.

151. Melzer RS, Visser CA, Fuster V. Intracardiac thrombi and systemic embolization. Ann Intern Med 104:689, 1986.

152. Veterans Administration Cooperative Study. Anticoagulants in acute myocardial infarction: Results of a cooperative clinical trial. JAMA 225:724, 1973.

153. Medical Research Council Group. Assessment of short-term anticoagulant administration after cardiac infarction: Report of the Working Party on Anticoagulant Therapy in Coronary Thrombosis. Br Med J 1:335, 1969.

154. Drapkin A, Merskey C. Anticoagulant therapy after acute myocardial infarction. JAMA 222:541, 1972.

155. Cairns JA, Hirsh J, Lewis HD Jr, et al. Antithrombotic agents in coronary artery disease. Chest 102:456S, 1992.

156. Goldberg RJ, Gore JM, Dalen JE, et al. Long term anticoagulant therapy after acute myocardial infarction. Am Heart J 109:616, 1985.

157. Leizorovicz A, Boissel JP. Oral anticoagulant in patients surviving myocardial infarction. Eur J Clin Pharmacol 24:333, 1983.

158. Chalmers TC, Matta RJ, Smith H Jr, Kunzler-A-M. Evidence favoring the use of anticoagulants in the hospital phase of acute myocardial infarction. N Engl J Med 297:1091, 1977.

159. Loeliger EA. Oral anticoagulation in patients surviving myocardial infarction: A new approach to old data. Eur J Clin Pharmacol 26:137, 1984.

160. Bjerkelund CJ. The effect of long term treatment with dicoumarol in myocardial infarction: A controlled clinical study. Acta Med Scand Suppl 330:13, 1957.

161. British Medical Reasarch Council. An assessment of long-term anticoagulant administration after cardiac infarction. Br Med J 2:837, 1964.

162. Aspenström G, Korsan-Bengsten K. A double blind study of dicumarol prophylaxis in coronary heart disease. Acta Med Scand 176:563, 1964.

163. Rozenberg MC, Kronenberg H, Firkin BG. "Thrombotest" and prothrombin time: A controlled clinical trial. Aust Ann Med 14:3, 1965.

164. Loeliger EA, Hensen A, Kroes F, et al. A double-blind trial of long-term anticoagulant treatment after myocardial infarction. Acta Med Scand 182:549, 1967.

165. Meuwissen OJ, Vervoon AC, Cohen O, Jordan FL, Nelemans FA. Double blind trial of long-term anti-

coagulant treatment after myocardial infarction. Acta Med Scand 186:361, 1969.

166. Sørensen OH, Friis T, Jørgensen AW, Jørgensen MB, Nissen NL. Anticoagulant treatment of acute coronary thrombosis. Acta Med Scan 185:65, 1969.

167. The Sixty Plus Reinfarction Study Research Group. A double-blind trial to assess long-term oral anticoagulant therapy in elderly patients after myocardial infarction. Lancet 2:989, 1980.

168. Mac Millan Rl, Brown KWG, Watt DL. Long-term anticoagulant therapy after myocardial infarction. Can Med Assoc J 83:567, 1960.

169. Harvald B, Hilden T, Lund E. Long-term anticoagulant therapy after myocardial infarction. Lancet 2:626, 1962.

170. Clausen J, Andersen PE, Andersen P, et al. Langtidsantikoagulansbehandling efter akut hjerteifarkt. Ugeskr Laeger 123:987, 1961.

171. Conard LL, Kyriacopoulos JD, Wiggins CW, Honick GL. Prevention of recurrences of myocardial infarction: A double-blind study of the effectiveness of long-term oral anticoagulant therapy. Arch Intern Med 114:348, 1964.

172. Lovell RR, Denborough MA, Nestel PJ, Goble AJ. A controlled trial of long-term treatment with anticoagulants after myocardial infarction in 412 male patients. Med J Aust 2:97, 1967.

173. Ebert RV. Long-term anticoagulant therapy after myocardial infarction: Final report of the Veterans Administration cooperative study. JAMA 207:2263, 1969.

174. Seaman AJ, Grisworld HE, Reaume RB, Ritzmann L. Long-tem anticoagulant prophylaxis after myocardial infarction: First report. N Engl J Med 281:115, 1969.

175. Ritland S, Lygern T. Comparison of efficacy of 3 and 12 months' anticoagulant therapy after myocardial infarction. Lancet 1:122, 1969.

176. Breddin K, Loew D, Lechner K, Uberla K, Walter E. Secondary prevention of myocardial infarction: A comparison of acetylsalicylic acid, placebo and phenprocoumon. Haemostasis 9:325, 1980.

177. The E.P.S.I.M. Research Group. A controlled comparison of aspirin and oral anticoagulants in prevention of death after myocardial infarction. N Engl J Med 307:701, 1982.

178. Goldman L, Feinstein AR. Anticoagulants and myocardial infarction: The problems of pooling, drowning, and floating. Ann Intern Med 90:92, 1979.

179. Yusuf S, Wittes J, Friedman L. Overview of results of randomized clinical trials in heart disease I. Treatments following myocardial infarction. JAMA 260:2088, 1988.

180. Smith P, Arnesen H, Holme I. The effect of warfarin in mortality and reinfarction after myocardial infarction. N Engl J Med 323:147, 1990.

181. ASPECT Research Group. Effect of long-term oral anticoagulant treatment on mortality and cardiovascular morbidity after myocardial infarction. N Engl J Med 323:147, 1990.

182. Kretschmer G, Wenzl E, Schemper M, et al. Influence of post-operative anticoagulant treatment of patient survival after femoropopliteal vein bypass surgery. Lancet 343:499, 1994.

183. Levine H, Pauker S, Eckman M. Antithrombotic therapy in valvular heart disease. Chest 108(Suppl.):360S, 1995.

184. Barnett HJM, Mc Donald JWD, Sacket L. Aspirin: Effective in mlaes threatened with stroke. Stroke 9:295, 1978.

185. Hirosowitz GS, Saffer D. Hemiplegia and billowing mitral leaflet syndrome. J Neurol Neurosurg Psychiatry 41:381, 1978.

186. Barnett HJM, Boughner DR, Taylow DW. Further evidence relating mitral valve prolapse to cerebral ischemic events. N Engl J Med 302:139, 1980.

187. Guthrie RB, Edwards JE. Pathology of myxomatous mitral valve: Nature, secondary changes and complications. Minn Med 59:637, 1976.

188. Geyer SJ, Franzini DA. Myxomatous degeneration of the mitral valve complicated by nonbacterial thrombotic endocarditis with systemic embolization. Am J Clin Pathol 72:489, 1979.

189. Fuster V, Gersh BJ, Guiliani ER, Tajik AJ, Brandenberg RO, Frye RL. The natural history of idiopathic dilated cardiomyopathy. Am J Cardiol 47:525, 1981.

190. Gottdiener JS, Gay JA, VanVoorhees L, Dibianco R, Fletcher RD. Frequency and embolic potential of left ventricular thrombus in dilated cardiomyopathy: Assessment by two-dimensional echocardiography. Am J Cardiol 52:1281, 1983.

191. Tobin R, Slutsky RA, Higgins CB. Serial echocardiograms in patients with congestive cardiomyopathies: Lack of evidence for thrombus formation. Clin Cardiol 7:99, 1984.

192. Lapeyre AC, Steele PP, Kazmier FJ, et al. Systemic embolism in chronic left ventricular aneurysm: Incidence and role of anticoagulation. J Am Coll Cardiol 6:534, 1985.

193. Meltzer R, Visser CA, Fuster V. Intracardiac thrombi and systemic embolization. Ann Intern Med 104:689, 1986.

194. Hamby RJ, Wisoff G, Davison ET, Hartstein ML. Coronary artery disease and left ventricular mural thrombi: Clinical, hemodynamic, and angiocardiographic aspects. Chest 66:488, 1974.

195. Simpson MT, Oberman A, Kouchoukos NT, Rogers WJ. Prevalence of mural thrombi and systemic embolization with left ventricular aneurysm: Effect of anticoagulation therapy. Chest 77:463, 1980.

196. Reeder GS, Lengyel M, Tajik AJ, Seward JB, Smith HC, Danielson GK. Mural thrombus in left ventricular aneurysm: Incidence, role of angiography, and relation between anticoagulation and embolization. Mayo Clin Proc 80:118, 1981.

197. de Iturbe Allesio I, Carmen Fonesca M, Mutchinik O, et al. Risks of anticoagulant therapy in pregnant women with artificial heart valves. N Engl J Med 315:1390, 1986.

198. Ezekowitz MD. Systemic Cardiac Embolism, New York: Marcel Dekker, 308, 1994.

199. Altman R, Rouvier J, Gurfinkel E, et al. Comparison of two levels of anticoagulant therapy in patients with substitute heart valves. J Thorac Cardiovasc Surg 101:427, 1991.

SECTION XII: HEMORRHAGIC COMPLICATIONS

Patrick T. O'Gara

The efficacy of thrombolytic, anti-coagulant and anti-platelet therapy in the management of a wide spectrum of cardiovascular disorders has been well established in multiple large scale clinical trials. The aggressive use of such medications, either alone or in conjunction with invasive reperfusion strategies, must be tempered by perceived risks of bleeding. Although the clinician's ability to predict hemorrhagic risk is imperfect, increasing experience gained from additional investigations and more relevant reporting have provided further insights from which rational recommendations can be made. In this section, we will review the relevant patient characteristics and laboratory parameters that enable stratification of hemorrhagic risk and provide clinical practice guidelines for the use of thrombolytic, anti-coagulant, and anti-platelet agents.

39. HEMORRHAGIC COMPLICATIONS

Cynthia M. Thaik and Patrick O'Gara

Introduction

Over the past decade there has been a marked increase in the use of thrombolytic, anticoagulant, and antiplatelet agents in a wide variety of clinical settings, including the prophylaxis and treatment of deep venous thrombosis (DVT) and pulmonary emboli (PE), the prevention of embolic strokes in atrial fibrillation (AF), and the management of acute myocardial infarction (MI). In very high-risk patients, the incidence of calf vein thrombosis may range from 40% to 80%, proximal vein thrombosis from 10% to 20%, and clinical PE from 4% to 10% [1]. Atrial fibrillation develops annually in over two million people in the United States and affects 3–10% of the adult population over the age of 65 years [2]. An estimated 1.5 million people in the United States suffer an acute MI yearly [3].

Approximately 30% of such patients who reach the hospital are candidates for thrombolytic therapy, which may establish reperfusion in approximately 75% of treated individuals and is associated with an approximate 25% survival benefit [4–19]. Improved survival has been observed among several patient cohorts, including those with inferior MI, the elderly (age >75 years), and those patients whose symptoms have persisted for up to 12 hours prior to presentation [4]. At experienced centers, primary angioplasty for acute MI compares favorably with the best outcomes reported from thrombolytic trials with similar short- and intermediate-term survival [5]. There is a higher patency rate achieved with angioplasty, as reflected in a lower incidence of reinfarction and recurrent angina. Recent studies have evaluated the use of more aggressive and innovative reperfusion regimens, and have included direct antithrombin agents, such as hirudin and hirulog, and antiplatelet agents, such as glycoprotein 2B3A (GPIIb/IIIa) receptor antagonists. As the use of these aggressive therapies becomes even more widespread and as invasive procedures are performed earlier in the course of ischemic syndromes, improved patient selection and greater vigilance are necessary to minimize the associated hemorrhagic complications.

Major hemorrhagic complications can be defined as intracranial or retroperitoneal bleeding; episodes that require hospitalization, surgery, or transfusion; or those that result in death or impairment in sight or hearing. Minor bleeding complications might include all other events. The extrapolation of observations made in large clinical trials to practice is hampered by (1) patient variability, (2) the different criteria used for the classification of hemorrhagic complications, (3) the varying use of invasive procedures, and (4) the frequency of under-reporting.

This chapter reviews briefly the mechanisms of hemostasis and fibrinolysis, the mechanism of action of the various thrombolytic, anticoagulant, and antiplatelet agents, and the clinical patient characteristics and laboratory parameters that might predict hemorrhagic risk. We summarize the efficacy and safety data from the available clinical trials on the use of these agents in the treatment of unstable angina, acute myocardial infarction, cerebral vascular disease, atrial fibrillation, deep venous thrombosis, and pulmonary embolism, and offer some recommendations for clinical practice.

Mechanisms of Hemostasis and Fibrinolysis

Hemostasis involves injury to the endothelial surface, release of vasoactive substances and tissue factors, platelet recruitment and activation, and initiation of the coagulation cascade. Platelets adhere to macromolecules on the subendothelial surface of injured blood vessels, aggregate to form the primary hemostatic plug, and stimulate local activation of plasma coagulation factors. The final step in the coagulation pathway is the conversion of fibrinogen to fibrin monomers via the action of thrombin, followed by crosslinking to form a fibrin polymer meshwork, thus generating a fibrin clot to reinforce the platelet aggregate [20].

Fibrinolysis involves the conversion of plasminogen to plasmin by naturally occurring or exogenous tissue plasminogen activators. Plasmin, an enzyme that digests fibrin, then binds to the fibrin surface and promotes the breakdown of the hemostatic plug. In the fluid phase, plasmin catalyzes fibrinogenolysis as well as the degradation of factors V and VIII, which leads, in turn, to a decrease in the generation of thrombin and a systemic lytic state. The proteolysis of fibrin and fibrinogen leads to an elevation in the levels of fibrin(ogen) degradation products, which also act as thrombin inhibitors and interfere with fibrin polymerization. In addition, plasmin interferes with platelet adhesion and aggregation by cleaving the platelet surface receptors, GPIb and GPIIb/IIIa. There are naturally occurring inhibitors of plasmin, including plasminogen activator inhibitor-1 (PAI-1) and α_2-antiplasmin, which serve to keep the fibrinolytic pathway in check [21].

Mechanisms of Action

THROMBOLYTIC AGENTS
All currently available thrombolytic agents act via the conversion of plasminogen to plasmin [22]. Streptokinase is a 47-kd protein produced by β-hemolytic streptococci, which has no intrinsic enzymatic activity. It forms a stable noncovalent 1:1 complex with plasminogen, inducing a conformational change in the plasminogen molecule and exposing it to cleavage to form free plasmin. Anisoylated plasminogen streptokinase activator complex (APSAC) has an acylated group on the catalytic site of the lys-plasminogen. This modification allows the complex to bind to fibrin prior to its activation via spontaneous deacetylation and may theoretically confer greater fibrin specificity. It is administered as a single bolus. Urokinase (UK) is a two-chain serine protease, which lacks fibrin specificity and readily induces a systemic lytic state.

Tissue plasminogen activator (t-PA) is a serine protease, which is a poor plasminogen activator in the absence of fibrin. It is produced in either the active double-chain form (duteplase) or in the less active single-chain form (alteplase), which, in turn, is immediately cleaved in the circulation to the more active form. t-PA binds fibrin and activates bound plasminogen several hundredfold more rapidly than free plasminogen in the circulation. The greater catalytic activity of t-PA on the fibrin surface confers greater fibrin specificity than that associated with SK or UK. While it was originally postulated that such fibrin specificity would result in less bleeding with t-

PA, this has not proved to be the case in major trials or clinical practice [16,19,36].

NEWER THROMBOLYTIC AGENTS
TNK-tissue plasminogen activator (TNK-tPA) is a genetically engineered variant of the wild type activator, with amino acid substitutions at three sites. These changes have led to a slower plasma clearance, greater fibrin specificity, and a greater (80-fold) resistance to plasminogen activator inhibitor-1 (PAI-1), with more rapid arterial recanalization and greater clot lysis compared with front-loaded alteplase in experimental models [23]. Reteplase (r-PA) is a nonglycosylated deletion mutant of the wild-type t-PA, consisting of the kringle-2 and protease domain, but lacking the kringle-1 finger and growth factor domain of t-PA. It has a longer half-life than alteplase, thus allowing bolus administration [24]. Staphylokinase is a 136 amino-acid single-chain protein without disulfide bridges, normally secreted by strains of *Staphylococcus aureus*, and reproduced by rDNA technology. It has demonstrate greater thrombolytic potential and fibrin specificity than other currently available plasminogen activators [25].

ANTITHROMBIN AGENTS

Heparin. Standard unfractionated heparin is a heterodisperse mixture of polysaccharides of molecular weights ranging between 3 and 40 kd [26]. Heparin acts as a cofactor for the naturally occurring antithrombin III (AT III) and serine proteases of the coagulation pathway. AT III is a glycosylated, single-chain polypeptide synthesized in the liver that rapidly inhibits thrombin only in the presence of heparin. It inhibits activated coagulation factors of the intrinsic and common pathways, including thrombin; factors XIIa, XIa, Xa, and IXa; and kallikrein. Heparin acts as a catalytic template to which both thrombin and the inhibitor bind and increases the rate of the thrombin–antithrombin reaction by at least a thousandfold. Heparin can also stimulate the inhibition of thrombin by PAI-1, protein C inhibitor, protease nexin-1, as well as the inhibition of factor Xa by tissue factor pathway inhibitor (TFPI). These four inhibitors are present in the plasma in less than one-hundredth the concentration of antithrombin III. In addition, high-dose heparin (>5 U/mL) induces thrombin inhibition through heparin cofactor II and can interfere with platelet aggregation and prolong the bleeding time [22].

The theoretical disadvantages of heparin compared with direct antithrombin inhibitors include (1) its failure to inactivate the thrombin that is bound to fibrin or to the exposed subendothelial matrix; (2) its inactivation by platelet factor-4 and heparinases released by activated platelets; (3) its variable effect between and among patients due to its binding with vitronectin, fibronectin, and other plasma proteins; and (4) a not-inconsequential (5–15%) incidence of thrombocytopenia [22,30,44,67].

Low Molecular Weight Heparins. Low-molecular weight heparins (LMWHs) are fragments of standard heparin formed by chemical or enzymatic depolymerization to approximately one-third the size of standard heparin, averaging 4–5 kd. Various commercial preparations of LMWH can differ in their molecular weight distribution, specific activity, clearance rates, and optimal dosing. A minimal chain length of eight saccharides (including the pentasaccharide sequence, composed of three N-acetyl 6-O-sulfate, glucuronic acid, and iduronic acid 2-O-sulfate) is required to serve as a template for thrombin (factor IIa), factor Xa, and antithrombin binding.

LMWHs bind less avidly to heparin binding plasma proteins and to endothelium than standard unfractionated heparin, and thus exhibit more complete absorption from subcutaneous sites, better bioavailability, a longer elimination half-life, and a more predictable anticoagulant response. LMWHs are slightly less effective than standard unfractionated heparin as antithrombotic agents in experimental models of venous thrombosis but are also associated with much less bleeding in models measuring blood loss from standard injury for any given level of anticoagulant efficacy [27,28].

In contrast to the inhibition of thrombin, inactivation of factor Xa by AT III requires fewer bound heparin molecules. As a result, various commercially available LMWHs exhibit a relative 2:1 to 4:1 anti–factor Xa to antithrombin (anti–factor IIa) activity, compared with a 1:1 ratio for standard heparin. LMWHs exhibit little or no effect on the aPTT or whole-blood clotting time, but have a major effect on assays for anti–factor Xa activity. When necessary, the clinical efficacy of the LMWHs can be related to serum heparin levels. In addition, LMWHs have less interaction with platelet factor-4 because platelet affinity for heparin is dependent on the length of the heparin polysaccharide chain [29].

Direct Antithrombins. The direct thrombin inhibitors include hirudin, synthetic hirudin fragments (hirugen and hirulog), and low molecular weight inhibitors that react with the active site of thrombin

(PPACK and argatroban). These inhibitors act directly on the thrombin molecule, blocking its catalytic and/or substrate recognition sites, and are potent, specific inhibitors of thrombin's biologic actions. Natural hirudin, a peptide found in medicinal leeches, acts by forming a tight stoichiometric, slowly reversible complex with thrombin and is the most potent inhibitor of thrombin found in nature [30].

The recombinant hirudins are severalfold less potent, with reduced affinity for thrombin. Hirugen is a synthetic dodecapeptide fragment of hirudin, which binds to the substrate recognition site (but not to the active catalytic site) on thrombin, blocking its interaction with fibrinogen, the thrombin receptor on platelets, and other physiologic substrates. The addition of the sequence D-Phe-Pro-Arg-Pro-(Gly)$_4$ to the amino terminus of hirugen converts this weak competitive inhibitor of thrombin to a potent bivalent inhibitor of both the active site and the substrate recognition site, known as hirulog.

D-Phe-Pro-ArgCH$_2$Cl (PPACK) is a low molecular weight thrombin inhibitor, the structure of which closely resembles fibrinopeptide A. It recognizes the active site and irreversibly inhibits thrombin. Argatroban is a synthetic arginine derivative of PPACK that competitively blocks the active site of thrombin. Hirudin and its congeners inhibit both bound and fluid-phase thrombin, and thus are more potent and specific in their actions than heparin.

ORAL ANTICOAGULANTS

Oxidation of vitamin K is coupled to the γ-carboxylation of the coagulation factors II, VII, IX, and X, and the anticoagulant proteins C and S. The carboxylation of the amino-terminal glutamic acid is essential for the assembly of the coagulation factors into an efficient catalytic complex. Reduced vitamin K must be regenerated to sustain the carboxylation and synthesis of these compounds. There are various orally available vitamin K antagonists; warfarin is the most widely used because of its intermediate metabolism ($t_{1/2}$ = 35 hours) and good bioavailability. Warfarin inhibits vitamin K by blocking the action of the specific reductase(s) needed to recycle the vitamin. Therapeutic doses of warfarin decrease hepatic synthesis of each vitamin K–dependent factor by 30–50%. In addition, the secreted coagulation factors are undercarboxylated, thus resulting in a diminished biological activity (10–40% normal) [22]. The therapeutic dose response to warfarin is dependent on a variety of factors, including the use of concomitant medications, dietary vitamin K intake, hepatic function, metabolic state, and age (Table 39-1) [31].

TABLE 39-1. Some factors that potentiate
or inhibit the anticoagulant effect of warfarin

Potentiate	Inhibit
Drugs	Drugs
Metronidazole	Cholestryamine
Trimethoprim/	Barbituates
sulfamethoxazole	Rifampin
Amiodarone	Carbamazepine
Erythromycin	Penicillin
Cimetidine	Other
Omeprazole	Increased vitamin K
Thyroxine	intake
Ketoconazole	Alcohol
Isoniazid	
Fluconazole	
Tamoxifen	
Quinidine	
Vitamine E (megadose)	
Phenytoin	
Other	
Low vitamin K intake	
Reduced vitamin K	
absorption	
Liver disease	
Hypermetabolic states	
(thyrotoxicosis)	

Modified, with permission, from Hirsh [31].

ANTIPLATELET AGENTS

Antiplatelet therapy is a critical component of the
management of the acute coronary syndromes [32].
Aspirin, the most widely use antiplatelet agent,
works via the irreversible inhibition of cyclooxygenase, the enzyme that produces the cyclic endoperoxide precursor of thromboxane A_2, a labile inducer of
platelet aggregation and a potent vasoconstrictor.
Because platelets cannot synthesize new proteins,
aspirin's effect on platelet cyclooxygenase is permanent and complete at doses of 160 mg taken daily.

Platelets, however, can continue to be activated
via thromboxane A_2–independent pathways. Recent
studies have included agents that inhibit platelet activation via a variety of mechanisms — thromboxane
A_2 receptor antagonists, serotonin receptor antagonists, prostanoids, and inhibitors of the proaggregatory platelet glycoprotein integrin receptor, GPIIb/
IIIa. GPIIb/IIIa receptors undergo conformational
changes after platelet adhesion and activation. These
receptors have high binding affinity for fibrinogen,
von Willebrand factor, and other glycoproteins, and
are a natural target for the prevention of platelet-
thrombus formation [32].

c7E3 is a chimeric human–murine monoclonal antibody Fab fragment directed against the glycoprotein IIb/IIIa receptor. Its mechanism of action is
thought to involve steric hindrance and/or conformational effects to block access to the receptor, rather
than direct interaction with the RGD (arginine-
glycine-aspartic acid) binding site of the GPIIb/IIIa
receptor. A bolus injection (0.25 mg/kg) achieves
>80% platelet receptor blockage with full inhibition
of platelet aggregation [156].

Integrelin is a synthetic cyclic heptapeptide that
includes a lysine-glycine-aspartate (KGD) sequence.
It exhibits a high affinity and specificity for the
GPIIb/IIIa integrin receptor and acts as a competitive
antagonist with a short (1.5–2 hours) half-life and
rapid onset of action [162]. Tirofiban (MK 383) is a
nonpeptide tyrosine derivative antagonist of the
RGD binding site within the platelet GPIIb/IIIa receptor with demonstrated antithrombotic efficacy.
Tirofiban demonstrates a dose-dependent inhibition
of in vivo platelet aggregation that is rapid in action
and sustained with continuous infusion of the drug
[165].

Dipyridamole interferes with platelet function by
increasing the intracellular levels of adenosine 3′,5′-
monophosphate (cyclic AMP) through inhibition
of phosphodiesterase activity [33]. Clinically,
dipyridamole provides no additional benefit to aspirin
alone in the treatment or prophylaxis of cerebrovascular and coronary thrombotic events or saphenous vein
bypass graft occlusion. It may be beneficial in combination with warfarin in the prevention of systemic
embolism in some patients with prosthetic heart
valves.

Ticlopidine (Ticlid) inhibits platelet function by
inducing a thrombasthenia-like state. Its mechanism
of action is unclear, but it is postulated to affect
platelet receptor signal transduction or to block expression of the platelet fibrinogen receptor, GPIIb/
IIIa, thus inhibiting platelet aggregation and clot
retraction. Some of its activity may be due to membrane abnormalities produced by megakaryocyto-
poiesis because ticlopidine is ineffective in vitro and
requires several days to demonstrate its maximal effect in vivo [34].

Clinical and Laboratory Predictors of Bleeding Risk

CLINICAL CHARACTERISTICS

Because thrombolytic and anticoagulant agents cannot differentiate between "bad" clot (i.e., coronary
thrombosis) and "good" clot (i.e., hemostatic plugs at

TABLE 39-2. Major risk factors for
intracranial and hemorrhage with thrombolytic therapy

Intracranial hemorrhage	Systemic hemorrhage
Intracranial tumor	Major surgery (<6 weeks)
Prior neurosurgery	Organ biopsy (<6 weeks)
Recent stroke (<6 months)	Major trauma (<6 weeks)
Head trauma (<1 months)	GI or GU bleeding (<6 months)
Acute severe hypertension	Significant bleeding diathesis
Recent transient ischemic attack	Puncture of a noncompressible vessel
	Prolonged CPR (>10 minutes)

GI = gastrointestinal; GU = genitourinary; CPR = cardiopulmonary resuscitation.
Modified, with permission, from Califf et al. [35].

TABLE 39-3. Strokes in the elderly

	n		Overall strokes (%)				Hemorrhagic strokes (%)			
			<70–75 years		>70–75 years		<70–75 years		>70–75 years	
	t-PA	SK	t-PA	SK	t-PA	SK	t-PA	SK	t-PA	SK
GISSI 2 [16]	10,028	10,067	0.7	0.8	2.7	1.6				
GUSTO I [36]	10,268	20,023	1.2	1.1	3.9	3.1	0.5	0.4	2.1	1.2

Pooled data not performed given different dosing regimen of t-PA.
t-PA = tissue plasminogen activator; SK = streptokinase.

sites of vascular injury), it is imperative to identify risk factors for hemorrhage. Significant risk factors for intracranial (ICH) and systemic hemorrhage with thrombolytic therapy are listed in Table 39-2 [35].

The risk of bleeding is consistently higher among older patients. In both the GISSI 2 and GUSTO 1 studies, total and hemorrhagic strokes were more common among the elderly and for patients who received t-PA (Table 39-3) [16,36,74]. This age-related increased susceptibility to stroke and ICH is due in part to the brittle, leaky vessels seen with amyloid angiopathy, a condition frequently observed in the elderly [37].

TIMI 2 showed a strong trend toward an increased risk of ICH in patients with chronic hypertension, although conclusive data are lacking [38]. The Thrombolytic Predictive Instrument (TPI) project collected original data from 12 clinical trials and registries and compared 19 patients with thrombolytic-related ICH to 175 matched controls. A significant relationship between advanced age, systolic blood pressure, mean arterial pressure, pulse pressure, and the occurrence of ICH was found. For example, the mean pulse pressure for patients with ICH was 63 mmHg versus 47 mmHg for those without hemorrhage ($P < 0.001$) [39].

Simoons et al. collected individual patient data from five sources, including registries from seven large thrombolytic trials involving greater than 28,000 patients and compared 150 patients with documented intracranial bleeds with 294 matched controls. Multivariate analysis identified four independent predictors of ICH: age >65 years (odds ratio [OR] 2.2, 95% confidence interval [CI] 1.4–3.5), body weight <70 kg (OR 2.1; CI 1.2–3.2), hypertension on hospital admission (OR 2.0; 95% CI 1.2–3.2), and administration of alteplase (OR 1.6; 95% CI 1.0–2.5) [40].

A major risk factor for bleeding with thrombolytic therapy is the performance of invasive procedures (i.e., cardiac catheterization, percutaneous transluminal coronary angioplasty [PTCA], intra-aortic balloon counterpulsation [IABP], and coronary artery bypass grafting [CABG]). Studies with routine early (up to 48 hours post-thrombolysis) cardiac catheterization have reported major bleeding rates of 11–20%, compared with 1–12% when catheterization has been deferred [14,41,42]. The vast majority of such complications occur at sites of vascular access.

Comorbidities such as preexisting vascular lesions, cerebral vascular disease, previous gastrointestinal bleed, trauma, renal insufficiency, alcoholism or liver failure, and cancer are additional risk factors for bleeding with thrombolytic therapy [35,40,43]. In TIMI 2, the use of calcium channel blockers was associated with an increased risk of ICH, whereas beta-blocker therapy was associated with a lower incidence of intracranial bleeding [15].

Similar patient characteristics contribute to the risk of bleeding with heparin alone. Older age, female gender, renal failure, platelet dysfunction, concomitant use of aspirin and nonsteroidal antiinflammatory drugs, and comorbidities such as recent surgery, trauma, or gastrointestinal hemorrhage, have all been implicated as risk factors for heparin-induced bleeding [44–46].

There are conflicting data on the role of age, hypertension, and the indication for warfarin as risk factors for bleeding [47–52]. The intensity of anticoagulation is the predominant risk factor. For each 0.5 increase in the prothrombin time ratio (PTR), the risk of ICH doubles (OR 2.1; 95% CI 1.4–2.9). After controlling for the intensity of anticoagulation, other independent clinical markers include a history of cerebrovascular disease (odd ratio 3.1; 95% CI 1.7–5.6) and the presence of a prosthetic heart valve (OR 2.8; 95% CI 1.3–5.8) [52]. Additional factors associated with bleeding include recent initiation of therapy, poor nutrition, liver disease, and the use of medications that potentiate the effect of coumadin or inhibit platelet function [31,47–52].

Gastrointestinal bleeding with aspirin appears to be a dose-related phenomenon. Hemorrhagic gastritis is due to local mucosal erosion and is uncommon with doses ≤100 mg/day. Pre-existent peptic ulcer disease and the concomitant use of other gastric irritants such as NSAIDs are additional risk factors [151].

LABORATORY PARAMETERS

As discussed earlier, hemostasis depends on a complex series of events, involving interactions among coagulation factors, platelets, and the vascular wall. Thrombolytic, anticoagulant, and antiplatelet therapies interrupt this process at several critical steps. While it seems intuitive that standard measurements of the products of the coagulation and fibrinolytic pathways (i.e., fibrin, fibrinogen, fibrin(ogen) degra-

dation products, plasminogen, t-PA, α_2-antiplasmin, and D-dimer) might predict bleeding risk in an individual patient, these tests do not offer the sensitivity and specificity required for routine clinical use [53,57].

Thrombolytic Therapy. Although it is true that t-PA is associated with relatively less fibrinogen depletion and hypofibrinogenemia, the incidence of bleeding in clinical trials of t-PA has been similar to that reported with SK, a non–fibrin-selective agent [16,19,36]. In fact, there is a slightly greater risk of ICH with t-PA [19,36]. Hypofibrinogenemia and elevation of fibrin(ogen) degradation products have been weakly correlated with the risk of hemorrhage. However, most hemorrhagic events during thrombolytic therapy are not associated with fibrinogen breakdown per se. The TIMI I, TIMI II, and TAMI studies showed a relationship between bleeding and peak plasma rt-PA and fibrinogen levels when major and minor bleeding events were combined [38,54–56]. These associations were too weak to be useful for monitoring individual patients. Hemorrhagic stroke was not associated with fibrinogen, fibrin(ogen) degradation product, plasminogen, or peak rt-PA levels. Fibrinogen depletion rarely results in levels low enough to cause significant bleeding and might simply serve as a marker of plasmin activity [57].

The fibrinolytic system is modulated by PAI-1, α_2-antiplasmin, and other inhibitors. Factors that decrease PAI-1 levels (high triglyceride levels, occult carbohydrate intolerance, or insulin resistance) can enhance fibrinolysis and predispose the patient to an increased risk of ICH. Similarly, the association between diabetes mellitus and occult cerebrovascular disease might also increase such risk [58].

Consumption of factors V and VIII in a lytic state might contribute to bleeding risk. However, in clinical trials, no consistent change in these levels has been documented with thrombolysis. Topol [59] reported no significant change in factor V and VIII levels with t-PA, whereas Collen [60] demonstrated a decline in the levels of these factors that was more significant with SK than with t-PA. It appears that some patients may develop significant depletion of factor V and VIII during thrombolytic therapy, the contribution of which to hemorrhagic complications is uncertain. Finally, the development of thrombocytopenia following thrombolysis, independent of its possible relation to heparin, may also contribute to hemorrhagic risk and excess mortality [69].

Anticoagulant Therapy. There is an association between the incidence of bleeding and the intensity of anticoagulation. The likelihood of bleeding is higher in those patients with an exaggerated anticoagulant response as measured by an in vitro test of coagulation. In the Urokinase Pulmonary Embolism Trial, bleeding occurred in 20% of the patients whose whole-blood clotting time was greater than 60 minutes compared with 5% in those patients whose clotting time was less than 60 minutes [61].

The activated partial thromboplastin time (aPTT) is used to monitor and adjust heparin dosing. TIMI II showed that patients with an aPTT >90 seconds had an increased frequency of major and minor bleeding [38]. Yet, this level of anticoagulation did not separate patients with from those without ICH. GUSTO I also showed that a higher aPTT was associated with a greater risk of moderate or severe bleeding and hemorrhagic strokes, with the risk dramatically increasing beyond an aPTT of 70 seconds. For aPTTs between 60 and 100 seconds, there was an approximate 1% increase in the risk of bleeding for every 10-second increase in the aPTT [63]. GUSTO 2A confirmed the association between the aPTT level and the risk of bleeding [75].

Standard clinical laboratory measurement of the aPTT is cumbersome and prone to multiple potential sources of error [64]. A prolonged laboratory turnaround time may also contribute to the common observation that therapeutic anticoagulation is rarely achieved rapidly and is often not maintained over time. Bedside aPTT monitoring has been validated [65] and has been shown to decrease the time from sample collection to data availability (3 vs. 126 minutes, $P < 0.001$) and the time to decision regarding heparin dose adjustment (14.5 minutes vs. 3 hours, $P < 0.001$) compared with standard laboratory testing [66]. More widespread use of this simple technique could lower the cumulative risk from a nontherapeutic aPTT, whether it is too low or too high.

The reliability of warfarin monitoring and reporting has improved with the development of the international normalized ratio (INR) as a method to account for the use of various thromboplastins by different laboratories. The predominant risk factor for ICH is the intensity of anticoagulation (prothrombin time ratio >2; equivalent INR >4.6–5.3; RR 3.0; 95% CI 1.9–4.7) [50]. Recent initiation of warfarin therapy (RR for the first 3 months compared with the first year, second year, and thereafter of 1.9 [95% CI 1.3–3.0], 3.0 [1.8–4.8], and 5.9 [3.8–9.3], respectively) and the variability of the prothrombin time ratio over time (RR 1.6; 95% CI 1.2–2.7) may also contribute [50].

Overall, while laboratory monitoring of thrombolytic, anticoagulant, and antiplatelet therapies has

theoretical benefit, in practice, there are several limitations. Several assays pertaining to the fibrinolytic system are not readily available, and the patient's hemostatic status is changing rapidly during therapy. In-vitro activation of the fibrinolytic system might occur, resulting in falsely lower levels of factors V and VIII, fibrinogen, plasminogen, and α_2-antiplasmin. The accuracy of any test result is greatly dependent on the method utilized. Clinically, the value of these laboratory parameters for predicting bleeding risk is extremely low [57]. The aPTT and activated clotting time (ACT), while used extensively to monitor anticoagulation, do not accurately reflect the level of anticoagulation in vivo. More elaborate testing of in vivo function of the coagulation system is being developed with assays for fibrinopeptide A (FPA), prothrombin fragment (F1.2), and thrombin-antithrombin complex (TAT) [70]. Platelet function can be evaluated by assays of proteins released by platelet activation (β-thromboglobulin, platelet factor-4) and by measuring changes in the conformation of surface glycoproteins and the bleeding time [71]. The clinical utility of such in vivo assays, however, has not been established.

Summary of Experience with Agents

THROMBOLYTIC THERAPY

Ischemic Heart Disease. Bleeding is the major complication of thrombolytic therapy; more than 70% of the hemorrhagic complications occur at vascular puncture sites [54]. Hemorrhagic stroke, the most devastating outcome, occurs relatively infrequently, with an incidence of 0.2–1% [4–19]. In the prethrombolytic era, the total stroke rate in acute MI was reported at 1.7–3.2%. Central nervous system (CNS) events typically occur within the first week of the infarct and are most commonly associated with anterior or apical infarct, large infarct size, atrial arrhythmia, cardiac pump failure (Killip class IV), or prior history of stroke [72].

In the thrombolytic era, the overall stroke rate has not changed, although the etiologies of the strokes have shifted. Limitation of infarct size and preservation of systolic function with early reperfusion have likely resulted in a decreased incidence of mural thrombi and embolic strokes. Currently, parenchymal ICH, hemorrhagic transformation of bland embolic infarcts, and subarachnoid and subdural hemorrhage constitute the major fear. The majority of such hemorrhages occur in multiple sites in the cortical and subcortical white matter (atypical of "hypertensive" strokes), usually during or within 24 hours of thrombolysis [72]. Strokes associated with acute MI can be devastating, with related mortality of 37% (range 22–50%) in thrombolytic-treated patients. The overall mortality rate is as high as 38% for cerebral infarction and as high as 60% for intracerebral hemorrhage [73]. There is a high morbidity associated with ICH, with only 31% of the patients regaining full or partial recovery (minor residual). The vast majority of patients with no lasting neurologic improvement succumb within 60 days of the ICH.

Levine recently reviewed several clinical trials comparing thrombolytic agents with conservative therapy in the treatment of acute MI [74]. The incidence of major bleeds was reported to range from 0.3% to 6% for SK, 0% to 7% for APSAC, and 0% to 10% for t-PA. For intracranial bleeds, the incidence was 0–1.3% for SK, 0–1% for APSAC, and 0–1.4% for t-PA. The incidences of major bleeds and intracranial bleeds in the conrtol population were 0–7% and 0–0.3%, respectively. Overall, the incidence of ICH appears to be slightly lower for those patients treated with SK, compared with those treated with APSAC or t-PA. These observations were confirmed by a large comparative trial (ISIS-3) involving over 40,000 patients randomized to SK, APSAC, or rt-PA [19]. The incidence of ICH was 0.2%, 0.6%, and 0.7%, respectively. The increased risk of hemorrhagic strokes associated with t-PA is more pronounced in patients over the age of 75 years [36] and demonstrates a dose-dependent effect. Patients treated with 150 mg t-PA have a 1.3% incidence of ICH compared with a 0.4% incidence in those patients receiving 100 mg rt-PA ($P < 0.01$) [14].

The GISSI-2 study compared SK ± subcutaneous heparin (12,500 U BID) with t-PA ± subcutaneous heparin. Surprisingly, there was less transfusion requirement with t-PA (RR 0.57, 95% CI 0.38–0.85) but a slightly higher incidence of minor bleeding. Overall stroke rates were similar for the two thrombolytic regimens. Subcutaneous heparin therapy was not associated with an increase in either hemorrhagic or total strokes [16].

The Global Use of Strategies to Open Occluded Arteries (GUSTO I) trial, which randomized over 40,000 patients with acute MI to one of four treatment strategies using SK, t-PA, or their combination, plus subcutaneous or intravenous heparin, found the incidence of major hemorrhage to range from 5.4% to 6.3% and the incidence of ICH from 0.49% to 0.94% [36]. In the analysis of the three strategies using intravenous heparin, there was a significant association between the level of the aPTT achieved and the incidence of moderate or severe hemorrhage, hemorrhagic stroke, and mortality [63].

GUSTO IIA studied the effect of intravenous heparin (5000 U bolus, 1000–1300 U/h to an aPTT of 60–90 seconds) versus hirudin (0.6 mg/kg bolus, 0.2 mg/kg/h without aPTT monitoring) for the treatment of acute coronary syndromes (unstable angina, non–Q-wave myocardial infarction, and ST-segment elevation MI) [75]. Patients with ST-segment elevation were eligible for thrombolytic therapy (SK or accelerated t-PA) at the discretion of the attending physician. The trial was terminated early after enrollment of 2564 patients because of excessive ICH. The overall incidence of hemorrhagic strokes was higher for patients receiving hirudin (1.3%) compared with heparin (0.7%), although this difference was not significant. The incidence of ICH was higher in patients treated with thrombolytic therapy compared with those who did not receive thrombolytic therapy (1.8% vs. 0.3%, $P < 0.001$). Of the patients receiving thrombolysis, the hemorrhagic stroke rate was similar, irrespective of whether they received heparin or hirudin (1.5% and 2.2%, respectively; $P = 0.34$) [75] (Table 39-4).

The stroke rate with heparin and thrombolysis in GUSTO IIA (2.7% with SK, 0.9% with t-PA) was higher than that reported for heparin in conjunction with SK (0.5%) or t-PA (0.7%) in GUSTO I [36], possibly reflecting the 20% higher heparin dose used in GUSTO IIA. The mean aPTT of patients with hemorrhagic stroke was 110 ± 46 seconds compared with 87 ± 36 seconds in patients without hemorrhagic stroke. GUSTO IIA also enrolled a significantly higher proportion of older patients, female patients, and those with a higher mean systolic blood pressure compared with patients enrolled in the GUSTO I study. These differences could account for the higher bleeding rates observed.

The Thrombolysis and Thrombin Inhibition in Myocardial Infarction (TIMI) 9A trial used an identical thrombolytic and antithrombotic regimen as GUSTO IIA for patients with acute MI [76]. The trial was suspended after the enrollment of 757 patients due to increased ICH compared with prior studies (1.7% hirudin, 1.9% heparin; see Table 39-4). Major spontaneous hemorrhage at nonintracranial sites occurred in 7% of hirudin-treated patients and 3% of heparin-treated patients ($P = 0.02$), whereas the incidence of major hemorrhage at instrumented sites was similar (5.2% both groups). Patients with major bleeds were older (68 vs. 61 years, $P < 0.01$), had a lower body weight (74 vs. 81 kg, $P < 0.01$), and had a higher aPTT at 12 hours after thrombolytic therapy (100 vs. 85 seconds; $P = 0.001$) [76].

TABLE 39-4. Hemorrhagic events in recent thrombolytic trials with adjuvant heparin versus hirudin

Trials	n	Year	Heparin		Hirudin	
			t-PA	SK	t-PA	SK
Major hemorrhage (%)						
HIT [108]	302	1994	1.9		6.8	
GUSTO IIA [75]	2,564	1994				
GUSTO IIB [109]	12,142	1996		1.1		1.2
TIMI-9A [76]	757	1994	4.9	4.9	7.9	12.7
TIMI-9B [77]	3,002	1996	6.1	3.9	4.9	3.9
Intracranial hemorrhage (%)						
HIT			0		3.4	
GUSTO IIA			0.9	2.7	1.7	3.2
GUSTO IIB				0.2		0.3
TIMI-9A				1.9		1.7
TIMI-9B				0.9		0.4

t-PA = tissue plasminogen activator; SK = streptokinase.

TIMI 9B modified the dose of heparin (5000 U bolus, 1000 U/h infusion) and hirudin (0.1 mg/kg bolus, 0.1 mg/kg/h infusion) and titrated both antithrombin regimens to a target aPTT of 55–85 seconds [77]. The study involved 3002 patients with acute MI treated with aspirin and either accelerated t-PA or SK. There was a significantly lower incidence of major and intracranial bleeding with this less aggressive regimen compared with the earlier TIMI 9A study. In the heparin-treated patients, the incidence of ICH was 0.9%, of major spontaneous nonintracranial bleed was 1.1%, and of major instrumented site bleed was 3.3%, compared with their respective 1.9%, 3.0%, and 5.2% incidences in TIMI 9A. The rate of major hemorrhage was lower with SK (3.9% with heparin or hirudin) compared with t-PA (6.1% with heparin, 4.9% with hirudin; see Table 39-4).

In the hirudin-treated patients, the incidence of ICH was 0.4%, of spontaneous nonintracranial bleed was 1.8%, and of major instrument site bleed was 2.4%, compared with their respective 1.7%, 7.0%, and 5.2% incidences in TIMI 9A. The dose of hirudin administered in the TIMI 9B was more effective than heparin at maintaining the aPTT in the therapeutic range but did not confer any greater benefit over heparin as adjunctive therapy to t-PA or SK in the primary endpoint (death, recurrent nonfatal MI, congestive heart failure, or cardiogenic shock by 30 days) [77].

GUSTO IIB was a continuation of the GUSTO IIA trial at a significantly lower dose of heparin (5000 U

bolus, 1000 U/h infusion) and hirudin (0.1 mg/kg bolus, 0.1 mg/kg/h infusion) in an attempt to minimize the bleeding complication [109]. In total, 12,142 patients with acute coronary syndromes were randomized. At 24 hours, the risk of death or MI was significantly lower in the hirudin group versus heparin (1.3% vs. 2.1%, P = 0.001). By 30 days, however, the benefit was less obvious (odd ratio 0.89, 95% CI 0.79–1.0, P = 0.06). There was an improved safety profile with the lower doses of heparin and hirudin, with an incidence of severe or life-threatening bleeding of 1.1% for heparin and 1.2% for hirudin, an incidence of stroke of 0.8% for heparin and 0.9% hirudin, and an incidence of ICH of 0.2% for heparin and 0.3% for hirudin (see Table 37-4) [109].

There is a wide variability in the incidence of hemorrhagic complications reported from the major trials. For instance, the rates of major bleeding for SK reported in the GISSI 1 and ISIS-2 trials were 0.3% and 0.6%, respectively, with a low incidence of ICH (0–0.3%) [4,8]. These rates are contrast with those reported from the ISAM study, in which major and intracranial bleeding were observed among 5.9% and 0.5% of the study population, respectively [9]. Such discrepancies may reflect differences in reporting or in the assiduousness with which bleeding complications were monitored and verified.

There have been several recent trials investigating newer thrombolytic agents. A small phase-I dosc-ranging (5–50 mg bolus) study of TNK-tPA demonstrated encouraging rates of 90-minute TIMI grade 3

TABLE 39-5. Intracerebral hemorrhage associated with thrombolytic therapy in acute ischemic stroke

Trial	Rx	n	Year	Spontaneous or parenchymal hemorrhage (%)		Disability or mortality	
				Thrombolytic	Control	Thrombolytic	Control
MAST-E [168]	SK	270	1994	18[b]	3.0	na	na
ASK [169]	SK	200	1995	na	na	62[c]	43
MAST-I [167]	SK	622	1995	6[a]	0.6	62	68
ECASS [170]	rt-PA	620	1995	20[b]	6.5	64	71
NINDS [166]	rt-PA	624	1995	6.4[b]	0.6	59[b]	71

[a] $P < 0.01$ versus control.
[b] $P < 0.001$ versus control.
[c] $P < 0.005$ versus control.
na = not available; Rx = treatment; SK = streptokinase; rt-PA = recombinant tissue plasminogen activator.
Modified from Adams [165], with permission.

patency (57–64%) at the 30–50 mg doses [23]. This was achieved with a relatively low rate of major hemorrhage (6.2%) compared with the 11–23% in other angiographic studies using front-loaded t-PA [34,35]. Two trials have compared the recombinant plasminogen activator (reteplase, 10 mg double bolus) to SK (INJECT) or rt-PA (RAPID II) [78,79]. The INJECT trial of 6010 patients found equivalent efficacy in the treatment of acute MI, with a non-significant excess of intracerebral events (37 vs. 30) and similar rates of overall bleeding events and need for transfusion with reteplase compared with SK [78].

RAPID II found a significantly higher rate of total patency (TIMI grade 2 or 3 flow) at 90 minutes with reteplase (83.4%) compared with alteplase (73.3%). The rates of total and hemorrhagic strokes were similar for reteplase (1.8%, 1.2%) and alteplase (2.3%, 1.9%), respectively. There were similar transfusion rates [79]. Recombinant staphylokinase (20 or 30 mg infusion over 30 minutes) achieved comparable 90-minute (62% vs. 59%) and 24-hour (89% vs. 68%) TIMI grade 3 patency as accelerated weight-adjusted rt-PA in the STAR trial [25]. Hemorrhagic complications did not differ between the two treatments, although a higher trend toward adverse bleeding was observed with rt-PA. Staphylokinase demonstrated significantly greater fibrin specificity, with no evidence of systemic fibrinogen degradation, α_2-antiplasmin consumption, or plasminogen activation during therapy [25].

Cerebrovascular Disease. There have been five randomized placebo-controlled trials of the use of intravenous thrombolytic agents (three involving 1.5

million U SK, two involving 0.9–1.1 mg/kg rt-PA) for the management of acute ischemic strokes within 4–6 hours of presentation [165–170]. All trials involving SK were stopped after interim analysis revealed a significantly higher rate of symptomatic or parenchymal hemorrhage and death in the SK patients compared with controls (Table 39-5). Use of intravenous rt-PA is also associated with a significantly higher rate of symptomatic or parenchymal hemorrhage. The NINDS trial was the only study to show a beneficial effect of rt-PA, when given very early and within 3 hours of the onset of symptoms in carefully selected patients, on death and severe disability at 24 hours and 3-month follow-up [166]. Symptomatic ICH within 36 hours after the onset of stroke occurred in 6.4% of patients given t-PA and in 0.6% patients receiving placebo ($P < 0.001$). The use of acetysalicylic acid (ASA) (300 mg) in addition to SK (1.5 million U) in the MAST-1 study was associated with a 10% incidence of ICH, compared with 6.5% with SK, 2% with ASA, and 0.6% with placebo [167].

Thromboembolic Disease. The risk of bleeding with thrombolytic therapy in the setting of venous thromboembolism is difficult to quantify given the relatively small number of patients entered into published trials. The incidence of major hemorrhage ranges from 2.7% to 30%, a threefold greater incidence than with heparin alone, although these observed differences are not statistically significant [74]. Goldhaber performed a pooled analysis of six randomized trials of SK versus heparin for the treatment of acute DVT, and reported a 3.7-fold greater efficacy of SK versus heparin ($P = 0.001$) [80]. In the three studies reporting complications, SK was associated with a threefold greater risk for major hemorrhage, defined as blood loss >1 L, transfusion requirement, or ICH. The higher incidence of bleeding in patients receiving therapy for DVT compared with patients receiving thrombolysis for acute MI probably reflects the prolonged period of lytic therapy and associated patient comorbidities, such as malignancy [74].

The initial multicenter urokinase pulmonary embolism trials (UPET1,2) reported rates of major hemorrhage of 31–45% with UK, 22% with SK, and 27% with heparin [61,62]. In more recent trials using rt-PA (100 mg over 2 hours), a lower incidence of major hemorrhage has been observed (0–25%). In these latter trials, the use of heparin alone was associated with only a 0–6% incidence of major hemorrhage [74]. Most of the major hemorrhage associated with thrombolytic therapy for pulmonary embolism occurs at sites of vascular puncture for diagnostic pulmonary angiography.

HEPARIN

Heparin can be administered in low doses subcutaneously for the prophylaxis of venous thrombosis, in higher doses intravenously to treat venous thromboembolism and acute coronary syndromes, or in very high doses during percutaneous transluminal coronary angioplasty (PTCA) or bypass surgery. The risk of bleeding is dependent on the dose, formulation, and method of heparin administration; the patient's clinical status and anticoagulant response; and the concomitant use of aspirin or thrombolytic agents [45,81]. The major mechanism of bleeding with heparin is related to its anticoagulant effect. However, heparin also interacts with platelets and can prolong bleeding time [82], induce thrombocytopenia [67,68], and increase capillary permeability [83].

Thromboembolic Disease. Although there have been no randomized trials comparing different doses of heparin, Levine et al. reviewed studies using different 24-hour dosing regimens and found a significant relationship between heparin dose and bleeding [44]. A meta-analysis of six randomized trials comparing continuous intravenous infusion with intermittent intravenous injection of heparin, and five randomized trials comparing continuous infusion to twice-daily subcutaneous injection, found an average incidence of major bleeding of 6.8% in the continuous-infusion group compared with 14.2% in the intermittent intravenous heparin group [81]. These data are confounded by the fact that the patients randomized to

intermittent intravenous injection received higher doses of heparin than the continuous-infusion group; thus, the increased bleeding could have been explained by differences in dosing. There was no difference in the incidence of bleeding between the subcutaneous heparin group (4.3%) and the continuous-infusion group (4.4%), in which total heparin doses were comparable.

The reported risks of major bleeding in trials using heparin at varying doses and methods of administration for the treatment of venous thromboembolism range from 1% to 33% [81]. The occurrence of major bleeding in contemporary studies, using weight-adjusted heparin or the standard clinical approach (5000 U bolus, 1000 U/h infusion) and monitoring of continuous infusion with either the activated partial thromboplastin time (aPTT) or heparin assay, is much less (median rate 1.8%) [81,84,85]. The weight-based heparin nomogram individualizes heparin dosing with more rapid achievement of the therapeutic range, while avoiding excess anticoagulation.

Ischemic Heart Disease. In trials comparing intravenous heparin to placebo or aspirin in patients with unstable angina (without concurrent use of thrombolytic therapy), there is no increased risk of major bleeding with heparin, and there is a nonstatistical trend toward increased minor bleeding, especially at sites of vascular access [86,87]. In the Montreal Heart Study of patients with unstable angina, the addition of ASA to heparin had no greater protective effect on the prevention of recurrent angina, MI, or death but was associated with slightly more serious bleeding (3.3% vs. 1.9%) [86].

The use of heparin as an adjunct to thrombolysis is associated with an increased risk of bleeding. In the SCATI study, patients with MI who received SK plus a 2000 U intravenous heparin bolus followed by 12,500 U subcutaneous injection twice daily had a higher incidence of bleeding compared with patients not receiving heparin (4.4% vs. 0.6%, control) [88]. In ISIS-3, adjunctive subcutaneous heparin did not increase the incidence of total stroke, but did increase the absolute incidence of cerebral hemorrhage by 0.2% [19]. GISSI z showed that subcutaneous heparin, in conjunction with SK or t-PA, caused more major bleeds, defined as blood transfusions greater than 2 units (RR 1.64; 95% CI 1.09–2.45), and minor bleeds (RR 1.88; 95% CI 1.64–2.14) compared with the non–heparin-treated patients, although there was no difference in the rate of hemorrhagic stroke [16]. In a study by Bleich and colleagues, patients randomized to intravenous heparin in addition to t-PA experienced a greater incidence of moderate or severe bleeding compared with t-PA alone (12% vs. 2%, respectively) [89]. Similar findings were observed in GUSTO 1 [36]. Other studies, however, have not demonstrated an additional risk of bleeding with heparin as an adjunct to thrombolysis [90,91].

Thrombocytopenia is often seen after heparin utilization and thrombolytic therapy, and may contribute to excess hemorrhage and mortality in patients with MI [60,67,69]. In TIMI 1, thrombocytopenia (<150,000/μL) was observed in 8% of patients treated with rt-PA and in 2% treated with SK [54]. In an analysis of the 1001 patients enrolled in parts 2, 3, and 5 of the Thrombolysis and Angioplasty in MI (TAMI) trial and in a urokinase trial of acute MI, thrombocytopenia (<100,000/μL or half baseline platelet counts) occurred in 16.4%, irrespective of the thrombolytic regimen [69]. Thrombocytopenia in patients with MI treated with heparin and thrombolytic therapy was associated with a greater drop in hematocrit, a greater need for transfusion, and a higher in-hospital mortality. Similarly, Bovill and colleagues found in the TIMI II study that thrombocytopenia after thrombolytic therapy was associated with a significant amount of excess hemorrhage, independent of other important variables such as bypass surgery, intra-aortic balloon counterpulsation (IABP), or age [38].

This form of heparin-induced thrombocytopenia is to be distinguished from the clinical syndrome of heparin-induced thrombocytopenia with associated thrombosis (HIT-T), which is characterized by a high incidence of heparin resistance, disseminated intravascular coagulation, and arterial and venous thromboembolic events. This is a life-threatening complication of heparin administration and is an immune-mediated process. The substitution of LMWH is not predictably safe in preventing this complication.

Prophylactic low-dose subcutaneous heparin is associated with a low incidence of bleeding. Collins reviewed 25 trials of heparin prophylaxis in patients undergoing thoracic, abdominal, or pelvic surgery and found a 2% absolute increase in minor bleeds, and no increase in fatal bleeds [92]. In four double-blinded randomized trials comparing heparin prophylaxis with placebo in patients undergoing surgery for hip fracture, the incidence of postoperative wound hematomas, hemoglobin depletion, or blood transfusions was similar and there were no fatal bleeds [44,92]. Other studies have suggested that there is an increase in minor bleeds and total blood loss with heparin prophylaxis [44].

LOW MOLECULAR WEIGHT HEPARINS

Low molecular weight heparins have been studied extensively for the prevention and treatment of venous thromboembolism in high-risk patients, with established safety and efficacy. In patients undergoing total knee replacement, postoperative subcutaneous twice-daily dosing of LMWH is the most effective anticoagulant-based prophylaxis regimen, superior even to low-intensity warfarin. Current data suggest a 2–9% incidence of bleeding with LMWH for regimens with equal or greater efficacy than other forms of therapy [93].

More recently, experience with LMWH has been gained in unstable angina, silent ischemia, and MI. A study of 219 patients with unstable angina randomized to aspirin (200 mg/day), aspirin plus regular heparin (400 IU/kg body weight IV), or aspirin plus LMWH (214 UIC/kg anti-Xa twice daily SC) found a significant decrease in the combined endpoint of recurrent angina, MI, urgent revascularization, major bleeding, or death with LMWH (59% vs. 63% vs. 22% incidence, respectively; $P < 0.00001$) [94]. Two episodes of major bleeding (decrease in hemoglobin >2 g/dL or the need for transfusion) occurred in two patients on standard intravenous heparin. Minor bleeds occurred in 10 patients (14.5%) on standard heparin and in one patient (1.5%) receiving LMWH ($P = 0.01$). There were no strokes in the entire cohort. A smaller study using high-dose anti-Xa (Fragmin; 240–360 U/kg/24 h SC) in 72 patients with acute anterior MI reported one ischemic cerebral stroke and three minor bleeds, all in patients receiving SK and aspirin in addition to Fragmin [95].

A large multicenter trial of 1506 patients with unstable angina or non–Q-wave MI (FRISC study group) compared subcutaneous LMWH (dalteparin, Fragmin, 120 IU/kg body weight BID for 6 days, then 7500 IU QD for 35–45 days) with placebo injection [96]. The rate of the combined endpoint (death, new MI, revascularization, or need for intravenous heparin) was lower in the dalteparin group (5.4% vs. 10.3%; RR 0.52; 95% CI 0.37–0.75). There was no difference in the incidence of major bleeds, defined as a decrease in hemoglobin >2 g/dL with associated symptoms, ICH, or bleeding leading to transfusion, interruption of treatment, or death (0.8% dalteparin vs. 0.5% placebo). There was a higher rate of minor bleeds with dalteparin, especially during the acute phase (8.2% vs. 0.3% placebo).

Of note, the initial study dose of 150 IU/kg body weight twice daily was discontinued after enrollment of 116 patients, when an interim safety analysis revealed an excess incidence of major (6%) and minor (14%) hemorrhage during the first 6 days of dalteparin therapy. A follow-up study (FRIC) compared LMWH (dalteparin, 120 IU/kg BID) with weight-adjusted unfractionated intravenous heparin during the acute open phase (day 1–6) and dalteparin (7500 IU qd) versus placebo in the prolonged treatment phase (days 6–45) in 1482 patients with unstable angina or non–Q-wave MI [97]. There was no difference in the incidence of the combined clinical endpoint of death, MI, or recurrent angina during the first 6 days of therapy and over the next 39 days (6–45 days). A possible explanation for the discrepancy in outcome from the earlier FRISC study is the use of unfractionated heparin during the acute phase in the active control group of the current study. There was no difference in the incidence of major bleeds (approximately 1% for both), but a greater number of minor bleeding events occurred with dalteparin (5.1%) compared with placebo (2.8%) during the second phase of follow-up.

ANTITHROMBINS
Theoretically, the bleeding risk associated with the direct thrombin inhibitors should be lower than that of the indirect antithrombins because of their greater specificity, shorter half-life, and lack of antiplatelet effects. Several phase I studies have reported low bleeding rates using hirulog, [98], hirudin [99], and argatroban [100]. Several phase II and III trials have examined the role of thrombin inhibitors in unstable angina, as adjuncts to thrombolysis in MI, during PTCA, and in the treatment of venous thrombosis.

Ischemic Heart Disease. Lidon and colleagues used three escalating doses of hirulog given over 72 hours in 55 patients with unstable angina and reported no deaths, infarctions, or bleeding complications [101]. TIMI 7 randomized 410 patients with unstable angina to four escalating doses of hirulog, given with aspirin, and found a significant reduction in death or nonfatal MI in those patients treated with the higher dose of hirulog (1 mg/kg/h × 72 hours) at hospital discharge and at the 6-week follow-up. Hirulog therapy had to be discontinued prematurely in only one patient due to major hemorrhage [102]. Gold and colleagues studied the effects of argatroban in 43 patients and found a dose-dependent prolongation of the aPTT and suppressed fibrinopeptide A levels (a measure of thrombin activity), without an effect on bleeding time or the rate of spontaneous bleeding. No clinical bleeding occurred during or 24 hours after drug infusion [103]. Topol et al. compared escalating doses of hirudin (0.05, 0.10, 0.20, and 0.30 mg/kg/h) with two doses of heparin (target aPTT of 65–90 or 90–110 seconds) in 163 patients with unstable an-

gina and a baseline angiogram indicating a 60% or greater stenosis in the culprit coronary artery. There were seven major bleeds, with no more than two occurring in any treatment group. All were procedure related or occurred in association with CABG. There were three spontaneous bleeds, none requiring transfusion, and no ICH [104].

In a pilot angiographic study, Lidon and colleagues randomized 42 patients to heparin or hirulog after streptokinase for acute MI and found greater 90-minute (77% vs. 47%, $P < 0.05$) and 120-minute (87% vs. 47%, $P < 0.01$) TIMI 2 or TIMI 3 patency with hirulog versus heparin. Total bleeding complications were the same, although there was a trend toward a higher incidence of severe bleeding with heparin (27%) compared with hirulog (13%) [105]. The TIMI 5 trial compared hirudin with heparin in 246 MI patients treated with aspirin and accelerated rt-PA [106]. Major spontaneous bleeding occurred more frequently in patients given heparin versus hirudin (4.7% vs. 1.2%; $P = 0.09$), whereas major hemorrhage at sites of instrumentation occurred with similar frequency (18.6% vs. 16.4%). Total major hemorrhage was not statistically different between the two treatments (23.3%, heparin vs. 17.5%, hirudin), although the incidence of hemorrhage at the highest (0.6 mg/kg bolus followed by 0.2 mg/kg/h fixed infusion for 5 days) hirudin dose (29.4%) was significantly higher than the 12.2% incidence of all other hirudin doses combined [106]. In this study, the hirudin infusion was not adjusted on the basis of the aPTT; as a safety measure, however the infusion rate was halved if the aPTT was >150 seconds after 24 hours.

The Hirudin for the Improvement of Thrombolysis (HIT) study evaluated three escalating doses of hirudin in conjunction with aspirin and accelerated t-PA for the treatment of ST-segment elevation MI. There were only three spontaneous bleeds in the entire study group, but an increase in puncture-site bleeding in the highest dose (0.4 mg/kg bolus followed by 0.15 mg/kg/h for 48 hours) hirudin group (5 of 83 patients) [107]. A larger phase 3 trial (HIT III), comparing high-dose hirudin (0.4 mg/kg bolus, 0.15 mg/kg/h infusion for 48–72 hours) with heparin therapy following thrombolysis, was stopped prematurely due to excessive intracranial bleeding (5 hemorrhagic strokes/148 patients) in the hirudin-treated group (vs. heparin, 0/154 patients). After considering other major bleeding events, the total rates of major hemorrhage in the hirudin- and heparin-treated groups were 6.8% and 1.9%, respectively (see Table 39-4) [108].

Similarly alarming results were obtained in GUSTO IIA and TIMI 9A; as a result, GUSTO IIB and TIMI 9B both used a substantially lower dose of hirudin (described earlier). Although it would appear that a survival benefit was not realized at this lower dose of hirudin, a recent prospective meta-analysis of the GUSTO IIB and TIMI 9B trials demonstrated a significant reduction in reinfarction at 24 hours (odds ratio 0.63; 95% CI 0.43–0.9, $P = 0.018$) and a persistent 14% reduction at 30 days ($P = 0.024$).

Interventional Trials. Hirudin and hirulog, as a replacement for heparin, have been found to be safe and effective in patients undergoing diagnostic angiography and angioplasty [110–112]. In a dose-escalating study of hirulog (0.15 mg/kg bolus, 0.6 mg/kg/h infusion to a maximum dose of 0.55 mg/kg bolus, 2.2 mg/kg/h infusion) in 291 patients pretreated with 325 mg aspirin undergoing elective angioplasty, only one patient (0.34%) had a significant bleeding complication requiring 2-unit RBC transfusion, although there were minor bleeds in 25% [112]. A 24-hour infusion of hirudin or heparin, adjusted to the aPTT, in 113 patients with chronic stable angina at the time of elective angioplasty resulted in no spontaneous bleeding and four puncture site bleeds, all in the hirudin-treated patients [113].

A large-scale European multicenter trial, Hirudin in a European Restenosis Prevention Trial Versus Heparin Treatment in PTCA Patients (HELVETICA), compared hirudin with heparin in patients with unstable angina undergoing coronary angioplasty and found similar rates of major and minor bleeding for the two groups [114]. Only one patient (IV plus SC heparin cohort) in this study developed an intracranial bleed. In a large trial of 4312 patients undergoing angioplasty for unstable or postinfarct angina, hirulog-treated patients (vs. heparin-treated) demonstrated a lower incidence of vascular puncture site bleeds (29.1% vs. 61.6%; $P < 0.001$), hematuria (16.6% vs. 20.6%; $P < 0.001$), bleeds requiring packed red cell transfusion (3.7% vs. 8.6%; $P < 0.001$), and hematemesis (0.8% vs. 1.9%; $P = 0.001$) [115].

Venous Thrombosis Prophylaxis. A dose-escalating study of subcutaneous hirulog (ranging from 0.3 mg/kg q12h to 1 mg/kg q8h) in 222 patients undergoing major orthopedic surgery for prophylaxis of venous thrombosis reported a blee-ding event rate of less than 5% in all doses examined [116]. A similar dose-escalating trial using hirudin (10, 15, 20, or 40 mg SC q12h for 8–10 days) in patients undergoing elective hip replacement recorded no intracerebral, intraocular, intraspinal, or retroperitoneal bleeds [117].

Five patients, including all three patients given the highest dose of hirudin, experienced major bleeding, defined as either a decrease in hemoglobin of 5 g/dL or total blood loss or transfusion >3500 mL. A larger randomized multicenter trial comparing hirudin (10, 15, and 20 mg SC BID) with heparin (5000 U SC TID) in 1120 patients undergoing elective total hip replacement revealed a similar median blood loss in all treatment groups [118]. In two small phase 2 studies evaluating hirudin and hirulog in the treatment of acute DVT, there was no clinically overt bleeding or major adverse experience [119,120].

ANTICOAGULANTS

Oral anticoagulation with warfarin is used for the treatment of ischemic heart disease, ischemic cerebral vascular disease, and venous thrombosis, and for the prevention of thromboembolism in patients with atrial fibrillation and prosthetic heart valves. A strong correlation exists between the level of anticoagulation and bleeding (Table 39-6) [121]. Those patients managed with moderate-intensity warfarin (targeted INR = 2–2.5) have a bleeding rate of 4–6%, compared with patients with higher intensity anticoagulation (targeted INR = 2.5–4.5), whose bleeding rate is 14–22% [122,124]. Independent clinical markers of an increased risk of bleeding include a history of cerebrovascular disease and the presence of a prosthetic heart valve [52]. The roles of age, hypertension, and the indication for anticoagulation remain controversial.

Ischemic Heart Disease. In patients anticoagulated for ischemic heart disease, the risk of bleeding has ranged from 3.8% to 36.5%, with the incidence of major bleeding ranging from 0% to 10% and fatal bleeding ranging from 0% to 2.9% [81]. In the Sixty Plus study, 878 patients post MI were randomized to continue oral anticoagulation (INR 2.7–4.5) or to substitute a placebo. There was a significant reduction in the 2-year incidence of total mortality (7.6% vs. 13.4%, $P = 0.017$) and reinfarction (5.9% vs. 15.9%, $P < 0.001$) with anticoagulation, without a concomitant increase in the rate of ICH [138]. Major extracranial hemorrhage (leading to protocol deviation) was observed in 3 placebo patients and in 27 patients on anticoagulation. The Warfarin-Reinfarction Study (WARIS) reported a 24% reduction in total mortality, a 34% reduction in reinfarction, and a 55% risk reduction in total cerebrovascular accidents in warfarin-treated (target INR 2.8–4.8) patients compared with control patients following acute MI ($P < 0.05$). Serious bleeding was noted in 0.6%/y warfarin-treated patients [139]. The

TABLE 39-6. Bleeding as a function of INR

Indication	Follow-up (months)	Patients with bleeding complications (%)			
		INR 2.0–3.0	INR 1.9–3.6	INR 2.0–4.5	INR 7.4–10.8
DVT treatment [122]	3	4.3	—	22.4	—
Tissue valve replacement [123]	3	5.9	—	13.9	—
Mechanical valve replacement [137]	—	—	21.3	—	42.4
Mechanical valve replacement [125]	11[a]	3.9	—	20.8	—

[a] Plus aspirin and dipyridamole.
INR = International Normalized Ratio; DVT = deep venous thrombosis.
Reproduced with permission from Douketis et al. [121].

ASPECT research group randomized over 3400 patients to placebo or oral anticoagulation with warfarin (target INR 2.8–4.8) following an acute MI and found a statistically significant increased rate of major bleeding with warfarin (1.5%/y vs. 0.2%/y, control; hazard ratio 9.05, 95%, CI 3.9–21) [140].

Atrial Fibrillation. Six randomized controlled trials (RCTs) have examined the role of long-term oral anticoagulation (INR range 1.5–4.5) in the treatment of AF (Table 39-7) [128–133]. Analysis of pooled data revealed an annual stroke rate of 4.5% for the control patients and 1.4% for the warfarin-treated patient (risk reduction 68%, 95% CI 50–79%) [134]. The annual rate of major bleeding (ICH or bleed requiring hospitalization) in the first five trials was 1.0% for control, 1.0% for aspirin, and 1.3% for the warfarin-treated patients. The reported annual incidence of major bleeding ranged from 0.5% to 1.8% for control, from 0.9% to 1.4% for aspirin, and from 0.6% to 2.5% for warfarin in the individual trials (target anticoagulation INR 2–4.2; PTR 1.2–1.8) [81]. Overall, the median rates of major bleeding and fatal bleeding were 1.7%/y and 0.2%/y, respectively for warfarin therapy. SPAF II reported a significantly higher rate of major hemorrhage in older patients (>75 years) compared with a younger age group (<75 years) receiving warfarin (4.2% vs. 1.7%, respectively) or aspirin therapy (1.6% vs. 0.9%, respectively) [133,135]. For the older patients, the incidence of ICH was 0.8%/y for the aspirin-treated group compared with 1.8%/y for the warfarin-treated group (P = 0.05). The ICH rate in patients ≥75 years old is substantially higher than the pooled annual rate of 0.3% reported from the other trials. The higher bleeding rate in SPAF II could be explained in part by the higher intensity of anticoagulation (upper range of INR of 4.5).

Heart Valve Replacement. Studies of long-term anticoagulation with warfarin for patients with mechanical heart valves or high-risk patients with tissue valves (AF or a history of thromboembolism) confirmed the correlation between the intensity of therapy and the incidence of bleeding complications. Trials using less intense anticoagulation regimens (INR 2–2.5) have reported substantially less bleeding complication without loss of antithrombotic efficacy [122,136,137]. In the trials of oral anticoagulation for heart valve replacement, the median rate of major bleeding was 2.4%/y, with a median rate of fatal bleeds of 0.7%/y [81].

Turpie et al. reported on the efficacy and safety of adding ASA (100 mg aspirin) to high-intensity (INR 3–4.5) warfarin therapy in patients with a mechanical heart valve or with a tissue valve plus AF or a history of thromboembolism. The combined therapy reduced the incidence of major systemic emboli, nonfatal ICH, or death from hemorrhage or vascular causes by 61% (P = 0.005). The addition of ASA reduced all-cause mortality, particularly mortality from vascular causes. Aspirin, however, increased the incidence of major hemorrhage (12.9% vs. 10.3%, P = NS) and total hemorrhage (38.7% vs. 26.1%, P < 0.05) over warfarin alone [124].

Antman et al. demonstrated the efficacy of low-intensity anticoagulation in patients with heart valve replacement. High-dose antiplatelet therapy with ASA (660 mg) plus dipyridamole (150 mg) in conjunction with low-intensity anticoagulation (INR 2–3) lowered thromboembolic complications, with less bleeding (3.9% vs. 20.8%, P < 0.05) than in combination with high-intensity anticoagulation (INR 3–4.5) [125]. This same group of investigators recently reported that low-dose ASA (100 mg) with low-intensity anticoagulation (INR 2–3) is as effective as high-dose ASA (650 mg) in preventing systemic

TABLE 39-7. Hemorrhage events associated with antithrombotic therapy in atrial fibrillation trials

	No. patients	Mean yr F/U	Target INR	Major bleed %/y		
				Warfarin	ASA	Placebo
AFASAK [130]	1007	1.2	2.8–4.2	0.6	0.3	0
SPAF [129]	1330	1.3	2.0–4.5	1.5	1.4	1.6
BAATAF [128]	420	2.2	1.5–2.7	0.9		0.4
CAFA [132]	383	1.3	2.0–3.0	2.5		0.5
SPINAF [131]	525	1.8	1.4–2.8	1.3		0.9
SPAFII [133]	1100	2.7	2.0–4.5	1.7	0.9 (<75 y)	
				4.2	1.6 (>75 y)	

F/U = follow-up; ASA = acetylsalicylic acid; INR = International Normalized Ratio.

emboli, with a significant decrease in total bleeding events (15.9% vs. 24.3%, $P = 0.035$) [126]. A recent multicenter prospectively randomized trial (AREVA) compared low-dose (INR 2–3) with standard-dose (INR 3–4.5) anticoagulation for mechanical prosthetic heart valves (95% in aortic position). This trial demonstrated similar protection from thromboembolic events, with a significant decrease in all hemorrhagic events (34 vs. 56 events, $P < 0.01$) and a trend toward lower major hemorrhagic events (13 vs. 19 events, $P = 0.29$) in the low-intensity regimen [127].

Thromboembolic Disease. In patients receiving anticoagulation for venous thromboembolism, the incidence of major hemorrhage is low, especially if less intense therapy is used. Of the trials reported, the median rate of major bleeding was 0.9%.

Among 1283 patients in seven trials examined, there was only one fatal bleed [81]. This is in contradistinction to those patients receiving oral anticoagulation therapy for cerebrovascular disease, in which the highest bleeding rates are reported. The risk of total bleeds range from 12% to 39%, with major bleeds (mostly intracerebral) occurring in 2–13%, and fatal hemorrhage occurring in 2–7% [141–143].

ANTIPLATELET AGENTS

Aspirin. Aspirin alone rarely causes significant bleeding, except in patients with a bleeding diathesis or those being treated with anticoagulants. In primary prevention studies evaluating cardiovascular endpoints, a small increase in hemorrhagic strokes of borderline significance (relative risk 2.14, $P = 0.06$)

has been demonstrated [144,145]. In secondary prevention, aspirin clearly reduces the risk of stroke [146–148]. A large meta-analysis from the Antiplatelet Trialist's Collaboration group reported on vascular events in 145 randomized trials involving over 100,000 patients treated with a variety of antiplatelet regimens [149]. Overall, there was a reduction in nonfatal MI of 34%, nonfatal strokes among high-risk patients of 31%, and vascular death of 17% in the treated patients. Aspirin in conjunction with thrombolytic therapy prolongs the bleeding time and increases the risk of minor bleeds [4,6]. Aspirin in combination with warfarin does increase the risk of minor hemorrhage and shows a trend toward increased risk of major hemorrhage in patients with unstable angina, mechanical heart valves, or tissue valve with additional risk factors for thromboembolic complication [121,124,150]. Aspirin has been shown to produce a dose-related increase in acute gastric bleeding, due to its direct effect on the gastric mucosa [151].

Ticlopidine. The Ticlopidine Aspirin Stroke Study, a blinded multicenter trial, compared the effects of ticlopidine (250 mg BID) with aspirin (650 mg BID) on the risk of stroke or death in 3069 patients with recent transient or mild persistent focal cerebral or retinal ischemia [152]. There was a 12% risk reduction in the 3-year event rate for nonfatal strokes or death and a 21% reduction in the risk of subsequent fatal or nonfatal strokes with ticlopidine compared with aspirin. Nine percent of patients treated with ticlopidine and 10% of aspirin-treated patients reported some evidence of bleeding (bruising, petechiae, epistaxis, microscopic hematuria, gastrointestinal) [152]. In an older trial, combination therapy with 81 mg aspirin and 100 mg ticlopidine for cerebral ischemia significantly improved the inhibition of platelet aggregation induced by arachidonic acid, adenosine diphosphate, and platelet activating factor compared with aspirin (300 mg) or ticlopidine (200 mg) alone [153]. Minor bleeding complications tended to occur sooner, more often, and were more prolonged with combination therapy for cerebral ischemia.

In a study of ticlopidine versus placebo added to conventional therapy (not including aspirin) in the treatment of unstable angina, there was a 46.3% (P = 0.009) reduction in the primary endpoint of vascular death and nonfatal MI, and a 53.2% (P = 0.006) decline in the incidence of fatal and nonfatal MI. There were only four minor bleeding episodes reported in the 314 patients receiving ticlopidine [154].

Currently, the major role for ticlopidine is the prevention of intracoronary stent thrombosis. In a randomized comparison of antiplatelet therapy (250 mg BID ticlopidine for 4 weeks, 100 mg aspirin) versus anticoagulant therapy (heparin infusion 5–10 days, phenprocoumon to INR 3.5–4.5, 100 mg aspirin), antiplatelet therapy reduced the risk of MI by 82%, the need for repeat intervention by 78%, and peripheral vascular complication by 87% compared with anticoagulation (P < 0.02). Stent occlusion occurred in 0.8% of the antiplatelet therapy group and in 5.4% of the anticoagulant therapy group (RR 0.14; 95% CI 0.02–0.62). There were no severe hemorrhagic events (bleeds requiring transfusion or surgery, or associated with organ dysfunction) in the antiplatelet group and 17 (6.5%) events in the anticoagulant group. One patient in the antiplatelet group had an ischemic stroke [155].

Glycoprotein IIb/IIIa Receptor Antagonists. A large clinical angiographic trial, Evaluation of c7E3 for the Prevention of Ischemic Complications (EPIC), randomized 2099 patients undergoing coronary angioplasty or atherectomy and felt to be at high risk for abrupt vessel closure, as defined by (1) acute evolving MI within 12 hours after onset of symptoms necessitating direct or "rescue" percutaneous intervention, (2) early postinfarction angina or unstable angina with at least two episodes of angina at rest associated with changes on the resting ECG despite medical therapy, or (3) clinical or angiographic characteristics indicating high risk for PTCA. Patients were randomized to placebo bolus and placebo infusion, c7E3 bolus (0.25 mg/kg) and placebo infusion, or c7E3 bolus (0.25 mg/kg) and infusion (10 μg/min). All patients received bolus heparin (ACT 300–350)

during the procedure and a continuous 12-hour infusion after the procedure to an aPTT 1.5–2.5× control.

The GPIIb/IIIa antagonist, c7E3 (bolus and infusion), reduced the frequency of a composite endpoint (death, nonfatal MI, repeat revascularization, and procedural failure requiring stent or IABP) by 35% at 30 days (8.3 vs. 12.8% control, P = 0.008), but at a cost of increased bleeding complications, mostly at the vascular access site. Major bleeding complications unrelated to bypass surgery occurred in 3.3%, 8.6%, and 10.6%, and blood product transfusion was required in 7.5%, 14.0%, and 16.8% of patients treated with placebo, c7E3 bolus, and c7E3 bolus plus infusion, respectively. Overall, there was a 112% relative increase in major bleeds (from 6.6% to 14%, P < 0.001), a 74% relative increase in minor bleeds (from 9.8% to 16.9%, P < 0.001), as well as a 125% relative increase in transfusion requirement (from 7.5% to 16.8%, P < 0.001) with c7E3 [157,158]. Most major bleeding complications occurred at the femoral access site (71% of the nonspontaneous hemorrhagic complications). Access site complications also accounted for 78% of the total minor bleeds. Spontaneous major organ bleeding (1.3%) and nonspontaneous bleeding (6.2%) events occurred in more patients receiving c7E3, and were more common in those patients receiving bolus plus infusion. Strokes (0.7%), ICH (0.3%), and death (0.9%) as a result of major bleeding were rare. Among patients undergoing CABG <24 hours after study drug infusion, the estimated blood loss was 6.9, 7.3, and 8.5 units in the placebo, bolus, and bolus plus infusion therapy groups, respectively. Risk factors for major bleeding complications with c7E3 included age, female sex, lower weight, and duration and complexity of procedure [158].

A preliminary study, PROLOG, examined c7E3 bolus and infusion in 103 patients undergoing angioplasty, with randomization to high-dose (100 U/kg) or low-dose (70 U/kg) heparin, and found similar rates of major and minor bleeds. Patients randomized to the low-dose heparin and early sheath removal had no transfusion requirement or major bleed, and demonstrated no compromise in efficacy [159]. A larger 4500 patient trial, EPILOG (Evaluation of PTCA to Improve Long-term Outcome by c7E3 GP11b/IIIa Receptor Blockade), examined the safety and efficacy of weight-adjusted c7E3 Fab (0.25 mg/kg bolus, 0.125 μg/kg/min infusion) plus standard-dose (100 U/kg bolus, titrated ACT >300s) or lower dose (70 U/kg, ACT >200s) weight-adjusted heparin in both high- and low-risk patients undergoing coronary angioplasty. This trial was terminated prematurely after enrollment of 2792 patients when an interim analysis revealed a highly significant 68% reduction in the combined endpoint of death or MI in patients receiving c7E3 plus low-dose heparin (2.6%) or c7E3 plus standard heparin (3.6%) versus standard heparin alone (8.1%) [160,161]. In contrast to the relatively high incidence of bleeding in the EPIC study (14% for c7E3), the incidence of bleeding was markedly reduced (1.8% low-dose heparin plus c7E3, 3.5% standard heparin plus c7E3, 3.1% standard heparin). The treatment strategy using weight-adjusted, low-dose heparin had the greatest efficacy and safety.

The IMPACT trial studied the GPIIb/IIIa antagonist, Integrelin (90 μg/kg bolus, 1 μg/kg/min infusion for 4 or 12 hours), in 150 patients undergoing elective percutaneous coronary intervention [162]. Major bleeding occurred in 5% of patients treated with Integrelin compared with 8% for placebo. Minor bleeding, primarily at vascular access sites, occurred in 40% of the Integrelin group and 14% of the placebo group. A greater proportion of the patients receiving Integrelin required transfusion of fresh-frozen plasma or platelets. IMPACT II randomized 4010 patients undergoing coronary intervention to placebo versus bolus/low-dose 24-hour infusion Integrelin versus bolus/high-dose 24-hour infusion Integrelin. Weight-adjusted heparin was used during intervention and was stopped 4 hours prior to sheath removal. At 24 hours, there was a significant relative reduction of 30–35% in the composite endpoint of death, MI, CABG, repeat urgent/emergent angioplasty, or stent for abrupt closure with both integrelin dosing strategies. This benefit was lower, but still present, at 30 days (13–19%) [160]. Moderate to severe vascular access site bleeding occurred in more Integrelin-treated patients (8.8% vs. 5.3% placebo; $P = 0.001$). Early sheath removal (5.6% vs. 9.6% sheath >12 hours, $P = 0.001$) and avoidance of venous sheaths (5.7% vs. 8.4% with sheaths; $P = 0.002$) reduced the risk of vascular complication. Overall, the need for surgical repair was rare (1%) and did not correlate with treatment, arterial sheath size, removal time, or use of a venous sheath [163]. Major bleeding (according to TIMI criteria) was the same in all three treatment groups.

A pilot study (TAMI 8) examined the safety of m7E3 after t-PA in 70 patients with acute MI. Improved patency with less recurrent ischemia and without an increased risk of bleeding was demonstrated [164]. Blood transfusion was required in 20% of the patients receiving c7E3 Fab compared with 40% of the control patients. Major bleeds occurred in 25% of the c7E3 Fab-treated patients and in 50% of

the control patients and minor bleeds occurred in 22% of the treated patients compared with 10% of the control. There was a dose-dependent increase in minor and major bleeds from 0.1 mg/kg to 0.25 mg/kg c7E3 Fab.

The CAPTURE study examined the role of c7E3 (0.25 mg/kg bolus, 10 μg/kg/min infusion) in refractory unstable angina patients undergoing angioplasty [161]. The trial was stopped early after an interim analysis of 1050 patients revealed a reduction in the combined endpoint of death, MI, or urgent reintervention from 16.4% in the placebo group to 10.8% in patients receiving c7E3. c7E3 was associated with an increased risk of major bleeding complication (from 1.7% incidence to 2.9%). Strokes were observed in 3 of 532 placebo-treated patients and in only 1 of 518 c7E3-treated patients.

An initial dose-ranging study of Tirofiban (MK-383) platelet IIb/IIIa blockage in 93 high-risk patients undergoing coronary angioplasty demonstrated relative safety with this drug [165]. There was no corrective vascular surgery, ICH, or retroperitoneal hemorrhage reported in the trial. The overall incidences of bleeding events was 4.8%, 3.3%, and 13.6% for the three escalating dose regimens. A large randomized, double-blind, placebo-controlled trial of Tirofiban (RESTORE) enrolled 2100 patients undergoing angioplasty for acute coronary syndromes [160,161]. At 2 days, the composite endpoint of death, nonfatal MI, revascularization due to recurrent ischemia, or insertion of stent for abrupt closure was reduced by 38% ($P < 0.005$). Major bleeding (defined as a decrease in hemoglobin >5 g/dL, transfusion >2 units, retroperitoneal hemorrhage or ICH) occurred in 4.2% of the placebo- and 5.4% of the Tirofiban-treated patients (RR 1.29, 95% CI 0.88–1.89, $P = 0.225$). In patients undergoing early CABG, there were equivalent rates of major hemorrhage.

Recommendation for Clinical Use

The beneficial effects of thrombolytic, anticoagulant, and antiplatelet therapy for the acute coronary syndromes and thromboembolic diseases have been well established. Bleeding continues to be the major risk involved with their clinical use. Much has been learned by both investigation and clinical experience regarding the optimal use of these agents and the final balance between efficacy and bleeding. Therapies that combine agents from different classes can be powerfully effective, yet the hemorrhagic cost must be justified.

The risk of major systemic hemorrhage is essentially the same among the most commonly used thrombolytic agents (SK, APSAC, t-PA), despite their varying properties and fibrin specificity. There appears to be a slight excess of total stroke and ICH with t-PA. Patient characteristics that confer an increased risk of bleeding have been identified and include: age, female gender, low body weight, presenting hypertension, and a prior history of cerebrovascular disease. Aggressive adjunctive therapy with heparin and hirudin increases the risk of ICH associated with thrombolytic therapy, and in a dose-dependent manner. This adverse interaction highlights the need for vigilant assessment of patient risk factors, close monitoring of anticoagulant effect, and careful delineation of the optimal dosing and duration of therapy of the specific anticoagulant and thrombolytic agent chosen. Consideration should be given to the use of weight-adjusted heparin with diligent (possibly bedside) monitoring of the aPTT. Similarly the dose of hirudin should be the lowest possible to achieve a target aPTT of 65–80 seconds.

Despite the relative risk, thrombolytic therapy should be considered in eligible patients presenting within 12 hours of the onset of symptoms compatible with an acute MI. If timely and expert primary PTCA is not available, SK might be considered for those patients deemed at relatively higher risk for hemorrhagic complications on the basis of their clinical characteristics and for patients with small anterior or inferior MI who present relatively late (6–12 hours).

Accelerated t-PA has otherwise become the standard thrombolytic regimen. There are currently no convincing clinical data to support the need for intravenous heparin as an adjunct to SK. Intravenous heparin should be used in conjunction with t-PA, but the duration should be limited to 24–48 hours in the absence of a specific indication for its longer use. Given the lack of compelling advantage over heparin at conventional doses, hirudin is not currently recommended as conjunctive therapy for MI.

The use of t-PA for acute ischemic stroke should be restricted to patients who present within 3 hours of symptom onset to centers with neurological and neurosurgical expertise. Thrombolytic therapy can be life saving in the treatment of a hemodynamically compromising massive pulmonary embolus. The incidence of significant hemorrhage is high when thrombolytic therapy has been used for the treatment of DVT and PE, possibly related to the dose and duration of the infusion and the need for invasive pulmonary angiography. Current experience with t-PA (100 mg over 2 hours) has improved on the complication. Careful selection of candidates for thrombolytic therapy with exclusion of patients with associated comorbidities known to increase the risk of bleeding might minimize these complications.

The risk of bleeding associated with intravenous heparin for the treatment of venous thromboembolism is less than 5%. This risk is increased with higher heparin doses, intermittent intravenous boluses, and prolonged therapy. The use of heparin alone in patients with acute coronary syndromes does not increase the hemorrhagic risk. However, its use in association with aspirin or thrombolytic agents magnifies the risk. Thrombocytopenia is associated with increased risk of bleeding and death, when observed in patients with acute MI treated with heparin and thrombolytic therapy. Prophylactic low-dose subcutaneous heparin is associated with an increased in minor bleeding at the operative site of patients undergoing orthopedic surgery.

LMWH has proven efficacy in unstable angina, non–Q-wave MI, and venous thromboembolism. It is currently the recommended prophylactic treatment of choice for patients undergoing orthopedic procedures and has been used extensively in the long-term treatment of DVT. Its advantages over standard unfractionated heparin include better bioavailability, longer elimination half-life, more predictable anticoagulant response, greater anti–factor Xa activity, and a safety and efficacy profile not requiring laboratory monitoring.

The risk of oral anticoagulants in patients with atrial fibrillation, venous thromboembolism, or mechanical heart valves is predominantly dependent on the intensity of anticoagulation. Evidence suggests that low-intensity therapy (INR 2–3) is effective and is associated with a lower risk of bleeding. Other contributors to the risk of bleeding include patient characteristics, concomitant drugs interfering with hemostasis or warfarin metabolism, and the length of therapy. Aspirin and other antiplatelet agents increase the risk of bleeding. Their routine use in conjunction with oral anticoagulation is not recommended. Consideration of the addition of low-dose aspirin can be made if there is evidence of ongoing thromboembolism despite adequate oral anticoagulation. Careful instruction to patients regarding their diet, concomitant medication, reporting of their symptoms, and monitoring of anticoagulation levels is critical, given the long-term nature of the therapy.

Aspirin has proven efficacy both in primary and secondary prevention of cardiovascular events. Aspirin is indicated in patients with coronary artery disease, acute MI, transient cerebral vascular ischemia, thrombotic stroke, and peripheral artery disease. The bleeding risk associated with aspirin is low and dose dependent. Doses as low as 75–100 mg are efficacious for long-term use, although an initial dose of 160–325 mg is recommended in the acute setting. The bleeding risk is increased in conjunction with thrombolytic, antithrombotic, and anticoagulant agents and the lowest effective aspirin dose should be used.

The weight of evidence suggests that a GPIIb/IIIa receptor antagonist should be used in all interventional patients deemed at high risk for abrupt vessel closure as defined in the EPIC trial. The GPIIb/IIIa receptor antagonists substantially reduce the risk of death, reinfarction, and the need for repeat revascularization in patients undergoing coronary angioplasty, but does carry a high risk of bleeding. The EPILOG trial extended the observed benefit to other angioplasty patients, including those patients at low risk for abrupt closure. However, given the enormous cost of this therapy and the increased hemorrhagic risk, selective use is still recommended. Based on the EPIC and EPILOG trials, the recommended regimen for c7E3 is currently 0.25 mg/kg bolus and a 0.125 µg/kg/min 12-hour infusion with low-dose weight-adjusted heparin (70 U/kg, ACT >200s). This regimen and the early removal of vascular sheaths have demonstrated improved safety.

References

1. Salzman EW, Hirsh J. Prevention of venous thromboembolism. In Coleman RW, Hirsh J, Marder VJ, et al. (eds). Hemostasis and Thrombosis: Basic Principles and Clinical Practice, 3rd ed. Philadelphia: JB Lippincott, 1994:1332.

2. Feinberg WM, Blackshear JL, Laupacis A, et al. Prevalence, age distribution, and gender of patients with atrial fibrillation. Arch Intern Med 155:469, 1995.

3. Heart and Stroke Facts, American Heart Association, 1996.

4. ISIS-2 (Second International Study of Infarct Survival) Collaborative Group. Randomized trial of intravenous streptokinase, oral aspirin, both, or neither among 17,187 cases of suspected acute myocardial infarction: ISIS-2. Lancet 1:349, 1988.

5. Brodie BR, Grines CL, Ivanhoe R, et al. Six-month clinical and angiographic follow-up after direct angioplasty for acute myocardial infarction. Final results from the primary angioplasty registry. Circulation 90:156, 1994.

6. Guerrci AD, Gerstenblith G, Brinker JA, et al. A randomized trial of intravenous tissue plasminogen activator for acute myocardial infarction with subsequent randomization to elective coronary angioplasty. N Engl J Med 317:1613, 1987.

7. European Cooperative Study Group for Streptokinase Treatment in Acute Myocardial Infarction. Streptokinase in acute myocardial infarction. N Engl J Med 301:797, 1979.

8. Gruppo Italiano per lo Studo della Sopravvivenza nell' Infarto Miocardico. (GISSI). Long-term effects of intravenous thrombolysis in acute myocardial infarction: Final report of the GISSI study. Lancet 2:871, 1987.

9. The ISAM Study Group. A prospective trial of intravenous streptokinase in acute myocardial infarction. N Engl J Med 314:465, 1986.

10. Collen D, Topol CJ, Tefenbrunn AJ, et al. Coronary thrombolysis with recombinant human tissue-type plasminogen activator: A prospective, randomized placebo-controlled trial. Circulation 70:1012, 1984.

11. Verstraete M, Brower RW, Witten D, et al. Double blind randomized trial of intravenous tissue-type plasminogen activator: A prospective, randomized placebo-controlled trial. Lancet 2:965, 1985.

12. Wilcox RG, Olsson CG, Skene AM, et al. Anglo-Scandinavian study of early thrombolysis (ASSET): Trial of tissue plasminogen activator for mortality reduction in acute myocardial infarction. Lancet 2:525, 1985.

13. The TIMI Study Group. The thrombolysis in myocardial infarction (TIMI) trial: Phase 1 findings. N Engl J Med 312:932, 1985.

14. TIMI Study Group. Comparison of invasive and conservative strategies after treatment with intravenous tissue plasminogen activator in acute myocardial infarction (TIMI) phase II trial. N Engl J Med 320:618, 1990.

15. Roberts R, Rogers WJ, Meuller HS, et al. Immediate versus deferred beta-blockade following thrombolytic therapy in patients with acute myocardial infarction; results of the thrombolysis in myocardial infarction (TIMI II-B study). Circulation 83:422, 1991.

16. Gruppo Italiano per lo Studo della Sopravvivenza nell' Infarto Miocardico. GISSI-2. A factorial randomized trial of anistreplase versus streptokinase and heparin versus no heparin among 12,490 patients with acute myocardial infarction. Lancet 336:65, 1990.

17. AIMS Trial Study Group. Long-term effects of intravenous anistreplase in acute myocardial infarction: Final report of the AIMS study. Lancet 335:427, 1990.

18. The International Study Group. In-hospital mortality and clinical course of 20,891 patients with suspected acute myocardial infarction randomized between alteplase and streptokinase with or without heparin. Lancet 336:71, 1990.

19. ISIS-3 (Third International Study of Infarct Survival) Collaborative Group. ISIS-3: A randomized comparison of streptokinase vs. tissue plasminogen activator vs. anistreplase and of aspirin plus heparin vs. aspirin alone among 41,299 cases of suspected acute myocardial infarction. Lancet 329:673, 1992.

20. Colman RW, Marder VJ, Salzman EW, Hirsh J. Overview of hemostasis. In Colman RW, Hirsh J, et al. (eds). Hemostasis and Thrombosis: Basic Principles and Clinical Practice. Philadelphia: JB Lippincott, 1994:1.

21. Stump D, Collen D. The fibrinolytic system: Implications for thrombolytic therapy. In Califf R, Mark D, Wagner G (eds). Acute Coronary Care in the Thrombolytic Era. St. Louis, MO: Yearbook Medical, 1988:58.

22. Majerus PW, Broze GJ, Miletich JP, et al. Anticoagulant, thrombolytic, and antiplatelet drugs. In Hardman JG, Limbird LE (eds). Goodman & Gilman's The Pharmacological Basic of Therapeutics. New York: McGraw Hill, 1996:1341.

23. Cannon CP, McCabe CH, Gibson M, et al. TNK-tissue plasminogen activator in acute myocardial infarction: Results of the Thrombolysis In Myocardial Infarction (TIMI) 10A dose-ranging trial. Circulation 1997, in press.

24. Bode C, Kohler B, Smalling RW, et al. Reteplase (r-PA): A novel recombinant plasminogen activator. Fibrinolysis 9(Suppl. 1):97, 1995.

25. Vanderschueren S, Barrios L, Kerdsinchai P, et al. A randomized trial of recombinant staphylokinase versus alteplase for coronary artery patency in acute myocardial infarction. Circulation 92:2044, 1995.

26. Salzman EW, Hirsh J, Marder VJ. Clinical use of heparin. In Coleman RW, Hirsh J, et al. (eds). Hemostasis and Thrombosis: Basic Principles and Clinical Practice. Philadelphia: JB Lippincott, 1994:1584.

27. Carter CJ, Kelton JG, Hirsh J, et al. The relationship between the hemorrhagic and antithrombotic properties of low-molecular weight heparins and heparin. Blood 59:1239, 1982.

28. Harker LA. Antiplatelet and Anticoagulant therapy. In Handin RI, Lux SE, Stossel TP (eds). Blood: Principles and Practice of Hematology. Philadelphia: JB Lippincott, 1995.

29. Verstraete M. Pharmacotherapeutic aspects of unfractionated and low molecular weight heparins. Drugs 40:498, 1990.

30. Lefkovits J, Topol EJ. Direct thrombin inhibitors in cardiovascular medicine. Circulation 90:1522, 1994.

31. Hirsh J. Optimal intensity and monitoring warfarin. Am J Cardiol 1995:39B.

32. Moran N, Fitzgerald GA. Mechanism of action of antiplatelet drugs. In Coleman RW, Hirsh J, et al. (eds). Hemostasis and Thrombosis: Basic Principles and Clinical Practice. Philadelphia: JB Lippincott, 1994:1623.

33. FitzGerald GA. Dipyridamole. N Engl J Med 316:1247, 1987.

34. Saltiel E, Ward A. Ticlopidine. A review of its pharmacodynamics and pharmacokinetic properties, and therapeutic efficacy in platelet dependent disease states. Drugs 34:222, 1987.

35. Califf RM, Fortin DF, Tenaglia AN, Sane DC. Clinical risks of thrombolytic therapy. Am J Cardiol 69:12A, 1992.

36. The GUSTO investigators. An international randomized trial comparing four thrombolytic strategies for acute myocardial infarction. N Engl J Med 329:673, 1993.

37. Leblanc R, Haddad G, Robitaille Y. Cerebral hemorrhage from amyloid angiopathy and coronary thrombolysis. Neurosurgery 31:586, 1992.

38. Bovill EG, Terrin ML, Stump DC, et al. Hemorrhagic events during therapy with recombinant tissue-type plasminogen activator, heparin, and aspirin for acute myocardial infarction: Results of the Thrombolysis in Myocardial Infarction (TIMI), phase II trial. Ann Intern Med 115:256, 1991.

39. Selker HP, Beshansky JR, Schmid CH, et al. Presenting pulse pressure predicts thrombolytic therapy-related intracranial hemorrhage. Thrombolytic Predictive Instrument (TPI) project results. Circulation 90:1657, 1994.

40. Simoons ML, Maggioni AP, Knatterud G, et al. Individual risk assessment for intracranial haemorrhage during thrombolytic therapy. Lancet 342:1523, 1993.

41. TIMI Research Group. Immediate vs. delayed catheterization and angioplasty following thrombolytic therapy for acute myocardial infarction. JAMA 260:2849, 1988.

42. SWIFT (Should We Intervene Following Thrombolysis?) Trial Group. SWIFT trial of delayed elective intervention vs. consecutive treatment after thrombolysis with anistreplase in acute myocardial infarction. Br Med J 302:555, 1991.

43. Boks AL, Brommer EJ, Schaim SW, et al. Hemostasis and fibrinolysis in severe liver failure and their relationship to hemorrhage. Hepatology 6:79, 1986.

44. Levine MN, Hirsh J, Kelton JG. Heparin-induced bleeding. In Lane DA, Lindahl U (eds). Heparin: Chemical and Biological Properties Clinical Applications. London: Edward Arnold, 1989:517.

45 Yett HS, Skillman JJ, Salzman EW. The hazards of heparin plus aspirin. N Engl J Med 298:1092, 1978.

46. Jick H, Slone D, Borda IT, et al. Efficacy and toxicity of heparin in relation to age and sex. N Engl J Med 279:284, 1968.

47. Landefeld CS, Goldman L. Major bleeding in outpatients treated with warfarin: Incidence and prediction by factors known at the start of outpatient therapy. Am J Med 187:144, 1989.

48. Van Der Meer FJ, Rosendaal FR, Van Den Broucke JP, et al. Bleeding complications in oral anticoagulant therapy: An analysis of risk factors. Arch Intern Med 153:1557, 1993.

49. Isaacs C, Paltiel O, Blake G, et al. Age-associated risks of prophylactic anti-coagulation in the setting of hip fracture. Am J Med 96:487, 1994.

50. Fihn SD, McDonnell M, Martin D, et al. Risk factors for complications of chronic anticoagulation. Ann Intern Med 118:511, 1993.

51. Beyth RJ, Landefeld CS. Anticoagulants in older patients. A safety perspective. Drug Aging 6:45, 1995.

52. Hylek EM, Singer DE. Risk factors for intracranial hermorrhage in outpatients taking warfarin. Ann Intern Med 120:897, 1994.

53. Tracy RP, Bovill EG. Fibrinolytic parameters and hemostatic monitoring: Identifying and predicting patients at risk for major hemorrhagic events. Am J Cardiol 69:52A, 1992.

54. Rao AK, Pratt C, Berke A, et al. Thrombolysis in Myocardial Infarction (TIMI) Trial-Phase I: Hemorrhagic manifestations and changes in plasma fibrinogen and fibrinolytic system in patients treated with recombinant tissue plasminogen activator and streptokinase. J Am Coll Cardiol 11:1, 1988.

55. Califf RM, Topol EJ, George BS, et al. Hemorrhagic complications associated with the use of intravenous tissue plasminogen activator in treatment of acute myocardial infarction. Am J Med 85:353, 1988.

56. Mueller HS, Rao AK, Forman SA. Thrombolysis in myocardial infarction (TIMI): Comparative studies of coronary reperfusion and systemic fibrinogenolysis with two forms of recombinant tissue-type plasminogen activator. J Am Coll Cardiol 10:479, 1987.

57. Sane DC, Califf RM, Topol EJ, et al. Bleeding during thrombolytic therapy for acute myocardial infarction: Mechanisms and management. Ann Intern Med 111:1010, 1989.

58. McGill JB, Schneider DJ, Arfken Cl, et al. Factors responsible for impaired fibrinolysis in obsese subjects and NIDDM patients. Diabetes 43:104, 1994.

59. Topol EJ, Bell WR, Weisfeldt ML. Coronary thrombolysis with recombinant tissue-type plasminogen activator. A hematologic and pharmacologic study. Ann Intern Med 103:837, 1985.

60. Collen D, Bounameaux H, De Cock F, et al. Analysis of coagulation and fibrinolysis during intravenous infusion of recombinant human tissue-type plasminogen activator in patients with acute myocardial infarction. Circulation 73:511, 1986.

61. Urokinase Pulmonary Embolism Trial Study Group. Urokinase pulmonary embolism trial: Phase 1 results. JAMA 214:2163, 1970.

62. Urokinase Pulmonary Embolism Trial Study Group. Urokinase/streptokinase embolism trial: Phase 2 trials results. JAMA 229:1606, 1974.

63. Granger CB, Hirsh J, Califf RM, et al. Activated partial thromboplastin time and outcome after thrombolytic therapy for acute myocardial infarction — results from the GUSTO-I trial. Circulation 93:870, 1996.

64. Shapiro Ga, Huntzinger SW, Wilson JE. Variation among commercial activated partial thromboplastin time reagents in response to heparin. Am J Clin Pathol 67:477, 1977.

65. Vacek JL, Kazuhira H, Rosamond TL, et al. Validation of a bedside method of activated partial thromboplastin time measurement with clinical range guidelines. Am J Cardiol 68:557, 1991.

66. Becker RC, Cyr J, Corrao JM, Ball SP. Bedside coagulation monitoring in heparin-treated patients with active thromboembolic disease: A coronary care unit experience. Am Heart J 128:719, 1994.

67. Kelton J, Warkentin T. Heparin-induced thrombocytopenia. In Coller BS (ed). Progress in Hemostasis and Thrombosis, Vol. 10. Philadelphia: W.B. Saunders, 1991:1.

68. Aster RH. Heparin-induced thrombocytopenia and thrombosis. N Engl J Med 332:1314, 1995.

69. Harrington RA, Sane DC, Califf RM, et al. Clinical importance of thrombocytopenia occurring in hospital phase after administration of thrombolytic therapy for acute myocardial infarction. J Am Coll Cardiol 23:891, 1994.

70 Bauer KA, Weitz JI. Laboratory markers of coagulation and fibrinolysis. In Coleman RW, Hirsh J, et al. (eds). Hemostasis and Thrombosis: Basic Principles and Clinical Practice. Philadelphia: JB Lippincott, 1994:1197.

71. Kaplan KL. Laboratory markers of platelet activation. In Coleman RW, Hirsh J, et al. (eds). Hemostasis and Thrombosis: Basic Principles and Clinical Practice. Philadelphia: JB Lippincott, 1994:1180.

72. Sloan MA, Gore JM. Ischemic stroke and intracranial hemorrhage following thrombolytic therapy for acute myocardial infarction: A risk-benefit analysis. Am J Cardiol 69:21A, 1992.

73. Gore JM, Sloan M, Price TR, et al. Intracerebral hemorrhage, cerebral infarction and subdural hematoma after acute myocardial infarction and thrombolytic therapy in the thrombolysis in myocardial infarction study. Circulation 83:448, 1992.

74. Levine MN, Goldhaber SZ, Gore JM, et al. Hemorrhagic complications of thrombolytic therapy in the treatment of myocardial infarction and venous thromboembolism. Chest 108:291S, 1995.

75. GUSTO IIA investigators. Randomized trial of intravenous heparin versus recombinant hirudin for acute coronary syndromes. Circulation 90:1631, 1994.

76. Antman EM. Hirudin in acute myocardial infarction: Safety report from the thrombolysis and thrombin inhibition in myocardial infarction (TIMI) 9A trial. Circulation 90:1624, 1994.

77. Antman EM for the TIMI 9B investigators. Hirudin in acute myocardial infarction: Final results of the Thrombolysis and Thrombin Inhibition in Myocardial Infarction. (TIMI) 9B Trial. Circulation 94:911, 1996.

78. International joint efficacy comparison of thrombolytics. Randomised, double-blind comparison of reteplase double-bolus administration with streptokinase in acute myocardial infarction (INJECT): Trial to investigate equivalence. Lancet 346:329, 1995.

79. Bode C, Smalling RW, Berg G, et al. Randomized

comparison of coronary thrombolysis achieved with double-bolus reteplase (recombinant plasminogen activator) and front-loaded, accelerated alteplase (recombinant tissue plasminogen activator) in patients with acute myocardial infarction. Circulation 94:891, 1996.

80. Goldhaber SZ, Buring JE, Lipnick RJ, et al. Pooled analyses of randomized trials of streptokinase and heparin in phlebographically documented acute deep vein thrombosis. Am J Med 76:393, 1984.

81. Levine MN, Raskob G, Landefeld S, Hirsh J. Hemorrhagic complications of anticoagulant treatment. Chest 108:276S, 1995.

82. Fernandez F, Nguyen P, van Ryn J, et al. Hemorrhagic doses of heparin and other glycosaminoglycans induce a platelet defect. Thromb Res 43:491, 1986.

83. Blajchman MA, Young E, Ofosu FA. Effects of unfractionated heparin, dermatan sulfate, and low molecular weight heparin on vessel wall permeability in rabbits. Ann N Y Acad Sci 556:245, 1989.

84. Raschke RA, Reilly BM, Gguidry J, et al. The weight-based heparin nomogram compared with a "standard card" nomogram: A randomized controlled trial. Ann Intern Med 119:874, 1993.

85. Levine MN, Hirsh J, Gent M, et al. A randomized trial comparing activated thromboplastin time with heparin assay in patients with acute venous thromboembolism requiring large daily doses of heparin. Arch Intern Med 154:49, 1994.

86. Theroux P, Ouimet H, McCans J, et al. Aspirin, heparin, or both to treat acute unstable angina? N Engl J Med 319:1105, 1988.

87. Serneri GGN, Roveli F, Gensini GF, et al. Effectiveness of low-dose heparin in prevention of myocardial reinfarction. Lancet 1:937, 1987.

88. The SCATI Group. Randomized controlled trial of subcutaneous calcium-heparin in acute myocardial infarction. Lancet 2:182, 1989.

89. Bleich SD, Nichols T, Schumacher R, et al. The role of heparin following coronary thrombolysis with tissue plasminogen activator. Circulation 80(Suppl. 1):113, 1989.

90. Topol EJ, George BS, Kereiakes DJ, et al. A randomized controlled trial of intravenous tissue plasminogen activator and early intravenous heparin in acute myocardial infarction. Circulation 79:281, 1989.

91. Hsia J, Hamilton WP, Kleiman N, et al. A comparison between heparin and low dose aspirin as adjunctive therapy with tissue plasminogen activator for acute myocardial infarction. N Engl J Med 323:1433, 1990.

92. Collins R, Scrimgeour A, Yusuf S, et al. Reduction of fatal pulmonary embolism and venous thrombosis by perioperative administration of subcutaneous heparin. N Engl J Med 318:1162, 1988.

93. Clagett GP, Anderson FA, Heit J, et al. Prevention of venous thromboembolism. Chest 108:312S, 1995.

94. Gurfinkel EP, Manos EJ, Mejail RI, et al. Low molecular weight heparin versus regular heparin or aspi-

rin in the treatment of unstable angina and silent ischemia. J Am Coll Cardiol 26:313, 1995.

95. Nesvold A, Kontny F, Abildgaard, et al. Safety of high doses of low molecular weight heparin (fragmin) in acute myocardial infarction. A dose-finding study. Thromb Res 64:579, 1991.

96. Fragmin During Instability in Coronary Artery Disease (FRISC) Study Group. Low-molecular-weight heparin during instability in coronary artery disease. Lancet 347:561, 1996.

97. Klein W, Buchwald A, Hillis SE, et al. Comparison of low molecular weight heparin with unfractionated heparin acutely and with placebo for 6 weeks in the management of unstable coronary artery disease — The Fragmin In Unstable Coronary Artery Disease study (FRIC). Circulation, 1997, in press.

98. Fox I, Dawson A, Loynds P, Eisner J, Findlen K, Lenn E, Hanson D, Mant T, Wagner J, Maraganore J. Anticoagulant activity of hirulog, a direct thrombin inhibitor, in humans. Thromb Haemost 69:157, 1993.

99. Verstraete M, Nurmohamed M, Kienast J, Siebeck M, Silling-Engelhardt G, Buller H, Hoet B, Bichler J, Close P, on behalf of the European Hirudin in Thrombosis Group. Biologic effects of recombinant hirudin (CGP 39393) in human volunteers. J Am Coll Cardiol 22:1080, 1993.

100. Clarke RJ, Mayo G, Fitzgerald GA, Fitzgerald DJ. Combined administration of aspirin and a specific thrombin inhibitor in man. Circulation 83:1510, 1991.

101. Lidon R, Theroux P, Juneau M, Adelman B, Maraganore J. Initial experience with a direct antithrombin, hirulog, in unstable angina: Anticoagulant, antithrombotic and clinical effects. Circulation 88:1495, 1993.

102. Fuchs J, McCabe CH, Antman EM, Borzak S, Palisaitis D, Herson S, Daum R, Palmeri S, Sequeira R, Sharma G, et al. for the TIMI 7 Investigators. Hirulog in the treatment of unstable angina: Results of the TIMI 7 trial (abstr). J Am Coll Cardiol 23:56, 1994.

103. Gold HK, Torres FW, Garabedian HD, Werner W, Jang IK, Khan A, Hagstrom JN, Yasuda T, Leinbach RC, Newell JB, Bovill EG, Stump DC, Collen D. Evidence for a rebound coagulation phenomenon after cessation of a 4-hour infusion of a specific thrombin inhibitor in patients with unstable angina pectoris. J Am Coll Cardiol 21:1039, 1993.

104. Topol EJ, Fuster V, Harrington RA, Califf RM, Kleiman NS, Kereiakes DJ, Cohen M, Chapekis A, Gold HK, Tannenbaum MA, Rao AK, Debowey D, Schwartz D, Henis M, Chesebro J. Recombinant hirudin for unstable angina pectoris: A multicenter, randomized angiographic trail. Circulation 89:1557, 1994.

105. Lidon RM, Theroux P, Bonan R, et al. A pilot early angiographic patency study using a direct thrombin inhibitor as adjunctive therapy to streptokinase in

acute myocardial infarction. Circulation 89:1567, 1994.

106. Cannon CP, McCabe CH, Henry TD, et al. A pilot trial of recombinant desulfatohirudin compared with heparin in conjunction with tissue-type plasminogen activator and aspirin for acute myocardial infarction (TIMI 5) trial. J Am Coll Cardiol 23:993, 1994.

107. Neuhaus KL, Niederer W, Wagner J, et al. HIT (Hirudin for the Improvement of Thrombolysis): Results of a dose escalation study (abstr). Circulation 88:I292, 1993.

108. Neuhaus KL, Essen RV, Tebber U, et al. Safety observations from the pilot phase of the randomized r-hirudin for improvement of thrombolysis (HIT III) study. Circulation 90:1638, 1994.

109. The Global Use of Strategies To Open Occluded Coronary Arteries (GUSTO) IIb Investigators. A comparison of recombinant hirudin with heparin for the treatment of acute coronary syndromes. N Engl J Med 335:775, 1996.

110. Cannon CP, Maraganore JM, Loscalzo J. Anticoagulant effects of hirulog, a novel thrombin inhibitor, in patients with coronary artery disease. Am J Cardiol 71:778, 1993.

111. Zoldhelyi P, Webster MWI, Fuster V, et al. Recombinant hirudin in patients with chronic stable coronary disease: Safety, half life and effect on coagulation parameters. Circulation 88:2015, 1993.

112. Topol EJ, Bonan R, Jewitt D, et al. Use of a direct antithrombin, hirulog, in place of heparin during coronary angioplasty. Circulation 87:1622, 1993.

113. van den Bos AA, Deckers JW, Heyndricks GR, et al. Safety and efficacy of recombinant hirudin (CGP 39 393) versus heparin in patients with stable angina undergoing coronary angioplasty. Circulation 88:2058, 1993.

114. Serruys PW, Herrman JP, Simon R, et al. A comparison of hirudin with heparin in the prevention of restenosis after coronary angioplasty. HEVETICA Investigators. N Engl J Med 333:757, 1995.

115. Bittl JA on behalf of the Hirulog Angioplasty Study Investigators. Comparative safety profiles of hirulog and heparin in patients undergoing coronary angioplasty. Am Heart J 130:658, 1995.

116. Ginsberrg JS, Nurmohamed MT, Gent M, et al. Use of hirulog in the prevention of venous thrombosis after major hip or knee surgery. Circulation 90:2385, 1994.

117. Eriksson BI, Kalebo P, Ekman S, et al. Direct thrombin inhibition with rec-hirudin CGP 39393 as prophylaxis of thromboembolic complications after total hip replacement. Thromb Haemost 72:227, 1994.

118. Eriksson BI, Kalebo P, Ekman S, et al. Effective prevention of thromboembolic complications after total hip replacement with three different doses of recombinant hirudin, CGP 39393 (abstr). Circulation 90:I569, 1994.

119. Ginsberrg JS, Nurmohamed MT, Gent M, et al. Effects on thrombin generation of single injections of hirulog in patients with calf vein thrombosis. Thromb Haemost 72:523, 1994.

120. Parest F, Bridey F, Dreyfus M, et al. Treatment of severe venous thrombo-embolism with intravenous hirudin (HBW023): An open pilot study. Thromb Haemost 70:386, 1993.

121. Douketis JD, Turpie AGG. Combined antiplatelet-anticoagulant therapy: Rationale and safety considerations. In Ezekowitz MD (ed). Long-Term Antithrombotic Antiplatelet Therapy in the Post-infarct Patient. American Journal of Cardiology Continuing Education Series. 1994:16.

122. Hull R, Hirsh J, Jay R, et al. Different intensities of oral anticoagulant therapy in the treatment of proximal vein thrombosis. N Engl J Med 307:1676, 1982.

123. Turpie AGG, Hirsh J, Gunstensen J, et al. Randomized comparison of two intensities of oral anticoagulant therapy after tissue heart valve replacement. Lancet 1:1242, 1988.

124. Turpie AGG, Gent M, Laupacis A, et al. A comparison of aspirin with placebo in patients treated with warfarin after heart valve replacement. N Engl J Med 329:524, 1993.

125. Altman R, Rouvier J, Gurfinkel E. Comparison of two levels of anticoagulant therapy in patients with substitute heart valves. J Thorac Cardiovasc Surg 101:427, 1991.

126. Altman R, Rouvier J, Gurfinkel E, et al. Comparison of high dose with low dose aspirin in patients with mechanical heart valve replacement treated with oral anticoagulant. Circulation 94:2113, 1996.

127. Acar J, Iung B, Boissel JP, et al. AREVA: Multicenter randomized comparison of low-dose versus standard-dose anticoagulation in patients with mechanical prosthetic heart valves. Circulation 94:2107, 1996.

128. The Boston Area Anticoagulation Trial for Atrial Fibrillation Investigators. The effect of low dose warfarin on the risk of stroke in patients with non-rheumatic atrial fibrillation. N Engl J Med 323:1505, 1990.

129. Stroke Prevention in Atrial Fibrillation Investigators. Stroke Prevention in Atrial Fibrillation Study: final results. Circulation 84:527, 1991.

130. Peterson P, Boysan G, Godtfredsen J, et al. Placebo-controlled randomized trial of warfarin and aspirin for prevention of thromboembolic complications in chronic atrial fibrillation: The Copenhagen AFASAK study. Lancet 1:175, 1989.

131. Ezekowitz MD, Bridgers SI, James KE, et al. Warfarin in the prevention of stroke associated with non-rheumatic atrial fibrillation. N Engl J Med 327:1406, 1992.

132. Connolly SJ, Laupacis A, Gent M, et al. Canadian atrial fibrillation anticoagulation study. J Am Coll Cardiol 18:349, 1991.

133. Stroke Prevention in Atrial Fibrillation Investigators.

Warfarin versus aspirin for prevention of thromboembolism in atrial fibrillation: Stroke Prevention in Atrial Fibrillation II Study. Lancet 343:687, 1994.

134. Atrial Fibrillation Investigators. Risk factors for stroke and efficacy of anti-thrombotic therapy in atrial fibrillation: Analysis of pooled data from five randomized controlled trials. Arch Intern Med 154:1449, 1994.

135. The Stroke Prevention in Atrial Fibrillation Investigators. Bleeding during anti-thrombotic therapy in patients with atrial fibrillation. Arch Intern Med 156:409, 1996.

136. Antman R, Rouvier J, Gurfinkel E. Comparison of two levels of anticoagulant therapy in patients with substitute heart valves. J Thorac Cardiovasc Surg 101:427, 1991.

137. Saour JN, Sieck JO, Marno LAR, et al. Trial of different intensities of anticoagulation in patients with prosthetic heart valves. N Engl J Med 322:428, 1990.

138. Report of the Sixty Plus Reinfarction Study Research Group. A double-blind trial to assess long-term oral anticoagulant therapy in elderly patients after myocardial infarction. Lancet 2:989, 1980.

139. Smith P, Arnesen H, Holme I. The effect of warfarin on mortality and reinfarction after myocardial infarction. N Engl J Med 323:147, 1990.

140. ASPECT Research Group. Effect of long-term anticoagulant treatment on mortality and cardiovascular morbidity after myocardial infarction. Lancet 343:499, 1994.

141. Olsson JE, Brechter C, Backlund H, et al. Anticoagulant us antiplatelet therapy as prophylactic against cerebral infarction in transient ischemic attacks. Stroke 11:4, 1980.

142. Baker RN. An evaluation of anticoagulant therapy in the treatment of cerebrovascular disease: Report of the Veterans Administration Cooperative study of atherosclerosis. Neurology 11:132, 1961.

143. Hill AB, Marshall J, Shaw DA. Cerebrovascular disease: Trial of long term anticoagulant therapy in cerebrovascular disease. Q J Med 29:597, 1960.

144. Steering Committee of the Physicians' Health Study Research Group. Final report on the aspirin component of the ongoing Physicians' Health Study. N Engl J Med 321:129, 1989.

145. Peto R, Gray R, Collins R, et al. Randomised trial of prophylactic daily aspirin in British male doctors. Br Med J 296:313, 1988.

146. The SALT Collaborative Group. Swedish Aspirin Low-Dose Trial (SALT) of 75 mg aspirin as secondary prophylaxis after cerebrovascular ischemic events. Lancet 338:1345, 1991.

147. Sze PC, Reitman D, Pincus MM, et al. Antiplatelet agents in the secondary prevention of stroke: Meta-analysis of the randomized control trials. Stroke 19:436, 1988.

148. Goldstein LB, Bonito AJ, Matchar CB, et al. US national survey of physician practices for the second-

ary and tertiary prevention of ischemic stroke. Carotid endarterectomy. Stroke 27:801, 1996.

149. Antiplatelet Trialists' Collaboration. Collaborative overview of randomised trials of antiplatelet therapy I: Prevention of death, myocardial infarction, and stroke by prolonged antiplatelet therapy in various categories of patients. Br Med J 308:81, 1994.

150. Meade TW, Miller GJ. Combined use of aspirin and warfarin in primary prevention of ischemic heart disease in men at high risk. Am J Cardiol 75:23B, 1995.

151. Prichard PJ, Kitchingman GK, Walt RP, et al. Human gastric mucosal bleeding induced by low dose aspirin, but not warfarin. Br Med J 298:493, 1989.

152. Hass WK, Easton JD, Adams HP, et al. A randomized trial comparing ticlopidine hydrochloride with aspirin for the prevention of stroke in high-risk patients. N Engl J Med 321:501, 1989.

153. Uchiyama S, Sone R, Nagayama T, et al. Combination therapy with low-dose aspirin and ticlopidine in cerebral ischemia. Stroke 20:1643, 1989.

154. Balsano F, Rizzon P, Violi F, et al. Antiplatelet treatment with ticlopidine in unstable angina. A controlled multicenter clinical trial. Circulation 82:17, 1990.

155. Schomig A, Neumann FJ, Kastrati A, et al. A randomized comparison of antiplatelet and anticoagulant therapy after the placement of coronary-artery stents. N Engl J Med 334:1084, 1996.

156. Tcheng J, Ellis SG, George BS. Pharmacodynamics of chimeric glycoprotein IIb/IIIa integrin antiplatelet antibody Fab 7E3 in high risk coronary angioplasty. Circulation 90;1757, 1994.

157. The EPIC Investigators. Use of a monoclonal antibody directed against the platelet glycoprotein IIb/IIIa receptor in high-risk coronary angioplasty. N Engl J Med 330:956, 1994.

158. Aguirre FV, Topol EJ, Ferguson JJ, et al. Bleeding complications with the chimeric antibody to platelet glycoprotein IIb/IIIa Integrin in patients undergoing percutaneous coronary intervention. Circulation 91:2882, 1995.

159. Lincoff AM, Tcheng JE, Bass TA, et al. A multicenter, randomized, double blind pilot trial of standard versus low dose weight adjusted heparin in patients treated with the platelet GPIIb/IIa receptor antibody c7E3 during percutaneous coronary angioplasty (abstr). J Am Coll Cardiol 25:80A, 1995.

160. Tcheng JE. Glycoprotein IIb/IIIa receptor inhibitors: Putting the EPIC, IMPACT II, RESTORE, and EPILOG trials into perspective. Am J Cardiol 7B(Suppl. 3A):35, 1996.

161. Ferguson JJ. Meeting highlights: ACC 45th annual scientific session. Circulation 94:1, 1996.

162. Tcheng JE, Harrington RA, Kandice KM, et al. Multicenter, randomized, double-blind, placebo-controlled trial of the platelet integrin glycoprotein, IIb/IIIa blocker, Integrelin in elective coronary intervention. Circulation 91:2151, 1995.

163. Blankenship J, Mandak J, Aguirre F, et al. Vascular access site complications during angioplasty with glycoprotein IIb/IIIa receptor inhibition in the IMPACT II trial (abstr). J Am Coll Cardiol 27:360, 1996.

164. Kleinman NS, Ohman ME, Califf RM, et al. Profound inhibition of platelet aggregation with monoclonal antibody 7E3 Fab following thrombolytic therapy: Results of the TAMI 8 pilot study. J Am Coll Cardiol 22:381, 1993.

165. Kereiakes DJ, Kleiman NS, Ambrose J, Cohen M. Randomized, double-blind, placebo-controlled dose-ranging study of tirofiban (MK-383) platelet IIb/IIIa blockade in high risk patients undergoing coronary angioplasty. J Am Coll Cardiol 1996:536.

165. Adam HP, Brott TG, Furlan AJ, et al. Guidelines for thrombolytic therapy for acute stroke: A supplement to the guidelines for the management of patients with acute ischemic stroke. Circulation 94:1167, 1996.

166. The National Institute of Neurological Disorders and Stroke rt-PA Stroke Study Group. Tissue plasminogen activator for acute ischemic stroke. N Engl J Med 333:1581, 1995.

167. Multicentre Acute Stroke Trial-Italy (MAST-I) Group. Randomised controlled trial of streptokinase, aspirin, and combination of both in treatment of acute ischaemic stroke. Lancet 346:1509, 1995.

168. Hommel M, Boissel JP, Cornu C, et al. Termination of trial of streptokinase in severe acute ischaemic stroke [letter]. Lancet 345:57, 1994.

169. Donnan GA, Davis SM, Chambers BR, et al. Trials of streptokinase in severe acute ischaemic stroke. Lancet 345:578, 1995.

170. Hacke W, Kaste M, Fieschi C, et al. Intravenous thrombolysis with recombinant tissue plasminogen activator for acute hemispheric stroke: The European Cooperative Acute Stroke Study (ECASS). JAMA 274:1017, 1995.

SECTION XIII: GENE THERAPY IN VASCULAR DISEASE

Douglas W. Losordo

The application of modern molecular techniques to the study of vascular pathologies has begun to change our understanding of the underlying mechanisms involved in these processes. Akin to the evolution of antibiotic therapy after the discovery of the bacterial etiology of infectious diseases, the mechanistic insights yielded from studying the genetic and molecular basis of vascular disease will ultimately revolutionize their treatment. This section provides an overview of this nascent field and a glimpse of some of the early strategies for gene therapy for the prevention of pathologic vascular thrombosis.

40. GENE THERAPY FOR THE VULNERABLE PLAQUE

Jeffrey M. Isner

Introduction

Rupture of coronary atherosclerotic plaque and subsequent formation of an occlusive intracoronary thrombus (Figure 40-1) are the major events precipitating acute coronary syndromes [1–6]. The vulnerable plaque is smaller in size [7], richer in lipids [1,2], and more infiltrated with macrophages [2,3,8–10] than the stable, fibromuscular lesion. Therefore, lowering the lipid and/or macrophage pools stored in the plaque may "stabilize" the plaque and reduce the incidence of plaque rupture [2,4–6]. Indeed, cholesterol-lowering trials have yielded a significant reduction in acute cardiac events [11–18]. Antithrombotic therapies may further prevent acute coronary syndromes by altering the consequences of plaque rupture [4].

Recent advances in the field of molecular biology, combined with the development of efficient vectors to perform in vivo gene transfer, have led to the emergence of new therapies to prevent acute coronary syndromes. Because gene therapy, in contrast to drug therapy, implies a variable and currently undetermined time interval for the transgene to be expressed, certain gene therapy approaches may ultimately not prove appropriate for treatment of patients with acute infarction. Genetic interventions that are designed to stabilize the vulnerable plaque and/or to inhibit thrombus formation (Table 40-1), however, hold considerable promise and are the subject of this review.

Gene Therapy for the Vulnerable Plaque

Lowering the level of plasma cholesterol may reduce the progression, and even induce regression, of atherosclerotic lesions [11–19]. This result appears to represent the consequence of reducing plasma low-density lipoprotein (LDL) levels as well as increasing plasma high-density lipoprotein (HDL) levels. Even modest changes in coronary luminal diameter observed in patients, as a result of lipid-lowering interventions, have been associated with a significant reduction in the incidence of acute coronary syndromes [11–18]. It is likely that this beneficial effect was due to the regression of plaques rich in cholesterol and macrophages, that is, plaques prone to rupture [4,19]. Therefore, therapeutic strategies aimed at (1) lowering plasma LDL, (2) increasing plasma HDL, and/or (3) mitigating macrophage infiltration hold promise for reducing the mortality and morbidity associated with coronary atherosclerosis.

FAMILIAL HYPERCHOLESTEROLEMIA: A MODEL FOR LDL-TARGETED GENE THERAPY
Familial hypercholesterolemia (FH) is caused by a genetic deficiency in the hepatic receptors for LDL cholesterol and is associated with severe hypercholesterolemia and premature coronary artery disease [20]. The observation that orthotopic liver transplantation from donors who express normal LDL receptor activity may lead to complete correction of the dyslipidemia in homozygotes [21] set the stage for a genetic strategy, first articulated by Goldstein et al. [22], targeted toward introduction into the liver of normal LDL receptor genes.

Two different approaches to gene therapy have been developed for FH. In the first approach, referred to as ex vivo (or indirect) gene transfer, cells are removed, transduced ex vivo with the LDL receptor gene, then transplanted back into the liver. In the second approach, referred to as in vivo (or direct) gene transfer, the LDL receptor gene is directly introduced into the liver during a one-step procedure. Although FH accounts for only a small minority of patients, the promise of genetically increasing LDL receptor abundance in the liver may have implications for treating more common forms of hypercholesterolemia, and thereby potentially reducing the incidence of acute coronary syndromes in these patients [23].

TABLE 40-1. Potential targets for genetic
interventions to prevent acute coronary syndromes

Target gene	Intervention	Mechanisms
LDL receptor	Augmentation	Plaque stabilization
HDL	Augmentation	Plaque stabilization
eNOS	Augmentation	Plaque stabilization
		Inhibition of SMC proliferation
		Inhibition of thrombus formation
sVCAM-1	Augmentation	Plaque stabilization
Metalloproteinases	Inhibition	Plaque stabilization
t-PA	Augmentation	Inhibition of thrombus formation
scu-PA	Augmentation	Inhibition of thrombus formation
VEGF	Augmentation	Inhibition of thrombus formation
		Inhibition of SMC proliferation

LDL = low-density lipoprotein; HDL = high-density lipoprotein; eNOS = constitutive endothelial nitric
oxide synthase; SMC = smooth muscle cells; sVCAM-1 = soluble vascular cell adhesion molecule 1; t-PA =
tissular plasminogen activator; scu-PA = single-chain urokinase plasminogen activator; VEGF = vascular
endothelial growth factor.

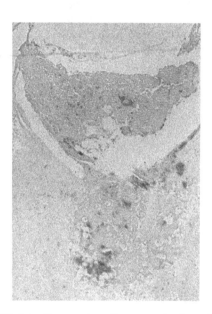

FIGURE 40-1. Cross-section of a ruptured atherosclerotic
plaque from an infarct-related coronary artery. R = plaque
rupture; T = intraluminal thrombus; H = intraplaque hemorrhage; L = lumen.

EX VIVO GENE THERAPY FOR FAMILIAL
HYPERCHOLESTEROLEMIA
Wilson et al. [24] and Chowdhury et al. [25] used
an animal model for FH, the Watanabe heritable
hyperlipidemic (WHHL) rabbit, to isolate hepatocytes following partial hepatectomy, to transfect these
cells ex vivo with replication-defective retroviruses
including an LDL receptor cDNA, and to implant the
transduced hepatocytes into the liver of recipient

WHHL rabbits. Stable expression of the recombinant
LDL receptor gene as well as a consistent decrease
in serum cholesterol could be detected for several
months after autologous transplantation [25].

Based on these encouraging results, the first clinical trial of gene therapy to treat patients with homozygous FH was initiated in 1992 [26]. In this
protocol, an ex vivo approach similar to the one used
in the WHHL rabbit was adopted. After partial
hepatectomy, hepatocytes were released and transfected ex vivo with recombinant retroviruses expressing a human LDL-receptor cDNA. Transduced
hepatocytes were subsequently infused directly into
the portal circulation to allow engraftment of LDL
receptor–expressing hepatocytes in the liver. Preliminary results on the first patient enrolled in this trial
were recently published [27]. The patient tolerated
the surgical procedure well, and expression of the
transfected LDL receptor gene was documented 4
months after gene transfer in $1:10^3$ to $1:10^4$ liver
cells. This was paralleled by a 17% decrease in serum
LDL that persisted for at least 18 months.

These results, although remarkable, require further
analysis. Brown et al. have outlined three major concerns that remain to be addressed before the promise
of gene therapy for FH can be fulfilled [28]. First, it
is unclear whether the observed reduction in serum
LDL was due to an actual increase of LDL receptor
activity or a reduction in LDL production in response
to liver surgery. Study of LDL clearance, rather than
LDL levels, may help to answer this question. Second,
it must be established that the reduction in serum
LDL resulted from expression of the exogenous LDL
receptor gene, rather than from upregulation of the

patient's own residual LDL-receptor activity induced, in this case, by the surgical procedure itself [29] and/or lovastatin therapy [28]. Third, clinical application of ex vivo gene therapy is limited by the surgical hazard, the costly and time-consuming procedures required for ex vivo transfection, and the fact that most hepatocytes lose their capacity for reintroduction following ex vivo transfection.

IN VIVO GENE THERAPY FOR FAMILIAL HYPERCHOLESTEROLEMIA

According to the ideal paradigm for in vivo gene therapy, a vector expressing a normal LDL receptor gene would be directly injected into the liver as an atraumatic, one-step procedure. Efficient gene transfer in vivo, however, has been difficult to achieve using retroviral vectors because mitotic activity is required to facilitate retrovirus-mediated transfection [30] and hepatocytes are typically quiescent under normal physiological conditions. Therefore, vectors capable of transducing nondividing cells, namely, recombinant adenoviruses and molecular conjugates, have been investigated for this purpose.

Several features of recombinant adenoviruses suggest that they might be appropriate vehicles for human gene therapies in general, and for liver-directed gene therapy in particular [23]. Indeed, recombinant adenoviruses can be rendered defective for replication by deleting the early sequences E1A and E1B from their genome. They do not integrate into the genome of transfected cells, thus reducing the risk of insertional mutagenesis. They can be produced at high titers, and they accommodate relatively large cDNA inserts (up to 7.5 kb).

These theoretical considerations have been translated into successful experimental studies. Indeed, intravenous or intraportal introduction of adenoviruses expressing a human LDL receptor cDNA — in normal mice [31], knockout mice lacking functional LDL receptor genes [32], and WHHL rabbits [33] — results in extremely efficient liver transfection, as well as increased LDL clearance and/or decreased LDL levels. This effect, however, was transient, lasting less than 3 weeks. The relatively rapid diminution in transgene expression may involve a T-lymphocyte–mediated immune response toward certain viral proteins [34]. In the case of hypercholesterolemia, such transient expression of the therapeutic gene is a major drawback of gene transfer strategies based on "first-generation" adenoviruses. Repeated administration of the same vector may not represent a simple solution to more protracted expression, given the additional evidence of antibody-mediated reduction in gene expression on subsequent exposures to the adenovirus [33]. Recent reports suggest that insertion of a temperature-sensitive mutation within the E2A region of the adenoviral genome results in less immunogenic vectors and prolonged transgene expression at permissive temperatures [35,36]. The effect of further deletions within the E2 and E4 regions on the time course of gene expression is currently under investigation.

Molecular conjugates have been recently used to perform liver-directed gene transfer in vivo [37]. A DAN–protein complex containing an LDL receptor cDNA complexed to a protein conjugate was injected systemically into WHHL rabbits. The protein conjugate incorporates a ligand (asialoorosomucoid) for the hepatocyte-specific asialoglycoprotein receptor covalently attached to the polycation poly-L-lysine. In this system, referred to as *receptor-mediated gene transfer*, liver transfection is mediated by the interaction between asialoorosomucoid and its receptor. Total serum cholesterol was decreased significantly after gene transfer, but returned to baseline in less than 6 days. The nonviral nature of the DNA–protein complex, as well as the noninvasive approach for gene delivery, nevertheless, remain attractive features for clinical application. Alternatively, the coupling of molecular conjugates to adenoviral particles has been shown to increase the efficiency of in vitro hepatocyte gene transfer as obtained by conjugates alone, by promoting DNA escape from lysosomal hydrolysis [38].

HDL CHOLESTEROL: A NEW TARGET FOR GENE THERAPY

Previous studies have established an inverse correlation between plasma levels of HDL and the incidence of coronary artery disease [39–41]. In several lipid-lowering clinical trials, an increase in serum HDL was correlated with a reduction in the incidence of acute coronary syndromes, and sometimes with a reduction in progression and/or slight regression of angiographic evidence of coronary atherosclerosis [12,14,16,42]. Taken together, these results suggest that therapies that increase serum HDL may have an antiatherogenic effect. Indeed, Badimon et al. showed that intravenous administration of HDL not only inhibited the formation [43] but also induced regression [44] of established fatty streaks.

More recently, Rubin et al. have developed a transgenic mouse that overexpresses apo-A1, the major protein component of HDL, and is protected from the development of early atherosclerotic lesions [45,46]. The mechanism of the protective effect of HDL is still unclear. It has been postulated that HDL may reduce the amount of cholesterol entering the plaque and promote the clearance of cholesterol deposits from the plaque [47]. Alternatively, intravenous injection of apo-A1 in the hypercholesterolemic rabbit reduces intimal thickening induced by arterial injury and is associated with a 50% reduction in neointimal macrophage content [48,49]. Therefore, high serum HDL might be expected to induce regression of lipid- and macrophage-rich plaques, and ultimately to reduce the risk of plaque rupture. Overexpression of apo-A1 by means of gene therapy has been recently reported in mice in which intravenous injection of an apo-A1–expressing adenovirus transiently increased serum HDL to a level comparable with that shown to be protective in humans [50]. Such an approach holds promise for the future development of gene therapy strategies targeted toward stabilization of the vulnerable plaque through HDL-mediated lipid and/or macrophage removal.

FUTURE DIRECTIONS: TARGETING THE MACROPHAGE

Certain studies have suggested that unstable plaque may be composed of abundant macrophages [10] (Figure 40-2), especially at the margins of the plaque [3]. Macrophages release lytic enzymes as well as matrix metalloproteinases [51,52] (Figure 40-3), which may be responsible for fibrous cap weakening and subsequent plaque rupture [6,10,53]. The association between macrophages and plaque rupture has

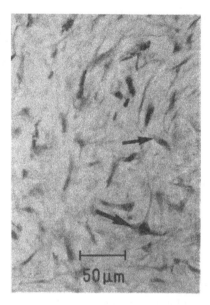

FIGURE 40-3. Atherectomy specimen obtained from patient with unstable angina and immunostained for 92-kd gelatinase. Arrows indicate sites of positive intracellular staining (200×).

been strengthened by the recent observations that activity of a 92 kd metalloproteinase is more frequently found in macrophages from coronary lesions of patients with unstable versus stable angina [52], and incubation of human atherosclerotic fibrous caps with macrophages in vitro increased collagen breakdown [54]. It is therefore conceivable that reducing macrophage infiltration may potentially reduce the risk of plaque rupture.

A first approach has been developed by Chen et al. in which a recombinant adenovirus expressing a soluble form of the endothelial adhesion molecule VCAM-1 (sVCAM-1) is transferred into porcine vein grafts ex vivo [55]. Vein grafts, interposed as vascular grafts in the carotid arteries, were shown to express high levels of sVCAM-1 3 days postimplantation. These findings suggest the possibility that high-level sVCAM-1 expression may be exploited to competitively inhibit interaction between endothelial VCAM-1 and its VLA-4 counterpart at the surface of circulating monocytes, and thereby to prevent macrophage infiltration of the graft.

Alternatively, preliminary findings indicate that nitric oxide (NO) inhibits monocyte chemotactic activity of the endothelium by downregulating the cytokine monocyte chemoattractant protein 1 (MCP-1) at the transcriptional level [56]; if these data are confirmed, it is likely that secretion of high levels of NO in the vicinity of an atherosclerotic plaque may

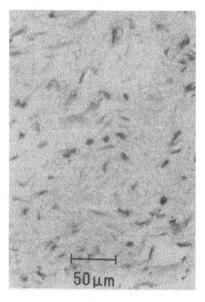

FIGURE 40-2. Immunohistochemical staining with monoclonal antibody to HAM56, a macrophage marker, of an atherectomy specimen from a patient with unstable angina (200×).

reduce macrophage recruitment into the plaque. In this case, the antithrombotic, antiproliferative, and vasorelaxing activities of NO [57] may also facilitate plaque passivation.

One way to increase local levels of NO is to transfer into the atherosclerotic lesion the gene encoding constitutive endothelial nitric oxide synthase (eNOS) [58]. It has been recently reported that the transfer of a eNOS cDNA packaged into a liposome–Sendai virus carrier inhibits neointima formation after balloon injury of the rat carotid artery [59]. It is still speculative, however, whether such a strategy may limit macrophage recruitment through downregulation of MCP-1 because many other cytokines as well as oxidized LDLs may act as monocyte chemoattractants and participate in upregulation of monocyte and/or endothelial cell adhesion molecules [5]. Moreover, the potential toxicity associated with local secretion of high levels of NO in the arterial wall, resulting in further LDL oxidation, remains to be addressed [5].

Arterial Gene Transfer: Contribution to Antithrombotic Strategies

When plaque ruptures, the development of an occlusive thrombus plays a major part in determining the clinical presentation in acute coronary syndromes [1,53,60–62]. Indeed, antithrombotic agents, such as aspirin, have been shown to reduce the risk of myocardial infarction [63,64]. Administration of antithrombotic therapies in the past has been conventionally achieved via a systemic route, enhancing the risk of hemorrhagic complications. Because of the focal nature of atherosclerosis, local delivery of antithrombotic agents at the site of the culprit lesion constitutes a logical alternative to systemic antithrombotic therapies. High concentrations of a pharmacologic agent can thus be achieved in the vicinity of the atherosclerotic lesion with a reduced risk of systemic toxicity [65,66]. Pharmacologic agents with antithrombotic activity, however, do not address the biologic mechanisms of thrombosis. Certain of these mechanisms involve aberrant endothelial gene expression [67]. Specifically, increased expression of prothrombotic molecules, such as plasminogen activator inhibitor type 1 (PAI-1) [68], and/or decreased expression of antithrombotic compound, such as tissue-type plasminogen activator (t-PA) [69], by the diseased endothelium may facilitate the development of an occlusive thrombus at the site of plaque rupture. These observations suggest a rationale for the application of gene therapy to restore and/or augment antithrombotic endothelial cell function [70].

FEASIBILITY OF ARTERIAL GENE TRANSFER TARGETED TOWARD THE ENDOTHELIUM

As previously described in the liver, two different approaches have been used to perform arterial gene transfer. Ex vivo gene transfer has been used to seed endothelium-denuded arteries, prosthetic vascular grafts, and stents with genetically modified endothelial cells. In vivo gene transfer, in contrast, involves direct introduction of genetic material into the arterial wall.

Ex Vivo Gene Transfer

EX VIVO GENE TRANSFER TO VASCULAR PROSTHETIC DEVICES. Nabel et al. first demonstrated that genetically engineered endothelial cells could be introduced into the arterial wall and express a recombinant gene [71]. In this study, porcine endothelial cells were transfected in vitro with a retroviral vector expressing a recombinant β-galactosidase gene. Successfully transfected cells were then introduced into denuded iliofemoral arteries of syngenic animals using a double-balloon catheter. Following this procedure, 2–11% of transduced endothelial cells attached to the arterial wall. Of these cells, 20–100% expressed β-galactosidase up to 4 weeks following gene transfer.

EX VIVO GENE TRANSFER TO VASCULAR PROSTHETIC DEVICES. Conventional use of grafts and stents has been compromised by the risk of acute thrombosis, predominantly during the first weeks following implantation [72], the time window required for endothelialization of the prosthetic material. Endothelial cells genetically engineered to produce antithrombotic molecules were therefore investigated as a means of favorably influencing the patency of such prosthetic devices.

Wilson et al., for example, employed dacron grafts coated with genetically modified endothelial cells as carotid interposition grafts in a canine model [73]. In this model, endothelial cells were transfected in vitro using a retroviral vector expressing a β-galactosidase gene prior to graft coating. By 5 weeks postimplantation, the luminal aspect of the graft was covered by a monolayer of endothelial cells, some of which expressed the β-galactosidase gene. Based on these results, the authors proposed that endothelial cells may be genetically modified to secrete antithrombotic proteins and thereby to improve vascular graft patency. Successful implantation of in vitro endothelialized polytetrafluoroethylene femoro-tibial grafts in four patients, resulting in 100% patency 3 months following implantation [74], suggests the feasibility of employing this strategy to bypass medium-sized arteries.

The risk of acute or subacute thrombosis after implantation of coronary stents remains a major issue for the interventional cardiologist [72]. Aggressive systemic antithrombotic treatment may not be optimal for prevention of stent occlusion because it is accompanied by increased bleeding complications, an extended hospital stay, and increased cost [75]. Seeding of arterial stents with endothelial cells prior to implantation has been proposed as an alternative strategy [76]. Because the antithrombotic activity of seeded endothelial cells may be altered, Dichek et al. seeded stents with endothelial cells genetically engineered to express a human tissue plasminogen activator (t-PA) gene. A significant percentage of transfected endothelial cells remained adherent to the stent after in vitro balloon-mediated stent expansion [77] and subsequent exposure to pulsatile flow [78]. Long-term adherence of the seeded cells under variable in vivo flow conditions, however, remains a concern.

EX VIVO GENE TRANSFER TO VEIN GRAFTS. Early vein graft thrombosis as well as accelerated graft atherosclerosis limits the long-term efficacy of aortocoronary bypass surgery [79]. Systemic delivery of antiplatelet agents has been shown to reduce by nearly one half the incidence of graft occlusion [80]. Ex vivo manipulation of vein grafts, however, provides a unique opportunity for local therapy to be applied to the graft prior to implantation. One attractive approach would be to transfect freshly explanted vein grafts with a foreign gene encoding an antithrombotic protein. As indicated previously, ex vivo, adenovirus-mediated vein-graft transfection is feasible and results in relatively high level recombinant protein secretion [55]. Successful introduction of antithrombotic genes in vein grafts, however, has not yet been reported.

IN VIVO ARTERIAL GENE TRANSFER. Since the first demonstration by Nabel et al. that direct introduction of a foreign gene into a specific arterial segment could be performed in live animals [81], the field of in vivo arterial gene transfer has evolved rapidly. As recently depicted by Leclerc and Isner [82], strategies aimed at introducing foreign genetic material into the arterial wall in live animals involve a macrodelivery system (the "gun") to transport the foreign gene to the arterial target site, a vector of gene transfer (the "bullet) to facilitate the cellular uptake of the transgene, and a molecular mechanism (the "target") with which the product of the transgene will ultimately interact.

THE GUNS. Earlier techniques designed to perform arterial gene transfer included those that relied on direct introduction of the transgene in a surgically exposed, isolated arterial segment [83–87]. Although this method is likely to optimize the efficiency of gene transfer, the invasive nature of this approach clearly limits its clinical applicability. An alternative approach involves catheter-based local delivery of the foreign gene to a specific arterial segment. In their seminal work, Nabel and her colleagues introduced a double-balloon catheter in porcine iliofemoral arteries via a side branch under direct vision [81]. Sequential inflation of the two balloons isolates an arterial segment in which a solution containing retroviral vectors or liposomes is instilled, allowed to incubate, and then retrieved before restoration of flow. Since these pioneering experiments, other delivery catheters have been developed [66], and different groups have reported entirely percutaneous approaches [88–91].

THE BULLETS. Several vectors have been used to facilitate cellular uptake of the transgene into the arterial wall. Cationic liposomes [81,83,92,93] and retroviruses [81,94] were first used to demonstrate that arterial gene transfer was feasible. Transfection efficiencies using these vectors, however, were extremely low (typically, less than $1 : 10^6$ cells expressed the transgene). Similar results were reported when DNA with no vehicle ("naked" DNA) was used (Figure 40-4) [95].

Replication-defective, recombinant adenoviruses represent an alternative to liposome- or retrovirus-based arterial gene transfer [23]. Several groups have recently reported highly efficient adenovirus-mediated arterial transfection, using either an intraoperative route [85,86,96] or a percutaneous approach [88–91,97–99]. Transfection efficiencies achieved using adenoviruses are at least three logs higher than those reported using liposomes [93,99] and retroviruses [81]. Important drawbacks of adenoviral vectors, however, include transient transgene expression, typically limited to 2–3 weeks post–gene transfer (see earlier) and the risk of systemic dissemination facilitated by the amphotropic character of the adenovirus. Reports have varied with regard to extra-arterial distribution of adenoviral vectors following percutaneous local delivery [90,91,97–99]. These discrepancies may be related to the specific local delivery device used for gene transfer. Indeed, extra-arterial transfection has been reported with the double-balloon [90,98] and the porous-balloon catheters [97,99], but not with the hydrogel-balloon catheter [90]. Finally, we recently reported that the efficiency of adenovirus-mediated gene transfer is

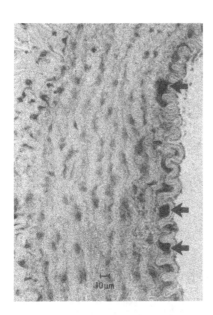

FIGURE 40-4. Gene transfer to the rabbit iliac artery using DAN alone (naked DNA). A plasmid coding for nuclear-specific β-galactosidase was applied onto the surface of a hydrogel-coated balloon and expressed into the arterial wall during balloon inflation. Double labeling for nuclear β-galactosidase (blue) and cytoplasmic smooth muscle α-actin (brown). Only rare medial smooth muscle cells show evidence of successful transfection (blue). (From Riessen et al. [95], with permission.)

reduced in atherosclerotic versus normal arteries [91]. Transfection efficiency achieved in atherosclerotic arteries with adenoviruses, however, is still several orders of magnitude higher than that achieved using liposomes [99].

In vivo transfection of the endothelium has been achieved using intraoperative [85,86,88] or catheter-based [81,88–90,100,101] delivery of retroviral [81] or adenoviral [85,86,88–90,101] vectors. Interestingly, exposure of a non-denuded, normal peripheral artery to adenoviral vectors results in gene expression, which is limited to the endothelium [85,86,88–90,101] (Figure 40-5A). Conversely, arterial de-endothelialization at the time of adenovirus-mediated gene transfer results in efficient medial smooth muscle cell transfection (Figure 40-5B) (86–88,90,98,102,103). Taken together, these findings suggest that (1) cell-specific gene transfer targeted toward the endothelium is feasible when adenoviruses are used as vectors, and (2) an intact endothelium constitutes a potential physical barrier to adenovirus penetration into the media of peripheral arteries. A recent report by Barr and his colleagues suggests, however, that intracoronary infusion of adenoviral vectors results in significant medial as well as myocardial transfection, in addition to predominant endothelial transfection [100]. This discrepancy may be due to structural differences between peripheral and coronary arteries. In contrast, very low-level gene transfer to all the layers of the arterial wall was observed after local delivery of liposomes or retroviral vectors using a double-balloon catheter [81]. Therefore, recombinant adenoviruses currently appear to be the most appropriate vector with which to perform endothelium-specific arterial gene transfer.

CURRENT APPROACHES FOR A GENETIC INTERVENTION TO PREVENT THROMBUS FORMATION

The demonstration that site-specific gene transfer to the vascular endothelium is feasible set the stage for the development of genetic strategies aimed at preventing acute coronary syndromes. Dichek et al. [104] proposed that arterial thrombosis might be prevented by altering certain endothelial functions at the site of endothelial injury or dysfunction. One approach by which normal antithrombotic activity of the endothelium might be restored involves transfection of the t-PA gene [77,104]. In vitro transfection of endothelial cells with a retrovirus expressing a human t-PA gene resulted in high-level secretion of t-PA [77,104].

One of the main limitations of this strategy, however, is the inactivation of recombinant t-PA resulting from binding of t-PA molecules to plasminogen activator inhibitor type 1 (PAI-1). A single-chain urokinase (scu-PA) cDNA, which encodes an enzyme that does not bind to PAI-1, has been used to circumvent this limitation [96,105]. Taken together, these data suggest that endothelial cells genetically engineered to produce fibrinolytic compounds such as t-PA may express high levels of thrombolytic agent in vitro and, presumably, in vivo. Hence, a gene transfer protocol in which endothelial cells would be directly transfected in vivo using catheter-based local delivery of adenoviral vectors expressing fibrinolytic molecules may augment endothelial antithrombotic activity and ultimately prevent thrombus formation at the site of endothelial injury or dysfunction.

Other potential candidates for endothelium-targeted gene therapy await experimental evidence that they may confer protection against arterial thrombosis. For example, secretion of NO contributes to the nonthrombogenic surface of the normal endothelium [57]. Therefore, successful transfection of a vulnerable atherosclerotic plaque with a cDNA encoding the constitutive eNOS (see earlier) [58] may reduce the likelihood of arterial thrombosis.

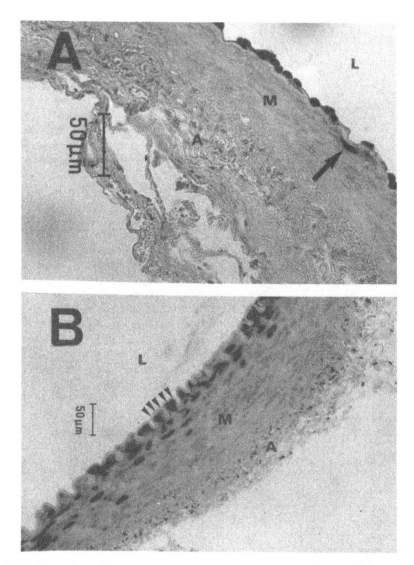

FIGURE 40-5. Percutaneous adenovirus-mediated arterial gene transfer. A recombinant adenovirus expressing a nuclear-specific β-galactosidase was delivered locally into the rabbit iliac artery using either a double-balloon (A) or a hydrogel-coated balloon catheter (B). β-galactosidase activity is revealed by X-gal staining (blue). A: Double-balloon catheter. Gene transfer is confined to the endothelium when the artery is intact. Note the presence of one superficial medial cell expressing β-galactosidase (black arrow) just below a site of focal disruption of the endothelium. B: Hydrogel-coated balloon catheter. In this case, the endothelial layer is removed at the time of transfection. A nearly continuous, superficial layer of transfected medial smooth muscle cells is observed below a well-preserved internal elastic lamina (black arrowheads). (Adapted from Steg et al. [90], with permission.)

Other potential candidates for endothelium-targeted gene therapy await experimental evidence that they may confer protection against arterial thrombosis. For example, local delivery of the endothelium-specific mitogen vascular endothelial growth factor (VEGF) at the site of arterial injury accelerates re-endothelialization and attenuates intimal thickening [106]. Therefore, it is possible that restoration of a potentially antithrombotic endothelial layer can be facilitated by transferring the VEGF gene to the endoluminal surface of a vulnerable atherosclerotic plaque. Successful transfer to the arterial wall of a VEGF-expressing plasmid from the surface of a hydrogel-coated balloon catheter has been recently reported [107].

This genetic strategy has several potential advantages over protein therapy. First, the prolonged synthesis and local release of VEGF following gene

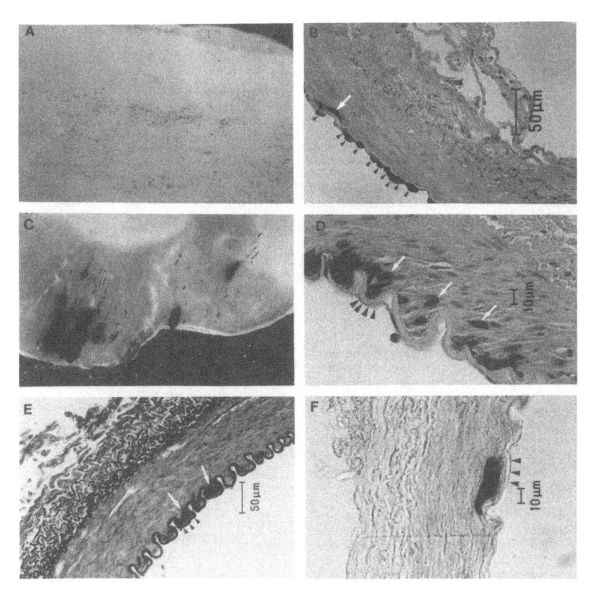

FIGURE 40-6. X-Gal staining of a rabbit iliac artery showing β-galactosidase activity 3 days after adenovirus-mediated transfer of the *nlslacZ* gene in vivo using the double-balloon technique without (A and B) or with (D, D, E, and F) previous de-endothelialization. A: Normal artery; macroscopic view of the luminal aspect of the artery. Blue staining identifies foci of transfected cells (original magnification ×25). B: Light-microscopic appearance of A after hematoxylin-eosin counterstaining. X-Gal staining is confined to the nuclei of the endothelial layer (black arrowheads). Note the presence of one superficial medial cell expressing β-galactosidase (white arrow) just below a site of focal disruption of the endothelium. C: Injured artery. Macroscopic view shows a mottled blue appearance of the luminal aspect of the artery (original magnification ×40). D: Light-microscopic appearance of C after hematoxylin-eosin counterstaining. Sparse medial cells, underlying an apparently intact internal elastic lamina (black arrowheads), express β-galactosidase (white arrows). E: Photomicrograph of C after Richardson's elastic trichrome counterstaining. Note the apparent integrity of the internal elastic lamina (black arrowheads). Some superficial medial cells, below the internal elastic lamina, express β-galactosidase (white arrows). F: Photomicrograph of C after immunohistochemical staining with monoclonal anti–α-actin antibody. High-power view of a superficial medial cell that coexpresses β-galactosidase (nucleus, blue) and α-actin (cytoplasm, brown), identifying it as a vascular smooth muscle cell expressing the *nlslacZ* transgene. Black arrowheads indicate internal elastic lamina. (Adapted from Steg et al. [90], with permission.)

transfer may constitute a more effective means of stimulating endothelium regrowth than a single bolus of VEGF protein. Second, relatively inexpensive expression plasmids encoding a secreted form of VEGF can be designed that may ultimately reduce the high costs associated with production of recombinant proteins. Direct introduction of DNA with no vehicle (naked DNA) into the arterial wall has been shown to be feasible, although with low efficiency [95]. In the case of VEGF, however, even a low efficiency may prove sufficient to induce re-endothelialization because the VEGF gene product is in this case secreted, and therefore capable of modulating neighboring cells via a paracrine effect. Further studies are warranted to investigate whether the favorable effect of VEGF on abluminal endothelial cells is associated with deleterious intraplaque neoangiogenesis, which might predispose to plaque hemorrhage.

Conclusions

Prevention of acute coronary syndromes represents a major target for cardiovascular research. Pharmacologic interventions aimed at lowering serum cholesterol or inhibiting thrombus formation have proved efficient in reducing mortality related to acute coronary events. Recent progress in the field of gene transfer, as well as a better understanding of the pathophysiology of plaque rupture and thrombus formation, have established new avenues for a molecular approach to acute coronary syndromes. Preliminary results of the first ex vivo gene therapy for FH suggest that genetically engineered hepatocytes expressing the human LDL receptor can be introduced into the liver and induce in some patients a significant reduction in serum LDL. Development of more practical protocols using direct administration of the LDL receptor gene in vivo are warranted, however, before the promise of this technology can be realized. Genetic modification of endothelial cells to improve endothelial antithrombotic activity is a viable alternative. Ultimately, strategies simultaneously addressing the concepts of atherosclerotic plaque stabilization and restoration of physiologic endothelial functions represent an opportune field for future research.

Acknowledgments

We gratefully acknowledge the contribution of Dr. David Brown, who initiated the investigations of the 92-kd gelatinase illustrated in this manuscript.

References

1. Richardson PD, Davies MJ, Born GVR. Influence of plaque configuration and stress distribution on fissuring of coronary atherosclerotic plaques. Lancet 2:941, 1989.
2. Falk E. Why do plaques rupture? Circulation 86(Suppl. III):30, 1992.
3. Lendon CL, Davies MJ, Born GVR, Richardson PD. Atherosclerotic plaque caps are locally weakened when macrophages density is increased. Atherosclerosis 87:87, 1991.
4. Fuster V, Badimon L, Badimon JJ, Chesebro JH. The pathogenesis of coronary artery disease and the acute coronary syndromes (Second part). N Engl J Med 326:310, 1992.
5. Ross R. The pathogenesis of atherosclerosis: A perspective for the 1990s. Nature 362:801, 1993.
6. MacIsaac AI, Thomas JD, Topol EJ. Toward the quiescent coronary plaque. J Am Coll Cardiol 22:1228, 1993.
7. Nobuyoshi M, Tanaka M, Nosaka H, et al. Progression of coronary atherosclerosis: Is coronary spasm related to progression? J Am Coll Cardiol 18:904, 1991.
8. van der Wal AC, Becker AE, van der Loos CM, Das PK. Site of intimal rupture or erosion of thrombosed coronary atherosclerotic plaques is characterized by an inflammatory process irrespective of the dominant plaque morphology. Circulation 89:36, 1994.
9. Alexander RW. Inflammation and coronary artery disease. N Engl J Med 331:468, 1994.
10. Moreno PR, Falk E, Palacios IF, Newell JB, Fuster V, Fallon JT. Macrophage infiltration in acute coronary syndromes. Implications for plaque rupture. Circulation 90:775, 1994.
11. Kane JP, Malloy MJ, Ports TA, Phillips NR, Diehl JC, Havel RJ. Regression of coronary atherosclerosis during treatment of familial hypercholesterolemia with combined drug regiment. JAMA 264:3007, 1990.
12. Brown G, Albers JJ, Fisher LD, et al. Regression of coronary artery disease as a result of intensive lipid-lowering therapy in men with high levels of apolipoprotein B. N Engl J Med 323:1289, 1990.
13. Ornish D, Brown SE, Scherwitz LW, et al. Can lifestyle changes reverse coronary heart disease? The Lifestyle Heart Trial. Lancet 336:129, 1990.
14. Blankenhorn DH, Nessim SA, Johnson RL, Sanmarco M, Azen SP, Cashin-Hemphill I. Beneficial effects of combined colestipol-niacin therapy on coronary atherosclerosis and coronary venous bypass grafts, JAMA 257:3233, 1987.
15. Brensike JF, Levy RI, Kesley SF, et al. Effects of therapy with cholestyramine on progression of coronary arteriosclerosis: Results of the NHLBI Type II Coronary Intervention Study. Circulation 69:313, 1984.

16. Buchwald H, Varco RL, Matts JP, et al. Effect of partial ileal bypass surgery on mortality and morbidity from coronary heart disease in patients with hypercholesterolemia: Report of the Program on the Surgical Control of the Hyperlipidemias (POSCH). N Engl J Med 323:946, 1990.

17. Cashin-Hemphill L, Mack WJ, Pagoda JM, Sanmarco ME, Azen SP, Blankenhorn DH. Beneficial effects of colestipol-niacin on coronary atherosclerosis. JAMA 264:3013, 1990.

18. Watts GF, Lewis B, Brunt JN, et al. Effects on coronary artery disease of lipid-lowering diet, or diet plus cholestyramine, in the St. Thomas' Atherosclerosis Regression Study (STARS). Lancet 339:563, 1992.

19. Badimon JJ, Fuster V, Chesebro JH, Badimon L. Coronary atherosclerosis. A multifactorial disease. Circulation 87(Suppl. II):3, 1993.

20. Brown MS, Goldstein JL. A receptor-mediated pathway for cholesterol homeostasis. Science 232:34, 1986.

21. Bilheimer DW, Goldstein JL, Grundy SM, Starzl TE, Brown MS, Liver transplantation to provide low-density-lipoprotein receptors and lower plasma cholesterol in a child with homozygous familial hypercholesterolemia. N Engl J Med 311:1658, 1984.

22. Goldstein JL, Kita T, Brown MS. Defective lipoprotein receptors and atherosclerosis. Lessons from an animal counterpart of familial hypercholesterolemia. N Engl J Med 309:288, 1983.

23. Schneider MD, French BA. The advent of adenovirus. Gene therapy for cardiovascular disease. Circulation 88:1937, 1993.

24. Wilson JM, Chowdhury NR, Grossman M, et al. Temporary amelioration of hyperlipidemia in low density lipoprotein receptor-deficient rabbits transplanted with genetically modified hepatocytes. Proc Natl Acad Sci USA 87:8437, 1990.

25. Chowdhury JR, Grossman M, Gupta S, Chowdhury NR, Baker JR, Wilson JM. Long-term improvement of hypercholesterolemia after ex vivo gene therapy in LDLR-deficient rabbits. Science 254:1802, 1991.

26. Wilson JM. Clinical protocol: Ex vivo gene therapy of familial hypercholesterolemia. Hum Gene Ther 3:179, 1992.

27. Grossman M, Raper SE, Kozarsky K, et al. Successful ex vivo gene therapy directed to liver in a patient with familial hypercholesterolaemia. Nature Genet 6:335, 1994.

28. Brown MS, Goldstein JL, Havel RJ, Steinberg D. Gene therapy for cholesterol. Nature Genet 7:349, 1994.

29. Dichek DA, Bratthauer GL, Beg ZH, et al. Retroviral vector-mediated in vivo expression of low-density-lipoprotein receptors in the Watanabe heritable hyperlipidemic rabbit. Somat Cell Mol Genet 17:287, 1991.

30. Miller DG, Adam MA, Miller AD. Gene transfer by retrovirus vectors occurs only in cells that are actively replicating at the time of infection. Mol Cell Biol 10:4239, 1990.

31. Herz J, Gerard RD. Adenovirus-mediated transfer of low density lipoprotein receptor gene acutely accelerates cholesterol clearance in normal mice. Proc Natl Acad Sci USA 90:2812, 1993.

32. Ishibashi S, Brown MS, Goldstein JL, Gerard RD, Hammer RE, Herz J. Hypercholesterolemia in low density lipoprotein receptor knockout mice and its reversal by adenovirus-mediated gene delivery. J Clin Invest 92:883, 1993.

33. Kozarsky KF, McKinley DR, Austin LL, Raper SE, Stratford-Perricaudet LD, Wilson JM. In vivo correction of low-density lipoprotein receptor deficiency in the Watanabe heritable hyperlipidemic rabbit with recombinant adenoviruses. J Biol Chem 269:13695, 1994.

34. Yang Y, Nunes FA, Berencsi K, Furth EE, Gönczöl E, Wilson JM. Cellular immunity to viral antigens limits E1-deleted adenoviruses for gene therapy. Proc Natl Acad Sci USA 91:4407, 1994.

35. Yang Y, Nunes FA, Berencsi K, Gönczöl E, Engelhardt JF, Wilson JM. Inactivation of E2A in recombinant adenoviruses improves the prospect for gene therapy in cystic fibrosis. Nature Genet 7:362, 1994.

36. Engelhardt JF, Ye X, Doranz B, Wilson JM. Ablation of E2A in recombinant adenoviruses improves transgene persistence and decreases inflammatory response in mouse liver. Proc Natl Acad Sci USA 91:1994.

37. Wilson JM, Grossman M, Wu CH, Chowdhury NR, Wu GY, Chowdhury JR. Hepatocyte-directed gene transfer in vivo leads to transient improvement of hypercholesterolemia in low-density lipoprotein receptor-deficient rabbits. J Biol Chem 267:963, 1992.

38. Cristiano R, Smith L, Kay M, Brinkley B, Woo S. Hepatic gene therapy: Efficient gene delivery and expression in primary hepatocytes utilizing a conjugated adenovirus–DNA complex. Proc Natl Acad Sci USA 90:11548, 1993.

39. Castelli WP, Doyle JT, Gordon T, et al. HDL cholesterol and other lipids in coronary heart disease: The cooperative lipoprotein phenotyping study. Circulation 55:767, 1977.

40. Gordon T, Castelli WP, Hjortland MC, Kannel WB, Dawber TR. High density lipoprotein as a protective factor against coronary heart disease: The Framingham study. Am J Med 62:707, 1977.

41. Heiss G, Johnson NJ, Reiland S, Davis CE, Tyroler HA. The Lipid Research Clinics Program Prevalence Study: Summary. Circulation 62(Suppl. IV):116, 1980.

42. Frick MH, Elo O, Haapa K, et al. Helsinki Heart Study primary prevention trial with gemfibrozil in middle-aged men with dyslipidemia: Safety of treatment, changes in risk factors, and incidence of coronary heart disease. N Engl J Med 317:1237, 1987.

43. Badimon JJ, Badimon L, Galvez A, Dische R, Fuster V. High density lipoprotein plasma fraction inhibit aortic fatty streaks in cholesterol-fed rabbits. Lab Invest 60:455, 1989.

44. Badimon JJ, Badimon L, Fuster V. Regression of atherosclerotic lesions by high density lipoprotein plasma fraction in the cholesterol-fed rabbit. J Clin Invest 85:1234, 1990.

45. Rubin EM, Krauss RM, Spangler EA, Verstuyft JG, Clift SM. Inhibition of early atherogenesis in transgenic mice by human apolipoprotein A1. Nature 353:265, 1991.

46. Pászty C, Maeda N, Verstuyft J, Rubin EM. Apolipoprotein A1 transgene corrects apolipoprotein E deficiency-induced atherosclerosis in mice. J Clin Invest 94:899, 1994.

47. Reichl D, Miller NE. Pathophysiology of reverse cholesterol transport: Insights from inherited disorders of lipoprotein metabolism. Arteriosclerosis 9:785, 1989.

48. Ameli S, Hultgardh-Nilsson A, Cercek B, et al. Recombinant apolipoprotein A-1 Milano reduces intimal thickening after balloon injury in hypercholesterolemic rabbits. Circulation 90:1935, 1994.

49. Soma MR, Donetti E, Parolini C, Sirtori CR, Fumagalli R, Franceschini G. Recombinant apolipoprotein A-I Milano dimer inhibits carotid intimal thickening induced by perivascular manipulation in rabbits. Circ Res 76:405, 1995.

50. Kopfler WP, Willard M, Betz T, Willard JE, Gerard RD, Meidell RS. Adenovirus-mediated transfer of a gene encoding human apolipoprotein A-I into normal mice increases circulating high-density lipoprotein cholesterol. Circulation 90:1319, 1994.

51. Welgus HG, Campbell EJ, Cury JD, et al. Neutral metalloproteinases produced by human mononuclear phagocytes. J Clin Invest 86:1496, 1990.

52. Brown DI, Hibbs MS, Kearney M, Topol EJ, Loushin C, Isner JM. Expresssion and cellular location of 92 kDa gelatinase in coronary lesions of patients with nustable angina. Circulation, in press.

53. Fuster V, Badimon L, Badimon JJ, Chesebro JH. The pathogenesis of coronary artery disease and the acute coronary syndromes (First part). N Engl J Med 326:242, 1992.

54. Shah PK, Falk E, Badimon JJ, et al. Human monocyte-derived macrophages express collagenase and induce collagen breakdown in atherosclerotic fibrous caps: Implications for plaque rupture (abstr). Circulation 88(Suppl. I):I254, 1993.

55. Chen S-J, Wilson JM, Muller DWM. Adenovirus-mediated gene transfer of soluble vascular cell adhesion molecule to porcine interposition vein grafts. Circulation 89:1922, 1994.

56. Zeiher AM, Schray-Utz B, Busse R. Nitric oxide modulates monocyte chemoattractant protein 1 in human endothelial cells: Implications for the pathogenesis of atherosclerosis (abstr). Circulation 88(Suppl. I):I367, 1993.

57. Moncada S, Higgs A. The L-arginine-nitric oxide pathway. N Engl J Med 329:2002, 1993.

58. Sessa WC, Harrison JK, Barber CM, et al. Molecular cloning and expression of a cDNA encoding endothelial cell nitric oxide synthase. J Biol Chem 267:15274, 1992.

59. von der Leyen H, Gibbons GH, Morishita R, et al. Gene therapy inhibiting neointimal vascular lesion: In vivo transfer of endothelial cell nitric oxide synthase gene. Proc Natl Acad Sci USA 92:1137, 1995.

60. DeWood MA, Stifter WF, Simpson CS, et al. Coronary arteriographic findings soon after non-Q-wave myocardial infarction. N Engl J Med 315:417, 1986.

61. DeWood MA, Spores J, Notske R, et al. Prevalence of total coronary occlusion during the early hours of transmural myocardial infarction. N Engl J Med 303:897, 1980.

62. Falk E. Unstable angina with fatal outcome: Dynamic coronary thrombosis leading to infarction and/or sudden death: Autopsy evidence of recurrent mural thrombosis with peripheral embolization culminating in total vascular occlusion. Circulation 71:699, 1985.

63. Steering Committee of the Physicians' Health Study Research Group. Final report on the aspirin component of the ongoing Physicians' Health Study. N Engl J Med 321:129, 1989.

64. Juul-Möller S, Edvardsson N, Jahnmatz B, et al. Double-blind trial of aspirin in primary prevention of myocardial infarction in patients with stable chronic angina pectoris. Lancet 340:1421, 1992.

65. March KL, Wilensky RL, Hathaway DR. Novel drug and device combinations for targeted prevention of restenosis. Cardiol Intervention 2:11, 1992.

66. Riessen R, Isner JM. Prospects for site-specific delivery of pharmacologic and molecular therapies. J Am Coll Cardiol 23:1234, 1994.

67. Gimbrone MA. Vascular endothelium: Nature's blood container. In Gimbrone MA (ed). Vascular Endothelium in Hemostasis and Thrombosis. NewYork: Churchill Livingstone, 1986:1

68. Quax PHA, van den Hoogen CM, Verheijen JH, et al. Endotoxin induction of plasminogen activator and plasminogen activator inhibitor type 1 mRNA in rat tissues in vivo, J Biol Chem 265:15560, 1990.

69. Loscalzo J, Braunwald E. Tissue plasminogen activator. N Engl J Med 19:925, 1988.

70. Dichek DA. Interventional approaches to the introduction of genetic material into the vasculature. In Topol EJ (ed). Textbook of Interventional Cardiology. Philadelphia: WB Saunders, 1993:989.

71. Nabel EJ, Plautz G, Boyce DM, Stanley JC, Nabel GJ. Recombinant gene expression in vivo within endothelial cells of the arterial wall. Science 244:1342, 1989.

72. Sutton JM, Ellis SG, Roubin GS, et al. Major clinical events after coronary stenting. The Multicenter Registry of Acute and Elective Gianturco-Roubin Stent Placement. Circulation 89:1126, 1994.

73. Wilson JM, Birinyi LK, Salomon RN, Libby P, Callow AD, Mulligan RC. Implantation of vascular grafts lined with genetically modified endothelial cells. Science 244:1344, 1989.

74. Kadletz M, Magometschnigg H, Minar E, et al. Implantation of in vitro endothelialized polytetrafluoroethylene grafts in human beings. A preliminary report. J Thorac Cardiovasc Surg 104:736, 1992.

75. Leon MB, Wong SC. Intracoronary stents. A breakthrough technology or just another small step? Circulation 89:1323, 1994.

76. van der Giessen WJ, Serruys PW, Visser WJ, et al. Endothelialization of intravascular stents. J Intervent Cardiol 1:109, 1988.

77. Dichek DA, Neville RF, Zwiebel JA, Freeman SM, Leon MB, Anderson WF. Seeding of intravascular stents with genetically engineered endothelial cells. Circulation 80:1347, 1989.

78. Flugelman MY, Virmani R, Leon MB, Bowman RL, Dichek DA. Genetically engineered endothelial cells remain adherent and viable after stent deployment and exposure to flow in vitro. Circ Res 70:348, 1992.

79. Fitzgibbon GM, Leach AJ, Kafka HP, Keon WJ. Coronary bypass graft fate: Long-term angiographic study. J Am Coll Cardiol 17:1075, 1991.

80. Antiplatelet Trialists' Collaboration. Collaborative overview of randomised trials of antiplatelet therapy-II: Maintenance of vascular graft or arterial patency by antiplatelet therapy. Br Med J 308:159, 1994.

81. Nabel EG, Plautz G, Nabel GJ. Site-specific gene expression in vivo by direct gene transfer into the arterial wall. Science 249:1285, 1990.

82. Leclerc G, Isner JM. Percutaneous gene therapy for cardiovascular disease. In Topol EJ (ed). Textbook of Interventional Cardiology. Philadelphia: WB Saunders, 1993:1019.

83. Lim CS, Chapman GD, Gammon JB, et al. Direct in vivo gene transfer into the coronary and peripheral vasculatures of the intact dog. Circulation 83:578, 1991.

84. Barbee RW, Stapleton DD, Perry BD, et al. Prior arterial injury enhances luciferase expression following in vivo gene transfer. Biochem Biophys Res Commun 190:70, 1993.

85. Lemarchand P, Jones M, Yamada I, Crystal RG. In vivo gene transfer and expression in normal uninjured blood vessels using replication-deficient recombinant adenovirus vectors. Circ Res 72:1132, 1993.

86. Guzman R, Lemarchand P, Crystal RG, Epstein SE, Finkel T. Efficient and selective adenovirus-mediated gene transfer into vascular neointima. Circulation 88:2838, 1993.

87. Lee SW, Trapnell BC, Rade JJ, Virmani R, Dichek DA. In vivo adenoviral vector-mediated gene transfer into balloon-injured rat carotid arteries. Circ Res 73:797, 1993.

88. Willard JE, Landau C, Glamann DB, et al. Genetic modification of the vessel wall. Comparison of surgical and catheter-based techniques for delivery of recombinant adenovirus. Circulation 89:2190, 1994.

89. Rome JJ, Shayani V, Flugelman MY, et al. Anatomic barriers influence the distribution of in vivo gene transfer into the arterial wall. Modeling with microscopic tracer particles and verification with a recombinant adenoviral vector. Arterioscler Thromb 14:148, 1994.

90. Steg PG, Feldman LJ, Scoazec J-Y, et al. Arterial gene transfer to rabbit endothelial and smooth muscle cells using percutaneous delivery of an adenoviral vector. Circulation 90:1648, 1994.

91. Feldman LJ, Steg PG, Zheng LP, et al. Low-efficiency of percutaneous adenovirus-mediated arterial gene transfer in the atherosclerotic rabbit. J Clin Invest, in press.

92. Leclerc G, Gal D, Takeshita S, Nikol S, Weir L, Isner JM. Percutaneous arterial gene transfer in a rabbit model. Efficiency in normal and balloon-dilated atherosclerotic arteries. J Clin Invest 90:936, 1992.

93. Takeshita S, Gal D, Leclerc G, et al. Increased gene expression after liposome-mediated arterial gene transfer associated with intimal smooth muscle cell proliferation. In vitro and in vivo findings in a rabbit model of vascular injury. J Clin Invest 93:652, 1994.

94. Flugelman MY, Jaklitsch MT, Newman KD, Casscells W, Brathauer GL, Dichek DA. Low level in vivo gene transfer into the arterial wall through a perforated balloon catheter. Circulation 85:1110, 1992.

95. Riessen R, Rahimizadeh H, Takeshita S, Gal D, Barry JJ, Isner JM. Successful vascular gene transfer using a hydrogel coated balloon angioplasty catheter. Hum Gene Ther 4:749, 1993.

96. Lee SW, Kahn ML, Dichek DA. Control of clot lysis by gene transfer. Trends Cardiovasc Med 3:61, 1993.

97. March KL, Gradus-Pizlo I, Wilensky RL, Yei S, Trapnell BC. Cardiovascular gene therapy using adenoviral vectors: Distant transduction following local delivery using a porous balloon catheter (abstr). J Am Coll Cardiol 23:177, 1994.

98. Ohno T, Gordon D, San H, et al. Gene therapy for vascular smooth muscle cell proliferation after arterial injury. Science 265:781, 1994.

99. French BA, Mazur W, Ali NM, et al. Percutaneous transluminal in vivo gene transfer by recombinant adenovirus in normal porcine coronary arteries, atherosclerotic arteries, and two models of coronary restenosis. Circulation 90:2402, 1994.

100. Barr E, Carroll J, Kalynych AM, Tripathy SK, Kozarsky K, Wilson JM. Efficient catheter-mediated gene transfer into the heart using replication-defective adenovirus. Gene Ther 1:51, 1994.

101. Muller DWM, Gordon D, San H, et al. Catheter-mediated pulmonary vascular gene transfer and expression. Circ Res 75:1039, 1994.
102. Guzman RJ, Hirschowitz EA, Brody SL, Crystal RG, Epstein Se, Finkel T. In vivo suppression of injury-induced vascular smooth muscle cell accumulation using adenovirus-mediated transfer of the herpes simplex virus thymidine kinase gene. Proc Natl Acad Sci USA 91:10732, 1994.
103. Chang MW, Barr E, Seltzer J, et al. Cytostatic gene therapy for vascular proliferative disorders with a constitutively active form of the retinoblastoma gene product. Science 267:518, 1995.
104. Dichek DA, Nussbaum O, Degen SJF, Anderson WF. Enhancement of the fibrinolytic activity of sheep endothelial cells by retroviral vector-mediated gene transfer. Blood 77:533, 1991.
105. Lee SW, Kahn ML, Dichek DA. Expression of an anchored urokinase in the apical endothelial cell membrane. J Biol Chem 267:13020, 1992.
106. Asahara T, Bauters C, Pastore C, et al. Local delivery of vascular endothelial growth factor accelerates reendothelialization and attenuates intimal hyperplasia in balloon-injured rat carotid artery. Circulation, in press.
107. Takeshita S, Zheng LP, Asahara T, et al. In vivo evidence of enhanced angiogenesis following direct arterial gene transfer of the plasmid encoding vascular endothelial growth factor. Proc Natl Acad Sci USA, in press.

41. GENE THERAPY: VECTOR DESIGN AND CURRENT CHALLENGES

Elizabeth G. Nabel

Prospects for Gene Therapy for Thrombotic Disorders

Gene transfer is an approach to the treatment of human diseases based on the delivery and expression of genetic material into somatic cells. Gene delivery can be achieved in vivo through direct introduction into cells or ex vivo through manipulation of cells in culture. In this sense, gene therapy is a new form of drug delivery, in which the drug is recombinant protein synthesized by transduced cells. Gene therapy can be viewed as an extension of conventional medical therapies in which the genetic material is the therapeutic agent. Gene therapy is being applied to many human diseases, and it offers the potential to cure diseases, either as a single treatment modality or as an adjuvant to existing treatments. However, gene therapy is still in its infancy, and many of these promises have not yet been fulfilled.

The field of gene transfer for cardiovascular disease has progressed significantly during the past decade. The feasibility of introducing recombinant genes into blood vessels using catheter-mediated gene delivery has been demonstrated by a number of laboratories in many animal models [1]. Furthermore, investigators have used recombinant gene transfer as a tool to study the pathophysiology of vascular diseases [2–5]. We now are poised to apply this technology to treat human vascular diseases. Indeed, several protocols have been initiated to stimulate angiogenesis in peripheral vascular disease and to treat restenosis following peripheral angioplasty [6,7]. Vascular gene transfer, however, faces certain challenges before widespread application can be made to many vascular diseases. These challenges include the type and design of the vector best suited for vascular diseases, the best methods of gene delivery, optimization of gene expression, and minimizing toxicities of vectors to host cells.

An increasing number of vector systems have been developed and evaluated. Viral vectors, including retrovirus, adenovirus, adeno-associated virus, and herpes virus, have been the predominant vectors used for the delivery of genes into cells for ex vivo and in vivo gene delivery. Because of concerns about the safety of viral vectors for human use, a number of investigators have optimized nonviral vectors, such as naked DNA, DNA–lipsome complexes, and biolistics, for gene delivery.

Both viral and nonviral vectors are used for vascular gene transfer studies (Table 41-1). Each vector has advantages and disadvantages, and unfortunately none of the current vectors is completely satisfactory for vascular gene transfer. Retroviruses were initially studied, but retroviral gene expression in vascular cells is low, and cell proliferation is required for integration of recombinant gene sequences into the host genome [8,9]. Because of low-level gene expression, investigators more recently have utilized adenoviral vectors in vascular studies. Adenoviruses are attractive vectors because they can be purified to high titer and efficiently infect vascular cells [10]. Recently there has been concern about host immune responses to adenoviral proteins, but it is presently unknown whether these will limit applications to human diseases [11,12]. Modifications in adenoviral vectors are being made in many laboratories to minimize toxicities to host cells. Likewise, substantial efforts have been made in the refinement of nonviral vectors. Plasmid DNA coated onto balloon catheters is currently being used in two clinical protocols for angiogenesis and restenosis [6,7]. Improvements in liposomes have been made that result in increased gene expression within vascular cells [13]. There are many possibilities for combining naked DNA or DNA–liposome complexes with mechanical devices, such as stents. Opportunities for advances in these

TABLE 41-1. Comparison of somatic gene transfer systems

Vector	Advantages	Disadvantages	Applications
Viral			
Retrovirus	Biology well understood Stable integration into host cells Efficient entry No viral genes in vector	Low titer Infection limited to dividing cells Expression difficult to control and stabilize Expensive and complex to prepare	Marker studies, ex vivo treatments, vaccines
Adenovirus	High titers Efficient entry into most cell types High level of expression Infection of nondividing cells	Vectors contain viral genes Immunogenic, stimulating T- and B-cell responses Generation of replication-competent virus Factors controlling tropism not well understood	Localized in vivo treatments: cystic fibrosis, short-term treatments such as cancer and cardiovascular disease
Adeno-associated virus	Integration at specific sites	Requires replicating adenovirus to grow No helper cell line Limited insert size	Similar to adenovirus
Herpesvirus	High titers May be neurotropic	Complex construction No packaging cell lines	Neurological diseases
Psseudotyped retrovirus	High titers Higher efficiency of retrovirus infection Broader host range	Similar to retrovirus	Not established; may be similar to retrovirus
Nonviral			
Naked DNA	Easy to prepare No size constraints High level of safety No viral genes Lack of integration High level of safety Lack of integration	Inefficient entry and uptake Limited persistence and lack of stability	Topical and/or mechanical applications, including skin and vasculature
DNA liposomes	Same as naked DNA More efficient uptake of DNA	Limited persistence and lack of stability	Direct in vivo applications, cancer, cardiovascular disease, cystic fibrosis
Adenoviral polylysine DNA conjugates	Same as DNA liposomes Targetable to specific cell types	Requires adenovirus Complex to construct	Same as DNA liposomes

Reprinted with permission from Nabel [10].

areas are great, and this technology requires more development.

Two critical steps are necessary for successful vascular gene therapy: delivery of genes to vascular cells and maintenance of gene expression. Gene delivery is being pursued through surgical and percutaneous approaches. Catheter-mediated gene transfer is likely to be used for multiple vascular applications. An area of important research is the combination of vectors with mechanical devices. Expression of transferred genes is also critical for successful gene therapy. While much is known about DNA sequences that regulate gene expression in cultured cells, relatively little is known about gene regulation in vivo. Additional studies are required in order to define and enhance sequences within constructs that optimize gene expression, to identify cell specific promoters that direct gene expression to specific vascular cells, and to stabilize gene expression within cells. The complexity of interactions between vector systems and vascular tissues is not completely understood. These complexities must be taken into consideration in the development of animal models. For example, while expression of recombinant genes within the vasculature of animal models may be helpful in dissecting disease pathophysiology, species variation and phenotypic differences are likely to exist between animal models and human patients. Principles of disease pathogenesis may vary between species. Nonetheless, animal models are useful in the elucidation of disease pathophysiology and the development of therapeutic modalities.

At the present time, there are no clinical gene therapy trials for coronary thrombosis and thrombolysis. However, several candidate genes have been identified and animal models have been developed [14,15]. Local thrombolysis can be achieved by overexpression of components of the plasminogen system, such as plasminogen, tissue plasminogen activator (t-PA), and/or urokinase plasminogen activator (u-PA). Thrombosis may also be inhibited by antagonists to thrombin and other procoagulant proteins. Many of these approaches are discussed within this section. It is possible that these genetic approaches may be used in combination with other thrombolytics, antiplatelet agents, or anticoagulants to diminish focal thrombosis.

While the promise of gene therapy is great, technical development will be required for full application to human vascular diseases. Nonetheless, substantial progress has been made, even in these early stages. The possibilities of using genetic approaches to treat thrombotic disorders are considerable, and the work described in the subsequent chapters represents important advances in this field.

References

1. Nabel EG. Gene therapy for cardiovascular diseases. Circulation 91:541, 1995.
2. Nabel EG, Yang Z, Plautz G, Forough R, Zhan X, Haudenschild CC, Maciag T, Nabel GJ. Recombinant fibroblast growth factor-1 promotes intimal hyperplasia and angiogenesis in arteries in vivo. Nature 362:844, 1993.
3. vonderLeyen HE, Gibbons GH, Morishita R, Lewis NP, Zhang L, Nakajima M, Kaneda Y, Cooke JP, Dzau VJ. Gene therapy inhibiting neointimal vascular lesion: In vivo transfer of endothelial cell nitric oxide synthase gene. Proc Natl Acad Sci USA 92:1137, 1995.
4. Geary RL, Clowes AW, Lau S, Vergel S, Dale DC, Osborne WR. Gene transfer in baboons using prosthetic vascular grafts seeded with retrovirally transduced smooth muscle cells: A model for local and systemic gene therapy. Hum Gene Ther 5:1211, 1994.
5. Chang MW, Barr E, Seltzer J, Jiang J-Q, Nabel GJ, Nabel EG, Parmacek MS, Leiden JM. Cytostatic gene therapy for vascular proliferative disorders using a constitutively active form of Rb. Science 267:518, 1995.
6. Isner JM, Walsh K, Symes J, Pieczek A, Takeshita S, Lowry J, Rossow S, Rosenfield K, Weir L, Brogi E, Shainfield R. Arterial gene therapy for therapeutic angiogenesis in patients with peripheral artery disease [news]. Circulation 91:2687, 1995.
7. Isner JM, Pieczek A, Schainfeld R, Blair R, Haley L, Asahara T, Rosenfield K, Razvi S, Walsh K, Symes JF. Clinical evidence of angiogenesis after arterial gene transfer of ph VEGF 165 in patient with ischaemic limb. Lancet 348:370, 1996.
8. Nabel EG, Plautz G, Nabel GJ. Site-specific gene expression in vivo by direct gene transfer into the arterial wall. Science 249:1285, 1990.
9. Miller AD. Retroviral vectors. Curr Top Microbiol 158:1, 1992.
10. Nabel EG. Vectors for gene therapy. In Current Protocols in Human Genetics. New York: John Wiley, 1996: 12.0.1.
11. Yang Y, Nunes FA, Berencsi K, Furth EE, Gonczol E, Wilson JM. Cellular immunity to viral antigens limits E1-deleted adenoviruses for gene therapy. Proc Natl Acad Sci USA 91:4407, 1994.
12. Yang Y, Nunes FA, Berencsi K, Gonczol E, Engelhardt JF, Wilson JM. Inactivation of E2a in recombinant adenoviruses improves the prospect for gene therapy in cystic fibrosis. Nature Genet 7:362, 1994.
13. Stephan D, Yang ZY, San H, Simari RD, Wheeler CJ, Felgner PL, Gordon D, Nabel GJ, Nabel EG. A new cationic liposome DNA complex enhances the efficiency of arterial gene transfer in vivo. Hum Gene Ther 7:1803, 1996.
14. Carmeliet P, Collen D. Gene targeting and gene transfer studies of the biological role of the plasminogen/plasmin system. Thromb Haemost 74:429, 1995.
15. Rade JJ, Schulick AH, Virmani R, Dichek DA. Local adenoviral-mediated expression of recombinant hirudin reduces neointima formation after arterial injury. Nature Med 2:293, 1996.

PART C: NEW DIMENSIONS

SECTION XIV: FUTURE DIRECTIONS FOR BASIC INVESTIGATIONAL AND CLINICAL RESEARCH

Paul R. Eisenberg

The importance of interaction of the hemostatic system with inflammatory mechanisms and estrogen has recently been appreciated. This section provides an overview of the importance of inflammatory mechanisms and their interaction with hemostasis and the consequences of coronary thrombosis. In addition, a perspective on potential interactions of estrogen with hemostasis and its role in cardiovascular disease in women is explored.

42. ROLE OF INFLAMMATION FOLLOWING MYOCARDIAL ISCHEMIA AND REPERFUSION

Nikolaos G. Frangogiannis and Mark L. Entman

Introduction

The purpose of this chapter is to discuss the potential mechanisms by which neutrophil-mediated inflammatory injury may complicate myocardial infarction. It should be emphasized that no one seriously proposes that the primary injury associated with myocardial infarction is inflammatory in nature. Rather, our goal is to describe mechanisms of reaction to injury and to present evidence suggesting that this secondary reaction might extend and complicate cardiac injury associated with ischemia.

Recently the development of effective reperfusion techniques of the previously ischemic myocardium has underlined the importance of a better understanding of the inflammatory reaction in both the acute myocardial injury and the healing phase. Numerous clinical trials have established the tremendous benefit of early reperfusion during a myocardial infarction. However, the reinstitution of coronary flow in previously ischemic areas markedly augments the influx of leukocytes and potentiates the inflammatory reaction to injury, leading to damage of potentially viable myocardium. Recognition that neutrophils play an important role in ischemia/reperfusion injury increased interest in defining the mechanisms responsible for leukocyte-mediated tissue injury.

This chapter summarizes the information derived from in vivo and in vitro experiments on the cellular and molecular mediation of the secondary inflammatory response occurring following myocardial ischemia and reperfusion. We begin with a brief general description of reperfusion injury as a concept and define the cellular and molecular mechanisms by which the inflammatory reaction ensues in response to myocardial ischemia and reperfusion. In the remainder of the chapter we propose a working hypothesis describing the events mediating the postreperfusion inflammatory injury.

Pathological Basis of Ischemia/Reperfusion Injury

The concept that a reaction to injury may extend a disease process is fundamental in pathology; however, its application to myocardial ischemia is relatively recent [1]. Early descriptions of the inflammatory process associated with myocardial infarction by Mallory and colleagues [2] concluded that "polymorphonuclear leukocytes are attracted and infiltrate around and into the necrotic muscle" and that "the infiltration is much more active . . . in those portions adjacent to the uninvolved muscle." However, these early descriptive studies focused on the role of inflammation in the healing phase of myocardial infarction and failed to consider the possibility that this reaction to injury may function in a deleterious way. Only in the past 20 years has the potential role of this inflammatory response been studied.

In both clinical and experimental models, the initial insult resulting in injury is in all cases ischemia. Coronary artery occlusion critically reduces the blood flow to the portion of the myocardium subserved, markedly impairing the energy metabolism, leading to cell death. In occlusions of the coronary arteries as short as 5 minutes, functional abnormalities of the reperfused myocardium are observed for as long as 24–48 hours [3]. These abnormalities are not attended by lethal injury to the ischemic myocardium, which ultimately recovers. Clearly this transient functional abnormality (*stunned myocardium*) is not associated with neutrophil infiltration; rather, it is related to reactive oxygen formation. The absence of any neutrophil response under these circumstances emphasizes that neutrophil-induced injury is only seen secondary to lethal injury of the myocardium resulting from previous ischemic insult.

The functional abnormalities seen during reperfusion consequent to lethal myocardial injury can be grouped into three general categories: myocardial dysfunction, endothelium-related vasomotor dysfunction, and increased microvascular permeability with associated flow abnormalities. In addition, it has been demonstrated that rapid neutrophil localization occurs during reperfusion within regions of previous myocardial ischemia, with the highest rates seen in the first hour of reperfusion [4]. This observation has led to a number of investigations to elucidate the role of the neutrophil in reperfusion-associated myocardial injury. Two general strategies have been applied to study this problem. The first approach involves the use of antiinflammatory therapy to mitigate both the functional and pathological changes associated with ischemia and reperfusion. The second strategy involves the study of the cellular and molecular mechanisms by which neutrophil localization and neutrophil-mediated myocardial injury occur. Both subjects are discussed here; however, the bulk of this chapter deals with the latter approach.

Use of Antiinflammatory Strategies in the Study of Myocardial Ischemia and Reperfusion

The first major body of evidence for a role of inflammation and neutrophil infiltration in the extension of myocardial ischemic injury came as result of a generalized effort to develop strategies to minimize the size of myocardial infarcts. Enormous resources were used in an attempt to interfere with a putative inflammatory mechanism associated with myocardial ischemia. Thus, strategies aimed at reducing the generation of chemotactic factors, such as complement depletion [5], lipoxygenase inhibitors [6], and leukotriene B_4 antagonists, were successful in limiting infarct size in some experimental models. Other experiments utilizing prostacyclin analogs [7] and adenosine [8] to alter neutrophil function were likewise successful. Approaches that reduced neutrophil number, such as antineutrophil antibodies [9], neutrophil-depleting antimetabolites [10], and neutrophil filters [11], were also successful in reducing ischemia-related injury in some models. Finally, free radical scavengers, expected to protect against neutrophil-derived reactive oxygen species, were also effective in reducing infarct size or sensitivity to ischemia [12,13]. All these experiments pointed to a potential role of inflammation in myocardial ischemia. These early experimental data were sufficiently compelling that a potential benefit from an antiinflammatory agent was suggested in patients with acute myocardial infarction.

The subsequent methylprednisolone [14] trial resulted in catastrophic results, increasing the incidence of ventricular aneurysm and cardiac rupture [15]. It also emphasized the need for a better understanding of the cellular and molecular events associated with myocardial ischemia and reperfusion in order to develop more site-specific interventions that could mitigate inflammatory injury during early reperfusion without interfering with myocardial healing.

In the remainder of this chapter we deal specifically with the mechanisms through which this inflammatory injury is mediated and attempt to propose potential targets through which it can be modified. We hope that the insights reviewed herein will promote the design of better experiments to assess the potential significance of reperfusion injury.

Neutrophil Chemoattractants Initiate Inflammation in Myocardial Ischemia and Reperfusion

COMPLEMENT ACTIVATION
Hill and Ward [16] were the first to demonstrate that ischemic myocardial injury can activate the complement cascade using a rat model of myocardial ischemia. Subsequently Pinckard and colleagues [17,18] suggested that myocardial cell necrosis results in the release of subcellular membrane constituents rich in mitochondria, which are capable of triggering the early-acting components (C1, C4, C2, and C3) of the complement cascade. The mechanism by which complement activation occurs has been actively studied. Rossen et al. [19] reported an increase in C1q binding molecules in the circulation of patients with acute myocardial infarction. In a canine model of ischemia/reperfusion, experimental coronary occlusions lasting from 15 to 45 minutes were sufficient to provide a stimulus on reperfusion for the accumulation of C1q in previously ischemic myocardium. C1q localization correlated with neutrophil accumulation in the same segments.

In subsequent experiments, C1q binding proteins of mitochondrial origin were demonstrable in the cardiac lymph during the first 4 hours of reperfusion [20]. Recently, Rossen and colleagues [21] have suggested that during myocardial ischemia, mitochondria, extruded through breaks in the sarcolemma, unfold and release membrane fragments rich in cardiolipin and protein. By binding C1 and supplying sites for the assembly of later-acting complement components, these subcellular fragments provide the means to disseminate the complement-mediated inflammatory response to ischemic injury.

Dreyer and coworkers [22] showed that postischemic cardiac lymph contains leukocyte chemotactic activity that is maximal during the first hour of reperfusion, with washout within the next 3 hours. Neutralizing antibodies to C5a completely inhibited the chemotactic activity of postischemic cardiac lymph during that period [23]. Furthermore, agents such as cobra venom factor [5], soluble complement receptor-1 [24], or C1 esterase inhibitor [25], which deplete or inactivate complement, have been shown to attenuate myocardial necrosis in animal models.

These experiments provide compelling evidence for a role for complement activation in the chemotaxis associated with myocardial ischemia/reperfusion. However, the potential importance of other chemotactic stimuli, such as leukotrienes and chemokines, cannot be ruled out. Most of the data concerning the time course of neutrophil chemotactic factors in myocardial ischemia come from experiments performed in a canine model of ischemia/reperfusion. Unlike in humans, in the dog the 5-lipoxygenase system for production of leukotrienes is not a prominent feature of the inflammatory response. In addition, canine neutrophils respond poorly to leukotriene B_4 (LTB$_4$). Thus, elucidation of the role of lipid-derived autacoids in myocardial ischemia/reperfusion will require study in other species. On the other hand, chemotactic factors that act when bound firmly to a cell or extracellular surface (such as interleukin-8) would not be found soluble in the cardiac lymph and could not be studied using these methods.

TABLE 42-1. Nomenclature of the chemokines

C-X-C chemokines	C-C chemokines
A. With ELR motif	
Interleukin-8	MCP-1, -2, -3
ENA-78	RANTES
GCP-2	MIP-1 α, -1 β
GRO-α, -β, -γ (rodent homologues:	TCA3
KC, MIP-2 α, -2 β)	LAG-1
β-Thromboglobulin	I-309
CTAP-III	Murine C10
NAP-2	
B. Without ELR motif	
Platelet factor-4 (PF-4)	
Inducible protein-10 (IP-10)	
MIG	

ENA-78: Epithelial cell-derived neutrophil-activating protein-78; GCP-2: Granulocyte chemotactic protein-2; GRO: Growth related protein; MIP: Macrophage inflammatory protein; CTAP-III: Connective tissue-activating peptide III; NAP-2: Neutrophil-activating peptide; MIG: Monokine induced by interferon-gamma; MCP: Monocyte chemotactic protein; RANTES: Regulated on activation, normal T cells, expressed and secreted; TCA: T-cell activated gene; LAG: Lymphocyte activation gene.

INTERLEUKIN-8 AND OTHER CHEMOKINES

An additional fundamental mechanism associated with leukocyte chemotaxis has only recently been investigated, involving a family of structurally related proteins, with chemotactic, proinflammatory, and reparative functions, which have been termed *chemokines* [26] (Table 42-1). They are small proteins of 70–80 amino acids, with four conserved cysteines that form two disulfide bonds, a short amino-terminal and a longer carboxy-terminal sequence. The disulfides confer to the chemokines the biologically active configuration and are, therefore, essential for biological activity. The chemokine family has been subdivided into two subfamilies, based on the arrangement of the first two cysteines, which are either separated by one amino acid (C-X-C chemokines) or adjacent (C-C chemokines) [27,28]. Members of the C-X-C chemokine subfamily (e.g., IL-8, NAP-2, GRO-α, GRO-β, GRO-gamma, and ENA-78) exert predominantly neutrophil-activating and chemotactic properties. On the other hand, C-C subfamily chemokines (e.g., MIP-1a, MIP-1β, MCP-1, MCP-2, MCP-3, and RANTES) generally mediate mononuclear cell activation and recruitment.

Interleukin [IL]-8 is the most prominent of the chemotactic and proinflammatory chemokines and is more selective for neutrophils than leukotriene B_4 (LTB), C5a, or platelet activating factor (PAF) [29,30]. Its importance in ischemia and reperfusion was first suggested by the ability of anti–IL-8 antibodies to reduce lung parenchymal injury in lung ischemia/reperfusion [31]. Utilizing a canine model of myocardial ischemia and reperfusion, Kukielka and colleagues [32] demonstrated that IL-8 mRNA is markedly and consistently induced in the ischemic and reperfused myocardium, peaking in the first 3 hours of reperfusion. IL-8 mRNA was not found in normally perfused myocardial segments. In contrast to the ischemic and reperfused segments, nonreperfused segments, after 3 or 4 hours of ischemia, demonstrated only minimal induction of IL-8 mRNA, despite severe ischemia. In vitro experiments showed that recombinant canine IL-8 markedly increased adhesion of neutrophils to isolated cardiac myocytes through a CD18-dependent mechanism, resulting in direct cytotoxicity for cardiac myocytes. Thus IL-8 constitutes a molecular signal that could contribute to neutrophil localization in early reperfusion and could participate in inflammatory myocardial injury by serving as a stimulus for activation of neutrophil adhesiveness and cytotoxic behavior. It is interesting to speculate that, under circumstances in which blood flow may preclude the establishment of a stable soluble chemotactic gradient, a surface-bound chemoattractant may represent an effective mechanism of chemotactic agent presentation (*haptotaxis*) and neutrophil activation.

Recently, Ivey and colleagues [33] investigated, in a rabbit model of myocardial infarction, the generation of neutrophil chemoattractants. Their observations suggested a sequential release of chemoattractants: The first, C5a, was generated in interstitial fluid, followed by IL-8 generation by infiltrating neutrophils.

LIPID-DERIVED AUTACOIDS

Leukotriene B_4 is the major product of the oxidative metabolism of arachidonic acid by the enzyme 5-lipoxygenase in neutrophils. In many species it is potently chemotactic for PMNs, and an increased generation of LTB_4 ex vivo in activated PMN from both acute myocardial infarction and unstable angina patients has been described [34]. A recent study [35] demonstrated increased urinary excretion of leukotriene E_4, the major urinary metabolite of peptide leukotrienes in humans, in patients with acute coronary syndromes, providing clinical evidence for involvement of 5-lipoxygenase in acute myocardial infarction and unstable angina. In addition to 5-lipoxygenase, there is also a 12-lipoxygenase and 15-lipoxygenase isozyme found in neutrophils, with relative quantities varying among species.

Thus the major product of dog neutrophils is 12-hydroxyisomers (12-HETES), which are weakly chemotactic [36]; whereas in the rabbit, in addition to LTB_4, neutrophils contain 15-hydroxyisomers (15-HETES) under higher arachidonic acid concentrations. These species variations and differences in the sensitivity of neutrophils to these products are probably responsible for the differences in therapeutic effectiveness of various antileukotriene strategies in ischemic models from different species. The relative absence of 5-lipoxygenase products in the dog and the insensitivity of dog neutrophils to LTB_4 may explain the ineffectiveness of LTB_4 receptor antagonists in limiting canine myocardial infarction size [37]. On the other hand, a similar LTB_4 receptor antagonist was capable of reducing infarct size in a rabbit model of myocardial ischemia [38]. It is possible that lipoxygenase derivatives may not be important chemotactic factors until after neutrophils have been localized to the ischemic and reperfused areas as part of their activation by a primary stimulus because their production depends on initial activation of their synthesis.

Platelet activating factor is another lipid-derived molecule that has been suggested as an important chemotactic factor in myocardial ischemia/reperfusion. PAF is formed by endothelial cells in response to thrombin [39] and, in addition to its potent platelet activating ability, is also an important chemotactic factor, which promotes neutrophil adhesion to endothelial cells. PAF is also involved in other adherence dependent processes, such as advanced production of reactive oxygen [39]. Its role in myocardial ischemia/reperfusion has not been elucidated yet. A recent study in a rat model of ischemia/reperfusion [40] demonstrated release of PAF in the plasma in early reperfusion and a reduction in infarct size with the use of a specific PAF receptor antagonist. However, another study in a canine model of myocardial ischemia/reperfusion failed to limit ischemia and reperfusion-induced myocardial damage. The role of PAF in myocardial ischemia/reperfusion requires careful investigation because of its potential implications in clinical reperfusion, which is undoubtedly associated with high concentrations of thrombin, a potent stimulator of PAF synthesis.

REACTIVE OXYGEN SPECIES AS CHEMOTACTIC ACTIVATORS

It has been suggested that oxygen-derived free radicals produced by activated neutrophils is a major mechanism by which neutrophils might injure other cells. However, the relationship of reactive oxygen and neutrophil function may be more complex. Evidence suggests that neutrophil-generated superoxide reacts with an extracellular precursor to generate a *neutrophil activating factor* in the serum [41]. This factor has not been identified; however, it may be related to enzymatic or nonenzymatic generation of lipid-derived autacoids. Granger and colleagues [42,43] have provided evidence for a potential role of reactive oxygen in chemotaxis, including studies that demonstrated free radical scavengers reduced neutrophil infiltration in the ischemic and reperfused intestine [44]. Similar studies have not been performed in the heart.

Potential mechanisms by which reactive oxygen may generate a leukotactic stimulus are as follows:

1. Complement activation. In whole human serum the H_2O_2 system induces generation of C5a activity [45] via pathways that have not been elucidated.
2. Induction of P-selectin expression [46].
3. Production of PAF and PAF analogs derived from oxidatively fragmenting phospholipids [47]. PAF and P-selectin may interact in the trapping and transmigration of neutrophils.

4. Increase of endothelial intracellular adhesion molecule (ICAM)-1's ability for binding neutrophils without detectable upregulation [48].

Neutrophil Localization and the Role of Adhesion Molecules

NEUTROPHIL TRAPPING IN MICROVESSELS AND THE "NO REFLOW" PHENOMENON

The first step in neutrophil localization involves neutrophil trapping in the microvasculature, specifically in capillaries and veins; a similar localization is seen within the first hour of reperfusion in an experimental myocardial infarction. Engler and coworkers [11] demonstrated that entrapment of leukocytes in the microcirculation precedes their role in an inflammatory reaction. Neutrophils are large and stiff cells, and may adhere to capillary endothelium, preventing reperfusion of capillaries following coronary ischemia. The mechanism by which neutrophil trapping occurs in the microvessels is likely to be multifactorial. Chemotactic factors rapidly induce neutrophils to change shape and to become less deformable. At higher concentrations of chemotactic factors, neutrophils also undergo homotypic aggregation, which may further contribute to obstruction. Neutrophils also release a variety of autacoids, which induce vasoconstriction and platelet aggregation, such as thromboxane B_2 [49] and LTB_4 [50]. Neutrophil interaction with endothelial cells via specific adhesion molecules results in neutrophil margination and adhesion to the endothelium. It has been suggested that this neutrophil localization may alter both endothelium-derived vasomotor functions and microvascular permeability, mediating ischemia/reperfusion-induced microvascular injury [51,52].

The most dramatic and pathologically significant microvascular abnormality is known as the no-reflow phenomenon [53] and has also been directly linked to neutrophil localization. Ambrosio and coworkers [54] demonstrated in a canine model that the occurrence of areas of markedly impaired perfusion in postischemic myocardium is related only in part to an inability to reperfuse certain areas on reflow. A more important factor was represented by a delayed progressive fall in flow to areas that initially received adequate reperfusion. This phenomenon develops in regions receiving no collateral flow during ischemia and is associated with neutrophil accumulation and capillary plugging during late reperfusion.

While changes in cell shape and deformability and vasoconstriction are important mechanisms for neutrophil accumulation in the ischemic and reperfused myocardium, the bulk of evidence suggests that the more specific interactions between adhesion molecules are the most critical factors in the control of neutrophil-induced pathophysiological changes.

NEUTROPHIL–ENDOTHELIAL INTERACTIONS AND NEUTROPHIL TRANSMIGRATION FOLLOWING MYOCARDIAL ISCHEMIA AND REPERFUSION

A better understanding of the molecular interactions between leukocytes and the endothelium has given rise to a consensus model of how leukocyte recruitment into tissues is regulated [55]. There is increasing evidence that leukocyte–endothelial interactions are regulated by a cascade of molecular steps that correspond to the morphological changes that accompany adhesion. This adhesion cascade can be divided into three sequential steps:

1. The initial "rolling" step involves overcoming the shear stress associated with laminar flow in the venules. The flowing leukocyte is tethered and brought into contact with the endothelial wall by selectin-mediated interactions. Rolling is hypothesized to allow leukocytes to interact with locally released inflammatory mediators and chemokines, such as IL-8.
2. The firm adhesion step is mediated through the integrins (such as CD11a/CD18 and CD11b/CD18) binding to ICAM-1 (CD54) on endothelial cells.
3. Transmigration of the neutrophil, in part mediated by platelet–endothelium cell adhesion molecule (PECAM-1; CD31).

NEUTROPHIL ROLLING: THE ROLE OF THE SELECTINS

The selectin family of adhesion molecules mediates the initial attachment of leukocytes to endothelial cells before their firm adhesion and diapedesis at sites of tissue injury and inflammation [56–59]. The selectin family consists of three closely related cell-surface molecules: L-selectin (MEL-14, LAM-1, CD62L), E-selectin (ELAM-1, CD62E), and P-selectin (PADGEM, GMP-140, CD62P) (Table 42-2). L-selectin expression is limited to hematopoietic cells, with most classes of leukocytes constitutively expressing L-selectin at some stage of differentiation. The majority of circulating neutrophils, monocytes, eosinophils T cells, and B cells express L-selectin, which is rapidly shed from the surface of these cells following their activation. The broad expression of L-selectin allows it to play a role in the trafficking of all leukocyte lineages. In contrast, E-selectin is expressed only following de novo synthesis 4–6 hours after activation of endothelial cells by cytokines (such as tumor recrosis factor [TNF]-α, IL-1β) or by bacterial endotoxin.

P-selectin is constitutively found in Weibel-Palade bodies of endothelial cells and in alpha granules of platelets. Within minutes after activation by thrombogenic and inflammatory mediators, P-selectin is mobilized to the cell surface without the need for new protein synthesis. Inducing agents include thrombin, histamine, complement fragments, oxygen-derived free radicals, and cytokines. Cell-surface expression of P-selectin is generally short lived, which makes it an ideal candidate for mediating early leukocyte–endothelial cell interactions. However, in vivo studies of P-selectin function suggest that it may also be important at later time points as a cytokine-induced adhesion molecule.

One important property of the selectins is that they promote leukocyte rolling under flow conditions. Each selectin recognizes specific carbohydrate sequences on either leukocytes (E-selectin or P-selectin) or the endothelium (L-selectin). In most venules, leukocyte rolling begins within minutes after tissue injury, reaching a peak 20–40 minutes later and remaining fairly constant over at least 2 hours. P-selectin mobilized from Weibel-Palade bodies is likely to be involved in the early phases of rolling. Blocking P-selectin function in vivo substantially reduces the initial spontaneous rolling of leukocytes in venules of exteriorized mesentery. However, rolling is progressively restored after a period of 10–15 minutes, reflecting the participation of L-selectin during subsequent stages of the process. Selectins are ideally suited to this tethering role because they have a long molecular structure that extends above the surrounding glycocalyx and allows them to capture passing leukocytes that express the appropriate receptor. Furthermore, L-selectin has been found on the tips of leukocyte microvilli, which are the first points of contact with the endothelium. These studies demonstrate that selectins mediate the initial interactions of leukocytes with endothelial cells, which slow the leukocyte as a prerequisite to stable adhesion and diapedesis.

The role of selectins in ischemia and reperfusion is not well defined at present and represents an area of active investigation. L-selectin is constitutively expressed in neutrophils in a highly specific distribution and is critical to neutrophil–endothelial adhesion under shear stresses found in venules [60]. Studies have suggested that it is obligatory for margination, although its counterligands have not been yet defined [61]. There is evidence that, under the proper circumstances, E-selectin or P-selectin may serve as a counterligand, but, because E-selectin must be synthesized de novo by endothelial cells, it would be projected to play only a minor role in early postreperfusion myocardial injury [62].

In contrast, P-selectin surface expression occurs rapidly on endothelial cells under circumstances likely to be seen during ischemia and reperfusion. It is stored in the Weibel-Palade bodies [63] and is rapidly translocated to the endothelial surface in response to thrombin and/or oxidative stress [64], both of which would be likely to be found on reperfusion and initiated by thrombolytic agents, and to histamine, which is rapidly released in the ischemic and reperfused myocardium by degranulating mast cells [65] (see discussion of mast cell degranulation later).

Recent work has suggested that P-selectin may, in part, constitute the counterligand to L-selectin to effect margination under these circumstances [66]. However, it is likely that additional inducible counterligands will be found significant in this reac-

TABLE 42-2. Nomenclature and structural characteristics of the selectins

Selectin	Location	Expression
L-selectin (MEL-14, Leu-8 TQ1, LAM-1, LECCAM-1)	Leukocytes (constitutive)	Decreases on cell activation
E-selectin (ELAM-1, LECCAM-2)	Endothelium (transcriptionally regulated)	Increases 4–6 hours after activation with LPS or cytokines (IL-1, TNF)
P-selectin (CD62P, PADGEM, GMP-140, LECCAM-3)	Platelets (α granules) Endothelium (Weibel-Palade bodies)	Increases minutes after activation with thrombin, histamine, substance P, free radicals, cytokines through increased surface expression

ELAM: Endothelial-leukocyte adhesion molecule; IL: Interleukin; TNF: Tumor necrosis factor.

tion. Recent studies have suggested that monoclonal antibodies against L-selectin [67] and P-selectin [68] were effective in reducing myocardial necrosis, preserving coronary endothelial function, and attenuating neutrophil accumulation in ischemic myocardial tissue in a feline model of ischemia/reperfusion.

Thus, current concepts of myocardial ischemia and reperfusion suggest a role for selectins in supporting margination under shear stress. The transient nature of this adhesive interaction is important because it allows leukocytes to "sample" the local endothelium for the presence of specific trigger factors that can activate leukocyte integrins and allow the cascade to proceed.

CD18 AND THE LEUKOCYTE β2 INTEGRINS

Although rolling appears to be a prerequisite for eventual firm adherence to blood vessels under conditions of flow, selectin-dependent adhesion of leukocytes does not lead to firm adhesion and transmigration unless another set of adhesion molecules is engaged. Activation of the leukocytes, mediated through the locally derived chemoattractants IL-8, PAF, or MCP-1, dramatically increases the adhesiveness of leukocytes for endothelium, primarily by upregulated surface expression of β_2 integrins. These models are based primarily on observations with neutrophils, and until recently the extent to which monocytes and lymphocytes conform to this paradigm had not been tested. For neutrophils, firm adhesion requires activation of the β_2 (CD18) integrin subfamily, resulting in binding to one of the intercellular adhesion molecules on the surfaces of endothelial cells [69].

Integrins are a family of heterodimeric membrane glycoproteins that consist of an α and β subunit [70]; these subunits are associated through noncovalent bonds and transported to the cell surface as a complex. The cell modulates its interaction with other cells and with the extracellular matrix by modifying the structure and function of the integrins. The most important of these subfamilies for neutrophils is the β_2

integrins (also known as leukocyte cell adhesion molecules), which share the β chain CD18 paired with CD11a (LFA-1), CD11b (Mac-1), or CD11c (p150,95) [71]. The structure and ligands of these proteins are summarized in Table 42-3.

LFA-1, Mac-1, and p150,95 have different and yet overlapping roles in adhesion, partly due to their characteristics of expression on leukocytes. LFA-1 is expressed on all immune cells, with the exception of some tissue macrophages. The distribution of Mac-1 is somewhat more limited and is predominantly expressed on myeloid cells, including macrophages and granulocytes. It is also expressed on large granular lymphocytes and a subset of CD5+ B cells. A similar distribution exists for p150,95. Three members of the immunoglobulin gene family, including ICAM-1, ICAM-2, and ICAM-3, are defined as functional ligands for LFA-1, but ICAM-1 appears to play the primary role in leukocyte trafficking.

In striking contrast to the cellular distribution of β_2 integrins, ICAM-1 is widely distributed on nonhematopoietic cells, including endothelial cells, fibroblasts, dendritic cells, keratinocytes, and certain epithelial cells. Constitutive expression of ICAM-1 in nonhematopoietic cells is low, but surface expression is markedly upregulated by a variety of inflammatory mediators, including TNF-α, IL-1, IL-6, and endotoxin. These characteristics of ICAM-1 account for its involvement in a wide range of pathologic disorders. Substantial evidence suggests that Mac-1, in addition to LFA-1, is capable of binding to ICAM-1. Smith and coworkers [72] demonstrated that adhesion of stimulated neutrophils to endothelial cells depends on both Mac-1 and LFA-1, whereas adhesion of unstimulated neutrophils is largely an LFA-1–dependent phenomenon. Because anti–ICAM-1 MAbs inhibited adhesion of both stimulated and unstimulated neutrophils to endothelial cells, it was concluded that both LFA-1 and Mac-1 interact with ICAM-1 [72]. The significance of the Mac-1–ICAM-1 interaction in inflammatory reperfusion injury is discussed later in this chapter.

TABLE 42-3. Nomenclature and ligands of the β_2 integrins

Name	Heterodimers	Ligands
LFA-1 (CD11a/CD18)	$a_L b_2$	ICAM-1, ICAM-2, ICAM-3
Mac-1 (CD11b/CD18)	$a_M b_2$	Fibrinogen, fibronectin iC3b, factor X, Leishmania gp63 Bordetella FHA ICAM-1, ICAM-2, ICAM-3(?)
p150, 95 (CD11c/CD18)	$a_X b_2$	Fibrinogen, iC3b ICAM-1,2

ICAM: Intercellular adhesion molecule.

The iC3b fragment of complement was the first ligand to be demonstrated for Mac-1 [73]. Several recent reports suggested the potential of Mac-1 to interact with a broad spectrum of ligands. These include fibrinogen, fibronectin, and polysaccharide determinants of bacterial capsules or yeast; the significance of these interactions remains unknown, however.

In a variety of cardiovascular-related inflammatory models, monoclonal antibodies against the CD11/CD18 complex reduced the pathophysiologic consequences. Simpson and colleagues showed in a canine model that a monoclonal antibody against CD11b substantially reduced myocardial necrosis after 90 minutes of coronary ischemia and 6 hours of reperfusion [74]. Later experiments suggested that inhibition of Mac-1–mediated neutrophil adhesion may provide sustained limitation of myocardial necrosis by demonstrating substantial benefit in a canine model of 90 minutes of coronary ischemia and 72 hours of reperfusion [75] when an F(ab')2 fragment of a monoclonal antibody against CD11b was tested.

Administration of anti-CD18 antibodies has reduced myocardial infarct size in a rabbit model of 1-hour ischemia and 5 hours of reperfusion when administered systemically before the coronary occlusion [76]. In another study in rabbits [77], a different anti-CD18 monoclonal antibody was applied to radiolabeled rabbit neutrophils before they were introduced into a rabbit undergoing a 30-minute occlusion and 3-hour reperfusion protocol, resulting in decreased accumulation of neutrophils. In canine models anti-CD18 antibodies have been shown to reduce neutrophil accumulation after 1 hour of ischemia and 1 hour of reperfusion [4]. Anti-CD18 antibodies have also been shown to reduce infarct size in a feline [78] and in a primate [79] model of myocardial ischemia/reperfusion. However, in another study in the dog they failed to reduce infarct size, although they were effective in reducing neutrophil accumulation and preserving microvascular blood flow [80].

In addition to myocardial injury, there is evidence that CD18-dependent adhesion may be important in injury to the endothelium in large vessels as well as in the microvasculature. Indeed, CD18 antibodies have been shown to prevent depression of endothelium-derived relaxation in postischemic vessels [81]. There is evidence that neutrophil migration into the subendothelial layer of the vascular wall may be important in this injury, and it is prevented by anti-CD18 antibodies. Finally, anti-CD18 antibodies have prevented alterations in microvascular permeability

in both ischemic and reperfused small intestine [52] and in skeletal muscle [82]. In addition to altering neutrophil–endothelial interaction, anti-integrin antibodies alter neutrophil adhesion to parenchymal cells. As discussed later in this chapter, this latter property may be a critical factor in limiting tissue injury.

An important characteristic of the neutrophil integrins is that under baseline conditions they exist in a relatively inactive conformation, rendering the leukocyte nonadhesive. A key event of the adhesion cascade is the activation and deactivation of these integrins at the proper times and places. Mac-1 is primarily stored in secondary granules of neutrophils and secretory granules in monocytes, with approximately 10% of the total protein found on the surface [83]. Recent evidence suggests that an initial leukotactic stimulus qualitatively activates the Mac-1 on the surface of the cell and markedly increases its affinity for its counterligand [83]. Good evidence to support the importance of surface activation in white cell emigration has been presented for two inflammatory mediators: PAF and IL-8 [69]. Both are present in the ischemic and reperfused myocardium. Thus activation and deactivation of the high-avidity state may be an important factor in neutrophil-induced cell injury.

Transendothelial cell migration does not necessarily accompany leukocyte adherence to the endothelium. The process of transendothelial migration of neutrophils has been shown to involve neutrophil β_2 integrins and endothelial cell platelet–endothelium cell adhesion molecule (PECAM-1; CD31) [84,85]. Recent studies implicate integrin-associated protein (IAP, CD47) as a third molecule essential for neutrophil migration through endothelium into sites of inflammation [86]. The significance of these findings and their possible implications in the pathogenesis of myocardial ischemia/reperfusion remain unclear.

Mechanisms of Neutrophil-Induced Myocardial Injury

The focus of the previous sections of this chapter has been the mechanism by which neutrophils are attracted to and activated in the ischemic and reperfused myocardium. The mechanism by which neutrophil-induced myocardial injury occurs has only recently been investigated. In addition to the potential role of neutrophil-mediated microvascular obstruction cited earlier, there is also substantial evidence suggesting that neutrophils may directly injure parenchymal cells through release of specific toxic products. Obviously neutrophils accumulating in the ischemic and reperfused areas might release proteolytic enzymes or reactive oxygen species to injure surrounding myocytes. However, under conditions found in vivo, these toxic products are almost exclusively secreted by adherent neutrophils [87,88]. Thus, it appears that a ligand-specific adhesion of the neutrophils to the cardiac myocytes may be critical for the mediation of ischemia-induced myocyte injury.

ADHESION-DEPENDENT CYTOTOXICITY

ICAM-1 is one of the primary ligands for the CD18 integrins. However, in contrast to the restricted cellular distribution of the β_2 integrins, ICAM-1 can be expressed by most tissue cells under certain circumstances. Recent studies from our laboratory examined the potential mechanisms of neutrophil adhesion to isolated adult canine cardiac myocytes. Intercellular adhesion occurred only if the myocytes were stimulated with cytokines inducing ICAM-1 expression [89] and when the neutrophils were stimulated to show Mac-1 activation. In vitro, myocyte ICAM-1 induction could be effected by the cytokines IL-1, TNF-α, and IL-6 [89,90]; neutrophil activation could be effected by zymosan-activated serum (a source of C5a) PAF and IL-8. The binding of neutrophils to activated cardiac myocytes was found to be specific for Mac-1–ICAM-1 interaction [88,91] and was completely blocked by antibodies to ICAM-1, CD11b, and CD18. This interaction was unaffected by antibodies to CD11a, which are capable of blocking neutrophil adhesion to an endothelial cell monolayer. Adhering neutrophils were apparently cytotoxic, as indicated by the sustained contraction often observed in myocytes after neutrophil adhesion.

In other experiments, the mechanisms of neutrophil-induced cytotoxicity were studied [88]. Either neutrophils or cardiac myocytes were loaded with 2',7'-dichlorofluorescein (DCFH), and the adherence-dependent oxidation of this marker to DCFH was monitored under fluorescence microscopy. Using zymosan-activated serum to activate the neutrophils in the presence of cytokine-stimulated cardiac myocytes, neutrophil–myocyte adhesion ensued as described earlier. When neutrophils were loaded with DCFH, fluorescence appeared almost immediately on adhesion of the neutrophil to a myocyte, suggesting a rapid adhesion-dependent activation of the NADP oxidase system of the neutrophil. In contrast, fluorescence of the cardiac myocytes appeared after several minutes and was rapidly followed by irreversible myocyte contracture.

The iron chelator desferrioxamine and the hydroxyl radical scavenger, dimethylthiourea, did not inhibit neutrophil adherence, but completely inhibited the fluorescence and contracture seen in the cardiac myocyte, preventing the neutrophil-mediated injury. In contrast, extracellular oxygen radical scavengers, such as superoxide dismutase and catalase, or extracellular iron chelators such as starch-immobilized desferrioxamine did not inhibit fluorescence, adhesion, or cytotoxicity. Under these experimental conditions, no superoxide production could be detected in the extracellular medium during the neutrophil–myocyte adhesion.

These data suggest that Mac-1/ICAM-1 adherence activates the neutrophil respiratory burst, resulting in a highly compartmentalized iron-dependent myocyte oxidative injury. Obviously, neutrophils are capable of secreting a variety of potentially toxic enzymes [92], and the ability of reactive oxygen scavengers to prevent toxicity completely only applies to a 2- to 3-hour period in vitro. The possibility of a later toxicity mediated by other toxic products of neutrophils cannot be ruled out.

INFLAMMATORY MYOCARDIAL INJURY IN VIVO: POSSIBLE ROLE OF ICAM-1

The pertinence of the in vitro neutrophil-mediated myocyte injury to ischemia/reperfusion injury was suggested by experiments with postischemic cardiac lymph that demonstrate the appearance of C5a activity present during the first 4 hours of reperfusion along with neutrophils showing upregulation of Mac-1 on their surface [22,93]. Postischemic cardiac lymph also contained cytokine activity that upregulated ICAM-1 in isolated cardiac myocytes; this latter activity was neutralized by antibodies to human IL-6 [90]. Further studies were designed to directly evaluate the role of ICAM-1 in myocardial inflammation associated with ischemia and reperfusion.

These investigations used the canine model of myocardial ischemia and reperfusion in which a coronary artery was occluded for 1 hour, during which time coronary blood flow was assessed with radiolabeled microspheres. At varying times thereafter, in the presence or absence of reperfusion, myocardial tissues were taken and processed for blood flow determinations, histologic studies, and mRNA isolation and analysis. Using this model, Kukielka and coworkers [94] demonstrated ICAM-1 mRNA expression in ischemic myocardial segments as early as 1 hour after reperfusion, with marked elevations after longer time intervals. No detectable ICAM-1 mRNA was found in segments with normal blood flow, while in the previously ischemic areas ICAM-1 mRNA appeared as an inverse function of coronary blood flow.

At later time points, such as 24 hours, however, mRNA was found in all myocardial samples (although tissue expression of protein remains confined to the viable border zone), suggesting that circulating cytokines (most likely IL-6) are inducing ICAM-1 mRNA in normal as well as in ischemic areas. The actual expression of ICAM-1 protein was not seen until 3–6 hours and was almost exclusively seen in the ischemic area at all time points, implying the possibility of a post-transcriptional regulation of ICAM-1 expression in cardiac myocytes, or more likely, proteolytic solubilization of surface ICAM-1 on normal cells that may be defective in the jeopardized zone, allowing the presence of surface ICAM-1.

Recently Youker and coworkers [95] examined the induction of ICAM-1 mRNA with respect to cells of origin as a function of time of reperfusion after a 1-hour ischemic event. Using in situ hybridization techniques, substantial message for ICAM-1 was detected in much of the previously ischemic viable myocardium by 1 hour of reperfusion, adjacent to areas of contraction band necrosis. At 3 hours ICAM-1 mRNA expression occurred in cells in the jeopardized area that appeared viable histologically. In contrast, under circumstances in which reperfusion did not occur, ischemic segments did not express ICAM-1 mRNA or ICAM-1 protein in areas of occlusion for periods up to 24 hours. It is important to point out that the layers of myocardial cells directly adjacent to the endocardium are spared injury, conserve glycogen, and do not express ICAM-1 mRNA in early reperfusion, probably as a result of diffusion across the endocardium from the left ventricular chamber. In addition, this area of induction of ICAM-1 mRNA on the viable border zone region of the infarct is the area where the most intense neutrophil margination and infiltration occur [95].

Based on these observations, it is reasonable to propose that ICAM-1 facilitates both the emigration of neutrophils in reperfused myocardium and their adherence-dependent cytotoxic behavior. Constitutive levels of ICAM-1 on endothelial cells may be sufficient to support CD18-dependent adhesion and subsequent transendothelial migration in response to chemotactic stimuli, whereas newly expressed ICAM-1 may participate in the myocardial injury associated with reperfusion only under circumstances where a leukotactic gradient and neutrophil activation are present.

Recently Gottlieb and coworkers [96] identified elements of apoptosis (programmed cell death) in myocytes as a response to myocardial reperfusion. Using a rabbit model of ischemia/reperfusion, they

detected the hallmark of apoptosis, nucleosomal ladders of DNA fragments in ischemic and reperfused rabbit myocardial tissue, but not in normal or ischemic-only' rabbit hearts. One interesting suggestion from these findings is that persistence of cellular ICAM-1 in the jeopardized border zone allows apoptotic myocytes to be cleared by phagocytes, converting apoptosis to necrosis by neutrophil adherence and activation. This role for ICAM-1 becomes a potential source for injury when an intense inflammatory process is rapidly induced by reperfusion.

MECHANISM OF ICAM-1 INDUCTION: THE CYTOKINE CASCADE

Because of the capacity of IL-6, present in postischemic cardiac lymph, to induce myocyte ICAM-1 expression, the expression of IL-6 mRNA in the ischemic and reperfused myocardium was investigated. In these experiments it was demonstrated that IL-6 was rapidly expressed in the same ischemic segments in which ICAM-1 mRNA was found [97], with a peak preceding that of ICAM-1 mRNA. Again, a clear reverse relationship between blood flow during the ischemic period and the induction of IL-6 message was demonstrated. Finally, as with ICAM-1, the expression of IL-6 mRNA appeared to be dependent on reperfusion.

These observations are consistent with the hypothesis that reperfusion initiates a cascade of cytokine-related events, leading to IL-6 expression and subsequent induction of ICAM-1 mRNA in the ischemic and reperfused myocardium. It appears that IL-6 synthesis is rapidly induced in cells found within the ischemic and reperfused areas. In recent studies we investigated the factors responsible for IL-6 upregulation in the previously ischemic myocardium. We demonstrated the presence of resident cardiac mast cells along small vessels in control canine myocardium, containing significant stores of preformed TNF-α [65]. Mast cell degranulation in the previously ischemic myocardium was documented by demonstrating a rapid release of histamine and TNF-α in the cardiac lymph following myocardial ischemia, with a peak in the first 30 minutes of reperfusion [65].

Furthermore, IL-6 protein was immunolocalized in leukocytes infiltrating the previously ischemic myocardium. TNF-α of mast cell origin may be a crucial factor in upregulating IL-6 in infiltrating cells and in initiating the cytokine cascade responsible for myocyte ICAM-1 induction and subsequent neutrophil-induced injury. Parenthetically, release of histamine is a potent stimulator of P-selectin surface expression from the Weibel-Palade bodies of venular endothelium.

In addition, IL-6 effects may extend beyond the induction of ligand-specific adhesion of neutrophils to cardiac myocytes. IL-6 is devoid of a direct effect on neutrophils, but it has been shown to prime and enhance the neutrophil oxidative burst in response to chemotactic stimulation [98]. This priming effect represents a potential complementary mechanism for IL-6 to facilitate neutrophil cytotoxic behavior in reperfused myocardium, in which the presence of complement-derived chemotactic factors and IL-8 has been demonstrated [32,93].

A Cell Biological Approach to Therapeutic Interventions

Obviously, the goal of any therapeutic strategy should be to control postreperfusion inflammatory injury without interfering with the healing phase. Of course, at this point one can only speculate on what type of target may be appropriate; however, it is possible to categorize the potential approaches as follows:

1. Complement (complement receptor-1)
2. Cycloxygenase and lipoxygenase inhibitors and LTB$_4$ antagonists
3. Anti–IL-8 approaches (anti–IL-8 monoclonal antibodies)
4. Selectin antagonism (monoclonal antibodies to P-selectin and L-selectin
5. Antiadhesion approaches (monoclonal antibodies to CD11b, CD18, and ICAM-1)
6. Anticytokine approaches (anti–IL-6 antibodies)

It appears that the complement cascade would be an unlikely place to intervene because it is independent of reperfusion and it would be difficult to get an agent to the area at risk until complement activation has already proceeded. However, interventions aimed at the complement receptor may have some practical application, because recombinant DNA technology has allowed the production of a soluble form of complement receptor 1 (CR1) [24].

The rest of the cell biological targets suggested earlier are induced or accelerated with reperfusion. However, in order to better define the potential therapeutic approaches, it will be critical to fully understand the relationship of the healing process to the acute inflammatory response. It is possible that limiting the intervention to the first 3 hours of reperfusion, during which the complement gradient exists and neutrophil influx into the intracellular space occurs,

may be sufficient to separate the effect on acute inflammation from that on the more chronic healing phase. However, better understanding of the specific mechanisms involved in the healing and remodeling phase of the infarct is needed because the influx of leukocytes that enter the ischemic myocardium during reperfusion may be crucial for the mediation of ongoing biological events.

Infiltrating leukocytes may change their pattern of cytokine and/or growth factor secretion both qualitatively and quantitatively in response to changes in molecular signals. For example, it is possible that, during later reperfusion periods, infiltrating mononuclear cells may secrete growth factors and fibrogenic cytokines capable of regulating fibroblast proliferation, which is critical for scar formation. The possible importance of monocytes as a source of fibrogenic or growth signals may explain the significant benefit seen with late reperfusion (after 6 hours) in the TAMI-6 and LATE trials. Late reperfusion would not be expected to salvage myocardium; however, it could accelerate mononuclear cell influx and promote healing.

Recent animal studies have demonstrated that reperfusion (early or late) is associated with an increased presence of macrophages compared with the nonreperfused myocardium. Birdsall and coworkers [99] have presented evidence that mononuclear leukocytes rapidly localize in the reperfused myocardium and transmigrate into the extracellular fluid within the first hour of reperfusion. They also suggested the presence of noncomplement monocyte chemoattractants (TGF-β_1 and MCP-1) that appear in the cardiac lymph in the second and third hour of reperfusion when C5a is rapidly disappearing. In other studies, Kumar et al. [100] demonstrated induction of MCP-1 mRNA in the previously ischemic myocardium, peaking at 3 hours of reperfusion and persisting throughout the first day of reperfusion. In the absence of reperfusion, no significant MCP-1 induction was seen.

Cellular and Molecular Biology of the Inflammatory Injury in Ischemia/ Reperfusion: A Working Hypothesis

We propose the following working hypothesis, which describes the events that mediate inflammatory reaction to myocardial ischemia/ reperfusion. This construct deals specifically with the inflammatory component, making the assumption that neutrophils are the principal determinant of this injury.

1. Leukotactic factors cause neutrophil influx in the ischemic myocardium.

The initial chemotactic event occurs when the injured myocardial cell releases complement-activating macromolecules of mitochondrial origin, initiating the production of C5a. This chemotactic mechanism is not dependent on reperfusion. An additional leukotactic factor, appearing in the previously ischemic myocardium with reperfusion, is IL-8, which participates in neutrophil-mediated myocardial injury by activating neutrophil adhesiveness and motility. Other C-X-C chemokines may have a role as neutrophil chemoattractants following myocardial ischemia and reperfusion. It is likely that specific lipoxygenase products, such as LTB$_4$, may be important leukotactic factors in some species.

2. Activated neutrophils adhere to the endothelium and emigrate to the extravascular space.

Selectins appear to be critical to early neutrophil margination by promoting neutrophil "rolling." Firm adhesion of the neutrophil to the endothelium follows, mediated through CD11b/CD18 adhesion to ICAM-1, which is constitutively expressed at low levels in the unstimulated endothelium. This step is associated with neutrophil Mac-1 activation. Subsequently, the neutrophil transmigrates to the extracellular space.

3. Cytokines induce ICAM-1 expression in cardiac myocytes in the ischemic and reperfused myocardium

IL-6 appears to be the critical cytokine involved in the induction of ICAM-1 in myocardial cells in the ischemic and reperfused areas. ICAM-1 has a highly specific localization to ischemic but viable myocardium, demarcating a "border zone" susceptible to neutrophil-induced injury. It is likely that release of preformed cytokines, possibly TNF-α of mast cell origin, stimulates IL-6 synthesis and secretion by infiltrating cells in the previously ischemic areas. The augmentation of infiltrating cells by reperfusion may explain the reperfusion dependence of induction of IL-6 and, as a result, ICAM-1.

4. Neutrophils mediate myocyte injury through CD11b/CD18/ICAM-1–dependent adhesion and subsequent compartmentalized transfer of reactive oxygen.

Once neutrophils have migrated into the extracellular space, they are capable of adherence to vulnerable myocytes that express ICAM-1 on their surface. Neutrophils are capable of mediating acute myocyte injury through reactive oxygen products. Other neutrophil-derived proteolytic and lipolytic products may also be important in inducing cytotoxic injury.

Conclusions

We have attempted to present the basic cellular and molecular mechanisms by which the inflammatory reaction associated with myocardial ischemia and reperfusion may occur. Understanding of the basic mechanisms initiating this reaction to injury is crucial for the development of site-specific cell biological strategies of intervention. Obviously, there is great hazard in completely inhibiting the process, and the ultimate goal of our investigations should be to identify specific molecular targets and to devise practical methods for intervention.

Acknowledgments

This study was supported by HL 42,550 from the National Institutes of Health and the DeBakey Heart Center.

References

1. Hillis LD, Braunwald E. Myocardial ischemia. N Engl J Med 296:1093, 1977.
2. Mallory GK, White PD, Salcedo-Salgar J. The speed of healing of myocardial infarction. A study of the pathologic anatomy in seventy-two cases. Am Heart J 18:647, 1939.
3. Hearse DJ, Bolli R. Reperfusion-induced injury: Manifestations, mechanisms and clinical relevance. Trends Cardiovasc Med 1:233, 1993.
4. Dreyer WJ, Michael LH, West MS, Smith CW, Rothlein R, Rossen RD, Anderson DC, Entman ML. Neutrophil accumulation in ischemic canine myocardium: Insights into the time course, distribution, and mechanism of localization during early reperfusion. Circulation 84:400, 1991.
5. Maroko PR, Carpenter CD, Chiariello M, Fishbein MC, Radvany P, Knostman JD, Hale SL. Reduction by cobra venom factor of myocardial necrosis after coronary artery occlusion. J Clin Invest 61:661, 1978.
6. Shappell SB, Taylor AA, Hughes H, Mitchell JR, Anderson DC, Smith CW. Comparison of antioxidant and nonantioxidant lipoxygenase inhibitors on neutrophil function. Implications for pathogenesis of myocardial reperfusion injury. J Pharmacol Exp Ther 252:531, 1990.
7. Simpson RJ, Mickelson J, Fantone JC, Gallagher KP, Lucchesi BR. Iloprost inhibits neutrophil function in vitro and in vivo and limits experimental infarct size in canine heart. Circ Res 60:666, 1987.
8. Olafsson B, Forman MB, Puett DW, Pou A, Cates CU, Friessinger GC, Virmani R. Reduction of reperfusion injury in the canine preparation by intracoronary adenosine: Importance of the endothelium and the no-reflow phenomenon. Circulation 76:1135, 1987.
9. Romson JL, Hook BG, Kunkel SL, Abrams GD, Schork MA, Lucchesi BR. Reduction of the extent of

ischemic myocardial injury by neutrophil depletion in the dog. Circulation 67:1016, 1983.

10. Mullane KM, Read N, Salmon JA, Moncada S. Role of leukocytes in acute myocardial infarction in anesthesthized dogs. Relationship to myocardial salvage by anti-inflammatory drugs. J Pharmacol Exp Ther 228:510, 1984.

11. Engler RL, Dahlgren MD, Morris DD, Peterson MA, Schmid-Schonbein GW. Role of leukocytes in response to acute myocardial ischemia and reflow in dogs. Am J Physiol 251:H314, 1986.

12. Jolly SR, Kane WJ, Bailie MB, Abrams GD, Lucchesi BR. Canine myocardial reperfusion injury: Its reduction by the combined administration of superoxide dismutase and catalase. Circ Res 54:277, 1984.

13. Lucchesi BR, Mullane KM. Leukocytes and ischemia induced myocardial injury. Ann Rev Pharm Tox 26:201, 1986.

14. Roberts R, DeMello V, Sobel BE. Deleterious effects of methylprednisolone in patients with myocardial infarction. Circulation 53(Suppl. I):204, 1976.

15. Hammerman H, Kloner RA, Hale S, Schoen FJ, Braunwald E. Dose-dependent effects of short-term methylprednisolone on mycardial infarct extent, scar formation, and ventricular function. Circulation 68:446, 1983.

16. Hill JH, Ward PA. The phlogistic role of C3 leukotactic fragment in myocardial infarcts of rats. J Exp Med 133:885, 1971.

17. Pinckard RN, Olson MS, Kelley RE, Detter DH, Palmer JD, O'Rourke RA, Goldfein S. Antibody-independent activation of human C1 after interaction with heart subcellular membranes. J Immunol 110:1376, 1973.

18. Pinckard RN, Olson MS, Giclas PC, Terry R, Boyer JT, O'Rourke RA. Consumption of classical complement components by heart subcellular membranes in vitro and in patients after acute myocardial infarction. J Clin Invest 56:740, 1975.

19. Rossen RD, Swain JL, Michael LH, Weakley S, Giannini E, Entman ML. Selective accumulation of the first component of complement and leukocytes in ischemic canine heart muscle: A possible initiator of an extra myocardial mechanism of ischemic injury. Circ Res 57:119, 1985.

20. Rossen RD, Michael LH, Kagiyama A, Savage HE, Hanson G, Reisbery JN, Moake JN, Kim SH, Weakly S, Giannini E, Entman ML. Mechanism of complement activation following coronary artery occlusion: Evidence that myocardial ischemia causes release of constituents of myocardial subcellular origin which complex with the first component of complement. Circ Res 62:572, 1988.

21. Rossen RD, Michael LH, Hawkins HK, Youker K, Dreyer WJ, Baughn RE, Entman ML. Cardiolipin-protein complexes and initiation of complement activation after coronary artery occlusion. Circ Res 75:546, 1994.

22. Dreyer WJ, Smith CW, Michael LH, Rossen RD, Hughes BJ, Entman ML, Anderson DC. Canine neutrophil activation by cardiac lymph obtained during reperfusion of ischemic myocardium. Circ Res 65:1751, 1989.

23. Dreyer WJ, Michael LH, Rossen RD, Nguyen T, Anderson DC, Smith CW, Entman ML. Evidence for C5a in post-ischemic canine cardiac lymph (abstr). Clin Res 39:271, 1991.

24. Weisman HF, Barton T, Leppo MK, Marsh HC Jr, Carson GR, Concino MF, Boyle MP, Roux KH, Weisfeldt ML, Fearon DT. Soluble human complement receptor type 1: In vivo inhibitor of complement suppressing post-ischemic myocardial inflammation and necrosis. Science 249:146, 1990.

25. Buerke M, Murohara T, Lefer AM. Cardioprotective effects of a C1 esterase inhibitor in myocardial ischemia and reperfusion. Circulation 91:393, 1995.

26. Miller MD, Krangel MS. Biology and biochemistry of the chemokines: A family of chemotactic and inflammatory cytokines. Crit Rev Immunol 12:17, 1992.

27. Baggiolini M, Moser B, Clark-Lewis I. Interleukin-8 and related chemotactic cytokines. The Giles Filley Lecture. Chest 105:95S, 1994.

28. Baggiolini M, Dewald B, Moser B. Interleukin-8 and related chemotactic cytokines–CXC and CC chemokines. Adv Immunol 55:97, 1994.

29. Baggiolini M, Dewald B, Walz A. Interleukin-8 and related chemotactic cytokines. In Gallin JI, Goldstein IM, Snyderman R (eds). Inflammation: Basic Principles and Clinical Correlates. New York: Raven Press, 1992:247.

30. Baggiolini M, Walz A, Kunkel SL. Neutrophil-activating peptide-1/interleukin 8, a novel cytokine that activates neutrophils. J Clin Invest 84:1045, 1989.

31. Sekido N, Mukaida N, Harada A, Nakanishi I, Watanabe Y, Matsushima K. Prevention of lung reperfusion injury in rabbits by a monoclonal antibody against interleukin-8. Nature 365:654, 1993.

32. Kukielka GL, Smith CW, LaRosa GJ, Manning AM, Mendoza LH, Hughes BJ, Youker KA, Hawkins HK, Michael LH, Rot A, Entman ML. Interleukin-8 gene induction in the myocardium following ischemia and reperfusion in vivo. J Clin Invest 95:89, 1995.

33. Ivey CL, Williams FM, Collins PD, Jose PJ, Williams TJ. Neutrophil chemoattractants generated in two phases during reperfusion of ischemic myocardium in the rabbit. J Clin Invest 95:2720, 1995.

34. Mehta J, Dinerman J, Mehta P, Saldeen TG, Lawson D, Donnelly WH, Wallin R. Neutrophil function in ischemic heart disease. Circulation 79:549, 1989.

35. Carry M, Korley V, Willerson JT, Weigelt L, Ford-Hutchinson AW, Tagari P. Increased urinary leukotriene excretion in patients with cardiac ischemia. In vivo evidence for 5-lipoxygenase activation. Circulation 85:230, 1992.

36. Mullane KM, Salmon JA, Kraemer R. Leukocyte-derived metabolites of arachidonic acid in ischemia-induced myocardial injury. Fed Proc 46:2422, 1987.

37. Hahn RA, MacDonald BR, Simpson PJ, Potts BD, Parli CJ. Antagonism of leukotriene B4 receptors does not limit canine myocardial infarct size. J Pharmacol Exp Ther 253:58, 1990.

38. Taylor AA, Gasic AC, Kitt TM, Shappell SB, Rui J, Lenz ML, Smith CW, Mitchell JR. A specific leukotriene B^4 antagonist protects against myocardial ischemia-reflow injury (abstr). Clin Res 37:528, 1989.

39. Zimmerman GA, McIntyre TM, Mehra M, Prescott SM. Endothelial cell-associated platelet-activating factor: A novel mechanism for signaling intercellular adhesion. J Cell Biol 110:529, 1990.

40. Stahl GL, Terashita Z, Lefer AM. Role of platelet activating factor in propagation of cardiac damage during myocardial ischemia. J Pharmacol Exp Ther 244:898, 1988.

41. Petrone WF, English DK, Wong K, McCord JM. Free radicals and inflammation: Superoxide-dependent activation of a neutrophil chemotactic factor in plasma. Proc Natl Acad Sci USA 77:1159, 1980.

42. Granger DN. Role of xanthine oxidase and granulocytes in ischemia-reperfusion injury. Am J Physiol 255:H1269, 1988.

43. Inauen W, Granger DN, Meininger CJ, Schelling ME, Granger HJ, Kvietys PR. Anoixa/reoxygenation-induced, neutrophil-mediated endothelial cell injury: Role of elastase. Am J Physiol 259:H925, 1990.

44. Suzuki M, Onauen W, Kiretys PR, Grisham MB, Meininger C, Schelling ME, Granger HJ, Granger DN. Superoxide mediates reperfusion-induced leukocyte-endothelial cell interactions. Am J Physiol H1740, 1989.

45. Shingu M, Nobunaga M. Chemotactic activity generated in human serum from the fifth component on hydrogen peroxide. Am J Pathol 117:210, 1984.

46. Patel KD, Zimmerman GA, Prescott SM, McEver RP, McIntyre TM. Oxygen radicals induce human endothelial cells to express GMP-140 and bind neutrophils. J Cell Biol 112:749, 1991.

47. Smiley PL, Stremler KE, Prescott SM, Zimmerman GA, McIntyre TM. Oxidatively fragmented phosphatidylcholines activate human neutrophils through the receptor for platelet-activating factor. J Biol Chem 266:11104, 1991.

48. Sellak H, Franzini E, Hakim J, Pasquier C. Reactive oxygen species repidly increase endothelial ICAM-1 ability to bind neutrophils without detectable upregulation. Blood 83:2669, 1994.

49. Michael LH, Zhang Z, Hartley CJ, Bolli R, Taylor AA, Entman ML. Thromboxane B2 in cardiac lymph: Effect of superoxide dismutase and catalase during myocardial ischemia and reperfusion. Circ Res 66:1040, 1990.

50. Mullane KM, Westlin W, Kraemer R. Activated neutrophils release mediators that may contribute to myocardial dysfunction associated with ischemia and reperfusion. In Biology of the Leukotrienes. New York: New York Academy of Sciences, 1988:103.

51. Engler RL, Dahlgren MD, Peterson MA, Dobbs A, Schmid-Schonbein GW. Accumulation of polymorphonuclear leukocytes during 3 h experimental myocardial ischemia. Am J Physiol 251:H93, 1986.

52. Hernandez LA, Grisham MB, Twohig B, Arfors KE, Harlan JM, Granger DN. Role of neutrophils in ischemia-reperfusion-induced microvascular injury. Am J Physiol 238:H699, 1987.

53. Ambrosio G, Weisman HF, Baker LC. The no-reflow phenomenon: A misnomer. Circulation 74:II260, 1986.

54. Ambrosio G, Weisman HF, Mannisi JA, Becker LC. Progressive impairment of regional myocardial perfusion after initial restoration of post ischemic blood flow. Circulation 80:1846, 1989.

55. Adams DH, Shaw S. Leukocyte-endothelial interactions and regulation of leukocyte migration. Lancet 343:831, 1994.

56. Bevilacqua MP, Butcher E, Furie B, Gallatin M, Gimbrone MA, Harlan JM, Kishimoto TK, Lasky LA, McEver RP, Paulson JC, Rosen SD, Seed B, Siegelman M, Springer TA, Stoolman LM, Tedder TF, Varki A, Wagner DD, Weissman IL, Zimmerman GA. Selectins: A family of adhesion receptors. Cell 67:233, 1991.

57. Lasky LA. Selectins: Interpretors of cell-specific carbohydrate information during inflammation. Science 258:964, 1992.

58. Tedder TF, Steeber DA, Chen A, Engel P. The selectins: Vascular adhesion molecules. FASEB J 9:866, 1995.

59. Lasky LA, Presta LG, Erbe DV. Structure-function aspects of selectin-carbohydrate interactions. Molecular definition to therapeutic potential. In Metcalf BW, Dalton BJ, Poste G (eds). Cellular Adhesion. New York: Plenum Press, 1994:37.

60. Kishimoto TK, Jutila MA, Berg EL, Butcher EC. Neutrophil Mac-1 and MEL-14 adhesion proteins inversely regulated by chemotactic factors. Science 245:1238, 1989.

61. Smith CW, Kishimoto TK, Abbassi O, Hughes BJ, Rothlein R, McIntire LV, Butcher E, Anderson DC. Chemotactic factors regulate lectin adhesion molecule 1 (LECAM-1)-dependent neutrophil adhesion to cytokine-stimulated endothelial cells in vitro. J Clin Invest 87:609, 1991.

62. Bevilacqua MP, Stengelin S, Gimbrone Jr, Seed B. Endothelial leukocyte adhesion molecule 1: An inducible receptor for neutrophils related to complement regulatory proteins and lectins. Science 243:1160, 1989.

63. Altieri DC, Edgington TS. The saturable high affinity association of Factor X to ADP-stimulated monocytes defines a novel function of the Mac-1 receptor. J Biol Chem 263:7007, 1988.

64. Geng JG, Bevilacqua MP, Moore KL, McIntyre TM, Prescott SM, Kim JM, Bliss GA, Zimmerman GA,

McEver RP. Rapid neutrophil adhesion to activated endothelium mediated by GMP-140. Nature 343:757, 1990.

65. Frangogiannis NG, Youker KA, Kukielka GL, Breasler RB, Michael LH, Spengler RN, Smith CW, Entman ML. Resident cardiac mast cells degranulate and release preformed TNF-α during ischemia/reperfusion injury. J Invest Med 43:313, 1995.

66. Picker LJ, Warnock RA, Burns AR, Doerschuk CM, Berg EL, Butcher EC. The neutrophil selectin LECAM-1 presents carbohydrate ligands to the vascular selectins ELAM-1 and GMP-140. Cell 66:921, 1991.

67. Ma X-L, Weyrich AS, Lefer DJ, Buerke M, Albertine KH, Kishimoto TK, Lefer AM. Monoclonal antibody to L-selectin attenuates neutrophil accumulation and protects ischemic reperfused cat myocardium. Circulation 88:649, 1993.

68. Weyrich AS, Ma X-L, Lefer DJ, Albertine KH, Lefer AM. In vivo neutralization of P-selectin protects feline heart and endothelium in myocardial ischemia and reperfusion injury. J Clin Invest 91:2620, 1993.

69. Albelda SM, Smith CW, Ward PA. Adhesion molecules and inflammatory injury. FASEB J 8:504, 1994.

70. Luscinskas FW, Lawler J. Integrins as dynamic regulators of vasular function. FASEB J 8:929, 1994.

71. Anderson DC. The role of beta-2 integrins and intercellular adhesion molecule type I in inflammation. In Granger DN, Schmid-Schonbein GW (eds). Physiology and Pathophysiology of Leukocyte Adhesion. New York: Oxford University Press, 1995:3.

72. Smith CW, Marlin SD, Rothlein R, Toman C, Anderson DC. Cooperative interactions of LFA-1 and Mac-1 with intercellular adhesion molecule-1 in facilitating adherence and transendothelial migration of human neutrophils in vitro. J Clin Invest 83:2008, 1989.

73. Fehr J, Moser R, Leppert D, Groscurth P. Antiadhesive properties of biological surfaces are protective against stimlated granulocytes. J Clin Invest 76:535, 1985.

74. Simpson PJ, Todd III, Fantone JC, Mickelson JK, Griffin JD, Lucchesi BR. Reduction of experimental canine myocardial reperfusion injury by a monoclonal antibody (anti-Mo1. anti-CD11b) that inhibits leukocyte adhesion. J Clin Invest 81:624, 1988.

75. Simpson PJ, Todd III, Mickelson JK, Fantone JC, Gallagher KP, Lee KA, Tamura Y, Cronin M, Lucchesi BR. Sustained limitation of myocardial reperfusion injury by a monoclonal antibody that alters leukocyte function. Circulation 81:226, 1990.

76. Seewaldt-Becker E, Rothlein R, Dammgen JW. CDw18 dependent adhesion of leukocytes to endothelium and its relevance for cardiac reperfusion. In Springer TA, Anderson DC, Rosenthal AS, Rothlein R (eds). Leukocyte Adhesion Molecules: Structure, Function, and Regulation. New York: Springer-Verlag, 1989:138.

77. Williams FM, Collins PD, Nourshargh S, Williams TJ. Suppression of 111In-neutrophil accumulation in rabbit mycoardium by MoA isechmic injury. J Mol Cell Cardiol 20:S33, 1989.

78. Lefer DJ, Suresh ML, Shandelya ML, Serrano CV, Becker LC, Kuppusamy P, Zweier JL. Cardioprotective actions of a monoclonal antibody against CD-18 in myocardial ischemia-reperfusion injury. Circulation 88:1779, 1993.

79. Aversano T, Zhou W, Nedelman M, Nakada M, Weisman H. A chimeric IgG4 monoclonal antibody directed against CD18 reduces infarct size in a primate model of myocardial ischemia and reperfusion. J Am Coll Cardiol 25:781, 1995.

80. Ballantyne CM, Smith CW, Beaudet A, Yagita H, Dai XY. Endothelial-leukocyte cell adhesion molecules in cardiac allograft rejection (abstr). Circulation 88:I419, 1993.

81. Ma XL, Tsao PS, Lefer AM. Antibody to CD18 exerts endothelial and cardiac protective effects in myocardial ischemia and reperfusion. J Clin Invest 88:1237, 1991.

82. Carden DL, Smith JK, Korthuis RJ. Neutrophil-mediated microvascular dysfunction in postischemic canine skeletal muscle. Role of granulocyte adherence. Circ Res 66:1436, 1990.

83. Hughes BJ, Hollers JC, Crockett-Torabi E, Smith CW. Recruitment of CD11b/CD18 to the neutrophil surface and adherence-dependent cell locomotion. J Clin Invest 90:1687, 1992.

84. Muller WA. The role of PECAM-1 (CD31) in leukocyte emigration: Studies in vitro and in vivo. J Leukoc Biol 57:523, 1995.

85. Muller WA, Weigl SA, Deng X, Phillips DM. PECAM-1 is required for transendothelial migration of leukocytes. J Exp Med 178:449, 1993.

86. Cooper D, Lindberg FP, Gamble JR, Brown EJ, Vadas MA. Transendothelial migration of neutrophils involves integrin-associated protein (CD47). Proc Natl Acad Sci USA 92:3978, 1995.

87. Shappell SB, Toman C, Anderson DC, Taylor AA, Entman ML, Smith CW. Mac-1 (CD11b/CD18) mediates adherence-dependent hydrogen peroxide production by human and canine neutrophils. J Immunol 144:2702, 1990.

88. Entman ML, Youker KA, Shoji T, Kukielka GL, Shappell SB, Taylor AA, Smith CW. Neutrophil induced oxidative injury of cardiac myocytes: A compartmented system requiring CD11b/CD18-ICAM-1 adherence. J Clin Invest 90:1335, 1992.

89. Smith CW, Entman ML, Lane CL, Beaudet AL, Ty TI, Youker KA, Hawkins HK, Anderson DC. Adherence of neutrophils to canine cardiac myocytes in vitro is dependent on intercellular adhesion molecule-1. J Clin Invest 88:1216, 1991.

90. Youker KA, Smith CW, Anderson DC, Miller D, Michael LH, Rossen RD, Entman ML. Neutrophil adherence to isolated adult cardiac myocytes: Induc-

tion by cardiac lymph collected during ischemia and reperfusion. J Clin Invest 89:602, 1992.

91. Entman ML, Youker KA, Shappell SB, Siegel C, Rothlein R, Dreyer WJ, Schmalstieg FC, Smith CW. Neutrophil adherence to isolated adult canine myocytes: Evidence for a CD18-dependent mechanism. J Clin Invest 85:1497, 1990.

92. Weitz JI, Huang AJ, Landman SL, et al. Elastase-mediated fibrinogenolysis by chemoattractant-stimulated neutrophils occurs in the presence of physiologic concentrations of anti-proteinases. J Exp Med 166:1836, 1987.

93. Dreyer WJ, Michael LH, Nguyen T, Smith CW, Anderson DC, Entman ML, Rossen RD. Kinetics of C5a release in cardic lymph of dogs experiencing coronary artery ischemia-reperfusion injury. Circ Res 71:1518, 1992.

94. Kukielka GL, Hawkins HK, Michael LH, Manning AM, Lane CL, Entman ML, Smith CW, Anderson DC. Regulation of intercellular adhesion molecule-1 (ICAM-1) in ischemic and reperfused canine myocardium. J Clin Invest 92:1504, 1993.

95. Youker KA, Hawkins HK, Kukielka GL, Perrard JL, Michael LH, Ballantyne CM, Smith CW, Entman ML. Molecular evidence for induction of intercellular adhesion molecule-1 in the viable border zone associ-ated with ischemia-reperfusion injury of the dog heart. Circulation 89:2736, 1994.

96. Gottlieb RA, Burleson KO, Kloner RA, Babior BM, Engler RL. Reperfusion injury induces apoptosis in rabbit cardiomyocytes. J Clin Invest 94:1621, 1994.

97. Kukielka GL, Smith CW, Manning AM, Youker KA, Michael LH, Entman ML. Induction of Interleukin-6 synthesis in the myocardium: Potential role in post-reperfusion inflammatory injury. Circulation 92:1866, 1995.

98. Kharazmi A, Mielsen H, Rechnitzer C, Bendtzen K. Interleukin 6 primes human neutrophil and mono-cyte oxidative burst response. Immunol Lett 21:177, 1989.

99. Birdsall HH, Green DM, Trial JA, Youker KA, Entman ML, Michael LH, Rossen RD. Reperfusion of ischemic myocardium releases TGF-beta, MCP-1 and C5a into cardiac extracellular fluids and stimu-lates transendothelial migration of TNF-alpha and IL-1 secreting monocytes (abstr). Circulation I-711, 1995.

100. Kumar AG, Ballantyne CM, Ty MT, Kukielka GL, Michael LH, Entman ML. Cardiac reperfusion ini-tiates the induction of monocyte chemoattractant molecule-1 and vascular cell adhesion molecule-1. Circulation 90:1427, 1994.

43. ESTROGEN AND CARDIOVASCULAR DISEASE

Linda R. Peterson

Introduction

Cardiovascular disease (CVD) is the number one cause of death in women in industrialized countries. Estimates show that a 50-year-old white woman has a 46% probablilty of developing heart disease in her lifetime and a 31% probablilty of dying as a result. Treatment of CVD in women is estimated to cost at least $11 billion dollars per year [1]. However, clinical evidence of coronary artery disease in women is unusual until after menopause. Moreover, premenopausal women who have undergone oopherectomy are at increased risk for atherosclerotic disease when compared with premenopausal women who have not [2].

These observations have led to the hypothesis that estrogen replacement therapy (ERT) may be protective against the development of atherosclerotic disease and may be useful in its treatment. Supporting this idea are results of human epidemiologic studies, several animal studies, in vitro studies, and human in vivo studies on estrogen's beneficial effect on CVD. In epidemiologic studies, ERT has been associated with a 40% reduction in the rate of cardiovascular death in postmenopausal women [3]. However, to date only one prospective, randomized, placebo-controlled, double-blind study on the effects of ERT in postmenopausal women has been completed, and too few patients were enrolled to allow any definitive conclusions to be drawn [4]. In addition, although there are data that support the hypothesis that ERT is beneficial with regard to reducing CVD events, there is also evidence that oral contraceptive pills (OCPs), most of which contain synthetic estrogen, are associated with a slightly increased overall risk of CVD events; possible explanations for this apparant contradiction will be discussed in detail later.

There are now several ongoing studies, including the Women's Health Initiative and the ERA study, that should provide enough data to conclusively determine whether ERT does have a protective effect, and if it does, to what degree it protects against CVD. These prospective studies should also provide more definitive data on the true long-term effect of ERT on the risk of breast cancer and other diseases.

The possible mechanisms of estrogen's protective effect in postmenopausal women, and of its mild adverse effects in premenopausal women on OCPs, is also the subject of much research. ERT has a beneficial effect on the lipoprotein profile of postmenopausal women, but it is too modest to account for estrogen's overall protective effects [5]. Thus, research on estrogen's effects on lipid profiles, atherogenesis, oxidative metabolism of lipoproteins, vasomotor tone, hemostasis, and exercise training is currently underway. Regarding the potential negative effects of OCPs, there appear to be important differences between the effects of OCPs on the coagulation system of premenopausal women and the effects of ERT on the coagulation system of postmenopausal women (see Estrogen and Coagulation: Oral Contraceptives, later).

Epidemiologic Studies

ESTROGEN REPLACEMENT THERAPY AND CARDIOVASCULAR DISEASE

Results of many epidemiologic studies support the hypothesis that ERT protects against CVD and that menopause is associated with an increase in CVD. The Framingham Study, a long-term prospective investigation of the incidence of CVD, has shown that men under the age of 60 years develop CVD at twice the rate of women of the same age; however, by age 70, the rate of CVD in men in the study was only 1.4 times that of the women [6]. As Figure 43-1 shows, there is clearly an increase in the incidence of CVD in women after menopause [6]. Further supporting this hypothesis are data from a comprehensive review of over 30 epidemiologic studies on postmenopausal

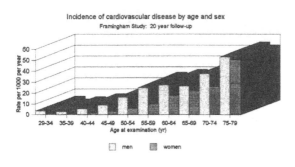

FIGURE 43-1. Incidence of cardiovascular disease in men and women in the Framingham Study 20 year follow-up. (Data from Kannel and Vokonas [6], with permission.)

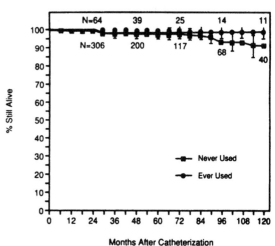

FIGURE 43-2. Ten-year cumulative survival of control patients with normal coronary angiograms in the study of Sullivan et al. Actuarial methods were used to calculate survival. The number of persons still being followed up is indicated by numbers on the survival curves. (Reprinted, with permission, from Sullivan et al. [11]. Copyright 1990, American Medical Association.)

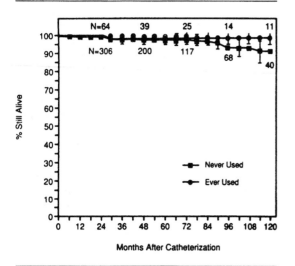

FIGURE 43-3. Ten-year survival of patients in the study of Sullivan et al. whose coronary stenoses were between "detectable" and 67%. (Reprinted, with permission, from Sullivan et al. [11]. Copyright 1990, American Medical Association.)

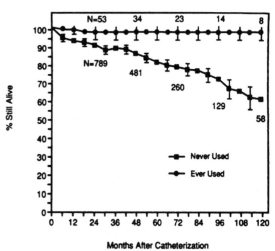

FIGURE 43-4. Ten-year survival of patients in the study of Sullivan et al. with left main coronary stenosis of 50% or greater or other stenoses of 70% or greater. (Reprinted, with permission, from Sullivan et al. [11]. Copyright 1990, American Medical Association.)

women that was conducted by Grady et al. [7]. In nearly all of the studies they reviewed, postmenopausal women on ERT proved to be at lower risk of coronary heart disease than those who did not. The calculated estimate of relative risk of coronary heart disease for women who had ever used ERT was between 0.55 and 0.65 when compared with that for those who had never used ERT [7–9]. The relative risk of death from coronary heart disease for women who had ever used ERT was estimated at 0.63 [7]. It

TABLE 43-1. Lifetime probabilities of selected conditions for
a 50-year-old white woman treated with long-term hormone replacement

Variable	Lifetime probability[a]			
	No treatment	Estrogen	E + P[b]	E + P[c]
Coronary heart disease (%)	46.1	34.2	34.4	39.0
Stroke (%)	19.8	20.2	20.3	19.3
Hip fracture (%)	15.3	12.7	12.8	12.0
Breast cancer (%)	10.2	13.0	13.0	19.7
Endometrial cancer (%)	2.6	19.7	2.6	2.6
Life expectancy (yr)	82.8	83.7	83.8	82.9

[a] Estimated lifetime probability of developing the condition.
[b] Assuming that the addition of progestin to the estrogen regimen does not alter any of the relative risks for disease from estrogen therapy, except to prevent the increased risk due to endometrial cancer (relative risk for endometrial cancer estimated to be 1.0).
[c] Assuming that the addition of a progestin to the estrogen regimen provides only two thirds of the coronary heart disease risk reduction afforded by estrogen therapy (relative risk for coronary heart disease estimated to be 0.8) and the relative risk for breast cancer in treated women is 2.0.
E + P = estrogen plus progestin.
Reprinted, with permission, from Grady D et al. [7].

is not clear whether the addition of progestins affects this relative risk. The risk of stroke did not appear to be affected by ERT [7].

There is also evidence from results of The Cardiovascular Health Study that ERT may lower rates of subclinical CVD [10]. In this study, after accounting for possible confounding factors such as age and smoking, estrogen use was still statistically significantly associated with less thickening of the carotid intimal-medial layer, a lower incidence of carotid stenoses, and left ventricular hypertrophy (by ECG criteria). After including for the effect of ERT on lipid profiles, however, the significance of the benefit of ERT on these measures of subclinical CVD was borderline. Estrogen use was also associated with a more favorable left ventricular diastolic filling, as evidenced by mitral valve Doppler flow patterns [10].

There are also epidemiologic data showing that estrogen may have a role in secondary prevention of coronary events because ERT is associated with a decrease in coronary events in women who already had evidence of CAD [11]. In a 13-year study done by Sullivan et al., there was evidence to suggest that the women who may benefit the most from ERT are those who have the most significant coronary stenoses on angiogram (Figures 43-2 to 43-4) [11]. In addition, there is evidence that ERT is associated with improved survival in women who have undergone coronary artery bypass grafting (CABG). Five-year

survival was 98.8% in women who used ERT at the time of surgery or afterward versus 80.7% in nonusers, and 10-year survival was 69.3% in users in comparison with 46.3% in nonusers. The women on ERT in this study, on average, were younger, had fewer vessels with significant stenoses, less left main disease, higher ejection fractions, and a lower incidence of diabetes, but after a Cox proportional hazards model was used to account for the above-mentioned differences in baseline characteristics, ERT was still an incidendent predictor of survival [12].

Clearly ERT is associated with a decreased risk of CVD, but this has still not been adequately tested in randomized, prospective trials. As mentioned earlier, the one such trial to date, the 10-year, double-blinded study by Natchigall et al., was not large enough to have sufficient power to allow determination of a statistically significant difference in mortality due to CVD or other causes [4]. The study results did suggest that the incidence of complications from ERT is not high. Of interest is the fact that, although the incidence of myocardial infarction was less in the treatment group, this difference did not reach statistical significance, but the incidence of breast cancer was statistically significantly lower in the estrogen-treated group [4].

The effect of ERT on risk of breast cancer and other diseases must, of course, be taken into account when a physician considers prescribing ERT for a postmenopausal woman for prevention of CVD,

TABLE 43-2. Lifetime probabilities of selected conditions
for a 50-year-old white woman at risk for coronary
artery disease treated with long-term hormone replacement[a]

Variable	Lifetime probability[b]			
	No treatment	Estrogen	E + P[c]	E + P[d]
Coronary heart disease (%)	71.2	59.6	59.8	64.4
Stroke (%)	15.4	16.9	17.0	15.6
Hip fracture (%)	11.3	10.2	10.2	9.2
Breast cancer (%)	9.1	11.9	12.0	17.9
Endometrial cancer (%)	2.4	18.6	2.5	2.4
Life expectancy (yr)	79.6	81.1	81.2	80.2

[a] Relative risk of developing or dying of coronary heart disease was estimated as 2.5, the same as for a woman who smokes, has hypertension, or has diabetes.
[b] Estimated lifetime probability of developing the condition.
[c] Assuming that the addition of progestin to the estrogen regimen does not alter any of the relative risks for disease from estrogen therapy, except to prevent the increased risk due to endometrial cancer (relative risk for endometrial cancer estimated to be 1.0).
[d] Assuming that the addition of a progestin to the estrogen regimen provides only two thirds of the coronary heart disease risk reduction afforded by estrogen therapy (relative risk for coronary heart disease estimated to be 0.8) and the relative risk for breast cancer in treated women is 2.0.
E + P = estrogen plus progestin.
Reprinted, with permission, from Grady D et al. [7].

osteoporosis, or treatment of menopausal symptoms. Relative risk, calculated from results of epidemiologic studies, of a postmenopausal woman developing and dying from breast cancer is approximately 1.25 in comparison with those not on ERT [7]. Grady et al. examined the effect ERT on the relative risk of breast cancer, coronary artery disease, and other diseases. As is shown in Tables 43-1 and 43-2, if progestins (which are often added to estrogen replacement) do not change the beneficial effects of ERT on CVD and if they remove the risk of endometrial cancer due to unopposed estrogen, ERT is associated with a 1-year increase in life expectancy for a 50-year-old white woman with no risk factors, and a 1.5-year increase in a woman with risk factors for coronary artery disease [7]. However, if a pessimistic estimate is made, assuming that progestins reduce the benefit of ERT on CAD by a third and increase the risk of breast cancer, the expected increase in life span afforded by ERT would be only 0.1 years [7].

In summary, epidemiologic studies suggest that ERT decreases the risk of CVD development and is probably helpful in the treatment of coronary disease. However, if a woman is at increased risk for breast cancer, has lupus, has a history of venous thromboses, or has another disease that may be negatively affected by ERT, her overall risk/benefit ratio of ERT may indicate that she would not benefit from ERT. An individual woman's fear that ERT may increase her risk of breast cancer must also be addressed when discussing ERT with her. A recent survey done of well-educated, perimenopausal women showed that 73% believed that their risk of heart disease was less than 1%; 52%, however, perceived their risk of breast cancer as 10% or more [13]. Also, the major health concern in 63% of the women was breast cancer, and only 31% of the women reported that their first concern was heart disease [13]. These perceptions must be taken into account, along with scientific data and the risk of coronary artery disease, breast cancer, and other diseases in the counseling of women on the advisability of ERT. The American College of Physicians has published guidelines on this subject [14].

ORAL CONTRACEPTIVES AND CARDIOVASCULAR DISEASE

The risk of CVD, in general, is increased in premenopausal women on OCPs in comparison with those not taking contraceptives; women over 35 years old who smoke are at a particularly high risk of having a cardiovascular event [15–21]. The risk is relatively low and not statistically significant in healthy women under age 35 who do not smoke, and the increased risk of cardiovascular events does not appear to persist once OCPs are discontinued. This lack of a persistent effect was documented by Stampfer et al. in an analysis of the data from the Nurses' Health Study [22].

These authors also found no evidence of an increase in risk of CVD associated with an increase in duration of therapy, and in a meta-analysis of 13 studies discovered no difference in the rate of CVD in women who never used and past users of OCPs.

The risk of myocardial infarction in women who are currently taking OCPs has not been definitively shown to be greater than that in women not on OCPs [21]. Realini et al. reviewed the case-control, cohort, and mortality data on this subject gathered up to 1985, and the results were mixed: Some studies showed a positive correlation with myocardial infarction and some did not [21]. Whether past OCP use increases the risk of myocardial infarction was addressed in studies was addressed in the study by Stampfer et al., mentioned earlier [22]. In their meta-analysis of 13 studies, only 2 suggested that there may be an increased risk of myocardial infarction with past OCP use, and the study designs of these two studies were flawed [21–24]. The overall conclusion reached by the authors of this meta-analysis and that done by Realini et al. is there is no good, consistent evidence that past OCP use is associated with an increase in myocardial infarction [21,22,25].

There is, however, evidence that current OCP use is associated with an increased risk of deep vein thrombosis (DVT) and/or pulmonary embolism (PE). Realini et al. have thoroughly reviewed the studies on this subject, and although the designs of many of these are flawed, the finding that the risk of DVT and/or PE is increased in OCP users is consistent and generally accepted by the medical community [21]. There is also evidence that the risk of DVT and/or PE is dependent on the dose of estrogen in the OCP. Thus, it is likely that the lower the dose of estrogen in an OCP, the lower the risk of venous thromboembolic disease [26,27].

Current OCP use by itself is not clearly associated with an increased risk of cerebrovascular events (either thrombotic or hemorrhagic) [21]. There may, however, be an increased risk of thrombotic stroke or subarachnoid hemorrhage in women on OCPs who are older than 35 years and who smoke [28–32]. Women who are hypertensive and on OCPs are also at an increased risk for cerebrovascular events. In the study by the Collaborative Group for the Study of Stroke in Young Women, the age-adjusted relative risk of thrombotic strokes among OCP users was 3.1 for normotensive women, 4.2 for those who smoked ≥1 pack/day, and 13.6 for users with severe hypertension [28]. The age-adjusted relative risk of hemorrhagic strokes among OCP users was 1.2 for nonsmokers, 6.1 for smokers (≥1 pack/day), and 25.7 for those with severe hypertension. There is also no clear evidence that past OCP use in associated with an increased risk of cerebrovascular events.

In summary, there is epidemiologic evidence that the risk of CVD is increased in women who use OCPs and who are over 35 years old and smoke. There is also evidence that current OCP use increases a woman's risk of DVT and/or PE [33]. However, OCP use, by itself, is not clearly associated with an increase in myocardial infarction or cerebrovascular events [21]. Consequently, premenopausal women who are considering taking oral contraceptives should be advised of the risk posed by the combination of cardiovascular risk factors (such as smoking and hypertension) and OCP use. Alternative means of contraception should be discussed with women with any of these other risk factors.

ANTIESTROGENS AND CARDIOVASCULAR DISEASE

Because there is evidence that ERT may provide some protection against coronary disease, the question arises as to how drugs that have some antiestrogenic properties, such as tamoxifen (used primarily in the treatment of breast cancer), affect CVD rates. Tamoxifen is not a pure antiestogen because it has some estrogen agonist properties, depending on the target site [34]. There are not much data on the effects of tamoxifen on CVD, but the Scottish Breast Cancer Committee has published results of their retrospective study comparing 1070 postmenopausal women who had operable breast cancer and who received tamoxifen for 5 years after diagnosis or for at least 6 weeks after the first recurrence of disease with those who did not receive any tamoxifen [35]. They found that women who received tamoxifen were significantly less likely ($P = 0.0087$) to die of a myocardial infarction than those who did not. There was no difference in the rates of death due to other CVD processes, such as congestive heart failure, stroke, mitral valve disease, and chronic ischemic heart disease [35]. A firm conclusion about tamoxifen's effect on CVD cannot be reached based on this single retrospective study, but it appears that tamoxifen does not increase rates of CVD.

Hormones and Risk Factors for Cardiovascular Disease

LIPIDS

Estrogen Replacement Therapy. In women as well as men, total cholesterol tends to rise with age. High-density lipoprotein (HDL) levels, in contrast, stay

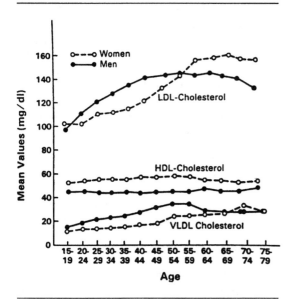

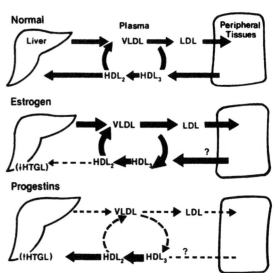

FIGURE 43-5. Age trends in lipoprotein cholesterol fractions. Framingham Study. (Reprinted, with permission, from Kannel [36].)

FIGURE 43-6. A general model of lipoprotein metabolism. Top: Normal flow of cholesterol to and from peripheral tissues. Middle and bottom: Known or postulated effects of estrogen and progestin on lipoprotein transport. Estrogen and progestin have opposing actions on very low-density lipoprotein (VLDL) secretion and hepatic triglyceride lipase (HTGL) activity. HDL and LDL are high-and low-density lipoproteins, respectively. (Reprinted, with permission, from Knopp [155].)

relatively constant throughout life in both sexes, although women's HDL levels are approximately 10 mg/dL higher than men's. Low-density lipoprotein (LDL) levels increase in both sexes with age, but women have a much more marked rise in LDL after menopause, and LDL levels in women over age 60 are higher than those in men of the same age (Figure 43-5) [36]. These data suggest that there is an effect of menopause, and the consequent decrease in estrogen levels, on lipid levels. As alluded to earlier, this idea is further supported by reports on the effect of postmenopausal ERT on the lipid levels in women.

Estrogen has a beneficial effect on most components of the lipid profile [37,38]. It is one of the few medications that has been shown to increase HDL levels, particularly the subfraction HDL2, as well as levels of the major apoprotein of HDL, apoprotein A-I. Because estrogen also decreases the levels of the atherogenic lipoproteins LDL and LP(a), the result is an improved LDL/HDL ratio [39]. One potentially negative effect of estrogen on the lipid profile is that it increases very low-density lipoprotein (VLDL) levels, and thus increases triglyceride levels. Whether this effect is atherogenic is a matter of debate, but if a patient already has markedly elevated triglyceride levels, estrogen (especially oral estrogens) may exacerbate this problem [40–42].

The route of administration, potency, and chemical structure of estrogen also have an impact on its effects on lipids. Oral estrogen formulations, such as oral conjugated equine estrogens (CEE), in general, are much more potent in this regard than are transdermal estrogens such as Estraderm, because oral preparations induce achieve a higher concentration in the liver from the portal circulation [43]. However, the synthetic estrogen, ethinyl estradiol, is so potent that even if given topically it may cause lipoprotein changes similar to those seen with oral estrogens [44]. In general, synthetic estrogens tend to be more potent than the standard doses of natural estrogens. Thus, the physician prescribing either oral contraceptives or ERT should take into account the different effects of the various formulations on the lipid profile. For example, in the patient with moderately elevated triglyceride levels, a transdermal preparation may be preferable to an oral one.

How estrogen causes changes in lipoprotein levels is not completely known, but there are some data on how estrogen affects lipoprotein metabolism. First, it

TABLE 43-3. Effects of nonoral estrogens on lipoproteins

Study	n	Duration	Estrogen	Dose/day	Route	LDL-c (% Δ from baseline)	HDL-c (% Δ from baseline)
Mandel [143]	20	1 mo	CEE	0.3 mg	Vaginal cream	0	0
Goebelsmann [44]	3	25 days	EE	50 μg	Vaginal suppository	−20	25
Lobo [144]	22	3 mo	Estradiol	25 mg	Pellet	3	48
Farish [145]	14	6 mo	Esradiol	50 mg	Pellet	−6	7
Sharf [146]	8	3 mo	Estradiol	100 mg	Pellet	−31	32
Jensen [147]	20	12 mo	Estradiol	5 mg	Abdominal cream	10	6[a]
Fahraeus [148]	17	6 mo	Estradiol	3 mg	Abdominal gel	—	4
Chetkowski [149]	23	4 mo	Estradiol	0.2 mg	Patch	0	0

[a] Percent change from placebo group.
EE = ethinyl estradiol; CEE = conjugated equine estrogen; LDL-c = low-density lipoprotein cholesterol; HDL-c = high-density lipoprotein cholesterol.
Reprinted, with permission, from Miller and LaRosa [48].

inhibits the catabolism of HDL, and it increases that of LDL [45,46]. One mechanism by which estrogen increases LDL catabolism is by inducing an increase in the number of LDL receptors in the liver [47]. In addition, it decreases the size of LDL particles and the apoprotein E/B ratio, both of which may have an effect on LDL's atherogenicity. Overall cholesterol excretion is enhanced by estrogen because it stimulates the function of 7-alpha-hydroxylase enzyme, which is important in the production of bile acids. Even though estrogen increases triglyceride levels by increasing the production of VLDL, the major carrier of triglycerides in the blood, it also increases catabolism of VLDL, leading to an overall increased rate of its turnover. This increased rate of turnover may lead to improved transfer of cholesterol to HDL, facilitating reverse cholesterol transport, but this is still under investigation [48]. A depiction of the mechanisms by which estrogen and progestins affect lipid metabolism is shown in Figure 43-6 [49].

Studies demonstrate that the synthetic estrogens (most commonly found in OCPs) increase HDL by 26%–38%, and natural estrogens (most commonly used for ERT in the United States) increase HDL by 9%–24%. In the PEPI trial, CEE therapy induced increases in HDL levels in first 6–12 months of therapy that were not evident in the following 24 months [38]. Table 43-3 shows the effect of nonoral estrogen preparations on lipoprotein profiles [48]. These beneficial changes in the lipoprotein profile induced by estrogen probably contribute to its protective effect against coronary disease, but when the magnitude of these changes are compared with that of changes with other lipid-lowering therapy, the

TABLE 43-4. Progestogens and progestins

19-Nortestosterone-related progestogens
Gonanes
    Levonorgestrel
    Desogestrel
    Gestodene
    Norgestimate
Estranes
    Norethindrone
    Norethindrone acetate
    Ethynodiol diacetate
    Lynestranol
    Norethynodrel
17-α-Hydroxyprogesterone-related progestins
Pregnanes
    Medroxyprogesterone
    Chlormadinone acetate
    Megestrol acetate
    Cyproterone acetate
    Natural progesterone

Reprinted, with permission, from Miller and LaRosa [48].

benefits of estrogen are out of proportion to the rather modest effect on lipids.

Progestin Replacement. Because progestins are often used to nullify the negative effects that ERT can have on uterine tissue in postmenopausal women who have not had a hysterectomy, it is important to consider the effects of progestins on lipid levels as well. In general, the effects of progestins on the lipid profile are opposite those of estrogen. Progestins decrease HDL, increase LDL, and decrease VLDL levels; the more androgenic a particular progestin is, the greater these effects on lipids will be. Thus, norethindrone is a synthetic progestin that exerts a greater amount of androgenic activity than medroxyprogesterone acetate (MPA), so that norethindrone decreases HDL (particularly HDL2) and VLDL, and increases LDL, to a greater degree than does MPA. Table 43-4 lists progestins (and progestogens) and their chemical classification [48]. In general, estranes have a greater androgenic effect than pregnanes. Norgestimate and levonorgesterel are moderately androgenic. The newer gonanes, desogesterel and gestodene, and MPA are the least androgenic of those listed [50].

Desogestrel even has a beneficial effect on total HDL levels, although HDL2 levels tend to decrease slightly [51–54]. Of the progestins typically used for hormone replacement, natural progesterone has the least negative effect on HDL levels, as was shown in the PEPI Trial [38,55]. However, even when natural progesterone was given with CEE, there was a slight attenuation of the beneficial effects on lipids of CEE therapy alone. The magnitude of the changes in LDL, total cholesterol, and triglyceride levels due to the addition of different progestins to 0.625 mg CEE seen in the PEPI trial is shown in Figure 43-7 [38].

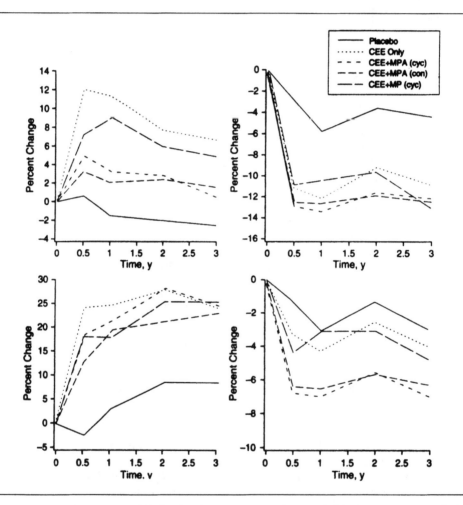

FIGURE 43-7. Mean percentage change from baseline by treatment arm for high-density lipoprotein (**top left**), low-density lipoprotein (**top right**), triglycerides (**bottom left**), and total cholesterol (**bottom right**). Three-year treatment groups were as follows: (1) placebo; (2) conjugated equine estrogen (CEE), 0.625 mg/day; (3) CEE, 0.625 mg/day, plus cyclic medroxyprogesterone acetate (MPA), 10 mg/day for 12 days/month; (4) CEE, 0.625 mg/day, plus consecutive MPA, 2.5 mg/day; or (5) CEE, 0.625 mg/day, plus cyclic micronized progesterone (MP), 200 mg/day for 12 days/mo. (Reprinted, with permission, from Writing Group for the PEPI Trial. [38]. Copyright 1995, American Medical Association.)

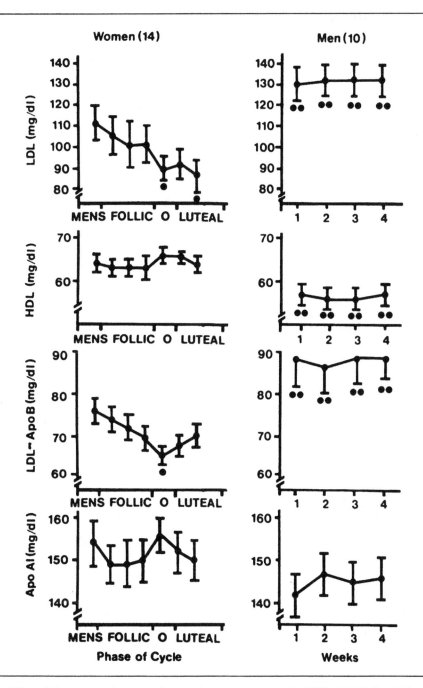

FIGURE 43-8. Effect of the menstrual cycle on lipoproteins. Apo = apoprotein; HDL-C, LDL-C = high- and low-density lipoprotein cholesterol; follic = follicular phase; luteal = luteal phase; mens = menses; O = ovulation. (Reprinted, with permission, from Kim and Kalkoff [57].)

TABLE 43-5. Percent change of lipids and lipoproteins due to oral contraceptives

Reference	Ethinyl estradiol (μg)	Progestogen Name	mg	Total cycle dose (mg)	HDL-c	HDL₂	HDL₃	Apo A-I	LDL-c	Apo B	Total trig.
Lipson [150]	50	Norgestrel	0.5	10.5	−13	−27	5	−9	18	—	32
Powell [151]	30	Levonorgestrel	0.15	3.15	−12.2	—	—	—	11.8	—	26
Burkman [152]	30	Levonorgestrel	0.15	3.15	−8.7	—	—	3.2	15.6	28.9	17.5
Krauss [153]	30	Levonorgestrel	0.15[a]	3.15	−4.3	—	—	—	4.2	—	18.2
Powell [151]	30	Ethynodiol acetate	2.0	42	−6.3	—	—	—	8.8	—	25
Burkman [152]	35	Ethynodiol acetate	1.0	21	2.4	—	—	19.3	10	28.8	38
Lipson [150]	50	Ethynodiol acetate	1.0	21	1	4	5	11	10	—	57
Powell [151]	50	Ethynodiol acetate	1.0	21	−0.5	—	—	—	12.5	—	—
Lipson [150]	50	Norethindrone acetate	1.0	21	3	−3	11	9	6	—	45
Burkman [152]	35	Norethindrone	1.0	21	−2.6	—	—	12.3	14.9	30	24.4
Burkman [152]	35	Norethindrone (biphasic)	0.5, 1.0	16	−4.6	—	—	12.2	10	24.8	45.3
Krauss [153]	35	Norethindrone	0.4	8.4	10.9	—	—	—	11.9	—	11.7
Percival-Smith [154]	Triphasics (30, 40, 30)	Levonorgestrel	0.05, 0.075, 0.125	1.925	−1.7	—	—	—	18.5	—	50
Havengt [51]	Triphasics (30, 40, 30)	Levonorgestrel	0.05, 0.075, 0.125	1.925	−1.6	−51.5	—	0	8.7	3.3	14.6
Kloosterboer [52]	Triphasics (30, 40, 30)	Levonorgestrel	0.05, 0.075, 0.125	1.925	0.0	−22	1.6	2.7	−6.3	22.5	—
Gaspard [53]	Triphasics (30, 40, 30)	Levonorgestrel	0.05, 0.075, 0.125	1.925	0.0	—	—	13.2	0.9	2.3	29.7
März [54]	30	Desogestrel	0.15	3.15	8.3	−1.3	14.2	21.1	2.1	0.1	35.1
Harvengt [51]	30	Desogestrel	0.15	3.15	13	−4.5	—	22.6	−1.9	0	46.3
Kloosterboer [52]	30	Desogestrel	0.15	3.15	11.8	−4.4	9.8	18.1	−8.1	19.4	35
Gaspard [53]	30	Desogestrel	0.15	3.15	5.4	—	—	14.5	−3.2	−19.2	21.4

[a] Actually dl-norgestrel 0.3 mg.

trig. = triglycerides; HDL-c = high-density lipoprotein cholesterol; LDL-c = low-density lipoprotein cholesterol; Apo = apoprotein.
Reprinted, with permission, from Miller and LaRosa [48].

Exactly how progestins cause these changes in the lipid profile remains speculative. It is known that they increase the activity of lipoprotein lipase, which helps to rid the blood of triglyceride-rich particles such as VLDL and chylomicrons [56]. Progestins also decrease concentrations of VLDL (and, therefore, triglyceride levels) by decreasing its production. The increases in levels of LDL that occur in patients on these drugs is at least in part due to decreasing LDL receptor synthesis because this receptor is necessary for LDL uptake and clearance [49].

Menstrual Cycle. Many studies have documented that LDL decreases in the second half of the menstrual cycle in normally ovulating women [58–61]. HDL and triglyceride levels, on the other hand, remain relatively stable throughout the cycle (Figure 43-8) [49]. Only in the study by Woods et al. was this pattern not apparent [62].

Oral Contraceptives. The changes in the lipid profile that are due to oral contraceptives are more difficult to document because there are many different formulations, and because some are biphasic and some are triphasic, so that delivered doses of estrogen and progestins vary with the stage of the menstrual cycle. Table 43-5 shows the effects of various OCPs on lipid levels [48]. The studies are listed so that those in

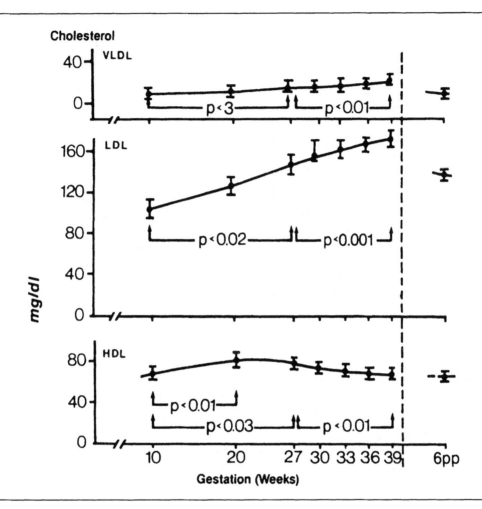

FIGURE 43-9. Lipoprotein cholesterol concentrations (mean ± SE) in normal women in the study of Knopp et al. pp = lipoprotein cholesterol level at 6 weeks postpartum; HDL, LDL, and VLDL = high-, low- and very-low–density lipoprotein cholesterol. (Reprinted, with permission, from Knopp et al. [156].)

which a more androgenically potent progestin was used are listed first. It is important to note in interpreting these data that the laboratories performing blood tests and the length of treatment varied from study to study. Also, as was shown in the PEPI study, the same estrogen/progestogen combination could produce different lipid effects over time. Thus, although these studies are not completely comparable, they do illustrate that overall the dose and potency of the progestogen is the most important factor that determines the effects on lipids of a particular contraceptive.

Pregnancy. Lipid levels increase substantially throughout pregnancy, triglyceride levels by 250% and total cholesterol by 25%, the latter reflecting increases in both LDL and HDL [63]. LDL increases to 1.6 times the prepregnancy level and HDL to approximately 1.5 times the prepregnancy level by midterm, but the increase in HDL drops to about 1.15 times the pregestational level by the end of pregnancy (Figure 43-9) [49]. Levels of the main apoprotein of HDL, apoprotein AI, also increase, and they remain elevated throughout pregnancy [64].

These increases in lipoprotein levels appear to be necessary for the maturation of the fetus because over half the fetal cholesterol supply is derived from the maternal circulation. In vitro studies suggest that higher cholesterol levels also may be necessary for the production of placental steroids. Moreover, higher apoprotein AI levels have been associated with increased birthweight.

Thus, the marked increase in maternal cholesterol levels is probably necessary for fetal health, but this temporary increase does not appear to be detrimental to the mother with regard to her risk of atherosclerotic disease. One study has found an association between parity and angina; however, no other "hard" endpoints, such as myocardial infarction or cardiovascular death, were found to correlate with parity, confirming the findings of Oliver, who found no correlation between CVD, in general, and giving birth [65,66]. Therefore, unless a woman has marked hyperlipidemia, such as heterozygous hypercholesterolemia or hypertriglyceridemia, that could put her at risk of a clinical event (such as pancreatitis) during her pregnancy, it is probably not necessary to check her routine lipid levels routinely: They will return to baseline levels by approximately 6 weeks postpartum.

BLOOD PRESSURE

Estrogen Replacement Therapy. The PEPI trial results have helped clarify the effect of ERT on blood pressure. This trial enrolled postmenopausal women who had a systolic blood pressure less than 160 mmHg and a diastolic pressure less than 95 mmHg. Although previous shorter trials led to conflicting results about the effect of estrogen on blood pressure, results from the PEPI trial showed that after 3 years there was no difference in systolic or diastolic blood pressure of subjects treated with estrogen, those on estrogen and medroxyprogestreone acetate, those receiving estrogen and micronized progesterone, and those on placebo. Although mean systolic pressures decreased during the first year of treatment, they increased in years 2 and 3 in all groups [38,67,68]. A recent prospective trial of ERT in postmenopausal women who were hypertensive at baseline also found no increase in blood pressure due to the estrogen [69]. Although occasional increases in blood pressure have been attributed to idiosyncratic reactions to estrogen, in general, ERT, with or without progesterone therapy, does not increase blood pressure in postmenopausal women.

Oral Contraceptive Pills. Unlike ERT, therapy with OCPs has been associated with an increase in blood pressure in premenopausal women [70]. Although in most women the increase is slight, approximately 5% develop hypertension within 5 years of OCP use, which is more than double the incidence in women who use other methods of birth control [70]. The risk

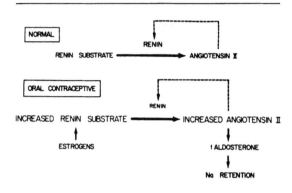

FIGURE 43-10. Changes in the renin-angiotensin system induced by oral contraceptives containing estrogen. The dashed lines show the feedback inhibition of renin release by angiotensin II. (Reprinted, with permission, from Kaplan [157]. Copyright 1990, Williams and Wilkins.)

of hypertension with OCP use is increased in women who are over age 35, who are obese, who drink large amounts of alcohol, or who have had pregnancy-induced hypertension [71,72]. In half of patients with an increase in blood pressure with OCP, this effect disappears within 6 months after the OCP has been discontinued [72]. If this does not occur, a workup for another secondary cause of hypertension should be considered. All women on OCPs should have their blood pressure closely monitored. There is no difference in the incidence of hypertension between those who formerly used OCPs and those who never used OCPs [73].

The mechanism by which OCPs increase blood pressure is diagrammed in Figure 43-10 [72,74]. Both estrogen and the synthetic progestins in OCPs contribute to this effect, which causes an increase in the amount of renin substrate, angiotensin II levels, and aldosterone levels, which leads to sodium retention [75]. Although these same processes are noted in postmenopausal women on ERT, as was mentioned earlier, these women do not appear to be at increased risk of hypertension [73]. Therapy for oral contraceptive–induced hypertension includes stopping their use, and a diuretic may be helpful for attenuation of increased sodium retention and plasma volume.

INSULIN RESISTANCE

Estrogen Replacement Therapy. Results from the PEPI trial have also helped to answer some of the questions about the effect of ERT and progesterone replacement therapy on insulin resistance in nondiabetic women. Insulin levels, obtained 2 hours after a glucose challenge, did not vary between treatment and placebo groups, and levels in both groups tended to decrease over the 3-year follow-up period [38]. Fasting insulin levels tended to be lower in the treatment groups when compared with the placebo group, though not statistically significantly so. Fasting glucose levels were also decreased in all the treatment groups compared with levels in the placebo group, but levels drawn 2 hours after a glucose challenge increased in the treatment versus the placebo group. The patients who experienced the largest increase in these levels were those taking conjugated equine estrogens and cyclic medroxyprogesterone acetate, or congugated equine estrogens and continuous medroxyprogesterone acetate, Thus, ERT has various effects on the markers of insulin resistance. If fasting insulin levels are better markers of insulin resistance than 2-hour postchallenge levels, as has been hypothesized, results of the PEPI trial indicate a beneficial effect of ERT on glucose tolerance [76].

Oral Contraceptive Pills. In contrast to the effects of ERT, OCP use in premenopausal women is associated with a slightly increased insulin resistance. In a prospective study by Kasdorf and Kalkhoff, plasma insulin levels are increased for at least 6 months after the initiation of OCP use [77]. As in the case of hypertension, it appears that the clinical effects of ERT on insulin resistance are qualitatively different from those of OCPs.

Estrogen and Atherogenesis

There is epidemiologic evidence that suggests estrogen can inhibit atherosclerosis formation more than would be expected from its lipid-lowering effects alone. Many studies have been done to investigate this in a more controlled manner.

Specifically, there have been studies in different mammalian models that show oopherectomized animals administered ERT have less atherosclerosis than those not given ERT [78,79]. In the study by Haarbo et al., ovariectomized rabbits on high-cholesterol diets that were also on ERT had one-third the aortic accumulation of cholesterol of control animals [78]. Adams et al. also found that the antiatherogenic effects of estradiol were independent of changes in total plasma cholesterol, apoprotein A-1 (a lipoprotein in HDL) and B (a lipoprotein in LDL) concentrations, HDL subfraction heterogeneity, and LDL molecular weight [79]. These investigators also found that when

some animals were given cyclic progesterone, there was no blunting of the beneficial effect on atherogenesis seen with ERT alone [78,79].

The mechanism(s) by which estrogen may alter the course of atherosclerosis has been the subject of much investigation. There is now evidence in nonhuman primates that estrogen affects some of the earliest events in atherogensis: LDL accumulation in the arterial wall and the degradation of LDL [80]. Remarkably, ERT-induced decreases in LDL deposition and degradation are "independent of changes in cholesterol, lipoprotein cholesterol, apo A1 and B concentrations, HDL subfraction heterogeneity, and LDL molecular weight" [80]. Also, early in atherogenesis, endothelial cells become cuboidal; later they exhibit degenerative changes. Estrogen has been shown to help to prevent this change in endothelial cells in a rabbit model of accelerated atherosclerosis [81].

Oxidation of LDL is also one of the critical early events in atherogenesis because oxidized LDL is ingested by macrophages initially via the normal LDL receptor and later, after continued oxidation, via scavenger receptors in an uncontrolled manner [82,83]. As a result, these macrophages become stuffed with lipids and evolve into foam cells, the cells that make up fatty streaks, and are the earliest grossly visible evidence of atherogenesis. Oxidized LDL is a chemoattractant that recruits more monocytes to the arterial wall, and it induces the endothelium to produce monocyte chemoattractant protein 1 [83,84]. Oxidized LDL also facilitates the three stages of monocyte binding to endothelial cells: tethering, activation, and attachment [83,85]. In addition, as LDL becomes more oxidized it can exert a direct cytotoxic effect. As will be discussed later, there is evidence that estrogen can act as an antioxidant and could therefore prohibit the formation of oxidized LDL. Results of the study by Jacobsson et al. support this hypothesis: They found that estradiol inhibited foam cell formation in rabbits with aortic allografts that were on a high-cholesterol diet [81]. Thus, there is evidence that estrogen can inhibit some of the early events in atherogenesis.

There is also evidence that ERT can inhibit some of the later events in atherosclerosis, such as smooth muscle cell proliferation, excess collagen deposition, and an increase in thickness in the arterial wall. In Jacobsson's study, the thickness of the intima of the arterial wall in estradiol-treated rabbits on a high-cholesterol diet was significantly reduced in comparison with wall thickness in those animals not on estradiol [81]. This intimal thickening consisted of smooth muscle cells in addition to foam cells, as observed by transmission electron microscopy.

Estradiol may act on smooth muscle cells via an estrogen receptor–mediated pathway because these receptors have been found on the vascular smooth muscle cells of many species, including humans [86,87]. Smooth muscle cells are primarily responsible for the formation of a more advanced "sclerotic" plaque from the more benign fatty streaks, because these cells deposit collagen in the arterial wall. There is also evidence in animal models that estradiol prevents this collagen deposition, leading to a higher ratio of elastin to collagen, which probably makes arteries more distensible [88,89]. Estradiol does not, however, appear to protect vein grafts from smooth muscle cell proliferation and consequent intimal hyperplasia [90].

Of interest is the fact that estrogen appears to facilitate one of the later processes in atherosclerotic plaque development: calcium deposition. Capillary pericytes are probably responsible for calcium deposition in vessels, and these cells do respond to estradiol. Estradiol appears to cause more bone formation and deposition in the arterial wall [91].

In summary, estrogen's antiatherogenic effects are out of proportion to its effect on lipid levels. There is evidence that estrogen may protect arteries from many early and late events in the progression of atherosclerosis, although it does facilitate calcium deposition in the arterial wall.

Estrogen and Oxidation

One possible reason that estrogen is associated with a decrease in progession of atherosclerosis is that it has antioxidant properties. As detailed earlier, lipid oxidation, and LDL oxidation in particular, is thought to be one of the critical events in atherosclerosis initiation and progression. Thus, many substances, including estrogen, have been tested to determine if they act as antioxidants.

There is reason to suspect that estrogen may be an antioxidant because, like the antioxidant α-tocopherol (vitamin E), estradiol has a phenolic hydroxyl group that can donate a hydrogen atom and thus inhibit further oxidative reactions [92]. In solution, estradiol reacts with lipid peroxyl radicals and neutralizes them [93]. It also inhibits cell membrane phospholipid oxidation [94]. Estradiol may also help restore the antioxidant properties of other antioxidants such as vitamin E, and there have been reports that it inhibits LDL oxidation [93,95]. To determine whether estrogen has an effect on the cell that mediates LDL oxidation in vivo, Rifici and Khachadurian incubated mononuclear cells with estradiol (at a concentration of 1 μmol/L) and LDL, and found that

estradiol decreased LDL oxidation by 52% at a ratio of one molecule of estradiol to two particles of LDL [96]. Moreover, they observed that not all estrogens had the same capacity to inhibit oxidation: Specifically, estradiol had a significant antioxidant effect on LDL oxidation, but estriol and estrone did not. Extending these studies, Subbiah tested the antioxidant capacity of different equine estrogens in comparison with the human estrogens estradiol and estrone. They found that the equine estrogens, especially equilin, had a more potent antioxidant effect than did either estrone or estradiol [97]. However, the concentration of estradiol used in the above-mentioned studies was much higher than that in a normal premenopausal woman or a postmenopausal woman on ERT. In fact, many of the studies on the antioxidative effects of estrogen in vitro have used supraphysiologic concentrations.

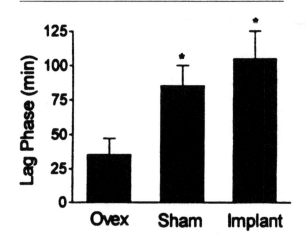

FIGURE 43-11. Plot illustrating ex vivo low-density lipoprotein (LDL) susceptibility to oxidation by aqueous peroxyl radicals in swine after 16 weeks of an atherogenic diet. Animals were subjected to ovariectomy (Ovex), sham procedure (Sham), or ovariectomy with 17β-estradiol implant (Implant) followed by an atherogenic diet. After 16 weeks, LDL was harvested as described in "Methods" and assayed for susceptibility to oxidation by incubation (0.05 mg/mL LDL protein) with 10 μmol/L 2,2'-azobis-(2-amidinopropane) hydrochloride, and lipid peroxidation was monitored by absorbance at 234 nm. The lag phase represent the time preceding the propagation of conjugated dienes as described by Esterbauer et al. [158]. Values represent mean ± SEM of four animals per group. *P < 0.05 versus ovariectomy group. (Reprinted, with permission, from Keaney et al. [106].)

Results of animal studies have also suggested that estrogen has some antioxidant properties. Keaney et al. showed that LDL from hypercholesterolemic swine that were given 17-β estradiol and had undergone ovariectomy was significantly more resistant to ex vivo oxidation. This increased resistance to oxidation is shown by an increase in the *lag phase*, which is the time that precedes the propogation of conjugated dienes, that is, the time before oxidation can take place (Figure 43-11) [98].

In vivo studies in human subjects, both short-term intravenous infusions of estradiol and longer term estradiol administration by transdermal patch (0.1 mg/day), have been shown to inhibit LDL oxidation [99]. In addition, the antioxidant effect of estradiol disappeared 1 month after it was discontinued. To determine whether estradiol helps restore other agents to their full antioxidant potential in vivo, Guetta et al. conducted an experiment wherein postmenopausal women were treated with either vitamin E, 17-β estradiol, or both. They found that estradiol significantly inhibited LDL oxidation, and vitamin E also inhibited it, but that there was no evidence of a synergistic benefit when both were given. Thus, it does not appear that estradiol significantly regenerates vitamin E's antioxidant effect in vivo [92].

In summary, there is evidence that estrogen acts as an antioxidant, and that certain estrogens, such as equilin, may have more potent antioxidant effects than others. However, most of the in vitro studies on the antioxidant effects of estrogen have used supraphysiologic doses, and the in vivo human studies described earlier used the highest dose of commercially available, transdermal 17-β estradiol. The conclusions of these studies regarding estrogen's antioxidant capacity, therefore, may not apply to postmenopausal women on lower doses of ERT.

Estrogen and Vasomotor Tone

There is a growing body of literature on the vasomotor effects of estrogen. Published results of in vitro and in vivo studies show that estrogen can cause vasodilation in many different arterial beds [100]. Conversely, a lack of estrogen has been shown to cause vasomotor instability [101]. Thus ERT's overall cardioprotective effect is likely, in part, to be the result of its beneficial effect on vasomotor tone.

The mechanism by which estrogen causes vasodilation has not been fully elucidated. In vitro, 17-β estradiol causes relaxation of animal coronary artery rings that have been denuded of endothelium, apparently because it attenuates the contractile response of the ring caused by endothelin-1 [102]. Estrogen may

also enhance vasodilation by decreasing calcium influx into coronary rings [103]. It is known that estrogen increases the basal release of the potent vasodilator nitric oxide (NO) in vitro [104]. This is likely due to an increase in the activity of NO synthase, the enzyme that produces NO [105]. In another in vitro study, estrogen was shown to preserve normal endothelial-dependent relaxation in response to bradykinin and substance P, and estrogen also has been shown to cause vasodilation of canine coronary arteries in an endothelial-independent manner when it is given in supraphysiologic doses [106,107]. There are conflicting data regarding whether or not estrogen affects prostaglandin synthesis, which may influence vasomotor tone [108,109].

Results of many in vivo animal studies have supported these in vitro findings. Short-term, systemic administration of 17-β estradiol was shown to increase uterine blood flow and to decrease uterine vascular resistance in sheep, a vasodilative effect that appears to be dependent on endothelial funtion in some animal models [110]. Williams et al. studied the effect of ethinyl estradiol on the vasomotor tone of the coronary arteries of ovariectomized, cynomologous monkeys with atherosclerosis [111]. To determine whether the vasodilation caused by estrogen is endothelial dependent, these investigators first administered intracoronary acetlycholine before the intravenous administration of ethinyl estradiol.

Acetylcholine administration can help delineate endothelial function because it has a vasodilative effect when it causes endothelial cells to release NO, but a direct vasoconstrictive effect when it acts on vascular smooth muscle cells via a muscarinic receptor [112]. In normal arterial segments, the vasodilative effect of acetlycholine predominates, but in segments that are atherosclerotic or those that are denuded of endothelium, the vasoconstrictor effect predominates [113]. In Williams' study, ethinyl estradiol caused a reversal of the acetylcholine-induced vasoconstriction in the atherosclerotic arteries, indicating that the ethinyl estradiol acted via an endothelial-dependent mechanism. Another interesting finding in this study was that vasodilation occurred within 20 minutes of the start of the ethinyl estradiol infusion, suggesting that estrogen does not act by increasing NO synthesis alone, because this would probably require more time [111,114]. In another study, Williams' group found that the atherosclerotic coronary arteries of monkeys on long-term estrogen vasodilated in response to after acetylcholine [115].

Results of in vivo human studies also supported the hypothesis that estrogen is a vasodilator. Gangar et al. showed that the *pulsatility index* of the carotid artery

TABLE 43-6. Mean age-adjusted clotting factor and cholesterol levels during 6-year follow-up by menopausal status

| | Continued periods (n = 136) | | Menopause | | | |
| | | | Natural (n = 69) | | Artificial (n = 28) | |
	Entry	Follow-up	Entry	Follow-up	Entry	Follow-up
Factor VII$_c$ (%)	102.8	101.9	107.4	121.2	99.5	106.6
Fibrinogen (g/L)	2.76	2.8	2.84	3.31	2.81	3.03
Cholesterol (mmol/L)	5.46	5.34	6.05	6.69	5.5	5.55

All changes with natural menopause, $P < 0.0001$.
Reprinted, with permission, from Meade and Berra A [125].

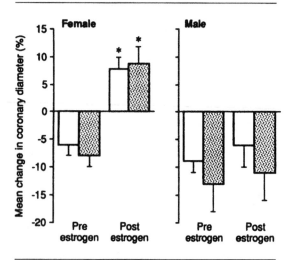

FIGURE 43-12. Change in the diameters of coronary arteries from women (left) produced by an intracoronary infusion of acetylcholine (1.6 μmol/min, open bars; 16 μmol/min, stippled bars) before and after 2.5 μmol of intracoronary 17β-estradiol. Net constriction before estrogen. *$P < 0.01$ before vs. after estrogen. Change in the diameter of coronary arteries from men (right) produced by an intracoronary infusion of acetylcholine (1.6 μmol/min, open bars; 16 μmol/min, stippled bars) before and after 2.2 μmol of intracoronary 17β-estradiol. P = NS before vs. after estrogen. (Reprinted, with permission, from Collins et al. [121].)

(which is thought to represent impedance to blood flow) correlated with time since menopause, and that there was a negative correlation between this index and administration of transdermal ERT in postmenopausal women [116]. Several studies of the effect of short-term ERT on forearm blood flow have also been done [117,118]. When 1 mg sublingual 17-β estra-

diol was given to healthy postmenopausal women, it caused a decrease in the resistance in the vascular bed of the forearm, as tested by venous occlusion plethysmography. However, it should be noted that the blood levels of estradiol achieved by the dose used in this study were higher than those in normal premenopausal women. Gilligan et al. also studied the short-term vasodilator effects of short-term estrogen on forearm arteries, but the dose used in this study resulted in estradiol concentrations typical of premenopausal women at midcycle [117]. They also study found that estradiol potentiated the vasodilation induced by acetylcholine, both in women who had risk factors for vascular dysfunction and in those who did not. Thus, estradiol potentiated endothelial-dependent vasodilation. Estradiol also potentiated endothelial-independent vasodilation in the women with risk factors for vascular dysfunction. In contrast, Lieberman's study of the effects of long-term estradiol on the vasomotor tone of the forearm found that only endothelial-dependent vasodilation was enhanced by estradiol [119].

The vasomotor response of the coronary arteries to a short-term infusion of estrogen has also been tested [114,120,121]. Gilligan et al. observed that short-term infusion of estradiol to premenopausal levels caused an enhancement of endothelial-dependent vasodilation in both large epicardial coronary arteries and coronary microvascular resistance arteries [114]. In contrast to the findings of studies of forearm vascular resistance, it did not cause endothelial-independent vasodilation. Also, estradiol alone did not cause vasodilation in the absence of acetylcholine.

There is also evidence to suggest that the coronary arteries of men and women with atherosclerosis do not react in the same way to estrogen [121]. The coronary arteries of postmenopausal women increase in diameter after estrogen administration and pretreatment with acetylcholine, but the atherosclerotic coronary arteries of men are not affected (Figure 43-12) [121]. Estradiol also potentiated the increase in flow caused by acetylcholine in women but not in men. Thus, preexisting risk factors for vascular dysfunction — dose of estrogen used, vascular bed studied, duration of ERT, and gender — may all have an effect on the type and degree of vascular response to estrogen.

Estrogen and Coagulation

ESTROGEN REPLACEMENT THERAPY

Epidemiologic evidence suggests that postmenopausal women on ERT have a decreased risk of arterial thrombotic disease, which is in contrast with the increased risk of venous thromboembolic disease in premenopausal women on OCPs. While these two facts initially appear to be incongruous, the contradiction can be explained by changes that occur in the coagulation and fibrinolytic pathways with menopause and with administration of different formulations of hormones.

With menopause, levels of key elements in the coagulation–anticoagulation balance change. Factor VIIc and fibrinogen levels increase slightly, but there is a marked increase in the levels of the natural anticoagulant, antithrobin III (Table 43-6 and Figure 43-13) [122–126]. Consequently, postmenopausal women on low-dose ERT may not be at increased risk

for thrombotic disease because of their high levels of antithrombin III.

These natural changes in the coagulation and fibrinolytic systems become more pronounced with the institution of ERT, which appears to tip the system balance in favor of anticoagulation as opposed to coagulation. For example, fibrinogen levels decrease in postmenopausal women who begin taking ERT; this decrease is especially important because an elevated fibrinogen level is a predictor of CVD [38,127]. In fact, the levels of fibrinogen in postmenopausal women on ERT are not significantly different from levels in premenopausal women [124]. In addition, levels of protein C and plasminogen, a precursor in the fibrinolytic pathway, are increased in postmenopausal women on ERT [124,128]. On the other hand, ERT does not appear to affect levels of factor VIII and von Willebrand factor [128].

Markers of thrombin and Xa activity also do not appear to be adversely affected by ERT, as shown by Saleh et al. [129]. In their study, prothrombin fragment 1 + 2, which is a marker of factor Xa generation and thrombin–antithrombin III complexes, were measured in postmenopausal women on HRT and in those not on HRT. There were no differences between these two groups with regard to these clotting parameters between the women not on ERT and those on ERT; moreover, there were no differences in these parameters between women on estrogen replacement only and those on estrogen and progesterone replacement. One of the only coagulation factors that has been studied that is increased in postmenopausal women on ERT, as compared with those not on it, is factor VII, but this does not appear to cause a hypercoagulable state in the face of all of the other changes in the coagulation cascade mentioned earlier [128]. As was alluded to earlier, in the United States the dose and potency of the estrogens and progestins most commonly used for replacement therapy are lower than those used in oral contraceptives. Also, premenopausal women have higher endogenous levels of estrogen and lower levels of antithrombin III than postmenopausal women. Thus, the low rates of thrombotic disease in postmenopausal women on ERT may also be due, in part, to the lower levels and potencies of hormones in the blood and higher levels of antithrombin III of these women as compared with premenopausal women on OCPs.

In summary, there is no evidence that ERT increases thrombotic risk in postmenopausal women. Still, in women who have had previous thromboembolic disease and who may have a condition that predisposes them to clot, it may be prudent to avoid ERT unless the possible

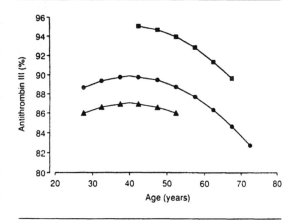

FIGURE 43-13. Antithrombin III levels in participants in the Northwick Park Heart Study. ▲ = premenopausal women; ■ = postmenopausal women; • = men. (Reproduced, with permission, from Meade et al. [123].)

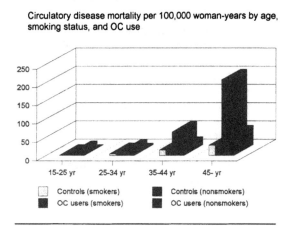

Circulatory disease mortality per 100,000 woman-years by age, smoking status, and OC use

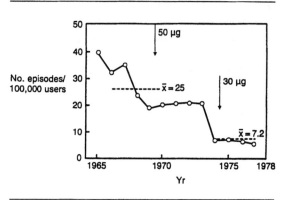

FIGURE 43-14. Circulatory disease mortality in the Royal College of Practitioners Oral Contraception Study per 100,000 women-years by age, smoking status, and oral contraceptive (OC) use. (Data from Layde and Beral [130].)

FIGURE 43-15. Thromboembolic episodes reported to the Swedish Adverse Drug Reaction Committee, 1965–1977. Broken lines indicate mean numbers for 1966–1970 and 1974–1977; arrows indicate switch to oral contraceptives with a lower estrogen content. (Reprinted, with permission, from Meade et al. [26]. Copyright 1977, The Lancet Ltd.)

increased risk of thrombosis is outweighed by the benefits of ERT.

ORAL CONTRACEPTIVE PILLS

As was mentioned in the section on oral contraceptives and CVD, it has been shown that OCPs, particularly those that provide high doses of estrogen, increase the risk of CVD, especially in women over 35 years of age who smoke (Figure 43-14) [19–21,130]. Epidemiologic studies also suggest that the risk of DVT and/or PE is increased with OCP use, and that the lower the dose of estrogen in an OCP, the lower the risk of thromboembolic disease [26,27,131]. Indeed, with a decrease in the average estrogen dose in OCPs came a decrease in the frequency with which thromboembolic disease was reported as an "adverse drug reaction" (Figure 43-15) [26]. In addition, in their Michigan Medicaid study, Gerstman et al. found that when they assigned the relative risk of DVT or PE in women taking low-dose estrogen OCPs (those containing less than 50 μg) to be 1.0, the women taking "intermediate-dose" OCPs (those with 50 μg of estrogen) and the group of women taking "high-dose" OCPs (those containing more than 50 μg of estrogen) had relative risks of 1.5 and 1.7, respectively [132]. Interpretation of these findings is somewhat confounded by the fact that patients were assigned to a group on the basis of estrogen dose and not potency, but the study provides some evidence that lower doses of estrogen correlate with a decreased risk of DVT and PE [132]. Consequently, the

percentage of women taking OCPs with high doses of estrogens has decreased. In 1968, less than 1% of oral contraceptives contained less than 50 μg of estrogen, whereas in 1987, 75% of OCPs contained less than 50 μg of estrogen [132]. The increased risk of DVT associated with higher dose OCPs has led to the withdrawl of OCPs that contained 100 μg of estrogen from the market [27].

There is no consensus as to the mechanism by which contraceptive steroids may increase the risk of thromboembolic disease, despite much research on the subject. It is known that the synthetic estrogens, ethinyl estradiol and mestranol (which in vivo is converted to ethinyl estradiol) both increase the clotting factors VII and X, and that these increases are dose dependent [133,134]. Fibrinogen levels also appear to be increased in women on OCPs, but two studies found no independent effect of these drugs on fibrinogen levels [135,136]. With OCP use, levels of anticoagulation factors increase, protein C levels and protein S levels decrease, and antithrombin III levels and thrombin–antithrombin III levels remain the same (Table 43-7) [136]. Thus, OCPs may facilitate thrombosis because levels of some factors that promote thrombosis are increased but the low levels of antithrombin III in premenopausal women are not [136]. Fibrinolytic factors are also affected by OCPs, but in a manner that would favor fibrinolysis. Plasminogen activator inhibitor (PAI), an inhibitor of the fibrinolytic system that therefore promotes coagulation, decreases in both level and activity with

TABLE 43-7. Impact of two monophasic oral contraceptive formulations on coagulation factors

	20 µg EE/150 µg DSG		30 µg EE/75 µg GSD	
	Pretherapy	12 mo	Pretherapy	12 mo
Factor VII (%)				
Median	80	126	87	137
Range	66–113	98–163	73–119	96–198
Fibrinogen (µmol/L)				
Median	7.2	8.7	7.7	8.4
Range	5.6–10.8	5.7–11.4	6.4–11.1	7.2–11.2
Antithrombin III (%)				
Median	96	99	101	100
Range	86–108	87–111	85–121	84–109
Protein C (%)				
Median	86	103	88	93
Range	59–127	66–158	63–118	72–131
Protein S (%)				
Median	94	84	101	84
Range	67–134	67–124	80–129	67–131
Thrombin–antithrombin III (µg/L)				
Median	2.7	3.1	2.9	3.0
Range	2.0–5.9	2.4–10.7	1.9–6.8	2.2–6.5

EE = ethinyl estradiol; DSG = desogestrel; GSD = gestodene.
Reprinted, with permission, from Samsioe [27].

administration of OCPs, whereas levels of plasminogen antigen (the precursor of plasmin, a fibrinolytic enzyme) increase [136].

The mechanism of the apparent synergistic effect of smoking and OCP use on thrombosis is also not completely understood. Data from two studies suggest that platelet aggregation is increased by the combination of smoking and OCP use [137,138]. The data from the study by Mileikowski et al. also support the hypothesis that this synergy may be due to a decrease in prostacyclin formation. In this study, women who smoked and who were taking OCPs had a much lower level of prostacyclin production (as evidenced by a lower urinary level of 6-keto-PGF1α) in comparison with women who smoked but were not on OCPs and with nonsmokers who used OCPs [137].

Thus, although the exact mechanism(s) by which OCPs increase the risk of venous thromboembolic events is not known, OCPs clearly affect clotting and fibrinolytic factors. Inherently low antithrombin III levels in premenopausal women also probably contribute to the increased risk of thromboembolic events in OCP users. In addition, other risk factors for thrombotic or hemorrhagic events (such as smoking) appear to have a synergistic effect with OCP use, perhaps through the effects of the combination of smoking and OCP use on prostacyclin synthesis.

Estrogen and Exercise Capacity

Estrogen may affect the adaptive response to training in women because in studies of healthy subjects, young women and young men exhibit the same adaptations to training, but postmenopausal women and age-matched men do not. With training, young men and women experience an increase in maximal oxygen uptake (VO2 max), cardiac output, maximal oxygen extraction by the working skeletal muscles, and left ventricular size [139]. However, postmenopausal women not taking ERT experience no increase in maximal cardiac output in response to training, and the increase with training in VO2 max seen in these women is solely based on an improvement in maximal oxygen extraction [140,141]. Postmenopausal women also do not have an increase in left ventricular size in response to training, in contrast to older men [141]. Studies are now underway to assess the effect of ERT on adaptations to training. Preliminary evidence suggests that healthy postmenopausal women on ERT do increase their cardiac output as well as their oxygen extraction in response to training.

There have been few studies to assess the effect of ERT on exercise capacity in postmenopausal women who have known coronary disease. One double-blinded, crossover study of the effects of short-term ERT in this subset of postmenopausal women showed

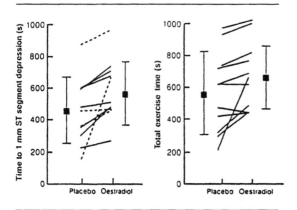

FIGURE 43-16. Effect of estradiol-17β on time to 1-mm ST-segment depression and total exercise time. Broken lines indicate patients who, after estradiol-17β, did not experience 1-mm ST-segment depression; total exercise time is given instead in these patients. (Reprinted, with permission, from Romano et al. [159]. Copyright 1993, The Lancet Ltd.)

that in those women on ERT, total exercise time, and time to 1-mm ST-segment depression was significantly increased as compared with those in women on placebo (Figure 43-16) [142]. The increase in total exercise time in this subset of postmenopausal women may be due to an antiischemic effect and/or to an increase in cardiac output.

Conclusions

Estrogen has many different effects on the cardiovascular system of women, and these effects depend on their menopausal status and possibly on the type of estrogen and/or progestin being used, if any. ERT is associated with a decreased risk of death from CVD, but oral contraceptive use is accociated with a small increase in risk of CVD. This seeming paradox can be explained by examining estrogen's mechanisms of action in premenopausal and postmenopausal women. ERT in postmenopausal women improves lipid profiles, but this effect does not appear to account for all of its cardioprotective effect. ERT probably retards atherogenesis directly and has antioxidant effects, and it also improves vasomotor function. Moreover, it does not increase the risk of hypertension or thromboembolic events in general. Finally, there is some evidence that estrogen has a role in a woman's response to exercise training, and it may improve myocardial perfusion.

ERT should be considered for postmenopausal patients, especially if they have risk factors for or evidence of CVD. When counseling a woman about ERT, a physician must consider the individual's risk of developing CVD or other conditions on which estrogen may have salutary effects (such as postmenopausal symptoms and osteoporosis), and her risk of developing a disease that may be negatively affected by ERT (such as breast cancer). Obviously, if a woman already has such a condition, her risk/benefit ratio may dictate that she would be better served by refraining from ERT. An individual's fears about developing breast cancer as a result of ERT must also be taken into account in the counseling process.

Current OCP use, on the other hand, is associated with an increased risk of hypertension and venous thromboembolic events. The incidence of the latter is particularly increased in older women on OCPs who smoke or who have other cardiovascular risk factors, and these women should be made aware of their increased risk, and alternative means of contraception should be discussed with them.

References

1. Harlan WR. Cardiovascular disease care for women: Service utilization, disability, and costs from the National Medical Care Utilization and Expenditure Survey. In Eaker ED, Packard B, Wenger NK, Clarkson TB, Tyroler HA (eds). Coronary Heart Disease in Women. New York: Haymarket Doyma, 1986:55.
2. Parrish HM, Carr CA, Hall DG, King TM. Time interval from castration in premenopausal women to development of excessive coronary atherocslerosis. Am J Obstet Gynecol 99:155, 1967.
3. Green A, Bain C. Epidemiological overview of oestrogen replacement and cardiovascular disease. Bailleres Clin Endocrinol Metab 7:95, 1993.
4. Natchigall LE, Natchigall RH, Natchigall RD, Beckman EM. Estrogen replacement therapy II: A prospective study in the relationship to carcinoma and cardiovascular and metabolic problems. Obstet Gynecol 54:74, 1979.
5. Bush T, Cowan LD, Barrett-Connor E, Criqui MH, Karon JM, Wallace RB, Tyroler HA, Rifkind BM. Estrogen use and all-cause mortality: Preliminary results from the Lipid Research Clinics Program follow-up study. JAMA 249:903, 1983.
6. Kannel WB, Vokonas PS. Menopause and the risk of cardiovascular disease: The Framingham Study. Ann Intern Med 85:447, 1976.
7. Grady D, Rubin SM, Petitti DB, Fox CS, Black D, Ettinger B, Ernster V, Cummings SR. Hormone therapy to prevent disease and prolong life in postmenopausal women. Ann Intern Med 117:1016, 1992.

8. Bush TL. Noncontraceptive estrogen use and risk of cardiovascular disease: An overview and critique of the literature. In Korenman SG (ed). The Menopause. Biological and Clinical Consequences of Ovarian Failure: Evolution and Management. Norwell, MA: Serono Symposia, 1990:211.

9. Stampfer MJ, Colditz GA. Estrogen replacement therapy and coronary heart disease: A quantitative assessment of the epidemiologic evidence. Prev Med 20:47, 1991.

10. Manolio TA, Furberg CD, Shemanski L, Psaty BM, O'Leary DH, Tracy RP, Bush TL. Associations of postmenopausal estrogen use with cardiovascular disease and its risk factors in older women. Circulation 88:2163, 1993.

11. Sullivan JM, Vander Zwaag R, Hughes JP, Maddock V, Kroetz FW, Ramanathan KB, Mirvis DM. Estrogen replacement and coronary artery disease. Effect on survival in postmenopausal women. Arch Intern Med 150:2557, 1990.

12. Sullivan JM, El-Zeky F, Vander Zwaag R, Ramanathan KB. Estrogen replacement therapy after coronary artery bypass surgery: Effect on survival (abstr). J Am Coll Cardiol February (Special issue):7, 1994.

13. Pilote L, Hlatky M. Hormone replacement after menopause: Importance of heart disease in women's decision making (abstr). J Am Coll Cardiol February (Special issue):51, 1994.

14. American College of Physicians. Guidelines for counseling postmenopausal women about preventive hormone therapy. Ann Intern Med 117:1038, 1992.

15. Mann JI, Vessey MP, Thorogood M, Doll R. Myocardial infarction in young women with special reference to oral contraceptive practice. Br Med J 2:241, 1975.

16. Mann JI, Inman WHW. Oral contraceptives and death from myocardial infarction. Br Med J 2:245, 1975.

17. Mann JI, Inman WHW, Thorogood M. Oral contraceptive use in older women and fatal myocardial infarction. Br Med J 2:445, 1976.

18. Ory H. Association between oral contraceptives and myocardial infarction: A review. JAMA 237:2619, 1977.

19. Inman WHW, Vessey MP, Weterholm B, Engelund A. Thromboembolic disease and the steroidal content of oral contraceptives: A report to the Committee on Safety of Drugs. Br Med J 2:203, 1970.

20. Vessey MP, Doll R. Investigation of relation between use of oral contraceptives and thromboembolic disease. Br Med J 2:199, 1968.

21. Realini JP, Goldzieher JW. Oral contraceptives and cardiovascular disease: A critique of the epidemiologic studies. Am J Obstet Gynecol 152:729, 1985.

22. Stampfer MJ, Willet WC, Colditz GA, Speizer FE, Hennekens CH. Past use of oral contraceptives and cardiovascular disease: A meta-analysis in the context of the Nurses' Health Study. Am J Obset Gynecol 163:285, 1990.

23. Sloane D, Shapiro S, Kaufman DW, Rosenberg L, Miettinen OS, Stolley PD. Risk of myocardial infarction in relation to current and discontinued use of oral contraceptives. N Engl J Med 305:420, 1981.

24. Jick H, Dinan B, Rothman KJ. Oral contraceptives and nonfatal myocardial infarction. JAMA 239:1403, 1978.

25. Adam SA, Thorogood M. Oral contraception and myocardial infarction revisited: The effects of new preparations and prescribing patterns. Br J Obstet Gynaecol 88:838, 1981.

26. Meade TW, Haines AP, North WR, Chakrabarti R, Howarth DJ, Stirling Y. Haemostatic, lipid, and blood-pressure profiles of women on oral contraceptives containing 50 microgram of 30 microgram oestrogen. Lancet 2:948, 1977.

27. Samsioe G. Coagulation and anticoagulation effects of contraceptive steroids. Am J Obstet Gynecol 170:1523, 1994.

28. Collaborative Group for the Study of Stroke in Young Women: Oral Contraceptives and stroke in young women: Associated risk factors. JAMA 231:718, 1975.

29. Collaborative Group for the Study of Stroke in Young Women: Oral contraception and increased risk of cerebral ischemia or thrombosis. N Engl J Med 288:871, 1973.

30. Petitti DB, Wingerd J. Use of oral contraceptives, cigarette smoking, and risk of subarachnoid hemorrhage. Lancet 2:234, 1978.

31. Inman WH. Oral contraceptives and fatal subarachnoid hemorrhage. Br Med J 2:1468, 1979.

32. Royal College of General Practitioners' Oral Contraceptive Study. Further analysis of mortality in oral contraceptive users. Lancet 1:541, 1981.

33. Vessey M, Mant D, Smith A, Yeates D. Oral contraceptives and venous thromboembolism: Findings of a large prospective study. Br Med J (Clin Res Ed) 292:526, 1986.

34. Furr BJA, Jordan VC. The pharmacology and clinical uses of tamoxifen. Pharmacol Ther 25:127, 1984.

35. McDonald CC, Stewart HJ. Fatal myocardial infarction in the Scottish adjuvant tamoxifen trial. The Scottish Breast Cancer Committee. BMJ 303:435, 1991.

36. Kannel WB. Metabolic risk factors for coronary heart disease in women: Perspective from the Framingham Study. Am Heart J 114:413, 1987.

37. La Rosa JC. The varying effects of progestins on lipid levels and cardiovascular disease. Am J Obstet Gynecol 158:1621, 1988.

38. The Writing Group for the PEPI trial. Effects of estrogen or estrogen/progestin regimens on heart disease risk factors in postmenopausal women. JAMA 273:199, 1995.

39. Kim CJ, Min YK. Apolipoprotein(a)-lowering effect

of hormone replacement therapy in postmenopausal women may be one mechanism of cardioprotective effect of estrogen (abstr). J Am Coll Cardiol February (Special issue):431, 1994.

40. Kannel WB, D'Agostino RB, Belanger AJ. New insights on cholesterol-lipoprotein profiles: The Framingham Study. Presented at the 61st Scientific Sessions of the American Heart Association, November, 1988.

41. Freedman DS, Gruchow HW, Anderson AJ, Rimm AA, Barboriak JJ. Relation of triglyceride levels to coronary artery disease: The Milwaukee Cardiovascular Data Registry. Am J Epidemiol 127:1118, 1988.

42. Farmer JA, Gotto AM. Risk factors for coronary artery disease. In Braunwald E (ed). Heart Disease: A Textbook of Cardiovascular Medicine. Philadelphia: WB Saunders, 1992:1125.

43. Belchetz PE. Hormonal treatment of postmenopausal women. N Engl J Med 330:1062, 1994.

44. Goebelsmann U, Maschak CA, Mishell DR. Comparison of hepatic impact of oral and vaginal administration of ethinyl estradiol. Am J Obstet Gynecol 151:868, 1985.

45. Applebaum DM, Goldberg AP, Pykalisto OJ, Brunzell JD, Hazzard WR. Effect of estrogen on postheparin lipolytic activity. Selective decline in hepatic triglyceride lipase. J Clin Invest 59:601, 1977.

46. Wagner JD. Effect of estrogens on arterial LDL metabolism. Presented at the AHA Scientific Conference on Hormonal Metabolism and Cellular Influence on Cardiovascular Disease in Women, San Diego, CA, 1995.

47. Kovanen PT, Brown MS, Goldstein JL. Increased binding of low-density lipoprotein to liver membrane from rats treated with 17 alpha-ethinyl estradiol. J Biol Chem 254:1376, 1979.

48. Miller VT, La Rosa JC. Sex steroids and lipoproteins. In Redmond GP (ed). Lipids and Women's Health. New York: Springer-Verlag, 1990:48.

49. Knopp RH. Cardiovascular effects of endogenous and exogenous sex hormones over a woman's lifetime. Am J Obstet Gynecol 158:1630, 1988.

50. Runnebaum B, Rabe TR. New progestogens in oral contraceptives. Am J Obstet Gynecol 157:1059, 1987.

51. Harvengt C, Desager JP, Gaspard U, Lepot M. Changes in lipoprotein composition in women receiving two low-dose oral contraceptives containing ethinylestradiol and gonane progestins. Contraception 37:565, 1988.

52. Kloosterboer HJ, van Wayjen RGA, van den Ende A. Comparative effects of monophasic desogesterel plus ethinyl estradiol and triphasic levonorgestrel plus ethinyloestradiol on lipid metabolism. Contraception 34:135, 1986.

53. Gaspard UJ, Buret J, Gillain D, Romus MA, Lambotte R. Serum lipid and lipoprotein changes induced by new oral contraceptives containing ethinylestradiol plus levonorgestrel or desogestrel. Contraception 31:395, 1985.

54. März W, Gross W, Gahn G, Romberg G, Taubert HD, Kuhl H. A randomized crossover comparison of two low-dose contraceptives: effects on serum lipids and lipoproteins. Am J Obstet Gynecol 153:287, 1985.

55. Ottosson UB, Johansson BG, Von Schoultz B. Subfractions of high density lipoprotein cholesterol during estrogen replacement: A comparison between progestogens and natural progesterone. Am J Obstet Gynecol 151:746, 1985.

56. Kim H-J, Kalkoff RK. Sex steroid influence on triglyceride metabolism. J Clin Invest 56:888, 1975.

57. Kim H-J, Kalkhoff RK. Changes in lipoprotein composition during the menstrual cycle. Metabolism 28:663, 1979.

58. Basdevant A, De Lignieres B, Bigorie B, Guy-Grand B. Estradiol, progesterone, and plasma lipids during the menstrual cycle. Diabetes Metab 7:1, 1981.

59. Hemer HA, de Bourges VV, Ayala JJ, Brito G, Diaz-Sanchez V, Garza-Flores J. Variations in serum lipase and lipoproteins throughout the menstrual cycle. Eur J Obstet Gynecol Reprod Biol 44:80, 1984.

60. Mattson L A, Silfverstolpe G, Samsioe G. Lipid composition of serum lipoproteins in relation to gonadal hormone during the normal menstrual cycle. Eur J Obstet Gynecol Reprod Biol 17:327, 1984.

61. Tikkanen MJ, Kuusi T, Nikkila EA, Stenman U-H. Variation of postheparin plasma hepatic lipase by menstrual cycle. Metabolism 35:99, 1986.

62. Woods M, Schaefer EJ, Morrill A, Goldin BR, Longcope C, Dwyer JD, Gorbach SL. Effect of menstrual cycle phase on plasma lipids. J Clin Endocrinal Metab 65:321, 1987.

63. Herrera E, Lasuncion MA, Gomez-Coronado D, Aranda P, Lopez-Luna P, Maier I. Role of lipoprotein lipase activity on lipoprotein metabolism and the fate of circulating triglycerides in pregnancy. Am J Obstet Gynecol 158:1575, 1988.

64. Desoye G, Schweditsch M, Pfieffer KP, Zechner R, Kostner GH. Correlation of hormones with lipid and lipoprotein levels during normal pregnancy and postpartum. J Clin Endocrinol Metab 64:704, 1987.

65. Bengtsson B, Rybo G, Westerberg H. Number of pregnancies, use of oral contraceptives and menopausal age in women with ischaemic heart disease, compared to a population sample of women. Acta Med Scand 549(Suppl.):75, 1973.

66. Oliver MF. Ischaemic heart disease in young women. Br Med J 4:253, 1974.

67. Maschak CA, Lobo RA. Estrogen replacement therapy and hypertension. J Reprod Med 30:805, 1985.

68. Barrett-Connor E. Putative complications of estrogen replacement therapy: Hypertension, diabetes, thrombophlebitis, and gallstones. In Koernman SG (ed). The Menopause: Biological and Clinical Conse-

quences of Ovarian Failure; Evolution and Management. Norwell, MA: Serono Symposia, 1990:199.

69. Lip GYH, Beevers M, Churchill D, Beevers DG. Hormone replacement therapy and blood pressure in hypertensive women. J Hum Hypertens 8:491, 1994.

70. Woods JW. Oral contraceptives and hypertension. Hypertension 11(Suppl. II):11, 1988.

71. Wallace RB, Barrett-Connor E, Criqui M, Wahl P, Hoover J, Hunninghake D, Heiss G. Alteration in blood pressures associated with combined alcohol and oral contraceptive use — the lipid research clinics prevalence study. J Chronic Dis 35:251, 1982.

72. Kaplan NM. Systemic hypertension: Mechanisms and diagnosis. In Braunwald E (ed). Heart Disease: A Textbook of Cardiovascular Medicine. Philadelphia: W.B. Saunders, 1992:817.

73. Hassager C, Riis BJ, Strom V, Guyene TT, Christiansen C. The long-term effect of oral and percutaneous estradiol on plasma renin substrate and blood pressure. Circulation 76:753, 1987.

74. Kaplan NM (ed). Clinical Hypertension. Baltimore, MD: Williams and Wilkins, 1990:346.

75. McAreavey D, Cumming AM, Boddy K, Brown JJ, Praser R, Leckie BJ, Lever AF, Morton JJ, Robertson JI, Williams ED. The renin-angiotensin system and total body sodium and potassium in hypertensive women taking oestrogen-progestagen oral contraceptives. Clin Endocrinol Oxf 18:111, 1983.

76. Laakso M. How good a marker is insulin level for insulin resistance? Am J Epidemiol 137:959, 1993.

77. Kasdorf G, Kalkhoff RK. Prospective studies of insulin sensitivity in normal women receiving oral contraceptive agents. J Clin Endocrinol Metab 66:846, 1988.

78. Haarbo J, Leth-Espensen P, Stender S, Christiansen C. Estrogen monotherapy and combined estrogen-progestogen replacement therapy attenuate aortic accumulation of cholesterol in ovariectomized cholesterol-fed rabbits. J Clin Invest 87:1274, 1991.

79. Adams MR, Kaplan JR, Manuck SB, Koritnik DR, Parks JS, Wolfe MS, Clarkson TB. Inhibition of coronary atherosclerosis by 17-beta estradiol in ovariectomized monkeys. Arteriosclerosis 10:1051, 1990.

80. Wagner JD, Clarkson TB, St. Clair RW, Schwenke DC, Shively CA, Adams MR. Estrogen and progesterone replacement therapy reduces low density lipoprotein accumulation in the coronary arteries of surgically postmenopausal cynomologous monkeys. J Clin Invest 88:1995, 1991.

81. Jacobsson J, Cheng L, Lyke K, Kuwahara M, Kagan E, Ramwell PW, Foegh ML. Effect of estrodiol on accelerated atherosclerosis in rabbit heterotopic aortic allografts. J Heart Lung Transplant 11:1188, 1992.

82. Brown MS, Goldstein JL. Scavenging for receptors. Nature 343:508, 1990.

83. Berliner JA, Navab M, Fogelman AM, Frank JS, Demer LL, Edwards PA, Watson AD, Lusis AJ. Atherosclerosis: basic mechanisms. Oxidation,

84. Cushing SD, Berliner JA, Valente AJ, Territo MC, Navab M, Parhami F, Gerrity R, Schwartz CJ, Fogelman AM. Minimally modified low density lipoprotein induces monocyte chemotactic protein 1 in human endothelial cells and smooth muscle cells. Proc Natl Acad Sci USA 87:5134, 1990.

85. McEver RP. Leukocyte-endothelial interactions. Curr Opin Cell Biol 4:840, 1992.

86. Losordo DW, Kearney M, Kim EA, Jekanowski J, Isner JM. Variable expression of the estrogen receptor in normal and atherosclerotic coronary arteries of premenopausal women. Circulation 89:1501, 1994.

87. Karas RH, Patterson BL, Mendelsohn ME. Human vascular smooth muscle cells contain functional estrogen receptor. Circulation 89:1943, 1994.

88. Fischer GM, Swain ML. Effect of sex hormones on blood pressure and vascular connective tissue is castrated and noncastrated male rats. Am J Physiol 232:H617, 1977.

89. Fischer GM, Cherian K, Swain ML. Inreased synthesis of aortic collagen and elastin in experimental atherosclerosis. Inhibition by contraceptive steroids. Atherosclerosis 39:463, 1981.

90. Calgano D, Bei M, Ross SA, Klein A, Foegh ML. Effects of estrogen on vein grafts. J Cardiovasc Surg 33:579, 1992.

91. Demer LL. Estrogen and arterial wall calcification. Presented at the American Heart Association Scientific Conference on Hormonal Metabolism and Cellular Influence on Cardiovascular Disease in Women, San Diego CA, 1995.

92. Guetta V, Panza JA, Waclawiw MA, Cannon RO. Effect of combined 17-β estradiol and vitamin E on low-density lipoprotein oxidation in postmenopausal women. Am J Cardiol 75:1274, 1995.

93. Mukai K, Daifuku K, Yokoyama S, Nakano M. Stopped-flow investigation of antioxidant activity of estrogens in solution. Biochim Biophys Acta 1035:348, 1990.

94. Sugioka K, Shimosegawa Y, Nakano M. Estrogens as natural antioxidants of membrane phospholipid peroxidation. FEBS Lett 210:37, 1987.

95. Huber LA, Scheffler E, Poll T, Ziegler R, Dresel HA. 17 beta-estradiol inhibits LDL oxidation and cholesteryl ester formation in cultured macrophages. Free Radic Res Commun 8:167, 1990.

96. Rifici VA, Khachadurian AK. The inhibition of low-density lipoprotein oxidation by 17-β estradiol. Metabolism 41:1110, 1992.

97. Subbiah MTR, Kessel B, Agrawal M, Rajan R, Abplanalp W, Rymaszewski Z. Antioxidant potential of specific estrogens on lipid peroxidation. J Clin Endocinol Metab 77:1095, 1993.

98. Keaney JF, Shwaery GT, Aiming X, Nicolosi RJ, Loscalo J, Foxall TL, Vita JA. 17-β estradiol preserves endothelial vasodilator function and limits low-den-

sity lipoprotein oxidation in hypercholesterolemic swine. Circulation 89:2251, 1994.

99. Sack MN, Rader DJ, Cannon RO. Oestrogen and inhibition of oxidation of low-density lipoproteins in postmenopausal women. Lancet 343:269, 1994.

100. Sarrel PM. Effects of ovarian steroids on the cardiovascular system. In Ginsberg J (ed). Circulation in the Female. Park Ridge, NJ: Parthenon, 1989:117.

101. Sarrel PM, Lindsay D, Rosano GM, Poole-Wilson PA. Angina and normal coronary arteries in women: Gynecologic findings. Am J Obstet Gynecol 167:467, 1992.

102. Jiang C, Sarrel PM, Poole-Wilson PA, Collins P. Acute effect of 17-β estradiol on rabbit coronary artery contractile responses to endothelin-1. Heart Circ Physiol 263:H271, 1992.

103. Collins P, Rosano GMC, Jiang C, Lindsay D, Sarrel PM, Poole-Wilson PA. Hypothesis: Cardiovascular protection by oestrogen: A calcium antagonist effect? Lancet 341:1264, 1993.

104. Hayashi T, Fukoto JM, Ignarro LJ, Chaudhuri G. Basal release of nitric oxide from aortic rings is greater in female rabbits: Implications for atherosclerosis. Proc Natl Acad Sci USA 89:11259, 1992.

105. Weiner CP, Lizasoain I, Baylis SA, Knowles RG, Charles IG, Moncada S. Induction of calcium-dependent nitric oxide synthases by sex hormones. Proc Natl Acad Sci USA 91:5212, 1994.

106. Keaney JF, Shwaery GT, Xu A, Nicolosi RJ, Loscalzo J, Foxall TL, Vita JA. 17-β estradiol preserves endothelial vasodilator function and limits low-density lipoprotein oxidation in hypercholesterolemic swine. Circulation 89:2251, 1994.

107. Sudhir K, Chou TM, Mullen WL, Hausmann D, Collins P, Yock PG, Chattergee K. Mechanisms of estrogen-induced vasodilation. In vivo studies in canine coronary conductance and resistance arteries. J Am Coll Cardiol 26:807, 1995.

108. Jiang C, Sarrel PM, Lindsay DC, Poole-Wilson PA, Collins P. Endothelium-independent relaxation of rabbit coronary artery to 17-β estradiol in vitro. Br J Pharmacol 104:1033, 1991.

109. Chang WC, Nakao J, Orimo H, Murota S. Stimulation of prostacyclin biosynthetic activity by estradiol in rat aortic smooth muscle cells in culture. Biochim Biophys Acta 619:107, 1980.

110. Magness RR, Rosenfeld CR. Local and systemic effects on uterine and systemic vasodilation. Am J Physiol 256:E536, 1989.

111. Williams JK, Adams MR, Herrington DM, Clarkson TB. Short-term administration of estrogen and vascular responses of atherosclerotic coronary arteries. J Am Coll Cardiol 20:452, 1992.

112. Vanhoutte PM (ed). Vasodilation: Vascular Smooth Muscle, Peptides, Autonomic Nerves, and Endothelium. New York: Raven Press, 1988.

113. Ludmer PL, Selwyn AP, Shook TL, Wayne RR, Mudge GH, Alexander W, Ganz P. Paradoxical vaso-

constriction induced by acetylcholine in atherosclerotic coronary arteries. N Engl J Med 315:1046, 1986.

114. Gilligan DM, Quyyumi AA, Cannon RO. Effects of physiological levels of estrogen on coronary vasomotor function in postmenopausal women. Circulation 89:2545, 1994.

115. Williams JK, Adams MR, Klopfenstein HS. Estrogen modulates responses of atherosclerotic coronary arteries. Circulation 81:1680, 1990.

116. Gangar KF, Vyas S, Whitehead M, Crook D, Meire H, Campbell S. Pulsatility index in internal carotid artery in relation to transdermal oestrogen and time since menopause. Lancet 338:839, 1991.

117. Gilligan DM, Badar DM, Panza JA, Quyyumi AA, Cannon RO. Acute vascular effects of estrogen in postmenopausal women. Circulation 90:786, 1994.

118. Volterrani M, Rosano G, Coats A, Beale C, Collins P. Estrogen acutely increases peripheral blood flow in postmenopausal women. Am J Med 99:119, 1994.

119. Lieberman EH, Gerhard MD, Uehata A, Walsh BW, Selwyn AP, Ganz P, Yeung AC, Creager MA. Estrogen improves endothelium-dependent, flow-mediated vasodilation in postmenopausal women. Ann Intern Med 121:936, 1994.

120. Reis SE, Gloth ST, Blumenthal RS, Resar JR, Zacur HA, Gerstenblith G, Brinker JA. Ethinyl estradiol acutely attenuates abnormal coronary vasomotor responses to acetylcholine in postmenopausal women. Circulation 89:52, 1994.

121. Collins P, Rosano GMC, Sarrel PM, Ulrich L, Adamopoulos S, Beale CM, McNeill JG, Poole-Wilson PA. 17-β estradiol attenuates acetylcholine-induced coronary arterial constriction in women but not men with coronary heart disease. Circulation 92:24, 1995.

122. Meade TW, Haines AP, Imeson JD, Stirling Y, Thompson SG. Menopausal status and haemostatic variables. Lancet I:22, 1983.

123. Meade TW, Dyer S, Howarth DJ, Imeson JD, Stirling Y. Antithrombin III and procoagulant activity: Sex differences and effects of the menopause. Br J Haematol 74:77, 1990.

124. Meilahn EN, Kuller LH, Matthews KA, Kiss JE. Hemostatic factors according to menopausal status and use of hormone replacement therapy. Ann Epidemiol 4:445, 1992.

125. Meade TW, Berra A. Hormone replacement therapy and cardiovascular disease. Br Med Bull 48:276, 1992.

126. Meilahn E, Kuller ME, Kiss LH, Matthews JE, Lewis KA. Coagulation parameters among pre- and post-menopausal women. Am J Epidemiol 28:908, 1990.

127. Kannel WB, Wolf PA, Castelli WP, D'Agostino RB. Fibrinogen and risk of cardiovascular disease — The Framingham Study. JAMA 258:1183, 1987.

128. Nabulsi AA, Folsom AR, White A, Patsch W, Heiss

G, Wu KK, Szklo M. Association of hormone-replacement therapy with various cardiovascular risk factors in postmenopausal women. The Atherosclerosis Risk in Communities Study Investigators. N Engl J Med 328:1069, 1993.

129. Saleh AA, Dorey LG, Dombrowski MP, Ginsburg KA, Hirokawa S, Kowalczyk C, Hirata J, Bottoms S, Cotton DB, Mammen EF. Thrombosis and hormone replacement therapy in postmenopausal women. Am J Obstet Gynecol 169:1554, 1993.

130. Layde PM, Beral V. Further analyses of mortality in oral contraceptive users: Royal College of General Practitioners' Oral Contraception Study. Lancet 1:541, 1981.

131. Comp PC, Zacur HA. Contraceptive choices in women with coagulation disorders. Am J Obstet Gynecol 168:1990, 1993.

132. Gerstman BB, Piper JM, Tomita DK, Ferguson WJ, Stadel BV, Lundin FE. Oral contraceptive estrogen dose and the risk of deep venous thromboembolic disease. Am J Epidemiol 133:32, 1991.

133. Lobo RA. Estrogen and the risk of coagulopathy. Am J Med 92:283, 1992.

134. Poller L, Thompson JM. Clotting factors during oral contraception: Further report. Br Med J 2:23, 1966.

135. Lee AJ, Lowe GDO, Smith WCS, Tunstall-Pedoe H. Plasma fibrinogen: Its relationship with oral contraception, the menopause and hormone replacement therapy. Clin Biochem 25:403, 1992.

136. Petersen KR, Sidelmann J, Skouby SO, Jespersen J. Effects of monophasic low-dose oral contraceptives on fibrin formulation and resolution in young women. Am J Obstet Gynecol 168:32, 1993.

137. Mileikowsky GM, Nadler JL, Huey F, Francis R, Roy S. Evidence that smoking alters prostacyclin formation and platelet aggregation in women who use oral contraceptives. Am J Obstet Gynecol 159:1547, 1988.

138. Pan JQ, Hall ER, Wu KK. Alteration of platelet responses to metabolites of arachadonic acid by oral contraceptives. Br J Haematol 58:317, 1984.

139. Spina RJ, Ogawa T, Martin WH, Coggan AR, Holloszy JO, Ehsani AA. Exercise training prevents decline in stroke volume during exercise in young subjects. J Appl Physiol 72:2458, 1992.

140. Spina RJ, Ogawa T, Miller TR, Kohrt WM, Ehsani AA. Effect of exercise training on left ventricular performance in older women free of cardiopulmonary disease. Am J Cardiol 71:99, 1993.

141. Spina RJ, Ogawa T, Kohrt WM, Martin WH, Holloszy JO, Ehsani AA. Differences in cardiovascular adaptations to endurance exercise training between older men and women. J Appl Physiol 75:849, 1993.

142. Rosano GMC, Sarrel PM, Poole-Wilson PA, Collins P. Beneficial effect of oestrogen on exercise-induced myocardial ischaemia in woman with coronary disease. Lancet 342:133, 1993.

143. Mandel FP, Geola FL, Meldrum DR, Lu JH, Eggena P, Sambhi MP, Hershman JM, Judd HL. Biological effects of various doses of vaginally administered conjugated equine estrogens in postmenopausal women. J Clin Endocrinol Metab 57:133, 1983.

144. Lobo RA, March CM, Goebelsmann U, Krauss RM, Mishell DR Jr. Subdermal estradiol pellets following hysterectomy and oophorectomy. Effect upon serum estrone, estradiol, luteinizing hormone, follicle-stimulating hormone, corticosteroid binding globulin-binding capacity, testosterone-estradiol binding globulin-binding capacity, lipids, and hot flushes. Am J Obstet Gynecol 138:714, 1980.

145. Farish E, Fletcher CD, Hart R, et al. The effects of hormone implants on serum lipoproteins and steroid hormones in bilaterally oopherectomized women. Acta Endocrinol (Copenhagen) 106:116, 1984.

146. Sharf M, Oettinger M, Lanir A, Kahana L, Yeshurun D. Lipid and lipoprotein levels following pure estradiol implantation in post-menopausal women. Gynecol Obstet Invest 19:207, 1985.

147. Jensen J, Riis BJ, Strom V, Nilas L, Christiansen C. Long-term effects of percutaneous estrogens and oral progesterone on serum lipoproteins in post-menopausal women. Am J Obstet Gynecol 156:66, 1987.

148. Fahraeus L, Larsson-Cohn U, Wallentin L. Lipoproteins during oral and cutaneous administration of estradiol-17 beta to menopausal women. Acta Endocrinol 101:597, 1982.

149. Chetkowski RJ, Meldrum DR, Steingold KA, Randle D, Lu JK. Eggena P, Hershman JM, Alkjaersig NK, Fletcher AP, Judd HL. Biological effects of transdermal estradiol. N Engl J Med 314:1615, 1986.

150. Lipson A, Stoy DB, LaRosa JC, et al. Progestins and oral contraceptive-induced lipoprotein changes: A prospective study. Contraception 34:121, 1986.

151. Powell MC, Hedlin AM, Cerkus I, et al. Effects of oral contraceptives on lipoprotein lipids: A prospective study. Obstet Gynecol 63:764, 1966.

152. Burkman RT, Robinson JC, Kruszon-Moran D, Kimball AW, Kwiterovich P, Burford RG. Lipid and lipoprotein changes associated with oral contraceptive use: a randomized clinical trial. Obstet Gynecol 71:33, 1988.

153. Krauss RM, Roy S, Mishell DR Jr, et al. Effects of two low-dose oral contraceptives on serum lipids and lipoproteins: Different changes in high-density lipoprotein subclasses. Am J Obstet Gynecol 145:446, 1983.

154. Percival-Smith RK, Morrison BJ, Sizto R, Abercrombie B. The effects of triphasic and biphasic oral contraceptive preparations on HDL-cholesterol and LDL-cholesterol in young women. Contraception 35:179, 1987.

155. Knopp RH. Arteriosclerotic risk. The roles of oral contraceptives and postmenopausal estrogens. J Reprod Med 31:913, 1986.

156. Knopp RH. Metabolic adjustments in normal and diabetic pregnancy. Clin Obstet Gynecol 24:21, 1981.
157. Kaplan NM. Clinical Hypertension, 5th ed. Baltimore, MD: Williams and Wilkins, 1990:346.
158. Esterbauer H, Striegl G, Puhl H, Rotheneder M. Continuous monitoring of in vitro oxidation of human low density lipoprotein. Free Radic Res Commun 6:67, 1989.
159. Rosano GM, Sarrel PM, Poole-Wilson PA, Collins P. Beneficial effect of oestrogen on exercise-induced myocardial ischaemia in women with coronary artery disease. Lancet 342:133, 1993.

PART D: EVOLUTION OF THROMBOCARDIOLOGY

SECTION XV: CLINICAL TRIAL DESIGN AND DRUG DEVELOPMENT

Robert A. Harrington

Given the importance of both platelets and thrombin in the pathophysiology of acute ischemic coronary events, intense research efforts have focused on developing novel antithrombotic agents for clinical use. A number of antiplatelet and antithrombin drugs have been investigated in clinical trials in the last decade. The appropriately designed randomized clinical trial has become increasingly important in the drug development process in that it provides the necessary evidence to introduce new drugs into clinical practice.

This section provides a broad review of the antithrombotic agents presently under development and includes a detailed discussion of the rationale for their possible use. Basic concepts of clinical trials design and methodology are discussed, with a focus on the development of the platelet glycoprotein IIb/IIIa receptor inhibitors. A glossary of commonly used terms in thrombocardiology is included in this section.

44. DRUGS IN DEVELOPMENT

Mark C. Thel and Robert A. Harrington

Introduction

The prevention and treatment of intracoronary thrombosis has assumed greater priority as our understanding of the pathogenesis of ischemic heart disease has increased [1,2]. The appearance of layered thrombi in healed and acute coronary plaques implies that recurrent fissuring and thrombosis lead to plaque growth and fibrosis [3–7]. Platelet-derived growth factors contribute to the cellular response by inducing neointimal proliferation [8,9]. Platelet deposition and thrombus formation at the site of plaque disruption are basic to atherosclerotic progression and eventual occlusion, with thrombosis at the site of atherosclerotic plaque rupture being the fundamental step in the acute coronary syndromes of unstable angina (UA) and acute myocardial infarction (AMI). Fresh thrombi in these lesions have been confirmed by angioscopic, angiographic, and histologic studies [4,5,10–13]. While thrombolytic agents restore complete arterial patency (Thrombolysis in Myocardial Infarction [TIMI] grade 3 flow) in up to 54% of patients at 90 minutes, residual thrombus and ongoing thrombin generation and platelet activation contribute to vessel reocclusion and subsequently increase myocardial dysfunction and mortality [14–27].

Thrombosis also occurs at the site of vascular injury following percutaneous transluminal coronary angioplasty (PTCA) [6,28–32]. Platelet activation and aggregation and thrombus formation lead to abrupt closure and, more importantly, to clinical ischemic complications [33–40]. The same processes promote restenosis, the major chronic limitation of PTCA [41–46]. In fact, the relatively controlled and predictable events following PTCA and the ability to time pharmacologic interventions in this setting provide a useful model to investigate antithrombotic and antiplatelet agents. Animal and human studies suggest that suppression of ADP-induced platelet aggregation to <20% of baseline (>80% inhibition of platelet aggregation) may be an appropriate ex vivo marker because it correlates with reduced thrombosis and fewer ischemic events following PTCA [47–50].

The pathologic generation of thrombus in the setting of UA, AMI, and PTCA proceeds identically to the appropriate protective mechanisms that minimize hemorrhage following other forms of vascular injury (Figure 44-1). The initial step in hemostasis and thrombus formation is platelet *adherence* to newly exposed subendothelial proteins via integrin receptors. Described by Hynes in 1987, integrins are a family of membrane heterodimers found on essentially all cell types that are responsible for cell–cell and cell–matrix interaction [51,52]. They are composed of noncovalently bound glycoprotein (GP) α and β transmembrane subunits. The extracellular portion of the subunit combination defines the receptor's specificity and affinity for ligands. The intracellular domain interacts with cytoplasmic constituents, producing a cellular response upon ligand binding. At least 16 α and 8 β subunits, forming 22 integrins, have been identified.

Inactivated resting platelets form a monolayer on the disrupted subendothelium by binding to von Willebrand factor (vWF) and collagen directly via their GPIb (not an integrin) and GPIa/IIa receptors, respectively. Once *activated* (by adenosine diphosphate [ADP], serotonin, epinephrine, thromboxane A_2 [TxA_2], vasopressin, plasmin, shear stress, or thrombin), the GPIIb/IIIa receptors undergo conformational changes, allowing them to bind soluble fibrinogen and vWF [53,54]. Because each platelet contains about 50,000 GPIIb/IIIa receptors, and the ligands themselves are multivalent, fibrinogen bridges are quickly formed that produce a platelet network, the final common pathway of platelet *aggregation*.

In 1984 Pierschbacher and Ruoslahti identified Arg-Gly-Asp (RGD) as the minimum recognition sequence in fibronectin for GPIIb/IIIa binding [55]. The same RGD sequence is responsible for GPIIb/IIIa binding to fibrinogen, vWF, thrombospondin, col-

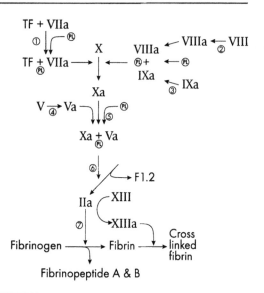

TF = Tissue Factor
2, 4, 5 = Stimulated by thrombin
1, 2, 6 = Inhibited by protein c/s
1, 3, 6, 7 = Inhibited by Antithrombin III–Heparin
7 = Inhibited by direct antithrombins

FIGURE 44-1. Generation of thrombus after vascular injury.

TABLE 44-1. Antiplatelet agents

I.   Cyclooxygenase inhibitors
     1. Aspirin
II. Thromboxane synthase inhibitors
III. Thromboxane A$_2$ receptor antagonists
     1. Sulotroban
     2. GR32191B
IV. Phosphodiesterase inhibitors
     1. Dipyridamole
V.   Anti-ADP
     1. Ticlopidine
     2. Clopidogrel
VI. GP IIb/IIIa antagonists
     1. Monoclonal antibody
        a. Abciximab/c7E3
     2. Cyclic RGD peptides
        a. Eptifibatide
        b. MK-852
        c. G-4120
     3. Pseudopeptides
        a. Lamifiban
        b. Tirofiban MK-383
     4. Orally active drugs
        a. Xemlofiban SC 54684
        b. BIBU-52
        c. GR 144,053
        d. L 703,014

lagen, laminin, and vitronectin [56]. Likewise, this RGD sequence also adheres to other integrins, for example, $\alpha_5\beta_1$ and $\alpha_v\beta_3$. The RGD sequence is necessary, but not sufficient, for ligand binding. Ironically, though fibrinogen contains four RGD sequences, its primary GPIIb/IIIa binding sequence appears to be a Lys-Gln-Ala-Asp-Val sequence on its γ chain [57–59].

Tissue factor is also expressed on disruption of the vascular endothelium and initiates the coagulation cascade simultaneously with the formation of the platelet network, which is initiated by exposure to collagen and vWF [60–62]. Tissue factor is a transmembrane glycoprotein that is normally shielded from the intravascular space. Once expressed on activated endothelial and smooth muscle cells and monocytes/macrophages, tissue factor acts in conjunction with factor VIIa to launch the extrinsic pathway of coagulation (see Figure 44-1). The coagulation cascade is amplified by activation of the factor IX/factor VIII–dependent intrinsic pathway. The participation of both pathways ensures adequate levels of factor Xa to stimulate thrombin (factor II) production. Thrombin cleaves fibrinogen to fibrin and fibrinopeptides A

TABLE 44-2. Antithrombin agents

I.   Indirect antithrombins (antithrombin III dependent)
     1. Heparin
     2. Low molecular weight heparin
     3. Heparinoids
II. Direct antithrombins
     1. Hirudin derivatives
        a. Desirudin (hirudin)
        b. Hirulog
        c. Hirugen
     2. Thrombin active site inhibitors
        a. PPACK
        b. Argatroban
III. Factor Xa inhibitors
     1. Recombinant tick anticoagulant peptide
     2. Antistatin
IV. Endogenous inhibitors
     1. Tissue factor pathway inhibitor
     2. Thrombomodulin
     3. Protein C
     4. Antithrombin III

TABLE 44-3. Selected trials and meta-analyses of antiplatelet agents

Agent	Population	Trial
Aspirin	Primary prevention	Physicians Health Study [76]
Aspirin	Primary prevention	British Doctors Trial [77]
Aspirin	Primary prevention	Nurses' Health Study In Progress [78]
Aspirin	Secondary prevention	Antiplatelet Trialists' Collaboration [80]
Aspirin	Secondary prevention	Antiplatelet Trialists' Collaboration [81]
Aspirin	UA	VA Cooperative Study [84]
Aspirin	UA	Theroux [82]
Aspirin	UA	Cairns [83]
Aspirin	UA	RISC [85]
Aspirin	AMI	ISIS-2 [86]
Aspirin	PTCA	Schwartz [43]
Aspirin	PTCA	Lembo [87]
Aspirin	CABG	Antiplatelet Trialists' Collaboration [81]
Sulotroban	PTCA	M-HEART II [107]
GR32191B	PTCA	CARPORT [109]
Ridogrel	AMI	RAPT [116]
Ticlopidine	UA	Balsano [144]
Ticlopidine	PTCA	Ticlopidine Multicenter Trial [147]
Ticlopidine	PTCA	TACT [311]
Ticlopidine	PTCA/stent	Hall [153]
Ticlopidine	PTCA/stent	ISAR [154]
Clopidogrel	Secondary prevention	CAPRIE, in progress
Abciximab	UA	Simoons [161]
Abciximab	PTCA	EPIC [45]
Abciximab	PTCA	EPILOG [165]
Abciximab	PTCA	CAPTURE [166]
Abciximab	Stent	ERASER, in progress
Abciximab	AMI	RAPPORT, in progress
Eptifibatide	UA	Schulman [172]
Eptifibatide	AMI	IMPACT-AMI [173]
Eptifibatide	PTCA	IMPACT II [176]
Eptifibatide	UA	PURSUIT, in progress
Lamifiban	UA	Theroux [177]
Lamifiban	UA	PARAGON, in progress
Lamifiban	AMI	PARADIGM, in progress
Tirofiban	PTCA	Kereiakes [178]
Tirofiban	UA	PRISM, in progress
Tirofiban	PTCA	RESTORE [179]
Xemlofiban	PTCA	ORBIT, in progress

UA = Unstable angina; AMI = Acute myocardial infarction; PTCA = percutaneous transluminal coronary angioplasty; CABG = coronary artery graft.

and B. Fibrin polymerization and crosslinking stabilize the platelet scaffolding by filling the gaps among the platelets and the subendothelial matrix.

The complexity and redundancy of hemostasis yield several potential mechanisms to inhibit intracoronary thromboembolism (Tables 44-1 and 44-2). Platelet *activation* can be inhibited through blockade of in vivo agonists and intraplatelet enzymes. Platelet *aggregation* can be interrupted by drugs that prevent GPIIb/IIIa recognition and binding to RGD sequences. Potential targets for interruption of the coagulation cascade include inhibition of naturally occurring procoagulants (e.g., tissue factor), thrombin generation, and thrombin activity, either directly or indirectly via antithrombin III. Fundamental to thrombosis, the inhibition of thrombin generation and activity has been a focus in drug development. Thrombin is directly responsible for fibrinogen cleavage, activation of factor XIII that crosslinks fibrin and secures the clot, activation of factors V and VIII that autoamplify its own production, vasoconstriction in the damaged vessel through endothelin release, platelet activation, neutrophil and monocyte chemotaxis, and the production of mitogens that enhance endothelial and smooth muscle cell proliferation [15,63,64].

This chapter reviews the use of novel antiplatelet and antithrombotic agents to minimize intracoronary thrombosis, both as primary and as adjunctive therapy, to stabilize the unstable plaque in the acute coronary syndromes, to accelerate and maintain coronary patency after thrombolytic therapy, and to reduce abrupt closure and restenosis following percutaneous coronary intervention.

Cyclooxygenase Inhibitors and Aspirin

While aspirin is hardly a novel drug, its efficacy proves the potential benefit of platelet inhibition and provides the benchmark for comparisons (Table 44-3) [65–67]. The initial step in the synthesis of all prostaglandins and thromboxane A_2 is the conversion of arachidonic acid from membrane phospholipids to the endoperoxide intermediate PGG_2 via cyclooxygenase. Aspirin irreversibly acetylates cyclooxygenase [68,69]. The nonsteroidal antiinflammatory agents only transiently inhibit cyclooxygenase and prolong the bleeding time [70–72]. The subsequent conversion of PGG_2 to PGH_2 is catalyzed by a hydroperoxidase [73]. These first two steps are generalized; the further metabolism of PGH_2 is cell specific. In platelets PGH_2 is converted to TxA_2, and in endothelial cells it is converted to prostacyclin (PGI_2). Thromboxane A_2 is a potent stimulator of vasoconstriction and platelet aggregation, while prostacyclin is a vasodilator that inhibits platelet aggregation [74].

Over 300 randomized trials have evaluated aspirin's therapeutic potential in ischemic heart disease [75]. The two large primary prevention trials yielded conflicting results. In the Physician's Health Study, practitioners assigned to alternate-day aspirin (325 mg) had a 44% relative reduction in the incidence of first acute myocardial infarction (AMI) at the cost of a statistically insignificant increased risk of stroke; there was no difference in mortality or the incidence of angina [76]. In the British Doctor's Trial (aspirin 500 mg daily), there was not a significant difference between the groups in total mortality or the incidence of fatal or nonfatal AMI or stroke [77]. The ongoing Nurses' Health Study is evaluating the use of aspirin in 40,000 nurses without known cardiovascular disease [78].

Because individual trials have been insufficiently powered, pooled data are necessary to demonstrate aspirin's efficacy in the secondary prevention of myocardial infarction. The 1988 Oxford Antiplatelet Trialists' Collaboration review of 25 secondary prevention trials found that, compared with placebo, treatment with antiplatelet agents reduced reinfarction by 32%, nonfatal stroke by 42%, and vascular mortality by 15% [79]. Their second analysis of 145 randomized trials involving 70,000 patients with prior cardiovascular disease found similar results [80]. Further analysis revealed an approximate 50% increase in vessel patency, with the use of aspirin in patients following coronary artery bypass surgery, PTCA, peripheral vascular surgery, and even placement of hemodialysis shunts [81].

Four randomized trials investigating the use of aspirin in unstable angina have shown about a 50% reduction in the incidence of death and myocardial infarction [82–85]. In the Second International Study of Infarct Survival (ISIS-2), patients assigned to treatment with aspirin had reduced reinfarction, stroke, and all-cause mortality [86]. Patients randomized to aspirin alone had a 23% reduction in vascular mortality compared with placebo at 5 weeks (95% CI 15–30%, $2P < 0.00001$), while patients randomized to aspirin in combination with streptokinase had a 42% reduction in total mortality (95% CI 34–50%, $2P < 0.00001$). Treating 1000 patients with suspected AMI with aspirin for 1 month would avoid 25 deaths and 10–15 nonfatal reinfarctions or strokes.

Several studies and reviews have documented aspirin's ability to decrease abrupt closure and acute ischemic complications following coronary angioplasty [43,87–90]. Schwartz et al. randomized 376 patients to aspirin and dipyridamole or placebo prior to PTCA. The incidence of Q-wave myocardial infarction was 1.6% in patients assigned to active treatment versus 6.9% in the placebo group ($P = 0.0113$) [43]. In Kent et al.'s retrospective analysis of 500 consecutive patients, those patients who received aspirin had a procedural success rate of 92% versus a success rate of 80% in those who did not receive aspirin ($P < 0.01$) [89]. Although several studies have evaluated the combination of aspirin and dipyridamole after PTCA, Lembo et al. found no additional benefit of dipyridamole to aspirin alone [87].

Although aspirin's role in the treatment of ischemic heart disease is accepted, its limitations and the persistence of ischemic events despite full doses have spurred the investigation of more effective agents. Aspirin's efficacy is limited by its inability to inhibit platelet adhesion to the subendothelial matrix; release of platelet-derived growth factor (PDGF) and secretory granules; and ADP, collagen, and thrombin-induced platelet aggregation [91–94]. Just as the initial successful thrombolytic trials led to other larger trials, aspirin's success has stimulated the development and investigation of novel antiplatelet agents to further decrease the complications of ischemic heart disease.

Thromboxane Synthase Inhibitors

Attempts to selectively inhibit TxA_2 and to spare prostacyclin production with various doses of aspirin have failed; even low-dose aspirin inhibits both TxA_2 and PGI_2 production [91,95]. Thromboxane synthase catalyzes the conversion of PGH_2 to TxA_2 in platelets. Selective inhibition of thromboxane synthase (rather than cyclooxygenase) not only decreases TxA_2 formation, but also increases endothelial prostacyclin and PGD_2 production due to the accumulation of PGH_2 [96–98]. Ideally, the increased production of these endogenous platelet inhibitors could be exploited to inhibit thrombosis. Unfortunately, this approach has failed to produce any clinical benefit. At least seven thromboxane synthase inhibitors have been evaluated in multiple disease processes with minimal effect on ex vivo platelet aggregation, bleeding time, and clinical course [99–102]. The ability of the accumulated PGH_2 to occupy the TxA_2 receptor and to activate platelets, the short half-life of these agents, and their incomplete inhibition of thromboxane synthase explain the disappointing results in human clinical trials [102–104].

Thromboxane Receptor Antagonists

Blockade of the thromboxane A_2 receptor offers the potential advantage of overcoming incomplete enzyme inhibition and blocking the action of both TxA_2 and the cyclic endoperoxide intermediates without interfering with prostacyclin's "protective" effect [73,105,106]. Sulotroban (BM 13,177) has been studied most extensively. In the first phase I study, Gresele et al. found that a single dose prolonged the bleeding time and inhibited arachidonic acid, low-dose collagen, and endoperoxide-mediated platelet aggregation [105]. The Multi-Hospital Eastern Atlantic Restenosis Trial (M-HEART II) investigators randomized 752 patients to aspirin, sulotroban, or placebo prior to planned PTCA [107]. Treatment with aspirin reduced the rate of the composite primary endpoint (death, myocardial infarction, or clinically significant restenosis) to 30%, compared with 44% in patients treated with sulotroban ($P < 0.05$) and 41% in the placebo group ($P < 0.05$). While

there was not a statistically significant difference in the rate of angiographic restenosis at 6 months in either active group compared with placebo, the 39% restenosis rate in the aspirin group was significantly less than the 53% rate in the sulotroban group ($P = 0.006$). In a placebo-controlled study (no aspirin) in 175 patients, Hacker et al. found that assignment to sulotroban produced a significant reduction in angiographically documented saphenous vein graft occlusion 21 days after surgery of 3.1% versus 11.5% in patients assigned to placebo ($P < 0.02$) [108]. In the Coronary Artery Restenosis Prevention on Repeated Thromboxane-Antagonism Study Group (CARPORT), 697 patients were randomly assigned to either the oral thromboxane A_2 antagonist GR32191B 1 hour prior to intervention, which was continued for 6 months, or a single dose of aspirin prior to the procedure followed by placebo for 6 months [109]. Despite minimal antiplatelet therapy in the control group, there was no difference in clinical events or angiographic restenosis between the groups. At least six other oral agents that effectively inhibited ex-vivo platelet aggregation have been evaluated in clinical trials, but none produced a clinical benefit [99.110]. Because these drugs are competitive inhibitors, they are displaced from receptors by high levels of the endogenous ligands, TxA_2 and PGH_2. In addition, like aspirin, they are limited by their inability to inhibit TxA_2-independent platelet aggregation [111].

Combined thromboxane synthase inhibition and TxA_2/PGH_2 receptor blockade overcomes some of the limitations of the selective agents. In a series of experiments in healthy subjects, the combination of the enzyme inhibitor dazoxiben and the receptor antagonist BM 13,177 produced a greater prolongation of the bleeding time and more complete inhibition of collagen-induced platelet aggregation than aspirin (high or low dose) or either drug alone [111]. The increased antiaggregatory effect compared with aspirin and indomethacin has been attributed to the accumulation of prostacyclin and PGD_2. Picotamide and ridogrel combine both actions and have been evaluated in multiple animal models of thrombosis and in phase I human trials [112–115]. Both agents prolong the bleeding time and inhibit ex vivo platelet aggregation more than aspirin. In the Ridogrel Versus Aspirin Patency Trial (RAPT), 907 patients with AMI were treated with streptokinase and either ridogrel or aspirin (no heparin) [116]. There was no difference in the primary endpoint, TIMI grade II or III flow at angiography performed 7–14 days after admission. The rates of in-hospital clinical events and markers of reperfusion at 2 hours were also similar in the two groups. Though not a prespecified endpoint, the incidence of new ischemic events (reinfarction, recurrent angina, and ischemic stroke) was less in patients treated with ridogrel than in those patients treated with aspirin (13% vs. 19%; $P < 0.025$).

ADP Antagonists

Two thienopyridine derivatives, ticlopidine and clopidogrel, are noncompetitive, irreversible antagonists of ADP-induced platelet aggregation [117–120]. They primarily inhibit pathways of platelet activation and aggregation that require amplification, or at least participation, by ADP. Their exact mechanism of action is incompletely understood [121–124]. Several investigators have demonstrated that ticlopidine interferes with fibrinogen binding to platelets [125–127]. Dunn et al. demonstrated that ticlopidine reduced fibrinogen binding to ADP-treated platelets by 68% [125]. Because ADP binding was not affected, ticlopidine appeared to act directly on the fibrinogen receptor. Di Minno et al. demonstrated that ticlopidine markedly reduced platelet aggregation, clot retraction, and fibrinogen and vWF binding [126]. They likened treatment with ticlopidine to a "functionally thrombasthenic state." Ticlopidine-treated platelets behaved similarly to the platelets of patients with Glanzmann's thrombasthenia, which do not bind fibrinogen after activation by ADP and lack the GPIIb/IIIa receptor. But ticlopidine does not appear to act directly on the GPIIb/IIIa receptor. Rather, it apparently produces a functional defect in ADP-induced fibrinogen binding. Gachet et al. confirmed the near-complete suppression of ADP-induced aggregation and fibrinogen binding, but demonstrated unchanged GPIIb/IIIa electrophoretic studies and monoclonal antibody binding [128]. In healthy volunteers, Hardisty et al. also demonstrated unchanged monoclonal antibody binding to the GPIIb/IIIa complex and suggested ticlopidine interfered with signal transduction between ADP and fibrinogen binding to their receptors [119]. Ticlopidine may also inhibit (reverse) platelet aggregation after the initiation of thrombosis. In what may prove to be a major advantage, ticlopidine has been shown to disassemble thombin-induced platelet aggregates [129].

TICLOPIDINE

Ticlopidine is rapidly absorbed orally and reaches peak plasma concentrations within 3 hours [130]. It is minimally active ex vivo and requires hepatic biotransformation to active metabolite(s). Platelet function is inhibited within hours of oral administration, although its maximum effect is delayed to about 5 days [131,132]. Ex vivo studies in platelets from healthy volunteers demonstrate that ticlopidine inhibits aggregation in response to ADP, epinephrine, thrombin, and collagen [118,126,132,133]. The antiplatelet effects persist about 4 days after drug discontinuation, resolving as new platelets are formed [132,134].

Much of the experience with ticlopidine comes from the two large secondary prevention trials in cerebrovascular disease. In the Canadian-American Ticlopidine Study (CATS), 1053 patients with a recent thromboembolic stroke were randomized to ticlopidine or placebo [135]. Patients randomized to ticlopidine had a 23% relative risk reduction ($P = 0.020$) in the occurrence of the primary endpoint (the composite of stroke, myocardial infarction, and vascular death) compared with placebo. In the Ticlopidine-Aspirin Stroke Study (TASS), 3069 patients with a history of a cerebrovascular event were randomized to ticlopidine or aspirin [136]. The 3-year event rate (all-cause mortality or nonfatal stroke) was 17% in patients randomized to ticlopidine and 19% in those randomized to aspirin ($P = 0.048$ for cumulative Kaplan-Meier estimates). Combining both trials, adverse effects occurred in about 50% of patients. Gastrointestinal symptoms were the most common: diarrhea occurred in about 20%, dyspepsia in 13%, and nausea in 11% of patients taking ticlopidine. Total cholesterol levels rose about 9%. Neutropenia (secondary to direct toxicity to the bone marrow suppression or an immunologic reaction) was the most serious adverse event, occurring in about 1% of patients and making close monitoring of blood counts necessary [137]. All adverse events were reversible within 3 weeks of discontinuation of ticlopidine. In a review of four randomized trials, including 2048 patients assigned to ticlopidine, Haynes et al. reported the incidence of ticlopidine-induced neutropenia was 2.4%, and was severe in 0.85% (absolute neutrophil count $<0.45 \times 10^9$/L) [138]. Reportedly, clopidogrel, which has a much faster onset of action, has not exhibited toxicity to the bone marrow in animal studies [139]. It is currently being evaluated in a secondary prevention trial of 18,000 patients, the CAPRIE study.

Four trials have evaluated the ability of ticlopidine to maintain patency of saphenous vein grafts [140–143]. In the largest study, which was started in 1982, Limet et al. randomized 173 patients to ticlopidine or placebo (not aspirin) postoperatively and assessed patency angiographically on postoperative days 10, 180, and 360 [141]. Treatment with ticlopidine increased the bleeding time and reduced ADP-induced platelet aggregation at each interval. Intention-to-treat analysis demonstrated at least a 37% relative risk reduction ($P < 0.05$) in graft occlusion in the ticlopidine group at each interval, when analyzed by either patient or number of grafts.

In a study started in 1986, Balsano et al. evaluated the efficacy of ticlopidine in patients with unstable angina [144]. In this unblinded, multicenter study, 652 patients with unstable angina were randomized to ticlopidine and conventional therapy (nitrates, calcium channel blockers, and beta blockers, but not aspirin) versus conventional therapy alone. By intention-to-treat analysis, the primary event (vascular death and nonfatal myocardial infarction) rate at 6 months was 7.3% in patients randomized to ticlopidine and 13.6% in patients randomized to conventional therapy alone, producing a 46.3% relative risk reduction ($P = 0.009$). The reduction in the primary event rate was largely driven by a reduction in the incidence of fatal and nonfatal myocardial infarction, with a relative risk reduction of 53%. The implications are limited due to the unblinded nature of the study, the absence of an aspirin control group, the lack of treatment with heparin, the use of calcium channel blockers in 86% of the patients, and the early termination of the study [145]. The Swedish Ticlopidine Multicenter Study randomized 687 patients with intermittent claudication to ticlopidine or placebo [146]. By intention-to-treat analysis, randomization to ticlopidine produced a trend toward a reduction in the specified composite primary endpoint: myocardial infarction, stroke, or transient ischemic attack (TIA). Though not a specified endpoint, all-cause mortality was reduced in the ticlopidine group compared with placebo.

Several studies have investigated the role of ticlopidine in the setting of PTCA. In the Ticlopidine Multicenter Trial, 333 patients were randomly assigned to aspirin and dipyridamole, ticlopidine, or placebo prior to PTCA [147]. Pretreatment with ticlopidine or the combination of aspirin and dipyridamole reduced the incidence of ischemic complications (abrupt occlusion, thrombosis, or major dissection) from 14% in patients assigned to placebo to 2% ($P < 0.005$) and 5% ($P < 0.005$), respectively. Bertrand et al. randomized 266 patients to ticlopidine or placebo following successful angioplasty [148]. Treatment with ticlopidine reduced the incidence of acute closure from 16.2% in the placebo group to 5.1% ($P < 0.01$). However, there was no difference in the incidence of restenosis assessed angiographically at 6 months.

Currently, ticlopidine is most frequently used to prevent thrombosis after placement of intracoronary stent(s). In the first of several observational studies, Barragan et al. treated 238 patients with intracoronary stents with ticlopidine 500 mg/d for 3–6 months and intravenous heparin for 20 hours, followed by subcutaneous heparin for 1 week [149]. At 30 days the thrombosis rate was 4.2%. In another study, Morice et al. treated 246 patients with ticlopidine 250 mg/d and aspirin for 1 month and intravenous heparin for 2 days followed by low molecular weight heparin for 1 month after stent deployment [150]. There were three subacute occlusions; in the first 30 days there were two deaths, five non–Q-wave myocardial infarctions, and two patients required coronary artery bypass graft (CABG).

Colombo et al. used high-pressure balloon inflation and ultrasound guidance to optimize stent deployment and to avoid warfarin anticoagulation in 359 patients, involving 864 stents in 452 lesions [151]. Of the 252 patients who received ticlopidine alone, two (0.8%) had acute stent thromboses. One of the 69 patients (1.4%) treated with aspirin alone had subacute stent thrombosis. Hall et al. randomized 226 patients to aspirin for 5 days and ticlopidine or aspirin alone following intravascular ultrasound-guided stent implantation [152]. At 1 month, the stent thrombosis rate was 2.9% in the aspirin-alone group and 0.8% in the combined aspirin-ticlopidine group ($P = 0.2$). The incidence of major clinical events (stent thrombosis, death, myocardial infarction, need for reintervention [CABG or PTCA], and significant medication side effects requiring termination) at 1 month was 0.8% in the ticlopidine-aspirin group and 3.9% in the aspirin group. Although the authors concluded there was no difference between the groups, there was a trend toward improved outcome in the combined group, suggesting the study may have been underpowered.

In the final phase of the Benestent-II pilot study, patients received a heparin-coated stent electively and were treated with single daily doses of aspirin and ticlopidine [153]. The rates of stent thrombosis, bleeding, angiographic restenosis at 6 months, and reintervention within 6 months were 0%, 0%, 6%, and 6%, respectively. In the Intracoronary Stenting and Antithrombotic Regimen (ISAR) trial, 517 patients were randomized to ticlopidine and aspirin or phenprocoumon and aspirin following successful stent implantation [154]. At 30 days, 1.6% of the patients assigned to antiplatelet therapy and 6.2% of the patients assigned to anticoagulant therapy reached the primary endpoint: the composite of cardiac mortality, myocardial infarction, bypass surgery, or repeated angioplasty. The 75% relative risk reduction was largely driven by a reduced incidence of myocardial infarction and reintervention in the antiplatelet group. Assignment to the antiplatelet group also resulted in a 16% relative risk (95% CI 0.06–0.36) in the combined clinical endpoint, composed of primary cardiac events and noncardiac events (including death, stroke, hemorrhagic events, and peripheral vascular events). Despite these encouraging results, the appropriate treatment after stent deployment, particularly for non-elective indications, awaits the results of ongoing randomized trials.

GPIIb/IIIa Antagonists

MONOCLONAL ANTIBODIES

Each of the antiplatelet agents discussed so far inhibits only a single pathway of platelet *activation*. The complexity of platelet activity, including activation by ADP, serotonin, epinephrine, thromboxane A_2, thrombin, collagen, and shear stress, precludes narrow-spectrum agents from adequately suppressing platelet function to minimize ischemic events. Clinical trials have confirmed that inhibition of the final common pathway of platelet *aggregation* (regardless of the activating stimulus) using antagonists to the GPIIb/IIIa receptors on platelets profoundly inhibits their function ex vivo, which translates into a marked reduction in ischemic events. The rapid, fascinating progress of these drugs from bench to bedside is a paradigm for future drug development [155].

Coller and his colleagues performed much of the original research on antagonists to the GPIIb/IIIa receptor using the antibody 7E3. This monoclonal antibody blocks access of vWF, fibrinogen, and other adhesive proteins to the GPIIb/IIIa receptor on activated platelets via steric hindrance or induced conformational changes. In 1985 Coller described activation-dependent binding of m7E3 to the GPIIb/IIIa receptor and, for the first time, near-complete inhibition of platelet aggregation using an in vivo agent [156,157]. The following year Coller et al. demonstrated that 7E3 inhibited cyclic flow reduction in an animal model of thrombosis that reproduces blood flow changes in humans following coronary angioplasty [158]. In 1988 Gold et al. used 7E3 to accelerate reperfusion and to reduce reocclusion following successful thrombolysis in dogs [17].

The antibody has been investigated as adjunctive therapy in humans in three settings: unstable angina, AMI, and PTCA. By 1990 Gold et al. published the first use of 7E3 in a phase II trial, demonstrating safety and dose-related inhibition of platelet function .without spontaneous bleeding in 16 patients with

unstable angina [159]. In a pilot study published in 1993, the Thrombolysis and Angioplasty in Myocardial Infarction (TAMI) Study Group investigated the combination of m7E3 with t-PA, aspirin, and heparin in patients with AMI [160]. The trial demonstrated profound inhibition of platelet aggregation and trends toward reduced recurrent ischemia and improved arterial patency, without a significant increase in bleeding. Ellis et al. were the first to use m7E3 in patients referred for elective angioplasty, and they demonstrated 93% occupancy of binding sites at the largest dose [48]. Using m7E3 Fab, 36% of the patients (8 of 22) exhibited an antimurine antibody response in this trial.

ABCIXIMAB

The currently used agent c7E3 (generic name *abciximab*) is a chimeric antibody consisting of murine and human components. Like m7E3, the Fc portion has been cleaved to reduce clearance by the reticuloendothelial system, but the Fab fragments are composed of a murine variable region and human constant region to avoid the formation of antimurine antibodies. The European Cooperative Study Group published the first phase II study of c7E3 in patients with refractory unstable angina [161]. Using the currently recommended dose (0.25 mg/kg bolus followed by a 10 μg/min infusion), they demonstrated >90% blockade of the GPIIb/IIIa receptors and >90% reduction in ex vivo platelet aggregation to ADP without excess bleeding. There was no difference in the number of ischemic episodes between the treatment and control groups. Randomization to study drug reduced the occurrence of major events (death, nonfatal AMI, and urgent intervention) from 23% in the placebo group to 3% in the c7E3 group (P = 0.03).

Tcheng et al. evaluated the pharmacodynamics and the initial safety and efficacy studies of c7E3 in the first phase II trial [162]. The optimal dose of 0.25 mg/kg bolus and infusion of 10 μg/min produced >80% platelet receptor blockade and inhibited platelet aggregation to <20% of baseline. The drug irreversibly binds to the receptor with a pharmacologic half-life of about 30 minutes and a biologic half-life of about 48 hours. This trial served as the dose-finding study for the Evaluation of c7E3 for the Prevention of Ischemic Complications (EPIC) trial, which began enrolling its 2099 patients at high risk for complications following coronary intervention in November 1991 [45]. Patients who received both bolus and infusion of c7E3 had a 35% relative reduction in the rate of the primary endpoint (death, nonfatal AMI, and unplanned revascularization) compared with patients who received placebo (8.3 vs.

12.8%, respectively; $P = 0.008$). After 6 months, randomization to the bolus and infusion group had resulted in a 26% reduction in the need for target vessel revascularization compared with placebo (16.5% vs. 22.3%, respectively; $P = 0.007$) [163]. The composite of death, nonfatal AMI, CABG, or repeat PTCA was reduced by 23% with c7E3 compared with placebo (27.0 vs. 35.1%; $P = 0.001$). The significant reduction in ischemic events was at the cost of an approximate doubling in the risk of bleeding, regardless of the definition used [45]. Aguirre et al. demonstrated an association between female gender, lower body weight, older age, procedure complexity, and the use of c7E3 in major bleeding in this trial [164].

The Evaluation in PTCA to Improve Long-term Outcome with abciximab/c7E3 GPIIb/IIIa Blockade (EPILOG) trial, which investigated the efficacy of abciximab in elective PTCA, was stopped early because of a marked reduction in the primary endpoint, death and myocardial infarction [165]. There was a 70% reduction in the rate of ischemic events at 30 days and a reduction in the rate of major bleeding in patients assigned to c7E3 and low-dose heparin (70 U/kg bolus with a target ACT of 200 seconds) compared with patients assigned to placebo and standard-dose heparin (100 U/kg bolus with an ACT goal of 300 seconds). Similarly, the CAPTURE trial, which investigated the use of abciximab for 24 hours prior to and 1 hour after PTCA in patients with refractory unstable angina, was stopped early because of improved outcome in patients assigned to active treatment [166].

RGD Peptides

The disintegrins are a family of peptides isolated from the venom of pit vipers that inhibit ligand binding to the GPIIb/IIIa receptor [167–169]. They share a homologous RGD sequence that served as a template for the synthetic RGD analogues, the second generation of GPIIb/IIIa antagonists [54]. In contrast to abciximab, these peptides and peptidomimetics are competitive antagonists that bind directly to the GPIIb/IIIa receptor with high specificity. Their reversible binding, and shorter plasma and biologic half-lives, which result in rapid onset and reversal of action, and lack of immunogenicity suggest a broader therapeutic index may be obtained with appropriate dosing strategies. Cyclic RGD peptides were synthesized to increase potency and resistance to enzymatic destruction relative to linear peptides [170]. Therapeutic agents in this class include MK-852, G-4120, and Eptifibatide.

EPTIFIBATIDE

Integrilin is a cyclic heptapeptide that contains a lysine for arginine substitution, producing a KGD sequence that confers even greater potency and specificity for the GPIIb/IIIa receptor [171]. Shulman et al. randomized 157 patients with unstable angina to placebo or one of two doses of Eptifibatide (bolus and infusion) [172]. Treatment with Integrilin decreased ischemia detected by Holter monitor in a dose-dependent fashion, with identical bleeding rates in the treatment and placebo groups. Ohman et al. investigated the combination of Eptifibatide with t-PA, confirming increased platelet aggregation in patients with AMI treated with a thrombolytic agent, and demonstrated Eptifibatide's ability to reduce platelet aggregation and to improve arterial patency in a dose-dependent fashion [173]. There was no increase in severe bleeding or intracranial hemorrhage, but the sample size was small.

Phase II studies have documented Eptifibatide's half-life to be approximately 1.5–2 hours and have established the dose used in the IMPACT II study, the largest clinical study of Eptifibatide to date [174,175]. In this double-blind, multicenter study, 4010 patients scheduled for elective, urgent, or emergency PTCA were randomized to placebo or one of two doses of Eptifibatide [176]. By intention-to-treat analysis, treatment with low-dose Eptifibatide (135 µg/kg bolus followed by a 0.5 µg/kg/min infusion for 20–24 hours) yielded a nonsignificant 19% reduction in the composite endpoint of 30-day mortality, myocardial infarction, unplanned revascularization, or implantation of a coronary stent for abrupt closure compared with placebo (9.2% vs. 11.4%, $P = 0.063$). Restricting analysis to those patients actually treated (efficacy analysis), treatment with the low-dose Eptifibatide regimen produced a 22% reduction in the primary composite endpoint compared with placebo (9.1% vs. 11.6%, $P = 0.035$). There was no difference in the incidence of serious bleeding or the need for red blood cell or platelet transfusion among the groups. Possible explanations for the lack of a statistically significant therapeutic effect include inadequate dose or duration of treatment or Eptifibatide's marked specificity for the GPIIb/IIIa receptor and the rapid reversal of effect (lower Kd) compared with abciximab. Ongoing and planned clinical trials have been designed to establish an optimal dosing strategy to maximize efficacy while maintaining a broad therapeutic index in the setting of acute coronary syndromes and coronary interventions.

PSEUDOPEPTIDES/PEPTIDOMIMETICS

Modification of the peptide bond and side chains was the second mechanism employed to increase resistance to enzymatic degradation and to prolong the survival of synthetic RGD analogues. Lamifiban (Ro 44-9883) and tirofiban (MK-383) are two pseudopeptides that are currently being investigated in phase III clinical trials. In a dose-escalation study, Theroux et al. randomized 365 patients with unstable angina to placebo or one of four doses of lamifiban [177]. The largest dose produced 100% and 76% inhibition of platelet aggregation in response to ADP and thrombin-receptor agonist peptide, respectively, and increased the bleeding time to more than 30 minutes. Treatment with the highest dose of lamifiban also produced a trend toward a reduction in the occurrence of the composite primary endpoint (death, nonfatal AMI, and recurrent angina). In the first tirofiban (MK-383) dose-finding study, Kereiakes et al. demonstrated dose-dependent inhibition of ex vivo platelet aggregation and prolongation of the bleeding time, which markedly resolved within 4 hours of stopping the infusion in patients undergoing high-risk coronary angioplasty [178]. In the RESTORE trial, 2110 patients who presented with unstable angina or AMI prior to PTCA were randomly assigned to tirofiban or placebo [179]. As in IMPACT II, there was a marked reduction in the rate of early ischemic events, but by 30 days there was not a statistically significant difference in the occurrence of the composite primary endpoint (death, (re)infarction, and urgent revascularization).

ORALLY ACTIVE DRUGS

At least five orally active RGD analogues have been developed, xemlofiban (SC-54684), BIBU-52, GR 144,053, DMP 728, and L 703,014. Their unique pharmacokinetics and pharmacodynamics, in principle, make them ideal candidates for extended outpatient therapy. The ability to prolong treatment at a reasonable cost may have a major impact on their role in primary and secondary prevention if serious bleeding is not an issue. Their potential is promising. Mousa et al. demonstrated a single oral dose of DMP 728 completely inhibited thrombosis in an electrolytically induced carotid artery thrombosis model in dogs and ex vivo platelet aggregation [180]. In a canine dose-escalation study, a single dose of oral xemlofiban completely inhibited collagen-induced platelet aggregation for more than 24 hours [181]. In a similar study, twice-daily oral xemlofiban maintained 75% inhibition of collagen-induced platelet aggregation for 14 days [182]. In a phase I study, a single dose of xemlofiban completely inhibited platelet aggregation in response to ADP and prolonged the bleeding time 5.6-fold [183]. It is currently being

evaluated in a phase II study in the setting of coronary angioplasty and acute coronary syndromes.

Anticoagulants

Platelet activation and aggregation and the coagulation cascade are fundamentally interdependent pathways. Just as thrombin is a potent platelet agonist, *activated* platelets, in turn, stimulate and accelerate the coagulation cascade. Activated platelets release α granules that contain factor Va and fibrinogen, while their phospholipid membranes bind factor VIII and permit the enzymatic cleavage of factor X and prothrombin itself [184–189]. This synergy between thrombin generation and platelet aggregation necessitates the combined use of antiplatelet and antithrombin agents to adequately suppress thrombosis, with agents from both of the artificial classes inhibiting each pathway.

As with aspirin, appreciation of heparin's mechanism of action, efficacy, and limitations is critical to understanding the newer agents [190]. Heparin is a heterogenous mixture of mucopolysaccharides collected from porcine intestines and bovine lungs that have molecular weights between 3000 and 30,000 daltons. Heparin chains with at least 18 saccharide residues provide a scaffold to appose thrombin and antithrombin III, and produce a 1000-fold increase in antithrombin III's ability to neutralize thrombin [191]. The heparin–antithrombin III complex inhibits thrombin production by inactivating factor Xa and, to a lesser extent, factors XIIa, XIa, and IXa [192,193]. Heparin also interferes with thrombin generation by inhibiting the thrombin positive-feedback loops — activation of factors V and VIII [194,195]. While an individual heparin molecule's ability to neutralize thrombin is directly proportional to its chain length, only a high-affinity pentasaccharide subunit is required for heparin to bind antithrombin III and to inactivate factor Xa [196,197].

Heparin's therapeutic potential is limited by its complex pharmacodynamics and pharmacokinetics. Because heparin is poorly absorbed, subcutaneous or intravenous injection is required. Its plasma and biologic half-life is about 90 minutes. Heparin binding to plasma proteins precludes a linear, predictable dose–response relationship and results in a disproportionate increase in both the intensity and duration at higher doses. Heparin is deactivated by endothelial cells, platelet factor-4, and other proteins, and is eliminated by poorly understood renal and hepatic pathways. Most importantly, thrombin bound to fibrin and fibrin degradation products is protected from the bulky heparin–antithrombin III complex, while the platelet membrane shields factor Xa from inactivation [198,199].

Hemorrhage is the most serious and common adverse effect of the anticoagulants. Even with frequent monitoring, measuring and adjusting heparin activity is particularly difficult and results in delays in producing a therapeutic effect and in an increase in bleeding complications. Nomograms have been produced to assist optimal dosing and to minimize bleeding [200–202]. Immunologic idiosyncratic thrombocytopenia occurs 3–14 days into heparin therapy but can occur within hours in previously exposed patients, and is more common from bovine lung than porcine gut preparations [203–206]. Therapeutic use of porcine heparin (rather than prophylactic use) produces thrombocytopenia in about 3% of patients; the incidence of arterial or venous thrombosis is about 0.4% [205]. Other adverse effects include osteoporosis, skin necrosis, alopecia, hypoaldosteronism, and hyperkalemia [207].

Despite these complications, heparin remains the most commonly used anticoagulant. In four studies of patients with unstable angina, heparin reduced the incidence of death, myocardial infarction, and recurrent refractory angina [82,85,208,209]. This benefit may be attenuated by "heparin rebound" and reactivation of ischemia on its discontinuation. Théroux et al. reported reactivation of unstable angina and myocardial infarction in 14 of 107 patients treated with heparin alone at a median of 9.5 hours after discontinuation of treatment [210]. In patients treated with aspirin or combined aspirin and heparin, 5 of 101 ($P < 0.01$) and 5 of 108 ($P < 0.01$) patients had reactivation at 21 and 30 hours after completing treatment, respectively. Logistic regression revealed that therapy with heparin alone was the most important predictor of reactivation of the disease process.

The additional benefit of heparin in patients with AMI treated with thrombolytic agents is controversial [211]. There are minimal data to support the use of heparin with streptokinase, but patency data suggest treatment with heparin improves the outcome in patients treated with t-PA, possibly because of its shorter half-life. In both the GISSI-2 and ISIS-3 trials, the mortality, reinfarction, and overall stroke rate were similar in patients treated with and without heparin [212–214]. The apparent lack of benefit from heparin may have been related also to a suboptimal dose and inappropriate delay and route of administration. In the Global Utilization of Streptokinase and t-PA for Occluded Arteries (GUSTO) trial, patients treated with accelerated t-PA and heparin had a 14% relative mortality reduction compared with patients treated with one of the two streptokinase-alone strategies (6.3% vs. 7.3% respectively; $P = 0.001$) [215]. In patients treated with streptokinase, the route of heparin administration had minimal effect. The adjunctive benefit of heparin to t-PA alone has not been examined in a clinical trial. Two smaller studies have shown an association between aPTTs at least twice the control value and improved infarct-vessel patency in patients treated with t-PA [216,217]. Yet in the GUSTO trial, excessively elevated aPTTs were associated with increased mortality, reinfarction, and bleeding [218].

Remarkably, heparin's ability to reduce ischemic complications following PTCA has not been subjected to a randomized trial. Several retrospective analyses have shown an association between the intensity of anticoagulation and the occurrence of abrupt closure and other ischemic complications after percutaneous coronary interventions [219–225]. Data from four studies indicate that an ACT of about 300 seconds is optimal for minimizing ischemic and hemorrhagic complications [223,226,227]. The fourth American College of Chest Physicians' Conference on Antithrombotic Therapy recommended the maintenance of an ACT at 300 seconds using a Hemo Tec machine and at 350 seconds using a Hemochron machine [229].

LOW MOLECULAR WEIGHT HEPARIN

The promise of low molecular weight heparins (LMWHs) to inhibit thrombosis while producing fewer bleeding complications and their favorable pharmacodynamics stimulated their development and evaluation in clinical trials. They are produced from standard heparin by enzymatic or chemical degradation, resulting in polysaccharide fractions with molecular weights between 3000 and 10,000 d. Each proprietary preparation has a distinct pharmacologic profile because of its different animal source and the depolymerization and extraction techniques used in production [230–232]. The complexes formed between antithrombin III and the LMWHs have weaker activity against thrombin than standard heparin because of the saccharide chain length dependence of this reaction. On the other hand, inhibition of factor Xa requires only a pentasaccharide subunit. So, unlike standard heparin, which has a 1:1 anti–factor Xa to antithrombin effect, the LMWHs generally have ratios between 2:1 and 4:1. Due to their smaller size, the LMWHs inactivate platelet-bound factor Xa equally well and neutralize platelet factor-4 (which inhibits standard heparin) [233–235]. Compared with standard heparin, the LMWHs bind less avidly to plasma proteins and endothelial cells, and thus have increased bioavailability and duration of action. Typically given as a weight-adjusted subcutaneous injection, the more predictable dose–response relationship obviates the need for laboratory monitoring.

The experience with the LMWHs is chiefly from clinical trials of the prophylaxis and treatment of deep venous thrombosis [236–239]. In sum, these trials indicate that treatment with LMWH is at least as effective as standard unfractionated heparin, causes fewer bleeding complications, costs less, does not require laboratory monitoring, and may be used for outpatient therapy. Given these advantages, the use of LMWH in cardiovascular disorders may increase in the coming years. Potential uses include the prevention of heparin rebound in unstable angina and prolonged therapy in patients with intracavity or intracoronary thrombus. In the first trial to examine the efficacy and safety of LMWHs in patients with unstable angina, Gurfinkel et al. compared aspirin, aspirin and standard heparin, and aspirin plus LMWH [240]. The incidence of recurrent angina, nonfatal myocardial infarction, urgent revascularization, silent myocardial ischemia, and bleeding was lowest in patients treated with aspirin and LMWH. The single-blinded design of the trial makes these subjective endpoints subject to bias and limits the validity of the results.

HEPARINOIDS

Heparinoids are a mixture of low molecular weight heparin and dermatan and chondroitin sulfates. Their antithrombotic effect appears to be mediated by inhibition of factors IX and X [241]. Their anticoagulation effect is generally monitored by measuring plasma anti–factor Xa activity. Unlike LMWH, the heparinoids produce minimal cross-reactivity during in vitro testing with sera containing heparin–associated antiplatelet antibodies. Organan/ Lomoparan (Org 10172) has been studied most extensively, principally as an alternative to heparin in patients with heparin-induced thrombocytopenia (HIT) who require anticoagulation for CABG, PTCA, or hemodialysis [242–244]. In an analysis of 67 patients with HIT, Organan exhibited cross-reactivity in 12% of sera containing the HIT antibody, compared with historical rates of 80–90% using LMWH [245]. In a review of 230 patients with heparin-induced thrombocytopenia, including 88 who had a thrombotic event attributed to heparin anticoagulation, Magnani reported successful therapy in 93% and a cross-reactivity in 10% of plasma samples [246]. Although decreased, persistent cross-reactivity makes in

vitro testing mandatory to minimize platelet aggregation in these patients.

Direct Thrombin Inhibitors

The therapeutic use of heparin is limited by its narrow therapeutic index, complex pharmacokinetics, unpredictable dose–response relationship, need for frequent laboratory monitoring, stimulation of life-threatening immune-mediated thrombocytopenia, and neutralization by proteins, particularly platelet factor-4. But its major limitation is its dependence on antithrombin III, precluding inhibition of thrombin bound to fibrin [198,199]. This enzymatically active thrombin reservoir continues to cleave fibrinogen to fibrin and to augment thrombogenesis by activation of factors V and VIII, despite "therapeutic" doses of heparin. The direct thrombin inhibitors act independently of antithrombin III and equally inactivate both free and clot-bound thrombin [198]. Their independent action inhibits thrombogenesis, clot formation, and thrombin-induced platelet activation [247–249].

DESIRUDIN

Desirudin (hirudin), derived from a leech salivary peptide, is the prototypic direct thrombin inhibitor. It suppresses all of thrombin's functions. The therapeutic use of the medicinal leech and desirudin dates to antiquity and reached its height of popularity with bloodletting in Europe in the early 19th century [250,251]. Desirudin, which was cloned in 1986 and is now produced via recombinant DNA technology in yeast and bacteria, is still the most potent and specific antithrombin identified [252,253]. It is a 65 amino acid peptide with no natural inhibitor that produces an essentially irreversible bond to thrombin avidly enough to displace it from platelet binding [254,255]. Desirudin has a biologic half-life of 2–3 hours, which produces a stable curvilinear, dose-related increase in the aPTT, prothrombin time (PT), and ACT [256–258].

Desirudin has been evaluated as adjunctive therapy in patients with AMI and unstable angina and as the primary anticoagulant for patients undergoing PTCA. The Thrombolysis in Myocardial Infarction (TIMI) 5 and Hirudin for the Improvement of Thrombolyis (HIT) trial were angiographic phase II dose-finding studies [259,260]. In the TIMI-5 trial 246 patients presenting within 6 hours of AMI were treated with front-loaded t-PA and aspirin, and either heparin or hirudin (CGP-39393) [260]. In patients assigned to hirudin, there was a trend toward improvement in the primary endpoint, TIMI 3 flow at 90 minutes and 18–36 hours without intervening

TABLE 44-4. Selected trials and
meta-analyses of antithrombotic agents

Agent	Population	Trial
Heparin	UA	Theroux [82]
Heparin	UA	RISC [85]
Heparin	UA	Telford [208]
Heparin	UA	Neri Serneri [209]
Heparin	AMI	GISSI-2 [212,213]
Heparin	AMI	ISIS-3 [214]
Heparin	AMI	GUSTO [215]
Heparin	PTCA	Ferguson [226]
Heparin	PTCA	Narins [227]
Heparin	PTCA	Mooney [228]
Heparin	PTCA	Satler [223]
LMWH	UA	Gurfinkel [240]
Hirudin	UA	TIMI 5 [260]
Hirudin	AMI	HIT [259]
Hirudin	AMI	HIT III [261]
Hirudin	UA/AMI	TIMI 9B [264]
Hirudin	UA/AMI	GUSTO IIb [265]
Hirudin	PTCA	HELVETICA [268]
Hirulog	UA	TIMI 7 [274]
Hirulog	AMI	Theroux [275]
Hirulog	AMI	HERO [276]
Hirulog	PTCA	Topol [277]
Hirulog	PTCA	Bittl [278]
Argatroban	UA	Gold [285]

UA = unstable angina; AMI = acute myocardial infarction; PTCA = percutaneous transluminal coronary angioplasty.

death or reinfarction. Restricting the analysis to clinical endpoints, the rate of in-hospital death or reinfarction in the hirudin group was 6.8% compared with 16.7% in the heparin group ($P = 0.02$). Finally, in the hirudin group there was a trend toward less reocclusion by 18–36 hours, with 1.6% in the hirudin group compared with 6.7% in the heparin group ($P = 0.07$). In the HIT trial, 143 patients with AMI were treated with front-loaded t-PA and one of three doses of hirudin (HBW 023) [259]. Treatment with hirudin exhibited dose-related improvement in the rates of TIMI 3 flow at the 30, 60, and 90 minute, and 36–48 hour angiograms and decreased rates of reocclusion. In the TIMI 6 trial, 193 patients were treated with streptokinase and aspirin, and either one of three doses of hirudin (CGP-39393) or heparin for 5 days [258]. In the patients treated with hirudin, there was a dose-related improvement in the incidence of death, AMI, severe congestive heart failure (CHF), and cardiogenic shock. The safety profile and dose-related improvement in ischemic events in these dose-escalation trials led to large-scale efficacy trials.

Hirudin has been evaluated in three phase III mortality trials of unstable angina and AMI. The HIT-III trial compared high-dose hirudin with heparin in patients treated with t-PA. The trial was stopped after 302 patients were enrolled because of higher than expected rates of intracranial bleeding [261]. There was also excessive intracranial bleeding in both thrombolysis treatment arms of the TIMI 9A and GUSTO IIa studies, necessitating reduction of both the heparin and hirudin doses and target aPTTs to 55–85 seconds [262,263]. In TIMI 9B, 3002 patients with AMI were treated with t-PA and randomly assigned to either heparin or hirudin [264]. There was no statistically significant difference in the incidence of the composite endpoint or hemorrhage between the groups. The composite endpoint of death, MI, and CHF occurred in 11.8% of patients assigned to heparin and in 12.8% of patients assigned to hirudin (P = NS). The incidence of "any hemorrhage" was 4.9% in the heparin group and 4.4% in the hirudin group (P = NS). In the GUSTO IIb trial 12,142 patients presenting within the spectrum of the acute coronary syndromes (chest pain with or without ST-segment elevation) were randomly assigned to heparin or desirudin, in addition to standard therapy [265]. Use of desirudin produced a marginal benefit that did not reach standard statistical significance compared with heparin, the rate of the 30-day composite endpoint of death and (re)infarction overall, for patients with ST-segment elevation, or for the "non–ST-segment" elevation group: 8.9% versus 9.8% ($P = 0.058$), 9.9% versus 11.3% ($P = 0.13$), and 8.3% versus 9.1% ((P = 0.22), respectively.

The results of two pilot studies in patients with stable and unstable angina prior to PTCA suggested hirudin had the potential to decrease thrombotic complications following percutaneous intervention [266,267]. The Hirudin in a European Trial versus Heparin in the Prevention of Restenosis after PTCA (HELVETICA) trial was designed to evaluate the ability of thrombin inhibition with hirudin to decrease restenosis following PTCA [268]. In this study 1141 patients with unstable angina scheduled for PTCA were randomly assigned to treatment with heparin or one of two dosing strategies of hirudin (CGP-39393), bolus and infusion versus bolus and infusion plus subcutaneous injection for 3 days. There was no difference in the rate of the primary endpoint, event-free survival at 7 months, which occurred in 67.3% of the patients in the heparin group, 63.5% in the intravenous-only hirudin group, and 68.0% in the group who received both intravenous and subcutaneous hirudin. Treatment with hirudin did produce a significant reduction in the incidence of cardiac events in the first 96 hours; the combined relative risk with hirudin was 0.61 (95% CI 0.41, 0.90; $P = 0.023$). There was not a significant difference in the incidence of overall, major, or minor bleeding among the groups. If the dose and duration of the infusion were adequate, the results dispute the significance of thrombin in the generation of intracoronary thrombosis and restenosis following PTCA and the ability of new antithrombins to improve outcomes, both acute and chronic, beyond standard use of heparin and aspirin.

HIRULOG

Hirulog (bivalirudin) is a 20 amino acid synthetic peptide that was designed by Maraganore et al. using the hirudin template [269,270]. Early phase II studies established hirulog's tolerability and its pharmacokinetics: Anticoagulation is produced within minutes of a bolus dose, the biologic half-life is approximately 40 minutes, and infusion maintains predictable, dose-dependent anticoagulation as measured by standard laboratory parameters [271–273]. In the TIMI 7 trial, 410 patients with unstable angina were randomized to aspirin and one of four doses of hirulog for 72 hours [274]. There was no difference in the development of the primary composite endpoint (death, nonfatal myocardial infarction, rapid clinical deterioration, or recurrent ischemia) among the groups. While there was no clear dose-response, patients treated with one of the three higher doses of hirulog had a decreased incidence of the secondary composite endpoint, death and nonfatal myocardial infarction.

The GUSTO angiographic substudy conclusively demonstrated the correlation between complete restoration of coronary flow and improvement of myocardial salvage and survival in patients with AMI [14]. Accordingly, restoration of TIMI 3 flow is a useful surrogate for dose-finding studies in this patient population. Theroux et al. randomized 68 patients with AMI to treatment with streptokinase and aspirin, and either heparin or one of two doses of hirulog in an angiographic study [275]. At the 90-minute catheterization, the relative risk of restoring TIMI 3 flow was 2.77 (95% CI 1.21–6.35, $P < 0.001$) and 1.4 (95% CI 1.00–1.51, $P = 0.04$) compared with heparin for the two doses of hirulog, 0.5 mg/kg/h and 1.0 mg/kg/h, respectively. The trial was not powered to produce reliable conclusions about clinical outcomes. Though not a prespecified endpoint, 5% of the patients treated with hirulog required a blood transfusion, compared with 31% of patients treated with heparin ($P < 0.02$). The Hirulog versus Heparin after Streptokinase trial (HERO) was the first to show improved patency with adjunctive therapy to a thrombolytic agent in patients with AMI [276]. In this trial 412 patients who presented within 12 hours of symptom onset of an AMI were treated with streptokinase and aspirin, and were randomized to heparin or hirulog. In patients assigned to hirulog, there was a 50% improvement in the rate of TIMI 3 flow ($P = 0.016$), the primary endpoint, without an increase in the rate of bleeding.

Hirulog's short half-life and potential for less bleeding may be particularly advantageous during coronary interventions. Topol et al. enrolled 291 patients in a dose-escalation study to determine the feasibility and optimal dose of hirulog in place of heparin in patients undergoing elective PTCA [277]. This trial was the first to demonstrate the safety of using an anticoagulant other than heparin in patients treated with aspirin during PTCA; only one patient required a red cell transfusion, and the rate of abrupt closure was 3.9%. Bittl et al. performed the only phase III trial of hirulog, in patients undergoing angioplasty for unstable angina or postinfarct angina [278]. At 121 sites 4098 patients were randomly assigned to treatment with heparin or hirulog prior to PTCA. Although the difference in the incidence of the primary endpoint between the groups was not statistically significant, patients assigned to hirulog had a reduced rate of bleeding, regardless of the parameter used. The incidence of the primary composite endpoint (death, AMI, abrupt vessel closure, or rapid clinical deterioration) was 11.4% in patients assigned to hirulog and 12.2% in patients assigned to heparin. The incidence of major hemorrhage, retroperitoneal hemorrhage, and need for transfusion was significantly lower in the hirulog group: 0.2%, 3.7%, and 3.8% compared with 0.7% ($P = 0.02$), 8.6% ($P < 0.001$), and 9.8% ($P < 0.002$) in the heparin group, respectively.

HIRUGEN

Hirugen is another synthetic hirudin derivative. It is composed of hirudin's 12 terminal amino acids, which bind to thrombin's substrate recognition sequence without interfering with its active site [279]. Hirugen has not undergone extensive clinical testing because its antithrombotic effect is considerably weaker than the other direct antithrombins, perhaps because it does not block thrombin's catalytic site [280,281].

ARGATROBAN

Argatroban is a synthetic competitive inhibitor of the thrombin catalytic site that suppresses both fibrinogen cleavage and platelet activation [282–284]. In a phase I study, argatroban produced dose-dependent prolongation of the aPTT and PT, without prolonging of the template bleeding time despite aspirin use [279]. Laboratory measures returned to baseline within 1 hour of drug discontinuation. Gold et al. infused argatroban for 4 hours into 43 patients with unstable angina [285]. Patients also received concomitant therapy with nitrates, calcium antagonists, and heparin or aspirin or both. Analysis of the laboratory data has been particularly informative. During drug infusion, concentrations of thrombin–antithrombin III were unchanged (indicating ongoing thrombin production), but levels of fibrinopeptide A decreased 2.3-fold (indicating decreased fibrinogen cleavage). Myocardial ischemia did not occur during infusion, but did occur in a dose-related fashion in 9 of the 43 patients a mean of 5.8 hours after the infusion was completed. Two hours after completion of the infusion, levels of thrombin–antithrombin III increased by a factor of 3.9 and fibrinopeptide A levels returned to baseline values. In a separate analysis on the same patients, the authors reported evidence of an actual increase in thrombin production during and after argatroban infusion by recording increased production of F1.2 fragments (released from prothrombin during conversion to thrombin) [286]. This rebound in unstable angina, thrombin generation, and fibrinogen cleavage may also have been related to cotreatment and simultaneous termination of heparin infusion [287]. The completed studies of hirudin and hirulog have not demonstrated rebound angina, but detailed analysis awaits further review of the results from the phase III TIMI 9B and GUSTO IIb studies [267,272,273].

Tabata et al. evaluated the efficacy of argatroban in preventing reocclusion in paitents with AMI [288]. Following successful thrombolysis, 22 patients received argatroban and 74 patients received heparin for 72 hours, to maintain an ACT between 150 and 200 seconds. At 1 month none of patients treated with argatroban had reocclusion of the infarct-related artery, whereas in the heparin group 15% had reocclusion ($P < 0.05$).

PPACK

PPACK is a tripeptide similar in structure to fibrinopeptide A, produced upon cleavage of fibrinogen to fibrin [289]. It is a noncompetitive inhibitor of the catalytic site on thrombin that irreversibly alkylates the histidine residue on free and clot-bound thrombin equally well. Its clinical usefulness may be limited by its specificity, toxicity, and extremely short biologic half life, although there may be a role for topical/local administration [290,291]. Orally active compounds similar to PPACK have been developed and await further testing.

Factor Xa Inhibitors

Unlike the direct thrombins, the factor Xa inhibitors, tick anticoagulant peptide and antistatin, suppress thrombin generation and its positive-feedback loops. These agents do not inhibit preformed thrombin. Tick anticoagulant peptide is a 60 amino-acid peptide isolated from the soft tick, *Ornithodoros moubata* [292]. Antistatin is a 119 amino-acid protein isolated from the Mexican leech *Hirudo officinalis* [293]. They are both produced using recombinant technology. Each inhibits both free factor Xa and factor Xa bound to the platelet surface and the prothrombinase complex, unlike antithrombin III [294,295]. Both agents have shown superiority to heparin when combined with t-PA in animal models of occlusion, decreasing clot lysis time and reocclusion [296,297]. Tick anticoagulant peptide, unlike antistatin, produces a minimal immunologic response and may prove to be particularly useful as an adjunct to thrombolytic therapy.

Future Considerations

Supplemental endogenous anticoagulants are only beginning to be tested in animal models and in phase I and II clinical trials. Tissue factor pathway inhibitor (TFPI), thrombomodulin, protein C, and antithrombin III are available through recombinant technology and plasma concentrates. Tissue factor is an endothelial membrane protein exposed on plaque rupture that initiates the extrinsic pathway of coagulation [60,298]. It is an essential cofactor for activation of factor VII and its substrate factor X. Tissue factor pathway inhibitor suppresses coagulation by first binding and inactivating factor Xa. This complex then binds and inactivates factor VIIa [299]. Thrombomodulin is a membrane protein on endothelial cells that binds and inactivates thrombin. Paradoxically, the thrombomodulin–thrombin complex activates antithrombin III and cleaves protein C to activated protein C [300,301]. Protein C, especially in the presence of protein S, inactivates plasminogen activator inhibitor and inhibits thrombin generation by degrading factors Va and VIIIa [302,303]. Again, antithrombin III inhibits thrombin; factors Xa, IXa, XIa, and XIIa; factor VIIa in the presence of tissue factor; and the formation of factors Va and VIIIa indirectly via thrombin inhibition [301]. Only antithrombin III has been evaluated in a large-scale clinical trial. Schachinger et al. randomized 615 patients undergoing PTCA to heparin or to heparin and intracoronary antithrombin III. Adjunctive antithrombin III did not affect procedural success or the incidence of complications overall or in any of the subgroups [304].

The platelet thrombin receptor was cloned by Vu et al. in 1991 [305]. Antagonists to this receptor now include monoclonal antibodies and synthetic peptides [306,307]. These antagonists will not necessarily be more efficacious than the direct thrombin inhibitors, which bind to the active and/or binding site, and determination of their clinical usefulness awaits clinical studies.

Conclusions

Intracoronary thrombosis is fundamental to the development and progression of the unstable coronary syndromes, reocclusion following successful thrombolysis, and ischemic complications following PTCA. The coagulation cascade and platelet activation and aggregation are completely interdependent pathways. Improved understanding of the physiology of these pathways and the pathogenesis of complications stimulated the development of multiple classes of new drugs and their testing in large-scale trials [54,247–249,308–309]. It is becoming increasingly clear that drugs from multiple classes will need to be combined to provide synergy and optimal regulation of thrombosis. Their role in the prevention and treatment of coronary thromboembolism needs to be determined by adequately powered randomized trials examining efficacy, adverse effects (principally bleeding), requirement for frequent laboratory monitoring, and cost. Future efforts will likely be targeted at improving specificity, decreasing the duration of action, and localizing their effect.

References

1. Fuster V, Badimon L, Badimon JJ, Chesebro JH. The pathogenesis of coronary artery disease and the acute coronary syndromes (1). N Engl J Med 326:242, 1992.
2. Fuster V, Badimon L, Badimon JJ, Chesebro JH. The pathogenesis of coronary artery disease and the acute coronary syndromes (2). N Engl J Med 326:310, 1992.
3. Roberts WC, Buja LM. The frequency and significance of coronary arterial thrombi and other observations in fatal acute myocardial infarction: A study of 107 necropsy patients. Am J Med 52:425, 1972.
4. Falk E. Unstable angina with fatal outcome: Dynamic coronary thrombosis leading to infarction and/or

sudden death. Autopsy evidence of recurrent mural thrombosis with peripheral embolization culminating in total vascular occlusion. Circulation 71:699, 1985.
5. Davies MJ, Bland JM, Hangartner JR, Angelini A, Thomas AC. Factors influencing the presence or absence of acute coronary artery thrombi in sudden ischaemic death. Eur Heart J 10:203, 1989.
6. Badimon L, Badimon JJ, Galvez A, Chesebro JH, Fuster V. Influence of arterial damage and wall shear rate on platelet deposition. Ex vivo study in a swine model. Arteriosclerosis 6:312, 1986.
7. Ross R. The pathogenesis of atherosclerosis: A perspective for the 1990s. Nature 362:801, 1993.
8. Ross R. The pathogenesis of atherosclerosis — an update. N Engl J Med 314:488, 1986.
9. Berk BC, Taubman MB, Cragoe EJ Jr, Fenton JWD, Griendling KK. Thrombin signal transduction mechanisms in rat vascular smooth muscle cells. Calcium and protein kinase C-dependent and -independent pathways. J Biol Chem 265:17334, 1990.
10. DeWood MA, Spores J, Notske R, et al. Prevalence of total coronary occlusion during the early hours of transmural myocardial infarction. N Engl J Med 303:897, 1980.
11. DeWood MA, Stifter WF, Simpson CS, et al. Coronary arteriographic findings soon after non-Q-wave myocardial infarction. N Engl J Med 315:417, 1986.
12. Ambrose JA, Winters SL, Stern A, et al. Angiographic morphology and the pathogenesis of unstable angina pectoris. J Am Coll Cardiol 5:609, 1985.
13. Ambrose JA, Winters SL, Arora RR, et al. Angiographic evolution of coronary artery morphology in unstable angina. J Am Coll Cardiol 7:472, 1986.
14. The GUSTO Angiographic Investigators. The effects of tissue plasminogen activator, streptokinase, or both on coronary-artery patency, ventricular function, and survival after acute myocardial infarction. N Engl J Med 329:1615, 1993. [Published erratum appears in N Engl J Med 330:516, 1994.]
15. Coller BS. Platelets and thrombolytic therapy. N Engl J Med 322:33, 1990.
16. Fitzgerald DJ, Catella F, Roy L, FitzGerald GA. Marked platelet activation in vivo after intravenous streptokinase in patients with acute myocardial infarction. Circulation 77:142, 1988.
17. Gold HK, Coller BS, Yasuda T, et al. Rapid and sustained coronary artery recanalization with combined bolus injection of recombinant tissue-type plasminogen activator and monoclonal antiplatelet GPIIb/IIIa antibody in a canine preparation. Circulation 77:670, 1988.
18. Golino P, Ashton JH, Glas-Greenwalt P, McNatt J, Buja LM, Willerson JT. Mediation of reocclusion by thromboxane A2 and serotonin after thrombolysis with tissue-type plasminogen activator in a canine

preparation of coronary thrombosis. Circulation 77: 678, 1988.

19. Fitzgerald DJ, Wright F, FitzGerald GA. Increased thromboxane biosynthesis during coronary thrombolysis. Evidence that platelet activation and thromboxane A2 modulate the response to tissue-type plasminogen activator in vivo. Circ Res 65:83, 1989.

20. Jang IK, Gold HK, Ziskind AA, et al. Differential sensitivity of erythrocyte-rich and platelet-rich arterial thrombi to lysis with recombinant tissue-type plasminogen activator. A possible explanation for resistance to coronary thrombolysis. Circulation 79:920, 1989.

21. Ohman EM, Califf RM, Topol EJ, et al. Consequences of reocclusion after successful reperfusion therapy in acute myocardial infarction. TAMI Study Group. Circulation 82:781, 1990.

22. Eisenberg PR, Sherman L, Rich M, et al. Importance of continued activation of thrombin reflected by fibrinopeptide A to the efficacy of thrombolysis. J Am Coll Cardiol 7:1255, 1986.

23. Chesebro JH, Fuster V. Dynamic thrombosis and thrombolysis. Role of antithrombins [editorial; comment]. Circulation 83:1815, 1991.

24. Winters KJ, Santoro SA, Miletich JP, Eisenberg PR. Relative importance of thrombin compared with plasmin-mediated platelet activation in response to plasminogen activation with streptokinase. Circulation 84:1552, 1991.

25. Meyer BJ, Badimon JJ, Mailhac A, et al. Inhibition of growth of thrombus on fresh mural thrombus. Targeting optimal therapy. Circulation 90:2432, 1994.

26. Lee CD, Mann KG. Activation/inactivation of human factor V by plasmin. Blood 73:185, 1989.

27. Verheugt FWA, Meijer A, Lagrand WK, Van Eenige M. Reocclusion: The flip side of coronary thrombolysis. J Am Coll Cardiol 27:766, 1996.

28. Marmur JD, Merlini PA, Sharma SK, et al. Thrombin generation in human coronary arteries after percutaneous transluminal balloon angioplasty. J Am Coll Cardiol 24:1484, 1994.

29. Uchida Y, Hasegawa K, Kawamura K, Shibuya I. Angioscopic observation of the coronary luminal changes induced by percutaneous transluminal coronary angioplasty. Am Heart J 117:769, 1989.

30. Johnson DE, Hinohara T, Selmon MR, Braden LJ, Simpson JB. Primary peripheral arterial stenoses and restenoses excised by transluminal atherectomy: A histopathologic study. J Am Coll Cardiol 15:419, 1990.

31. Ambrose JA, Almeida OD, Sharma SK, et al. Adjunctive thrombolytic therapy during angioplasty for ischemic rest angina. Results of the TAUSA Trial. TAUSA Investigators. Thrombolysis and Angioplasty in Unstable Angina trial. Circulation 90:69, 1994.

32. Minar E, Ehringer H, Ahmadi R, Dudczak R, Porenta G. Platelet deposition at angioplasty sites and platelet survival time after PTA in iliac and femoral arteries: Investigations with indium-111-oxine labelled platelets in patients with ASA (1.0 g/day)-therapy. Thromb Haemost 58:718, 1987.

33. Harker L. Role of platelets and thrombosis in mechanisms of acute occlusion and restenosis after angioplasty. Am J Cardiol 60:20B, 1987.

34. Wilentz JR, Sanborn TA, Haudenschild CC, Valeri CR, Ryan TJ, Faxon DP. Platelet accumulation in experimental angioplasty: Time course and relation to vascular injury. Circulation 75:636, 1987.

35. Arora RR, Platko WP, Bhadwar K, Simpfendorfer C. Role of intracoronary thrombus in acute complications during percutaneous transluminal coronary angioplasty. Cathet Cardiovasc Diagn 16:226, 1989.

36. Reeder GS, Bryant SC, Suman VJ, Holmes DR Jr. Intracoronary thrombus: Still a risk factor for PTCA failure? Cathet Cardiovasc Diagn 34:191, 1995.

37. Mabin TA, Holmes DR Jr, Smith HC, et al. Intracoronary thrombus: Role in coronary occlusion complicating percutaneous transluminal coronary angioplasty. J Am Coll Cardiol 5:198, 1985.

38. Neumann FJ, Ott I, Gawaz M, Puchner G, Schomig A. Neutrophil and platelet activation at balloon-injured coronary artery plaque in patients undergoing angioplasty. J Am Coll Cardiol 27:819, 1996.

39. Gasperetti CM, Gonias SL, Gimple LW, Powers ER. Platelet activation during coronary angioplasty in humans. Circulation 88:2728, 1993.

40. Kaplan AV, Leung LL, Leung WH, Grant GW, McDougall IR, Fischell TA. Roles of thrombin and platelet membrane glycoprotein IIb/IIIa in platelet-subendothelial deposition after angioplasty in an ex vivo whole artery model. Circulation 84:1279, 1991.

41. Willerson JT, Yao SK, McNatt J, et al. Frequency and severity of cyclic flow alternations and platelet aggregation predict the severity of neointimal proliferation following experimental coronary stenosis and endothelial injury. Proc Natl Acad Sci USA 88:10624, 1991.

42. Ip JH, Fuster V, Israel D, Badimon L, Badimon J, Chesebro JH. The role of platelets, thrombin and hyperplasia in restenosis after coronary angioplasty. J Am Coll Cardiol 17:77B, 1991.

43. Schwartz L, Bourassa MG, Lesperance J, et al. Aspirin and dipyridamole in the prevention of restenosis after percutaneous transluminal coronary angioplasty. N Engl J Med 318:1714, 1988.

44. Schwartz RS, Holmes DR Jr, Topol EJ. The restenosis paradigm revisited: An alternative proposal for cellular mechanisms [editorial]. J Am Coll Cardiol 20:1284, 1992.

45. The EPIC Investigators. Use of a monoclonal antibody directed against the platelet glycoprotein IIb/IIIa receptor in high-risk coronary angioplasty. N Engl J Med 330:956, 1994.

46. Liu MW, Roubin GS, King SBD. Restenosis after coronary angioplasty. Potential biologic determinants and role of intimal hyperplasia. Circulation 79:1374, 1989.

47. Ellis S, Bates E, Schaible T, Weisman H, Pitt B, Topol E. Prospects for the use of antagonists to the platelet glycoprotein IIb/IIIa receptor to prevent postangioplasty restenosis and thrombosis. J Am Coll Cardiol 17:89B, 1991.

48. Ellis SG, Tcheng JE, Navetta FI, et al. Safety and antiplatelet effect of murine monoclonal antibody 7E3 Fab directed against platelet glycoprotein IIb/IIIa in patients undergoing elective coronary angioplasty. Cor Art Dis 4:167, 1993.

49. Yasuda T, Gold HK, Fallon JT, et al. Monoclonal antibody against the platelet glycoprotein (GP) IIb/IIIa receptor prevents coronary artery reocclusion after reperfusion with recombinant tissue-type plasminogen activator in dogs. J Clin Invest 81:1284, 1988.

50. Bates ER, McGillem MJ, Mickelson JK, Pitt B, Mancini GB. A monoclonal antibody against the platelet glycoprotein IIb/IIIa receptor complex prevents platelet aggregation and thrombosis in a canine model of coronary angioplasty. Circulation 84:2463, 1991.

51. Hynes R. Integrins: A family of cell surface receptors. Cell 48:549, 1987.

52. Hynes RO. Integrins: Versatility, modulation, and signaling in cell adhesion. Cell 69:11, 1992.

53. Phillips D, Charo I, Parise L, Fitzgerald L. The platelet membrane glycoprotein IIb/IIIa complex. Blood 71:831, 1988.

54. Lefkovits J, Plow E, Topol E. Platelet glycoprotein IIb/IIIa receptors in cardiovascular medicine. N Engl J Med 332:1553, 1995.

55. Pierschbacher MD, Ruoslahti E. Cell attachment activity of fibronectin can be duplicated by small synthetic fragments of the molecule. Nature 309:30, 1984.

56. Marguerie GA, Plow EF, Edgington TS. Human platelets possess an inducible and saturable receptor specific for fibrinogen. J Biol Chem 254:5357, 1979.

57. Farrell DH, Thiagarajan P, Chung DW, Davie EW. Role of fibrinogen alpha and gamma chain sites in platelet aggregation. Proc Natl Acad Sci USA 89:10729, 1992.

58. Weisel JW, Nagaswami C, Vilaire G, Bennett JS. Examination of the platelet membrane glycoprotein IIb-IIIa complex and its interaction with fibrinogen and other ligands by electron microscopy. J Biol Chem 267:16637, 1992.

59. Farrell DH, Thiagarajan P. Binding of recombinant fibrinogen mutants to platelets. J Biol Chem 269:226, 1994.

60. Wilcox JN, Smith KM, Schwartz SM, Gordon D. Localization of tissue factor in the normal vessel wall and in the atherosclerotic plaque. Proc Natl Acad Sci USA 86:2839, 1989.

61. Jesty J, Nemerson Y. The pathway of blood coagulation. In Beutler E, Lichtman MA, Coller BS, Kipps TJ (eds). Williams Hematology, Vol. 1. New York: McGraw-Hill, 1995:1227.

62. Ruf W, Edgington TS. Structural biology of tissue factor, the initiator of thrombogenesis in vivo. FASEB J 8:385, 1994.

63. Harker LA, Hanson SR, Runge MS. Thrombin hypothesis of thrombus generation and vascular lesion formation. Am J Cardiol 75:12B, 1995.

64. Harlan JM, Thompson PJ, Ross RR, Bowen-Pope DF. Alpha-thrombin induces release of platelet-derived growth factor-like molecule(s) by cultured human endothelial cells. J Cell Biol 103:1129, 1986.

65. Vane JR, Flower RJ, Botting RM. History of aspirin and its mechanism of action. Stroke 21:IV12, 1990.

66. Patrono C. Aspirin as an antiplatelet drug. N Engl J Med 330:1287, 1994.

67. Willard JE, Lange RA, Hillis LD. The use of aspirin in ischemic heart disease. N Engl J Med 327:175, 1992.

68. Roth GJ, Calverley DC. Aspirin, platelets, and thrombosis: Theory and practice. Blood 83:885, 1994.

69. Vane JR, Anggard EE, Botting RM. Regulatory functions of the vascular endothelium. N Engl J Med 323:27, 1990.

70. Simon LS, Mills JA. Drug therapy: Nonsteroidal antiinflammatory drugs (first of two parts). N Engl J Med 302:1179, 1980.

71. Simon LS, Mills JA. Nonsteroidal antiinflammatory drugs (second of two parts). N Engl J Med 302:1237, 1980.

72. Buchanan GR, Martin V, Levine PH, Scoon K, Handin RI. The effects of "anti-platelet" drugs on bleeding time and platelet aggregation in normal human subjects. Am J Clin Pathol 68:355, 1977.

73. Oates JA, FitzGerald GA, Branch RA, Jackson EK, Knapp HR, Roberts LJD. Clinical implications of prostaglandin and thromboxane A2 formation (1). N Engl J Med 319:689, 1988.

74. Hamberg M, Svensson J, Samuelsson B. Thromboxanes: A new group of biologically active compounds derived from prostaglandin endoperoxides. Proc Natl Acad Sci USA 72:2994, 1975.

75. Underwood MJ, More RS. The aspirin papers [editorial; comment]. Br Med J 308:71, 1994.

76. Steering Committee of the Physicians' Health Study Research Group. Final report on the aspirin component of the ongoing Physicians' Health Study. N Engl J Med 321:129, 1989.

77. Peto R, Gray R, Collins R, et al. Randomised trial of prophylactic daily aspirin in British male doctors. Br Med J (Clin Res Ed) 296:313, 1988.

78. Manson JE, Stampfer MJ, Colditz GA, et al. A prospective study of aspirin use and primary prevention of cardiovascular disease in women. JAMA 266:521, 1991.

79. Antiplatelet Trialists' Collaboration. Secondary prevention of vascular disease by prolonged antiplatelet treatment. Br Med J (Clin Res Ed) 296:320, 1988.

80. Antiplatelet Trialists' Collaboration. Collaborative overview of randomised trials of antiplatelet therapy — I: Prevention of death, myocardial infarction, and

stroke by prolonged antiplatelet therapy in various categories of patients. Br Med J 308:81, 1994. [Published erratum appears in Br Med J 308:1540, 1994.]

81. Antiplatelet Trialists' Collaboration. Collaborative overview of randomised trials of antiplatelet therapy — II: Maintenance of vascular graft or arterial patency by antiplatelet therapy. Br Med J 308:159, 1994.

82. Theroux P, Ouimet H, McCans J, et al. Aspirin, heparin, or both to treat acute unstable angina. N Engl J Med 319:1105, 1988.

83. Cairns JA, Gent M, Singer J, et al. Aspirin, sulfinpyrazone, or both in unstable angina. Results of a Canadian multicenter trial. N Engl J Med 313:1369, 1985.

84. Lewis HD Jr, Davis JW, Archibald DG, et al. Protective effects of aspirin against acute myocardial infarction and death in men with unstable angina. Results of a Veterans Administration Cooperative Study. N Engl J Med 309:396, 1983.

85. The RISC Group. Risk of myocardial infarction and death during treatment with low dose aspirin and intravenous heparin in men with unstable coronary artery disease. Lancet 336:827, 1990.

86. (Second International Study of Infarct Survival) Collaborative Group. Randomised trial of intravenous streptokinase, oral aspirin, both, or neither among 17, 187 cases of suspected acute myocardial infarction: ISIS-2 Lancet 2:349, 1988.

87. Lembo NJ, Black AJ, Roubin GS, et al. Effect of pretreatment with aspirin versus aspirin plus dipyridamole on frequency and type of acute complications of percutaneous transluminal coronary angioplasty. Am J Cardiol 65:422, 1990.

88. Barnathan ES, Schwartz JS, Taylor L, et al. Aspirin and dipyridamole in the prevention of acute coronary thrombosis complicating coronary angioplasty. Circulation 76:125, 1987.

89. Kent KM, Ewels CJ, Kehoe MK, Lavelle JP, Krucoff MW. Effect of aspirin on complications during transluminal coronary angioplasty (abstrt). J Am Coll Cardiol 11:132, 1988.

90. Barry WL, Sarembock IJ. Antiplatelet and anticoagulant therapy in patients undergoing percutaneous transluminal coronary angioplasty. Cardiol Clin 12:517, 1994.

91. FitzGerald GA, Oates JA, Hawiger J, et al. Endogenous biosynthesis of prostacyclin and thromboxane and platelet function during chronic administration of aspirin in man. J Clin Invest 71:676, 1983.

92. Clowes AW, Karnovsky MJ. Failure of certain antiplatelet drugs to affect myointimal thickening following arterial endothelial injury in the rat. Lab Invest 36:452, 1977.

93. Cerletti C, Carriero MR, de Gaetano G. Platelet-aggregation response to single or paired aggregating stimuli after low-dose aspirin [letter]. N Engl J Med 314:316, 1986.

94. O'Brien J, Etherington MD. How much aspirin? [letter]. Thromb Haemost 64:486, 1990.

95. Kyrle PA, Eichler HG, Jager U, Lechner K. Inhibition of prostacyclin and thromboxane A2 generation by low-dose aspirin at the site of plug formation in man in vivo. Circulation 75:1025, 1987.

96. Deckmyn H, Van Houtte E, Verstraete M, Vermylen J. Manipulation of the local thromboxane and prostacyclin balance in vivo by the antithrombotic compounds dazoxiben, acetylsalicylic acid and nafazatrom. Biochem Pharmacol 32:2757, 1983.

97. Vermylen J, Deckmyn H. Reorientation of prostaglandin endoperoxide metabolism by a thromboxane synthetase inhibitor: In vitro and clinical observations. Br J Clin Pharmacol 15:17S, 1983.

98. Reilly IA, Doran JB, Smith B, FitzGerald GA. Increased thromboxane biosynthesis in a human preparation of platelet activation: Biochemical and functional consequences of selective inhibition of thromboxane synthase. Circulation 73:1300, 1986.

99. Fiddler GI, Lumley P. Preliminary clinical studies with thromboxane synthase inhibitors and thromboxane receptor blockers. A review. Circulation 81:I69; discussion I79, 1990.

100. Patrono C. Biosynthesis and pharmacological modulation of thromboxane in humans. Circulation 81:I12; discussion I22, 1990.

101 Vermylen J, Deckmyn H. Thromboxane synthase inhibitors and receptor antagonists. Cardiovasc Drugs Ther 6:29, 1992.

102. Verstraete M. Thromboxane synthase inhibition, thromboxane/endoperoxide receptor blockade and molecules with the dual property. Drugs Today 29:221, 1993.

103. Bartele V, Cerletti C, Schiepatti A, di Minno G, de Gaetano G. Inhibition of thromboxane synthetase does not necessarily prevent platelet aggregation [letter]. Lancet 1:1057, 1981.

104. Hornby EJ, Skidmore IF. Evidence that prostaglandin endoperoxides can induce platelet aggregation in the absence of thromboxane A2 production. Biochem Pharmacol 31:1158, 1982.

105. Gresele P, Deckmyn H, Arnout J, Lemmens J, Janssens W, Vermylen J. BM 13.177, a selective blocker of platelet and vessel wall thromboxane receptors, is active in man. Lancet 1:991, 1984.

106. Brittain RT, Boutal L, Carter MC, et al. AH23848: A thromboxane receptor-blocking drug that can clarify the pathophysiologic role of thromboxane A2. Circulation 72:1208, 1985.

107. Savage MP, Goldberg S, Bove AA, et al. Effect of thromboxane A2 blockade on clinical outcome and restenosis after successful coronary angioplasty. Multi-Hospital Eastern Atlantic Restenosis Trial (M-HEART II). Circulation 92:3194, 1995.

108. Hacker RW, Torka M, Yukseltan I, et al. Reduction of the vein graft occlusion rate after coronary artery bypass surgery by treatment with a thromboxane receptor antagonist. Z Kardiol 78:48, 1989.

109. Serruys PW, Rutsch W, Heyndrickx GR, et al. Prevention of restenosis after percutaneous transluminal coronary angioplasty with thromboxane A2-receptor blockade. A randomized, double-blind, placebo-controlled trial. Coronary Artery Restenosis Prevention on Repeated Thromboxane-Antagonism Study (CARPORT). Circulation 84:1568, 1991.

110. De Bono DP, Lumley P, Been M, Keery R, Ince SE, Woodings DF. Effect of the specific thromboxane receptor blocking drug AH23848 in patients with angina pectoris. Br Heart J 56:509, 1986.

111. Gresele P, Arnout J, Deckmyn H, Huybrechts E, Pieters G, Vermylen J. Role of proaggregatory and antiaggregatory prostaglandins in hemostasis. Studies with combined thromboxane synthase inhibition and thromboxane receptor antagonism. J Clin Invest 80:1435, 1987.

112. Gresele P, Deckmyn H, Arnout J, Nenci GG, Vermylen J. Characterization of N,N'-bis(3-picolyl)-4-methoxy-isophtalamide (picotamide) as a dual thromboxane synthase inhibitor/thromboxane A2 receptor antagonist in human platelets. Thromb Haemost 61:479, 1989.

113. Violi F, Ghiselli A, Iuliano L, Pratico D, Alessandri C, Balsano F. Inhibition by picotamide of thromboxane production in vitro and ex vivo. Eur J Clin Pharmacol 33:599, 1988.

114. De Clerck F, Beetens J, Van de Water A, Vercammen E, Janssen PA. R 68070: Thromboxane A2 synthetase inhibition and thromboxane A2/prostaglandin endoperoxide receptor blockade combined in one molecule — II. Pharmacological effects in vivo and ex vivo. Thromb Haemost 61:43, 1989.

115. Hoet B, Arnout J, Deckmyn H, Vermylen J. Synergistic antiplatelet effect of ridogrel, a combined thromboxane receptor antagonist and thromboxane synthase inhibitor, and UDCG-212, a cAMP-phosphodiesterase inhibitor. Thromb Haemost 70: 822, 1993.

116. The Ridogrel Versus Aspirin Patency Trial (RAPT). Randomized trial of ridogrel, a combined thromboxane A2 synthase inhibitor and thromboxane A2/prostaglandin endoperoxide receptor antagonist, versus aspirin as adjunct to thrombolysis in patients with acute myocardial infarction. Circulation 89:588, 1994.

117. Defreyn G, Bernat A, Delebassee D, Maffrand JP. Pharmacology of ticlopidine: A review. Semin Thromb Hemost 15:159, 1989.

118. Lips NP, Sixma JJ, Schiphorst ME. The effect of ticlopidine administration to humans on the binding of adenosine diphosphate to blood platelets. Thromb Res 17:19, 1980.

119. Hardisty RM, Powling MJ, Nokes TJ. The action of ticlopidine on human platelets. Studies on aggregation, secretion, calcium mobilization and membrane glycoproteins. Thromb Haemost 64:150, 1990.

120. Ito MK, Smith AR, Lee ML. Ticlopidine; A new platelet aggregation inhibitor. Clin Pharm 11:603, 1992.

121. Feliste R, Delebassee D, Simon MF, et al. Broad spectrum anti-platelet activity of ticlopidine and PCR 4099 involves the suppression of the effects of released ADP. Thromb Res 48:403, 1987.

122. Gachet C, Stierle A, Cazenave JP, et al. The thienopyridine PCR 4099 selectively inhibits ADP-induced platelet aggregation and fibrinogen binding without modifying the membrane glycoprotein IIb-IIIa complex in rat and in man. Biochem Pharmacol 40:229, 1990.

123. Nachman RL, Leung LL. Complex formation of platelet membrane glycoproteins IIb and IIIa with fibrinogen. J Clin Invest 69:263, 1982.

124. O'Brien J, Etherington MD, Shuttleworth RD. Ticlopidine — an antiplatelet drug: Effects in human volunteers. Thromb Res 13:245, 1978.

125. Dunn FW, Soria J, Soria C, Thomaidis A, Lee H, Caen JP. In vivo effect of ticlopidine on fibrinogen-platelet cofactor activity and binding of fibrinogen to platelets. Agents Actions Suppl 15:97, 1984.

126. Di Minno G, Cerbone AM, Mattioli PL, Turco S, Iovine C, Mancini M. Functionally thrombasthenic state in normal platelets following the administration of ticlopidine. J Clin Invest 75:328, 1985.

127. Lee H, Paton RC, Ruan C, Caen JP. The in vitro effect of ticlopidine on fibrinogen and factor VIII binding to human platelets. Thromb Haemost 46:590, 1981.

128. Gachet C, Cazenave JP, Ohlmann P, et al. The thienopyridine ticlopidine selectively prevents the inhibitory effects of ADP but not of adrenaline on cAMP levels raised by stimulation of the adenylate cyclase of human platelets by PGE1. Biochem Pharmacol 40:2683, 1990.

129. Cattaneo M, Akkawat B, Kinlough-Rathbone RL, Packham MA, Cimminiello C, Mannucci PM. Ticlopidine facilitates the deaggregation of human platelets aggregated by thrombin. Thromb Haemost 71:91, 1994.

130. Picard-Fraire C. Pharmacokinetic and metabolic characteristics of ticlopidine in relation to its inhibitory properties on platelet function. Agents Actions Suppl 15:68, 1984.

131. Ellis DJ, Roe RL, Bruno JJ, Cranston BJ, McSpadden MM. The effects of ticlopidine hydrochloride on bleeding time and platelet function in man. Thromb Haemost 46:176, 1987.

132. Knudsen JB, Gormsen J. The effect of ticlopidine on platelet function in normal volunteers and in patients with platelet hyperaggregability in vitro. Thromb Res 16:663, 1979.

133. Conard J, Lecrubier C, Scarabin PY, Horellou MH, Samama M, Bousser MG. Effects of long term administration of ticlopidine on platelet function and hemostatic variables. Thromb Res 20:143, 1980.

134. Thebault JJ, Blatrix CE, Blanchard JF, Panak EA.

Effects of ticlopidine, a new platelet aggregation inhibitor in man. Clin Pharmacol Ther 18:485, 1975.

135. Gent M, Blakely JA, Easton JD, et al. The Canadian American Ticlopidine Study (CATS) in thromboembolic stroke. Lancet 1:1215, 1989.

136. Hass WK, Easton JD, Adams HP Jr, et al. A randomized trial comparing ticlopidine hydrochloride with aspirin for the prevention of stroke in high-risk patients. Ticlopidine Aspirin Stroke Study Group. N Engl J Med 321:501, 1989.

137. Ono K, Kurohara K, Yoshihara M, Shimamoto Y, Yamaguchi M. Agranulocytosis caused by ticlopidine and its mechanism. Am J Hematol 37:239, 1991.

138. Haynes RB, Sandler RS, Larson EB, Pater JL, Yatsu FM. A critical appraisal of ticlopidine, a new antiplatelet agent. Effectiveness and clinical indications for prophylaxis of atherosclerotic events. Arch Intern Med 152:1376, 1992.

139. Herbert JM, Frehel D, Vallee E, et al. Clopidogrel, a novel antiplatelet and antithrombotic agent. Cardiovasc Drug Rev 11:189, 1993.

140. Rothlin ME, Pfluger N, Speiser K, et al. Platelet inhibitors versus anticoagulants for prevention of aortocoronary bypass graft occlusion. Eur Heart J 6:168, 1985.

141. Limet R, David JL, Magotteaux P, Larock MP, Rigo P. Prevention of aorta-coronary bypass graft occlusion. Beneficial effect of ticlopidine on early and late patency rates of venous coronary bypass grafts: A double-blind study. J Thorac Cardiovasc Surg 94:773, 1987.

142. Chevigne M, David JL, Rigo P, Limet R. Effect of ticlopidine on saphenous vein bypass patency rates: A double-blind study. Ann Thorac Surg 37:371, 1984.

143. Pfluger N, Goebel N, Turina M, Rothlin M. Influence of the antiaggregant ticlopidine on the patency of aorto-coronary bypass grafts. Eur Heart J 2:208, 1981.

144. Balsano F, Rizzon P, Violi F, et al. Antiplatelet treatment with ticlopidine in unstable angina. A controlled multicenter clinical trial. The Studio della Ticlopidina nell' Angina Instabile Group. Circulation 82:17, 1990.

145. FitzGerald GA. Ticlopidine in unstable angina. A more expensive aspirin? [comment]. Circulation 82:296, 1990.

146. Janzon L, Bergqvist D, Boberg J, et al. Prevention of myocardial infarction and stroke in patients with intermittent claudication; effects of ticlopidine. Results from STIMS, the Swedish Ticlopidine Multicentre Study. J Intern Med 227:301, 1990. [Published erratum appears in J Intern Med 228:659, 1990.]

147. White CW, Chaitman B, Lassar TA, et al. Antiplatelet agents are effective in reducing the immediate complications of PTCA. Circulation 76:1987, 1987.

148. Bertrand ME, Allain H, Lablanche JM. Results of a randomized trial of ticlopidine versus placebo for prevention of acute closure and restenosis after coronary angioplasty. Circulation 82:III190, 1990.

149. Barragan P, Sainsous J, Silvestri M, et al. Ticlopidine and subcutaneous heparin as an alternative regimen following coronary stenting. Cathet Cardiovasc Diagn 32:133, 1994.

150. Morice MC, Bourdonnec C, Lefevre T, et al. Coronary stenting without coumadin. Circulation 90:I125, 1994.

151. Colombo A, Hall P, Nakamura S, et al. Intracoronary stenting without anticoagulation accomplished with intravascular ultrasound guidance. Circulation 91:1676, 1995.

152. Hall P, Nakamura S, Maiello L, et al. A randomized comparison of combined ticlopidine and aspirin therapy versus aspirin therapy alone after successful intravascular ultrasound-buided stent implantation. Circulation 93:215, 1996.

153. Serruys PW, Emanuelsson H, van der Giessen W, et al. Heparin-coated Palmaz-Schatz stents in human coronary arteries. Early outcome of the Benestent-II pilot study. Circulation 93:412, 1996.

154. Schömig A, Neumann FJ, Kastrati A, et al. A randomized comparison of antiplatelet and anticoagulant therapy after the placement of coronary-artery stents. N Engl J Med 334:1084, 1996.

155. Coller BS. Blockade of platelet GPIIb/IIIa receptors as an antithrombotic strategy. Circulation 92:2373, 1995.

156. Coller BS. A new murine monoclonal antibody reports an activation-dependent change in the conformation and/or microenvironment of the platelet glycoprotein IIb/IIIa complex. J Clin Invest 76:101, 1985.

157. Coller BS, Scudder LE. Inhibition of dog platelet function by in vivo infusion of F(ab')2 fragments of a monoclonal antibody to the platelet glycoprotein IIb/IIIa receptor. Blood 66:1456, 1985.

158. Coller BS, Folts JD, Scudder LE, Smith SR. Antithrombotic effect of a monoclonal antibody to the platelet glycoprotein IIb/IIIa receptor in an experimental animal model. Blood 68:783, 1986.

159. Gold HK, Gimple LW, Yasuda T, et al. Pharmacodynamic study of F(ab')2 fragments of murine monoclonal antibody 7E3 directed against human platelet glycoprotein IIb/IIIa in patients with unstable angina pectoris. J Clin Invest 86:651, 1990.

160 Kleiman NS, Ohman EM, Califf RM, et al. Profound inhibition of platelet aggregation with monoclonal antibody 7E3 Fab after thrombolytic therapy. Results of the Thrombolysis and Angioplasty in Myocardial Infarction (TAMI) 8 Pilot Study. J Am Coll Cardiol 22:381, 1993.

161. Simoons ML, de Boer MJ, van den Brand MJ, et al. Randomized trial of a GPIIb/IIIa platelet receptor blocker in refractory unstable angina. European Cooperative Study Group. Circulation 89:596, 1994.

162. Tcheng JE, Ellis SG, George BS, et al. Pharmacodynamics of chimeric glycoprotein IIb/IIIa integrin antiplatelet antibody Fab 7E3 in high-risk coronary angioplasty. Circulation 90:1757, 1994.

163. Topol EJ, Califf RM, Weisman HF, et al. Randomised trial of coronary intervention with antibody against platelet IIb/IIIa integrin for reduction of clinical restenosis: Results at six months. The EPIC Investigators. Lancet 343:881, 1994.

164. Aguirre FV, Topol EJ, Ferguson JJ, et al. Bleeding complications with the chimeric antibody to platelet glycoprotein IIb/IIIa integrin in patients undergoing percutaneous coronary intervention. EPIC Investigators. Circulation 91:2882, 1995.

165. The EPILOG Investigators. Evaluation of PTCA to improve long-term outcome by c7E3 glycoprotein IIb/IIIa receptor blockade (EPILOG), 45th Annual Scientific Session of the American College of Cardiology, Orlando, Florida, March 27, 1996.

166. Simoons ML. Refractory unstable angina: Reduction of events by c-7E3: The CAPTURE study, 45th Annual Scientific Session of the American College of Cardiology, Orlando, FL, March 25, 1996.

167. Gould RJ, Polokoff MA, Friedman PA, et al. Disintegrins: A family of integrin inhibitory proteins from viper venoms. Proc Soc Exp Biol Med 195:168, 1990.

168. Scarborough RM, Rose JW, Naughton MA, et al. Characterization of the integrin specificities of disintegrins isolated from American pit viper venoms. J Biol Chem 268:1058, 1993.

169. Dennis MS, Henzel WJ, Pitti RM, et al. Platelet glycoprotein IIb-IIIa protein antagonists from snake venoms: Evidence for a family of platelet-aggregation inhibitors. Proc Natl Acad Sci USA 87:2471, 1990.

170. Barker PL, Bullens S, Bunting S, et al. Cyclic RGD peptide analogues as antiplatelet antithrombotics. J Med Chem 35:2040, 1992.

171. Scarborough RM, Naughton MA, Teng W, et al. Design of potent and specific integrin antagonists. Peptide antagonists with high specificity for glycoprotein IIb-IIIa. J Biol Chem 268:1066, 1993.

172. Schulman SP, Goldschmidt-Clermont PJ, Navetta FI, et al. Integrelin in unstable angina: A double-blind randomized trial. Circulation 88:I608, 1993.

173. Ohman EM, Kleiman NS, Talley JD, et al. Simultaneous platelet glycoprotein IIb/IIIa integrin blockade with accelerated tissue plasminogen activator in acute myocardial infarction. Circulation 90:I564, 1994.

174. Harrington RA, Kleiman NS, Kottke-Marchant K, et al. Immediate, reversible platelet inhibition after intravenous administration of a peptide glycoprotein IIb/IIIa inhibitor during percutaneous coronary intervention. Am J Cardiol 76:1222, 1995.

175. Tcheng JE, Harrington RA, Kottke-Marchant K, et al. Multicenter, randomized, double-blind, placebo-controlled trial of the platelet integrin glycoprotein IIb/IIIa blocker Integrelin in elective coronary intervention. IMPACT Investigators. Circulation 91:2151, 1995.

176. Tcheng JE, Lincoff AM, Sigmon KN, Kitt MM, Califf RM, Topol EJ for the IMPACT II Investigators. Platelet glycoprotein IIb/IIIa inhibition with Integrelin during percutaneous coronary intervention: The IMPACT II Trial. Circulation 92:I543, 1995.

177. Theroux P, Kouz S, Knudtson ML, et al. A randomized double-blind controlled trial with the non-peptide platelet GP IIb/IIIa antagonist Ro 44-9982 in unstable angina. Circulation 90:I232, 1994.

178. Kereiakes DJ, Kleiman NS, Ambrose J, et al. Randomized, double-blind, placebo-controlled dose-ranging study of tirofiban (MK-383) platelet IIb/IIIa blockade in high risk patients undergoing coronary angioplasty. J Am Coll Cardiol 27:536, 1996.

179. King III SB. Administration of tirofiban (MK-0383) will reduce the incidence of adverse cardiac outcome following PTCA/PCA (RESTORE), 45th Annual Scientific Session of the American College of Cardiology, Orlando, Florida, March 27, 1996, 1996.

180. Mousa SA, DeGrado WF, Mu DX, Kapil RP, Lucchesi BR, Reilly TM. Oral antiplatelet, antithrombotic efficacy of DMP 728, a novel platelet GP IIb/IIIa antagonist. Circulation 93:537, 1996.

181. Nicholson NS, Panzer-Knodle SG, Salyers AK, et al. SC-54684A: An orally active inhibitor of platelet aggregation. Circulation 91:403, 1995.

182. Szalony JA, Haas NF, Salyers AK, et al. Extended inhibition of platelet aggregation with the orally active platelet inhibitor SC-54684A. Circulation 91:411, 1995.

183. Anders RJ, Alexander JC, Hantsbarger GL, et al. Demonstration of potent inhibition of platelet aggregation with an orally active GP IIb/IIIa receptor antagonist. J Am Coll Cardiol 25:117, 1995.

184. Miletich JP, Jackson CM, Majerus PW. Interaction of coagulation factor Xa with human platelets. Proc Natl Acad Sci USA 74:4033, 1977.

185. Rosing J, van Rijn JL, Bevers EM, van Dieijen G, Comfurius P, Zwaal RF. The role of activated human platelets in prothrombin and factor X activation. Blood 65:319, 1985.

186. Tracy PB, Giles AR, Mann KG, Eide LL, Hoogendoorn H, Rivard GE. Factor V (Quebec): A bleeding diathesis associated with a qualitative platelet Factor V deficiency. J Clin Invest 74:1221, 1984.

187. Giles AR, Nesheim ME, Hoogendoorn H, Tracy PB, Mann KG. Stroma free human platelet lysates potentiate the in vivo thrombogenicity of factor Xa by the provision of coagulant-active phospholipid. Br J Haematol 51:457, 1982.

188. Walsh PN, Schmaier AH. Platelet-coagulant protein interactions. In Colman RW, Hirsh J, Marder VJ, Salzman EW (eds). Hemostasis and Thrombosis: Basic Principles and Clinical Practice. Philadelphia: JB Lippincott, 1994:629.

189. Bevers EM, Comfurius P, van Rijn JL, Hemker HC,

Zwaal RF. Generation of prothrombin-converting activity and the exposure of phosphatidylserine at the outer surface of platelets. Eur J Biochem 122:429, 1982.

190. Hirsh J. Heparin. N Engl J Med 324:1565, 1991.

191. Rosenberg RD, Damus PS. The purification and mechanism of action of human antithrombin-heparin cofactor. J Biol Chem 248:6490, 1973.

192. Rosenberg RD, Lam L. Correlation between structure and function of heparin. Proc Natl Acad Sci USA 76:1218, 1979.

193. Rosenberg JS, McKenna PW, Rosenberg RD. Inhibition of human factor IXa by human antithrombin. J Biol Chem 250:8883, 1975.

194. Ofosu FA, Sie P, Modi GJ, et al. The inhibition of thrombin-dependent positive-feedback reactions is critical to the expression of the anticoagulant effect of heparin. Biochem J 243:579, 1987.

195. Ofosu FA, Gray E. Mechanisms of action of heparin: Applications to the development of derivatives of heparin and heparinoids with antithrombotic properties. Semin Thromb Hemost 14:9, 1988.

196. Barrowcliffe TW, Johnson EA, Eggleton CA, Kemball-Cook G, Thomas DP. Anticoagulant activities of high and low molecular weight heparin fractions. Br J Haematol 41:573, 1979.

197. Casu B, Oreste P, Torri G, et al. The structure of heparin oligosaccharide fragments with high anti-(factor Xa) activity containing the minimal antithrombin III-binding sequence. Chemical and ^{13}C nuclear-magnetic-resonance studies. Biochem J 197:599, 1981.

198. Weitz JI, Hudoba M, Massel D, Maraganore J, Hirsh J. Clot-bound thrombin is protected from inhibition by heparin-antithrombin III but is susceptible to inactivation by antithrombin III-independent inhibitors. J Clin Invest 86:385, 1990.

199. Hogg PJ, Jackson CM. Fibrin monomer protects thrombin from inactivation by heparin-antithrombin III: Implications for heparin efficacy. Proc Natl Acad Sci USA 86:3619, 1989.

200. Flaker GC, Bartolozzi J, Davis V, McCabe C, Cannon CP. Use of a standardized heparin nomogram to achieve therapeutic anticoagulation after thrombolytic therapy in myocardial infarction. TIMI 4 investigators. Thrombolysis in Myocardial Infarction. Arch Intern Med 154:1492, 1994.

201. Hull RD, Raskob GE, Rosenbloom D, et al. Optimal therapeutic level of heparin therapy in patients with venous thrombosis. Arch Intern Med 152:1589, 1992.

202. Raschke RA, Reilly BM, Guidry JR, Fontana JR, Srinivas S. The weight-based heparin dosing nomogram compared with a "standard care" nomogram. A randomized controlled trial. Ann Intern Med 119:874, 1993.

203. Warkentin TE, Levine MN, Hirsh J, et al. Heparin-induced thrombocytopenia in patients treated with low-molecular-weight heparin or unfractionated heparin. N Engl J Med 332:1330, 1995.

204. Aster RH. Heparin-induced thrombocytopenia and thrombosis [editorial; comment]. N Engl J Med 332:1374, 1995.

205. Warkentin TE, Kelton JG. Heparin-induced thrombocytopenia. Annu Rev Med 40:31, 1989.

206. King DJ, Kelton JG. Heparin-associated thrombocytopenia. Ann Intern Med 100:535, 1984.

207. Fiore L, Deykin D. Anticoagulant therapy. In Beutler E, Lichtman MA, Coller BS, Kipps TJ (eds). New York: Williams Hematology. McGraw-Hill, 1995: 1562.

208. Telford AM, Wilson C. Trial of heparin versus atenolol in prevention of myocardial infarction in intermediate coronary syndrome. Lancet 1:1225, 1981.

209. Neri Serneri GG, Gensini GF, Poggesi L, et al. Effect of heparin, aspirin, or alteplase in reduction of myocardial ischaemia in refractory unstable angina. Lancet 335:615–618, 1990. [Published erratum appears in Lancet 335:868, 1990.]

210. Theroux P, Waters D, Lam J, Juneau M, McCans J. Reactivation of unstable angina after the discontinuation of heparin. N Engl J Med 327:141, 1992.

211. Mahaffey KW, Granger CB, Collins R, et al. Overview of randomized trials of intravenous heparin in patients with acute myocardial infarction treated with thrombolytic therapy. Am J Cardiol 77:551, 1996.

212. Gruppo Italiano per lo Studio della Sopravvivenza nell'Infarto Miocardico. GISSI-2: A factorial randomised trial of alteplase versus streptokinase and heparin versus no heparin among 12,490 patients with acute myocardial infarction. Lancet 336:65, 1990.

213. The International Study Group. In-hospital mortality and clinical course of 20,891 patients with suspected acute myocardial infarction randomised between alteplase and streptokinase with or without heparin. Lancet 336:71, 1990.

214. ISIS-3 (Third International Study of Infarct Survival) Collaborative Group. ISIS-3: A randomised comparison of streptokinase vs. tissue plasminogen activator vs. anistreplase and of aspirin plus heparin vs. aspirin alone among 41,299 cases of suspected acute myocardial infarction. Lancet 339:753, 1992.

215. The GUSTO investigators. An international randomized trial comparing four thrombolytic strategies for acute myocardial infarction. N Engl J Med 329:673, 1993.

216. Arnout J, Simoons M, de Bono D, Rapold HJ, Collen D, Verstraete M. Correlation between level of heparinization and patency of the infarct-related coronary artery after treatment of acute myocardial infarction with alteplase (rt-PA). J Am Coll Cardiol 20:513, 1992.

217. Hsia J, Kleiman N, Aguirre F, Chaitman BR, Roberts R, Ross AM. Heparin-induced prolongation of partial thromboplastin time after thrombolysis: Relation to coronary artery patency. HART investigators. J Am Coll Cardiol 20:31, 1992.

218. Granger CB, Hirsh J, Califf RM, et al. Activated partial thromboplastin time and outcome after

thrombolytic therapy for acute myocardial infarction: Results from the GUSTO-1 trial. Circulation 93:870, 1996.

219. McGarry TF Jr, Gottlieb RS, Morganroth J, et al. The relationship of anticoagulation level and complications after successful percutaneous transluminal coronary angioplasty. Am Heart J 123:1445, 1992.

220. Dougherty KG, Marsh KC, Edelman SK, Gaos CM, Ferguson JJ, Leachman DR. Relationship between procedural activated clotting time and in-hospital post-PTCA outcome. Circulation 82:III189, 1990.

221. Vaitkus PT, Herrmann HC, Laskey WK. Management and immediate outcome of patients with intracoronary thrombus during percutaneous transluminal coronary angioplasty. Am Heart J 124:1, 1992.

222. Rath B, Bennett DH. Monitoring the effect of heparin by measurement of activated clotting time during and after percutaneous transluminal coronary angioplasty. Br Heart J 63:18, 1990.

223. Satler LF, Leon MB, Kent KM, Pichard AD. Strategies for acute occlusion after coronary angioplasty. J Am Coll Cardiol 19:936, 1992.

224. Ogilby JD, Kopelman HA, Klein LW, Agarwal JB. Adequate heparinization during PTCA: Assessment using activated clotting times. Cathet Cardiovasc Diagn 18:206, 1989.

225. Gabliani G, Deligonul U, Kern MJ, Vandormael M. Acute coronary occlusion occurring after successful percutaneous transluminal coronary angioplasty: Temporal relationship to discontinuation of anticoagulation. Am Heart J 116:696, 1988.

226. Ferguson JJ, Dougherty KG, Gaos CM, Bush HS, Marsh KC, Leachman DR. Relation between procedural activated coagulation time and outcome after percutaneous transluminal coronary angioplasty. J Am Coll Cardiol 23:1061, 1994.

227. Narins CR, Hillegass WB, Nelson CL, et al. Relation between activated clotting time during angioplasty and abrupt closure. Circulation 93:667, 1996.

228. Mooney MR, Mooney JF, Goldenberg IF, Almquist AK, Van Tassel RA. Percutaneous transluminal coronary angioplasty in the setting of large intracoronary thrombi. Am J Cardiol 65:427, 1990.

229. Popma JJ, Coller BS, Ohman EM, et al. Antithrombotic therapy in patients undergoing coronary angioplasty. Chest 108:486S, 1995.

230. Wolf H. Low-molecular-weight heparin. Med Clin North Am 78:733, 1994.

231. Hirsh J, Levine MN. Low molecular weight heparin. Blood 79:1, 1992.

232. Levine MN, Hirsh J, Clinical use of low molecular weight heparins and heparinoids. Semin Thromb Hemost 14:116, 1988.

233. Beguin S, Mardiguian J, Lindhout T, Hemker HC. The mode of action of low molecular weight heparin preparation (PK10169) and two of its major components on thrombin generation in plasma. Thromb Haemost 61:30, 1989.

234. Vairel EG, Bouty-Boye H, Toulemonde F, Doutremepuich C, Marsh NA, Gaffney PJ. Heparin and a low molecular weight fraction enhances thrombolysis and by this pathway exercises a protective effect against thrombosis. Thromb Res 30:219, 1983.

235. Lane DA, Denton J, Flynn AM, Thunberg L, Lindahl U. Anticoagulant activities of heparin oligosaccharides and their neutralization by platelet factor 4. Biochem J 218:725, 1984.

236. Hirsh J. Overview of low molecular weight heparins and heparinoids: Basic and clinical aspects. Aust N Z J Med 22:487, 1992.

237. Hull RD, Raskob GE, Pineo GF, et al. Subcutaneous low-molecular-weight heparin compared with continuous intravenous heparin in the treatment of proximal-vein thrombosis. N Engl J Med 326:975, 1992.

238. Prandoni P, Lensing AW, Buller HR, et al. Comparison of subcutaneous low-molecular-weight heparin with intravenous standard heparin in proximal deep-vein thrombosis. Lancet 339:441, 1992.

239. Lensing AW, Prins MH, Davidson BL, Hirsh J. Treatment of deep venous thrombosis with low-molecular-weight heparins. A meta-analysis. Arch Intern Med 155:601, 1995.

240. Gurfinkel EP, Manos EJ, Mejail RI, et al. Low molecular weight heparin versus regular heparin or aspirin in the treatment of unstable angina and silent ischemia. J Am Coll Cardiol 26:313, 1995.

241. Ofosu FA. Anticoagulant mechanisms of Orgaran (Org 10172) and its fraction with high affinity to antithrombin III (Org 10849). Haemostasis 22:66, 1992.

242. Keeling DM, Richards EM, Baglin TP. Platelet aggregation in response to four low molecular weight heparins and the heparinoid ORG 10172 in patients with heparin-induced thrombocytopenia. Br J Haematol 86:425, 1994.

243. Ortel TL, Gockerman JP, Califf RM, et al. Parenteral anticoagulation with the heparinoid Lomoparan (Org 10172) in patients with heparin induced thrombocytopenia and thrombosis. Thromb Haemost 67:292, 1992.

244. Messmore HL, Griffin B, Koza M, Seghatchian J, Fareed J, Coyne E. Interaction of heparinoids with platelets: Comparison with heparin and low molecular weight heparins. Semin Thromb Hemost 17:57, 1991.

245. Chong BH, Magnani HN. Orgaran in heparin-induced thrombocytopenia. Haemostasis 22:85, 1992.

246. Magnani HN. Heparin-induced thrombocytopenia (HIT): An overview of 230 patients treated with orgaran (Org 10172). Thromb Haemost 70:554, 1993. [Published erratum appears in Thromb Haemost 70:1072, 1993.]

247. Weitz J, Hirsh J. New anticoagulant strategies. J Lab Clin Med 122:364, 1993.

248. Lefkovits J, Topol EJ. Direct thrombin inhibitors in cardiovascular medicine. Circulation 90:1522, 1994.

249. Muller TH, Binder K, Guth BD. Pharmacology of current and future antithrombotic therapies. Cardiol Clin 12:411, 1994.

250. Adams SL. The medicinal leech. A page from the annelids of internal medicine. Ann Intern Med 109:399, 1988. [Published erratum appears in Ann Intern Med 109:763, 1988.]

251. Adams SL. The medicinal leech: Historical perspectives. Semin Thromb Hemost 15:261, 1989.

252. Harvey RP, Degryse E, Stefani L, et al. Cloning and expression of a cDNA coding for the anticoagulant hirudin from the bloodsucking leech, *Hirudo medicinalis*. Proc Natl Acad Sci USA 83:1084, 1986.

253. Talbot M. Biology of recombinant hirudin (CGP 39393): A new prospect in the treatment of thrombosis. Semin Thromb Hemost 15:293, 1989.

254. Tam SW, Fenton JWD, Detwiler TC. Dissociation of thrombin from platelets by hirudin. Evidence for receptor processing. J Biol Chem 254:8723, 1979.

255. Stone SR, Hofsteenge J. Kinetics of the inhibition of thrombin by hirudin. Biochemistry 25:4622, 1986.

256. Cannon CP. Hirudin in acute myocardial infarction. J Thromb Thrombolys 1:259, 1995.

257. Zoldhelyi P, Webster MW, Fuster V, et al. Recombinant hirudin in patients with chronic, stable coronary artery disease. Safety, half-life, and effect on coagulation parameters. Circulation 88:2015, 1993.

258. Lee LV. Initial experience with hirudin and streptokinase in acute myocardial infarction: Results of the Thrombolysis in Myocardial Infarction (TIMI) 6 trial. Am J Cardiol 75:7, 1995.

259. Neuhaus KL, Niederr W, Wagner J, et al. HIT (Hirudin for the Improvement of Thrombolysis): Results of a dose escalation study. Circulation 88:I292, 1993.

260. Cannon CP, McCabe CH, Henry TD, et al. A pilot trial of recombinant desulfatohirudin compared with heparin in conjunction with tissue-type plasminogen activator and aspirin for acute myocardial infarction: Results of the Thrombolysis in Myocardial Infarction (TIMI) 5 trial. J Am Coll Cardiol 23:993, 1994.

261. Neuhaus KL, von Essen R, Tebbe U, et al. Safety observations from the pilot phase of the randomized r-Hirudin for Improvement of Thrombolysis (HIT-III) study. A study of the Arbeitsgemeinschaft Leitender Kardiologischer Krankenhausarzte (ALKK). Circulation 90:1638, 1994.

262. Antman EM. Hirudin in acute myocardial infarction. Safety report from the Thrombolysis and Thrombin Inhibition in Myocardial Infarction (TIMI) 9A Trial. Circulation 90:1624, 1994.

263. The Global Use of Strategies to Open Occluded Coronary Arteries (GUSTO) IIa Investigators. Randomized trial of intravenous heparin versus recombinant hirudin for acute coronary syndromes. Circulation 90:1631, 1994.

264. Antman EM. TIMI 9B Results, Scientific Sessions of the American Heart Association, Anaheim, CA, November 13, 1995, 1995.

265. The GUSTO IIb Investigators. A comparison of recombinant hirudin versus heparin for the treatment of acute coronary syndromes., 45th Annual Scientific Sessions American College of Cardiology, Orlando, Florida, March 26, 1996, 1996.

266. van den Bos AA, Deckers JW, Heyndrickx GR, et al. Safety and efficacy of recombinant hirudin (CGP 39393) versus heparin in patients with stable angina undergoing coronary angioplasty. Circulation 88:2058, 1993.

267. Topol EJ, Fuster V, Harrington RA, et al. Recombinant hirudin for unstable angina pectoris. A multicenter, randomized angiographic trial. Circulation 89:1557, 1994.

268. Serruys P, Herrman J, Simon R, et al. A comparison of hirudin with heparin in the prevention of restenosis after coronary angioplasty. N Engl J Med 333:757, 1995.

269. Maraganore JM, Bourdon P, Jablonski J, Ramachandran KL, Fenton JWD. Design and characterization of hirulogs: A novel class of bivalent peptide inhibitors of thrombin. Biochemistry 29:7095, 1990.

270. Maraganore JM. Pre-clinical and clinical studies on Hirulog: A potent and specific direct thrombin inhibitor. Adv Exp Med Biol 340:227, 1993.

271. Cannon CP, Maraganore JM, Loscalzo J, et al. Anticoagulant effects of hirulog, a novel thrombin inhibitor, in patients with coronary artery disease. Am J Cardiol 71:778, 1993.

272. Sharma GV, Lapsley D, Vita JA, et al. Usefulness and tolerability of hirulog, a direct thrombin-inhibitor, in unstable angina pectoris. Am J Cardiol 72:1357, 1993.

273. Lidon RM, Theroux P, Juneau M, Adelman B, Maraganore J. Initial experience with a direct antithrombin, Hirulog, in unstable angina. Anticoagulant, antithrombotic, and clinical effects. Circulation 88:1495, 1993.

274. Fuchs J, Cannon CP. Hirulog in the treatment of unstable angina. Results of the Thrombin Inhibition in Myocardial Ischemia (TIMI) 7 trial. Circulation 92:727, 1995.

275. Theroux P, Perez-Villa F, Waters D, Lesperance J, Shabani F, Bonan R. Randomized double-blind comparison of two doses of Hirulog with heparin as adjunctive therapy to streptokinase to promote early patency of the infarct-related artery in acute myocardial infarction. Circulation 91:2132, 1995.

276. White HD. Hirulog versus heparin after streptokinase (HERO), 45th Annual Scientific Session of the American College of Cardiology, Orlando, Florida, March 25, 1996.

277. Topol EJ, Bonan R, Jewitt D, et al. Use of a direct antithrombin, hirulog, in place of heparin during coronary angioplasty. Circulation 87:1622, 1993.

278. Bittl JA, Strony J, Brinker JA, et al. Treatment with bivalirudin (Hirulog) as compared with heparin during coronary angioplasty for unstable or postinfarction angina. Hirulog Angioplasty Study Investigators. N Engl J Med 333:764, 1995.

279. Maraganore JM, Chao B, Joseph ML, Jablonski J, Ramachandran KL. Anticoagulant activity of synthetic hirudin peptides. J Biol Chem 264:8692, 1989.

280. Cadroy Y, Maraganore JM, Hanson SR, Harker LA. Selective inhibition by a synthetic hirudin peptide of fibrin-dependent thrombosis in baboons. Proc Natl Acad Sci USA 88:1177, 1991.

281. Kelly AB, Maraganore JM, Bourdon P, Hanson SR, Harker LA. Antithrombotic effects of synthetic peptides targeting various functional domains of thrombin. Proc Natl Acad Sci USA 89:6040, 1992.

282. Knabb RM, Kettner CA, Timmermans PB, Reilly TM. In vivo characterization of a new synthetic thrombin inhibitor. Thromb Haemost 67:56, 1992.

283. Jang IK, Gold HK, Ziskind AA, Leinbach RC, Fallon JT, Collen D. Prevention of platelet-rich arterial thrombosis by selective thrombin inhibition. Circulation 81:219, 1990.

284. Okamoto S, Hijikata A, Kikumoto R, et al. Potent inhibition of thrombin by the newly synthesized arginine derivative No. 805. The importance of stereostructure of its hydrophobic carboxamide portion. Biochem Biophys Res Commun 101:440, 1981.

285. Gold HK, Torres FW, Garabedian HD, et al. Evidence for a rebound coagulation phenomenon after cessation of a 4-hour infusion of a specific thrombin inhibitor in patients with unstable angina pectoris. J Am Coll Cardiol 21:1039, 1993.

286. Garabedian H, Gold HK, Hagstrom JN, Collen D, Bovill EG. Accelerated thrombin generation accompanying specific thrombin inhibition in unstable angina pectoris. Circulation 88:I264, 1993.

287. Willerson JT, Casscells W. Thrombin inhibitors in unstable angina: Rebound or continuation of angina after argatroban withdrawal? [editorial; comment]. J Am Coll Cardiol 21:1048, 1993.

288. Tabata H, Mizuno K, Miyamoto A, et al. The effect of a new thrombin inhibitor (Argatroban) in the prevention of reocclusion after reperfusion therapy in patients with acute myocardial infarction. Circulation 86:I260, 1992.

289. Kettner C, Shaw E. D-Phe-Pro-ArgCH2Cl-A selective affinity label for thrombin. Thromb Res 14:969, 1979.

290. Hauptmann J, Markwardt F. Pharmacologic aspects of the development of selective synthetic thrombin inhibitors as anticoagulants. Semin Thromb Hemost 18:200, 1992.

291. Collen D, Matsuo O, Stassen JM, Kettner C, Shaw E. In vivo studies of a synthetic inhibitor of thrombin. J Lab Clin Med 99:76, 1982.

292. Waxman L, Smith DE, Arcuri KE, Vlasuk GP. Tick anticoagulant peptide (TAP) is a novel inhibitor of blood coagulation factor Xa. Science 248:593, 1990. [Published erratum appears in Science 248:1473, 1990.

293. Tuszynski GP, Gasic TB, Gasic GJ. Isolation and characterization of antistasin. An inhibitor of metastasis and coagulation. J Biol Chem 262:9718, 1987.

294. Vlasuk GP. Structural and functional characterization of tick anticoagulant peptide (TAP): A potent and selective inhibitor of blood coagulation factor Xa. Thromb Haemost 70:212, 1993.

295. Dunwiddie C, Thornberry NA, Bull HG, et al. Antistasin, a leech-derived inhibitor of factor Xa. Kinetic analysis of enzyme inhibition and identification of the reactive site. J Biol Chem 264:16694, 1989.

296. Sitko GR, Ramjit DR, Stabilito II, Lehman D, Lynch JJ, Vlasuk GP. Conjunctive enhancement of enzymatic thrombolysis and prevention of thrombotic reocclusion with the selective factor Xa inhibitor, tick anticoagulant peptide. Comparison to hirudin and heparin in a canine model of acute coronary artery thrombosis. Circulation 85:805, 1992.

297. Mellott MJ, Holahan MA, Lynch JJ, Vlasuk GP, Dunwiddie CT. Acceleration of recombinant tissue-type plasminogen activator-induced reperfusion and prevention of reocclusion by recombinant antistasin, a selective factor Xa inhibitor, in a canine model of femoral arterial thrombosis. Circ Res 70:1152, 1992.

298. Nemerson Y. Tissue factor and hemostasis. Blood 71:1, 1988. [Published erratum appears in Blood 71:1178, 1988.]

299. Rapaport SI. The extrinsic pathway inhibitor: A regulator of tissue factor-dependent blood coagulation. Thromb Haemost 66:6, 1991.

300. Esmon CT. The roles of protein C and thrombomodulin in the regulation of blood coagulation. J Biol Chem 264:4743, 1989.

301. Fenton JWD. Regulation of thrombin generation and functions. Semin Thromb Hemost 14:234, 1988.

302. Esmon CT. The regulation of natural anticoagulant pathways. Science 235:1348, 1987.

303. de Fouw NJ, de Jong YF, Haverkate F, Bertina RM. Activated protein C increases fibrin clot lysis by neutralization of plasminogen activator inhibitor — no evidence for a cofactor role of protein S. Thromb Haemost 60:328, 1988.

304. Schachinger V, Allert M, Kasper W, Just H, Vach W, Zeiher AM. Adjunctive intracoronary infusion of antithrombin III during percutaneous transluminal coronary angioplasty. Results of a prospective, randomized trial. Circulation 90:2258, 1994.

305. Vu TK, Hung DT, Wheaton VI, Coughlin SR. Molecular cloning of a functional thrombin receptor reveals a novel proteolytic mechanism of receptor activation. Cell 64:1057, 1991.

306. Coughlin SR, Vu TK, Hung DT, Wheaton VI. Characterization of a functional thrombin receptor. Issues and opportunities. J Clin Invest 89:351, 1992.

307. Vassallo RR Jr, Kieber-Emmons T, Cichowski K, Brass LF. Structure-function relationships in the activation of platelet thrombin receptors by receptor-derived peptides. J Biol Chem 267:6081, 1992.
308. Fiore LD, Deykin D. Use of antiplatelet agents and anticoagulants in post-myocardial infarction. Cardiol Clin 12:451, 1994.
309. Rihal CS, Flather M, Jirsh J, Yusuf S. Advances in antithrombotic drug therapy for coronary artery disease. Eur Heart J 16 (Suppl. D):10, 1995.
310. Fareed J, Hoppensteadt D, Walenga JM, Bick RL. Current trends in the development of anticoagulant and antithrombotic drugs. Med Clin North Am 78:713, 1994.
311. Bertrand M, Allain H, Lablanche J. Results of a randomized trial of ticlopidine versus placebo for prevention of actue closure and restenosis after coronary angioplasty (PTCA) The TACT study. Circulation 82:III190, 1990.

45. CLINICAL TRIALS OF NOVEL ANTITHROMBOTICS: BASIC CONCEPTS OF STUDY DESIGN AND METHODOLOGY

Melvin E. Tan and Robert A. Harrington

Overview of Hemostasis and Thrombosis

When the normally smooth endothelial surface of a blood vessel is denuded by the rupture of an atherosclerotic plaque or during the course of percutaneous coronary intervention, this triggers a cascade of events culminating in thrombus formation. Endothelial disruption leads to exposure of adhesive glycoproteins, such as collagen, von Willebrand factor (vWF), fibronectin, laminin, vitronectin, and subendothelial thrombospondin, to which circulating inactivated platelets adhere. This occurs largely through membrane glycoprotein (GP) Ib–factor IX binding to vWF immobilized onto subendothelial structures. These platelets are then activated by local agonists, which include epinephrine, adenosine diphosphate (ADP), collagen, serotonin, and thrombin. Platelet activation induces an active conformational change in the surface GPIIb/IIIa receptors; conferring on them a high affinity for fibrinogen, vWF, and other adhesive glycoproteins; and resulting in platelet aggregation and consequent thrombosis. This conformational change in the platelet GPIIb/IIIa receptor is believed to be the final common pathway by which all agonists act to initiate platelet aggregation.

Excessive deposition and aggregation of platelets and the ensuing formation of a platelet-rich thrombus results in vascular occlusion, leading to ischemia or infarction in the acute coronary syndromes, or to abrupt closure and restenosis after percutaneous coronary angioplasty [1,2]. This was first described by DeWood and colleagues almost 16 years ago [3], when they demonstrated the presence of thrombotic occlusion in early transmural myocardial infarction.

Thus, it would seem logical to make the platelet and thrombus the targets of interventions designed to manage unstable angina, acute myocardial infarction,

and ischemic complications after percutaneous transluminal coronary angioplasty (PTCA). Given the extensive amount of clinical research centering on the use of antiplatelet therapy over the last decade, this chapter focuses on these antiplatelet agents to explain the role of clinical trials in cardiovascular drug development. In particular, the clinical evolution of the platelet GPIIb/IIIa receptor inhibitors is highlighted as an example of novel antithrombotic drug development. In this chapter we present the clinical problem, discuss basic concepts of the randomized clinical trial, review typical cardiovascular drug development strategy, and cover the progress "from bench to bedside" of the GPIIb/IIIa inhibitors.

Overview of Antithrombotic Therapy

By definition, antithrombotics are drugs that block thrombus formation. They may be further classified as antiplatelet agents, antithrombin agents, and fibrinolytic agents. Aspirin and ticlopidine are currently the mainstay of oral antiplatelet therapy, while heparin and warfarin are established anticoagulant drugs. Although clinically effective and useful, all currently available antithrombotic agents have significant limitations to their use.

In the late 1950s and early 1960s, aspirin was shown to exhibit a mild hemostatic effect by inhibiting collagen-induced platelet aggregation and secondary aggregation to weak agonists such as ADP and epinephrine. While aspirin has been found to be a relatively weak inhibitor of platelet aggregation, principally because its effect is limited to blockade of thromboxane-A_2 formation through its irreversible acetylation of cyclooxygenase, it has been in widespread clinical use after clinical trials demonstrated its effectiveness in primary and secondary prevention of ischemic heart disease and cerebrovascular disease [4].

Resistance to heparin therapy reflects, at least in part, a failure to inactivate enzymatically active thrombin bound to fibrin and the subendothelial matrix, as well as its reduced availability due to neutralization from binding to proteins such as platelet factor-4 [5]. These limitations have galvanized the search for, and development of, newer, more specific antithrombotic strategies.

Understanding Clinical Trials: Basic Concepts

As with all therapeutic modalities, the contemporary management of many aspects of cardiovascular disease depends on the results of valid clinical trials. The randomized clinical trial (RCT) forms the foundation of our knowledge in understanding the role that novel therapies play in the management of complex disease processes. RCTs have provided the evidence required to practice rational, fact-based medicine. New therapeutics, techniques, and devices need to be exposed to the rigorous examination and scrutiny of the RCT if they are to be adopted into clinical practice. Nowhere is this more striking than in cardiovascular disease management, where a new therapy for unstable angina, for example, has the potential to be used on millions of new patients per year globally.

Traditionally, drug development originates with an understanding of a pathophysiologic pathway; then new agents are developed that affect that pathway. In such a pathophysiologic model, new therapeutics could then be used clinically after being tested in a relatively small number of actual patients with the disease process. Experience with antiarrhythmic agents to suppress premature ventricular contractions after myocardial infarction demonstrates the potential folly of this approach [6]. The new model for cardiovascular drug development will require large-scale RCTs, adequately powered, and needs to be designed to determine if the new therapy affects meaningful clinical outcomes (such as mortality or myocardial infarction) in large populations with the disease in question.

Cardiovascular Drug Development

Over the past 30 years, most therapeutic innovations in cardiovascular disease have been instituted only after careful consideration of the results of clinical trials. This attests to the importance, effectiveness, and clinical utility of these trials and the pivotal role

they have in clinical decision making. The development of any drug is a complicated process, because the drug undergoes an exhaustive sequence of stages prior to its approval for widespread clinical use.

The initial stage of drug development involves preclinical testing, when detailed investigations into the drug's pharmacologic and toxicological profile are undertaken. This includes descriptions of the drug's composition and source, manufacturing process, and toxicity, as well as its mutagenicity and carcinogenecity. Only after this stringent (preclinical testing) process has demonstrated that the investigational drug will pose no unreasonable risk to human subjects will it proceed to the clinical trial stages.

Traditionally, novel drugs have gone through three phases of clinical development, progressing from one phase to the next, with each phase providing the data required to proceed to the next one [7]. Each stage, therefore, has unique characteristics and goals; an appropriate study is designed with these goals in mind (Table 45-1).

Phase I clinical studies represent the initial use of an investigational drug in human subjects and is primarily focused on establishing the drug's clinical safety. These trials are typically conducted in normal volunteers or individuals with mild but stable disease, with enrollment typically numbering less than 100 participants. Phase I trials are designed to determine the metabolic and pharmacological actions of the drugs in humans, the side effects associated with increased doses, and, where possible, to gain early evidence of the drug's efficacy. Other aims of phase I trials are the study of a drug's pharmacokinetics, its structure–activity relationships, and mechanism of action in humans; in other phase I studies, investigational drugs are used as research tools to explore biological phenomena or disease processes.

Phase II trials are designed to assess the safety of the agent in patients who actually have the disease of interest. Additionally, these trials are designed to determine if the drug may be clinically effective. While not typically adequately powered to provide definitive clinical outcome data, these trials may provide trend evidence that a drug has effects making it worthwhile to pursue in a larger scale trial.

These trials include studies to evaluate the effectiveness of the drug for indications in patients with the relevant disease, and to determine the short-term side effects and risks associated with the drug. Phase II studies are controlled investigations, whereby the experimental drug is directly compared with a placebo or prevailing standard therapy. Because the safety and side-effect profiles of the drug are sill largely unknown, these trials are usually limited to a

TABLE 45-1. Completed clinical trials of
platelet glycoprotein IIb/IIIa receptor blockers

Name of trial/ Investigator	Agent	Patient population
EPIC	Abciximab	High-risk PTCA
EPILOG	Abciximab	PTCA
CAPTURE	Abciximab	PTCA in unstable angina
Schulman	Eptifibatide	Unstable angina
IMPACT	Eptifibatide	PTCA
IMPACT II	Eptifibatide	PTCA
IMPACT-AMI	Eptifibatide	Acute myocardial infarction
Theroux	Lamifiban	Unstable angina
Kereiakes	Tirofiban	High-risk PTCA
RESTORE	Tirofiban	PTCA

PTCA = percutaneous transluminal coronary angioplasty.

TABLE 45-2. Clinical trials of platelet
glycoprotein IIb/IIIa receptor blockers in progress

Name of Trial/ Investigator	Agent	Patient population
ERASER	Abciximab	Stent
RAPPORT	Abciximab	Acute myocardial infarction
PURSUIT	Eptifibatide	Unstable angina
PARAGON	Lamifiban	Unstable angina
PARADIGM4	Lamifiban	Acute myocardial infarction
PRISM	Tirofiban	Unstable angina
ORBIT	Xemlofiban	PTCA

PTCA = percutaneous transluminal coronary angioplasty.

Phase	Subjects	Goals	Numbers studied
I	Normal volunteers	Dose tolerability Toxicity	<10–50
II	Patients	Drug activity Understand biology Toxicity Efficacy	10s–100s
III	Patients	Efficacy Safety	100s–1000s

FIGURE 45-1. ••.

small subject group, usually 10 to several hundred subjects. Typically these small trials collect a large amount of information on each subject as an agent's safety profile develops.

Phase III clinical trials are definitive studies involving large numbers of patients and are designed to determine the effectiveness, safety, and optimal dosing regimen of the drug. These studies serve to gather the additional information needed to evaluate the overall benefit–risk relationship of the drug, and to form the basis for the regulatory approval process of an investigational agent. Definitive phase III randomized clinical trials may involve tens of thousands of patients, enrolled at hospitals around the world. Data collection on each patient is less extensive due to the number of patients and centers involved, but what these large trials lack in precision they make up by providing definitive answers to pertinent clinical questions. Typically these types of trials are directed at determining a treatment's effect on "hard" clinical endpoints, such as mortality or major morbid events, such as myocardial infarction.

Topol and Califf have described two types of clinical trial designs, each with distinctive characteristics and each with its own advantages and disadvantages: These are the smaller (mini-)trials and the larger (mega-)trials [8]. A distinct advantage of the megatrial is that the recruitment of large numbers of patients will obviate the need for in-depth data collection, measurement of pathophysiologic endpoints, and specification of ancillary therapy. This approach avoids unnecessary data and arrives at the crux of the matter, that is, the effect this new therapy has on the clinical outcomes of patients with the particular disease state.

The large thrombolytic trials performed in the mid-1980s paved the way for the concept of the large, simple trial [9,10]. These trials relied on large numbers of hospitals and investigators to enroll a broad spectrum of patients with acute myocardial infarction in randomized trials of thrombolysis versus placebo. Data collection was limited to recording some simple baseline variables and a reporting of mortality on a simple one-page form. The power of such studies is that a large number of patients randomly distributed among treatment groups can provide definitive evidence about the risks and effectiveness of a treatment in a commonly occurring disease, such as acute myocardial infarction. The limitation with these trials is that little information, other than that dealing with the primary endpoint, can be learned from the collected data.

Another type of large trial is exemplified by the Global Utilization of Streptokinase and t-PA for Occluded Coronary Arteries (GUSTO) trial [11]. In this multicenter international trial of four thrombolytic strategies for treating acute myocardial infarction, more than 40,000 patients were enrolled at approximately 1000 hospitals around the world. While overall simplicity was maintained, with a three-page case report form and limited on-site data monitoring, enough data were collected to address a number of interesting and potentially clinically pertinent questions of the study population. To date, more than 100 manuscripts have been written/submitted using the GUSTO dataset. Additionally, the GUSTO

angiographic substudy is an excellent example of how well-designed substudies conducted within a much larger trial can provide important mechanistic data that may help explain the overall trial treatment results. In GUSTO, the angiographic substudy clearly demonstrated that achieving brisk, TIMI 3 flow in the infarct vessel was associated with the best 30-day mortality rate, and that accelerated tissue plasminogen activator (t-PA) had the greatest likelihood of leading to TIMI 3 flow by 90 minutes [12,13].

Development of the Glycoprotein IIb/IIIa Inhibitors

Owing to the pivotal role it plays in the platelet-rich, thrombin-dependent coagulation process leading to thrombus formation, blockade of glycoprotech (GP) IIb/IIIa receptors has emerged as a powerful new therapeutic strategy in preventing platelet-dependent thrombosis. As such, GPIIb/IIIa inhibitors may play a role in the treatment of patients with acute coronary syndromes or those undergoing percutaneous coroanry intervention. The GPIIb/IIIa receptor is a calcium-dependent, noncovalently associated α/β heterodimer that belongs to the integrin family. This receptor interacts with ligands containing the tripeptide arginine-glycine-asparagine (Arg-Gly-Asp; RGD) recognition sequence, of which at least four are known: fibrinogen, vWF, fibronectin, and vitronectin.

The binding of fibrinogen to its binding sites on the GPIIb/IIIa receptor occurs only when the latter is in its conformational state; this requires the presence of extracellular Ca^{2+}, platelet agonist-mediated activation of phospholipase C, and the resultant increase in protein kinase C and intracellular Ca^{2+}. However, unlike intact fibrinogen, synthetic RGD-containing peptides bind to the GPIIb/IIIa receptor, even in its inactive state, thus allowing these agents to be used as competitive antagonists. Inhibitors of the GPIIb/IIIa receptor include laboratory-derived monoclonal antibodies against the receptor, naturally occurring RGD-containing peptides derived from snake venoms, and synthetic RGD-containing peptides and peptidomimetics that compete with fibrinogen for GPIIb/IIIa binding sites on the platelet surface [14–16].

Monoclonal Antibodies Against the GPIIb/IIIa Receptor

The development and discovery of the monoclonal antibody fragment abciximab (Reopro, Centocor,

Malvern PA; Eli Lilly, Indianapolis IN) have recently been detailed by Coller [17]. Coller and colleagues were the first to establish the cloned cell line for the monoclonal antibody 7E3 as a new and potentially valuable antiplatelet agent. The early murine antibody was felt to be too immunogenic to be useful as a human therapeutic agent; the Fc region of the antibody was subsequently cleaved off to produce an F(ab')2 fragment, which was then joined with the constant regions of human immunoglobulin to form the chimeric compound c7E3 (abciximab).

Coller and his colleagues were the first to describe virtually complete inhibition of platelet aggregation using this approach to GPIIb/IIIa inhibition in a canine model [17]. Early dose-finding/escalation and platelet aggregation and receptor occupancy studies in animal models suggested that significant platelet inhibition to <20% of baseline was achieved with blockade of >80% of platelet GPIIb/IIIa receptors. These biological findings formed the basis for subsequent testing of the drug in human clinical trials. The clinical development of abciximab might serve as a model of drug development in the antithrombotic arena. It was based on a solid basic science understanding of the role of GPIIb/IIIa in the process of platelet aggregation. From there, testing in animal models laid the groundwork for future trials by demonstrating that vascular thrombosis could be prevented or diminished using such an agent. A clinical problem was then identified that seemed to depend on platelet aggregation and subsequent coronary thrombus formation (i.e., percutaneous coronary intervention). Next, small dose-finding and feasibility studies were performed to look for evidence of the biological effects of the drug in a "real" clinical situation. Finally, a series of large, definitive phase III trials demonstrated the clinical utility of the drug in preventing the ischemic complications of coronary angioplasty.

Naturally Occurring RGD-Containing Peptides

Wile monoclonal antibody fragments directed against the GPIIb/IIIa receptor were the first agents to be developed as GPIIb/IIIa-specific platelet antagonists, there is a family of peptides that has been isolated from several varieties of snake venom. Known as the disintegrins, trigramin, bitistatin, echistatin, kirstin, and applaggin have been found to inhibit concentration-dependent ex vivo platelet aggregation. However, their clinical utility beyond the laboratory is limited by the fact that they are immunogenic and they cause transient thrombocytopenia. A similar polypeptide known as Barbourin, which was isolated from the southwestern pygmy rattlesnake (*Sistrurus m Barbouri*), was found to be more specific for binding to the GPIIb/IIIa receptor than are others in the disintegrin family. This specificity derives from a substitution of the arginine residue on the RGD sequence by lysine, forming a KGD recognition sequence. This important discovery formed the basis for the development of synthetic peptide GPIIb/IIIa inhibitors containing this tripeptide recognition sequence [18,19].

Synthetic GPIIb/IIIa Inhibitors

These compounds compete with fibrinogen for GPIIb/IIIa binding sites and produce concentration-dependent inhibition of platelet aggregation. When these agents are synthesized in a cyclical configuration, their affinity for the GPIIb/IIIa receptor is markedly increased and becomes similar to that of the naturally occurring compounds derived from snake venom [20]. When compared with the disintegrins and the monoclonal antibody compounds, the synthetic GPIIb/IIIa antagonists demonstrate a higher selectivity for the GPIIb/IIIa receptor, show less crossreactivity with the vitronectin receptors ($\alpha v \beta 3$) on endothelial cells, and are less immunogenic. The synthetic compounds also have a shorter half-life than c7E3, the prototypical monoclonal antibody GPIIb/IIIa inhibitor.

Another approach in the development of GPIIb/IIIa inhibitors has been the synthesis of nonpeptide compounds bearing the RGD recognition sequence. These include SC-5468A (Xemlofiban) [21], MK-383 (Tirofiban) [22], and RO-449583 (Lamifiban) [23]. Like the synthetic inhibitors, these peptidomimetic agents demonstrate high selectivity for the GPIIb/IIIa receptor and produce dose-dependent inhibition of these receptors. Because these compounds are not peptides, and therefore not subject to easy gastric enzymatic digestion, it is possible to configure the agents to be given orally.

GPIIb/IIIa Inhibitors in Coronary Angioplasty

Percutaneous coronary intervention provided the first clinical condition for safety and efficacy testing of this novel class of antithrombotics. This development path was chosen for several reasons. There are two major limitations of the angioplasty procedure: early abrupt vessel closure and late restenosis. These two complications account for most of the morbidity and mortality associated with PTCA, and exert a tremendous clinical and economic burden on the health care system [24]. Both abrupt closure and restenosis are at least partly mediated by platelet-dependent thrombosis, making them potentially affectable through platelet inhibition. The clinical development of abciximab exemplifies the study of a novel antithrombotic in a human disease state, and provides valuable information on not only the understanding of the drug's usefulness but also on the biology of the disease state as well.

Ellis and colleagues reported one of the first clinical trials of GPIIb/IIIa inhibition in patients undergoing elective coronary angioplasty [26]. This trial enrolled 28 patients, 23 of whom received the murine monoclonal antibody m7E3 Fab, while 5 received placebo. The patients were divided into groups of four to six patients, with each group receiving incremental doses of m7E3 of 0.15, 0.20, 0.25, 0.30, and 0.35 mg/kg immediately before angioplasty. The investigators found that no patient who received m7E3 Fab experienced a thrombotic complication after PTCA, while a single patient developed a small retroperitoneal and femoral hematoma, and another patient required red cell transfusion. Laboratory measurements of platelet function demonstrated that the degree of GPIIb/IIIa receptor blockade, as well as the ability to inhibit aggregation, increased with the dose and decreased with time after infusion. The promising conclusions of this study led to further investigations of this monoclonal antibody in the setting of percutaneous coronary intervention.

A subsequent dose-finding trial used the chimeric monoclonal antibody 7E3 Fab (c7E3 Fab, abciximab) [27]. This multicenter, open-label, dose-finding study enrolled 56 patients who were scheduled for elective coronary angioplasty and who were angiographically deemed to have high-risk lesions. The trial demonstrated that the blockade of platelet GPIIb/IIIa receptors is dose dependent; it also established that the effective suppression of platelet aggregation required a bolus dose of 0.25 mg/kg of c7E3 Fab, and that this suppression could be sustained for up to 24 hours by a continuous 12 hour infusion. These two trials paved the way for a large, definitive, phase III clinical trial of abciximab in high-risk coronary intervention.

EPIC Trial

The Evaluation of c7E3 Fab in the Prevention of Ischemic Complications (EPIC) trial was a landmark study, establishing the benefits of abciximab in preventing major ischemic complications in patients undergoing coronary angioplasty who were felt to be at risk for abrupt vessel closure [28]. This prospective, randomized, double-blind multicenter trial enrolled 2099 angioplasty patients who were at high risk of developing ischemic complications. The study's primary composite endpoint at 30 days was the occurrence of death, nonfatal myocardial infarction, coronary artery bypass grafting of repeat percutaneous intervention for acute ischemia, insertion of a coronary stent because of procedural failure, or placement of an intraaortic balloon pump for the treatment of refractory ischemia. The patients were assigned equally to one of three treatment groups: a 0.25 mg/kg bolus of c7E3 followed by a 12-hour infusion of 10 µg/min; a bolus dose of 0.25 mg/kg of c7E3, followed by a placebo infusion; or a placebo bolus and infusion. There was a statistically significant and clinically important 35% reduction of the primary endpoint event rate in the abciximab bolus and infusion group compared with placebo. A nonsignificant (10%) reduction in the composite event rate was observed with the abciximab bolus alone as compared with placebo, suggesting that when given at time of angioplasty, potent antiplatelet therapy must inhibit platelet aggregation for 20–24 hours if it is to exert a meaningful clinical effect. All components of the primary endpoint were positively affected by administration of abciximab, and the subset of patients with acute ischemic syndromes received the greatest overall benefit [29,30].

Not only were these impressive beneficial effects of abciximab sustained to 6 months, but there was an additional treatment effect conferred by abciximab to this secondary endpoint [31]. This has prompted some to call this a *passivation* of the arterial surface that takes place at the time of the initial procedure, with the antiplatelet agent positively affecting the clinical restenosis process.

There was, however, in EPIC a doubling of major bleeding events, including the need for red blood cell transfusions, in the patients treated with abciximab bolus plus infusion. Further analysis of these data revealed that certain clinical variables, such as age, gender (female), and body weight, were predictive of bleeding complications; excessive use of procedural heparin correlated with bleeding as well [32]. It was postulated that when giving GPIIb/IIIa inhibitors during coronary intervention, less concomitant heparin could be used while maintaining procedural efficacy and improving safety outcomes. Confirmation of the long-term effect, expansion of the eligible patient population, and resolution of the bleeding issue, were guiding principles in the design of the EPIC follow-up trials: PROLOG and EPILOG.

EPILOG Trial

After a small pilot trial (PROLOG) demonstrated the safety and feasibility of performing coronary intervention with lower heparin regimens than traditionally used, a larger clinical trial was undertaken [33]. The Evaluation of PTCA to Improve Long-term Outcome by c7E3 GPIIb/IIIa receptor blockade (EPILOG) trial was a multicenter, randomized, double-blind, placebo-controlled trial designed to compare the concomitant administration of abciximab and two different dosing regimens of heparin in all non–high-risk patients undergoing percutaneous coronary intervention. Patients were randomized to one of three treatment arms: a 0.25 mg/kg bolus and a 0.125 μg/kg/h infusion of c7E3 with standard-dose weight-adjusted heparin; a 0.25 mg/kg bolus and a 0.125 μg/kg/h infusion of c7E3 with low-dose weight-adjusted heparin; or placebo and standard-dose weight-adjusted heparin.

The primary efficacy endpoint of the study was a composite of death, myocardial infarction, and repeat revascularization (surgical or percutaneous) within 30 days or within 6 months of randomization. Although the study was initially scheduled to enroll 4500 patients, an independent Data and Safety Monitoring Board advised that it be stopped prematurely because of the overwhelming treatment benefit found in the abciximab-treated group in an analysis of the first 1500 patients enrolled in the trial [34]. Importantly, there was a greater than 60% reduction in the risk of death or myocardial infarction in patients treated with abciximab compared with placebo, with the lowest incidence of bleeding in the patients treated with abciximab and low-dose heparin. The final results of EPILOG are pending but these preliminary data speak to the overwhelming benefits of platelet GPIIb/IIIa inhibition with abciximab during coronary intervention.

CAPTURE Trial

In a pilot study, Simoons and colleagues reported the use of abciximab in the clinical setting of refractory unstable angina [35]. They enrolled 60 patients with at least one episode of angina and dynamic ST-segment–T-wave changes, and at least one other episode of angina occurring despite bed rest and aggressive medical therapy. These patients were randomized to receive a double-blinded bolus and infusion of either abciximab or placebo. All patients were also treated with aspirin, intravenous nitrates, and intravenous heparin. Despite the small numbers in this pilot feasibility trial, patients in the abciximab group had significantly lower in-hospital event rates of death, myocardial infarction, and recurrent ischemia requiring urgent intervention.

Following this pilot trial, the c7E3 Anti-Platelet Therapy in Unstable REfractory angina (CAPTURE) trial planned to enroll 1400 patients with refractory unstable angina scheduled to undergo PTCA. Patients were to be randomized to receive either abciximab or placebo, and the drugs were to be administered for approximately 24 hours prior to the intervention and continued for an hour after the procedure. Initially, two interim analyses were planned, to be conducted after enrollment reached 350 and 700 patients, but the independent Data and Safety Monitoring Committee recommended an additional analysis at 1050 patients. At this point the committee recommended that the trial be terminated prematurely because of the significant benefit demonstrated in patients who received abciximab [36]. When the study was stopped in December 1995, 1266 patients had been enrolled; a review of the preliminary data revealed that the primary composite endpoint of death, myocardial infarction, or urgent revascularization occurred in 16.4% placebo patients, compared with 10.8% of patients who received abciximab ($P = 0.0064$).

Thus it appears that abciximab, when given to a broad spectrum of patients undergoing percutaneous coronary intervention, is associated with very significant reductions (30–50+%) in the major ischemic complications of angioplasty, and with a continued improvement in clinical outcomes through at least 6 months of follow-up. Additionally, with careful attention to heparin dosing, these beneficial effects can be achieved without major increases in the risk of serious bleeding.

Peptide and Nonpeptide Inhibitors of GPIIb/IIIa

There are several synthetic peptide and peptidomimetic inhibitors of platelet GPIIb/IIIa in various stages of clinical development. Like abciximab, the focus of their early development has been in the setting of percutaneous coronary intervention. These agents are interesting in themselves, and also because of how they compare and contrast with abciximab. Whereas abciximab is a noncompetitive inhibitor of GPIIb/IIIa, and also acts against other cell receptors, the synthetic inhibitors are competitive inhibitors and highly selective against GPIIb/IIIa. Given the impressive clinical results of abciximab, one can postulate that comparisons among agents with differing mechanisms of action will lend some insight into the pathophysiology behind the acute and long-term complications of the angioplasty procedure.

Eptifibatide: A Peptide Inhibitor of GPIIb/IIIa

Eptifibatide, (Integrilin, Cor Therapeutics South Sea Franciso, CA) a cyclic heptapeptide containing a modified KGD sequence, has been extensively studied for use in preventing the ischemic complications of coronary angioplasty. The Integrilin to Minimize Platelet Aggregation in Coronary Thrombosis (IMPACT) study [37] was a multicenter, randomized, double-blind trial, enrolling 150 patients undergoing elective coronary angioplasty. Patients were randomly assigned to one of three treatment strategies: placebo; a 90 μg/kg bolus of Integrilin prior to commencement of angioplasty, followed by a 1.0 μg/kg/min infusion of the drug for 4 hours; and the 90 μ/kg bolus, followed by a 1.0 μg/kg/min infusion of the drug for 12 hours. IMPACT was a safety and feasibility pilot trial with a primary efficacy composite endpoint of all-cause mortality, myocardial infarction, urgent or emergency coronary intervention, stent implantation, or coronary artery bypass surgery for ischemia or threatened closure. Bleeding events, including transfusion requirements, were also recorded. Administration of the 90 μg/kg eptifibatide bolus resulted in an 86% inhibition of platelet aggregation, which was maintained by the 1.0 μg/kg/min infusion. There were no differences in the rate of major bleeding among the three groups, while there was a trend toward an increased incidence of minor bleeding in the eptifibatide-treated patients.

A second phase II trial on eptifibatide in coronary intervention, IMPACT HIGH/low, was carried out to better define the clinical pharmacokinetic and pharmacodynamic effects of the drug in the angioplasty population. The trial enrolled 73 patients and provided the information for the dose selection for the follow-up phase III trial: IMPACT II [38].

IMPACT II Trial

This was a multicenter, randomized, double-blind, placebo-controlled trial that enrolled 4010 low- and high-risk patients who underwent elective, urgent, and emergency percutaneous coronary intervention with any U.S. Food and Drug Administration (FDA)-approved device [39]. Patients were randomized to receive one of three treatment regimens: a 135 μg/kg bolus followed by a 0.75 μg/kg/min 24-hour infusion of eptifibatide, a 135 μg/kg bolus followed by a 0.5 μg/kg/min infusion of eptifibatide over 24 hours,

or placebo bolus plus infusion. All patients received aspirin and heparin. The primary endpoint was a composite at 30 days of death, myocardial infarction, repeat urgent or emergency intervention (percutaneous or surgical), or stent placement for threatened or actual abrupt vessel closure. Patients were followed for 6 months to record the occurrence of death, myocardial infarction, or any repeat procedure. Assessment of bleeding was the primary safety endpoint.

There was approximately a 19% reduction in primary endpoint events in the low-dose eptifibatide group compared with the placebo group (11.4% vs. 9.2%, $P = 0.063$) and a 13% reduction comparing the high dose with placebo (11.4% vs. 9.9%, $P = 0.22$). There was no increase in bleeding in the eptifibatide-treated patients compared with placebo, as measured by the TIMI criteria or transfusion requirement. The reduction in the clinical outcome events was consistent across all components of the composite endpoint. Additionally, the beneficial effects of eptifibatide, particularly its effect on reducing rates of death and myocardial infarction, were maintained at the 6-month follow-up point. Overall, the results of the IMPACT II trial confirm that platelet GPIIb/IIIa inhibition can improve acute ischemic complications of percutaneous coronary intervention. The more modest results seen with eptifibatide compared with abciximab can best be explained by lack of optimized dosing, an inadequate duration of the treatment effect, or the differing mechanism of action of the antibody versus either the peptide or nonpeptide inhibitors. Further investigation is required to determine the appropriate explanation for the findings.

Platelet GPIIb/IIIa Inhibitors: Acute Coronary Syndromes

In addition to use with coronary angioplasty, GPIIb/IIIa receptor blocker use has been extended to other clinical syndromes in which platelet-dependent thrombosis is thought to play a major role in pathogenesis. There is extensive clinical evidence supporting the role of antiplatelet therapy in improving outcomes in patients with both acute myocardial infarction and unstable angina.

In a phase II trial of the murine monoclonal antibody 7E3 [39], Gold and colleagues subdivided 16 patients with unstable angina into four groups, each of which received progressively escalating intravenous bolus doses of m7E3 F(ab')2 at 0.05, 0.10, 0.15, and 0.20 mg/kg. Patients were enrolled if they had rest angina lasting less than 30 minutes during the last 6 days before entry into the study, with electrocardiographic changes and angiographic evidence of at least a 50% diameter stenosis in the ischemia-related artery. They found that with the 0.2 mg/kg bolus, about 87% of GPIIb/IIIa receptors were blocked, with progressive recovery over time. Also, at this concentration of the bolus dose, the template bleeding time was significantly prolonged without significant clinical effects (bleeding).

Schulman and colleagues reported the first clinical trial results of eptifibatide in unstable angina [40]. This relatively small phase II trial found that patients who had received the higher dose eptifibatide had significantly fewer ischemic events (as determined by continuous Holter monitoring) than those in the placebo group, while the low-dose eptifibatide group had intermediate benefits compared with placebo-treated patients. A second dose-finding study of eptifibatide in unstable angina defined the pharmacodynamic and pharmacokinetic profiles of a broader range of eptifibatide [42]. These two trials formed the basis for pursuing the investigation of eptifibatide in unstable angina in a much larger, definitive clinical endpoint trial.

The PURSUIT (Platelet IIb/IIIa Unstable Angina Receptor Suppression Using Integrelin Therapy) trial will test the benefits of eptifibatide in patients with unstable angina and non–Q-wave myocardial infarction. All patients will be given aspirin and heparin, and will be randomized to receive a bolus and infusion of placebo, high-dose eptifibatide, or low-dose integrelin for up to 96 hours. The primary endpoint of PURSUIT is death or myocardial reinfarction at 30 days. Enrollment is ongoing and will continue until approximately 10,400 patients have been randomized. PURSUIT will be the first large-scale trial of a GPIIb/IIIa inhibitor in the broad spectrum of patients presenting with ischemic chest pain and without acute, persistent ST-segment elevation.

Theroux et al. have reported the preliminary experience of Lamifiban, a nonpeptide GPIIb/IIIa inhibitor, in patients with unstable angina [42]. This was a safety and dose-ranging study of four doses of Lamifiban bolus plus infusion compared with placebo. All patients received aspirin, and heparin was given at the discretion of the physician investigator. The results demonstrate the dose-dependent effect of Lamifiban in inhibiting ex-vivo platelet aggregation. Additionally, there were favorable trends toward the reduction of clinical ischemic events in the Lamifiban-treated patients compared with placebo. With this as a background, a large-scale effort to test the effectivess of Lamifiban in this patient population has been undertaken.

PARAGON will address the safety and efficacy of Lamifiban in patients with acute coronary syndromes without ST-segment elevation and will be divided into two independent but complementary studies. PARAGON-A will enroll approximately 2200 patients and randomize them to one of five treatment arms: heparin, low-dose Lamifiban with and without heparin, and high-dose Lamifiban with and without heparin. Patients in PARAGON-A will receive an infusion of the study drug for 72 hours and will not be eligible for catheterization in the first 24 hours of the treatment. In PARAGON-B, an optimal dosing regimen of Lamifiban with or without heparin will be chosen and compared directly to heparin in 7200 eligible patients. The PARAGON trials will thus address two important questions: Whether Lamifiban is effective and safe in patients with unstable angina, and whether concomitant heparin is required when treating patients with potent antiplatelet therapy.

There are several orally active GPIIb/IIIa inhibitors in various stages of clinical development. Many of these compounds are being evaluated for use in secondary prevention in patients with stabilized acute coronary syndromes. A number of issues with regard to dosing, level of required inhibition, duration of treatment, and safety will need to be addressed in carefully designed randomized clinical trials as part of the overall strategy to assess their effectiveness.

Use of platelet GPIIb/IIIa inhibitors is particulary attractive in the group of patients with acute ST-segment elevation myocardial infarction. Platelets seem to play a key role in the development of these syndromes, and antiplatelet therapy in the form of aspirin is a proven standard in these patients. Thrombolysis and primary angioplasty, the best-studied clinical strategies, are still associated with unacceptably high mortality rates for a disease with such high prevalence. Much of the early mortality benefit of reperfusion is related to the rapid achievement of normal coronary blood flow [44]. Additionally, the later problem of coronary reocclusion is associated with poor clinical outcomes. Potent antiplatelet therapy may attenuate these problems.

In an early animal study, Yasuda and colleagues analyzed the use of ^{125}I-labeled 7E3 F(ab')2 in preventing reocclusion in dogs with laboratory-induced coronary thrombosis who also received recombinant tissue-type plasminogen activator [44]. The infusion of rt-PA in eight dogs led to coronary artery reperfusion in all, but reocclusion occurred in all but one animal, despite anticoagulation with heparin. In contradistinction, the intravenous administration of 7E3 F(ab')2 prevented reocclusion in all 10 treated dogs.

Kleiman et al. have reported the results of the Thrombolysis and Angioplasty in Myocardial Infarction (TAMI 8) Pilot Study, which looked at the physiologic activity and safety of murine-derived monoclonal antibody 7E3 Fab in patients receiving recombinant tissue-type plasminogen activator (rt-PA) [45]. Sixty patients who fulfilled eligibility criteria for acute myocardial infarction were enrolled in the study and received rt-PA together with aspirin and heparin. They were subsequently randomized to receive either placebo or m7E3 Fab in escalating doses 3, 6, and 15 hours after the initiation of thrombolytic therapy. Effective blockade of the platelet receptor site and platelet inhibition were maximal at a dose of 0.25 mg/kg body weight of m7E3 Fab. Recurrent ischemia occurred in 13% of the m7E3-treated patients, compared with 20% of the patients who received placebo, while major bleeding occurred in 25% and 50% of the two groups, respectively. This study concluded that m7E3 Fab administration induced profound inhibition of platelet aggregation after thrombolysis, with a low rate of recurrent ischemic events, and a rate of bleeding comparable with that of control patients.

Lefkovitz reviewed the EPIC trial to look specifically at the subset of patients who underwent direct or rescue PTCA within 12 hours after the onset of an acute myocardial infarction [30]. The treatment benefit of the abciximab bolus plus infusion compared with placebo was greater in this group than in the overall trail cohort, suggesting an especially beneficial effect of the antiplatelet agent in this very high-risk patient group [••].

Dose-finding studies of both Integrilin and Lamifiban given in conjunction with thrombolysis have recently been completed [47,48]. The results of these smaller trials will form the underpinnings of larger, more definitive mortality trials of these agents. Issues that will require attention include optimal dosing, duration of treatment, thrombolytic dosage requirements, thrombolytic agent specificity, role in primary angioplasty, requirements for concomitant antithrombin therapy, and safety.

Conclusions

The use of the platelet GPIIb/IIIa receptor blockers has revolutionized the management of patients undergoing percutaneous coronary intervention, providing impressive acute and intermediate-term treatment benefits for a broad spectrum of patients. The development of the GPIIb/IIIa inhibitors might serve as a paradigm of antithrombotic drug development as an aid to understanding the application of basic laboratory findings to the clinical arena in the form of well-designed randomized clinical trials. Importantly, the lessons learned in the clinical trials have

spawned a series of new questions requiring further basic investigation. Feedback like this provides tremendous growth in the field and is an important part of the link between the basic and clinical investigative disciplines.

References

1. Steele PM, Chesebro JH, Stanson AW, Holmes DR Jr, Dewanjee MK, Badimon L, Fuster V. Balloon angioplasty. Natural history of the pathophysiological response to injury in a pig model. Circ Res 57:105, 1985.
2. Badimon L, Badimon JJ, Galvez A, Chesebro JH, Fuster V. Influence of arterial damage and wall shear rate on platelet deposition. Ex vivo study in a swine model. Arteriosclerosis 6:312, 1986.
3. DeWood MA, Spores J, Notske R, et al. Prevalence of total coronary occlusion during the early hours of transmural myocardial infarction. N Engl J Med 303:897, 1980.
4. Antiplatelet Trialists' Collaboration. Collaborative overview of randomised trials of antiplatelet therapy — II: Maintenance of vascular graft or arterial patency by antiplatelet therapy. Br Med J 308:159, 1994.
5. Hirsh J, Fuster V. Guide to anticoagulant therapy. Part 1: Heparin. American Heart Association. Circulation 89:1449, 1994.
6. Akiyama T, Pawitan Y, Greenberg H, Kuo CS, Reynolds-Haertle RA. Increased risk of death and cardiac arrest from encainide and flecainide in patients after non-Q-wave acute myocardial infarction in the Cardiac Arrhythmia Suppression Trial: CAST investigators. Am J Cardiol 68:1551, 1991.
7. Friedman LM, Furberg CD, DeMets DL. Fundamentals of Clinical Trials, 3rd ed. St. Louis, MO: Mosby-Year Book, 1996.
8. Topol EJ, Califf RM. Answers to complex questions cannot be derived from "simple" trials [see comments]. [Review] Br Heart J 68:348, 1992.
9. ISIS-2. Randomized trial of intravenous streptokinase, oral aspirin, both, or neither among 17,187 cases of suspected acute myocardial infarction: ISIS-2. J Am Coll Cardiol 12:3A, 1988.
10. GISSI. Effectiveness of intravenous thrombolytic treatment in acute myocardial infarction. Lancet 397, 1986.
11. The GUSTO Investigators. An international randomized trial comparing four thrombolytic strategies for acute myocardial infarction. N Engl J Med 329:673, 1993.
12. The GUSTO Angiographic Investigators. The effects of tissue plasminogen activator, streptokinase, or both on coronary-artery patency, ventricular function, and survival after acute myocardial infarction. N Engl J Med 329:1615, 1993.
13. Simes RJ, Califf RM, Mark DB, on behalf of the GUSTO Investigators. Tradeoffs between stroke and

mortality after acute myocardial infarction: Net clinical benefit of accelerated tissue plasminogen activator compared with streptokinase (abstr). Circulation 88(Suppl. I):I291, 1993.

14. Jang Y, Lincoff AM, Plow EF, Topol EJ. Cell adhesion molecules in coronary artery disease. J Am Coll Cardiol 24:1591, 1994.

15. Phillips DR, Charo IF, Parise LV, Fitzgerald LA. The platelet membrane glycoprotein IIb-IIIa complex. Blood 71:831, 1988.

16. Phillips DR, Charo IF, Scarborough RM. GPIIb-IIIa: The responsive integrin. Cell 65:359, 1991.

17. Coller BS, Scudder LE. Inhibition of dog platelet function by in vivo infusion of F(ab')2 fragments of a monoclonal antibody to the platelet glycoprotein IIb/IIIa receptor. Blood 66:1456, 1985.

18. Scarborough RM, Rose JW, Naughton MA, Phillips DR, Nannizzi L, Arfsten A, Campbell AM, Charo IF. Characterization of the integrin specificities of disintegrins isolated from American pit viper venoms. J Biol Chem 268:1058, 1993.

19. Tardiff BE, Miller J, Harrington RA, Tcheng JE, Califf RM. Integrilin (tm)-synthetic peptides against the platelet glycoprotein IIb/IIIa receptor. In Sasahara, Loscalzo (eds). New Therapeutic Agents in Thrombosis and Thrombolysis. New York: Marcel Dekker, in press.

20. Scarborough RM, Naughton MA, Teng W, Rose JW, Phillips DR, Nannizzi L, Arfsten A, Campbell AM, Charo IF. Design of potent and specific integrin antagonists. Peptide antagonists with high specifictity for glycoprotein IIb-IIIa. J Biol Chem 268:1066, 1993.

21. Kereiakes DJ, Runyon JP, Kleiman NS, Higby NA, Anderson LC, Hantsbarger G, McDonald S, Anders RJ. Differential dose response to oral Xemlofiban after antecedent intravenous abciximab: Administration for complex coronary Intervention. Circulation 94:906, 1996.

22. Theroux P, White H, David D, Van De Werf F, Nienaber CA, Charbonnier B, et al. A heparin-controlled study of MK-383 in unstable angina (abstr). Circulation 90(Suppl. I):I231, 1994.

23. Alig L, Edenhofer A, Hadvary P, Hurzeler M, Knopp D, Muller M, Steiner B, Trzeciak A, Weller T. Low molecular weight, non-peptide fibrinogen receptor antagonists. J Med Chem 35:4393, 1992.

24. Berdan LG, Holmes DR, Davidson-Ray L, Lam LC, Talley JD, Mark DB, for the CAVEAT Investigators. Economic impact of abrupt closure following percutaneous interrrvention: The CAVEAT experience. J Am Coll Cardiol 23:434A, 1994.

25. Mark DB, Talley JD, Topol EJ, Bowman L, Lam LC, Anderson KM, Jollis JG, Cleman MW, Lee KL, Aversano T, Untereker WJ, Davidson-Ray L, Califf RM, for the EPIC Investigators. Economic assessment of platelet glycoprotein IIb/IIIa inhibition for prevention of ischemic complications of high-risk coronary angioplasty. Circulation 94:629, 1996.

26. Ellis SG, Tcheng JE, Navetta FI, Muller DW, Weisman HF, Smith C, Anderson KM, Califf RM, Topol EJ. Safety and antiplatelet effect of murine monoclonal antibody 7E3 Fab directed against platelet glycoprotein IIb/IIIa in patients undergoing elective coronary angioplasty. Cor Art Dis 4:167, 1993.

27. Tcheng JE, Ellis SG, George BS, Keereiakes DJ, Kleiman NS, Talley JD, Wang AL, Weisman HF, Califf RM, Topol EJ. Pharmacodynamics of chimeric glycoprotein IIb/IIIa integrin antiplatelet antibody fab 7E3 in high-risk coronary angioplasty. Circulation 90:1757, 1994.

28. The EPIC Investigators. Use of a monoclonal antibody directed against the platelet glycoprotein IIb/IIIa receptor in high-risk coronary angioplasty. N Engl J Med 330:956, 1994.

29. Lincoff AM, Califf RM, Anderson K, Weisman HF, Topol EJ, for the EPIC Investigators. Striking clinical benefit with platelet GP IIb/IIIa inhibition by c7E3 among patients with unstabel angina: Outcome in the EPIC trial (abstr). Circulation 90(Suppl. I):I21, 1994.

30. Lefkovits J, Ivanhoe RJ, Califf RM, Bergelson BA, Anderson KM, Stoner GL, Weisman HF, Topol EJ. Effects of platelet glycoprotein IIb/IIIa receptor blockade by a chimeric monoclonal antibody (abciximab) on acute and six-month outcomes after percutaneous transluminal coronary angioplasty for acute myocardial infarction. EPIC investigators. Am J Cardiol 77:1045, 1996.

31. Topol EJ, Califf RM, Weisman HF, Ellis SG, Tcheng JE, Worley S, Ivanhoe R, George BS, Fintel D, Weston M, Sigmon K, Anderson KM, Lee KL, Willerson JT, on behalf of The EPIC Investigatiors. Randomised trial of coronary intervention with antibody against platelet IIb/IIIa integrin for reduction of clinical restenosis: Results at six months. Lancet 343:881, 1994.

32. Aguirre FV, Topol EJ, Ferguson JJ, Anderson K, Blankenship JC, Heuser RR, Sigmon K, Taylor M, Gottlieb R, Hanovich G, Rosenberg M, Donohue TJ, Weisman HF, Califf RM, for the EPIC Investigators. Bleeding complications with the chimeric antibody to paltelet glycoprotein IIb/IIIa integrin in patients undergoing percutaneous coronary intervention. Circulation 91:2882, 1995.

33. Lincoff AM, Tcheng JE, Bass TA, Popma JJ, Teirstein PS, Kleiman NS, Weisman HF, Musco MH, Cabot CF, Berdan LG, Califf RM, Topol EJ, PROLOG Investigators. A multicenter, randomized, double-blind pilot trial of standard versus low dose weight-adjusted heparin in patients treated with the platelet GP IIb/IIIa receptor antibody c7E3 during percutaneous coronary revascularization (abstr). J Am Coll Cardiol 25:80A, 1995.

34. Ferguson JJ. Meeting highlights: American College of Cardiology 45th Annual Scientific Session, Orlando, Florida, March 24 to 27, 1996. Circulation 94:1, 1996.

35. Simoons ML. Refractory unstable angina: Reduction of events by c-7E3: The CAPTURE study. Presented at

the 45th Annual Scientific Session of the American College of Cariology, Orlando, Florida, March 24, 1996.

36. Tcheng JE, Harrington RA, Kottke-Marchant K, Kleiman NS, Ellis SG, Kereiakes DJ, Mick MJ, Navetta FI, Smith JE, Worley SJ, Miller JA, Joseph DM, Sigmon KN, Kitt MM, du Mee CP, Califf RM, Topol EJ, for the IMPACT Investigators. Multicenter, randomized, double-blind, placebo-controlled trial of the platelet integrin glycoprotein IIb/IIIa blocker integrelin in elective coronary intervention. Circulation 91:2151, 1995.

37. Harrington RA, Kleiman NS, Kottke-Marchant K, Lincoff AM, Tcheng JE, Sigmon KN, Joseph D, Rios G, Trainor K, Rose D, Greenberg CS, Kitt MM, Topol EJ, Califf RM. Immediate and reversible platelet inhibition after intravenous administration of a peptide glycoprotein IIb/IIIa inhibitor during percutaneous coronary intervention. Am J Cardiol 76:1222, 1995.

38. Tcheng JE, Lincoff AM, Sigmon KN, Kitt MM, Califf RM, Topol FJ, for the IMPACT II Investigators. Platelet glycoprotein IIb/IIIa inhibition with integrelin™ during percutaneous coronary intervention: The IMPACT II trial (abstr). Circulation 92(Suppl. I):I543, 1995.

39. Gold HK, Gimple LW, Yasuda T, Leinbach RC, Werner W, Holt R, Jordan R, Berger H, Collen D, Coller BS. Pharmacodynamic study of F(ab')2 fragments of murine monoclonal antibody 7E3 directed against human platelet glycoprotein IIb/IIIa in patients with unstable angina pectoris. J Clin Invest 86:651, 1990.

40. Schulman SP, Goldschmidt-Clermont PJ, Navetta FI, Chandra NC, Guerci AD, Califf RM, Ferguson JJ, Willerson JT, Wolfe CL, Bahr R, Yakubov SJ, Nyggard TW, Mason SJ, Brashears L, Charo I, du Mee C, Kitt MM, Gerstenblith GG. Integrelin in unstable angina: A double-blind randomized trial (abstr). Circulation 88(Suppl. I):I608, 1993.

41. Harrington RA, Schulman SP, Kleiman NS, Lincoff AM, Goldschmidt-Clermont PJ, Joseph D, Sigmon KN, Parker J, Marchant K, Kitt MM. Profound, sustained and reversible platelet inhibition following ad-

ministration of a glycoprotein IIb/IIIa inhibitor with and without heparin in patients with unstable angina (abstr). Circulation 90(Suppl. I):I232, 1994.

42. Theroux P, Kouz, Roy L, Knudtson ML, Diodati JG, Marquis JF, et al. Platelet Membrane Receptor Glycoprotien IIb/IIIa Antagonism in Unstable Angina: The Canadian Lamifiban Study. Circulation 94:899, 1996.

43 Ohman EM, Califf RM, Topol EJ, Candela R, Abbottsmith C, Ellis S, Sigmon KN, Kereiakes D, George B, Stack R, the TAMI Study Group. Consequences of reocclusion after successful reperfusion therapy in acute myocardial infarction. Circulation 82:781, 1990.

44. Yasuda T, Gold HK, Fallon JT, Leinbach RC, Guerrero JL, Scudder LE, Kanke M, Shealy D, Ross MJ, Collen D, et al. Monoclonal antibody against the platelet glycoprotein (GP) IIb/IIIa receptor prevents corconary artery reocclusion after reperfusion with recombinant tissue-type plasminogen activator in dogs. J Clin Invest 81:1284, 1988.

45. Kleiman NS, Ohman EM, Kereiakes DJ, Ellis SG, Weisman HF, Topol EJ, for the TAMI 8 Investigators. Profound platelet inactivation with 7E3 shortly after thrombolytic therapy for acute myocardial infarction (abstr). Circulation 84:II522, 1991.

46. Ohman EM, Kleiman NS, Gacioch G, Talley D, Navetta FI, Worley S, Anderson RD, Cohen J, Kereiakes DJ, Sigmon KN, Krucoff MW, Califf RM, Topol EJ, for the IMPACT-AMI Investigators. Combined accelerated tissue plasminogen activator and platelet glycoprotein IIb-IIIa integrin blockade with Integrilin(TM) in acute myocardial infarction: Results from a randomized, placebo-controlled, dose-ranging trial. Circulation 1996, in press.

47. Moliterno DJ, Harrington RA, Califf RM, Rapold HJ, Topol EJ, for the PARADIGM Investigators. Randomized, placebo-controlled study of Lamifiban with thrombolytic therapy for the treatment of acute myocardial infarction: Rationale and design for the Platelet Aggregation Receptor Antagonist Dose Investigation and Reperfusion Gain in Myocardial Infarction (PARADIGM) study. J Thromb Thromboly 2:165, 1995.

46. A GLOSSARY OF TERMS IN THROMBOCARDIOLOGY

Patricia K. Hodgson and Robert A. Harrington

Abciximab Monoclonal antibody fragment inhibitor of the platelet glycoprotein IIb/IIIa receptor complex. Over a series of randomized clinical trials (EPIC, EPILOG, CAPTURE), it demonstrated its effectiveness in reducing ischemic complications of percutaneous coronary intervention. It is the first agent of its class approved for use in the setting of high-risk coronary angioplasty by the U.S. Food and Drug Administration.

Abrupt closure Coronary vessel occlusion following percutaneous coronary intervention, which typically occurs within 24 hours of the index procedure. The overwhelming majority of instances occur in the catheterization laboratory. It is associated with a marked increase in death, myocardial infarction, and the need for urgent bypass surgery.

Activation Process of platelet stimulation following adhesion to the vessel wall. It typically leads to expression of receptor proteins on the platelet surface, which are then responsible for binding adjacent platelets in the process called aggregation.

Acute coronary syndromes A number of disease states having the common denominator of atherosclerotic or plaque rupture and coronary thrombosis. Includes the spectrum ranging from unstable angina to acute myocardial infarction.

Adhesion Process of cells binding via various receptors to an injured vascular surface that has exposed a number of binding proteins.

Adhesive proteins Proteins responsible for cell-to-cell or cell-to-vessel wall interaction.

ADP (adenosine diphosphate) A relatively weak agonist of platelet aggregation.

Aggregation Process during which platelets bind to one another, creating thrombi. It is mediated by the binding of fibrinogen to the glycoprotein IIb/IIIa receptor complex on adjacent platelets. Aggrega-

tion is the final common pathway of platelet hemostasis.

Alteplase Tissue-plasminogen activator, a fibrinolytic agent. It is clinically useful in the management of acute myocardial infarction and large pulmonary embolism. Ongoing studies are examining its use in ischemic stroke.

Anticoagulant A nonspecific term that refers to any agent that inhibits thrombin generation or activity.

Antiplasmin Usually protein inhibitors of plasmin, which is the principal endogenous fibrinolytic agent.

APSAC (anisoylated plasminogen streptokinase activator complex) A nonspecific fibrinolytic agent.

Argatroban An arginine derivative, which is a direct thrombin inhibitor.

Bradykinin A mediator of the complement system.

CARS (Coumadin Aspirin Reinfarction Study) A randomized clinical trial of secondary prevention investigating Coumadin plus aspirin versus aspirin alone.

Coagulation Process of hemostasis, mainly focused on thrombin generation and subsequent fibrin formation.

Coagulation factors A series of circulating proteins necessary for the generation of thrombin and the formation of fibrin.

Collagen Extracellular matrix protein; also a weak agonist of platelet aggregation.

Dimers A byproduct of the fibrinolytic process.

Dipyridamole An orally active antiplatelet agent.

655

Duteplase   A recombinant tissue-type plasminogen activator.

ECSG (European Cooperative Study Group)   The sponsoring group of a number of small clinical trials that began in 1979 investigating thrombolytic agents with heparin in patients with acute myocardial infarction.

EPIC (Evaluation of 7E3 for the Prevention of Ischemic Complications trial)   A landmark randomized clinical trial that demonstrated the long-term effectiveness of abciximab in reducing the ischemic complications of high-risk coronary angioplasty.

Epinephrine   A potent agonist to platelet aggregation.

F1.2   A byproduct of the conversion of prothrombin to thrombin, and thus a measurable marker of thrombin generation.

Factor VII   A coagulation factor responsible for interacting with tissue factor, thus leading to stimulation of the prothrombinase complex, which leads to thrombin generation and fibrin formation.

Factor X   A coagulation factor responsible for the conversion of prothrombin to thrombin; along with factor V, calcium, and plospholipid, and essential part of the prothrombinase complex.

Factor XIII   A coagulation factor responsible for the crosslinking of fibrin, leading to a stable polymerized fibrin clot.

Fibrin   The end product protein of coagulation. It results from thrombin converting fibrinogen to fibrin.

Fibrinogen   A ubiquitous large circulating protein and the forerunner of fibrin. Its conversion to fibrin depends on the action of thrombin.

Fibronectin   An adhesive protein.

GISSI   A series of international randomized mortality trials using thrombolysis as well as antiplatelet and anticoagulant therapy for patients with acute myocardial infarction.

Glycoprotein IIb/IIIa   The most common integrin receptor on the surface of platelets. It is capable of binding fibrinogen between adjacent platelets and leading to platelet aggregation in the formation of a platelet ridge thrombus.

GUSTO (Global Use of Strategies To Open occluded coronary arteries)   A group of international randomized clinical trials of acute myocardial infarction and acute coronary syndromes testing —

singly and in combination — various thrombolytic, anticoagulant, and antiplatelet agents.

Hemostasis   A response to vascular injury. It includes both the platelet and the coagulant systems.

Heparin   A large molecule that requires an association with antithrombin III to inhibit thrombin. Currently the only intravenous anticoagulant available for clinical use.

Hirudin   A recombinant protein based on a protein found in the salivary gland of the medicinal leech. A potent direct thrombin inhibitor.

Hirugen   A synthetic peptide based on the hirudin molecule that acts as a direct thrombin inhibitor.

Hirulog   A synthetic peptide that acts as a direct thrombin inhibitor.

HIT (heparin-induced thrombocytopenia)   Platelet aggregation following the administration of heparin that results in prolongation of the bleeding time and a drop in the platelet count.

Homocysteinemin   A metabolic abnormality marked by high levels of homocysteine in the plasma and a risk factor for premature atherosclerosis.

Integrilin   A prototype peptide inhibitor of the platelet glycoprotein IIb/IIIa receptor complex.

Integrins   A family of cell surface receptor molecules.

ISIS (International Study of Infarct Survival)   The name given to a series of randomized clinical trials and the group of investigatiors who performed them. The ISIS group has studied patients with acute myocardial infarction, using several thrombolytic agents and adjunctive therapies.

Lamifiban   A peptidomimetic platelet plycoprotein IIb/IIIa inhibitor.

Leukocyte   A nonspecific term for white cells. They may be involved in the thrombotic process through platelet-leukocyte interactions.

Ligands   Circulation binding proteins.

MITI (Myocardial Infarction Triage and Intervention)   A series of trials coordinated in Seattle, Washington that looked at the advantages of early treatment of patients with acute myocardial infarction. Studies included the administration of thrombolytic agents by EMTs, and the use of thrombolytic therapy or direct coronary angioplasty.

PPACK Synthetic thrombin inhibitor used as an anticoagulant in certain blood collection tubes.

Plaque rupture Believed to be the initial step in the genesis of the acute coronary syndromes as well as in the progression of atherosclerotic disease. Can be triggered by a variety of neural, hormonal, and flow forces.

Plasmin An endogenous fibrinolytic protein that degrades fibrin into fibrinogen degradation products, which are soluble.

Plasminogen Forerunner of plasmin.

Platelet The blood cell responsible for the primary phase of hemostasis.

Platelet factor-4 A circulating platelet inhibitor.

Protein C An important part of the thrombin negative feedback loop, it inhibits thrombin formation through its effects on factors V and VIII.

Protein S Cofactor for the action of protein C.

Prothrombin Protein precursor that is converted to thrombin by the action of the prothrombinase complex.

Restenosis The process of renarrowing of a coronary artery segment following a successful intervention procedure. A major late complication of percutaneous interventional procedures, accounting for a large number of the repeart procedures needed following initially successful ones.

r-PA (recombinant plasminogen activator) A nonglycosylated plasminogen activator produced in *E. coli* by recombinant DNA techniques. It is a single-chain protein and has clower clearance and a longer half-life than wild-type t-PA.

Saruplase A single-chain, urokinase-type plasminogen activator.

Streptokinase A nonspecific thrombolytic agent first used in the treatment of acute myocardial infarction in the 1950s. It is an inexpensive agent with a low rate of reocclusion, but patency rates that are inferior to other thrombolytics, notably t-PA.

TAMI (Thrombolysis and Angioplasty in Myocardial Infarction) A series of 10 clinical trials (and the investigators who ran them) in the 1980s and early 1990s looking at pharmacological and mechanical ways to open an acutely occluded coronary artery.

TAT (thrombin–antithrombin III complex) An indirect marker of circulating thrombin.

TFPI (tissue factor pathway inhibitor) A protein inhibitor of the extrinsic coagulation system; mainly an inhibitor of the factor VII tissue factor system.

Ticlopidine An antiplatelet agent.

Thrombin the central enzyme of coagulation, reponsible for the conversion of fibrinogen to fibrin and activation of platelets. It plays a pivotal role in its own feedback regulation through its mediation of the protein C and S system.

Thrombomodulin A protein that combines with thrombin at the platelet surface to convert protein C to activated protein C.

TIMI (Thrombolysis In Myocardial Infarction) A series of randomized clinical trials, coordinated in Boston, that tested a variety of thrombolytic agents for patients with acute myocardial infarction.

TIMI flow A systematic visual method of expressing reperfusion success following administration of thrombolytic therapy to patients with acute myocardial infarction. TIMI 0 and 1 indicate no to little flow, TIMI 2 indicates partial flow, and TIMI 3 is normal coronary flow.

Tirofiban A nonpeptide inhibitor of the glycoprotein IIb/IIIa receptor inhibitor.

Tissue factor A protein found in the subendothelium that, when exposed following vascular injury to the circulation, is able to combine with factor VII and to initiate coagulation.

t-PA (tissue-plasminogen activator) A specific fibrinolytic agent with demonstrated value in the treatment of patients with acute myocardial infarction and plumonary embolism.

TRAP (thrombin receptor agonist peptide) A peptide that activates platelets in a manner similar to thrombin, but without the effect on coagulation.

Urokinase A nonspecific fibrinolytic agent.

Vitamin K An enzymatic cofactor necessary for the production of clotting factors II, VII, IX, and X, as well as proteins C and S.

Vironectin An adhesive protein capable of binding to cells such as platelets and perhaps mediating some elements of extracellular matrix formation following successful percutaneous coronary intervention.

vWF (von Willebrand factor)   An adhesive matrix protein that facilitates platelet adhesion by glycoprotein Ib. It also binds to platelet glycoprotein IIb/IIIa to play a role in platelet aggregation.

Warfarin   The only available oral anticoagulatnt approved for clinic use in the United States. It works through a depletion of the vitamin K–dependent clotting factors and is best measured and titrated by assessing its effect on prothrombin time (INR, international normalized ratio).

INDEX

CPSIA information can be obtained
at www.ICGtesting.com
Printed in the USA
LVHW061703161218
600668LV00002B/4/P